MERENSTEIN & GARDNER'S HANDBOOK OF
Neonatal Intensive Care

Eighth Edition

SANDRA L. GARDNER, RN, MS, CNS, PNP
Director, Professional Outreach Consultation
Editor, *Nurse Currents* and *NICU Currents*
Aurora, Colorado

BRIAN S. CARTER, MD, FAAP
Professor of Pediatrics
University of Missouri-Kansas City School of Medicine
Division of Neonatology & Bioethics Center
Children's Mercy Hospital-Kansas City
Kansas City, Missouri

MARY ENZMAN HINES, PhD, APRN, CNS, CPNP, APHN-BC
Professor Emeritus
Beth El College of Nursing and Health Sciences
University of Colorado at Colorado Springs;
Certified Pediatric Nurse Practitioner
Rocky Mountain Pediatrics
Lakewood, Colorado

JACINTO A. HERNÁNDEZ, MD, PhD, MHA, FAAP
Professor Emeritus of Pediatrics
Section of Neonatology
Department of Pediatrics
University of Colorado School of Medicine;
Chairman Emeritus Department of Neonatology
Children's Hospital Colorado
Aurora, Colorado

ELSEVIER

ELSEVIER

3251 Riverport Lane
St. Louis, Missouri 63043

MERENSTEIN & GARDNER'S HANDBOOK OF NEONATAL
INTENSIVE CARE, EIGHTH EDITION

ISBN: 978-0-323-32083-2

Notices

Library of Congress Cataloging-in-Publication Data

Merenstein & Gardner's handbook of neonatal intensive care / [edited by] Sandra L. Gardner, Brian S. Carter, Mary Enzman Hines, Jacinto A. Hernandez. -- Eighth edition.
    p. ; cm.
    Merenstein and Gardner's handbook of neonatal intensive care
    Preceded by Merenstein & Gardner's handbook of neonatal intensive care / [edited by] Sandra L. Gardner... [et al.]. 7th ed. c2011.
    Includes bibliographical references and index.
    ISBN 978-0-323-32083-2 (pbk. : alk. paper)
    I. Gardner, Sandra L., editor. II. Carter, Brian S., 1957- , editor. III. Hines, Mary Enzman, editor. IV. Hernandez, Jacinto A., editor. V. Title Merenstein and Gardner's handbook of neonatal intensive care.
    [DNLM: 1. Intensive Care, Neonatal. 2. Infant, Newborn, Diseases--therapy. WS 421]
    RJ253.5
    618.92'01--dc23   2015006347

Executive Content Strategist: Lee Henderson
Content Development Manager: Jean Sims Fornango
Senior Content Development Specialist: Tina Kaemmerer
Publishing Services Manager: Catherine Jackson
Senior Project Manager: Carol O'Connell
Design Direction: Renee Duenow

Printed in the U.S.A.

Last digit is the print number: 9 8 7 6 5 4 3 2 1

We dedicate this edition to the memory of Gerald B. Merenstein, MD—our friend, colleague, and mentor who was also a wonderful husband, father, and grandfather. As the inspiration for this text, Gerry contributed to the fields of neonatal and pediatric care through his dedication to nurses, nurse practitioners, child health associates, interns, residents, fellows, neonates, and their families. We miss him every day and know that his empathy, knowledge, teaching, and compassion influences all of us, as well as the newborns, children, and families that he and we serve.

SLG   BSC   MEH   JAH

In memory of Stephanie Marie Gardner, whose three days of life did have a purpose.

SLG

To my family: Angel, Sean, Yvonne, Rebecca, and Jacquelyn; my mentors and colleagues; and all of the children and families who have allowed me to share with them both joyous and difficult times in their lives.

BSC

To my family James, Jennifer, Sean, Finnoula, Steve, and Sarah for their enduring source of love, confidence, and encouragement and to all the families who have informed by practice and knowledge about caring for fragile infants.

MEH

To all the newborn infants, their families, and dedicated caregivers; my beloved wife Pam and sons Gabriel and Jacinto for their love and constant support.

JAH

In Memoriam
Jimmie Lynne Scholl Avery
L. Joseph Butterfield, MD
Lula O. Lubchenco, MD
William A. Silverman, MD

CONTRIBUTORS

Rita Agarwal, MD, FAAP
Professor of Anesthesiology
Director of Education, Pediatric Anesthesia
Pediatric Anesthesia Program Director
Director of the Colorado Review of Anesthesiology for
    Surgicenters and Hospital
Children's Hospital Colorado, University of Colorado
    Denver, School of Medicine
Aurora, Colorado

Marianne Sollosy Anderson, MD
Neonatologist
Sequoia Pediatrics
Kaweah Delta Medical Center
Visalia, California

Jaime Arruda, MD, FACOG
Assistant Professor, Obstetrics and Gynecology
University of Colorado Denver
Aurora, Colorado

James S. Barry, MD
Associate Professor of Pediatrics, Section of Neonatology
Department of Pediatrics
University of Colorado Denver School of Medicine
Medical Director, Neonatal Intensive Care Unit
University of Colorado Hospital Department of
    Neonatology Children's Hospital Colorado
Aurora, Colorado

Wanda Todd Bradshaw, MSN, RN, NNP-BC
Assistant Professor and Lead Faculty, NNP Specialty
Duke University School of Nursing
Durham, North Carolina;
Neonatal Nurse Practitioner
Moses Cone Health System
Greensboro, North Carolina

M. Colleen Brand, PhD, APRN, NNP-BC
Neonatal Nurse Practitioner
Texas Children's Hospital
Houston, Texas

Laura D. Brown, MD
Associate Professor of Pediatrics
Section of Neonatology
Department of Pediatrics
University of Colorado Denver School of Medicine
Aurora, Colorado

Jessica Brunkhorst, MD
Neonatology Fellow
Children's Mercy Hospital
Kansas City, Missouri

Brian T. Bucher, MD
Clinical Fellow
Pediatric Surgery
Department of Pediatric Surgery
Vanderbilt
Nashville, Tennessee

Deanne Buschbach, RN, MSN, NNP, PNP
Clinical Operations Director for Advanced Clinical
    Practice
Pediatric and Neonatal Critical Care APP Service
Pediatric Heart APP Service
Duke University Medical Center
Durham, North Carolina

Melissa A. Cadnapaphornchai, MD
Associate Professor of Pediatrics and Medicine
Pediatric Nephrology/The Kidney Center
University of Colorado Denver School of Medicine and
    Children's Hospital Colorado
Aurora, Colorado

Angel Carter, DNP, APRN, NNP-BC
Assistant Professor of Nursing
Assistant Chair—BSN Degree Completion Program
Park University
Kansas City, Missouri

Brian S. Carter, MD, FAAP
Professor of Pediatrics
University of Missouri-Kansas City School of Medicine
Division of Neonatology & Bioethics Center
Children's Mercy Hospital-Kansas City
Kansas City, Missouri

Susan B. Clarke, MS, RNC-NIC, RN-BC, CNS
Professional Development Specialist
Continuing Education and Outreach
NRP Regional Trainer
Children's Hospital Colorado
Aurora, Colorado

C. Michael Cotten, MD, MHS
Associate Professor of Pediatrics
Medical Director, Neonatology Clinical Research
Duke University
Durham, North Carolina

Heather Furlong Craven, MD
Associate Professor of Pediatrics
Division of Neonatology
Medical Director of Neonatal Transport Services
Wake Forest School of Medicine Brenner Children's
    Hospital
Winston-Salem, North Carolina

Jane Davis, RNC, BSN
Level III Permanent Charge Nurse
Neonatal Intensive Care Unit
University of Colorado Hospital
Aurora, Colorado

Jane Deacon, NNP-BC, MS
Neonatal Nurse Practitioner
Children's Hospital Colorado
Aurora, Colorado

David J. Durand, MD
Division of Neonatology
UCSF Benioff Children's Hospital-Oakland
Oakland, California

Jarrod Dusin, MS, RD
Clinical Dietitian Specialist
Children's Mercy Hospital
Kansas City, Missouri

Nancy English, PhD, RN
Fetal Concerns, Director and Coordinator
Colorado High Risk Maternity and Newborn Program
University of Colorado Health Sciences
The Children's Hospital
Aurora, Colorado

Mary Enzman Hines, PhD, APRN, CNS, CPNP, APHN-BC
Professor Emeritus
Beth El College of Nursing and Health Sciences
University of Colorado at Colorado Springs;
Certified Pediatric Nurse Practitioner
Rocky Mountain Pediatrics
Lakewood, Colorado

Lori Erickson, RN, CPNP, APRN
Fetal Cardiac and Cardiac High Acuity
    Monitoring APRN
Ward Family Heart Center
Children's Mercy Hospital
Kansas City, Missouri

Ruth Evans, MS, APRN, NNP-BC
Neonatal Nurse Practitioner
Children's Hospital Colorado and University of
    Colorado Hospital
Aurora, Colorado

Loretta P. Finnegan, MD
President, Finnegan Consulting, LLC
Perinatal Addiction and Women's Health
Avalon, New Jersey;
Founder and Former Director of Family Center
Jefferson Medical College of Thomas Jefferson University
Philadelphia, Pennsylvania

Sandra L. Gardner, RN, MS, CNS, PNP
Director, Professional Outreach Consultation
Editor, *Nurse Currents* and *NICU Currents*
Aurora, Colorado

Edward Goldson, MD
Professor, Department of Pediatrics
University of Colorado Denver School of Medicine
The Children's Hospital
Aurora, Colorado

Linda L. Gratny, MD
Associate Professor of Pediatrics
University of Missouri–Kansas City School of Medicine;
Neonatologist and Director, Infant Tracheostomy and
    Home Ventilator Program
Children's Mercy Hospital
Kansas City, Missouri

Marie Hastings-Tolsma, PhD, CNM, FACNM
Professor, Nurse Midwifery
Louis Herrington School of Nursing
Baylor University
Dallas, Texas;
Visiting Professor
University of Johannesburg
Johannesburg, South Africa

William W. Hay Jr., MD
Professor of Pediatrics, Section of Neonatology
Scientific Director, Perinatal Research Center
Co-Director for Child and Maternal Health and the
    Perinatal Research Center, Colorado Clinical and
    Translational Sciences Institute
University of Colorado School of Medicine and
    Children's Hospital Colorado
Aurora, Colorado

Kendra Hendrickson, MS, RD, CNSC, CSP
Clinical Dietitian Specialist
Neonatal Intensive Care Unit
University of Colorado Hospital
Aurora, Colorado

Carmen Hernández, MSN, NNP-BC
Neonatal Nurse Practitioner
Rocky Mountain Hospital for Children
Denver, Colorado

Jacinto A. Hernández, MD, PhD, MHA, FAAP
Professor Emeritus of Pediatrics
Section of Neonatology
Department of Pediatrics
University of Colorado School of Medicine;
Chairman Emeritus Department of Neonatology
Children's Hospital Colorado
Aurora, Colorado

Patti Hills, LMSW, LCSW
Fetal Health Center
NICU Social Worker
Children's Mercy Hospital
Kansas City, Missouri

Mona Jacobson, MSN, RN, CPNP-PC
Instructor in Pediatrics
Section of Child Neurology
University of Colorado School of Medicine
Children's Hospital Colorado
Aurora, Colorado

M. Douglas Jones, Jr., MD
Senior Associate Dean for Clinical Affairs
Professor, Section of Neonatology
Department of Pediatrics
University of Colorado Denver School of Medicine
Aurora, Colorado

Beena Kamath-Rayne, MD, MPH
Assistant Professor of Pediatrics
Perinatal Institute, Division of Neonatology
Global Health Center
Cincinnati Children's Hospital Medical Center
Cincinnati, Ohio

Rhonda Knapp-Clevenger, PhD, CPNP
Director, Research and Pediatric Nurse Scientist
Center for Pediatric Nurse Research and Clinical Inquiry;
Clinical Research Director, Pediatric and Perinatal
    Clinical Translational Research Centers
University of Colorado Denver, College of Nursing
Children's Hospital Colorado
Aurora, Colorado

Ruth A. Lawrence, MD, DD(Hon), FAAP, FABM
Distinguished Alumna Professor of Pediatrics and
    Obstetrics/Gynecology
Northumberland Trust Chair in Pediatrics
Director of the Breastfeeding and Human Lactation
    Study Center
University of Rochester School of Medicine and Dentistry
Rochester, New York

Mary Kay Leick-Rude, RNC, MSN, PCNS
Clinical Nurse Specialist
Children's Mercy Hospital
Kansas City, Missouri

Harold Lovvorn III, MD, FACS, FAAP
Assistant Professor of Pediatric Surgery
Vanderbilt University Children's Hospital
Nashville, Tennessee

Carolyn Lund, RN, MS, FAAN
Neonatal Clinical Nurse Specialist
ECMO Coordinator
Neonatal Intensive Care Unit
UCSF Benioff Children's Hospital-Oakland
Oakland, California;
Associate Clinical Professor
Department of Family Health Care Nursing
University of California
San Francisco, California

Marilyn Manco-Johnson, MD
Professor of Pediatrics, Section of Hematology
University of Colorado Denver and The Children's
    Hospital Colorado
Hemophilia and Thrombosis Center
Aurora, Colorado

Anne Matthews, RN, PhD, FACMG
Professor
Genetics and Genome Sciences
Director, Genetic Counseling Training Program
Case Western Reserve University
Cleveland, Ohio

Jane E. McGowan, MD
Professor of Pediatrics
Associate Chair for Research
Drexel University College of Medicine
Medical Director, NICU
St. Christopher's Hospital for Children
Philadelphia, Pennsylvania

Christopher McKinney, MD
Fellow, Pediatric Hematology
Center for Cancer and Blood Disorders
Children's Hospital Colorado
University of Colorado-Denver
Aurora, Colorado

Mary Miller-Bell, PharmD
Clinical Research Pharmacist
Duke University Hospital
Durham, North Carolina

Susan Niermeyer, MD, MPH, FAAP
Professor of Pediatrics and Epidemiology
University of Colorado School of Medicine and
    Colorado School of Public Health
Aurora, Colorado

Priscilla M. Nodine, PhD, CNM
Assistant Professor, Midwifery
College of Nursing
University of Colorado Anschutz Campus
Aurora, Colorado

Michael Nyp, DO, MBA
Assistant Professor of Pediatrics
University of Missouri-Kansas City
Division of Perinatal-Neonatal Medicine
Children's Mercy Hospital
Kansas City, Missouri

Steven L. Olsen, MD
Associate Professor of Pediatrics
University of Missouri-Kansas City
Division of Neonatology
Children's Mercy Hospital
Kansas City, Missouri

Annette S. Pacetti, RN, MSN, NNP-BC
Neonatal Nurse Practitioner
Monroe Carell, Jr. Children's Hospital at Vanderbilt
Nashville, Tennessee

Eugenia K. Pallotto, MD, MSCE
Associate Professor
University of Missouri-Kansas City School of Medicine
Medical Director, NICU
Children's Mercy Hospital
Kansas City, Missouri

Mohan Pammi, MD, PhD, MRCPCH
Associate Professor
Baylor College of Medicine
Houston, Texas

Alfonso Pantoja, MD
Neonatologist
Saint Joseph's Hospital
Denver Colorado

Julie A. Parsons, MD
Associate Professor of Pediatrics and Neurology
Haberfield Family Endowed Chair in Pediatric
    Neuromuscular Disorders
Child Neurology Program Director
University of Colorado School of Medicine
Children's Hospital Colorado
Aurora, Colorado

Webra Price-Douglas, PhD, CRNP, IBCLC
Maryland Regional Transport Program
Baltimore, Maryland

Daphne A. Reavey, PhD, RN, NNP-BC
Neonatal Nurse Practitioner
Children's Mercy Hospital
Kansas City, Missouri

Nathaniel H. Robin, MD, FACMG
Professor of Genetics and Pediatrics
University of Alabama at Birmingham
Birmingham, Alabama

Mario A. Rojas, MD, MPH
Professor of Pediatrics
Division of Neonatal-Perinatal Medicine
Wake Forest University School of Medicine
Winston Salem, North Carolina

Jamie Rosterman, DO
Neonatology Fellow
Children's Mercy Hospital
Kansas City, Missouri

Paul Rozance, MD
Associate Professor of Pediatrics
Section of Neonatology
University of Colorado Denver School of Medicine
Children's Hospital Colorado
Aurora, Colorado

Tamara Rush, MSN, RN, C-NPT, EMT
Nurse Manager
Brenner Children's Hospital-Wake Forest Baptist Health
Winston-Salem, North Carolina

Mary Schoenbein, BSN, RN, CNN
Perinatal Dialysis Nurse/The Kidney Center
Children's Hospital Colorado
Aurora, Colorado

Alan R. Seay, MD
Professor of Pediatrics and Neurology
University of Colorado School of Medicine
Children's Hospital Colorado
Aurora, Colorado

Danielle E. Soranno, MD
Assistant Professor of Pediatrics and Bioengineering
Pediatric Nephrology/The Kidney Center
University of Colorado Denver School of Medicine and
    Children's Hospital Colorado
Aurora, Colorado

John Strain, MD, FACR, CAQ Pediatric Radiology, Neuroradiology
Professor of Radiology
Department of Radiology
University of Colorado School of Medicine;
Chairman, Department of Radiology
Children's Hospital Colorado
Anschutz Medical Campus
Aurora, Colorado

Julie R. Swaney, MDiv
Manager, Spiritual Care Services
Associate Clinical Professor, Department of Medicine
University of Colorado Denver Anschutz Medical Campus
Aurora, Colorado

Tara M. Swanson, MD
Assistant Professor of Pediatrics
University of Missouri-Kansas City School of Medicine;
Director of Fetal Cardiology
Children's Mercy Hospital
Kansas City, Missouri

David Tanaka, MD
Professor of Pediatrics
Neonatologist
Duke University Medical Center
Durham, North Carolina

Elizabeth H. Thilo, MD
Associate Professor of Pediatrics
Section of Neonatology
University of Colorado Denver School of Medicine;
Neonatologist
University of Colorado Hospital and Children's Hospital
    Colorado
Aurora, Colorado

Kristin C. Voos, MD
Neonatologist
Children's Mercy Hospital;
Associate Professor of Pediatrics
University of Missouri-Kansas City School of Medicine
Kansas City, Missouri

Susan M. Weiner, PhD, MSN, RNC-OB, CNS
Perinatal Clinical Nurse Specialist
Assistant Clinical Professor/Retired
Freelance Author/Editor
Philadelphia, Pennsylvania

Jason P. Weinman, MD
Assistant Professor of Radiology
University of Colorado School of Medicine
Medical Director Computed Tomography
Children's Hospital Colorado
Aurora, Colorado

Leonard E. Weisman, MD
Professor of Pediatrics
Section of Neonatology
Baylor College of Medicine
Texas Children's Hospital
Houston, Texas

Rosanne J. Woloschuk, RD
Clinical Dietitian
The Kidney Center
Children's Hospital Colorado
Aurora, Colorado

REVIEWERS

Nancy Blake, PhD, RN, NEA-BC, CCRN
Patient Care Services Director
Critical Care Services
Children's Hospital Los Angeles
Los Angeles, California

Fran Blayney, RN-C, BSN, MS, CCRN
Education Manager
Pediatric Intensive Care Unit
Children's Hospital Los Angeles
Los Angeles, California

Karen C. D'Apolito, PhD, NNP-BC, FAAN
Professor & Program Director
Neonatal Nurse Practitioner Program
Vanderbilt University School of Nursing
Nashville, Tennessee

Mary Dix, BSN, RNC-NIC
Staff Nurse
Neonatal Intensive Care Unit
PIH Health Hospital–Whittier
Whittier, California

Sharon Fichera, RN, MSN, CNS, NNP-BC
Neonatal Clinical Nurse Specialist
Children's Hospital Los Angeles
Los Angeles, California

Joyce Foresman-Capuzzi, MSN, RN
Clinical Nurse Educator
Lankenau Medical Center
Wynnewood, PA

Delores Greenwood, MSN, RNC-NIC
Education Manager, Newborn and Infant Critical
    Care Unit
Children's Hospital Los Angeles
Los Angeles, California

Nadine A. Kassity-Krich, MBA, BSN, RN
Clinical Professor
Hahn School of Nursing
University of San Diego
San Diego, California

Lisa M. Kohr, RN, MSN, CPNP- AC/PC, MPH, PhD(c), FCCM
Pediatric Nurse Practitioner
Cardiac Intensive Care Unit
Children's Hospital of Philadelphia
Philadelphia, Pennsylvania

Carie Linder, RNC-NIC, MSN, APRN-BS
Neonatal Nurse Practitioner
Integris Baptist Medical Center
Oklahoma City, Oklahoma

Twila Luckett, BSN, RN-BC
Pediatric Pain Service
Monroe Carell Jr. Children's Hospital at Vanderbilt
Nashville, Tennessee

Erin L. Marriott, MS, RN, CPNP
Pediatric Cardiology Nurse Practitioner
American Family Children's Hospital
Watertown Regional Medical Center
Madison, Wisconsin

Andrea C. Morris, DNP, RNC-NIC, CCRN
Neonatal Clinical Nurse Specialist
Citrus Valley Medical Center-NICU
West Covina, California

Mindy Morris, DNP, NNP-BC, CNS
Neonatal Nurse Practitioner
Extremely Low Birth Weight Program Coordinator
Children's Hospital of Orange County
Orange, California

Tracy Ann Pasek, RN, MSN, DNP, CCNS, CCRN, CIMI
Clinical Nurse Specialist
Pain/Pediatric Intensive Care Unit
Children's Hospital of Pittsburgh
University of Pittsburgh Medical Center
Pittsburgh, Pennsylvania

Patricia Scheans, DNP, NNP-BC
Clinical Support for Neonatal Care
Legacy Health
Portland, Oregon

Peggy Slota, DNP, RN, FAAN
Associate Professor
Director, DNP and Nursing Leadership Programs
Carlow University
Pittsburgh, Pennsylvania

Nicole Van Hoey, PharmD
Medical Writer/Editor
Consultant
Arlington, Virginia

Winnie Yung, MN, RN
Registered Nurse
Lucile Packard Children's Hospital at Stanford
Palo Alto, California

PREFACE

The concept of the team approach is important in neonatal intensive care. Each health care professional must not only perform the duties of his or her own role but must also understand the roles of other involved professionals. Nurses, physicians, other health care providers, and parents must work together in a coordinated and efficient manner to achieve optimal results for patients in the neonatal intensive care unit (NICU).

Because this team approach is so important in the field of neonatal intensive care, we believe it is necessary that this book contain input from major fields of health care—nursing and medicine. Both nurses and physicians have edited and co-authored every chapter.

The book is divided into six units, all of which have been reviewed, revised, and updated for the eighth edition. Unit One presents evidence-based practice and the need to scientifically evaluate neonatal therapies, emphasizing randomized controlled trials as the ideal approach. Units Two through Five are the clinical sections, which have been fully updated for this edition. The chapters within these sections include highlighted clinical directions for quick reference, Parent Teaching boxes to aid in discharge instructions, and Critical Findings boxes to prioritize assessment data.

The combination of physiology and pathophysiology and separate emphasis on clinical application in this text is designed for neonatal intensive care nurses, nursing students, medical students, and pediatric, surgical, and family practice housestaff. This text is comprehensive enough for nurses and physicians, yet basic enough to be useful to families and all ancillary personnel.

Unit Six presents the psychosocial aspects of neonatal care. The medical, psychological, and social aspects of providing care for the ill neonate and family are discussed in this section. This section in particular will benefit social workers and clergy, who often deal with family members of neonates in the NICU.

In this handbook we present physiologic principles and practical applications and point out areas as yet unresolved. **Material that is clinically applicable is set in purple type so that it can be easily identified.**

INTRODUCTION

In 1974 as the Perinatal Outreach Educator at The Children's Hospital in Denver, Colorado, I took a folder to Gerry Merenstein, MD, at Fitzsimmons Army Medical Center to discuss his lectures for the first outreach education program in La Junta, Colorado. When we finished, he removed from his desk drawer a 1-inch thick compilation of the neonatal data, graphs, nomograms, and diagrams he had created for the medical housestaff during his fellowship. Giving the document to me, he asked that I review it and let him know what I thought. Several weeks later, I told him it was good *except* there was no nursing care or input, which is essential in every NICU. So Gerry asked, "Want to write a book?"—and the idea for the *Handbook* was born!

With this eighth edition in 2015, we celebrate 30 years of publication of the *Handbook of Neonatal Intensive Care*. Gerry and I co-edited this book for 21 years until his death in December 2007. To fulfill my promise that Gerry's name would always be on the book, the seventh and all subsequent editions will be known as *Merenstein & Gardner's Handbook of Neonatal Intensive Care*. Instead of editing this edition alone or with another physician, I decided to convene an editorial team consisting of myself, a nurse colleague, and two neonatologists. Together we bring 170 years of clinical practice, research, teaching, writing, and consulting in neonatal, pediatric, and family care to this eighth edition.

We have the distinction in this new edition of translation into Spanish for our colleagues in Central and South America and Spain. This was an ongoing wish of Gerry Merenstein, and after much negotiation it is finally a reality. Welcome to all our Spanish-reading colleagues! In addition, the eighth edition is available on multiple e-platforms to facilitate use at the bedside.

For our new audience, and for our continuing loyal readers, this is my opportunity to introduce myself and all the members of the editing team.

I am currently Editor of *Nurse Currents* and *NICU Currents* (www.anhi.org) and the Director of Professional Outreach Consultation (www.professionaloutreachconsultation.com), a national and international consulting firm established in 1980. I plan, develop, teach, and coordinate educational workshops on perinatal/neonatal/pediatric topics. I graduated from a hospital school of nursing in 1967 with a diploma, obtained my BSN at Spalding College in 1973 (magna cum laude), completed my MS at The University of Colorado School of Nursing in 1975 and my PNP in 1978. I have worked in perinatal/neonatal/pediatric care since 1967 as a clinician (37 years in direct bedside care), practitioner, teacher, author, and consultant. In 1974, I was the first Perinatal Outreach Educator in the United States funded by the March of Dimes. In this role I taught nurses and physicians in Colorado and the seven surrounding states how to recognize and stabilize at-risk pregnancies and sick neonates. I also consulted with numerous March of Dimes grantees to help them establish perinatal outreach programs. In 1978 I was awarded the Gerald Hencmann Award from the March of Dimes for "outstanding service in the improvement of care to mothers and babies in Colorado." I am a founding member of the Colorado Perinatal Care Council, a state advisory council to the Governor and the State Health Department on perinatal/neonatal health care issues, and I am the Treasurer and a member of the Executive Committee. I am also an active member of the Colorado Nurses Association/American Nurses Association, the Academy of Neonatal Nurses, and the National Association of Neonatal Nurses.

Mary Enzman Hines, RN, PhD, CNS, CPNP, AHN-BC, is currently Professor Emeritus at Beth-El College of Nursing at the University of Colorado in Colorado Springs and certified Pediatric Nurse Practitioner at Rocky Mountain Pediatrics, Lakewood, Colorado. Early in her nursing career, Mary worked in the NICU and PICU as a staff nurse, charge nurse, and nurse manager. After completing her PNP/CNS program and her master's degree at the University of Colorado, Mary became the Neonatal and Pediatric Clinical Nurse Specialist at Denver Health and Hospital, where she created a beginning, intermediate, and advanced orientation for nurses in the NICU and PICU. At the University of Colorado, Mary accepted the practitioner/teacher role in maternal-child services, providing clinical care and mentorship in the NICU and pediatric units where nursing students were placed from the CU nursing program. When University Hospital and The Children's Hospital combined their pediatric services, Mary became the Clinical Nurse Specialist in Research and Education and consulted in the NICU, PICU, and pediatric medical-surgical areas. In this role she was a founding member of the interdisciplinary Pain Management Team and provided consultation throughout The Children's Hospital for pain management issues. In 1996 Mary became a nursing faculty member at Beth-El College of Nursing and Health Sciences, where she created a student health center at the University and a school-based clinic for schoolchildren in Fountain, Colorado, while maintaining an active pediatric practice at Colorado Springs Health Partners. Currently Mary provides pediatric care at Rocky Mountain Pediatrics and continues to teach courses to DNP students at the University of Northern Colorado as an adjunct faculty. Mary is well published in the areas of pediatric, neonatal, and family health care, as well as in legal issues in maternal-child nursing. Mary is also a nurse researcher in the areas of pain, chronic illness, caring/healing praxis, pediatric pain, holistic nursing, and technology in health care.

Brian S. Carter, MD, FAAP, is a graduate of David Lipscomb College in Nashville, Tennessee, and of the University of Tennessee's College of Medicine in Memphis, Tennessee. Brian completed his residency in pediatrics at Fitzsimmons Army Medical Center in Aurora, Colorado. He completed his fellowship in neonatal-perinatal medicine at the University of Colorado Health Sciences Center in Denver. During the "Baby Doe" era, Brian trained in bioethics and, in addition to clinical neonatology and neonatal follow-up, he has dedicated most of his academic career to the advancement of clinical ethics in neonatology and pediatric palliative care. Brian has been recognized nationally for his efforts in both of these fields. Currently he is Professor of Pediatrics at the University of Missouri-Kansas City School of Medicine, where he serves on the Ethics Committee and mentors students, residents, and fellows in the areas of clinical ethics, neonatology, pain management, and palliative care. Brian, Marcia Levetown, MD, and Sarah Friebert, MD, co-edit the book *Palliative Care for Infants, Children, and Adolescents: A Practical Handbook,* whose second edition published in 2011 by Johns Hopkins University Press.

Jacinto A. Hernández, MD, PhD, MHA, FAAP, is currently Professor Emeritus of Pediatrics and Neonatology at the University of Colorado Denver and Chairman Emeritus of the Department of Neonatology at Children's Hospital Colorado, Aurora Colorado. He is a graduate of the School of Medicine of the University of San Marcos in Lima, Peru. Jacinto's postgraduate education includes a specialty in pediatrics and a subspecialty in neonatology from the Children's Hospital National Medical Center and George Washington University in Washington, DC, and from the University of Colorado Denver School of Medicine; a PhD from the University of San Marcos; and a Master's in Health Administration from the University of Colorado Denver School of Business. Jacinto has spent all of his professional life in academic medicine, first at the University of San Marcos as Associate Professor of Pediatrics, and subsequently at the University of Colorado Denver School of Medicine as Professor of Pediatrics. As a physician and professor, his professional activities have been carried out at The Children's Hospital of Denver in Aurora, Colorado, where he has been Director of the Newborn Intensive Care Unit, Chairman of the Department of Neonatology, an active staff neonatologist, and President of the Medical Staff. During his career, Jacinto has distinguished himself both clinically and academically, has written numerous publications in the field of neonatal medicine, and has participated as an invited professor at innumerable international events. Jacinto has been recognized with numerous awards, including the Career Teaching and Scholar Award, for his scientific achievements, professional qualities, and fruitful work as a superb clinical physician.

Borrowing from the words of Brian Carter in the introduction to the sixth edition of the *Handbook:*

> *The goals of care should be patient- and family-centered. It is the patient we treat, but it is the family, of whatever construct, with whom the baby will go home. Indeed, it is the family who must live with the long-term consequences of our daily decisions in caring for their baby.*

These goals include the provision of skilled professional care. An effective neonatal intensive care team consists of educated professionals of many disciplines—none of us can do it alone.

It has been my honor and privilege to work with these co-editors, who are all patient- and family-centered, and with the amazing editing team of Tina Kaemmerer, Lee Henderson, and Carol O'Connell for this eighth edition.

Sandra L. Gardner RN, MS, CNS, PNP
Senior Editor

CONTENTS

1

EVIDENCE-BASED CLINICAL PRACTICE

ALFONSO F. PANTOJA AND MARY ENZMAN HINES

Globally, health care systems are experiencing challenges when evaluating therapies, quality of care, and the risk of adverse events in clinical practice. Often health care systems fail to optimally use evidence. This failure is either from underuse, overuse, or misuse of evidence-based therapies and/or system failures.[75] Evidence-based practice (EBP) requires the integration of the best research evidence with our clinical expertise and each patient's unique values and circumstances.[75] EBP approaches in all fields of health care could prevent therapeutic disasters resulting from the informal "let's-try-it-and-see" methods of testing new therapies that are not recognized as risky. The epidemic of retinopathy attributable to the indiscriminate use of supplemental oxygen; gray baby syndrome attributable to the administration of chloramphenicol; kernicterus attributable to the introduction of sulfonamides[65]; and death due to liver toxicity of 40 premature newborns attributable to the administration of a parenteral form of vitamin E (E-Ferol)[71] are examples of these therapeutic misadventures in the field of neonatal care. Silverman described how painfully slow health care providers were to embrace a culture of skepticism and emphasizes, "We must insist on the highest standards of evidence in studies involving the youngest human beings; and, since there is no short route to this goal, we must prepare to be patient."[64] The use of experimentation and the scientific method has ultimately led to our present views of how to ask and answer clinical questions.[56]

Mistakes have also occurred at the other extreme, as well, resulting in a failure to adopt therapies that are of proven benefit or an assumption that the risks associated with changing practice justify complacency about current treatments. The significant delay in the adoption of antenatal corticosteroids by the obstetric community to promote fetal lung maturation[19,68] is a good example of failure to use the available evidence. One of the most important benefits of EBP is the constant questioning: "Have our current clinical practices been studied in appropriately selected populations, of sufficient size to accurately predict their efficacy, benefit, safety, side effects, and cost?"

EBP is a systematic way to integrate the best patient-centered, clinically relevant research with our clinical expertise and with the unique preferences, concerns, and expectations that each patient brings to a clinical encounter.[75] Furthermore, EBP presents an opportunity to enhance patient health and illness outcomes, increase staff satisfaction, and reduce health care expenses. There is great interest in identifying barriers and facilitators that could help in closing the knowledge-to-practice gap that is inherent to the acceptance and adoption of EBP by all providers.[76]

FINDING HIGH-QUALITY EVIDENCE

As new therapies are integrated into neonatal care, health care providers must continue to increase existing knowledge of the health and health problems of newborns. Providers need to formulate

PURPLE type highlights content that is particularly applicable to clinical settings.

well-designed questions about the specific clinical encounter and learn how to evaluate the quality of evidence regarding risks and benefits of new practices. Most clinical questions arise through daily practice and often involve knowledge gaps in background (general knowledge) and foreground (specific knowledge to inform clinical decisions or actions). The knowledge needs will vary according to the experience of the clinician.[75]

It is not the purpose of this chapter to provide a detailed review of the various research designs that permit reliable scientific inference. Rather, our purpose is to promote the propositions that (1) challenge clinical observations and wisdom by finding the current best evidence and (2) careful assessment and critique of research that supports or challenges the use of new and established clinical practices.

Clinical observations, although valuable in shaping research questions, are limited by selective perception—a desire to see a strategy work or fail to work. At times, a single case or case study may prompt us to question whether we should consider changing current practice. In some situations, much can be learned from carefully maintained databases. Such knowledge is gained only when we have formed databases with clear intentions and have collected the necessary data.

Sinclair and Bracken[67] described four levels of clinical research used to evaluate safety and efficacy of therapies, based on their ability to provide an unbiased answer. In ascending order, these are (1) single case or case series reports without controls, (2) nonrandomized studies with historical controls, (3) nonrandomized studies with concurrent controls, and (4) randomized controlled trials (RCTs). RCTs test hypotheses by using randomly assigned treatment and control groups of adequate size to examine the efficacy and safety of a new therapy. In theory, random assignment of the treatment balances unknown or unmeasured factors that might otherwise bias the outcome of the trial. A *meta-analysis* is a systematic review of the current literature that uses statistical methods to combine the results of individual studies and summarizes the results (http://neonatal.cochrane.org).[18] Tyson[79] has suggested criteria for identifying proven therapies in current literature (Box 1-1). Ideally, therapeutic recommendations are supported by evidence from systematic reviews of RCTs; however, such evidence is

BOX 1-1   PROVEN THERAPIES

Reported to be beneficial in a well-performed meta-analysis of all trials

or

Beneficial in at least one multicenter trial or two single-center trials

Modified from Tyson JE: Use of unproven therapies in clinical practice and research: how can we better serve our patients and their families? *Semin Perinatol* 19:98, 1995.

TABLE 1-1   LEVELS OF EVIDENCE

LEVEL OF EVIDENCE	THERAPY/PREVENTION/ETIOLOGY/HARM
1a	Systematic reviews of RCTs
1b	Individual RCT with narrow confidence interval
1c	All or none
2a	Systematic review of cohort studies
2b	Individual cohort study (including low-quality RCT [less than 80% follow-up])
3a	Systematic review of case-control study
3b	Individual case-control study
4	Case-controlled studies
5	Expert opinion without critical appraisal

From Straus SE, Richardson WS, Haynes RB: *Evidence-based medicine: how to practice and teach it*, ed 4, London, 2011, Harcourt.
RCT, Randomized controlled trial.

not always available. It is then important to have a system to grade the strength of the quality of the evidence found. An international collaboration has developed GRADE, providing an explicit strategy for grading evidence and the strength of recommendations.[36] GRADE classifies the evidence into one of four levels: high, moderate, low, and very low (Table 1-1). The strength of the recommendation is graded as strong or weak. Factors that influence the strength of the recommendation include desirable or undesirable effects, values, preferences, and economic implications (Figure 1-1).

Although conclusions drawn from quantitative studies (RCTs, meta-analysis of RCTs) are regarded as the strongest level of evidence, evidence from descriptive and qualitative studies should be factored

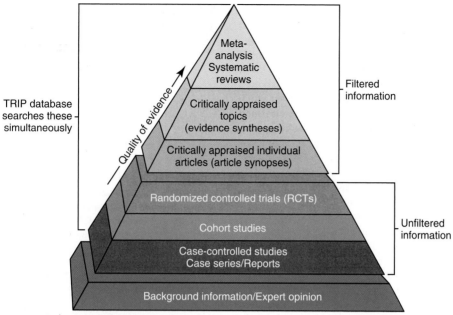

FIGURE 1-1 **Evidence appraisal.** (Adapted from DiCenso A, Bayley L, Haynes RB: Accessing pre-appraised evidence: fine-tuning the 5S model into the 6S model, *Evid Based Nurs* 12:99, 2009.)

into clinical decisions. Qualitative research provides guidance in deciding whether the findings of quantitative studies could be replicated in various patient populations. Qualitative research can also facilitate an understanding of the experience and values of patients. The validity, importance, and applicability of qualitative studies need to be evaluated in a similar way as quantitative studies.

PRESSURES TO INTERVENE

RCTs of appropriate size are cited as providing the best evidence for guiding clinical decisions; however, many take years to complete and publish. Providers find it difficult to delay introduction of promising therapies. Bryce and Enkin[12] discussed myths about RCTs and rationales for not conducting them. One myth is that randomization is unethical. This might be true in rare instances when an intervention is dramatically effective and lifesaving. The more common situation is one where there is limited evidence for a current or alternative strategy.

Pressure to intervene is, however, often overpowering. Believing that an infant is in trouble, interventions occur through a cascade of interventions,[49] one

leading to the next and each carrying risk. One of the most frequently cited examples is the epidemic of blindness associated with the unrestricted use of oxygen in newborns.[63,64] Oxygen, used since the early 1900s for resuscitation and treatment of cyanotic episodes, was noted in the 1940s to "correct" periodic breathing in premature infants. After World War II and introduction of new gas-tight incubators, an epidemic of blindness occurred, resulting from retrolental fibroplasia (RLF). Silverman[63] pointed out that although many causes were suspected, it was not until 1954 that a multicenter, controlled trial confirmed the association between high oxygen concentrations and RLF. Frequently forgotten, however, is that in subsequent years, mortality was increased in infants cared for with an equally experimental regimen of strict restriction of oxygen administration and many survivors had spastic diplegia. In the 1960s, the introduction of micro techniques for measuring arterial oxygen tension permitted better monitoring of oxygen therapy, with a reduction in mortality, spastic diplegia, and RLF, now called *retinopathy of prematurity* (ROP). Severe ROP is currently limited to extremely low-birth-weight (ELBW) infants.[63] Research continues to explore causes, preventive measures, and treatments (see Chapter 31).

Large multinational, pragmatic RCTs to resolve the uncertainty surrounding the most appropriate levels of oxygen saturation in premature infants have been recently conducted and the results published.[60,77,78] The publication of the results of the SUPPORT trial[77] brought about a significant debate about the ethical aspects of comparative effectiveness research and parental informed consent when one of the elements of the composite outcome was death before discharge.[63] The practice of allowing very-low-birth-weight (VLBW) infants to maintain lower O_2 saturations during the first weeks of life had been widely disseminated throughout the United States and the world due to anecdotal reports of a significant decrease in the severity of ROP and blindness with this approach.[17] The SUPPORT[77] and BOOST II[78] trials showed a significant decrease in the frequency of severe ROP and an increase in mortality rate in the low-saturation group. However, another study with a similar design[60] showed no significant effect on the rate of death or disability at 18 months.

The desire to see an intervention "work" encourages practitioners and investigators to seek early signs of benefit. Long-term effects are frequently overlooked. One reason is that they may not be foreseen. Consider the example of diethylstilbestrol (DES). DES administration to pregnant women was introduced in 1947 without clinical trials to prevent miscarriage, fetal death, and preterm delivery.[12,30] It was thought to be effective after uncontrolled studies despite controlled trials summarized in an overview (meta-analysis) by Goldstein et al[34] (Table 1-2) that showed the opposite. Clearly, DES was not effective, but it continued to be used until the 1970s, when the Food and Drug Administration (FDA) finally disapproved its use. The unforeseen result was that female children born to mothers who were given DES had structural abnormalities of the genital tract, pregnancy complications, decreased fertility, and an increased risk for vaginal adenocarcinoma in young women. Male children had epididymal cysts. This is not the only example of physicians continuing to use therapies that have been shown in RCTs to be of no benefit.[15]

The costs of long-term studies and follow-up surveillance are numerous. However, when effects are measured later in life (e.g., psychological problems, ability to function in school), the cost cannot determine study design. Even when randomized trials are conclusive, unanswered questions remain: Will

	TABLE 1-2	EFFECTS OF DIETHYLSTILBESTROL (DES) ON PREGNANCY OUTCOMES
	TYPICAL ODDS RATIO*	95% CONFIDENCE LIMITS
Miscarriage	1.20	0.89-1.62
Stillbirth	0.95	0.50-1.83
Neonatal death	1.31	0.74-2.34
All three	1.38	0.99-1.92
Prematurity	1.47	1.08-2.00

Data from Goldstein PA, Sacks HS, Chalmers TC: Hormone administration for the maintenance of pregnancy. In Chalmers I, Enkin M, Keirse M, editors: *Effective care in pregnancy and childbirth,* New York, 1989, Oxford University Press.

*An odds ratio is an estimate of the likelihood (or odds) of being affected by an exposure (e.g., a drug or treatment), compared with the odds of having that outcome without having been exposed. Women receiving DES did not have fewer stillbirths, premature births, or miscarriages than women who were untreated.

a technology or treatment have the same effect in all settings? Has an "appropriate" target population been selected? Are there long-term unforeseeable consequences?

EVALUATION OF THERAPIES

The major cause of death in premature infants is respiratory failure from respiratory distress syndrome (RDS) (see Chapter 23). Previously called *hyaline membrane disease,* this syndrome of expiratory grunting, nasal flaring, chest wall retractions, and cyanosis unresponsive to high oxygen concentrations was a mystery until the 1950s.[64]

The evaluation of various therapies for RDS contrasts the value of controlled and uncontrolled trials. Sinclair[66] noted that uncontrolled studies were more likely to show benefit than controlled trials. In 19 uncontrolled studies, 17 popular therapies showed "benefit." In 18 controlled studies, only 9 demonstrated benefit. An untrained reviewer of the research might base clinical practice on faulty conclusions of uncontrolled trials.

Surfactant Therapy

In contrast to many proposed treatments, surfactant therapy in premature infants has been well studied in RCTs.[3,37] Studies have evaluated the use of surfactant in treatment of RDS, including the optimal source and composition of surfactant and prophylactic versus rescue treatment. Morbidity (including pneumothorax, periventricular or intraventricular hemorrhage, bronchopulmonary dysplasia [BPD], and patent ductus arteriosus) and mortality rates in treatment and control groups have been compared. Systematic reviews of surfactant therapy confirm the effect of surfactant therapy in reducing the risk of morbidity and mortality.[67,72] Although RCTs involving thousands of newborns have clearly demonstrated the benefits of surfactant therapy, unanswered questions remain. One of

these questions is if prophylactic administration of surfactant to an infant judged to be at risk of developing RDS was better than early selective use of surfactant to infants with established RDS. Early trials demonstrated a decreased risk of air leak and mortality with the prophylactic approach. However, recent RCTs that reflect current practice (i.e., greater utilization of maternal steroids and routine postdelivery stabilization on continuous positive airway pressure [CPAP]) do not support these differences and actually demonstrate less risk of chronic lung disease or death when using early stabilization on CPAP with selective surfactant administration to infants requiring intubation[59,77] (Figure 1-2).

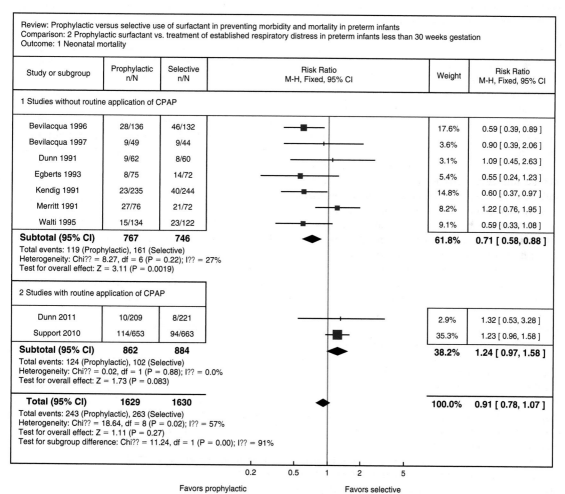

FIGURE 1-2 Table showing effect of prophylactic versus selective surfactant administration on morbidity and mortality rates in preterm infants. (From Rojas-Reyes X, Morley C, Soll R: Prophylactic versus selective use of surfactant in preventing morbidity and mortality in preterm infants, *Cochrane Database Syst Rev* 3:CD000510, 2012.)

Corticosteroid Therapy

Misuse of corticosteroids in perinatal medicine illustrates the consequences of failure to practice evidence-based medicine. Many practitioners initially declined to use antenatal steroids to promote maturation of the immature fetal lung and prevent RDS despite strong supportive evidence, demonstrating a failure to use a proven therapy.

ANTENATAL CORTICOSTEROID THERAPY: SINGLE COURSE

Antenatal administration of corticosteroids to pregnant women who threatened to deliver prematurely was first shown in 1972 to decrease neonatal mortality rate and the incidence of RDS and intraventricular hemorrhage (IVH) in premature infants.[44] In 1990, Crowley et al[21] used meta-analysis to evaluate 12 RCTs of maternal corticosteroid administration involving more than 3000 women. The data showed that maternal corticosteroid treatment significantly reduced the risk for neonatal mortality, RDS, and IVH. Sinclair,[68] using a "cumulative meta-analysis" approach of randomized trials, clearly demonstrated that the aggregate evidence that was sufficient to show that this treatment reduces the incidence of RDS and neonatal death was available for almost 20 years before the use of antenatal corticosteroids was widely accepted by the medical community.

This led to the National Institutes of Health (NIH) consensus development conference statement on "Effects of Corticosteroids for Fetal Maturation on Perinatal Outcomes."[50] Antenatal corticosteroid treatment of women at risk for preterm delivery between 24 and 34 weeks of gestation has been shown to be effective and safe in enhancing fetal lung maturity and reducing neonatal mortality. Yet adoption by caretakers was inexplicably slow.[42]

ANTENATAL CORTICOSTEROID THERAPY: REPEATED COURSES

At the same time, other practitioners administered repeated doses despite lack of evidence of additional benefit and questions about safety, representing unproven use of a proven therapy. Repeated courses of antenatal corticosteroids have been shown in humans and animals to improve lung function and the quantity of pulmonary surfactant.[22,35] They may also have adverse effects on lung structure, fetal somatic growth, and neonatal adrenocortical function, as well as poorly understood effects on blood pressure, carbohydrate homeostasis, and psychomotor development.[22,48] A 2000 NIH Consensus Development Conference found limited high-quality studies on the use of repeated courses of antenatal steroids.[51] The consensus statement discouraged routine use of repeated courses of antenatal corticosteroids. Published preliminary reports of infants exposed to multiple doses of antenatal steroids reaching school age are emerging.[6] A recent meta-analysis of infants exposed to more than one course of antenatal corticosteroids concluded that "although the short-term neonatal benefits of repeated courses of antenatal corticosteroids support their use, long-term benefits have not been demonstrated and long-term adverse effects have not been ruled out. The adverse effect of repeated doses of antenatal corticosteroids on birth weight and weight at early childhood follow-up is a concern. Caution should therefore be exercised to ensure that only those women who are at particularly high risk of very early preterm birth are offered treatment with repeated courses of antenatal corticosteroids."[23] The American College of Obstetricians and Gynecologists (ACOG) recommends a repeat course of antenatal steroids if the fetus is less than 34 weeks of gestation and the previous course of antenatal steroids was administered more than 14 days earlier.[4]

POSTNATAL STEROID THERAPY

Postnatal glucocorticoids, administered to the infant after birth, have been widely used despite weak evidence of long-term benefit and suggestions of possible harm, illustrating use of an uncertain therapy.[42] Despite early calls for caution in the use of postnatal corticosteroids to decrease the risk for chronic lung disease and limit ventilator time, they were used liberally in the 1990s.[70,74] A number of years passed before RCTs of postnatal corticosteroid administration included long-term follow-up. Taken together, these studies showed positive short-term effects on the lungs. Studies also showed increased blood pressure and blood glucose concentrations in the short term; increased incidence of septicemia and gastrointestinal perforation in the intermediate term; and with dexamethasone administered soon after birth, abnormal neurodevelopmental outcome, including cerebral palsy, in the long term.[25,37,43,74] An increased risk for septicemia should have been anticipated, because it was first identified in an RCT by Reese et al[58] over 50 years earlier.

In 2002, the American Academy of Pediatrics (Committee on Fetus and Newborn) and the Canadian Paediatric Society (Fetus and Newborn Committee) advised against the use of systemic dexamethasone and suggested that "outside the context of a RCT that include assessment of long-term development, the use of corticosteroids should be limited to exceptional clinical circumstances (e.g., an infant on maximal ventilator support and oxygen requirement)."[2] A 2005 reanalysis of many of the same data by Doyle et al[25] suggests that relative risks and benefits of postnatal corticosteroids vary with level of risk for BPD. When the risk for BPD or death is high, the risk for developmental impairment from postnatal corticosteroids might be outweighed by benefit.[27,29] Watterberg et al[83] suggested that hydrocortisone might have the benefits of dexamethasone on the lungs without adverse neurologic effects. Following these statements, the exposure of at-risk prematures decreased dramatically.[81,82]

QUALITATIVE RESEARCH EVALUATING EXPERIENCES IN THE NEONATAL INTENSIVE CARE UNIT

The contribution of qualitative research to EBP is evident when "best evidence from RCTs" may or may not work within the context of specific neonatal intensive care unit (NICU) environments. The context can be quite variable and influenced by practitioners and staff, the unit leadership, and family influence within the unit. The implementation of family-centered care in the NICU has shown promising outcomes, including minimizing parental stress related to the technology and complex care of a tiny, fragile preterm infant.[46] An environment of family-centered care has also contributed in a positive way to the success of the implementation of clinical practice guidelines and evaluating outcomes.[26] Qualitative studies are useful when limited information exists about a phenomenon or a deficiency is evident in the quality, depth, or detail of research in a specific area of clinical practice. Qualitative research contributes to EBP in several areas: (1) descriptions of patient needs and experiences; (2) providing the groundwork for instrument development and evaluation; and (3) elaborating on concepts relative to theory development.[47]

Systematic reviews and meta-analyses are emerging in qualitative literature researching parental experiences in the NICU.[33,52] In neonatology, qualitative studies provide in-depth views of parental and provider experiences within the NICU setting to humanize the health care of fragile infants. Parents of infants who require NICU care begin an experience of parenthood in an unfamiliar and intimidating environment that results in delayed attachment[38,62]; high levels of stress, including anxiety, depression, trauma symptoms, and isolation (both physical and emotional) from their infant[13,31]; lack of disclosure of their infant's condition; and a lack of control.[16] Mothers often experience feelings of ambivalence, shame, guilt, and failure that the infant is in the NICU.[61] Parents also experience the tension between exclusion and participation in their infant's care.[84] In contrast, parents describe factors that contribute to parental satisfaction in the NICU, including assurance, caring communication, provision of consistent information, education,[20] environmental follow-up care, appropriate pain management,[31] parental participation in care, and emotional, physical, and spiritual support.[20] Conversely, health care professionals' experiences of parental presence and participation in the NICU revealed similar findings to those described by parents: the need to develop a caring environment for parents to be present and take care of their child by guiding parents and giving parents' permission to care for their child, a need for personnel training in the art of dealing with parents in crisis, identifying a balance between closeness and distance, and dealing with parental worry.[85,86]

Quality care is a major issue currently evaluating the delivery of health care services, yet little research has been conducted on what parents of premature infants perceive as quality nursing care. Price[57] used a qualitative approach to reveal the meaning of quality nursing care from parents' perspectives and identified concepts inherent in the process of receiving quality nursing care. Four stages were identified: (1) maneuvering, (2) a process of knowing, (3) building relationships, and (4) quality care. For parents, nontechnical aspects of care, such as comforting infants after painful procedures, were as important as the technical aspects of care. Another qualitative study revealed seven categories that influence changes in practice: (1) staffing issues, (2) consistency in practice, (3) the approval process for change, (4) a multidisciplinary approach to care, (5) frequency and consistency of communication, (6) rationale for change, and (7) the feedback process. Three categories further delineate quality care: human resources, organizational structure, and communications.[73]

SYSTEMATIC REVIEW IN PERINATAL CARE AND EVIDENCE-BASED PRACTICE

Evidence-based practice is the integration of the best possible research evidence with clinical expertise and patient needs.[56,75] Examples from the literature, such as those cited in the preceding sections, illustrate how the application of the principles of EBP offer a strong argument countering those who assert that EBP is nothing more than "typical practice using good clinical judgment." Proponents of EBP argue that the principal four steps of evidence-based practice—formulating a clinical question, retrieving relevant information, critically appraising the relevant information, and applying the evidence to patient care—provide a foundation for practice that leads to improved newborn outcomes and avoidance of repeating medical disasters.

Believing that the results of perinatal controlled trials had to be summarized in a manner useful to practitioners, Chalmers[14] and other perinatal professionals from various countries developed a registry of RCTs. They reviewed a vast amount of literature from published trials, sought out unpublished trials, and encouraged those who had begun, but not completed, studies to make them known to the registry. Once gathered, the studies' findings were summarized in "overviews."

A *meta-analysis* is a systematic review of the current literature that uses statistical methods to combine the results of individual studies (preferably well-conducted RCTs with similar characteristics of the participants and the treatments) and summarizes the results.[75] These results produce unbiased estimates of the effect of an intervention on clinical outcomes and are distinguished from nonsystematic reviews in which author opinions often are reported along with the evidence. Table 1-1 and Figure 1-2 were developed after pooling the results of different studies.

From these systematic reviews, practitioners can learn the strengths or weakness of clinical trials and evaluate the claims of benefit for

implementing a strategy. The result of the efforts of Chalmers et al was the 1989 publication of a remarkably useful book, *Effective Care in Pregnancy and Childbirth.*[15] At the end of the book, the authors reported their own views of the reviewed treatments based on conclusions formed in the preceding articles. They found that although some strategies and forms of care were useful, others were questionable. Some interventions believed to be useful were not useful, of little benefit, or, in fact, harmful. In 1991 a companion publication, *Effective Care of the Newborn Infant,*[67] compiled and reviewed neonatal RCTs.

Multiple networks have been developed to perform multicenter RCTs. This is particularly useful, providing an opportunity to see whether treatments have similar effects in different practice settings. It is also useful in that practitioners in individual settings may not always see enough cases to reach robust conclusions. Rare conditions and rare outcomes are better understood when trials are replicated or their findings are pooled. Systematic reviews provide the opportunity to understand these findings in the context of clinical practice.

About the same time the Chalmers et al book was published, the Cochrane Collaboration was established, again largely through the efforts of Ian Chalmers (www.cochrane.org/index0.htm). The Cochrane Collaboration is a worldwide group with 53 Collaborative Review Groups whose members prepare, maintain, and disseminate systematic reviews based primarily on the results of RCTs. These reviews are published electronically in the Cochrane Library, which contains the Cochrane Database of Systematic Reviews (CDSR: www.cochrane.org/reviews/index.htm), along with editorial comments on these reviews. Comments come from an international group of individuals and institutions dedicated to summarizing RCTs relevant to health care. In addition to the Collaborative Review Groups, there are now 14 Cochrane Centers in the world. These centers provide support for the review groups. The Neonatal Group is based at the University of Vermont.[51] Cochrane Neonatal Reviews are available at the National Institute of Child Health and Human Development (NICHD) Cochrane Neonatal Internet home page; approximately 260 overviews are listed (http://neonatal.cochrane.org).[50]

Additional sources of high-grade integrative literature are also available to the practicing clinician. Critical appraisal of published research takes considerable time, and several groups assemble high-grade literature using a uniform methodology that is typically described to readers as a supplementary article.[9,10] Reading this article once can inform the practitioner if the method used to assemble a review or guideline is sufficiently rigorous. Also, a number of sites do not produce integrative literature but collect it from a number of sources. Some of these sites discuss the quality of the information presented. If we cannot appraise the method used to collect this information, we should always proceed with caution. Additional reliable sites include the following:

- The Database of Abstracts of Reviews of Effectiveness (DARE) (www.crd.york.ac.uk/CRDWeb), a collection of international reviews including those from the Cochrane Collaboration. Reviewers at the National Health Service Centre for Reviews and Dissemination at the University of York, England, provide quality oversight, including detailed structured abstracts that describe the methodology, results, and conclusions of the reviews. The quality of the reviews is discussed along with implications for health care.
- The National Guidelines Clearinghouse (www.guideline.gov), maintained by the U.S. Department of Health and Human Services, Agency for Healthcare Research and Quality (AHRQ), that was originally created in partnership with the American Medical Association (AMA) and the American Association of Health Plans (AAHP). This site provides a wide range of clinical practice guidelines from institutions and organizations. Structured abstracts facilitate critical appraisal, and abstracts on the same topic can be compared on a side-by-side table, allowing comparisons of relevance, generalizability, and rigor of research findings. Links also are provided to the full text of each guideline, when available.

Conducting systematic reviews is time consuming; thus not many are available. Often, the power of RCTs, especially in neonatology, is low. The evidence in published studies does not always apply to our specific patient. In addition, locating relevant evidence is time consuming and may require access to online resources and a higher level of information-seeking skills than are available. Finally, although recognizing that medical expertise and scientific knowledge are crucial components of neonatal care, these rigorous, objective, scientific evaluations create the potential to overlook valuable experiential knowledge of the NICU provided by practitioners and parents.

Reasons to use an evidence-based approach have been well documented. According to Asztalos,[5] there are basically two reasons to try to keep up with the literature: (1) to maintain clinical competence, and (2) to solve specific clinical problems. Phillips and Glasziou[56] suggest that clinicians seek information "just in time" (as a clinician seeing patients) and "just in case" (an almost impossible task to keep up with information pertinent to a particular clinical specialty). The former can be achieved by actively searching for information in filtered, summarized clinical point-of-care resources. FirstConsult (www.firstconsult.com/php/437124517-76/home.html), DynaMed (https://dynamed.ebscohost.com), and UpToDate (www.uptodate.com/home) fall into this category. The latter, "just in case" learning, also called surveillance of the literature, is best achieved by using technology tools to survey the current original literature. These tools include Evidence-Updates from the BMJ (http://group.bmj.com/products/evidence-centre/evidence-updates), auto-alerts, and RSS feeds in PubMed or online databases and journals. Learning about these ever-changing resources is a challenge. Many hospitals and clinics are beginning to include a clinical librarian or informationist as part of the health care team.[7-9,45,69,80]

Newer and practical resources to support evidence-based health care decisions are rapidly evolving. Large multicenter RCTs answer important clinical questions and provide more robust evidence synthesis and synopsis services that are currently integrated into electronic medical records. DiCenso et al[24] propose a hierarchic organization of preappraised evidence linking evidence-based recommendations with individual patients. This 6S model describes the levels of evidence building from *original single studies* at the foundation, and building up from *syntheses* (systematic reviews, such as Cochrane reviews); *synopses* (succinct descriptions of selected individual studies or systematic reviews, such as those found in the evidence-based journals); *summaries,* which integrate the best available evidence from the lower layers to develop practice guidelines based on a full range of evidence (e.g., Clinical Evidence, National Guidelines Clearinghouse); to the peak of the model, *systematic reviews,* where the individual patient's characteristics are automatically linked to the current best evidence that matches specific circumstances. Practitioners should start by looking at the highest-level resources available for the problem that prompts research. These resources have gone through a filtering process to generate evidence that is rigorous and exhibited over multiple studies. Evidence-based clinical information systems integrate and concisely summarize all relevant and important research evidence about a clinical problem, are updated as new research evidence becomes available, and automatically link (through an electronic medical record) specific patient circumstances to the relevant information. Figure 1-1 depicts elements of the 6S model.

At the end of this chapter is a list of additional evidence-based practice resources. To use these resources effectively, individuals must become familiar with the principles and value of evidence-based patient care.

TRANSLATING EVIDENCE INTO PRACTICE

Literature demonstrates that EBP interventions can produce changes in clinicians' knowledge and skills. Even when it is difficult to demonstrate, EBP may induce changes in health care provider behaviors and attitudes.[75] Changes in clinical outcomes are more difficult to demonstrate. In neonatology, the extent to which Cochrane reviews are used and are in agreement with clinical practice guidelines have been found to be disappointingly low.[11] A quality chasm of evidence exists in NICUs.[28] Enormous variations in the use of established therapies exist, so it is not surprising that multiple neonatal networks throughout the world have demonstrated an unexplained center-to-center variability in outcomes.[32,40,41] There are reports of how EBP can be practiced successfully at the single NICU level.[53] However, the implementations of "bundles" of evidence-based practices by multiple NICUs using collaborative quality improvement efforts have reported meaningful results.[54,55] Cluster randomized trials performed at regional or national levels using different strategies have led to significant changes in practice.[1,39]

CLINICAL PRACTICE GUIDELINES

Clinical practice guidelines are systematically defined statements that assist providers and patients

---

> ### BOX 1-2 THE KILLER Bs
>
> **Burden:** Is the *burden* of illness (frequency in our community, or our patient's pretest probability or expected event rate [PEER]) too low to warrant implementation?
>
> **Beliefs:** Are the *beliefs* of individual patients or communities about the value of the interventions or their consequences incompatible with the guideline?
>
> **Bargain:** Would the opportunity cost of implementing this guideline constitute a bad *bargain* in the use of our energy or our community's resources?
>
> **Barriers:** Are the *barriers* (geographic, organizational, traditional, authoritarian, legal, or behavioral) so high that it is not worth trying to overcome them?

From Straus SE, Richardson WS, Haynes RB: *Evidence-based medicine: how to practice and teach it,* ed 4, London, 2011, Harcourt.

---

with decisions about appropriate health care for specific clinical circumstances.[75] Valid clinical guidelines create components from evidence derived from systematic reviews and all relevant literature. Two essential components should be considered when considering the use of select guidelines: evidence and detailed instructions for application. In addition, "killer Bs" affect the instructions for application (Box 1-2). Detailed guides for assessing the validity of clinical guidelines have been developed. The AGREE Collaboration has developed an instrument for assessing the validity of the clinical guidelines, including items focusing on six domains: (1) scope and purpose, (2) stakeholder involvement, (3) rigor of development, (4) clarity of presentation, (5) applicability, and (6) editorial independence (www.agreecollaborative.org).

As stated by Silverman[65]:

> *Since ours is the only species on the planet that has achieved rates of newborn survival which exceed 90 percent, it seems to me we must demand the highest order of evidence possible before undertaking widespread actions that may affect the full lifetimes of individuals in the present, as well as in future generations. Here a strong case can be made for a slow and measured pace of medical innovation.*

REFERENCES

For a full list of references, scan the QR code or visit http://booksite.elsevier.com/ 9780323320832.

2

PRENATAL ENVIRONMENT
Effect on Neonatal Outcome

PRISCILLA M. NODINE, MARIE HASTINGS-TOLSMA, AND JAIME ARRUDA

The human fetus develops within a complex maternal environment. Structurally defined by the intrauterine/intraamniotic compartment, the character of the prenatal environment is determined largely by maternal variables. The fetus depends totally on the maternal host for respiratory and nutritive support and is significantly influenced by maternal metabolic, cardiovascular, and environmental factors. In addition, the fetus is limited in its ability to adapt to stress or modify its surroundings. This creates a situation in which the prenatal environment exerts a tremendous influence on fetal development and well-being. This influence lasts well beyond the period of gestation, often affecting the newborn in ways that have profound significance for both immediate and long-term outcome.

There is great utility in identifying maternal factors that adversely affect the condition of the fetus. Providers of obstetric care have long used this information to identify the "at-risk" population and design interventions that prevent or reduce the occurrence of fetal and neonatal complications. It is equally important that neonatal care providers obtain a clear picture of the prenatal environment and use this information before birth to anticipate the newborn's immediate needs and make appropriate preparations for resuscitation and initial nursery care. After birth, an awareness of the likely sequelae of environmental compromise helps focus ongoing assessment and aids in clinical decision making.

The purpose of this chapter is to help neonatal care providers evaluate maternal influences on the prenatal environment, identify significant environmental risk factors, and anticipate the associated neonatal problems. Maternal factors and environmental influences are important determinants in neonatal outcome.

PHYSIOLOGY

Two variables have a critical influence on fetal well-being throughout gestation: uteroplacental functioning and inherent maternal resources. The interplay of these factors is a major determinant of fetal oxygenation, metabolism, and growth. Alterations in the development and function of the placenta also influence fetal growth and development. The fetus may be affected to the point that survival is threatened. Likewise, extrauterine well-being may be compromised.

The placenta has a dual role in providing nutrients and metabolic fuels to the fetus. First, placental secretion of endocrine hormones, chiefly human chorionic somatomammotropin, increases throughout pregnancy, causing progressive changes in maternal metabolism. The net effect of these changes is an increase in maternal glucose and amino acids

PURPLE type highlights content that is particularly applicable to clinical settings.

available to the fetus, especially in the second half of pregnancy. Second, the placenta is instrumental in the transfer of these (and other) essential nutrients from the maternal to the fetal circulation and, conversely, of metabolic wastes from the fetal to the maternal system. Adequate maternal and fetal blood flow through the placenta is essential throughout the entire pregnancy.

Fetal respiration also depends on adequate placental function. Respiratory gases (oxygen and carbon dioxide) readily cross the placental membrane by simple diffusion, with the rate of diffusion determined by the Po_2 (or Pco_2) differential between maternal and fetal blood.

Although the placenta mediates the transport of respiratory gases, carbohydrates, lipids, vitamins, minerals, and amino acids, the maternal reservoir is their source. Maternal-fetal transfer depends on the characteristics and absolute content of substances within the maternal circulation, the relative efficiency of the maternal cardiovascular system in perfusing the placenta, and the function of the placenta itself. The fetal environment can be disrupted by inappropriate types or amounts of substances (e.g., ethanol) in the maternal circulation, decreases or interruptions in placental blood flow (e.g., placental abruption), or abnormalities in placental function (e.g., small placenta). Maternal nutrition, exercise, and disease can impair placental uptake and transfer of substances across the placenta to the fetus.

COMPROMISED FETAL ENVIRONMENT

Maternal Disease

DIABETES

The prevalence of diabetes mellitus and gestational diabetes mellitus (GDM) is increasing worldwide. Diabetes is the most common endocrine disorder affecting pregnancy, having doubled in the past decade with approximately 4% to 10% of pregnant women in the United States diagnosed with GDM annually.[21] This increase is likely fueled by the obesity epidemic. Despite major reductions in mortality rates over the past several decades, the infant of a diabetic mother (IDM) continues to have a considerable perinatal disadvantage. The physiologic changes in maternal glucose use that accompany pregnancy, coupled with either a preexisting hyperglycemia

(as found in types 1 and 2 diabetes) or an inability to mount an appropriate insulin response (as seen in patients with gestational diabetes), result in a significantly abnormal fetal environment. This is because of the increased level of maternal glucose, often in concert with episodic hypoglycemia, as well as high levels of triglycerides and free fatty acids. Early in pregnancy, this environment may have a teratogenic effect on the embryo, accounting for the dramatic increase in spontaneous abortions and congenital malformations in the offspring of diabetic women with poor metabolic control.[7] During the second and third trimesters, the mechanics of placental transport dictate that fetal glucose levels depend on, but are slightly less than, maternal levels.[11] Assuming adequate placental function and perfusion, elevations in maternal glucose lead to fetal hyperglycemia and increased fetal insulin production. Repeated or continued elevations in blood glucose result in fetal hyperinsulinism, alterations in the use of glucose and other nutrients, and altered patterns of growth and development.[7,11]

Fetal macrosomia (greater than the 90th percentile for weight) occurs in 25% to 42% of diabetic pregnancies because of hyperinsulinemia. These macrosomic infants suffer increased morbidity and mortality rates from unexplained death in utero, birth trauma, hypertrophic cardiomyopathy, vascular thrombosis, neonatal hypoglycemia, hyperbilirubinemia, erythrocytosis, and respiratory distress.[54] Although intrauterine fetal death (IUFD) is at an increased risk for those pregnant women with preexisting or overt diabetes, the most contemporary literature does not support an increased risk for IUFD for those with true GDM.[54] Macrosomic infants have increased risk for shoulder dystocia during vaginal birth, as well as brachial plexus injury, facial nerve palsy, dysfunctional labor patterns, and operative vaginal birth.

In addition to the basic metabolic disturbances, diabetes predisposes the pregnant woman to several other complications, including gestational hypertension, preeclampsia, renal disease, and vascular disease. As a consequence, the fetus may be compromised further by chronic hypoxia and other insults, which can lead to intrauterine demise, prematurity, growth restriction, cardiovascular problems, respiratory distress syndrome (RDS), and long-term neurologic problems.[7] In terms of predicting perinatal morbidity and mortality, the **prognostically bad signs of pregnancy** include diabetic ketoacidosis, hypertension, pyelonephritis, and maternal noncompliance, though risk of adverse neonatal outcome occurs on a continuum with no clear threshold.[7]

In preparing for the delivery of an IDM, the neonatal team should consider the classification of maternal diabetes (type 1 or 2, or gestational). In addition, the quality of metabolic control throughout the pregnancy and labor, maternal complications, and the duration of the pregnancy should be considered, along with indicators of fetal growth and well-being. In cases where oral antihypertensive agents have been used, there should be careful assessment of the neonate because sulfonylurea (i.e., glyburide) may cause neonatal jaundice. Glyburide crosses the placenta, as does metformin, with the potential to affect neonatal physiology.[12] Both of these medications are thought to be safe for the neonate during lactation (see Chapter 18).

THYROID DISEASE

Thyroid disorders during pregnancy are relatively common. The thyroid hormones *triiodothyronine (T3)* and *thyroxine (T4)* cross the placenta in small amounts, though the significance of the transfer has not been well elucidated. The fetus depends on maternal T_4 in the first trimester of pregnancy. At 8 to 10 weeks' gestation, the fetal thyroid begins to concentrate iodine and produce T_4. During the second and third trimester, the fetus is independent of maternal status. At approximately 24 weeks, thyroid-stimulating immunoglobulins (TSIs) or thyroid-stimulating hormone (TSH) receptor *Abs,* which are classes of immunoglobulin G (IgG), cross the placenta and stimulate fetal thyroid. Iodine is readily transferred from mother to fetus. The fetal thyroid gland concentrates iodine and synthesizes its own hormones as early as 10 to 12 weeks' gestation; this is independent of maternal thyroid function. Maternal thyroid hormones are believed to be important for fetal neurologic development in the first trimester and untreated hypothyroidism has been associated with a decrease in intelligence quotient (IQ) of offspring.[44] Subclinical and overt hypothyroidism should be treated because they may result in increased neurodevelopmental delay in offspring, pregnancy loss, prematurity, preeclampsia, low birth weight, and placental abruption.[44] Treatment with replacement hormone during pregnancy is well tolerated by the fetus and reduces these risks.[1]

Maternal hyperthyroidism presents a different situation. Thyroid-stimulating antibodies, commonly found in patients with Graves' disease, as well as many of the drugs used to treat hyperthyroidism, cross the placenta and can have a significant effect on the fetus. Antibodies, including long-acting thyroid stimulant and TSI, can increase fetal thyroid hormone production. High levels are associated with fetal and neonatal hyperthyroidism. Untreated maternal thyrotoxicosis has been linked to preterm delivery, intrauterine growth restriction (IUGR), low birth weight, and stillbirth. In rare cases, the offspring of women with Graves' disease may themselves have this condition. In fetuses and newborns, this is evidenced by elevations in heart rate, growth restriction, prematurity, goiter, and congestive heart failure.[44] Administration of antithyroid medication to the mother can decrease thyroid hormone production in both the mother and the fetus but may result in fetal hypothyroidism and goiter.[1]

Another maternal antibody, TSH-binding inhibitor immunoglobulin, also crosses the placenta and can prevent the expected fetal thyroid response to TSH. The result is a transient fetal and neonatal hypothyroidism. Iodine deficiency in the mother is another cause of fetal and neonatal hypothyroidism and, in its severe form, leads to cretinism because of the fetus's dependence on maternal iodine reserves.[1]

PHENYLKETONURIA

Phenylketonuria (PKU) is an inherited disorder in which an enzymatic defect precludes conversion of the essential amino acid *phenylalanine* to *tyrosine.* This metabolic derangement is evidenced by an accumulation of excessive amounts of phenylalanine and alternative pathway byproducts in the blood, and these are toxic to the central nervous system. Historically, PKU resulted in virtually certain mental retardation; affected individuals often were institutionalized and rarely reproduced. With the advent of universal neonatal screening in the United States since the 1960s and effective dietary treatment to prevent hyperphenylalaninemia during infancy and early childhood, genetically affected persons may avoid the devastating effects of this disease, have relatively normal development, and become pregnant. For women who do conceive, PKU poses a significant environmental risk for their developing fetus. The care of these women and their infants presents a unique perinatal challenge.

An estimated 3000 healthy young women of childbearing age with successfully treated PKU are in the United States.[57] However, most discontinued their special diet in childhood because, at the time, most doctors believed it was safe to do so. Unfortunately, their blood phenylalanine levels are very high when they become pregnant if they are eating a normal diet. In up to 90% of such cases, the offspring will be microcephalic and/or have mental retardation. These babies also have an increased incidence of low birth weight, cardiac defects, and characteristic facial features regardless of whether they are themselves affected with PKU, as well as preterm birth and intrauterine fetal death.[68] They cannot be helped by the PKU diet, or they suffer from brain damage caused entirely by their mothers' high phenylalanine levels during pregnancy. To prevent such damage, these women should resume their special PKU diets during preconception. Studies have identified improved long-term outcomes when desirable phenylalanine levels (2 to 8 mg/dl) are achieved at least 3 months before pregnancy and maintained throughout gestation.[56] Phenylalanine levels drop quickly once dietary restrictions are instituted, and there is a strong correlation between maternal blood levels and neonatal outcome.[56,68]

PKU is an inborn error of metabolism and approximately 1 baby in 14,000 inherits PKU when both parents have the PKU gene and both pass it on to their baby. Neonatal blood screening will identify these PKU babies. If this screening is performed within the first 24 hours of life, the American Academy of Pediatrics recommends rescreening at 1 to 2 weeks of age to avoid missed cases of PKU. Once identified, PKU babies should be fed a special formula that contains protein but no phenylalanine, started within the first 7 to 10 days of life, and they must remain on an individualized, restricted diet throughout childhood/adolescence, and generally for life. In some instances, breastfeeding may be possible[49] (see Chapter 18). When treatment is discontinued too soon, risks include blindness, learning disabilities, behavioral disturbances, and a decrease in IQ. When no treatment is instituted at all, phenylalanine accumulates in the bloodstream and causes brain damage and mental retardation.[14]

RENAL DISEASE

Maternal adaptation to pregnancy involves major changes in renal function and structure. Renal hemodynamic changes begin early in pregnancy and before significant expansion of plasma volume. Renal blood flow increases in the first trimester by 35% to 60% and then decreases from the second trimester to term. Additional changes include an increase in the glomerular filtration rate and effective renal plasma flow, a decrease in renal vascular resistance, an activation of the renin-angiotensin-aldosterone system, and increased retention of sodium and water. These changes place unique demands on the renal system. Women with preexisting renal disease may have a successful pregnancy outcome with proper prenatal care; however, some women experience fetal loss and deterioration in renal function. Furthermore, moderate or severe renal dysfunction complicates pregnancy and increases maternal and fetal risks and adverse outcomes.[36]

Renal disease in pregnancy may occur as a result of urinary tract infections, glomerular disease, or severe hypertension or as a complication of systemic diseases, including diabetes and systemic lupus erythematosus. Regardless of the underlying etiologic factors, pregnancy outcome relates most closely to these factors: the presence of hypertension and the degree of renal insufficiency before and during pregnancy.[36] Many women with renal disorders are hypertensive before pregnancy, and they often develop a superimposed pregnancy-induced hypertension leading to preeclampsia.[48] Even those with previously normal blood pressures run an increased risk for developing hypertension during pregnancy. The presence of hypertension in these pregnancies represents a significant risk to the fetus and is strongly associated with IUGR, preterm delivery, and perinatal loss.

Drug therapy to control chronic hypertension has been shown to have a beneficial effect on fetal outcome and generally is continued throughout pregnancy. Renal insufficiency, as measured by creatinine clearance or serum creatinine level, also has implications for fetal outcome. Mild to moderate renal insufficiency (serum creatinine less than 1.5 mg/dl) is associated with a generally favorable outcome, whereas severe insufficiency (serum creatinine greater than 1.6 mg/dl) often carries an increased risk for perinatal death. Persistent proteinuria also may increase fetal loss, and a urinary protein excretion rate higher than 0.5 g per 24 hours may be an independent predictor of fetal outcome. As a rule, the number of preterm deliveries and growth-restricted infants increases with increasing blood pressure and decreasing renal function.[36]

Bacteriuria occurs in 2% to 7% of pregnancies. If untreated, asymptomatic bacteriuria may lead to pyelonephritis or acute cystitis. Risks for the fetus are preterm birth and IUGR. Fetal death is an additional risk with pyelonephritis. Prophylactic antibiotics (suppressive therapy) should be given to women with persistent or frequent recurrence of bacteriuria or a history of pyelonephritis in pregnancy.[88] Two special circumstances are dialysis during pregnancy and pregnancy after renal transplant. Women undergoing dialysis rarely become pregnant. When pregnancy does occur, it is associated with significant perinatal morbidity and mortality risks, with spontaneous abortions reaching 50%. Hemodialysis also is associated with numerous complications, including placental abruption, polyhydramnios, IUGR, preterm labor, and pregnancy loss. Pregnancy after transplantation is more common and has better prognosis than pregnancy managed by dialysis. Where maternal serum creatinine remains less than 1.5 mg/dl and the woman is on a stable immunosuppressive regimen, outcomes can be expected to be positive.[36] Neonatal outcomes are typically good unless there is maternal hypertension with impaired kidney functioning in which case rates of preterm birth, small for gestational age, and neonatal mortality increase.[36]

NEUROLOGIC DISORDERS

The risks that accompany pregnancies complicated by maternal neurologic disorders vary according to the individual disease entity and pertain to both the course of the mother's disease and pregnancy outcome. The physiologic and hormonal changes of pregnancy can influence the course of chronic neuromuscular disorders, such as epilepsy, multiple sclerosis, and myasthenia gravis. The medications used to control these disorders can be particularly problematic for the fetus.

The prevalence of *maternal seizure disorders* is about 4 in every 1000 pregnancies, and most are treated with antiepileptic drugs (AEDs). The disorders and/or the AEDs have been associated with increased fetal and neonatal risks, including spontaneous abortion, prematurity, small for gestational age, congenital defects, intrauterine demise, neonatal depression, and hemorrhage. Significant numbers of epileptic women experience an increase in seizure activity during pregnancy. This is probably because of decreased compliance with medication regimens, physiologic changes associated with pregnancy, and gestational changes in plasma levels of anticonvulsant drugs.[51,60] There is evidence that maternal seizures may compromise fetal oxygenation, possibly because of diminished placental blood flow or maternal hypoxemia resulting from postseizure apnea. For these reasons, control of maternal seizure activity with anticonvulsants is one of the primary goals of prenatal care.

Placental transport of anticonvulsants does occur, resulting in fetal levels that approximate or, in some cases, exceed maternal levels.[37] Although the majority of infants born to women with epilepsy are normal, these infants are at increased risk for poor outcomes.[85] There is an increased risk of congenital malformations and adverse cognitive outcomes in offspring of epileptic women treated with anticonvulsants.[37] The teratogenic potential of most individual AEDs remains unclear, but valproate seems to be consistently associated with the highest rates of congenital malformations and the use of other AEDs is recommended if possible during pregnancy.[16,37] There are many newer AEDs but they should be used with caution due to potential teratogenicity concerns. The most common major congenital malformations associated with AEDs are neural tube defects (e.g., spina bifida), orofacial defects (e.g., cleft lip, cleft palate), heart malformations (e.g., ventricular septal defect), urogenital defects (e.g., hypospadias), and skeletal abnormalities (e.g., radial ray defects, phalangeal hypoplasias).[60] The influence of the seizure disorder itself, as well as genetic makeup, cannot be ignored. Maternal folic acid supplementation has been shown to improve pregnancy outcomes for women taking AEDs, decreasing the risk of spontaneous abortion, lowered verbal IQ, and birth defects.[37]

Infants born to mothers treated with anticonvulsants, especially barbiturates, may exhibit signs of generalized depression, including decreased respiratory effort, poor muscle tone, and feeding difficulties. They also may have symptoms indicative of drug withdrawal (see Chapter 11). These symptoms are usually present in the first week of life and include tremors, restlessness, hypertonia, and hyperventilation.[18] In addition, abnormal clotting and hemorrhage in the offspring of women treated with phenytoin, phenobarbital, and primidone have been reported. This appears to be caused by a decrease in vitamin K–dependent clotting factors. Hemorrhage usually starts within the first 24 hours, is often severe, and may result in death. Infants born to these mothers should have cord blood clotting studies done, vitamin K prophylaxis soon after birth, and close observation. Breastfeeding should be encouraged though adverse effects may occur if the mother is taking phenobarbital[37] (see Chapter 18).

Multiple sclerosis (MS) frequently strikes women during their reproductive years. The onset of MS usually is insidious; the course is marked by a seemingly capricious cycle of exacerbation and remission. A wide range of sensory, motor, and functional changes is associated with this disease; the type and severity of symptoms vary dramatically from one individual to another and in any one patient over time. The disease is a T-cell–mediated autoimmune disease of the central nervous system triggered by unknown exogenous agents in individuals with specific genetics.[26] Pregnancy usually is well tolerated and may be associated with MS stability or improvement. The reported effects of the disease on pregnancy outcomes, including risk for malformations, cesarean section rates, newborn birth weight, and rate of preterm delivery, are inconsistent. Some report no increase in adverse pregnancy outcomes, whereas other groups report a higher cesarean rate and a greater number of low-birth-weight infants in mothers with MS.[28] Alterations in neural function, fatigue, and general weakness may play a role in pregnancy outcomes. During the postpartum period, a higher-than-expected relapse rate has been identified and is associated with hormonal changes.[89] However, in women with MS, the disease process itself is not a threat to fetal or neonatal well-being.[26] The priority for neonatal care providers is to determine the extent of the mother's disability, including her level of fatigue and her ability to care for her infant. The availability of appropriate support systems, both personal and professional, should be assessed, and needed follow-up and referrals should be made.

Even though the prognosis for these infants is excellent, some factors associated with MS are potentially problematic. Bladder dysfunction, common in women with MS, often results in urinary tract infections during pregnancy. Associated fetal and neonatal problems include preterm delivery and sepsis. Early identification and prompt treatment with appropriate antibiotics should minimize these risks. An additional area of concern is the variety of drugs administered to MS patients. Immunosuppressants are frequently used during severe exacerbations. The placental transport and fetal risk vary with the individual agent used. Prednisone and intravenous steroids generally are considered safe for use in pregnancy, and disease-modifying therapies (e.g., interferon, glatiramer acetate) can be considered for those with very severe or highly active MS.[26] Whereas the later part of pregnancy typically demonstrates a reduction in MS disease activity, there is often rebound above the pregnancy level during the first 3 months postpartum before a return to the prepregnancy state. A final consideration is the long-term one: The incidence of MS in offspring of a parent with the disease is about 2.5%, compared with 0.13% in the general population; the risk is even greater where a sibling has MS.[26]

Myasthenia gravis (MG) is a chronic autoimmune disease that causes neuromuscular dysfunction and is encountered rarely in pregnancy; only 1 in 20,000 pregnancies is complicated by MG.[47] Cells of the immune system make proteins called *antibodies* that block nerve impulses to the muscles. Antibodies to acetylcholine receptor (AchR) have been found in most affected persons. Distinguishing features include generalized weakness and muscle fatigue with activity. Pregnant women with MG also may experience respiratory compromise due to muscle weakness compounded by pressure of the fetus against the diaphragm,[59] as well as difficulty swallowing.[47] The course of MG during pregnancy is unpredictable and may vary in different pregnancies in the same woman.[32] Unmasking or exacerbations of MG occur in approximately 40% of pregnancies and remission in 30%, with the remaining 30% experiencing no change. During the first trimester and the first month postpartum, exacerbations are more likely.[47] Corticosteroids can be used to maintain the remissions of MG and should be continued on the lowest possible doses throughout the pregnancy and postpartum period. Immunosuppressive agents, such as methotrexate, cyclophosphamide, and mycophenolate mofetil, are contraindicated in pregnancy, but azathioprine and cyclosporine A are sometimes used and plasmapheresis and intravenous immunoglobulins can be effective in the treatment of myasthenic crises during pregnancy. Though uterine smooth muscle is not compromised during labor because it is not affected by AchR, patients with MG may become exhausted during the second stage of labor necessitating instrumental delivery.[47,59]

Infants born to myasthenic mothers may be affected by the drug therapy and the underlying immunologic dysfunction. Increased rates of premature rupture of membranes (PROM), preterm delivery, and cesarean birth have been reported.[32] An additional risk stems from transplacentally acquired anti–acetylcholine receptor antibodies, which cause approximately 12% of these newborns to experience a transient, self-limited course of MG. It is difficult to predict which pregnancies will result in an affected infant, although infants born to women with very high AchR antibody titers may be at highest risk.[47] Affected infants usually present at birth or within the first 24 hours of life with transient neonatal MG, demonstrating generalized weakness, a feeble cry, diminished suck and swallow, and a decreased respiratory effort that may require mechanical support.[32] Therefore plans should be made in advance for delivery of the mother with MG, and intensive care facilities for the newborn should be available immediately. Symptoms from neonatal MG generally subside within a few weeks after birth and do not recur.[32]

MG is not a contraindication to pregnancy and can usually be managed well with relatively safe and effective therapies, including maternal rest. Standard therapies for some obstetric complications, such as preeclampsia and preterm labor, may need to be altered in women with MG.[47] Vaginal delivery is recommended if possible. Breastfeeding is not contraindicated but depends on maternal medications and infant and maternal health postpartum (see Chapter 18).

SYSTEMIC LUPUS ERYTHEMATOSUS

Systemic lupus erythematosus (SLE) is an autoimmune disease that presents primarily in women of childbearing age. The pathogenesis involves the production of autoantibodies and immune complexes. The clinical effects of lupus range from mild or subclinical disease to serious illness affecting multiple organ systems. The leading causes of death are infections and renal failure. In pregnancy, SLE is associated with an increased incidence of preeclampsia, thrombotic events, spontaneous abortion, preterm delivery, IUGR, and stillbirths.[61,84] Outcome is best when infections, renal disease, and hypertension do not complicate pregnancy and when pregnancy occurs with prolonged disease remission.[31,73] A recent study suggests that

4 months of disease quiescence before pregnancy is enough to ensure a safe pregnancy.[67] A history of lupus nephritis or current disease is a predictor of poor pregnancy outcome.[67] Reported frequency of SLE flares in pregnancy is 15% to 60%.[2] When necessary, treatments used with pregnancies complicated by SLE include antiinflammatory, antimalarial, immunosuppressive, and biologic drugs and/or anticoagulants.[31]

The neonatal manifestations of SLE are rare and are attributed to the placental transfer of maternal antibodies to the fetus. Usual findings of neonatal lupus include a transient lupus-like rash (erythematous lesions of the face, scalp, and upper thorax), thrombocytopenia, and hemolysis.[2] These findings generally are transient and clear within a few months. A strong association has been established between maternal antibodies to the anti–Ro/SS-A and anti–La/SS-B antigens and congenital heart block, a rare manifestation of neonatal lupus syndrome.[2,67] The fetal heart block may be detected with antenatal testing; some authors believe that antenatal fetal surveillance with nonstress tests should begin at 28 weeks of gestation. Infants are treated with cardiac pacemakers after delivery; however, about one third of affected infants die within 3 years.[67]

HEART DISEASE

Significant changes in cardiovascular function accompany normal pregnancy. Plasma and red blood cell volumes rise, heart rate and cardiac output increase, and peripheral vascular resistance falls. These changes facilitate increased uterine blood flow, placental perfusion, and fetal oxygenation and growth. They also increase maternal oxygen consumption and cardiovascular workload and can further compromise the cardiovascular status of women with preexisting serious heart disease. Approximately 2% to 4% of childbearing-age women have concomitant heart disease.[74] Pregnancy creates a risk for maternal cardiovascular complications, but especially for those with underlying heart disease, and includes an increased incidence of thromboembolism and sudden death.[63] In some cases, such as Eisenmenger's syndrome and primary pulmonary hypertension, the risk to maternal survival is so great that pregnancy is contraindicated. In general, how well the woman with heart disease tolerates pregnancy depends on the specific disease process and the degree to which her cardiac status is compromised.

Maternal heart disease also affects the fetus. Fetal risks are the result of genetic factors, alterations in placental perfusion and exchange, and the effect of maternally administered drugs. The genetic risk is demonstrated by the increased incidence of congenital heart defects that occur in the offspring of parents who have such a defect. The exact risk depends on the specific parental lesion, mode of inheritance, and exposure to environmental triggers.[63,74]

Alterations in placental perfusion and gas exchange occur when the mother's condition involves chronic hypoxemia or a significant decrease in cardiac output. These factors increase the threat to the fetus, with fetal risk increasing as maternal cardiac status declines. Chronic maternal hypoxemia results in a decrease in oxygen available to the fetus and is associated with fetal loss, prematurity, and IUGR. Significant reductions in maternal cardiac output create decreased uterine blood flow and diminished placental perfusion with a resulting impairment in the exchange of nutrients, oxygen, and metabolic wastes. Possible fetal and neonatal consequences include spontaneous abortion; IUGR; neonatal asphyxia; central nervous system (CNS) damage; and intrauterine, intrapartum, or neonatal death.[63,74]

A wide variety of drugs are used in the management of maternal cardiovascular disease. Although sometimes it is difficult to differentiate drug effects from the effects of the underlying disease, some associations between drug administration and fetal outcomes can be made. Anticoagulants are used to decrease the risk for thromboembolism, especially in women with artificial valves, a history of thrombophlebitis, or rheumatic heart disease. Oral anticoagulants, specifically warfarin sodium (Coumadin), have been associated with fetal malformations, including nasal hypoplasia and epiphyseal stippling, when administered during the first trimester. They also have been associated with eye and CNS abnormalities when administered later in pregnancy. The incidence of warfarin embryopathy is estimated to be 15% to 25%. Warfarin also is associated with maternal and fetal hemorrhage. Because of these risks, warfarin is contraindicated in pregnancy except in special circumstances, such as pregnancy in women with prosthetic heart valves. Heparin is considered the preferred agent for anticoagulation therapy during pregnancy. Heparin does not cross the placenta; therefore it does not result in fetal anticoagulation or neonatal hemorrhage (although maternal hemorrhage still may occur), nor has it been associated with congenital defects. Low-molecular-weight heparin is another alternative for anticoagulation during pregnancy.[63,74] In general, patients being treated with low-molecular-weight heparin during pregnancy are converted to unfractionated heparin during the final weeks of pregnancy because of the ease of rapid reversal of anticoagulation for labor and delivery. Some studies, however, did not demonstrate any difference in bleeding complications for gravidas continued on low-molecular-weight heparin versus those who were converted to unfractionated heparin.[63]

Antiarrhythmic medications and cardiac glycosides used during pregnancy cross the placenta to varying degrees. They have not been implicated in fetal malformations and, although several have been associated with minor complications, generally are considered safe for use in pregnancy.[63] Reported complications include uterine contractions (quinidine, disopyramide), decreased birth weight (digoxin, disopyramide), and maternal hypotension with a sudden decrease in placental perfusion (verapamil).

Antihypertensives and diuretics also have been used in the treatment of cardiovascular disease during pregnancy. Labetalol and methyldopa are commonly used in pregnant women with chronic hypertension. These medications have been studied in prospective trials that revealed no adverse fetal or maternal outcomes, though methyldopa is not recommended postpartum because it is associated with increased incidence of depression.[63] Their use in the first trimester has also demonstrated safety. Atenolol has been associated with fetal growth restriction and abnormal placental growth.[63,74] Calcium channel blockers, such as nifedipine, are also safely used during pregnancy without an increase in major birth defects or adverse neonatal outcomes.[63,74] Diuretic use in pregnancy remains an area of some controversy. Fetal and neonatal compromise can result from diuretic-induced electrolyte and glucose imbalance and decreased placental perfusion caused by maternal hypovolemia. The use of thiazide diuretics has been linked to neonatal liver damage and thrombocytopenia. In general, diuretic use is restricted to women with pulmonary edema or acute cardiac or renal failure.[63]

Although a great number of complications are possible, remember that, with few exceptions, most of the drugs used in the treatment of maternal heart disease can be used in pregnancy if the maternal condition warrants it. Angiotensin-converting enzyme inhibitors are contraindicated in pregnancy because of an association with fetal injury (renal dysfunction, fetal oliguria, oligohydramnios, fetal skull hypoplasia) and fetal death.

RESPIRATORY DISEASE

Respiratory function is altered even in normal pregnancy. Changes include a decrease in lung volume and increases in oxygen consumption, tidal volume, and minute ventilation. Significant decreases in maternal respiratory function and oxygenation can result in fetal growth restriction and fetal hypoxia with negative outcomes, but careful management of respiratory disease during pregnancy generally results in a favorable outcome.

Asthma is the most common respiratory disease in pregnancy, occurring in 3% to 12% of women, and the prevalence among pregnant women is rising.[3] For about two thirds of pregnant women, the course of asthma worsens.[3] Infants born to women whose asthma is well controlled usually do well; unstable or worsening disease, especially status asthmaticus, increases fetal risk. Commonly used asthma medications (e.g., long-acting beta agonists, inhaled corticosteroids, oral corticosteroids, other bronchodilators, and cromones) are generally considered safe for use in pregnancy. Although children of women with asthma are 10% more likely to have malformations than those of nonasthmatic mothers, large controlled studies have concluded that most asthma medications had no impact on the overall risk for malformations.[81] The exception is cromone exposure, which slightly increases the risk of fetal musculoskeletal malformation.[81] Additional research is needed to determine whether a real risk exists and to guide asthma treatment during pregnancy. Presently, clinical evidence supports pharmacologic asthma control because the fetus is at greater risk from inadequate control of asthma than from asthma medications.[58]

Fetal risks related to maternal asthma depend on the severity of the condition. Controlled asthma carries few risks for the fetus. However, severe or uncontrolled asthma increases the risk for infant death and the incidence of low birth weight, IUGR, preterm birth (possibly influenced by steroid use), and the need for cesarean delivery.[58] Risks are higher in poorly controlled asthma patients.[9] Noncompliance with treatment, respiratory tract infections, allergens and irritants, smoking, gastroesophageal reflux, and exercise can lead to asthma exacerbations.[62]

Cystic fibrosis (CF) was once considered a lethal childhood disease, but the life expectancy of a person with CF has increased, and one study reports that those with CF in the year 2000 will have a life expectancy of around 50 years.[30] With careful planning and appropriate medical care, women with CF of childbearing age may conceive and have successful pregnancies with good neonatal outcomes, especially if their nutritional state and lung function remain good.[83] Women with severe disease may be cautioned to avoid conception because there is a risk for significant deterioration during gestation. Women who are positive for *Burkholderia cepacia* in sputum also have a worse prognosis.[83] Pregnancy in women with CF is likely to be associated with increased health care utilization and more antibiotic use compared with that of nonpregnant women with CF; high rate of gestational diabetes (14%) compared with non-CF pregnancies; and aggressive interventions to ensure weight gain, including the use of total parenteral nutrition for some.[83] Although pregnancy with CF does not increase maternal mortality risk, women with CF have a shorter life span and therefore their days as a parent may be limited. Twenty percent of mothers with CF will not live to see their child's tenth birthday and for those with severe CF, 40% will have died.

Fetal risks related to CF include prematurity, IUGR, and perinatal death, caused primarily by maternal hypoxemia and infection. Because all infants born to mothers with CF will be heterozygous carriers for CF (at least), genetic counseling and carrier testing of the father are important components of preconceptual care and early prenatal care.[83]

Maternal Behavior

Maternal health behavior is an important component of neonatal and childhood health and may even be the single most important factor for the overall health of a child.[65] Health behaviors evaluated here are smoking, substance abuse, and nutrition, but other maternal behaviors also influence pregnancy outcomes, such as sleep patterns and exercise. Appropriate preconceptual and prenatal counseling regarding maternal health behaviors can help optimize neonatal health.[65]

SMOKING

From 16% to 25% of women in the United States smoke during pregnancy,[66] with approximately 60% of smokers continuing to smoke through pregnancy. Of those who quit during pregnancy, half resume smoking by 6 months postpartum,[45] putting children at risk for secondhand smoke. It is well established that maternal smoking is a risk factor for stillbirths, IUGR, placental abruption, placental previa, PROM, and preterm labor.[23] Long-term effects include childhood obstructive airway disease, sudden infant death syndrome (SIDS), neurodevelopmental abnormalities, and childhood cancer,[23] and concerns about exposure to secondhand smoke continue to escalate. The exact mechanism by which fetal growth is restricted or fetal health is compromised is not entirely clear; reduced uterine artery blood flow, reduced placental blood flow resulting from vasoconstriction of smaller fetal capillaries in the placental capillary bed, elevated nicotine and carbon monoxide levels, and chronic fetal hypoxia all may play a role. Fetal risk increases with the number of cigarettes smoked, maternal anemia, and poor nutrition.[93] The babies of smokers may undergo withdrawal-like symptoms manifested by jittery movements and may be more difficult to soothe.[93]

Eliminating or reducing smoking, especially by the end of the first trimester, can improve fetal growth and health. Smoking cessation programs consistently implemented during prenatal visits have been shown to significantly improve smoking cessation rates.[17] The use of nicotine patches to facilitate smoking cessation during pregnancy is controversial. Smoking cessation during pregnancy must be a major priority in counseling women preconceptually and prenatally because these are times when women may be most receptive to quitting because of a strong desire for a healthy pregnancy and baby.[17]

SUBSTANCE ABUSE

Prenatal substance abuse rates vary greatly; however, it is estimated that about 11% of childbearing women have used illegal substances.[93] Use of drugs and alcohol by the mother places the fetus and newborn at risk for a plethora of structural, functional, and developmental problems. Perinatal morbidity is related to the direct effects of the abused substance on the developing fetus, its sudden withdrawal, the interactions of multiple abused substances, the nutritional effects of addiction on the mother, and the social and health care implications of substance abuse.[39,93]

Alcohol is one of the most commonly abused substances during pregnancy. Although known to be a teratogen since the 1970s, about 40% of women in the United States drink some alcohol during pregnancy and about 1% to 5% drink heavily throughout pregnancy.[46] Alcohol in the maternal circulation crosses the placenta, resulting in direct fetal exposure to alcohol and its metabolites.[46] There may be a wide range of effects on the exposed fetus; these include developmental and behavioral abnormalities, spontaneous abortion, stillbirth, craniofacial malformations, growth restriction, preterm birth, CNS dysfunction, and organ or joint abnormalities.[46,91] The mechanism of fetal injury is not entirely clear but is likely related to three main factors: a teratogenic effect, hypoxia as a result of increased oxygen consumption, and a diminished ability to use amino acids in protein synthesis.[19] The expression of fetal alcohol effects ranges from subtle to extreme and depends on the timing of exposure, the dose, and the genetic response of the mother and fetus to the effects of alcohol. Secondary factors, such as maternal age, nutritional status, general health, and the effects of other abused substances also may influence outcome.[91]

When the more severe effects are exhibited, the condition is known as *fetal alcohol syndrome (FAS)*. FAS is characterized by growth restriction; physical dysmorphic features, including facial anomalies (small palpebral fissures, low nasal bridge, indistinct philtrum, thin upper lip, shortened lower jaw); and neurologic dysfunction, including mental retardation and neurodevelopmental deficits.[91] Other physical abnormalities involve the heart, skeletal system, and ears. *Fetal alcohol spectrum disorders (FASD)* is an umbrella term for FAS and other less physically noticeable yet long-term effects of alcohol exposure on the fetus.[19] Infants with FASD also may exhibit problems with suck, tremors, irritability, and hypertonus related to alcohol withdrawal. Continued abnormalities in motor, behavioral, and intellectual development often persist into childhood. Safe levels of alcohol intake have not been established; therefore women should be advised to avoid alcohol intake during pregnancy.

Chemical dependency in pregnancy is a complex problem and creates a high-risk patient. The mother's reporting of drug use often is unreliable; frequently, more than one substance is involved, and there may be a cycle of drug use and periodic abstinence during pregnancy. In addition, a host of medical and social problems are associated with maternal drug abuse. Substance abusers generally have poor health; infectious diseases, such as pneumonia, sexually transmitted disease (including human immunodeficiency virus [HIV] infection and acquired immunodeficiency syndrome [AIDS]), urinary tract infections, and hepatitis are common.[10,39,93] Nutrition and prenatal care often are inadequate; anemia frequently is seen. These factors contribute to a poor pregnancy outcome and make it difficult to isolate the effects of any one drug on the fetus. However, several generalizations can be made. The majority of drugs used by the mother, including opiates (e.g., methadone, heroin), barbiturates, and sedative-hypnotic drugs, cross the placenta and affect the fetus. Fetal risks include growth restriction, malformations, intrauterine demise, prematurity, asphyxia, CNS dysfunction, and neurobehavioral abnormalities. Fetal drug dependence does occur and is associated with neonatal abstinence syndrome (NAS), which is manifested by CNS irritability and gastrointestinal dysfunction[79,93] (see Chapter 11).

Cocaine use by the mother merits special attention. Cocaine is a CNS stimulant that produces vasoconstriction, tachycardia, and hypertension in both the mother and the fetus. Its use during pregnancy has been linked to growth restriction, smaller head circumference, genitourinary tract anomalies, placental abruption, stillbirths, RDS, congenital infection, NAS, and cerebral infarcts, as well as impaired performance as measured with the Brazelton behavioral assessment tool.[20]

All prenatal care providers should thoroughly assess pregnant women for alcohol and substance abuse at each prenatal visit, and treatment interventions should be initiated when abuse is identified. Toxicology screening of maternal blood or urine can verify suspicions of abuse; however, universal screening is not currently recommended. Neonatal urine or meconium screening can provide an accurate indication of exposure when there are clinical indications of drug effect. Laws in some states consider prenatal drug exposure to be a form of child abuse; thus the practitioner may be required to report positive drug tests in pregnant women or their newborns. (See Chapter 11 for a more complete discussion of complications in drug-exposed neonates.)

MATERNAL NUTRITION, MALNUTRITION, AND OBESITY

Maternal nutritional status and placental function during pregnancy can significantly influence the growth, development, and health of the fetus and newborn. Nutritional problems that interfere with fetal cell division (increases in cell number) can have permanent consequences. If the fetus is at a stage in which cells are only enlarging (increases in cell size), nutritional deficits may be reversed if a healthy maternal dietary intake is resumed soon enough in the pregnancy. All women presenting for prenatal care should be questioned about their usual dietary intake and should have their weight and height assessed so that body mass index (BMI) can be determined and appropriate nutrition counseling initiated. BMI can be calculated by dividing a woman's prepregnancy weight in kilograms by her height in meters squared; it is the most frequently used single tool in determining obesity. If a woman's prepregnancy weight is unknown, the value obtained at the first prenatal visit should be used. Although the BMI values for classification vary, the Institute of Medicine (IOM) employs the relative weight classification and prepregnancy BMI values as follows[69]:

- Underweight: less than 18.5
- Healthy weight: 18.5 to 24.9
- Overweight: 25 to 29.9
- Obese: greater than or equal to 30

Optimal ranges for weight gain in singleton pregnancies are also based on the IOM recommendations. As a general rule, weight gain should be as follows: underweight women should gain 28 to 40 lb; normal-weight women, 25 to 35 lb; overweight women, 15 to 25 lb; obese women, 11 to 20 lb. The optimal weight gain for women carrying twins is 35 to 45 lb.[69] The IOM guidelines are continually being evaluated, but at least one study confirms that following these guidelines can improve pregnancy outcomes. However, fewer than half of women gain the recommended weight during pregnancy, with 43.3% of women gaining above the IOM guidelines.[77]

Prenatal nutrition involves more than appropriate weight gain; a variety of healthy foods should be consumed, providing essential nutrients. The dietary reference intakes increase for most nutrients during pregnancy. Protein, iron, vitamin A, and iodine requirements nearly double, yet some nutrient requirements do not change much.[86] Other maternal factors that should be considered when counseling women on nutrition include age, parity, preconceptual nutritional status, preexisting medical conditions, current medical conditions complicating the pregnancy, food likes and dislikes, and cultural influences. Each woman's counseling should be individualized, and referral to a nutrition specialist and other medical specialists may be indicated.

Malnourished and underweight mothers have more perinatal losses and preterm births, and their newborns have lower Apgar scores and more frequently are of low birth weight (less than 2500 g). This is especially true of significantly underweight women (low BMI) and women with eating disorders, such as anorexia and bulimia, who fail to gain adequate weight during pregnancy.[90] Small-for-gestational-age newborns, defined as below the tenth percentile birth weight for gestational age, have higher mortality rates in the perinatal period and are at risk for later problems, such as insulin resistance and poor school performance.[90] However, it may be difficult to draw direct correlations between inadequate maternal diet and fetal growth unless the nutritional disturbances are severe. Many fetuses grow well despite suboptimal maternal nutrition, in part because of the complexities of placental transport and the ability of the fetus to be preferentially supplied with some nutrients.

Although reduced birth weight is associated with inadequate carbohydrate, protein, and total caloric intake, inappropriate amounts of other nutrients may also affect the fetus. Vitamin and mineral deficiencies have been linked to miscarriage and stillbirth, congestive heart failure (thiamine), megaloblastic anemia (folic acid, vitamin B_{12}), congenital anomalies, including neural tube defects (folic acid, zinc, copper), and skeletal abnormalities (vitamin D, calcium).[34,87] Women pregnant after bariatric surgery are at increased risk for nutritional deficiencies and need close monitoring. Vitamin overdosage, especially of the fat-soluble vitamins, also has been implicated in fetal abnormalities. Vitamin A overdose has been associated with kidney malformations, neural or cranial defects, and hydrocephalus; vitamin D overdose has been linked with cardiac, neurologic, and renal defects.[25]

Obesity has become an epidemic in the United States and other developed countries. Public health officials now cite obesity as the leading health problem confronting women today. It is a complex problem resulting from a combination of genetic, cultural, behavioral, socioeconomic, and environmental influences. Obesity affects all organ systems and contributes to a multitude of physiologic complications, such as cardiovascular disease, gestational diabetes, infections, preeclampsia, and other adverse perinatal outcomes.[64]

Overweight, obese, and morbidly obese women (BMI greater than 40) are at risk for chorioamnionitis, preeclampsia, stillbirth, cesarean delivery, instrumental delivery, postpartum hemorrhage, perineal lacerations, and prolonged hospital stay. Their offspring may suffer macrosomia, shoulder dystocia, meconium aspiration, fetal distress, early neonatal death, complications from cesarean birth, and birth defects.[64] A 1% decrease in the number of obese pregnant women in the United States would result in 16,000 fewer cesarean births per year.[24]

In addition, obese women may be struggling with associated psychosocial problems, such as poor self-esteem, guilt about weight, depression, and ridicule from family and others. Some may not seek prenatal care until pregnancy is well into the second or third trimester. Thus obese women should be considered at high risk for childbearing complications, and these women and their fetus/newborn should be monitored closely throughout gestation and the perinatal period. Preconception or early pregnancy dietary counseling, taking into account the increased risk of gestational diabetes for women with obesity, and promoting routine exercise and sleep hygiene can improve maternal health and pregnancy outcomes. Women with obesity are less likely to stay within the gestational weight gain recommendations, yet staying within weight gain guidelines promotes normal birth weight (appropriate for gestational age) and improves perinatal outcomes.[64]

In conclusion, maternal health behavior, including smoking, problems with nutrition, and drug use, before and during pregnancy is associated with adverse outcomes for the newborn and also long-term health risks of the newborn well into adulthood. Supportive, informed prenatal care for pregnant women at risk is essential to improved newborn health.

Obstetric Complications

ANTEPARTUM BLEEDING

Maternal cardiovascular support is crucial to fetal well-being. Chronic blood loss can lead to maternal anemia and a related decrease in oxygen-carrying capacity. Uncompensated acute bleeding results in diminished blood volume, decreased systolic pressure, decreased cardiac output, and ultimately decreased placental perfusion. The net effect on the fetus is decreased oxygenation and impaired nutrient delivery.

Gestational bleeding in the first or second trimester of pregnancy has been linked to increased risks of preterm labor, preterm birth, PROM, and low birth weight.[27] The most common causes of hemorrhage late in pregnancy include placental abruption and placenta previa. In an abruption, a normally implanted placenta separates from the uterine wall before the time of delivery, resulting in maternal bleeding and a functional decrease in uteroplacental size. A relationship between hypertensive disorders, cocaine use, and cigarette smoking and an increased incidence of abruptions has been reported.[27] The risk for abruption was four times higher in women with preterm PROM. In the presence of an intrauterine infection, the relative risk increased ninefold. The separation may be partial or complete, involving peripheral and/or central portions of the placenta. Fetal compromise relates to the extent of the separation and to the frequent need for preterm delivery. When the abruption is small and bleeding is minimal, the pregnancy may continue without significant fetal compromise; however, remember that the decrease in uteroplacental surface area is irreversible and reduces the absolute placental capability. As the fetus grows or experiences additional stressors, its ability to tolerate the abruption may change. Extensive abruptions are poorly tolerated by both fetus and mother; the resulting maternal hemorrhage and decreased placental function lead to fetal asphyxia and, without immediate intervention, to intrauterine demise.

A *placenta previa* exists when the placenta lies abnormally low in the uterus and to some extent covers or encroaches on the internal cervical os. In the latter part of pregnancy, the normal elongation of the lower uterine segment and changes in the cervix disrupt the attachment of the overlying placenta. This generally presents as episodic, painless maternal bleeding, often accompanied by preterm labor. To avoid active labor with resulting maternal hemorrhage, fetal lung maturity is assessed at 36 to 37 weeks.[13] If the lungs are sufficiently mature, a cesarean section is scheduled before the onset of labor. Fetal compromise relates to the extent of the previa, severity of maternal hemorrhage, degree of the resulting fetal hypoxia, and gestational age at delivery.[27]

Other placental abnormalities leading to antepartum bleeding include velamentous insertion and vasa previa. A *vasa previa* occurs when naked fetal vessels traverse the cervical os below the level of the fetal presenting part; it is associated with a high perinatal mortality rate. A *velamentous insertion* is defined as the insertion of the umbilical cord into the chorioamnionic membranes rather than the mass of the placenta. These unprotected cord vessels have a higher rate of rupture. Rupture requires an emergency cesarean delivery to prevent fetal demise and maternal hemorrhage.

HYPERTENSIVE DISORDERS OF PREGNANCY

Chronic hypertension in pregnancy, defined as hypertension diagnosed before pregnancy or before 20 weeks of gestation, complicates 1% to 6% of births in the United States each year. Chronic hypertension is associated with IUGR, preterm birth, placental abruption, and stillbirth.[27] The degree of fetal compromise is related to the degree and control of maternal hypertension. Women with chronic hypertension have a 25% risk for developing superimposed preeclampsia.[71]

Gestational hypertension was defined by the Working Group on Research on Hypertension in Pregnancy as hypertension arising after 20 weeks in the absence of proteinuria.[71]

Preeclampsia, a type of pregnancy-induced hypertension, is a condition in which hypertension, accompanied by proteinuria and edema, develops during the second half of pregnancy in women with or without preexisting hypertensive disease. It is most common in primigravidae, obese women, and women with multiple gestations and molar pregnancies, family history of preeclampsia, and history of pregestational diabetes mellitus.[27] As a perinatal complication, preeclampsia is significant because of its high toll in terms of both maternal and fetal well-being.

Pregnancy is normally associated with vasodilation and decreased peripheral vascular resistance. The net effect is that, even though there is a significant increase in blood volume, maternal blood pressure does not increase during pregnancy. In contrast, pregnancy-induced hypertension is associated with vasoconstriction and an increase in peripheral vascular resistance and arterial pressure. The result is a reduction in blood flow to the vital organs, including the kidney, liver, brain, and uterus; reduced maternal blood volume; and a host of maternal hepatic, CNS, and coagulation abnormalities. Associated fetal and neonatal risks include IUGR, prematurity with all of its attendant problems, perinatal asphyxia, and perinatal death. The risk to the infant increases with earlier onset and increasingly severe maternal disease, such as chronic hypertension with superimposed preeclampsia. Maternal seizures (eclampsia) further compromise the fetus by promoting hypoxemia and acidosis, which can result in intrauterine demise.

HELLP syndrome, a severe form of pregnancy-induced hypertension manifested by **h**emolysis, **e**levated **l**iver enzymes, **l**ow **p**latelets, and renal function abnormalities, carries a high risk for fetal and maternal death. In mild cases of HELLP syndrome, conservative management may facilitate improvement in the condition before delivery, but the risk for IUGR remains. In many cases of HELLP syndrome, immediate delivery is indicated regardless of the gestational age of the fetus.[27] The use of steroids in HELLP syndrome has been shown to improve maternal oliguria, mean arterial pressure, mean increase in platelet count, mean increase in urinary output, and liver enzyme elevations. However, no evidence suggests an improvement in maternal and perinatal mortality or morbidity rates with the use of maternal corticosteroids except with regard to improvement in fetal lung maturity.[27]

Drugs commonly used to treat pregnancy-induced hypertension include magnesium sulfate, hydralazine, labetalol, nifedipine, and other antihypertensive agents. Magnesium sulfate is the most commonly used agent in the United States for the prevention of maternal seizures and has been shown to be more effective than other regimens.[27]

Hypotonia and CNS depression have been reported as neonatal side effects, but magnesium therapy appears to be safe for the fetus.[78] Hypotonia and CNS depression are more likely the result of coexisting complications, such as prematurity and asphyxia. Hydralazine and other antihypertensives are used in the treatment of severe maternal hypertension; actions include relaxation of the arterial bed, decreased vascular resistance, and decreased blood pressure. Maternal response to antihypertensives must be monitored carefully, because precipitous decreases in blood pressure reduce placental perfusion and further compromise the fetus.

INFECTION

Group B streptococcus (GBS) is a major cause of sepsis, meningitis, and death among newborn infants. It is estimated that 10% to 30% of all pregnant women are colonized with GBS in the vagina or rectum. The American College of Obstetricians and Gynecologists (ACOG) Committee on Obstetric Practice now recommends "vaginal or rectal group B streptococci screening cultures at 35 to 37 weeks of gestation for all pregnant women." Treatment for women with a positive culture, GBS bacteriuria in the current pregnancy, or a previously GBS-infected infant is usually penicillin.[4]

PRETERM LABOR

Preterm birth, defined as any birth before 37 weeks' gestation, poses an unparalleled threat to neonatal survival and well-being. Its cost, both human and economic, is staggering, and its prevention is a primary focus of modern obstetric care. Prevention is best accomplished through an aggressive effort to identify women at risk and close follow-up to achieve early recognition and appropriate intervention should preterm labor occur. Unfortunately, many women continue to receive inadequate prenatal care or no care at all. Even women who obtain early and ongoing care often fail to recognize the signs of preterm labor and delay reporting symptoms until intervention becomes difficult if not impossible.[27]

Risk assessment markers in clinical use today include measurements of cervical length and the biochemical marker fetal fibronectin. *Fetal fibronectin* is a glycoprotein secreted by fetal membranes. Its presence in cervical-vaginal secretions between 22 and 35 weeks' gestation has been associated with an increased risk for preterm labor and delivery. Its absence (high negative predictive value) can be used to identify patients who are at low risk for preterm delivery. *Cervical length* is assessed by three consecutive measurements using transvaginal ultrasound. The average length of the cervix varies with gestational change but is approximately 4 cm in length from 26 weeks. The length of the cervix has been inversely correlated to the risk for preterm birth. Thus a combination of fetal fibronectin and cervical length may be used to assess the risk for preterm delivery for a given patient.[29]

Depending on onset of short cervix in pregnancy, cervical cerclage, intramuscular progesterone, and vaginal progesterone have been used to prevent preterm labor with some encouraging success.[15] Generally in women with a history of preterm birth, there appears to be a beneficial effect of intramuscular progesterone to prevent recurrent preterm birth. Evidence supports the use of vaginal progesterone for women with short cervix and no prior history of preterm delivery and early cerclage with short cervix and history of preterm delivery.

Although in many specific instances a definitive cause cannot be identified, it is possible to identify several factors that generally are associated with preterm labor and delivery.[6] When preterm labor cannot be halted, it culminates in the delivery of a physiologically immature infant. The result is a host of neonatal problems that relate largely to the degree of immaturity and also to compounding problems, such as infant anomalies or maternal disease, and to the events that led to the preterm delivery (e.g., asphyxia resulting from a bleeding placenta previa). Problems commonly encountered in preterm infants include respiratory distress, asphyxia, hyperbilirubinemia, metabolic disturbances, fluid and electrolyte imbalances, neurologic and behavioral problems, infection, nutritional deficits and feeding problems, ineffective thermoregulation, cardiovascular disturbances, chronic respiratory disease, and hematologic disturbances.

Beta-sympathomimetic agents are sometimes used to prolong pregnancy in women having uterine contractions but no sign of infection. Mothers may experience tachycardia and dysrhythmias, hyperglycemia, hypokalemia, anxiety, nausea, and vomiting. Myocardial ischemia and pulmonary edema are rare but serious maternal side effects. The fetus also may develop tachycardia and hyperglycemia. Neonates born after beta-sympathomimetic therapy may develop a rebound hypoglycemia in response to in utero hyperglycemia and overproduction of insulin. Beta-sympathomimetic tocolytic agents increase fetal aortic blood flow and fetal cardiac output that might increase fetal systolic pressure and cerebral blood flow, which can lead to an increased incidence of intracranial bleeding in immature fetal brains. More recent studies show lower risk of side effects and improved prolongation of pregnancy from nifedipine compared with beta-sympathomimetic tocolytics (see paragraph on calcium channel blockers later).[42]

Magnesium sulfate has also been employed as a tocolytic. Magnesium sulfate decreases muscle contractility, thereby inhibiting uterine activity and effectively interrupting preterm labor. Neonatal consequences of maternal magnesium administration include decreased muscle tone and drowsiness, as well as decreases in serum calcium level.[50] A double-blind randomized control trial has suggested that magnesium sulfate given to preterm babies may decrease rates of gross motor dysfunction.[8]

Prostaglandins play an important role in the onset of labor. *Prostaglandin synthetase inhibitors,* such as indomethacin, are a class of pharmacologic agents that interfere with the body's synthesis of prostaglandin, thereby inhibiting prostaglandin-mediated uterine contractions. These drugs have been used to treat preterm labor. They can cause in utero constriction, or closure, of the ductus arteriosus with resulting development of fetal pulmonary hypertension and congestive heart failure. They also may lead to oligohydramnios and must be used with caution, especially late in the third trimester. Other neonatal risks include decreased platelet activity and gastrointestinal irritation.[50] Use of cyclooxygenase (COX-2) inhibitors in preterm labor treatment is being investigated.[55]

Calcium channel blockers, such as nifedipine, also have a demonstrated ability to interfere with the labor process. Uterine contractility is directly related to the presence of free calcium. Increased calcium concentration enhances muscle contractility, whereas decreased calcium levels inhibit contractility. Calcium antagonists block the entry of calcium into cells and inhibit uterine muscle contraction. In animal studies, these drugs have been associated with fetal acidosis. However, lower umbilical artery pH values or lower Apgar scores have not been associated with nifedipine.[50]

Corticosteroid treatment of pregnant women who are at sufficient risk to deliver prematurely was first introduced in 1972 to enhance fetal lung maturity. Human studies suggested possible benefits in reduction of the incidence and severity of RDS and the incidence of patent ductus arteriosus. Little or no evidence supported a reduction in mortality rate or reductions in the incidence of intraventricular hemorrhage, chronic lung disease, sepsis, necrotizing enterocolitis, or retinopathy of prematurity with repeated antenatal corticosteroid therapy. Some of the suggested fetal risks of repeated antenatal corticosteroid therapy include decreased somatic and brain growth, adrenal suppression, neonatal sepsis, chronic lung disease, and death. All pregnant women between 24 and 34 weeks of gestation who are at risk for preterm delivery within 7 days should be considered candidates for antenatal treatment with a single course, such as 2×12 mg of betamethasone administered intramuscularly, within 24 hours. The evidence to date is clearly against the routine administration of multiple antenatal steroid courses.[80]

ENVIRONMENTAL EFFECTS OF LABOR ON THE FETUS

Effects of Contractions

During labor, the dynamics of uterine contractions alter the intrauterine environment and influence the fetus. A "healthy" fetus is equipped to withstand the challenge of labor, but when the fetus is compromised or the labor is dysfunctional, the fetus can be taxed beyond its capacity, placing it at risk for further compromise, asphyxia, or intrauterine death.

Strong uterine contractions are characterized by decreased blood flow through the intervillous spaces in the placenta. As blood flow decreases, a corresponding decline in placental gas exchange occurs and the fetus must depend on its existing reserves to maintain oxygenation until placental blood flow is reestablished. The net effect is that fetal Pao_2 decreases as the consequence of uterine contraction. In the fetus with adequate reserves, the fall in Pao_2 is not drastic; the fetus remains adequately oxygenated and so can tolerate the stress of labor.

Fetal Reserve

The factors that influence fetal reserve fall into two general categories: those that diminish reserves and those that exhaust reserves. When fetal oxygen reserves are diminished, the fetus has less-than-optimal oxygenation at the onset of a contraction. This may occur as a consequence of any condition that decreases placental exchange, including reduced placental surface area caused by abruption, placenta previa, an abnormally small placenta, decreased placental perfusion caused by maternal hypotension or hypertension, or maternal hypoxemia. Oxygen reserves can be diminished also as a result of a reduction in fetal oxygen-carrying capacity, as in severe anemia or acute fetal hemorrhage.[43]

A fetal reserve that is adequate at the onset of labor can be exhausted by factors that place unusual demands on the fetus. Exhaustion of reserves occurs with contractions that last for a prolonged period, are of extremely high intensity, or occur with increased frequency and without an adequate recovery period between individual contractions.[43] This is often a consequence of the use of oxytocic agents to induce or augment labor.

Determination of cord gases at delivery can be used to determine the timing of a hypoxic or neurologic event. A base excess of equal to or less than 12 mmol/L generally is defined as the threshold that may be associated with hypoxic injury.[72] Fetal pulse oximetry may also be used. Decreased fetal pulse oximetry values, especially prolonged and recurrent recordings less than 30%, are correlated with abnormal fetal heart rate patterns, indicating an association with fetal compromise and metabolic acidosis.[82]

Another intrapartum fetal monitoring tool, continuous fetal electrocardiogram (ECG) monitoring, is being adopted in order to evaluate fetal well-being during labor. This electrode works through the fetal scalp electrode system and gives feedback on the fetal ECG during labor. Abnormal fetal ECG findings seem to be more closely associated with intrapartum fetal hypoxia than continuous fetal monitoring alone.[52]

Fetal Response to Contraction-Induced Hypoxia

When the fetal oxygen reserve is diminished or exhausted, uterine contractions can precipitate a significant fall in Pao_2. The fetus is quite limited in its ability to compensate for this hypoxemia. The adult mechanism, which involves increasing total cardiac output by increasing heart rate, does not play a major role in the fetal response. Instead, the fetus responds with a redistribution of cardiac output as a means of maintaining critical function; blood flow to the brain and heart increases, whereas perfusion of less critical organs is reduced.[5] This mechanism enables the fetus to survive brief episodes of hypoxia, but severe and prolonged hypoxic episodes are poorly tolerated.

Acute hypoxemia leads to the development of acidosis and also produces a reflex bradycardia as a result of vagal stimulation, both of which further compromise fetal oxygenation. In addition, myocardial hypoxia has a direct bradycardic effect.[5] These mechanisms give rise to one of the classic signs of fetal distress, the late deceleration, in which the peak of uterine pressure, which also represents the nadir of intervillous blood flow and the onset of fetal hypoxemia, is followed by a decline in fetal heart rate. Late decelerations are significant in that they help identify the fetus that cannot tolerate labor because of inadequate oxygen reserves and they allow for the implementation of measures to enhance fetal reserve, improve placental perfusion, or interrupt labor.[92]

Late decelerations are particularly ominous when accompanied by loss of fetal heart rate variability and/or fetal baseline tachycardia, because these findings are indicative of fetal acidosis. In the preterm infant, the findings of decreased variability and tachycardia, with or without late decelerations, correlate highly with acidosis, depression, and low Apgar scores.[92]

Other Factors That Evoke a Fetal Response during Labor

HEAD COMPRESSION

Pressure on the fetal head during labor, especially with pushing efforts in the second stage, also produces a vagal response and a reflex slowing of the fetal heart rate. In general, this does not indicate hypoxia or fetal compromise and often is seen in a healthy fetus. The deceleration that accompanies head compression, also called an *early deceleration,* is differentiated from the late deceleration of fetal asphyxia by its timing in relation to a contraction. In early deceleration, the heart rate begins to fall as a contraction builds, reaching its lowest point as the contraction peaks. As the contraction subsides, the heart rate returns to baseline. The result is a uniformly shaped dip that mirrors the shape of the contraction. In comparison, a late deceleration also has a uniform shape but lags behind the contraction, with the fall in heart rate beginning at or slightly after the contraction peak and continuing to fall as the contraction subsides. With a late deceleration, the heart rate does not return to baseline until well after the contraction has ended.

CORD COMPRESSION

Compression of the umbilical cord occurs when the cord is looped around fetal body parts, when it is knotted or prolapses, or when amniotic fluid is scant (oligohydramnios). During labor, cord compression

may be exacerbated by contractions and descent of the fetus, resulting in varying degrees of occlusion of the umbilical vessels and diminution of blood flow. Partial venous occlusion may be manifested by fetal heart rate acceleration, whereas significant occlusion precipitates a rapid fall in heart rate, caused at least in part by vagal reflex. *Variable decelerations* can be spontaneous, occurring at any time, or periodic, occurring with contractions. They typically have an abrupt descent in heart rate and may be V, U, or W shaped—hence the term *variable deceleration.* Periodic variable decelerations are identified by a decline in heart rate that generally begins before the contraction peaks but, unlike early decelerations, falls rapidly and does not mirror the shape of the contraction. Typically, recovery of the heart rate also is rapid. However, when the occlusion is severe or of long duration or if the fetus has diminished oxygen reserves, recovery may be slow, indicating fetal hypoxia and, in essence, incorporating a component of late deceleration within the variable deceleration.[92]

When variable decelerations are persistent and worsening during labor in the presence of oligohydramnios, intrapartum amnioinfusions have significantly decreased fetal heart rate abnormalities, acidemia at birth, and rates of cesarean birth.[40] An *amnioinfusion* involves infusion of fluid into the uterine cavity via an intrauterine pressure catheter. This fluid provides cushioning of the umbilical cord, which may reduce the frequency and severity of the cord compression. Amnioinfusions have also been used when thick meconium is present in amniotic fluid to provide a diluting effect that can reduce the amount of meconium present in the infant's trachea. However, one study showed no benefit of amnioinfusion on moderate to severe meconium aspiration syndrome or perinatal death.[33]

MATERNAL PAIN MEDICATION

Maternal anesthesia and/or analgesia has the potential to affect the infant, either during labor and delivery or in the newborn period. The risk is increased if the fetus is preterm or is otherwise compromised. This is not to say that there is no place for these drugs in obstetric care—only that they must be used judiciously and with a clear understanding of the risks and benefits involved. Table 2-1 summarizes the effects of commonly used analgesic and anesthetic agents on the fetus and newborn.[7,35]

TABLE 2-1	FETAL AND NEONATAL EFFECTS OF MATERNAL ANALGESIA AND ANESTHESIA DURING LABOR
DRUG	**POSSIBLE FETAL AND NEONATAL SIDE EFFECTS**
Narcotics	Fetal and neonatal effects are related to the dose, route, and timing of maternal administration and may be reversed by the administration of a narcotic antagonist (naloxone): • CNS depression • Fetal bradycardia • Depressed respiratory effort • Decreased muscle tone and reflexes • Decreased responsiveness
Paracervical block	Fetal bradycardia and asphyxia related to decreased uterine blood flow and direct fetal myocardial depression
Epidural and spinal block	Fetal bradycardia and asphyxia related to maternal hypotension Fetal/neonatal toxicity Neonatal respiratory depression after epidural containing fentanyl
General (inhalation) anesthesia	Fetal and newborn effects related to the duration and depth of maternal anesthesia include the following: • CNS depression • Respiratory depression • Decreased responsiveness

CNS, Central nervous system.

ASSESSMENT OF FETAL WELL-BEING

Over the past 30 years, the capability to assess fetal well-being has advanced from simple auscultation of the fetal heart to direct physiologic and biochemical measurement of fetal status. With these advances, an appreciation of the similarities between the fetus and newborn, as well as a more complete understanding of the unique features of fetal life, has been gained. This knowledge reinforces the importance of viewing fetal physiology as a precursor of neonatal function and especially as a significant influence on the success with which the fetus will complete the adaptations required by the birth process.

The goal of antepartum fetal surveillance is to answer the following questions: What is the safest environment for a fetus at the gestational age at which the testing is taking place? Is the fetus more likely to survive in utero for the week after testing, or does the fetus have a significant risk for in utero death based on the degree of environmental or intrinsic intolerance demonstrated through testing? In the case of preterm infants, this may mean delivery at a gestational age at which there is a high likelihood for respiratory, neurologic, cardiac, gastrointestinal, and immunologic immaturity that will require neonatal intensive care.

The obstetric practitioner has several tools available to help answer the preceding questions. First and foremost is the identification of maternal conditions that may predispose the fetus to in utero compromise. Examples of such conditions include type 1 diabetes mellitus, chronic hypertension, collagen vascular disease, antiphospholipid antibody disease, maternal cardiac or pulmonary disease, preeclampsia, blood group isoimmunization, in utero infection, PROM, and maternal substance abuse. This list is not all-inclusive but demonstrates several commonly encountered conditions for which antepartum fetal surveillance is warranted.

Once the decision is made to assess fetal well-being, four modalities are available in general practice to help the practitioner and patient answer questions about the optimal environment for the fetus at any given time—fetal movement counts, the contraction stress test, the nonstress test, and the fetal biophysical profile. Two additional tools often used by maternal-fetal medicine specialists in certain clinical situations are Doppler flow studies and percutaneous umbilical cord blood sampling (PUBS). None of these tools is used as the sole determinant for delivery; rather, each is used in conjunction with the entire clinical picture. The choice of testing method also is clinically driven; each method is useful in certain clinical settings, but no one method is the correct choice in all situations.

Although most of the procedures used to monitor fetal well-being are decidedly high-tech, the simple "kick count," or *fetal movement survey,* is a low-tech, low-cost screening tool. Many women with an intrauterine fetal demise have no identifiable risk factors that would place them in a fetal testing protocol. Fetal motor activity reflects the fetal condition in utero, and a decrease in or absence of fetal movements often presages fetal death. This is one reason that many institutions ask their patients to begin a fetal movement counting protocol at 26 to 32 weeks of gestation. Although there are continuing study results, some centers have demonstrated a significant decrease in the incidence of fetal mortality rates after the institution of a fetal movement counting protocol.

There are several different approaches to fetal movement counting. None has been shown to be superior.[5] One approach is to have the patient choose a certain time every day to rest in the lateral position and count fetal movements. The perception of 10 distinct fetal movements within 2 hours constitutes a reassuring session. The most important aspect of this type of testing is to emphasize to the patient the importance of notifying her practitioner immediately if the fetal movement counting has not met the established criteria. A system must be in place in which patients have immediate access to health care personnel 24 hours per day.

The *contraction stress test (CST)* is used in an attempt to evaluate fetal response to uterine contractions.[41] The principle behind the CST is that uterine contractions cause a transient interruption in uteroplacental perfusion. With normal fetal reserve, this intermittent interruption is well tolerated. With inadequate or exhausted reserve, late fetal heart rate decelerations appear. Because late decelerations during labor had been associated with fetal hypoxia and acidosis, it was reasoned that similar interpretations could be applied to contractions induced in the antepartum patient. Thus the CST is considered a test of uteroplacental reserve.

During a CST, uterine contraction activity is evoked with either the use of maternal nipple stimulation or an intravenous infusion of oxytocin. The fetal heart rate is charted using graph paper attached to a monitor that uses a continuous wave ultrasound transducer placed on the maternal abdomen over the uterus. The minimum number of spontaneous or evoked contractions necessary for adequate testing is three contractions of 40 seconds' duration in a 10-minute period. The results are interpreted as follows:

- A negative CST result is one in which no late fetal heart rate decelerations occur during the examination.
- In a positive CST result, late decelerations occur after 50% or more of the contractions, even if contraction frequency is fewer than three in 10 minutes.
- A suspicious or equivocal finding is one in which intermittent late or significant variable decelerations occur.

- A CST result is considered unsatisfactory if fewer than three contractions occur per 10 minutes or a poor-quality tracing is obtained.

In many clinical situations, a positive CST warrants delivery of the fetus because of suspected in utero hypoxemia during periods of uterine contraction. However, there are numerous exceptions to this rule. For example, if a positive CST is noted in the presence of maternal diabetic ketoacidosis, a correction of the underlying metabolic process may reverse the fetal acidosis and a negative CST may be obtained subsequently. Thus the delivery of a neonate who has metabolic acidosis and is preterm can be avoided.

The *nonstress test (NST)* is a tool used to indirectly assess the integrity of the fetal autonomic nervous system. The fetal heart is under the dual influences of the sympathetic and parasympathetic nervous systems. By approximately 28 weeks' gestation, 85% of fetuses demonstrate fetal heart rate accelerations in response to fetal movement. Lack of these intermittent fetal heart rate accelerations usually indicates a fetal sleep cycle. However, many other intrinsic and extrinsic factors, including fetal acidosis, may lead to an absence of these intermittent accelerations in heart rate. Examples include but are not limited to medication exposure, maternal smoking, uteroplacental insufficiency, and fetal structural or chromosomal anomaly. Factors leading to maternal acidosis (severe anemia, congenital heart disease, and sepsis) also can result in fetal acidosis and nonreactive NST.

The NST is performed with the patient in a semi-Fowler's or lateral tilt position. As in the CST, the fetal heart rate is monitored with an external transducer. NSTs are interpreted as either reactive or nonreactive. An accepted definition of a reactive NST is an increase in fetal heart rate of 15 beats/min for 15 seconds above the baseline heart rate occurring twice in a 20-minute period.[5] A nonreactive test is defined as lacking the necessary fetal heart rate accelerations during a 40-minute period. The following may be candidates for nonstress testing:

- Women who have diabetes that must be controlled with medication
- Women who have pregnancy-induced hypertension, preeclampsia, or intrinsic renal disease
- Women in whom fetal IUGR, oligohydramnios, or postdate pregnancy has been determined
- Women who have reported decreased fetal movement

The NST has certain advantages over the CST. It does not entail the production of uterine contractions, and so there are fewer potential problems or contraindications to the NST. Because the NST is quicker and easier to conduct, it is often the first-line screening test of fetal well-being. Its disadvantages are that it does not evaluate uteroplacental reserve and that it has a higher false-positive rate than the CST.

When the NST is nonreactive, an option that is often used in lieu of the CST or delivery of the fetus is the *biophysical profile* (BPP) (Table 2-2). This test combines the NST with real-time ultrasound evaluation of the fetus. Although there are several different BPP scoring systems, the one most generally accepted assigns a numerical score of 0 or 2 for the absence or presence, respectively, of five different parameters: fetal movement, tone, "breathing" movements, amniotic fluid volume, and the NST. One advantage to evaluation of several different fetal biophysical variables is enhanced specificity of testing with a diminished incidence of delivery for false-positive results. The presence or absence of acute markers (movement, tone, breathing, and NST) helps reflect fetal status at the time of testing. However, the absence of a given marker may be difficult to interpret, because it may simply reflect normal periodicity.

The biophysical activities that mature first in fetal development disappear last as acidosis worsens. Fetal tone (flexion and extension) is present at 7½ to 8½ weeks after the last menstrual period. This activity, as well as gross body movement, is mediated in the cortex and nuclei of the CNS. Fetal movement is present by 9 weeks. Fetal breathing movements (i.e., rhythmic breathing movements of 35 seconds or more) can be seen by 20 weeks' gestation. The CNS center responsible for control of this activity is the ventral surface of the fourth ventricle. The final acute marker to mature is fetal heart rate acceleration in response to movement (reactive NST) seen in the later second trimester. The posterior hypothalamus and medulla control this activity. Given that the first marker to appear in development is the last to disappear with worsening fetal acidosis, the absence of fetal tone has been found to be associated with high perinatal morbidity and mortality rates. Chronic sustained fetal hypoxia or acidosis may produce a protective redistribution of cardiac output away from less vital fetal organs (e.g., kidney, lung) toward the essential organs (e.g., brain, heart, adrenal glands). Redistribution of fetal blood flow may be so profound that renal perfusion decreases to the point that oligohydramnios is established. When the largest vertical amniotic fluid pocket within the uterus is less than 1 cm, the perinatal mortality rate is as high as 110 per 1000.[22,38]

A BPP score of 8 or 10 is normal; a score of 6 is equivocal, and the profile should be repeated in 12 to 24 hours. A score of 4 or less is abnormal. Management in the presence of an abnormal BPP depends on the gestational age and the maternal and/or fetal factors contributing to the altered state.

The BPP employs the advantages of real-time ultrasonography to observe fetal behavior.[27] One of its major advantages is as an intermediate step in the evaluation of a fetus with a nonreactive NST

TABLE 2-2 BIOPHYSICAL PROFILE SCORING		
BIOPHYSICAL VARIABLE	**NORMAL (2)**	**ABNORMAL (0)**
Fetal breathing—At least one episode of at least 30 seconds during a 30-minute observation	Present	Absent
Gross body movement—At least three body or limb movements during a 30-minute observation	≥3	≤2
Fetal tone—One episode of extension or flexion of limbs or trunk during a 30-minute observation	Present	Absent
Reactive nonstress test—At least two episodes of 15 beats/min fetal heart rate accelerations during 30-minute observation	Yes	No
Amniotic fluid volume—A pocket of fluid that measures at least 2 cm in two planes perpendicular to each other (2 × 2–cm pocket)	Present	Absent
Normal Score: 8–10		

before a time-consuming CST is performed. It is also a useful tool for patients with contraindications to the CST, such as premature labor, premature rupture of membranes, placenta previa, malpresentation, unexplained vaginal bleeding, or multiple gestations. The modified BPP, which combines an acute marker (NST) with the chronic marker of fetal well-being (amniotic fluid index [AFI]), has been shown by some centers to be as predictive of fetal well-being as the full BPP. Because evaluation of the AFI is less time consuming and requires less technical skill, this may be an acceptable alternative for many centers. Finally, it should be noted that though widely used, there is insufficient evidence from randomized trials to support the use of BPP as a test of fetal well-being in high-risk pregnancies.[53]

No matter which of these testing modalities is used, the patient should be counseled as to the predictive value of a "normal" test. The incidence of stillbirth within 1 week of a reactive NST is 1.9 per 1000; for a negative CST, it is 0.3/1000; and for a normal BPP, it is 0.8 per 1000.[5] Although some investigators have reported a decreased incidence of fetal mortality after initiation of a fetal movement counting program for "low-risk" patients,[75] more controlled studies are needed.

The role of *Doppler flow assessment* of the fetal arterial and venous systems in the prediction of in utero well-being is also accepted. Measurement of umbilical artery velocity is used as a method of fetal surveillance for growth-restricted fetuses.

Specifically, decreased or absent end-diastolic flow may appear days before conventional antenatal tests become abnormal. In cases such as these, at a minimum, intensive fetal surveillance is advised.[27] Reversal of diastolic flow is highly predictive of in utero fetal demise within 24 hours and warrants immediate intense investigation or delivery.[27]

The dramatic improvement in ultrasound image quality over the past 15 years also has made it possible to directly sample fetal blood and tissue. The technique of *percutaneous umbilical blood sampling (PUBS)* has given the obstetrician access to the fetal circulation with relative safety for both the fetus and mother. In this procedure, real-time ultrasonography is used to guide the insertion of a needle into the umbilical vein or artery. Samples of fetal blood can be obtained, or, as in the case of red cell isoimmunization, transfusions can be carried out. The fetal loss rate is generally quoted as 1% to 2%.[76]

REFERENCES

For a full list of references, scan the QR code or visit http://booksite.elsevier.com/ 9780323320832.

3

PERINATAL TRANSPORT AND LEVELS OF CARE

MARIO AUGUSTO ROJAS, HEATHER FURLONG CRAVEN, AND TAMARA RUSH

Perinatal transport is the timely and appropriate transfer of high-risk pregnant mothers to health care facilities in which expertise and resources for optimal care are available to improve mortality and morbidity of both the mother and her fetus. If transfer of the mother is not possible because of risk outweighing potential benefit, the objective then shifts to optimizing delivery and birth of the high-risk infant. In the latter situation, it is necessary to have adequately trained professionals to resuscitate and stabilize the infant before his or her transfer to a medical center that has the appropriate expertise and resources.

For perinatal transport to effectively support high-risk mothers and their fetuses, as well as sick newborn infants, each country, state, or region must identify its perinatal resources with respect to physical and human capabilities. This review should include classification of levels of care and expertise, as well as mapping of resources as they exist within specific geographic areas. Classification of perinatal resources according to the different levels of care as recommended by the American Academy of Pediatrics and the American College of Obstetricians and Gynecologists in their *Guidelines for Perinatal Care*[5] will direct organization, identification of resources, and roles of patient referral and retrieval centers, as well as reveal the natural elevation of care within the geographic area of question (Table 3-1). Historically, regionalization has been recommended as the most effective and cost-efficient use of perinatal resources.[10,13,14,39,48] The implementation of this important strategy is subject to qualitative variance depending on the characteristics of the health care system and resources where it is applied. In countries in which universal health care is the norm,

regionalization is more easily implemented, whereas in market-driven health care systems in which deregionalization is predominant, these provisions for care become more challenging.[*] Whatever the circumstances, perinatal providers must use innovative strategies to maintain high-quality perinatal transport systems.[21,24]

Because all hospitals cannot provide all levels of perinatal care, interhospital transport of pregnant women and neonates is an essential component of any regional perinatal effort. Women who are at risk for complications and pose significant risk for adverse outcomes or whose neonates are likely to require intensive care support should be considered candidates for referral during the antepartum period.[27] Similarly, it is accepted medical practice to transfer a neonate to a hospital that can provide the services needed or anticipated to be needed if the birth hospital cannot provide that level of service.[†]

Once resources are identified and classified, a model for integration of perinatal services may be constructed. Strategic planning at this level will direct the design of the organizational structure of the perinatal transport system, including identification of leadership functions, the different member nurseries/units and their roles, and the definition and process for perinatal elevation of care. This integration will then allow for the creation of a system for continuous data collection and analysis, facilitating a systems approach to problem solving and the implementation of quality improvement strategies within the system.[29]

---

[*]References 21, 24, 27, 39, 44, 61.
[†]References 10, 13, 14, 21, 27, 39, 44, 48, 61.

PURPLE type highlights content that is particularly applicable to clinical settings.

TABLE 3-1	LEVELS OF PERINATAL AND NEONATAL CARE AND THEIR EXPECTED CAPABILITIES	
	PERINATAL CARE	**PERSONNEL**
	All institutions providing perinatal care should be capable of neonatal resuscitation and stabilization.	
Basic	• Surveillance and care of all patients admitted to the obstetric service with an established triage system for identifying patients at high risk who should be transferred to a facility that provides specialty or subspecialty care • Proper detection and initial care of unanticipated maternal-fetal problems that occur during labor and delivery • Capability to begin an emergent cesarean delivery within an interval based on the timing that best incorporates maternal and fetal risks and benefits • Availability of appropriate anesthesia, radiology, ultrasonography, and laboratory and blood bank services on a 24-hour basis • Care of postpartum conditions • Ability to make transfer arrangements in consultation with physicians at higher-level receiving hospitals • Provision of accommodations and policies that allow families (including their other children) to be together in the hospital following the birth of an infant • Data collection, storage, and retrieval • Initiation of quality improvement programs, including efforts to maximize patient safety	Family physicians, obstetricians, laborists, hospitalists, certified nurse-midwives, certified midwives, nurse practitioners, advanced practice registered nurses, physician assistants, surgical assistants, anesthesiologists, radiologists
Specialty	• Provision of all basic care services plus care of appropriate women at high risk and fetuses both admitted and transferred from other facilities	All basic health care providers plus sometimes maternal-fetal medicine specialists
Subspecialty	• Provision of all basic and specialty care services plus evaluation of new technologies and therapies	All specialty health care providers plus maternal-fetal medicine specialists

Regional Subspecialty Health Care Center	• Provision of comprehensive perinatal health care services at and above those of subspecialty care facilities
	• Responsibility for regional perinatal health care service organization and coordination, including the following:
	  • Maternal and neonatal transport
	  • Regional outreach support and education programs
	  • Development and initial evaluation of new technologies and therapies
	  • Training of health care providers with specialty and subspecialty qualifications and capabilities
	  • Analysis and evaluation of regional data, including perinatal complications and outcomes
		All subspecialty health care providers plus other subspecialists, including obstetric and surgical subspecialists

	NEONATAL CARE	**PERSONNEL**
Level I	*Well Newborn Nursery* Provide neonatal resuscitation and stabilization (NRP; S.T.A.B.L.E.) Evaluate and provide postnatal care to stable term neonates Stabilize and provide care for infants born 35-37 weeks of gestation who remain physiologically stable Stabilize neonates who are ill and those <35 weeks of gestation until transfer to a higher level of care	Pediatrician Family physicians Certified nurse-midwife Nurse practitioner

Continued

TABLE 3-1	**LEVELS OF PERINATAL AND NEONATAL CARE AND THEIR EXPECTED CAPABILITIES — cont'd**	

	NEONATAL CARE	PERSONNEL
Level II	*Special Care Nursery* Level I capabilities AND Provide care for infants born ≥32 weeks of gestation and weighing ≥1500 g who have physiologic immaturity and who are moderately ill with problems expected to resolve rapidly and are not anticipated to need subspecialty services on an urgent basis Provide care for infants convalescing after intensive care Provide mechanical ventilation for brief duration (<24 hours) or continuous positive pressure or both Stabilize infants <32 weeks of gestation and weighing <1500 g until transfer to a neonatal intensive care facility	Level I health care providers *plus* Neonatologist Pediatric neonatal hospitalist Neonatal nurse practitioner
Level III	*NICU* Level II capabilities AND Provide sustained life support Provide comprehensive care for infants <32 weeks of gestation and weighing <1500 g and infants born at all gestational ages and birth weights with critical illness Provide prompt and readily available access to full range of pediatric medical subspecialists, pediatric surgical specialists, pediatric anesthesiologists, and pediatric ophthalmologists Provide full range of respiratory support that may include conventional and/or high-frequency ventilation and inhaled nitric oxide Perform advanced imaging, with interpretation on an urgent basis, including computed tomography, MRI, and echocardiography	Level II health care providers *plus* Pediatric medical subspecialists, pediatric anesthesiologists, pediatric surgeons, and pediatric ophthalmologists
Level IV	*Regional NICU* Level III capabilities AND Located within an institution with the capability to provide surgical repair of complex congenital or acquired conditions Maintain a full range of pediatric medical subspecialists, pediatric surgical subspecialists, and pediatric anesthesiologists at the site Facilitate transport and provide outreach education	Level III health care providers *plus* Pediatric surgical subspecialists

MRI, Magnetic resonance imaging; *NRP*, Neonatal Resuscitation Program; *S.T.A.B.L.E.*, S.T.A.B.L.E. Program.
Adapted from American Academy of Pediatrics, American College of Obstetricians and Gynecologists: Organization of perinatal health care. In *Guidelines for perinatal care*, ed 7, Elk Grove Village, Ill, 2012, The Academy.

REGIONAL PERINATAL REFERRAL AND TRANSPORT SYSTEM

Independent of the health care system with which one identifies (universal versus market driven), the referral system must identify a subspecialty care regional perinatal center, for which the responsibility of coordinating interfacility perinatal transfer lies. Although many different models provide clinical care in transport, the transport system should include the minimal components of (1) leadership (both medical and administrative), (2) communication, and (3) quality assurance (Figure 3-1).

Leadership

One proposed model is the implementation of a leadership team that comprises a medical director, administrative director, and quality director. This team approach enables collaborative and timely oversight of the transport system with potential for growth and quality improvement. The medical director should be a physician with expertise

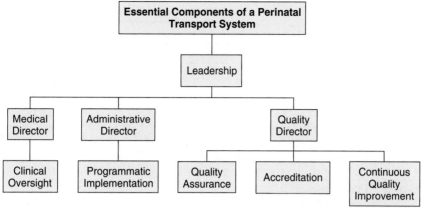

FIGURE 3-1 Organizational structure of neonatal/perinatal transport system.

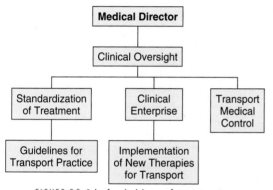

FIGURE 3-2 Role of medical director of transport services.

in transport medicine. The medical director's role includes overseeing the following[40] (Figure 3-2):

- Development, implementation, and monitoring of patient care and transport standards
- Scope of practice of team members
- Team selection
- Training and continuing education
- Support of perinatal partnerships and advocacy

The administrative director working in conjunction with the medical director oversees the budget and day-to-day management of the transport process, including maintenance of equipment. The administrative director should possess clinical transport knowledge paired with strong administrative qualities, because this role includes oversight of finance, human resources, and communication operations (Figure 3-3).[40] The quality director should be a health care provider with a professional background

in continuous quality improvement, process analysis, and management. In association with the medical director and administrator, the quality director is responsible for the development and maintenance of a transport database for operational management, quality assurance, and analysis. This administrator should also be able to apply the basic concepts of quality improvement and management to implement novel interventions aimed at improving the perinatal transport system (Figure 3-4).[29]

Communication

As indicated in Table 3-1, a regional subspecialty perinatal care center should be responsible for coordination of perinatal transport. Integral to the regional transport system is the creation of a centralized communication center with a perinatal regional hotline.[22] The communication center is responsible for coordinating maternal and neonatal transports within the different levels of care. Roles within this center include referring physician, dispatcher, bed locator, and transport medical control officer (obstetrician and neonatologist). The inclusion of specialized personnel in the initial communication process may support rendering institutions appropriate treatment strategies while decreasing diagnostic discordance.[49]

For purposes of basic communication, a central dedicated telephone line is recommended to provide direct, easy, and immediate access to the regional system. This access should be staffed 24 hours per day, 7 days per week and should be unencumbered. This model also includes the transfer of the referral call to the transport medical control officer, thereby greatly

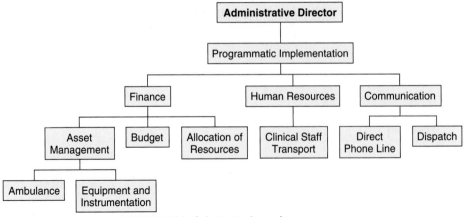

FIGURE 3-3 Role of administrative director of transport services.

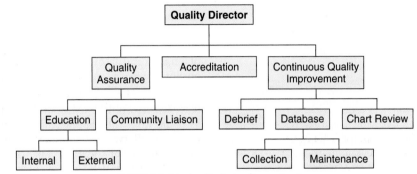

FIGURE 3-4 Role of quality director of transport services.

simplifying the process for the referral-consultation. The ability to support communication among the referring physician, the dispatcher, and the medical control officer simultaneously can speed up decision making and the initiation of transport. Once the transport is initiated, communication among the transport team, the referring physician, and the medical control officer becomes integral to the care provided (Figure 3-5). Changes in weather, patient status, equipment needs, and bed status need to be communicated in a timely manner. This information may demand a review of the transport plan and is best facilitated through a central communication center.[22,40] The organization of a perinatal regional hotline has been shown to increase significantly both in utero and neonatal transports, allowing for safe, 24-hour, on-call management of perinatal transports and the collection of epidemiologic indicators relative to perinatal transfers.[22]

The rapidly advancing field of telecommunications offers a wide variety of opportunities for transmitting medical information, subject to proper consideration of privacy and confidentiality requirements. This medium permits the use of satellite technology and video-conferencing equipment to conduct a real-time consultation between medical specialists in two geographically different areas. Store-and-forward telemedicine involves acquiring medical data (e.g., medical images, biosignals) and then transmitting these data to a medical specialist for assessment offline. It does not require the presence of both parties at the same time. These technologies may facilitate appropriate referral of patients according to complexity and may decrease incidence of inappropriate transfer or diagnostic discordance, allowing for optimal use of resources.[48,56] Furthermore, these innovative strategies have the potential to overcome deregionalization of services

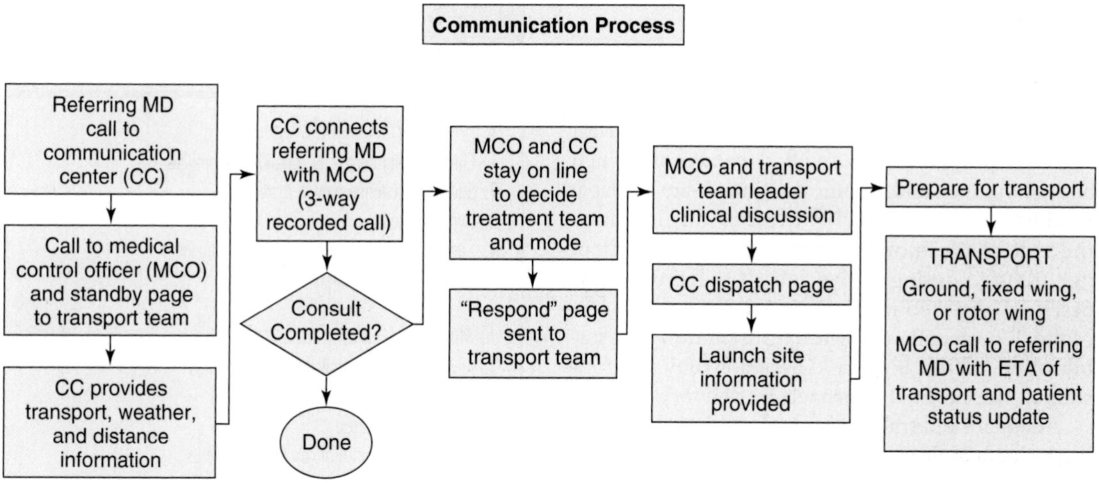

Communication Process

FIGURE 3-5 Working model of Vanderbilt Transport Communication Tool (unpublished), version September 2008. (Contributed by S. Brodtrick, D. Quinn, and M. Cortez.)

by creating virtual regional networks for perinatal transport.

Quality

The regional subspecialty perinatal care center, as noted in Table 3-1, is responsible for regional outreach support, education, and continuous quality oversight. Traditionally, quality improvement was assigned to the medical director. However, in light of current health care complexities and regulatory specifications surrounding the quality and safety of patient care, it is recommended that this role be assigned to an individual with the expertise to effectively evaluate programmatic performance at all levels of the organizational structure. This continuous evaluation of the process will facilitate modification of the transport system when potential problems are identified.[29]

The leadership team should oversee overall transport performance. The systematic collection and analysis of carefully selected performance indicators such as patient demographics, management and outcome data, safety standards, logistics, equipment malfunction, and cost will drive quality initiatives. A quality review of individual transports, incidence reports, and occurrence debriefs will enhance this process.[40,59] Using a transport validated physiologic score (e.g., the transport risk index of physiologic stability [TRIPS]) to evaluate patient status before, during, and after transport can assist team and transport performance.[37,40]

The Academy of Pediatrics Section on Transport Medicine has recently developed a database for neonatal/pediatric critical care transport quality metrics. The GAMUT database (**G**round and **A**ir **M**edical q**U**ality **T**ransport database) borrows its name from the expression "run the gamut." It welcomes all types of transport programs big or small, academic or corporate, adult or pediatric—all programs that wish to collaborate with others and use benchmarking to drive the quality of the care they provide. Tracking of data related to these quality metrics is just beginning. Teams' data contributions (kept anonymous from other teams) will help determine the performance benchmarking goals necessary to begin the quality improvement phase of this work.[1]

In addition, quality assurance may be implemented through continuing education both internally and externally. Transport programs must create individualized internal training programs that effectively provide current and continuous education to ensure maintenance of appropriate skills for high-quality perinatal transport. A similar program must be adapted to provide educational resources to the referring hospital where training in pretransport resuscitation and stabilization is imperative. Ensuring competence in these areas has the potential to improve short-term and long-term morbidity of sick infants, offsetting the negative effects of deregionalization and distance between interhospital transfer facilities.[9,40]

High-Risk Maternal Referral

The most effective method to decrease mortality and morbidity during the perinatal and neonatal period is the timely and appropriate referral of mothers with high-risk pregnancies to medical centers in which both the human and technical resources are available to address complications.[16,22] In situations in which the risk to the mother outweighs the benefit of her transfer during active labor, the timely dispatch of the neonatal transport team from the regional perinatal center for resuscitation and stabilization of the high-risk neonate may be considered the optimal approach to delivery of care.

Adequate referral of high-risk perinatal patients begins with high-quality antepartum surveillance.[51] Indications for referral to a regional center are shown in Box 3-1. Early identification of factors that can affect pregnancy outcome is important in developing appropriate diagnostic and treatment plans. Optimal perinatal care implies having well-trained and up-to-date obstetricians at all levels of care during both the antepartum and intrapartum period. These physicians should be experts in identifying maternal-fetal risk factors and complications through their knowledge, clinical skills, and expertise in prenatal ultrasound and fetal monitoring.[2,19,43,45] In situations in which this level of expertise is not available, medical and nursing personnel should be specifically trained to identify high-risk pregnancies with the objective of pursuing early referral. Consultation and referral decisions for the high-risk mother should be based on the results of a thorough evaluation of each patient and specific guidelines. Communication between the referral center and the regional perinatal center may be facilitated through the use of video-medicine technology.[20]

Neonatal Referral

Despite efforts to identify high-risk perinatal patients during the antepartum period, as many as 30% to 50% of infants who ultimately require additional neonatal care may not be recognized until the late intrapartum or early neonatal period.[36] For this reason, all hospitals that provide obstetric services must be prepared for the birth, resuscitation, stabilization, and treatment of premature or term sick infants. The Neonatal Resuscitation Program (NRP)[4,8,45] sponsored by the American Heart Association and the American Academy of Pediatrics is an excellent resource for training individuals and maintaining

> **BOX 3-1** **INDICATIONS FOR REFERRAL TO A REGIONAL PERINATAL CENTER**
>
> **A. Prenatal Ultrasound Diagnosis**
> 1. Complex fetal genetic or congenital anomalies
> 2. Severe intrauterine growth restriction[47]
> 3. Hydrops fetalis
> 4. Severe oligohydramnios and polyhydramnios
> 5. Fetal airway anomalies
>
> **B. Maternal Medical Complications**
> 1. Advanced or uncontrolled diabetes mellitus
> 2. Severe organic heart or lung disease
> 3. Severe renal disease
> 4. Maternal infection that can affect the fetus
> 5. Thyrotoxicosis
>
> **C. Maternal Surgical Complications**
> 1. Acute abdominal emergency
> 2. Trauma requiring intensive care
> 3. Thoracic emergency requiring intensive care
>
> **D. Obstetric Complications**
> 1. Premature onset of labor
> 2. Premature rupture of membranes
> 3. Third trimester bleeding
> 4. Severe preeclampsia or hypertension
> 5. Multiple gestations
> 6. Rh isoimmunization

resuscitation skills in both a regional program and an individual hospital setting. Certification (and renewal) of NRP training should be a universal standard for all delivery room and nursery staff. Beyond the immediate delivery room setting, supportive care should be offered and maintained until the transport team has arrived and assumed care (Box 3-2). This continuance of care is well standardized within the S.T.A.B.L.E. program.[30,55] This program is the only neonatal continuing education program to focus exclusively on the postresuscitation and/or pretransport stabilization care of neonates.

NEONATAL TRANSPORT

Stabilization of patients and preparation for transport should begin immediately on identification

BOX 3-2	S.T.A.B.L.E. PRETRANSPORT STABILIZATION OF THE NEWBORN

Sugar and safe care
Temperature
Airway
Blood pressure
Lab work
Emotional support for the family

Modified from Karlsen K: *The S.T.A.B.L.E. Program: post-resuscitation/pre-transport stabilization care of sick infants—guidelines for neonatal healthcare providers*, ed 6, Park City, Utah, 2013, S.T.A.B.L.E.

of a need for transport and before the transport team arrives. The S.T.A.B.L.E. curriculum provides a comprehensive set of generalized guidelines for the assessment and stabilization of sick infants in the postresuscitation/pretransport stabilization period. The "S.T.A.B.L.E." mnemonic was created to assist with information recall and to standardize and organize care in the pretransport/postresuscitation stabilization period. Prevention of adverse events and delivery of safe patient care are stressed throughout the program.[30] In consultation, the referring center (physician) and transport medical control officer (MCO) may address additional areas of attention based on specific patient clinical assessment and presumptive diagnosis. Although the reasons for neonatal referral may be quite diverse and based on needs of infants relative to the capabilities of the referring center, the most common indication is respiratory distress of the neonate.[30] Other common indications include prematurity, congenital anomalies (surgical and nonsurgical), and suspected congenital heart disease. Stabilization and support of these infants may require frequent interhospital communication (referring physician and transport MCO) to identify specific medical interventions. The importance of this form of continuing dialogue with respect to accuracy in diagnosis, management, and changes in patient status cannot be stressed enough. Again, the use of video-telemedicine may facilitate the accuracy of these interactions.[9,20]

Assumption of care of the neonate is a complex issue without a straightforward answer. However, transition of care should be seamless. Many health care professionals can have medical responsibility for a single patient at one time. The fact that one person has acquired medical responsibility does not automatically release someone else. On arrival of the transport team, collaborative management is of upmost importance. While the patient remains in the referring facility the referring physician cannot hand off the patient and proceed as if the patient has left the facility and his or her care. The referring facility allows the specialty team to provide care under the supervision and authority of the referring physician. The specialty team leads the effort to prepare the patient for transport. However, leading does not mean command or infer sole medical responsibility. The referring physician retains involvement and ultimate responsibility and signs the transfer certificate at the time of actual transfer. If at any time the referring physician deems it is in the best interest of the patient to intervene or cancel the transfer, it is the physician's right and responsibility to do so. Simultaneously the transport team has a medical responsibility to the patient. A team approach is in the best interest of the patient and should involve all participants in the process. Communication between the referring physician, the transport team, and the accepting physician is of great importance.[3] As long as the transport team is in the referring hospital, the ultimate responsibility lies with the referring physician. On leaving the referring facility, the transport team and receiving facility assume responsibility and control for medical decision making.[53] In the event that a community emergency medical service (EMS) is used for transport, the referring physician retains medical control until the patient reaches the regional referral center.

Pediatric and neonatal interfacility transport teams are unique entities. Provision of intensive care in the transport environment incorporates the philosophies of neonatal and pediatric critical care, but in a mobile environment with physical and environmental constraints of staff, space, mobility, and equipment. It is important to recognize that the physical requirements of team members are different from those who work solely in a hospital or clinic environment. Team members will be required to lift patients or carry equipment often with little or no help. The ability to function within the confines of a moving vehicle is important. Personnel should not be unusually prone to motion sickness or have mastered the techniques to mitigate the effects of motion sickness. Weight restrictions are a consideration in regard to aircraft. Personnel with chronic illness or disability may not be able to perform all expected duties. Pregnancy may pose a temporary limitation and medical clearance should be provided by the member's obstetrician at a minimum. In the event that a team member is unable to function, patient and crew safety may be compromised because there are few options should a team member be incapacitated while on duty. For this reason team members with certain medical conditions may be at least temporarily precluded from participation on a transport. Policies developed with human resources and legal counsel should be put into place and address the physical requirements for team members.[3]

Interfacility transport teams are a part of the continuum of care provided by the system of emergency medical services provided for neonates and children. Transition of care should be seamless without compromise of level of care or monitoring. Neonatal-pediatric interfacility transport teams do not "scoop and run" or "swoop and scoop" (limited evaluation at the scene with rapid stabilization and transport to an advanced care environment as the primary goal) as may be appropriate for the prehospital transport from an accident scene. Patients transported by neonatal-pediatric interfacility teams benefit from organized, coordinated, controlled transport that does not prioritize speed over thorough stabilization described as a " stay and play" philosophy. The exception to this principle is the patient whose outcome will be compromised without access to care not available at the referring hospital or in the transport environment.[3]

Team Composition and Configuration

Transport teams may be composed of a variety of medical personnel, including physicians, neonatal nurse practitioners, physician assistants, registered nurses (RNs), respiratory therapists (RTs), paramedics, and emergency medical technicians.[31,37,38] Karlson et al[31] conducted a Web-based national survey of 335 neonatal transport teams to describe the United States Neonatal Transport Team workforce. Published in 2011, variations in aspects of neonatal transport teams were described including team composition. The most common composition among unit-based and dedicated teams was the RN-RT composition. There were a total of 26 compositions reported.[31] Interfacility transport should be accomplished in the most efficient and

safe manner by qualified personnel. The composition of a neonatal-pediatric transport team should be tailored to meet the specific needs and resources of its patients and referral region.[3] Factors that can influence team composition include program resources, program design, unit-based versus dedicated teams, transport volume, and transport mode, as well as local, state, and regional regulation agencies.[53] As a general guideline, a transported infant or child should receive the same level of care en route as will be provided in the unit to which he or she will be admitted.[3]

There is considerable debate regarding the presence of physicians on transport. Traditionally pediatric teams have included a resident or attending physician. There is little evidence to support that such a composition results in better outcomes. Many neonatal teams have been led by nurse practitioners or advanced practice nurses, as described by Karlson et al.[31] Nurse-led teams have been shown (1) to provide better continuity of care, improved documentation, better maintenance of transport equipment, improved team availability, and stronger liaisons with referring hospitals and (2) to reduce overall operating costs.[40] Leslie and Stephenson[38a] evaluated physiologic parameters of infants stabilized and transported by neonatal nurse practitioners versus physicians. Though stabilization of the infants took longer by the nurse practitioners, physiologic conditions were improved for pH and Pao_2 in the pretransport period and temperature and oxygen saturations were improved in the posttransport period when transported by nurse practitioners. King et al[33] reported on the effects on patient outcomes when team composition was changed from RN-physician team to nurse only. There was no difference found in mortality rates between groups and team response times were significantly shorter for the RN team.[33] Limited research has demonstrated that providers such as RNs and RTs can function safely and effectively in the transport environment without the direct supervision of a physician.[3]

Team configuration has been categorized as *dedicated* and *unit based*. Dedicated teams are those whose members perform neonatal transport on a full-time basis. They generally are not assigned to any other major clinical responsibilities. However, between transports, team members may assist with procedures, attend deliveries, or have other responsibilities that do not involve patient care. Dedicated teams can be based in a receiving facility or in a freestanding transport service not affiliated with a hospital.[31] Unit-based teams are composed of members who, although available for transport, are primarily involved with other clinical duties. Institutional factors should drive the decision about which type of team to use. These factors often include the acuity of care level managed in the unit, annual volume of transports, financial support, and national, state, or local laws regulating the expanded role of nurses and respiratory therapists in health care.[25] Regardless of the team composition, the team must have the cumulative expertise to resuscitate, stabilize, and provide critical care throughout the transport.

Dedicated transport teams originated in the 1970s-1980s when regionalized perinatal care was established[31] and large metropolitan hospitals began to experience an increase in the demand for neonatal transports. These teams often are composed of a nurse designated as team leader and a respiratory therapist as a partner, with a physician or nurse practitioner added to the team when a neonate is critically ill and more advanced procedures may be anticipated.[18,19,33,38] The principal advantage to dedicated teams includes their immediate around-the-clock availability and their advanced training in neonatal resuscitation and stabilization procedures. However, the additional personnel necessary for dedicated teams may make these teams expensive to maintain. Dedicated neonatal teams were found to transport greater distances and to have larger transport volumes; were more likely to use all modes of transport; and were more rigorous with regard to orientation, annual skills maintenance, use of protocols, and quality assurance activities.[31]

Unit-based teams usually are made up of staff nurses and respiratory therapists within the neonatal intensive care unit (NICU).[18,38] The advantage to having a unit-based, nondedicated transport team is the large pool of trained personnel available around the clock. Qualifications of team members can be based on their daily bedside critical care experience and supplemental education, such as certification as a neonatal resuscitation provider. The primary disadvantage to this team design is that the transport nurse's patient assignments must be absorbed by the unit nursing staff until he or she returns. However, unit-based teams usually are very cost effective because critical care skills are maintained during regular patient care, advanced skill training may be more focused, and administrative oversight duties are diminished.[38]

The American Academy of Pediatrics' Section of Transport Medicine article "Pediatric and Neonatal Interfacility Transport: Results from a National Consensus Conference"[53] describes an additional method of categorizing transport teams. Four types of transport systems are described: hospital based, community based, EMS based, and a hybrid (mix of the previous three systems). Hospital-based teams are owned and operated by sponsoring institutions and serve the needs of these institutions. These systems often operate at a net loss. Indirect revenue is generated providing an overall profit. Community-based teams are most often owned and operated by private companies and are dependent on a mix of adult transports, high volumes, and low expenses. EMS-based teams are typically subsidized by local, regional, and state government funding, including taxpayer revenue. Hybrid teams are gaining popularity with an increased awareness of cost and resource sharing and increased collaboration.[53]

Transport Education and Training

The goal for training of transport teams should be the development of a program that ensures that members will have the combined expertise to effectively assess and manage actual and potential problems in the transport environment. The training program should enable team members to demonstrate their abilities to plan, implement, and evaluate ongoing stabilization efforts and interventions during transport. The scope of this training program should reflect the team member's job description, transport responsibilities, patient population, and modalities of travel.[3,53] Training is often begun during an orientation period but must continue throughout the career of the transport team member. Orientation is accomplished through participation on transport under the supervision of an experienced team member, as well as with the use of didactic and process curricula.[3,53] Cognitive knowledge should be demonstrated in transport and medical content areas as described in the American Academy of Pediatrics Section on Transport Medicine's *Guidelines for Air and Ground Transport of Neonatal and Pediatric Patients*.[3] Team members should be able to recognize and manage life-threatening conditions as appropriate for their transport population. New team members will need training designed to enhance their current knowledge base and will need to learn and interpret certain assessments, techniques, studies, and procedures not usually expected in their standard or previous positions.[3]

Procedural skills required by transport teams will be defined by patient population, program guidelines, and legal scope of practice. The American Academy of Pediatrics Section on Transport Medicine describes suggested skills and procedures.[3] Resourcefulness is required for the development of opportunities to attain and maintain the necessary skills. Laboratory simulations are available for certain skills. Electronic computer-linked simulators are additional resources but are limited by their availability and expense to purchase and maintain. Resources exist within the hospital for attainment and maintenance of procedures and skills and include the operating room, NICU and delivery room, pediatric intensive care unit, and emergency department. Each area provides unique opportunities for skill and knowledge development.[3]

Continual education for transport team members is vitally important because as technology changes, therapies will change. Procedural skills must be maintained because some skills are only performed occasionally if ever in actual practice. Continual learning of rare conditions allows team members to be prepared to initiate appropriate management of these conditions.[3] Multiple modalities are used for continuing education and can include quality improvement initiatives, case conferences, didactics, skills laboratory sessions, case simulation, literature review, computer-based activities, and peer performance.[53]

Simulation laboratories are an excellent adjunct to transport team education. Procedures can be performed in a safe, controlled environment. Patient care environments (transport vehicle workspace) can be simulated. Scenarios can be created to assess not only resuscitation skills but also team dynamics. Debriefing is a vital component to simulation. Through facilitated discussions participants review and critique their experiences.[53]

Variability among neonatal transport teams has been described by Karlson et al[31] with regard to length of orientation, readiness for independent transport, orientation content, procedures performed, and skills maintenance.[31] Competency assessment as used in medical education has been recommended by the American Academy of Pediatrics Section on Transport Medicine. This would allow teams to evaluate individual personnel, focus

on educational needs, and ensure acquisition of necessary knowledge and skills.[53]

A minimum of 2 years of level III neonatal critical care staff experience is a basic requirement for the nursing and respiratory therapy components of most neonatal transport services. Nurses and respiratory therapists who specialize in neonatal transport should have a basic understanding of neonatal pathophysiology, resuscitation and stabilization techniques, ventilatory management, and radiographic interpretation. In the event of a critically ill patient, a nurse practitioner or physician may serve as team leader with respect to high-level procedures and patient management.[32,33]

Programs using air transport should ensure that all providers, including physicians who may be involved occasionally, have education on air safety, survival methods, and flight physiology (including air transport effects of barometric pressure, g-force, humidity change, potential temperature loss, noise, and vibration).[40,52]

Mode of Transport

The optimal transport of a neonatal or pediatric patient is facilitated by the appropriate use of resources, including staff, equipment, and vehicles. Vehicles used in transport include surface (ground) and air (rotor-wing or fixed-wing) ambulances. A fully integrated transport system would include all three modalities.[3] When initiating a neonatal transport program, the first step should be to identify the geographic catchment area, total number and location of perinatal resources, distance in miles/kilometers, and duration of transport time (ground versus air) between the different levels of care. An important factor is the particular characteristics of the topography of the catchment area, which will help determine the ratio of ground-to-air transport resources required. In areas with good roads and low traffic volume, ground transport may be the only transport system required.[16,28,40,54]

Selecting the proper mode of transport (ground ambulance, helicopter, or fixed-wing aircraft) depends on many variables. However, safety of patient and crew must be the foremost consideration when determining the mode of transport. Careful consideration of risks should be made before any patient transport. Variables that affect mode of transport and benefits of ground versus helicopter include clinical status of the patient, medical care required by the patient before and during transport, urgency of the transport, and other logistical considerations. By shortening response time and transport time in a clinically unstable patient, the selection of one mode of transport over another may be lifesaving. Logistical concerns affect the appropriate selection of mode of transport and can include distance, weather, traffic, and accessibility of area.[3]

Potential advantages and disadvantages of the available modes of transport should be considered. Ground ambulances are the most common means for interfacility transport of neonatal and pediatric patients. Ground ambulances offer many advantages over air transport. Ground ambulances are routinely available, can operate in weather conditions that restrict safe air operations, may be more user-friendly and functional with regard to the transport environment, and provide door-to-door service without need for helipad, landing zone, or runway. There are limitations to ground transport. There is a high potential for a rough ride, as well as the possibility of motion sickness for patient, team members, or family. Ground ambulances have significant time, distance, and access constraints.[3]

Helicopters have strengths and weaknesses as well. Speed of travel is one of the unique characteristics of air transport. There is no need for a runway and helicopters are able to avoid common traffic delays and ground obstacles and fly into areas that are otherwise inaccessible to other modes of transport. The disadvantages associated with helicopter transport include limitation in cabin size, landing zone requirements, and weather considerations.[3]

Fixed-wing aircraft travel at a greater speed and cover a greater service area compared with ground ambulances and helicopters. Other advantages include a larger patient cabin than that of a helicopter and the ability to fly above or around inclement weather. The greatest limitation of fixed-wing aircraft is the need for an airport landing that may be a distance from the referral and receiving facilities. Ground transport is needed between referral and receiving facilities and the airport.[3]

Selection of the appropriate mode of transport is not a simple decision and no single vehicle is ideal for all patients or transport teams. The risks, benefits, advantages, and disadvantages of each mode should be considered, as well as the mission of the team and needs of the patient.[3]

In general, when transport time exceeds 2 hours, air transport is more appropriate.[40] However, local ground transport capabilities to-from a referring hospital and airport must be known when fixed-wing air transport is used.

Equipment and Medications

Transport teams should be self-sufficient with dedicated, organized supplies for quick, efficient access.[3] The equipment and medications necessary for neonatal transport are similar to those used in the NICU. Equipment must be light, compact, durable, and motion and g-force tolerant. All electronic equipment should have its own independent power supply (AC/DC capability), adequate visual and audio alarms, and lack of electromagnetic interference.[16,40] Compatibility of all equipment is of vital importance to prevent potential interruption in therapy. Maintenance of equipment should be scheduled on a routine basis and be performed by competent, well-trained biomedical technicians. Equipment should be secured in all transport vehicles by approved methods.[3]

Storage packs should be organized, maintained, and checked on a routine basis by transport team members. It should not be standard practice to rely on or plan to borrow equipment or medications from referral facilities.[3]

Medication storage is of the utmost importance for the delivery of safe care. Special considerations are needed for certain medications such as surfactant and prostaglandins that require refrigeration. Security of controlled substances must be maintained as mandated by institutional, state, and federal regulations.[3]

The American Academy of Pediatrics Section on Transport Medicine's *Guidelines for Air and Ground Transport of Neonatal and Pediatric Patients* provides sample supply lists for equipment and medications needed for ground and fixed-wing transports of neonates and pediatric patients.[3] Table 3-2 provides a list of common transport equipment and medications.

Novel Interventions

Because the objective of the perinatal transport team is to bring the intensive care environment to the newborn infant, it is fundamental that initial resuscitation and stabilization be performed

TABLE 3-2	EQUIPMENT AND MEDICATIONS FOR NEONATAL TRANSPORT*					
PHYSIOLOGIC MONITORING AND SAFETY	**AIRWAY AND SUCTION EQUIPMENT**	**RESPIRATORY EQUIPMENT**	**PROCEDURE EQUIPMENT**	**IV FLUID AND ACCESS**	**MEDICATIONS**	**REFRIGERATED MEDICATION**
BP cuffs, #2-#4 (2 each)*	Laryngoscope (2)	Anesthesia bags (2 per T-PICU infant resuscitator)	Sterile towels (1)	D_5W 50 m (2)	Epinephrine 1:10,000 (2)	Exogenous surfactant (1)
Electrodes (2 of each available size)	Laryngoscope blades (2 of each size)	Self-inflating bag (2)	UAC tray (1)	NS 250 m (1)	Naloxone 1 mg/1 m (2)	PGE (2)
Pulse oximeter probes (2)	Laryngoscope light bulbs (3)	Oxygen mask (2)	Single-lumen umbilical catheters (2 of each size)	$D_{10}W$ 500 m (1)	4.2% sodium bicarbonate (2)	
Dispensable thermometers (2)	AA batteries (4)	Facemasks (2 of each size)	Double-lumen umbilical catheters (2 of each size)	$D_{50}W$ 50 m (1)	Dopamine (2)	
Skin temperature probes (8)	Endotracheal tubes (3 of each size)	Infant nasal cannula (2)	Umbilical tape (2)	Heparin sodium 1000 mcg/m vial (3)	Dobutamine (2)	
Rectal probe (1)	Stylettes (4)	CPAP prongs (2 of each size)	Povidone-iodine (3)	Syringes, 3 m/1 m (6 each)	Acyclovir (1)	
Warming pad por table: chemical (2)	CO_2 detector (2 self-contained, sterile)	Neonatal flow sensor (2)	Scalpels #11 and #15 (1 each)	IV catheter, #22 and #24 gauge (5 each)	Ampicillin (2)	
4×4 gauze pads (2)	Closed suction catheter (2 of each size)	CPAP circuit (1)	4.0 silk suture (4)	Access kit, including dressing, tourniquet (2)	Gentamicin (2)	
Nonstick gauze pads (2)	Meconium aspiration device (2)	Ventilator circuit (1)	Dressing for umbilical line (2)	Butterfly needle (3 of each size)	Vitamin K for injection (1)	
Bowel bag (1)	Bulb suction (2)	Point-of-care blood gas equipment (1–2)	Needle aspiration/ chest tube kit (2)	Arm board (2)	Eye ointment (2)	
Sterile rolled gauze (2)	Suction catheters (2 of each size)		Transducer (2)	Heel warmers (2)	Lidocaine HCl (1)	
Ear protectors (2)	Saline bullets (4)		Chest tubes, 10 Fr/12 Fr (2 of each size)	Lancets (2 of infant and preemie size)	Adenosine (1)	
Hats (2)	Replogle (2 of each size)		Heimlich valve (2)	Syringes (5 of each size)	Vecuronium (1)	
Flashlight (2)	Orogastric tubes (2 of each size)		Sterile gloves (5 of each size)		Sterile saline for injection (2)	
Tape measures (2)					Abboject needle (2)	
					Fentanyl (2)	
					Midazolam (2)	
					Phenobarbital (2)	

*( ) designates numbers of pieces of equipment to be carried in transport kit.

BP, Blood pressure; *CPAP*, continuous positive airway pressure; *NS*, normal saline; *PGE*, prostaglandin E; *UAC*, umbilical artery catheter; *T-PICU*, T-piece infant care unit.

by skilled practitioners in order for the team to successfully continue to offer appropriate high-quality intensive care during the transport of the baby. Level II centers should be equipped with surfactant, nasal continuous positive airway pressure (NCPAP) systems, and oxygen–air blenders to give prompt and effective respiratory support while maintaining blood saturation levels within acceptable limits awaiting the arrival of the transport team. Adequate management of the premature infant with surfactant deficiency will include supporting adequate recruitment of the lung and minimizing barotrauma. Acquiring the requisite skills and education to intubate and administer

surfactant appropriately and to administer early NCPAP has the potential to improve patient survival, decrease the need for mechanical ventilation,[17,50,51,57,58] and decrease morbidity in situations in which duration of transport may be prolonged for hours because of unforeseen delays. Although the use of NCPAP in the delivery room is not a novel intervention,[60] its use as an early intervention in the delivery room for infants with respiratory failure is accepted as a common approach for the management of premature infants with respiratory distress syndrome and term infants with mild to moderate respiratory failure. Because surfactant is an expensive medication, level II centers can maintain one or two ampules in their pharmacy to be restocked by the perinatal transport team before transport. The use of NCPAP during transport has also been evaluated and has been shown to be a safe and efficacious intervention for respiratory support.[42]

The use of a resuscitation device such as the T-piece infant resuscitator (Neopuff™ Infant Resuscitator, Fisher & Paykel Healthcare) may help decrease the variability of pressures administered to the neonate during resuscitation, stabilization, or administration of surfactant. This device also has the potential to minimize lung damage while supporting lung recruitment with the use of positive end-expiratory pressure.[11,46] This system can also temporarily replace the need for mechanical ventilation if NCPAP is unsuccessful in maintaining respiratory stability.

Early mobilization of the transport team for an impending premature delivery or delivery of a sick neonate allows for earlier implementation of tertiary care in the community. There has been a change in philosophy regarding departure of the transport team. The patient need not be born to mobilize a team. Close monitoring of aborted or prolonged transports is necessary to avoid inappropriate use of resources in a region. Time spent awaiting the delivery must also be monitored.

Another important intervention for perinatal transport is the administration of prostaglandin E$_1$ (PGE$_1$) in patients in whom a suspicion of congenital heart diseases is supported with a positive hyperoxia test. Adequate knowledge of dosing and preparation is fundamental to the successful use of this medication, which can prevent patients with ductal dependent lesions from becoming clinically unstable and developing severe hypoxemia and metabolic acidosis before the arrival of the transport team. The need for intubation and ventilator support to prevent apnea varies depending on the anticipated length of transfer and the dose of PGE$_1$ necessary to maintain the infant asymptomatic.[12,23] Knowledge by the referring physician of the performance and interpretation of the hyperoxia test will facilitate the decision to start PGE$_1$ and should be part of the maintenance-of-skills program. It is recommended that level II nurseries maintain in stock a vial of PGE$_1$.

In recent years, inhaled nitric oxide (iNO) has been used on transport to support term and near-term infants with hypoxemic respiratory failure that does not respond to conventional mechanical ventilation.[34] It has become the standard of care in the NICU environment.[3] The use of this therapeutic gas can be lifesaving and may decrease associated morbidities. Its use during transport requires certain adaptations for both ground and air transport in order to use this gas safely and effectively, but the feasibility of administering iNO during ground and air transport has been established by Kinsella et al[34] and Jesse et al.[28a]

Another novel intervention is the use of whole-body cooling or head cooling during transport to minimize brain damage from severe hypoxic ischemic encephalopathy. The use of passive and active cooling before and during transport as a therapy for neonatal encephalopathy has been reported in the literature, but more studies are required to determine the safety and efficacy of this intervention.[7]

Patients managed during transport with other more-complex interventions such as high-frequency jet ventilation and extracorporeal membrane oxygenation have been reported in the literature. Their use for routine transport cannot be recommended because of the complexity of training, equipment, and logistics required to administer these interventions.[15,41] Every country and regional perinatal center must determine its priorities for transport based on epidemiologic studies conducted in its catchment area to support the demand with appropriate resources for adequate perinatal transport.

FAMILY-CENTERED CARE FOR TRANSPORT

Separation of the infant and mother is often the consequence of neonatal transport. This physical separation affects both bonding and attachment, increasing the stress surrounding the delivery of an ill infant.[30,35,55] Creative ways to minimize the negative effects of this separation must be incorporated into the transport process. Whenever possible, transport should allow for the presence of a family member.[3]

Principles of family-centered care used in the inpatient setting should apply to the transport environment. Despite the evidence of the benefits, there is not universal acceptance and implementation of family-centered care in transport. Transport members cite multiple reasons for excluding parents, including anticipated difficulty caring for the patient if the parent needs attention, potential difficulty dealing with distraught parents, difficulty controlling the child with the parent present, and general team member anxiety in providing care with parent(s) watching.[3]

Before departure from the referring facility the transport team should meet with the parents of the infant, communicating the plan for transport, providing information with regard to the receiving hospital (including phone numbers, directions, and unit-specific guidelines), and answering any questions the parents may have. The transport team should identify a phone number that may be used to communicate with the parents once the infant is transported. In addition, the transport team should enable the parents to see and touch the infant before departure and should provide the parents with a photograph of their infant.[40]

Offering for parents to be present during provision of critical care is the cornerstone of family-centered care. Family presence during resuscitation continues to gain support. Presence of family allows families to continue to act as allies in the care of their child and enables them to see firsthand that team members did their best and treated their child with respect, dignity, and empathy.[3]

With the presence of family on transport, safety should remain the priority. All vehicle occupants should wear appropriate restraints. Family members should be educated if it is unsafe for them to ride in the transport vehicle or in a particular location in the transport vehicle. It is the responsibility of the transport team to define a standard of family-centered care during the transport of sick neonates and pediatric patients.[3]

If family is unable to accompany child on transport, on arrival at the receiving medical center, a transport team member should call the parents to update them on the condition and the safe arrival of their child in the receiving facility. At this time, the transport team should give the parents the names of those who will be responsible for the care of the infant. Once the infant is admitted into the receiving unit, the receiving physician should communicate directly with the parents and referring physician. Engaging the parents in the caregiving process as soon as possible empowers parents

and assists the health care team in devising a care plan that will be mutually acceptable and in the best interest of the infant.

Facilitation of communication with parents may be improved with the use of video-telemedicine.[26] This technology enables parents to see their infant in the receiving center and speak directly with the nurses or physicians caring for their infant.

FUTURE OF NEONATAL TRANSPORT

Research, innovation, and maintenance of regionalization represent the future for perinatal transport. The mandate for highly motivated leadership able to apply epidemiologic, research, and quality-improvement methodology to the area of perinatal transport is essential for progress. The development and evaluation of new interventions, as well as the evaluation of what we consider "standard therapies," are imperative to better outcomes. The inclusion of continuous quality improvement at the top leadership level of the organizational structure of the perinatal transport system and the systematic collection of relevant data within an identified perinatal region represents the backbone for research in standing and new technologies. Special attention must be centered toward the community in order to improve resuscitation and stabilization efforts. In addition, benchmarking with regard to morbidity and mortality outcomes for transported patients will provide clarity for evaluation of the transport experience. The ultimate focus of this effort is to improve maternal and neonatal outcomes. Ultimate success will depend on the level of multidisciplinary participation of government, community, and private industry stakeholders.

REFERENCES

For a full list of references, scan the QR code or visit http://booksite.elsevier.com/ 9780323320832.

4 DELIVERY ROOM CARE

SUSAN NIERMEYER, SUSAN B. CLARKE, AND JACINTO A. HERNÁNDEZ

A GOLDEN OPPORTUNITY

The initial evaluation and management of the newly born infant must focus on promoting normal adaptation to extrauterine life and detecting significant medical problems so they can be evaluated and treated appropriately. In adjusting to extrauterine life, the newly born infant experiences a complex series of biologic, physiologic, and metabolic changes. These changes are evoked by a variety of processes, including perinatal surges in hormones, labor, delivery, ventilation and oxygenation of the lungs, umbilical cord occlusion, decreased environmental temperature, and activation of the sympathoadrenal system.

Such complex changes are essential for survival. Every infant must successfully complete this process of transition in order to survive in the extrauterine environment. For a small percentage of infants, transition is never achieved; for a slightly larger number, transition is delayed or complicated; however, for most infants, transition is so smooth it appears uneventful.[1] It has been estimated that in approximately 10% of live births, active intervention of a skilled individual or team is necessary to ensure a successful transition.[31] Consequently, the optimum care of the neonatal patient during this period needs to be prospective and anticipatory.

The purpose of immediate delivery room care is to support the newborn's respiratory and circulatory systems during the transition from fetal to neonatal life. Normal physiologic changes at birth include expansion of the lungs with air, initiation of gas exchange across the alveolar membrane, and closure of circulatory shunts that were necessary during intrauterine life. When delivery is complicated by perinatal conditions leading to perinatal depression, the aim of resuscitation is to reverse hypoxia, hypercarbia, and acidosis. The survival and outcome of distressed newborns depends on timely and effective intervention in the first few minutes after birth.

All resuscitation efforts begin with the basic techniques of thermal control, clearing of the airway if needed, and stimulation of breathing.[2,44] Advanced resuscitation includes assessment of oxygenation, supplemental oxygen administration (if needed), bag-and-mask ventilation, endotracheal intubation, chest compressions, and use of epinephrine and volume expansion. Delivery room emergencies may require resuscitation, as well as more advanced procedures during stabilization in the delivery room and transition to the neonatal care unit. Finally, truly successful resuscitation depends on care of the family, collaborative perinatal decision making, and teamwork and communication among health care professionals.

PHYSIOLOGY

At birth, rapid physiologic transition from the intrauterine to extrauterine environment must be made.[39,70] Effective, regular respirations should be initiated within the first minute after delivery[1,22] Environmental factors, such as a relatively cool ambient temperature and tactile stimulation, assist in initiating respiration. The changes in Pao_2 and $Paco_2$ during delivery affect chemoreceptors and aid in the reflexive initiation of respiration. The initial breath may generate from 20 to 70 cm H_2O of negative intrathoracic pressure to replace lung liquid with air inside the alveoli.[72] A rapid decrease

PURPLE type highlights content that is particularly applicable to clinical settings.

47

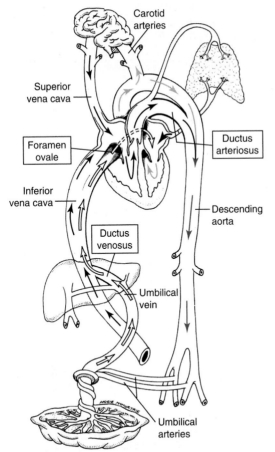

Carotid
arteries

Superior
vena cava

Foramen
ovale

Ductus
arteriosus

Inferior
vena cava

Descending
aorta

Ductus
venosus

Umbilical
vein

Umbilical
arteries

FIGURE 4-1 Circulatory pattern before birth. (From Goldsmith JP: Delivery room resuscitation of the newborn. In Martin RJ, Fanaroff AA, Walsh MC, editors: *Fanaroff and Martin's neonatal-perinatal medicine*, ed 9, St. Louis, 2011, Elsevier Mosby.)

in pulmonary vascular resistance and an increase in pulmonary blood flow occur after expansion of the lungs with air and filling of the pulmonary circuit with blood from the placenta. This results in increased pulmonary perfusion and oxygenation.[71] Resorption of fetal lung liquid across the respiratory epithelium accelerates during labor, resulting in net clearance of liquid from the potential airspaces.[10] Colloid osmotic pressure and the relatively lower postnatal hydrostatic pressure of blood within the pulmonary circuit assist in absorbing alveolar fluid after delivery. During this process, fetal right-to-left shunts through the ductus arteriosus and foramen ovale gradually close[21] (Figure 4-1; Table 4-1).

ASPHYXIA AND APNEA

Asphyxia is defined as inadequate tissue perfusion that fails to meet the metabolic demands of the tissues for oxygen and waste removal. Asphyxia is characterized by progressive hypoxemia ($\downarrow Po_2$), hypercarbia ($\uparrow Pco_2$), and acidosis ($\downarrow pH$). Hypoxic tissues convert from aerobic metabolism to anaerobic glycolysis, producing lactate and metabolic acidosis that is initially buffered by bicarbonate.[15] When the buffering capacity is exhausted, acidosis occurs. Acidosis and hypoxemia initially result in reflexive, compensatory cardiovascular changes. After early tachycardia, cardiac output decreases and generalized peripheral vasoconstriction occurs to maintain a blood pressure adequate for perfusion of the heart and brain. Prolonged asphyxia results in eventual bradycardia and hypotension as severe acidosis and cardiac failure occur.

Asphyxia may occur in utero or postnatally. In either circumstance, a well-defined series of respiratory events follows (Figure 4-2).[15] During *primary apnea*, respiratory movements cease after a brief period of rapid breathing. At the same time, heart rate falls and neuromuscular tone diminishes. Intrapartum-related events may result in the passage of meconium before birth. If the hypoxic-ischemic event continues, the heart rate falls further, blood pressure falls, hypotonia worsens, and a series of spontaneous deep gasps occurs. Gasping continues but becomes weaker and more irregular and then finally ceases. After the last gasp, a period of *secondary apnea* begins.[15,44] Another simple, functional definition of asphyxia used by the World Health Organization is the failure to establish effective breathing at birth.[75]

Delivery may occur at any point during an intrapartum-related hypoxic event and the progression to biochemical asphyxia. If an infant is born during primary apnea, stimulation will usually induce respirations. If delivery occurs during secondary apnea, the infant will not respond to stimulation. Spontaneous respirations will not resume until resuscitation is initiated with assisted ventilation.[15,44] In the clinical setting of birth, primary and secondary apnea are essentially indistinguishable. The infant who is not breathing may have a heart rate less than 100 beats/min and may be hypotonic. Thus any infant who is apneic at delivery must be assumed to be in secondary apnea, and intervention should begin immediately.

TABLE 4-1	COMPARISON OF VASCULAR AND PULMONARY FUNCTIONS BEFORE AND AFTER BIRTH	
BODY STRUCTURE	**FETAL FUNCTION**	**EXTRAUTERINE FUNCTION**
Aorta	Carries oxygenated blood from left ventricle and deoxygenated blood from pulmonary arteries to fetal organs and placenta	Carries oxygenated blood from left ventricle into systemic circulation
Ductus venosus	Shunts most of the oxygenated blood from placenta to inferior vena cava	Disappears within 2 weeks after birth; becomes ligamentum venosum
Foramen ovale	Connects right and left atria; permits oxygenated blood from right atrium to bypass right ventricle and pulmonary circuit and go directly into left atrium	Functionally closes soon after birth; anatomically seals during childhood
Ductus arteriosus	Shunts blood from pulmonary artery directly into aorta	Functionally closes soon after birth; eventually becomes ligamentum arteriosum
Umbilical arteries and vein	Carry blood to and from placenta, the organ of respiration before birth	Clamped at birth, obliterating placental connections; become ligaments
Lungs	Distended with fluid; minimal pulmonary circulation; fetal respiratory movements	Expanded and aerated; pulmonary circulation allows CO_2 and O_2 exchange; organ of respiration

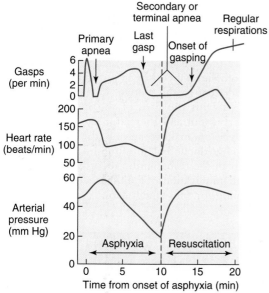

FIGURE 4-2 Changes in physiologic parameters during asphyxiation and resuscitation of rhesus monkey fetus at birth. (From Dawes GS: *Foetal and neonatal physiology: a comparative study of the changes at birth*, St Louis, 1968, Mosby.)

increases by about 2 minutes and the time to the onset of spontaneous breathing is prolonged by more than 4 minutes.[15] In the absence of effective resuscitation after delivery, apnea and decreased cardiac output result in progressive biochemical deterioration.[15]

Severe fetal and neonatal asphyxia impair the physiologic transitions to extrauterine life. The normally high fetal pulmonary vascular resistance may not decrease in the presence of pulmonary hypoexpansion, persistent acidosis, and hypoxemia. Pulmonary blood flow and oxygen transfer are impeded, perpetuating hypoxemia.[71] As part of persistent pulmonary hypertension of the newborn, normal closure of fetal shunts is delayed by high pulmonary vascular resistance and pulmonary hypoperfusion, hypoexpansion, and hypoxemia. This results in persistent right-to-left shunting through the ductus arteriosus and foramen ovale. Lung fluid clearance also may be delayed because of poor lung inflation or pulmonary hypoperfusion and hypoxemia. In addition, intraalveolar fluid may accumulate as a result of leakage from damaged pulmonary capillaries, resulting in pulmonary edema. With worsening hypoxemia and acidosis, myocardial function begins to fail, cardiac output falls, and systemic perfusion decreases to the brain, kidney, and intestine, setting the stage for postasphyxial injury of these organs.[5]

The longer the initiation of ventilation is delayed after an infant's last gasp in secondary apnea, the longer the time necessary during resuscitation for return of the infant's spontaneous respiration. For every 1-minute delay, the time to the first gasp

CLAMPING OF THE UMBILICAL CORD

The optimal timing for cord clamping remains a subject for debate, as it has been for decades, but only recently has the placental transfusion been considered as part of stabilization or resuscitation of the newly born infant.[55,56,95] The approach to timing of cord clamping is variable worldwide, even among formal practice guidelines.[4,65] Placental transfusion refers to the amount of blood that flows from the placenta to the infant at birth, before cord clamping or cessation of cord pulsations.[25] A delay in clamping the cord for 30 to 120 seconds after birth facilitates the transfer of an additional 30 to 150 ml of blood from the placenta to the newborn, with most of the transfer occurring in the first minute.[28,55,93] Maximal mean volume of placental transfusion has been reported between 24 and 32 ml/kg of body weight or an additional 30% to 40% of blood volume in the first 3 minutes after birth.[16,21,28a] Immediate clamping of the umbilical cord after delivery blocks the normal transfer of blood from the placenta to the infant resulting in a deficit of as much as 25% of normal blood volume.[55] The quantity of blood transferred to the infant appears to be influenced by the route of delivery (vaginal, cesarean), timing of cord clamping, initiation of respiration and cry, the position of the newborn relative to the placenta (gravity), manipulation of the cord (stripping), and intensity of uterine contractions at the end of the second stage of labor.[60,74] The definitions of *early cord clamping* (ECC) and *delayed cord clamping* (DCC) vary widely and may differ between term and preterm births. In term infants, ECC most often refers to clamping of the cord between delivery and 30 seconds (commonly within 10 to 20 seconds), whereas DCC refers to clamping of the cord anywhere between 30 and 90 seconds after delivery or after complete cessation of cord pulsations.[28,40,53,54] In preterm births, ECC refers to clamping of the cord immediately after delivery (commonly within 5 to 10 seconds), whereas DCC has been defined as any time beyond 30 seconds.[28,40,53,54] Experimental evidence suggests that onset of respirations is crucial in optimizing placental transfusion, and the physiologic definition of DCC is clamping after onset of respirations.[9]

Studies conducted in term infants suggest that ECC, compared with DCC, results in a greater risk of anemia in infancy.[50,55,67,93] Late clamping acts as a low-cost intervention to reduce anemia during the first 6 months of life.[29,33,56] Despite concerns that the increase in neonatal blood volume with DCC may result in volume overload, thus increasing the likelihood of respiratory distress,[94] neonatal jaundice, and polycythemia, randomized trials in term infants have not substantiated increased need for special care related to these diagnoses.[40,51,61] Several recent reviews evaluating the potential benefits and risks of late versus early cord clamping in the preterm and term population summarize the evidence that delaying cord clamping after birth is beneficial to both preterm and term infants.[28,40,54,68,79] In preterm infants these studies report benefits in terms of improved physiologic stability and reduction in the relative risk of intraventricular hemorrhage and the need for transfusion.

Although there may be physiologic benefits to delayed clamping, few studies have examined the timing of cord clamping with respect to the need for or response to resuscitation at birth.[7,43,60,74] In the event of fetal distress and neonatal depression, immediate clamping of the cord has usually been performed so the infant can be resuscitated. Alternatively, the initial steps of resuscitation and positive-pressure ventilation can be carried out with the cord intact by creating an area for resuscitation adjacent to the mother. Clinicians who are charged with the care of the newborn in the delivery room and thereafter should be part of the decision making around the time of cord clamping, document the time of cord clamping as part of the resuscitation record, and be aware of the implications of either early or delayed clamping for subsequent care.

RESUSCITATION OF THE NEWBORN

Preparation for Resuscitation

Immediate, effective resuscitation of the newborn infant can reduce or prevent morbidity and mortality. Much of neonatal resuscitation focuses on accurate assessment and initiation of ventilation. Basic interventions are often all that is necessary to successfully resuscitate a depressed infant.[32,57,64] However, effective resuscitation requires anticipation, adequate preparation of equipment and personnel, and teamwork.[27,86]

In the mid-1980s, the American Heart Association and the American Academy of Pediatrics addressed the need for a national training program for neonatal resuscitation in the United States by developing the **Neonatal Resuscitation Program (NRP)**. The NRP provides the training necessary for health care professionals to put into practice the scientific consensus established and updated periodically by the International Liaison Committee on Resuscitation (ILCOR). The ILCOR Consensus on Science is revised periodically based on a rigorous process of evidence evaluation.[65] Changes are then incorporated into regional guidelines and the *Textbook of Neonatal Resuscitation*.[44,47] The program's widespread acceptance ensures consistent awareness of current scientific consensus, use of proper equipment, and preparation of personnel to work as a team using shared knowledge and performance skills. *Helping Babies Breathe* shares the same evidence base as NRP; however, it emphasizes the initial steps of resuscitation through bag-and-mask ventilation with air for resource-limited settings where both mother and baby are cared for by a single birth attendant and advanced interventions are not universally available.[1,58]

The NRP recommends the following[44]:

At every delivery, there should be at least one person capable of initiating resuscitation whose only responsibility is the baby. Either that person or another who is immediately available should have the skills necessary to perform a complete resuscitation, including endotracheal intubation and administration of medications.

When a high-risk delivery is anticipated, *two* persons whose sole responsibility is resuscitation of the infant should be present and their roles designated in advance. Multiple births require a full team of personnel with complete equipment for each newborn.

The pediatric staff must be familiar with the prenatal and intrapartum history of the mother and fetus, because this information guides preparation for resuscitation. Preterm/postterm gestation, multiple gestation, meconium-stained amniotic fluid, and risk factors in medical, obstetric, intrapartum, and social history may identify the infant at risk for perinatal asphyxia (Box 4-1). However, any normal pregnancy may become high risk at the onset of previously unexpected or undetected intrapartum complications, including maternal hemorrhage, cord prolapse, and meconium staining of the amniotic

---

BOX 4-1 **CONDITIONS THAT MAY REQUIRE AVAILABILITY OF SKILLED RESUSCITATION AT DELIVERY**

Intrapartum Problems
- Fetal distress
  - Persistent late decelerations
  - Severe variable decelerations without baseline variability
  - Bradycardia
  - Meconium-stained amniotic fluid
  - Cord prolapse
- Prolonged, unusual, or difficult labor
- Emergency operative or assisted delivery
- Breech presentation with vaginal delivery
- Narcotic administration to mother within 4 hours of delivery

Medical/Obstetric/Genetic Problems
- Diabetes mellitus
- Suspected or confirmed maternal infection
- Substance abuse
- Third trimester bleeding
- Preeclampsia
- Abnormal amniotic fluid volume
- Prolonged rupture of membranes
- Multiple gestation
- Low-birth-weight infant
- Prematurity
- Isoimmunization
- Fetal congenital anomalies

---

fluid. Although prevention, detection, and treatment of fetal asphyxia are the responsibilities of the obstetric team, coordination between obstetric and neonatal services in a "prebriefing" before delivery is vital to ensure timely and effective resuscitation.

Resuscitation equipment, supplies, and drugs (Box 4-2) should always be readily available, functional, and assembled for immediate use in a designated location—ideally in a specific area of the delivery/birthing room or on a radiant warmer/intensive care bed equipped with easily accessible storage (Figures 4-3 and 4-4).

Prepare to facilitate normal transition or provide neonatal resuscitation by performing the following:

- Conduct a prebriefing to review pregnancy history and designate roles among the resuscitation team.

EQUIPMENT USED DURING NEONATAL RESUSCITATION

...... *Management*
- Radiant warmer
- Warmed blankets or towels
- Infant stocking cap
- Food-grade plastic wrap or polyethylene bags
- Chemically activated warming pad

Airway
- Bulb syringe
- Mechanical suction
- Suction catheters—5-6, 8, 10, 14 Fr
- 8-Fr feeding tube and 20-ml syringe
- Meconium aspirator/suction device
- Shoulder roll

Breathing
- Bag-and-mask ventilation
  - Oxygen source with flowmeter and tubing
  - Neonatal resuscitation bag with 21% to 100% oxygen capability and manometer or pressure release valve and/or T-piece device
  - Facemasks—newborn and premature sizes
  - Oral airways—newborn and premature sizes
  - Pulse oximeter with neonatal probe
  - Oxygen blender and compressed air source
- Intubation
  - Laryngoscope with extra batteries
  - Straight blades—No. 0 and No. 1 with extra bulbs
  - Endotracheal tubes—2.5, 3.0, 3.5, 4.0 mm internal diameter
  - Stylet
  - Tape, skin preparation
  - Scissors
  - CO_2 detector
  - Laryngeal mask airway

Circulation
- Stethoscope
- Wall clock or stopwatch
- Cord clamp
- Medications (epinephrine, normal saline)
- Sterile gloves
- Chlorhexidine sponges, povidone-iodine solution
- Umbilical vessel catheterization tray
- Umbilical catheters—3.5 and 5 Fr
- Three-way stopcocks
- Umbilical tape
- Suture material
- Intravenous catheters, tubing, fluid
- Needles—25, 23, 22, 20, 18 gauge
- Syringes—1, 3, 5, 10, 20 or 30, 50 or 60 ml
- Cardiorespiratory monitor and temperature probe (for prolonged stabilization)
- Procedure light

- Prepare the mother for skin-to-skin care and preheat the radiant warmer.
- Assemble basic supplies: warm linens, head covering for infant, suction device, cord clamp, and appropriate personal protection.
- Check suction equipment for function; set the vacuum regulator control not to exceed 100 mm Hg.
- Turn on the air/oxygen flow to the ventilation bag or T-piece device, and check all connections, flow-control valves, pressure-release valve, and manometer function to enable the ventilation device to deliver up to 30 to 40 cm H_2O pressure. Select the appropriate oxygen concentration for initiation of positive-pressure ventilation. Prepare an appropriate-size facemask and a pulse oximeter with neonatal probe.
- Check the laryngoscope for a bright light source and appropriate blades (size 0 for premature infants and size 1 for term infants); tighten the bulb.
- Check the availability of appropriate-size endotracheal tubes (2.5 to 4 mm internal diameter).
- Locate a stethoscope of appropriate size and confirm that it is functioning properly.
- Check the ancillary equipment (i.e., umbilical catheter supplies, intravenous solutions, unexpired resuscitation drugs).
- If the clinical situation warrants, draw up and label emergency medications for ready administration, using the estimated fetal weight, and obtain O-negative packed red blood cells for emergency transfusion.

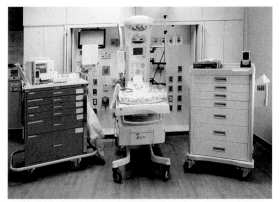

FIGURE 4-3 Labor/delivery/recovery (LDR) room resuscitation area prepared for high-risk delivery. Blended oxygen is available from wall outlets via T-piece device incorporated into the radiant warmer. Flow-inflating bag and manometer are prepared with self-inflating bag as backup. Bulb suction device and catheter for use with wall suction are available. Other supplies for airway suctioning and intubation are stored in the drawers of the supply cart. Resuscitation drugs and umbilical catheterization trays are kept in a separate resuscitation cart accessible from all LDR rooms. (Photo courtesy of Children's Hospital Colorado, Maternal Fetal Care Unit. Photo by Tia Brayman.)

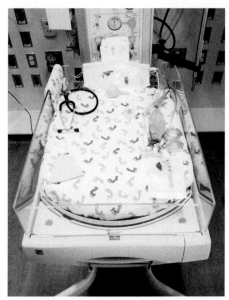

FIGURE 4-4 Patient area of radiant warmer prepared for a delivery. Supplies needed for initial steps and ventilation include warm blankets *(left rear)* for drying, overhead heater for warmth, head covering, suction devices, ventilation bag and masks, pulse oximetry probe and patient connector, stethoscope, and cord clamp. Temperature probe and cardiorespiratory monitor connector are available for prolonged stabilization. (Photo courtesy of Children's Hospital Colorado, Maternal Fetal Care Unit. Photo by Tia Brayman.)

TABLE 4-2	TIME-SPECIFIC SATURATION TARGETS AFTER BIRTH	
TIME AFTER BIRTH	**SATURATION**
1 min	60%-64%
2 min	65%-69%
3 min	70%-74%
4 min	75%-79%
5 min	80%-84%
10 min	85%-95%

Adapted from Kattwinkel J, editor: *Textbook of neonatal resuscitation*, ed 6, Elk Grove Village, Ill, 2011, American Academy of Pediatrics and American Heart Association.

The steps of transition and neonatal resuscitation follow the standard ABCs of resuscitation:

A—Airway

B—Breathing

C—Circulation

With the ABCs as an overall framework for neonatal resuscitation, the components of the procedure can be examined sequentially:

A—Establish an airway:

Position the infant.

Clear secretions from the mouth, nose, and trachea as needed.

Perform endotracheal intubation, if necessary.

B—Initiate breathing:

Dry thoroughly.

Provide specific tactile stimulation to breathe, if necessary.

Provide free-flow oxygen based on time-specific oxygenation targets (Table 4-2).

Provide positive-pressure ventilation.

C—Maintain circulation:

Delay umbilical cord clamping for at least 1 minute in term and preterm infants. Take steps to establish respirations before umbilical cord clamping.

Provide chest compressions.

Administer epinephrine, volume expander, if indicated.

Each step of the resuscitation procedure, whether uncomplicated or extended, is guided by the evaluation/decision/action cycle. Evaluation includes assessment of respirations, heart rate, and oxygen saturation (Figure 4-5).[44] The importance

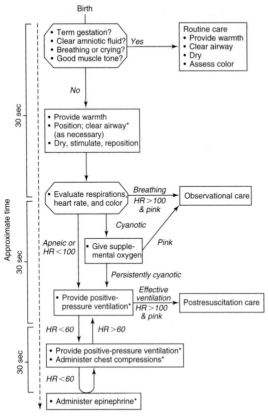

Birth

- Term gestation?
- Clear amniotic fluid?
- Breathing or crying?
- Good muscle tone?

Yes →

Routine care
- Provide warmth
- Clear airway
- Dry
- Assess color

No

- Provide warmth
- Position; clear airway* (as necessary)
- Dry, stimulate, reposition

- Evaluate respirations, heart rate, and color

Breathing HR > 100 & pink → Observational care

Cyanotic

Apneic or HR < 100 → Give supplemental oxygen

Pink

Persistently cyanotic

- Provide positive-pressure ventilation*

Effective ventilation HR > 100 & pink → Postresuscitation care

HR < 60   *HR > 60*

- Provide positive-pressure ventilation*
- Administer chest compressions*

HR < 60

- Administer epinephrine*

*Endotracheal intubation may be considered at several steps.

30 sec / 30 sec / 30 sec

Approximate time

FIGURE 4-5 Throughout resuscitation, the infant's respirations, heart rate (HR), and oxygen saturations are evaluated as a basis for decisions and actions. (From Kattwinkel J, editor: *Textbook of neonatal resuscitation*, ed 6, Elk Grove Village, Ill, 2011, American Academy of Pediatrics and American Heart Association, p. 12.)

of establishing an airway, drying, and stimulating the newly born to initiate breathing cannot be overemphasized in neonatal resuscitation. Expansion of the lungs with air and adequate ventilation are the keys to successful resuscitation. Successful performance of these steps often obviates the need for further intervention, but inadequate lung expansion and ventilation cannot be overcome by performing chest compressions or administering medications.

Apgar Score

The Apgar score provides a comprehensive, objective measure of the infant's condition in the first minutes after birth (Figure 4-6). The Apgar score does not serve as an indicator of the need for resuscitation;

rather, it quantifies an infant's response to the extrauterine environment and resuscitative measures. In term and preterm infants, the Apgar score remains a valuable predictor of infants who will need ongoing support in the immediate perinatal period and those who are at higher mortality risk in the neonatal period.[13]

Although perinatal asphyxia may be associated with low Apgar scores, it is possible for an infant to have a low Apgar score without having asphyxia.[48] For example, an infant born to a mother who received general anesthesia may be flaccid and have depressed reflexes and poor respiratory efforts. Such infants usually respond rapidly to bag-and-mask ventilation, and no further intervention is necessary. However, an infant may have an equally low Apgar score as a result of intrauterine asphyxia and may require prolonged resuscitative efforts. An infant with a midrange Apgar score between 6 and 7 may be using homeostatic mechanisms to maintain an adequate central blood pressure and cardiac output. Apgar scores should be assigned at 1 and 5 minutes, and every 5 minutes thereafter until the score is 7 or greater. A complete description of the timing and nature of resuscitative measures is vital to interpreting a low Apgar score.[3]

Although the Apgar score is not used to guide resuscitation, the experienced clinician performs a rapid visual assessment of an infant at the moment of birth. This rapid assessment incorporates two elements from the Apgar score, as well as a key question that influences the overall conduct of the resuscitation.

Rapid Assessment after Birth

In the first few seconds after birth, a rapid visual assessment of the baby should be performed to answer the following questions[47]:
- Is the baby term?
- Is the baby breathing or crying (respiratory effort)?
- Is there good muscle tone?

If the answer to all of these questions is "yes," the baby can remain with the mother to receive routine care as described in the Routine Care and Initial Steps of Resuscitation section that follows.

If the answer to any of the questions is "no," the infant may be evaluated under a radiant heat source during the initial steps of resuscitation.

Sign	0	1	2	1 min	5 min	10 min	15 min	20 min
Color	Blue or pale	Acrocyanotic	Completely pink					
Heart rate	Absent	Less than 100 min	Greater than 100 min					
Reflex irritability	No response	Grimace	Cry or active withdrawal					
Muscle tone	Limp	Some flexion	Active motion					
Respiration	Absent	Weak cry, hypoventilation	Good, crying					
Total								

Comments:		Resuscitation					
	Min	1	5	10	15	20
	Oxygen					
	PPV/NCPAP					
	ETT					
	Chest compressions					
	Epinephrine					

FIGURE 4-6 Expanded Apgar score. (From American College of Obstetricians and Gynecologists, ACOG Committee Opinion No. 333: The Apgar score, *Obstet Gynecol* 106:1141, 2005.)

If meconium is present, the vigor of the infant may alter the initial steps.

If meconium is present, evaluate the vigor of the infant:

- Does the baby have strong respiratory efforts?
- Is there good muscle tone?
- Is the heart rate greater than 100 beats/min?

If the answer to all of the questions is "yes," the airway may be cleared as described in the Position and Clear the Airway section. If the answer to any of the questions is "no," endotracheal suctioning may be performed.[44,89] In this circumstance, the initial steps of resuscitation should be completed after intubation for suctioning of meconium.

Routine Care and Initial Steps of Resuscitation

The care of every infant at birth includes (1) warmth, (2) clearing the airway (positioning and suctioning as necessary), and (3) support of breathing with drying and tactile stimulation.

Whether part of routine care or during the initial steps of resuscitation, many of the actions can be performed simultaneously, especially if more than one person is caring for the infant.

PROVIDE WARMTH

- Dry the infant thoroughly, and place him or her directly on the mother's abdomen/chest; cover both with warm linen (routine care).
  or
- Place the infant under a radiant heat source, dry thoroughly, and remove the wet linen.
  or
- Wrap preterm infants less than 28 weeks of gestation in a polyethylene sheet or bag of food-grade plastic from the shoulders to the toes (without drying), with the right arm exposed for pulse oximetry probe placement, and place under a radiant heat source.[85]

POSITION AND CLEAR THE AIRWAY (AS NECESSARY)

- Ensure that the infant's neck is slightly extended when positioning him or her on the mother's chest; wipe secretions from the mouth and nose or clear the airway with a bulb suction device if secretions are blocking the airway (routine care).

or

- Position the infant supine and flat with the neck slightly extended. A rolled blanket or towel may be used under the shoulders.
- Turn the head (or the head and body) to the side to allow secretions to pool in the cheek, and then remove with a suction device. Suction the mouth and then the nose to clear the airway. The mouth is suctioned first to clear the largest volume of secretions; when the nasopharynx is suctioned, a reflex cough, sneeze, or cry often results. Deep pharyngeal suction in an infant not requiring positive-pressure ventilation or intubation should not be performed during the first few minutes after birth to avoid vagal stimulation, resultant bradycardia, and delay in rise in PaO_2.[11,24]

or

- If meconium is present, evaluate the vigor of the infant before drying (as described earlier) to decide if endotracheal suction is needed.[89]

STIMULATE AND REPOSITION

- Provide tactile stimulation by briefly rubbing the back for infants who are not breathing or crying after drying.

or

- Continue gentle rubbing of trunk, extremities, or head to support early respiratory efforts in the newborn.
- Keep the head and neck in a slightly extended position to maintain an open airway.

Evaluate the Infant

Evaluation of the infant is a continuous, ongoing process. Subsequent action is guided by evaluation during each step of resuscitation and decisions about whether the response is adequate.

EVALUATE RESPIRATIONS

- Rate and depth of respirations (chest wall movement, air exchange) must be adequate; apnea and gasping respirations both require positive-pressure ventilation.

EVALUATE HEART RATE

- The heart rate should be greater than 100 beats/min. Feel the base of the umbilical cord or listen over the left side of the chest with a stethoscope to count the heart rate. Count the heart rate in 6 seconds and multiply by 10 for the beats per minute. Indicate each beat for other team members by tapping the forefinger on the bed or tapping the thumb and index finger together.

EVALUATE OXYGENATION

- Term, healthy babies may take more than 10 minutes to achieve a preductal oxygen saturation above 95% and nearly an hour to achieve the same level in the postductal circulation.[17,35,69,77]
- Give free-flow oxygen and place a pulse oximeter probe on the right hand/wrist if the infant is breathing but remains centrally cyanotic. Peripheral cyanosis (acrocyanosis) is *not* an indication for supplemental oxygen. The goal of oxygen administration should be normoxia based on time-specific oxygenation targets, not hyperoxia.[17,65]

Positive-Pressure Ventilation

Indications for positive-pressure ventilation in the newborn infant include the following:

- Apnea or gasping respirations despite a brief period of tactile stimulation
- A heart rate less than 100 beats/min
- Central cyanosis despite free-flow oxygen

Prolonged tactile stimulation or administration of supplemental oxygen to a baby who is not breathing effectively or who has a heart rate less than 100 beats/min only delays appropriate treatment. If supplemental oxygen is unavailable, positive-pressure ventilation should be provided with room air. When supplemental oxygen is available, it should be administered with the goal of achieving normoxia and avoiding hyperoxia.[17,65] Research in animals and humans has demonstrated that room air is equivalent to 100% oxygen for positive-pressure ventilation in many newly born infants. The exclusive use of 100% oxygen for postnatal resuscitation, as previously recommended, can result in hyperoxia and predisposition to changes induced by generation of oxygen free radicals.[80,82] The concentration and duration of supplemental oxygen administration should be individualized to patient needs. Pulse oximetry, initiated as soon as feasible, can help guide oxygen administration.[16] The ability to administer oxygen in concentrations from 21% to 100% in the delivery setting is now standard of care. This has special importance for preterm infants who are more vulnerable to oxygen injury yet may need concentrations greater than 21%.[23,81,84] Positive-pressure ventilation should be initiated with 21% oxygen for term infants. Preterm infants often require 30% to 50% oxygen initially to achieve target saturations; frequently, preterm infants who have received antenatal corticosteroids wean back to room air by admission to the neonatal intensive care unit (NICU).

IMPROVE VENTILATION
- The best indication of good mask seal and adequate lung inflation is a rising heart rate and bilateral breath sounds. Oxygen saturation should also rise and chest movement should be seen with each inflation.
- If heart rate and oxygenation do not improve, take steps to improve ventilation by (1) replacing the mask, (2) repositioning the airway, (3) opening the mouth, (4) increasing ventilation pressure, and (5) considering an alternative airway (endotracheal tube or laryngeal mask airway).

Chest Compressions

- If, after 30 seconds of effective positive-pressure ventilation, the heart rate is less than 60 beats/min, begin chest compressions and increase the oxygen concentration to 100% Fio_2. Consider intubation if not already performed, and call for help to prepare for possible umbilical venous catheter (UVC) placement and administration of emergency drugs.

Administration of Epinephrine and Volume Expansion

- If the heart rate remains below 60 beats/min despite ongoing positive-pressure ventilation and chest compressions, ensure that ventilation and chest compressions are being given effectively.

- If the heart rate remains below 60 beats/min after 45 to 60 seconds of coordinated chest compressions and effective ventilation, administer epinephrine.
- If the baby is not responding to resuscitation, including administration of epinephrine, and there is evidence of blood loss or hypovolemia, consider administration of a volume expander.

The initial steps in resuscitation should be accomplished rapidly so that the baby is breathing spontaneously or receiving positive-pressure ventilation by 1 minute. The initial rapid assessment can be performed in the first few seconds after birth to determine whether routine care can be provided to the infant, who remains with the mother, or whether more extensive evaluation and resuscitation will be necessary during the initial steps. The initial steps of resuscitation can be performed concurrently with evaluation of heart rate, respirations, and oxygen saturations, especially if more than one person is present to care for the infant. Positive-pressure ventilation should be performed for at least 30 seconds before moving to the next level of intervention. When oxygen concentrations less than 100% are used with positive-pressure ventilation and an adequate response in heart rate does not occur, steps to improve lung inflation should be taken and then the oxygen concentration can be increased before initiating chest compressions. Chest compressions should be continued for 45 to 60 seconds before pausing for assessment. If the resuscitation proceeds to use of epinephrine, reassessment should occur after 60 seconds to allow the epinephrine to circulate.

An infant who has received more than the initial steps of resuscitation will require close monitoring for additional or recurrent problems during the postnatal transition and may need supportive care such as continued oxygen administration. Infants who require more than brief positive-pressure ventilation should be monitored in a nursery setting in which they can receive ongoing care.[4]

Skills Necessary for Neonatal Resuscitation

INITIAL STEPS: SUCTIONING FOR MECONIUM-STAINED AMNIOTIC FLUID
Meconium-stained amniotic fluid is seen most often in infants who are more than 34 weeks of

gestational age, especially in term and postterm neonates. Passage of meconium may be associated with asphyxia. Severe fetal acidosis can result in fetal gasping, leading to in utero aspiration of meconium.[8] Suctioning the mouth and hypopharynx at delivery of the head and again after delivery is complete was advocated to help prevent meconium aspiration.[65] Current evidence no longer advises routine intrapartum suctioning for infants with meconium-stained amniotic fluid.[78]

Infants with meconium-stained amniotic fluid who are *not vigorous* at birth may receive tracheal intubation for suctioning. *Vigor* is defined by effective spontaneous respirations, a heart rate of greater than 100 beats/min, and good muscle tone. A large, multicenter, controlled trial examining management of vigorous infants with meconium-stained fluid found no difference in the incidence of respiratory distress (meconium aspiration or other respiratory distress) between groups who received routine airway management and endotracheal intubation for suctioning.[89] In that trial, infants were suctioned on the perineum, but results from a subsequent study suggest that intrapartum suctioning does not prevent the meconium aspiration syndrome.[78]

Nevertheless, any infant born with meconium-stained amniotic fluid who develops signs of airway obstruction or needs positive-pressure ventilation should first have the trachea suctioned and cleared of any meconium present.

If meconium is present in the amniotic fluid, perform the initial steps in the following manner:
- If the infant is vigorous, suction the mouth, posterior pharynx, and nose as necessary and proceed with drying, stimulation, and removal of wet linen.
- If the infant is depressed, clear the oropharynx with a large-bore catheter and suction the trachea under direct visualization using an endotracheal tube, adapter, and mechanical suction or a meconium suction device (Figure 4-7). Dry and stimulate the infant, and remove wet linen after the airway has been cleared.
- Suction the stomach when airway management is complete and vital signs are stable (usually after 5 minutes). Clearing meconium from the stomach decreases the risk for postnatal regurgitation and aspiration; however, suctioning too soon after birth can provoke apnea and bradycardia by vagal stimulation and complicate the initial resuscitation.

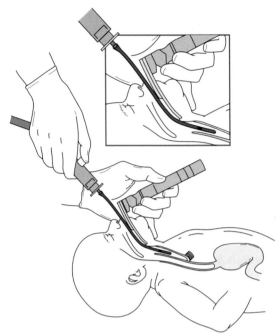

FIGURE 4-7 Equipment for suctioning meconium from the airway. Both meconium aspirator and meconium suction device connect to wall suction. (From Kattwinkel J, editor: *Textbook of neonatal resuscitation*, ed 6, Elk Grove Village, Ill, 2011, American Academy of Pediatrics and American Heart Association, p. 43.)

ADMINISTRATION OF FREE-FLOW OXYGEN

Supplemental oxygen should be administered after the initial steps if the infant remains centrally cyanotic.[47] The administration of oxygen is guided by pulse oximetry to achieve time-specific saturation targets (see Table 4-2).[17,47] Oxygen delivered at a flow rate of 5 L/min may be administered by mask or by holding the oxygen tubing in a cupped hand over the infant's face. The delivered oxygen concentration decreases rapidly as the tubing or mask is withdrawn from the face.

Once the target oxygen saturations are achieved, gradually withdraw the oxygen tubing or the mask from the infant's face. If cyanosis persists, reevaluate the quality of respirations and the heart rate; perform a brief physical examination; and consider bag-and-mask ventilation or intubation if there is evidence of respiratory distress.

BAG-AND-MASK VENTILATION

The indications for bag-and-mask ventilation include (1) apnea unresponsive to brief stimulation or gasping respirations, (2) heart rate less than 100 beats/min, and (3) persistently low oxygen saturation despite free-flow oxygen increased to 100%. The equipment for bag-and-mask ventilation can be either a self-inflating bag with an oxygen reservoir and pressure-release valve or pressure gauge, a flow-inflating bag (anesthesia bag) with a flow-control valve and pressure gauge, or a T-piece resuscitation device.

Although used widely, *self-inflating bags* do not deliver consistent tidal volumes or inflation pressures, even in the hands of providers who resuscitate frequently. Some data suggest, however, that self-inflating bags may offer advantages over flow-inflating bags when in the hands of inexperienced operators.[37] Self-inflating bags cannot be used reliably to deliver free-flow oxygen, and they require a special adapter to deliver continuous positive airway pressure (CPAP) (Figure 4-8). Ideally they would be fitted with a CPAP device and a manometer for use with newborns. *Flow-inflating bags* require a complete seal between mask and face to deliver a tidal volume. They offer the capability to achieve high peak pressures, deliver positive end-expiratory pressure (PEEP) and CPAP, and administer free-flow oxygen. The volume of the bag should generally be between 200 and 750 ml.[44] Larger bags are more difficult to handle and are predisposed to overly large tidal volumes, especially for preterm infants. A *T-piece resuscitation device,* as opposed to a bag, can achieve desired inflation pressures and respiratory times more consistently (at least in mechanical models) but requires setting the inspiratory pressure and PEEP before use and may be more difficult to adjust during resuscitation (see Figure 4-8).[18,26,37]

The facemask should be selected to ensure that it is the appropriate size to cover the chin, mouth, and nose but not the eyes. Masks are commonly available in term and premature sizes and may be obtained to fit even very low-birth-weight infants. Flexible, translucent masks with a cushioned rim generally provide the best seal with minimal trauma and allow monitoring of mouth position and secretions.[90,91]

Perform the following steps:

- Set the flowmeter to deliver 5 to 10 L/min. Flow rates at the higher end of the range are necessary to achieve higher pressures and faster ventilation rates with a flow-inflating bag.
- Test equipment before use. Equipment failure can cause resuscitation failure!

- Position the infant with the neck slightly extended, place the mask on the chin, and roll it over the mouth and nose (but not the eyes) to make a firm seal.[74] Avoid compression of soft tissues of the neck by holding the mask to the face with the thumb and index finger and providing gentle upward pressure with the third finger under the chin. Ventilate with initial pressures of 20 to 30 cm H_2O; pressure as high as 30 to 40 cm H_2O may be necessary in term infants not breathing spontaneously. Most apneic preterm infants respond to initial inflation pressures of 20 to 25 cm H_2O.[44]
- Ventilate at a rate of 40 to 60 breaths/min with pressures of 15 to 20 cm H_2O for normal lungs or up to 20 to 40 cm H_2O for diseased lungs. When surfactant is administered immediately after birth, rapid compliance changes may require equally rapid adjustment of ventilation pressures and oxygen concentration.
- Observe the heart rate. Prompt improvement in heart rate is the best indicator of adequate ventilation. If inadequate, (1) reapply the facemask for a better seal, (2) reposition the head, (3) suction secretions, (4) open the infant's mouth slightly, (5) increase pressure, and (6) consider an alternative airway.[44] The acronym MR SOPA will assist in remembering the order of steps to improve ventilation.
- Reevaluate respirations, heart rate, and oxygen saturation.
- Provide CPAP after spontaneous respirations have returned. End-expiratory pressure decreases lung injury and improves compliance and gas exchange.[42,76] CPAP may have a role in maintaining lung volumes in premature infants and aiding the absorption of lung fluid.[57]
- Insert an orogastric catheter (8-Fr feeding tube) after several minutes of bag-and-mask ventilation or if there is evidence of gastric distention.
- Measure the insertion depth of the catheter by holding the tip at the bridge of the nose and measuring to the earlobe and then midway between the xiphoid and the umbilicus.[44]
- Insert the catheter through the mouth, not the nose, because newborns are obligate nose-breathers.
- Aspirate gastric contents with a 20-ml syringe and leave the catheter open.
- Tape the catheter to the infant's cheek.

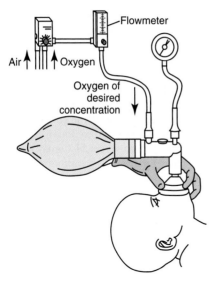

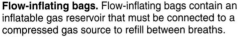

Flow-inflating bags. Flow-inflating bags contain an inflatable gas reservoir that must be connected to a compressed gas source to refill between breaths.
 Advantages:
  • Ability to deliver 21% to 100% oxygen, depending on the source
  • Ability to maintain a positive end-expiratory pressure and measure with manometer
  • Easy to determine when there is a seal around the neonate's face
  • Ability to deliver free-flow oxygen at concentrations up to 100% depending on the source
 Disadvantages:
  • Requires an external compressed gas source to inflate
  • Requires a tight seal between mask and face to remain inflated
  • Requires use of pressure gauge (manometer) to
 A   monitor pressure delivered with each breath.

Self-inflating bags. Self-inflating bags fill with ambient air and are independent on an external oxygen or compressed air source.
 Advantages:
  • Will always refill after being squeezed, even with no compressed gas source
  • Pressure-release valve makes overinflation less likely
 Disadvantages:
  • Will inflate even if there is not a seal between the mask and the neonate's face
  • Requires an oxygen reservoir to provide high concentration of oxygen
  • Cannot be used to deliver free-flow oxygen reliably through the mask
  • Cannot be used to deliver continuous positive airway pressure (CPAP) and can deliver positive end-expiratory pressure (PEEP) only when a PEEP
 B   valve is added and pressurized gas is entering the bag

FIGURE 4-8 **A,** Flow-inflating bag. **B,** Self-inflating bag. (From Kattwinkel J, editor: *Textbook of neonatal resuscitation,* ed 6, Elk Grove Village, Ill, 2011, American Academy of Pediatrics and American Heart Association.)

The adequacy of bag-and-mask ventilation must be continuously assessed by monitoring of heart rate, auscultation of breath sounds, visualization of chest wall movement, and oxygen saturations. Peak inspiratory pressure should be limited to that necessary to see an improvement in heart rate and chest wall movement and to hear good air exchange on auscultation of the chest. Inspiratory pressures cannot be judged clinically; bags fitted with in-line pressure manometers or T-piece devices are recommended in the delivery room.[44] The neonatal respiratory system responds slowly to mechanical inspiratory pressure; prolonged

inspiratory times are under active investigation as a means to more rapidly establish functional residual capacity and achieve adequate inspiratory volume.[59] Devices that more easily and consistently deliver targeted volumes during positive-pressure ventilation are the focus of much recent research.[73] Strategies to avoid intubation, especially continuous positive airway pressure with limited oxygen concentration, offer the promise of reduction in severity of chronic lung disease.[6,19] Further clinical trials will help establish the optimal method(s) for achieving lung expansion while minimizing the complications of positive-pressure ventilation.[66,83]

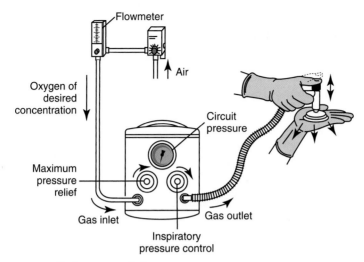

Flowmeter

Air

Oxygen of desired concentration

Circuit pressure

Maximum pressure relief

Gas inlet

Gas outlet

Inspiratory pressure control

T-piece resuscitator.
Advantages:
- Consistent pressure
- Reliable control of peak inspiratory pressure (PIP) and positive end-expiratory pressure (PEEP)
- Reliable delivery of 100% oxygen
- Operator does not become fatigued from bagging

Disadvantages:
- Requires compressed gas supply
- Requires pressures to be set prior to use
- Changing inflation pressure during resuscitation is more difficult
- Risk of prolonged inspiratory time

C

FIGURE 4-8, cont'd **C,** T-piece resuscitator. (From Kattwinkel J, editor: *Textbook of neonatal resuscitation*, ed 6, Elk Grove Village, III, 2011, American Academy of Pediatrics and American Heart Association.)

Potential complications of bag-and-mask ventilation include trauma to the eyes or face from improper size or position of the mask, lung injury (especially in preterm infants), air leak (pneumothorax, subcutaneous air), gastric distention elevating the diaphragm, and direct lung compression in the case of a diaphragmatic hernia (Table 4-3). Complications can be minimized by using gentle technique and equipment of correct size, careful monitoring of pressures, and insertion of an orogastric tube when indicated.

ENDOTRACHEAL INTUBATION

Endotracheal intubation may be performed at several points during neonatal resuscitation.[44] Intubation is indicated when (1) tracheal suctioning is needed, as with meconium-stained amniotic fluid in a nonvigorous infant; (2) bag-and-mask ventilation is ineffective or prolonged positive-pressure ventilation is needed; (3) chest compressions are necessary; or (4) epinephrine administration is necessary. Additional indications for endotracheal intubation include extreme prematurity, surfactant administration, and suspected diaphragmatic hernia. Equipment for intubation is listed in the "Airway" and "Breathing" sections in Box 4-2.

Select an uncuffed, uniform-diameter endotracheal tube of the correct size (Table 4-4). A variety of sizes (2.5- to 4-mm internal diameter) should be available, because estimated weights may be inaccurate or airway anomalies may exist. Orotracheal intubation is preferable to nasotracheal intubation during acute resuscitation because it can be performed rapidly and without additional equipment.

TABLE 4-3	COMPLICATIONS DURING RESUSCITATION AND STABILIZATION

PROBLEM	CAUSE	DIAGNOSIS	REMEDIES
Persistent cyanosis	Inadequate oxygenation		
	• Inadequate Fio_2	Check pulse oximetry saturation and blender setting	Always have available blended O_2
	• Disconnected O_2 line	Check all connections	Reconnect line
	• Empty O_2 cylinder	Check O_2 source	Replace O_2 cylinder
	Inadequate ventilation		
	• Inadequate facemask seal	Diminished breath sounds; little chest wall movement; air leak around mask	Readjust facemask; seal tightly against skin
	• Compression of airway	Diminished breath sounds; little chest wall movement	Apply upward force to mandible to counteract downward force holding facemask in place; extend neck slightly
	• Insufficient insufflation pressure	Diminished breath sounds; little chest wall movement	Increase insufflation pressure until breath sounds are audible and chest movement seen
	• Compression of lungs by distended stomach	Diminished breath sounds; little chest wall movement; visibly distended stomach	Place orogastric tube
	• Malpositioned ET tube	Check tube position with laryngoscope Check breath sounds	Reinsert into trachea Withdraw until breath sounds are bilaterally equal Tape ET tube in place
	Pneumothorax	Check breath sounds Check for chest asymmetry Transillumination Chest x-ray examination	Decompress tension pneumothorax
Bradycardia	Same as for persistent cyanosis	Auscultation of precordium or palpation of umbilical cord base; pulse oximeter or cardiac monitor	Same as for persistent cyanosis External cardiac compression if heart rate less than 60 beats/min after 30 sec of effective ventilation
	Vagal stimulation Perinatal myocardial ischemia	Lack of response to oxygenation, ventilation, and chest compressions	Stop oropharyngeal suctioning Emergency epinephrine/volume expander administration
Hypothermia	Evaporative heat loss; conductive heat loss	Specific signs overlap those of asphyxia and shock Low core temperature	Dry infant; remove wet linen Use polyethylene bags/warming mattress Cover wet hair Keep under radiant warmer
Hyperthermia	Excessive warming Maternal fever	Apnea High core temperature	Servocontrol of warming devices Removal of warming mattress
Hypoglycemia	Glucose stores used before birth or during resuscitation	Specific symptoms overlap those of asphyxia and shock Low blood sugar	Bolus 2 ml/kg of $D_{10}W$ Maintenance infusion of $D_{10}W$
Hemorrhage	Inadequately secured umbilical arterial or venous line	Pallor Poor capillary refilling Leakage of blood	Keep all intravascular tubing connection sites in plain view Tape UAC/UVC in place in addition to suturing lines
	Liver laceration		Perform chest compressions with correct position/depth

ET, Endotracheal; *UAC,* umbilical artery catheter; *UVC,* umbilical venous catheter.

TABLE 4-4	ENDOTRACHEAL TUBE SIZE AND DEPTH OF INSERTION		
WEIGHT (g)	GESTATIONAL AGE (wk)	TUBE SIZE (mm) (INSIDE DIAMETER)	DEPTH OF INSERTION (cm FROM UPPER LIP)
<1000	<28	2.5	<7
1000–2000	28–34	3.0	7
2000–3000	34–38	3.5	8
>3000	>38	3.5–4.0	9

Adapted from Kattwinkel J, editor: *Textbook of neonatal resuscitation,* ed 6, Elk Grove Village, Ill, 2011, American Academy of Pediatrics and American Heart Association.

Perform the following steps:
- Shorten the selected endotracheal tube to 13 cm (or the length appropriate for the fixation method used), and prepare the laryngoscope, tape, suction, oxygen, bag, and mask.
- Position the infant with the neck slightly extended.
- Provide free-flow oxygen as needed to achieve target saturations.
- Hold the laryngoscope with the left hand; open the mouth with the right index finger and gently insert the blade.
- Lift the laryngoscope upward and outward so that the blade is nearly parallel to the surface beneath the infant.
- Visualize landmarks; identify the epiglottis, vocal cords, and glottis (Figure 4-9). If the esophagus is seen, withdraw the blade until the epiglottis drops down. If only the tongue is visible, advance the blade further until it enters the vallecula or passes under the epiglottis.
- Apply gentle external pressure over the cricoid, which may help visualize the vocal cords. Pressure may be applied with the little finger of the hand holding the laryngoscope or by an assistant.
- Insert the endotracheal tube from the right corner of the mouth to the level of the vocal cord guideline at the tip of the tube.
- Limit each intubation attempt to 30 seconds to avoid hypoxia.
- Confirm endotracheal tube position by exhaled CO_2 detector and by auscultation for bilaterally equal breath sounds in the axillae and absence of breath sounds over the stomach. Observe chest wall movement. Note the centimeter marking at the lip (see Table 4-4).

- Secure the endotracheal tube and obtain a chest radiograph.
- Shorten the endotracheal tube to 4 cm beyond the lips, if necessary.

Complications of intubation include hypoxia caused by prolonged intubation attempts or lack of supplemental oxygen; tube malposition; apnea or bradycardia caused by hypoxia or vagal stimulation; and trauma to the oropharynx, trachea, vocal cords, or esophagus (see Table 4-3). Exhaled CO_2 detection devices, commonly used to confirm endotracheal tube position in children, may be helpful even in newborn infants weighing less than 2 kg.[92] Color change may be delayed in extremely preterm infants, especially if cardiac output is low, as during bradycardia. To prevent complications, provide free-flow oxygen during intubation, use gentle technique, and limit each intubation attempt to 30 seconds.

CHEST COMPRESSIONS

Indications for chest compressions include a heart rate less than 60 beats/min despite effective positive-pressure ventilation for 30 seconds. Follow the sequence of (A) airway, (B) breathing, and (C) circulation in providing resuscitative support. Even if the heart rate is less than 60 beats/min shortly after delivery, the airway should be cleared and positive-pressure ventilation should be given for 30 seconds before beginning chest compressions. Often, adequate ventilation alone will result in a rapid increase in heart rate.[64] Beginning chest compressions too early may interfere with the effectiveness of positive-pressure ventilation and actually delay an infant's response to resuscitation.

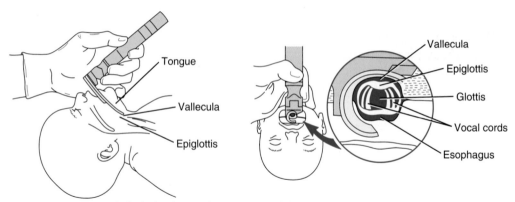

FIGURE 4-9 Anatomic landmarks that relate to intubation. (From Kattwinkel J, editor: *Textbook of neonatal resuscitation*, ed 6, Elk Grove Village, Ill, 2011, American Academy of Pediatrics and American Heart Association.)

Perform the following steps:
- Position the infant with the neck slightly extended.
- Provide firm support for the back.
- Perform compressions using the two-thumb (preferred) or two-finger technique (Figure 4-10).

Position: Lower third of sternum[47,74]

Rate: 90 times/min

Depth: One third of the anterior-posterior diameter of the chest

Support: Encircling fingers or hand under back

- Provide 90 compressions/min and interpose 30 breaths/min with a 3:1 ratio of compressions to breaths (120 events/min).[47]
- Evaluate the heart rate after 45 to 60 seconds.
- Continue chest compressions until the heart rate is greater than 60 beats/min.
- Administer epinephrine if the heart rate remains less than 60 beats/min after 45 to 60 seconds of coordinated and effective chest compressions.

When response to positive-pressure ventilation and chest compressions is poor, reevaluate for technical problems and conditions interfering with ventilation. Confirm that oxygen is connected properly and that oxygen has been increased to 100% (see Table 4-3). To ensure a patent airway, place an endotracheal tube and confirm proper position. Ventilate with pressures to expand the chest and breaths interposed between compressions. Evaluate the infant for pneumothorax, diaphragmatic hernia, or hypovolemia (see Delivery Room Emergencies later in this chapter).

Complications of chest compressions include liver laceration, rib fractures, and pneumothorax. To prevent complications, check the position of compressions, maintain contact with the chest during the release portion of the compression cycle, and avoid excessive force during compressions.

MEDICATIONS

The indications for drug administration during newborn resuscitation include the following:
- Epinephrine: Heart rate less than 60 beats/min despite 45 to 60 seconds of coordinated ventilation and chest compressions
- Volume expanders: Evidence of acute bleeding or signs of hypovolemia; poor response to other resuscitative measures

Perform the following steps:
- Calculate the correct dosage of each drug based on the newborn's weight.
- Prepare each drug for administration, draw up the appropriate concentration and volume, and label the syringe.
- Administer each drug by the correct route and at the proper rate.
- Reevaluate for desired effect and take follow-up action.

Epinephrine increases the rate and strength of cardiac contractions. Perhaps more important during resuscitation is its action as a peripheral vasoconstrictor, directing cardiac output to the central circulation and increasing coronary perfusion pressure.[87] Epinephrine is most effective when administered by umbilical venous catheter in a dose of 0.1 to 0.3 ml/kg of 1:10,000 concentration.

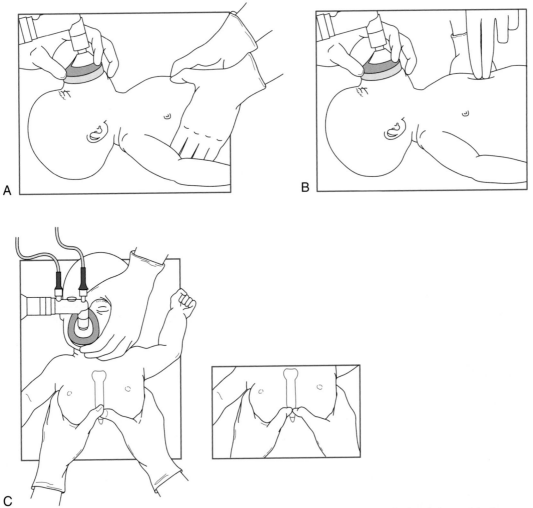

FIGURE 4-10 Two-thumb (**A**, preferred) and two-finger (**B**) methods of chest compression. **C**, The two-thumb method uses two thumbs placed one over the other or side by side (depending on the size of the baby) to compress the sternum; encircle the chest with the hands so that your fingers support the spine. Providing chest compressions from the head of the bed facilitates emergency UVC placement. (From Kattwinkel J, editor: *Textbook of neonatal resuscitation*, ed 6, Elk Grove Village, Ill, 2011, American Academy of Pediatrics and American Heart Association.)

Endotracheal administration in a one-time dose of 0.5 to 1 ml/kg can be considered while obtaining venous access. Expansion of plasma and blood volume may also be necessary to maintain cardiac output, blood pressure, and peripheral perfusion.

Volume expansion should be considered when there is evidence of acute blood loss (e.g., abruptio placentae, bleeding from placenta previa, fetal-maternal hemorrhage, umbilical cord tear, acute neonatal hemorrhage) or poor response to resuscitation (e.g., pallor, bradycardia, exaggerated tachycardia). Normal saline is the preferred solution for volume expansion in a dose of 10 ml/kg by umbilical venous catheter.

Complications of drug administration include extravasation with intravascular administration, hepatic injury with low umbilical venous catheters, and unpredictable absorption with endotracheal administration. The use of resuscitation drugs also may result in complications from their adverse pharmacologic effects. Epinephrine, administered in high doses, increases the risk for significant hypertension and a hyperadrenergic state, which may result in germinal matrix hemorrhage or myocardial damage. Absorption of epinephrine after endotracheal administration is erratic.[81] Volume overload may result from administration of repeated doses of volume expanders. Rapid volume expansion, resulting in acute elevation of systolic blood pressure, has been associated with intraventricular hemorrhage.[30]

Distressed newborns have impaired autoregulation of cerebral blood flow, with blood flow directly related to the systolic blood pressure. Increased cerebral blood flow and elevated systolic pressures may be responsible for intraventricular hemorrhage in the presence of a capillary bed insulted by acidosis and hypoxia.[52] Autopsy studies also suggest that increased cerebral venous capillary pressure can initiate intraventricular hemorrhage. Volume expansion should be performed cautiously in preterm or asphyxiated infants, infusing 10 ml/kg aliquots of fluid over a 5- to 10-minute period and evaluating the response before administering repeated aliquots of fluid. The exception to this rule is the infant who has experienced acute perinatal hemorrhage with hypovolemia. These infants should have the circulatory fluid volume restored as rapidly as possible. Complications of medication administration can be prevented by choosing the correct dose, rate, and route of administration and positioning umbilical lines carefully. The infant should be evaluated for adverse effects and response to fluid volume after each medication/volume dose.

Sodium bicarbonate is no longer recommended for use during resuscitation immediately after birth. Although acidosis frequently persists after a prolonged resuscitation, many infants correct an acidosis spontaneously once the asphyxiating circumstances are relieved and adequate ventilation is established. Metabolic correction of pH is a slow process that takes several hours, and treatment with sodium bicarbonate is not necessary. Sodium bicarbonate results in worsened acidosis in the setting of impaired ventilation; bicarbonate also may worsen intracellular acidosis. Furthermore, bicarbonate adds a high sodium load, which may directly depress myocardial performance.[6]

Naloxone hydrochloride is indicated during acute resuscitation only in the very specific circumstance of severe neonatal respiratory depression and narcotic administration to the mother in the last 4 hours. Naloxone is not part of the routine resuscitation of an apneic infant.[47] Establishment of gas exchange with positive-pressure ventilation is the first priority for any infant who does not have adequate spontaneous respirations after birth. No randomized controlled trials of naloxone for treatment of apnea have been conducted in the delivery room setting. Furthermore, naloxone hydrochloride is contraindicated in infants of narcotic-addicted mothers, because administration can result in severe abstinence syndrome, including seizures.

Calcium and atropine have little role in delivery room settings. Calcium is indicated for hypocalcemia or hyperkalemia, both of which are infrequent problems in the delivery room. Atropine may mask hypoxia-related bradycardia.

DELIVERY ROOM EMERGENCIES

Certain conditions can present as emergencies in the delivery room (Table 4-5). These conditions may require extensive resuscitation or result in a poor response to resuscitation. Some situations require special intervention immediately; most merit the involvement of a neonatal nurse practitioner, pediatrician, or neonatologist for management. Coordinated teamwork, with techniques and communication skills acquired through simulation training, can help ensure rapid and effective stabilization.[34,86] Surgical intervention is necessary to complete the treatment of diaphragmatic hernia, abdominal wall defects, and neural tube defects. See Box 4-3 for an outline of emergency procedures in the delivery room setting.

CARE DURING THE TRANSITION FROM THE DELIVERY ROOM TO THE NURSERY

After the infant is stabilized and vigorous, perform elective procedures, such as clamping and shortening the umbilical cord, footprinting and identification, applying ophthalmic prophylaxis, and weighing (see Chapter 5). A vigorous, stable infant may remain in skin-to-skin contact with the mother and breastfeed

TABLE 4-5   DELIVERY ROOM EMERGENCIES

CONDITION	SIGNS AND SYMPTOMS	ONGOING PROBLEMS	INITIAL RESPONSES
Pneumothorax	Cyanosis, respiratory distress, unequal breath sounds, bradycardia, displaced heart sounds	Continuing asphyxia, shock (poor venous return)	Transilluminate chest, perform needle thoracentesis, evaluate chest tube placement
Choanal atresia; oral/pharyngeal airway anomalies	Noisy respirations, pink when crying but cyanotic when quiet, cannot pass suction catheter per nares	Respiratory distress, intermittent hypoxemia and bradycardia	Supplemental oxygen, oral airway, and prone positioning; or intubation (lower airway anomalies may require emergency tracheostomy)
Extreme prematurity	Respiratory distress	Continuing hypoxemia, hypothermia, possible sepsis, hypovolemia	Intubate, place umbilical lines, evaluate for artificial surfactant, begin antibiotics, consider transport to neonatal center
Sepsis	Respiratory distress, hypotonia, poor perfusion, foul odor	Continuing hypoxemia, shock	Intubate, place umbilical lines, administer antibiotics
Severe asphyxia	Prolonged apnea, bradycardia, poor perfusion, pallor, hypotonia, seizures	Hypoxemia, shock, multiorgan system injury	Intubate, place umbilical lines, give volume expander and vasopressors for shock, consider transport to neonatal center
Hydrops fetalis	Body wall edema, ascites, pallor, poor perfusion, respiratory distress, possibly unequal breath sounds (pneumothorax), distant heart sounds (pericardial effusion)	Hypoxemia, anemia, shock, potential for multiorgan system injury	Intubate, perform posterolateral needle thoracentesis bilaterally if unable to ventilate; consider paracentesis if ascites compromises ventilation; place chest tube for pneumothorax, place umbilical lines, evaluate need for partial exchange transfusion, consider transport to neonatal center
Pulmonary hypoplasia and oligohydramnios	Respiratory distress; flattened, deviated nose; infraorbital creases; low-set, crumpled ears; small chin; deformities of the extremities	Hypoxemia, pneumothorax, pulmonary hypoplasia	Intubate, place umbilical lines, monitor closely for pulmonary air leak, consider transport to neonatal center
Congenital diaphragmatic hernia	Respiratory distress with asymmetric breath sounds, barrel chest and scaphoid abdomen, point of maximal cardiac intensity shifted to side opposite hernia	Hypoxemia, pulmonary hypertension, contralateral pneumothorax	Intubate, decompress bowel with orogastric tube to low intermittent suction, place umbilical lines, arrange transport to neonatal center
Abdominal wall defect	Midline abdominal wall defect at base of umbilical cord (omphalocele) or lateral to cord insertion (gastroschisis) with externalization of abdominal contents	Hypovolemia, respiratory distress, hypothermia, ischemic injury to externalized abdominal contents, infection	Protect exposed tissue with evaporative barrier; begin parenteral fluids at 1.5 times maintenance; place an orogastric tube to low intermittent suction, position infant side-lying with support of exposed organs, monitor temperature and urine output, arrange transport to a neonatal center with pediatric surgery
Neural tube defects	Open spinal defect (myelomeningocele), cranial defect with outpouching brain tissue (occipital or frontal encephalocele), failure of formation of skull and brain (anencephaly)	Prolonged apnea, infection, hypothermia	Provide supportive care unless prenatal diagnosis of lethal anomaly has allowed formation of a plan for limited support; protect exposed tissue with gauze soaked in warmed saline and evaporative barrier; arrange transport to a neonatal center with specialists in spinal defects

BOX 4-3   EMERGENCY PROCEDURES IN THE DELIVERY ROOM

A. Umbilical vessel catheterization (see Chapter 7)
B. Thoracentesis and chest tube placement (see Chapter 23)
C. Partial exchange transfusion for anemia (see Chapter 20)
1. Indications: Profound chronic anemia (hematocrit [Hct] <25%), as in the setting of hydrops. Distinct from situations of acute loss of blood volume, chronic anemia results in normal blood volume per kilogram, necessitating partial exchange transfusion to rapidly raise the hematocrit.
2. Procedure
  a. Obtain O-negative packed red blood cells (PRBCs) by emergency release if necessary. PRBCs should be as fresh as possible to minimize risk for hyperkalemia.
  b. Insert a low umbilical vein catheter, and attach a four-way stopcock (exchange set).
  c. Perform an isovolumetric exchange by alternating withdrawal and infusion of 5- to 10-ml aliquots of patient blood and PRBCs to a total exchange volume of approximately 20 ml/kg. The formula is as follows:

  Exchange volume = Estimated dry wt × Blood volume/kg
  (desired Hct − current Hct) ÷ Hct of PRBCs

  This equation can be used to estimate the rise in hematocrit for a given exchange volume and a given hematocrit of exchange blood.
  d. Alternatively, place both a low umbilical vein catheter (UVC) and an umbilical artery catheter (UAC). Withdraw from the UAC while infusing PRBCs per the UVC at the same rate to the total exchange volume.
3. Risks
  a. Thrombotic, embolic events
  b. Infection

  c. Bleeding (from mechanical complications or depletion of clotting factors)
  d. Hyperkalemia (consider use of washed PRBCs for nonemergent partial volume exchanges)
D. Prophylactic administration of exogenous surfactant (see Chapter 23)
1. Indications
  a. Prematurity
  b. Respiratory distress
  c. Presumed surfactant deficiency
2. Procedure
  a. Calculate the appropriate dose of surfactant based on birth weight.
  b. Confirm correct endotracheal tube position by centimeter markings at the lip (see Table 4-4) and careful auscultation. Chest x-ray film confirmation is ideal if surfactant is administered during stabilization in the nursery.
  c. Suction the endotracheal tube to clear secretions.
  d. Monitor heart rate and oxygen saturation with pulse oximetry.
  e. Administer surfactant according to manufacturer's directions. Administration options include rapid bolus and gradual infusion combined with positioning of the infant and hand or mechanical ventilation.
  f. Refrain from suctioning for at least 4 hours after surfactant administration.
  g. Monitor chest wall rise, saturations, and arterial blood gases, and adjust ventilator support accordingly.
3. Complications
  a. Hypoxemia
  b. Air leak
  c. Pulmonary hemorrhage

---

immediately. A head covering prevents heat loss from the large surface area of the head and wet hair. The stable infant may complete the transition period with the parents under appropriate observation.

The infant who has required more extensive resuscitation in the delivery room should be transferred to a special care or intensive care nursery when adequate spontaneous or controlled ventilation has been established, the heart rate is greater than 100 beats/min, and the infant has been dried and protected from excessive heat loss. Note the time of the infant's first respiratory effort and when sustained, regular respirations occur. Transfer the infant in a warmed transport incubator with necessary support measures such as supplemental oxygen or positive-pressure ventilation and pulse oximetry monitoring of heart rate and oxygen saturations.[38] Delay elective procedures until the infant is physiologically stable.[46] Depending on the level of care required by the infant and the level of care available in the institution, the infant may need to be transported from the birth setting to receive appropriate care after resuscitation (see Chapter 3).

In the intensive care nursery, place the infant on a preheated open warmer with servo control. Avoid overwarming, because hyperthermia may be associated with respiratory depression and worsened neurologic outcome after asphyxial insults.[49,63] Continue adequate cardiopulmonary monitoring, including electrocardiogram, respiratory rate and pattern, and monitoring of oxygen saturation with pulse oximetry (see Chapter 7). Obtain serum glucose by heelstick and blood pressure by a Doppler device and blood pressure cuff. If a UVC was inserted during the initial resuscitation for medication administration, remove this catheter. Begin a peripheral intravenous infusion if blood glucose is low or volume expansion is indicated; alternatively, consider rapid placement of a low UVC to administer glucose or volume expander. Evaluate for placement of a central umbilical venous line for maintenance fluid administration and/or an arterial line for blood sampling and continuous arterial pressure monitoring. Confirm endotracheal tube and umbilical line placement with an x-ray examination.

Debriefing after resuscitation and stabilization of the infant in the NICU gives those who attended the delivery an opportunity to have a conversation and reflect on their care, teamwork, and communication. Debriefing identifies aspects of the resuscitation that went well and those that could be improved with the goal of practice and systems change for continuous improvement.

CARE OF THE FAMILY AND PERINATAL DECISION MAKING

Encouraging the presence of the father or another mature support person in the delivery room is common obstetric practice and should not interfere with delivery room care. Ideally, members of the obstetric and neonatal resuscitation team should introduce themselves to the parents/birth companion before the delivery. Parents have a great deal of anxiety concerning procedures performed on their newborn; a few moments spent describing routine procedures will help allay their fears and avoid misinterpretation. When problems are anticipated, a calm, professional explanation of neonatal assessment and life support measures is necessary. Parental awareness that the medical and nursing staff have anticipated and prepared for possible problems can partially relieve their anxieties. Care must be taken, however, to avoid instilling undue alarm. Care providers should understand ethical principles and the impact of their personal moral and ethical beliefs on decisions made about resuscitation.[36]

If an infant requires resuscitation or prolonged assessment and support, the attending staff's primary obligation is to provide this care and communicate with the parents. Parents should be encouraged to have contact with their baby, but the presence of the father or a support person must not be allowed to interfere with or delay the delivery of care. The pediatric staff should tell the parents what is happening at the earliest possible opportunity, because lack of communication prolongs anxiety for the parents. A few brief statements to explain the status of the baby and procedures can relieve the anguish of silence. Especially when a difficult resuscitation is anticipated, it is ideal to designate, in advance, a team member who can keep parents informed.

When severe perinatal problems are suspected prenatally and confirmed after birth, such as extreme prematurity (gestational age less than 23 weeks, birth weight less than 400 g), anencephaly, or trisomy 13 or 18, discussions may be held in advance with obstetric care providers and the family about limiting the extent of resuscitative measures (see Chapter 32).[36,62] Current data suggest that resuscitation of these infants is very unlikely to result in survival or survival without disability.[14] When problems are unanticipated, information is uncertain, or there has been no time for decision making before delivery, intervention in the delivery room may be warranted.[20] This approach allows time for complete information to be gathered and discussed with the family. If appropriate, support measures can be withdrawn later in the nursery. When an infant fails to respond to intensive resuscitative measures in the delivery room, a decision, in consultation with the parents, must be made as to when to stop support. Survival is unlikely if no heart rate has been obtained after 10 minutes.[12,13,41,96] Discontinuation of resuscitation may be appropriate if, after 10 minutes of full resuscitative effort, there is no return of spontaneous circulation. The data for infants who have an inadequate response to resuscitation remain less clear. The probability of survival diminishes and the probability of cerebral palsy increases with the length of time during which Apgar scores remain below 4. For example, if the Apgar score remains below 4 at 20 minutes, the probability of cerebral palsy in surviving infants is greater than 50%.[45] It is essential to rapidly identify remediable causes of poor response to resuscitation.

Anticipation and recognition of fetal and neonatal problems indicating delivery room resuscitation depend on a knowledgeable and prepared staff working as a team to effectively and efficiently communicate and respond in a critical situation. By applying current evidence in performing the skills necessary for neonatal resuscitation, evaluating the infant's response, and taking the time to discuss resuscitation options and outcomes with the parents and resuscitation team, successful delivery room care and stabilization of the newborn is more likely.

REFERENCES

For a full list of references, scan the QR code or visit http://booksite.elsevier.com/ 9780323320832.

5

INITIAL NURSERY CARE

SANDRA L. GARDNER AND JACINTO A. HERNÁNDEZ

A neonate must demonstrate a condition of well-being before being considered a normal, low-risk infant. Neonatal intensive care professionals must understand the normal neonate to care for the sick neonate. This chapter discusses the initial assessment, transitional period, and gestational age characteristics that are of fundamental clinical importance for the provision of quality initial nursery care by all health care providers.

Physical, biologic, and physiologic changes occur so rapidly after birth that the assessment of the newly born can be divided into four distinctive periods: at delivery, during transition, during the first 24 hours of life, and at discharge. Each of these assessments has a specific purpose. One should consider these evaluations in relation to the age of the newborn infant (minutes, hours, days, and weeks) rather than to the location of the mother and infant in the hospital or to arbitrary nursery routines.

The evaluation at delivery is aimed at determining the condition of the infant at the time of birth and at detecting potentially life-threatening emergencies. The examination during the next few hours (*transition period*) is used to evaluate the infant's adjustment to extrauterine life. The complete newborn examination by a qualified health care provider should be performed at about 12 to 24 hours.[6] It is the most important examination, because many findings can be treated or complications can be avoided. Finally, the assessment/evaluation at discharge is of the utmost importance. Although it is not as detailed as the complete examination, it is aimed at establishing the infant's readiness to leave the hospital and to be cared for by the mother. During this examination, the health care professional demonstrates the

baby's unique abilities and answers the parents' questions. This is a good time to provide support and encouragement as the parents begin to incorporate the new member into their family.

ASSESSMENT AND CARE AT DELIVERY

Before the delivery, one should obtain pertinent facts about the pregnancy, such as parity, gravidity, fetal losses, estimated birth weight and gestational age of the fetus, and, of course, any problems present in the current pregnancy.[75] The results of prenatal screening tests should be available to the clinician at delivery. Health care providers should note whether the mother was screened for group B streptococcus and whether she received any antibiotic treatment.[6,28]

During labor, one can observe the frequency and duration of contractions and the mother's reaction to contractions. Passage of meconium, rupture of membranes, fetal distress, vaginal infections, and other signs will alert the attendants to impending problems.

At birth, the most common way to assess the infant's condition is to use the Apgar scoring system.[7,26] This score provides a comprehensive, objective measure of the state of an infant at given times after birth, traditionally at 1 and 5 minutes (see Chapter 4, Figure 4-6). The Apgar score standardizes initial newborn assessment and continues to be a predictor of neonatal survival.[7,26] The Apgar score should not be used as the primary indicator for resuscitation because it is not normally assigned until 1 minute of age. Assessment of the initial respiratory effort and heart rate, within the first 60 seconds, is paramount to begin timely resuscitative procedures if the infant is limp and not breathing

---

PURPLE type highlights content that is particularly applicable to clinical settings.

(see Chapter 4). If the baby is vigorous, the care provider may place him or her on the mother's abdomen or in her arms; Apgar assessment can be done there or in a bassinet or warmer. Scoring is repeated at 5 minutes. Between the 1- and 5-minute Apgar scores, one systematically evaluates the baby for potential or apparent medical emergencies.

Most infants are vigorous, cry at birth, and breathe easily thereafter. In most circumstances, a healthy, vigorous infant does not even require suctioning after birth. With appropriate training and oversight, most infants can be given directly to the mother after birth without compromising the infant.

Shortly after birth, a *quick estimate of gestational age* is done. Several tables, charts, and graphs have been developed over time to assist the clinician in performing this task. With practice and experience, the professional will be able to identify approximate gestational age from the physical appearance. Additional discussion on gestational age assessment will be covered later. Immediately following birth, *a brief but complete initial examination* should be performed on each newborn to assess the condition of the infant and to ensure that there are no major anomalies or birth injuries, that the infant is pink, and that breathing is normal. The entire body must be assessed, including overall size, proportionality and contour, respiratory pattern and presence of distress, posture, tone, and state of alertness. This usually allows the clinician to reassure parents that their infant is well and appears normal. A more detailed evaluation/examination is described later.

The most severely ill neonates are usually apparent after birth. Most of them will have been identified prenatally (e.g., serious congenital anomalies, extreme prematurity), their presence anticipated, and a management plan made before delivery (see Chapter 4).

EVALUATION AND CARE DURING THE TRANSITIONAL PERIOD

Physiologic Changes and Clinical Stages

The initial evaluation, assessment, and management of a newborn must be directed toward promoting and facilitating normal adaptation to extrauterine life and early detection of significant health problems so that they can be evaluated and treated promptly and appropriately.[59]

The obligatory change of environment at birth necessitates adjustment to the extrauterine environment so that the newborn experiences a complex series of biologic, physiologic, and metabolic changes. These changes are essential for survival. Every infant must complete this process of transition successfully to survive in the extrauterine environment. For a small percentage of newborns, transition is never achieved; for a slightly larger number, transition is delayed or complicated. For most newborns, transition is so smooth it appears uneventful.

With the first breath of life and the cutting of the umbilical cord, all neonates begin the transition from intrauterine to extrauterine life. Three major changes take place at birth. First, fluid in the alveoli is reabsorbed and air fills the alveoli, allowing for gas to diffuse into and out of the pulmonary blood vessels. Second, because the umbilical arteries and vein are clamped, the low-resistance placental circuit is gone and systemic blood pressure increases. Third, pulmonary vascular resistance is decreased as a result of mechanical distention of the alveoli and increased oxygen content in the alveoli. Oxygen is a potent pulmonary vasodilator.

During the first few hours after birth, the normal newborn progresses through a fairly predictable sequence of events, recovering from the stress of birth and adapting to extrauterine life. Intrapartum and immediate neonatal events result in sympathetic discharges reflected in changes in heart rate, color, respiration, motor activity, gastrointestinal function, and temperature. Awake and sleep states affect a neonate's behavior and ability to respond to the environment. A newborn may go from one state to another quite frequently in the nursery and at home (see Critical Findings: Newborn States and Considerations for Caregiving in Chapter 13). Figure 5-1 shows the classic description by Desmond of the transitional period, which includes the three stages shown in Box 5-1. Failure to establish this pattern of transition requires careful observation and investigation.

Management of the Newborn during Transition

Traditionally, care in "normal newborn" nurseries was based on the optimistic assumption that most

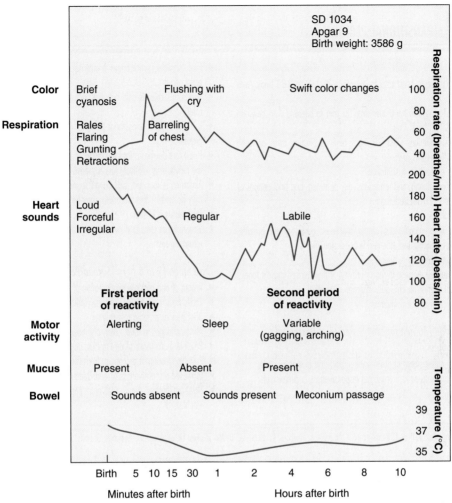

FIGURE 5-1 Critical findings: Neonatal transitional period. (From Desmond MM, Rudolph AJ, Phitaksphraiwan P, et al: The transitional care nursery: a mechanism for preventive medicine in the newborn, *Pediatr Clin North Am* 13:651, 1966.)

newborns have no difficulty with transition after birth and that term infants, in particular, do exceedingly well. With this philosophy, nursery care was geared toward the 85% to 90% of newborns who do well rather than the 10% to 15% with transitional complications.[59] Modern nursery care recognizes the complexity of transitioning to extrauterine life and the reality of serious disease even in term newborns.

NEWBORN SHOULD BE TREATED AS A RECOVERY PATIENT

During the immediate neonatal period, an "intensive care" concept has been introduced into care of the newly born. All newborns are to be cared for, regarded, and observed as recovering patients until they have successfully completed a smooth transition.

SKILLED PROVIDERS SHOULD CARE FOR THE NEWBORN

Current standards of care[6] require skilled health care providers (24 hours/day) to care for newborns during the first minutes after birth (e.g., in the delivery room; birth center) and in the follow-up period (e.g., in the birth room; mother-baby area; newborn nursery).[59] All personnel caring for the newborn must be familiar with the transitional

BOX 5-1 | TRANSITIONAL PERIOD

First Stage (0 to 30 min) = First Period of Reactivity
- Rapid increase in heart rate to the range of 160 to 180 beats/min (0 to 15 min)
- Gradual decrease in heart rate over 30 min to baseline rate between 100 and 120 beats/min
- Irregular respirations (first 15 min), peak respiratory rates between 60 and 80 breaths/min
  - Rales present on auscultation
  - Grunting, flaring, and retractions may be noted, and brief periods of apnea (<10 sec in duration)
  - Plethora
  - Alert with spontaneous startle reactions, gustatory movements, tremors, crying, and side-to-side head movements
  - Decrease in body temperature
  - Generalized increase in motor activity, with increased muscle tone
  - Bowel sounds absent, and abdomen distended
  - Production of saliva minimal

Second Stage (30 min to 2 hr) = Period of Decreased Responsiveness
- Newborn either sleeps or has a marked decrease in motor activity
- Muscle tone returns to normal, but responsiveness is diminished

- Fast, shallow, synchronous breathing (60 breaths/min) without dyspnea occurs
- Newborn's color is pale but pink with excellent perfusion and capillary refill
- Increase in anterior-posterior diameter (barreling) of the chest is usually present
- Heart rate decreases into the range of 100 to 120 beats/min or lower; the newborn is relatively less responsive to external stimuli
- Abdomen is rounded, and bowel sounds are audible; peristaltic waves may be visible, and meconium may be passed
- Oral mucus is absent
- Spontaneous jerks and twitches are common, but the newborn quickly returns to rest

Third Stage (2 to 8 hr) = Second Period of Reactivity
- Return of and possible exaggeration of responsiveness
- Labile heart rate: periods of tachycardia
- Brief periods of rapid respirations
- Abrupt changes in tone, color, and bowel sounds
- Possible prominence of oral mucus; gagging and vomiting not unusual
- Possible clearing of meconium from the bowel
- Increased responsiveness to endogenous and exogenous stimuli
- Newborn hunger cues; quiet alert periods when maternal bonding is established

Modified from Hernandez JA, Thilo E: Routine care of the full-term newborn. In Osborn LC, DeWitt TG, First LR, et al, editors: *Pediatrics,* St Louis, 2005, Mosby.

changes after birth and deviations from normal transitional events. After a normal, low-risk pregnancy and birth, primary evaluation and care of the newborn must be provided by educated neonatal-perinatal nurses who consult advanced practice nurses and/or physician(s) when appropriate.[6,59]

STANDARDS FOR ROUTINE CARE AND PHYSIOLOGIC MONITORING DURING TRANSITION MUST BE MAINTAINED

Parent-infant bonding, skin-to-skin care, early breastfeeding, and careful neonatal monitoring during the transition period should be addressed in delivery/birth room and nursery routines. After birth, the stable, pink newborn whose Apgar score is greater than 7 at 5 minutes can be placed skin-to-skin with the mother[100] or wrapped in warm, dry blankets and given to the parents to hold. Early breastfeeding and skin-to-skin contact is acceptable if the

neonate is stable and continuous observation is provided. After birth, at 15-minute intervals, *every* newborn must be assessed for general condition, respiratory effort, color, muscle tone, and temperature; all assessments must be documented.[59]

Routine care in Table 5-1 includes glucose screening, eye prophylaxis, and administration of vitamin K_1, which can be done at the mother's bedside. By 30 minutes of age, *every* newborn, regardless of where the baby is being cared for, must be examined by a neonatal-perinatal nurse. During the first 6 hours after birth, heart rate, respirations, blood pressure, degree of alertness, and color of skin and mucous membranes should be assessed frequently and the findings recorded. This period is when clinical signs of the most threatening infections, cardiopulmonary diseases, and major congenital abnormalities appear. Table 5-2 presents a useful scoring system for assessing the

TABLE 5-1 ROUTINE CARE DURING TRANSITION

ROUTINE CARE	TIME	DRUG/DOSE	COMMENTS
Glucose screening (see Chapter 15)	At 30-60 minutes of age	By POC glucometer device	Abnormal screen: glucose <40 mg/dl
Eye prophylaxis	Within 1 hour of age	Erythromycin (0.5%) or tetracycline (1%) eye ointment: apply ribbon in each conjunctival sac	Eye prophylaxis for ophthalmia neonatorum. Bactericidal effect depends on tissue concentration of drug and microorganisms.
Vitamin K_1	Within 1 hour of age	0.5-1 mg IM as a single dose for infants <1.5 kg or >1.5 kg *or*	Prophylaxis for hemorrhagic disease of the newborn. Vitamin K concentrations are physiologically low in breast milk so that exclusively breastfed infants are at increased risk for vitamin K deficiency, as are infants with fat malabsorption (e.g., biliary atresia, cystic fibrosis, alpha$_1$-antitrypsin deficiency) and prolonged treatment with antibiotics. Use sucrose, breastfeeding, kangaroo care,[69] and topical analgesia for pain relief during injections.
		2 mg PO	Repeated oral dosing (e.g., first feed, 1 week, 4 weeks, 8 weeks) is necessary; increased risk for late-onset hemorrhagic disease when infant receives only one dose. Oral intake is contraindicated in preterms, sick infants with diarrhea or cholestasis, or receiving antibiotics.

IM, Intramuscular; *PO*, orally; *POC*, point-of-care.
*Routine care is required wherever (e.g., labor-delivery-recovery; labor-delivery-recovery-postpartum; birth center; mother-baby unit; nursery) the newly born infant is cared for after birth.
Modified from Hernandez JA, Thilo E: Routine care of the full-term newborn. In Osborn LC, DeWitt TG, First LR, et al, editors: *Pediatrics*, St Louis, 2005, Mosby.

TABLE 5-2 CLINICAL RESPIRATORY DISTRESS SCORING SYSTEM*

	0	1	2
Respiratory rate (breaths/min)	60	60-80	>80 or apneic episode
Cyanosis	None	In room air	In 40% F_{IO_2}
Retractions	None	Mild	Moderate to severe
Grunting	None	Audible with stethoscope	Audible without stethoscope
Air entry[†]	Clear	Delayed or decreased	Barely audible

F_{IO_2}, Fraction of inspired oxygen; *RDS*, respiratory distress syndrome.
*The respiratory distress syndrome score is the sum of the individual scores for each of the five observations.
[†]Air entry represents the quality of inspiratory breath sounds as heard in the midaxillary line.
From Downes JJ, Vidyasager DD, Boggs TR, et al: Respiratory distress syndrome in newborn infants: I. New clinical scoring system (RDS score) with acid-base and blood-gas correlates, *Clin Pediatr* 9:325, 1970.

TABLE 5-3	MATERNAL, OBSTETRIC, NEONATAL CONDITIONS THAT INCREASE THE RISK OF ABNORMAL TRANSITION
Maternal Factors	Chronic hypertension
	Preeclampsia
	Diabetes mellitus
	Renal disease
	Infection
	Abuse of tobacco, alcohol, or illicit drugs
	Collagen vascular diseases
	Hemizygous hemoglobinopathies
	Certain maternal medications
Obstetric Factors	Rh or other isoimmunization
	Fetal growth restriction
	Decreased fetal movements
	Multiple gestation
	Oligohydramnios or polyhydramnios
	Premature rupture of membranes
	Third-trimester bleeding
	Delivery by cesarean section
Neonatal Factors	Prematurity (<37 weeks)
	Postmaturity (>42 weeks)
	Small for gestational age
	Large for gestational age
	Infection
	Metabolic abnormalities
	Birth trauma
	Major malformations
	Anemia
	Apgar 0-4 at 1 minute or need for resuscitation at delivery

From Hernandez JA, Thilo E: Routine care of the full-term newborn. In Osborn LC, DeWitt TG, First LR, et al, editors: *Pediatrics,* St Louis, 2005, Mosby.

pattern of respirations for signs of respiratory distress; findings should be documented. The range of blood pressure in term infants during the first few hours of life is 65 to 95 mm Hg systolic and 30 to 60 mm Hg diastolic, with an average mean blood pressure of 50 to 55 mm Hg. The blood pressure value will steadily increase from birth over the transitional period.[59]

Abnormal Transition

Regardless of gestational age or route of delivery, the sequence of clinical behavior just described is common to all well newborns. Preterm infants may exhibit variations in the duration of the transitional phases—shorter phase 1 or longer phase 2—but the patterns are similar. Knowledge of the normal changes occurring during transition enables early recognition of a newborn who is not making a normal extrauterine adaptation.[59]

Failure to make a normal transition to extrauterine life may result from obstetric anesthesia or analgesia, neonatal illness, or stress such as perinatal asphyxia and its sequelae. If the infant's pulse, respirations, color, and activity have not stabilized within the normal ranges *after 1 hour of life,* a problem should be suspected and investigated.

Observation for risk factors for abnormal transition is essential. A variety of conditions may result in significant deviation from the normal sequence of events during transition. Table 5-3 lists factors that may alter the sequence or pattern of changes expected to occur after birth and that result in either a healthy newborn or a newborn with significant illness. The health care provider's challenge is to discriminate between signs of diseases that produce an ill newborn from the dynamic, rapidly changing features that accompany the physiologic adjustments of normal or altered transition but that still result in a healthy neonate.[59] Box 5-2 lists clinical manifestations of abnormal transition.

PHYSICAL ASSESSMENT OF THE NEWBORN

Data Collection

HISTORY

Good perinatal care requires the identification of social, demographic, and medical-obstetric risk factors that correlate with fetal outcome. This must be an ongoing process, because high-risk patients may be identified on the first prenatal visit, during follow-up prenatal visits, or not until the intrapartum and postpartum periods. Review of the perinatal history is important in determining significant factors for neonatal health management. Identification of an at-risk maternal situation is essential to plan and organize care for an at-risk neonate. Review of the perinatal history includes antepartum and intrapartum events (see Chapter 2) and early neonatal events, both in the delivery room and during transition.

B O X 5-2	NEONATAL CLINICAL MANIFESTATIONS SIGNALING ABNORMAL TRANSITION

- Persistent tachypnea, flaring, grunting, and retractions (respiratory score >4; duration >first hour of life); fixed bradycardia
- Diffuse and persistent rales, retractions, flaring, and grunting (respiratory score >4; duration >first hour of life)
- Persistent cyanosis (persistent oxygen saturation <90% in room air) and prolonged requirements for supplemental oxygen (after 2 to 3 hr of age)
- Episodes of prolonged apnea (>20 sec) and bradycardia (<80 beats/min)
- Marked pallor or ruddiness
- Temperature instability, persistently (after 2 to 3 hr of age) low temperature (<36.5° C)
- Poor capillary filling (>3 sec) and blood pressure instability
- Unusual neurologic behavior (lethargy, decreased activity with marked and persistent hypotonia, irritability, excessive tremors and jitteriness)
- Excessive oral secretions, drooling, and choking/coughing spells, cyanosis

Modified from Hernandez JA, Thilo E: Routine care of the full-term newborn. In Osborn LC, DeWitt TG, First LR, et al, editors: *Pediatrics,* St Louis, 2005, Mosby.

SIGNS AND SYMPTOMS

Unlike the verbalizing adult patient, the nonverbal neonate communicates needs primarily by behavior. Through objective observations and evaluations, the neonatal care provider interprets this behavior into information about the individual infant's condition. Initial newborn assessment includes the following:

- Assessment of gestational age and fetal growth
- Newborn classification and neonatal mortality and morbidity risk
- Physical and neurologic examination
- Assessment of neurobiologic development

Assessment of Gestational Age and Fetal Growth. Optimal management of the pregnant woman and her fetus is entirely dependent on an accurate knowledge of the age of the fetus. An assessment of gestational age should be done on *all* newborns to establish maturity and pattern of fetal growth at birth.[75]

Pattern of Fetal Growth. With the use of anthropometric measurements, including weight, length, and head circumference, together with gestational age, fetal growth standards have been determined for different reference populations from various locations. From these data, it is apparent that there are variations in "normal" weight at any given gestational age from one locale to another. This variation is related to a number of factors, including sex, race, socioeconomic class, and even altitude. The Colorado intrauterine growth curves presented by Lubchenco and colleagues in the 1960s (Figure 5-2) are unique in that each anthropometric measurement was related to gestational age. The graphic display of this relationship provides a useful and simple method for determining the appropriateness of growth with respect to gestational age. Since then, other fetal weight curves have been published.[70] Even though such curves differ in details, all demonstrate nearly linear growth between 20 and 38 weeks of gestation, with slowing thereafter. In 1967, Battaglia and Lubchenco[12] used the gestational age/birth weight relationship to categorize those infants whose birth weights were less than the 10th percentile as *small for gestational age (SGA)*, those weighing more than the 90th percentile as *large for gestational age (LGA)*, and the remaining 80% as *appropriate for gestational age (AGA)* (Figure 5-3).

Gestational Age. Gestational age can be assessed by obstetric methods and by pediatric methods. The obstetric method considers that the best guide to an infant's gestational age is an early ultrasound evaluation combined with information about the mother's last menstrual period (LMP). Dating gestation based on mother's LMP could be the most accurate method if the mother is sure of the dates of her last menstrual period (see Chapter 2). Early antenatal ultrasonography appears to have 95% confidence intervals of less than 7 days.[118] Ultrasonography is preferred because it confirms conception, assesses gestation, and evaluates fetal growth. This way of determining maturity will have already been performed by the time the newborn reaches the nursery. All newborn care providers should be familiar with these methods.

Pediatric methods of determining gestational age are based on physical characteristics and neurologic examination. Within 2 hours after birth, every newborn should have an assessment of gestational age by physical characteristics.[6] Physical criteria are used because they progress in an orderly fashion with increasing gestation. Neurologic criteria involve the assessment of posture, passive and active tone, reflexes, and righting reaction.

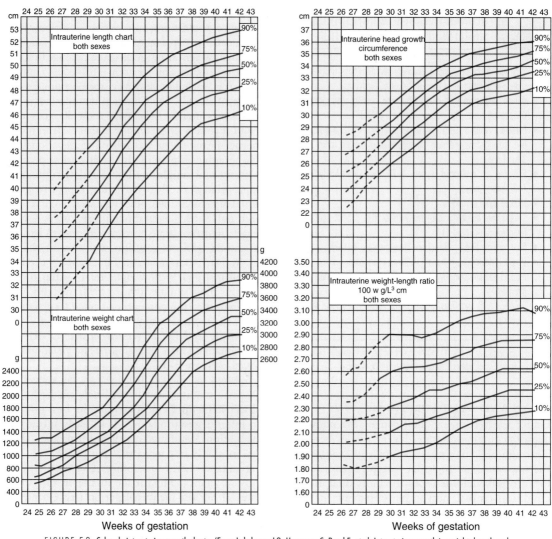

FIGURE 5-2 Colorado intrauterine growth charts. (From Lubchenco LO, Hansman C, Boyd E, et al: Intrauterine growth in weight, length and head circumference as estimated from live births at gestational ages from 26-43 weeks, *Pediatrics* 37:403, 1966.)

Numerous tables, charts, and graphs are available for determining gestational age.[9,24,40,99] Some tables are more subjective and laborious than others, and each has proponents and detractors. There is no perfect system and all require the examiner to be familiar with and have experience in their use. At least one form should be adopted and consistently used by each nursery.

Gestational age can be assessed most accurately by combining the physical criteria and the neurologic assessment. The revised Ballard system[9] displayed in Figure 5-4 is a combined scoring system. The Ballard incorporates physical maturity (six characteristics) and neuromuscular maturity (six criteria) on an equal basis, and includes assessment for extremely premature infants. The score for the neuromuscular and physical maturity is added and noted under the maturity rating column. Weeks of gestation are assigned according to the maturity rating score. This scoring system is easy to perform, accurate, and widely used in most nurseries.

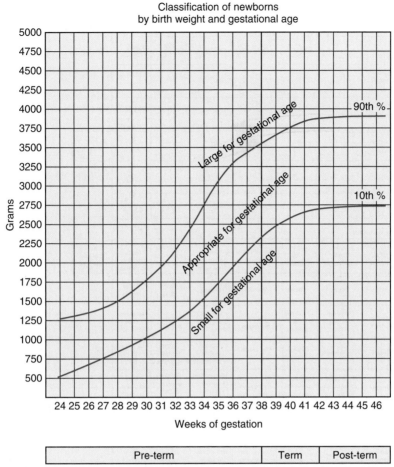

FIGURE 5-3 Classification of newborns by birth weight and gestational age. Birth weight of liveborn singleton white infants at gestational age from 24 to 42 weeks. (From Battaglia F, Lubchenco LO: A practical classification of newborn infants by weight and gestational age, *J Pediatr* 7:159, 1967.)

Assessment of Gestational Age in Very Low-Birth-Weight (VLBW) and Extremely Premature Infants. Accuracy in estimation of gestational age is important because, for VLBW and extremely premature infants, small differences in gestational age result in large differences in outcome and may be a criterion in decision making by parents and professionals as they decide whether comfort care or intensive care is used.[38] Research has shown that estimation of gestational age in very immature preterm infants is inaccurate. For preterm infants of 22 to 28 weeks of gestation, estimates of gestational age (by the scoring system shown in Figure 5-4) exceeded the gestational age (by dates) by 1.3 to 3.3 weeks.[38] These inaccuracies must be considered

in decision making, and better scoring systems are needed, particularly in the delivery room.

One quick and effective way to estimate gestational age in VLBW infants is by *measuring foot length*. Foot length of appropriate-for-gestational age preterm infants has been correlated with gestational age (Table 5-4). In short gestation (i.e., 24th to 34th week), there is a predictable increase in the mean foot length of 0.5 cm every 2 weeks. Measurement of foot length from the posterior prominence of the heel to the tip of the first (great) toe with a millimeter ruler is a rapid and simple method of assessing maturation of all newborns, even the very ill, VLBW, moderate intrauterine growth restriction infant. With this method, as with other physical

Neuromuscular maturity

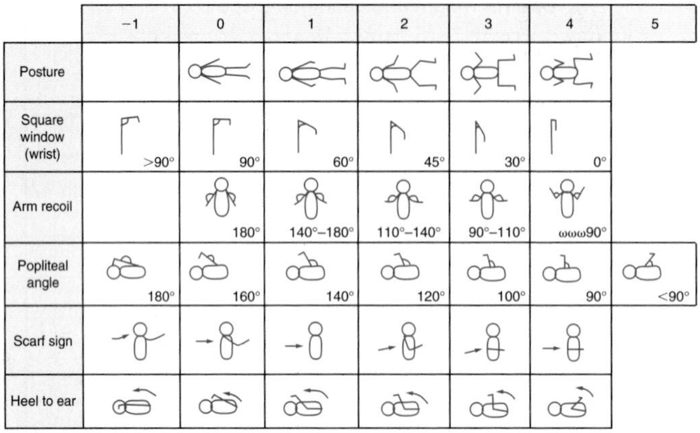

	−1	0	1	2	3	4	5
Posture							
Square window (wrist)	>90°	90°	60°	45°	30°	0°	
Arm recoil		180°	140°–180°	110°–140°	90°–110°	ωωω90°	
Popliteal angle	180°	160°	140°	120°	100°	90°	<90°
Scarf sign							
Heel to ear							

Physical maturity

									Maturity rating	
									Score	Weeks
Skin	Sticky, friable, transparent	Gelatinous red, translucent	Smooth pink, visible veins	Superficial peeling and/or rash; few veins	Cracking pale areas, rare veins	Parchment deep, cracking, no vessels	Leathery, cracked, wrinkled		−10	20
Lanugo	None	Sparse	Abundant	Thinning	Bald areas	Mostly bald			−5	22
									0	24
Plantar surface	Heel-toe 40–50 mm: −1 <40 mm: −2	>50 mm no crease	Faint red marks	Anterior transverse crease only	Creases ant. 2/3	Creases over entire sole			5	26
									10	28
Breast	Imperceptible	Barely perceptible	Flat areola, no bud	Stippled areola 1–2 mm bud	Raised areola, 3–4 mm bud	Full areola, 5–10 mm bud			15	30
									20	32
Eye/ear	Lids fused loosely: −1 tightly: −2	Lids open; pinna flat, stays folded	Sl. curved pinna; soft, slow recoil	Well-curved pinna; soft but ready recoil	Formed and firm, instant recoil	Thick cartilage, ear stiff			25	34
									30	36
Genitals male	Scrotum flat, smooth	Scrotum empty, faint rugae	Testes in upper canal, rare rugae	Testes descending, few rugae	Testes down, good rugae	Testes pendulous, deep rugae			35	38
									40	40
Genitals female	Clitoris prominent, labia flat	Prominent clitoris, small labia minora	Prominent clitoris, enlarging minora	Majora and minora equally prominent	Majora large, minora small	Majora cover clitoris and minora			45	42
									50	44

FIGURE 5-4 Clinical estimation of gestational age. (From Ballard JL, Khoury JC, Wedig K, et al: New Ballard score, expanded to include extremely premature infants, *J Pediatr* 119:417, 1991.)

measurements of gestational age, one must consider the standard deviation in interpreting results.

SIGNS OF PHYSICAL MATURITY

To use these charts accurately, the examiner must assess the following physical characteristics[75,113]:

Vernix. At 20 to 24 weeks, vernix is produced by sebaceous glands. Note the amount and distribution of vernix on the baby's skin (best done in the delivery room). Vernix is high in fat content and protects the skin from the aqueous amniotic fluid and bacteria. At 36 weeks, the white, cheeselike material begins to decrease and disappears by 41 weeks.

Skin. In early gestation, the skin of the fetus is very transparent and veins are easily seen. As gestation progresses, the skin becomes tougher, thicker, and less transparent. By 37 weeks, very few vessels are visible. From 36 weeks to delivery, fat deposits begin to form and grow. In a postterm infant, desquamation will be prominent at the ankles, wrists, and possibly palms and soles. As gestation progresses, the loss of vernix and subcutaneous tissue causes wrinkling. Note skin turgor, color, texture, and the prominence of vessels, especially on the abdomen.

Lanugo. At 20 weeks, fine, downy hair (lanugo) appears over the entire body of the fetus. At 28 weeks,

TABLE 5-4	FOOT LENGTH BY GESTATIONAL AGE*				

| | | FOOT LENGTH (cm) | | | |
GESTATIONAL AGE (wk)	NO. OF INFANTS	MEAN	MEDIAN	SD	RANGE
24	6	4.22	4.1	0.17	3.8-4.4
25	12	4.5	4.5	0.08	4.4-4.6
26	16	4.72	4.7	0.07	4.65-4.9
27	19	4.99	5.0	0.14	4.8-5.2
28	18	5.23	5.2	0.13	5.0-5.5
29	22	5.47	5.4	0.129	5.3-5.7
30	27	5.75	5.75	0.23	5.6-6.2
31	24	5.95	6.0	0.19	5.7-6.23
32	21	6.22	6.2	0.13	6.0-6.4
33	25	6.5	6.5	0.26	6.3-6.9
34	24	6.77	6.8	0.20	6.5-7.1
35	20	7.1	7.0	0.15	6.8-7.3
36	22	7.27	7.27	0.21	7.0-7.6
37	24	7.51	7.5	0.24	7.4-8.0
38	40	7.92	8.0	0.23	7.6-8.3
39	42	8.22	8.3	0.32	7.9-8.6
40	56	8.6	8.7	0.37	8.2-8.9
41	22	8.75	8.9	0.30	8.3-9.1
42	12	9.1	9.2	0.33	8.7-9.3
43	8	9.27	9.3	0.25	8.9-9.6

SD, Standard deviation.
*Applies to both male and female infants.
From Hernandez JA, Lazarte R, Pisano D, et al: Foot length and gestational age in the very-low-birth-weight infant, *The Children's Hospital Pediatric Update,* September 1987, p. 4.

it begins to disappear around the face and anterior trunk. At term, a few patches of lanugo may still be present over the shoulders. Note the distribution of lanugo, first on the face and anterior trunk and then on the rest of the body.

Hair on the Head. Hair appears on the head at 20 weeks. At 20 to 23 weeks, the eyelashes and eyebrows develop. From 28 to 36 weeks, the hair is fine and woolly and sticks together. It appears disheveled and sticks out in bunches from the head. At term, the hair lies flat on the head, it feels silky, and single strands are identifiable. Note the quality and distribution of the hair, and feel its texture. Scalp hair abnormalities (e.g., growth pattern, hypopigmentation, quantity, distribution, texture) may be external markers of genetic, metabolic, and neurologic disorders.

Sole Creases. Sole creases develop from toe to heel, progressing with gestational age. An infant with intrauterine growth restriction and early loss of vernix may have more sole creases than expected. By 12 hours after birth, the skin has dried to a point that sole creases are no longer a valid indicator of gestational age. Note the development of sole creases as they progress from the superior to inferior aspects of the foot (Figure 5-5).

Eyes. In the third month of fetal life, the eyelids fuse; they reopen between 26 and 30 weeks. In neonates of 27 to 34 weeks' gestation, examination of the anterior vascular capsule of the lens is useful in assessing gestational age. Gestational age is determined by assessing the level of remaining embryonic vessels on the lens (Figure 5-6). Before 27 weeks, the hazy cornea prevents visualization of the vascular system. After 34 weeks, only remnants of the vascular system are visible. Because rapid atrophy occurs in the vascular system, an ophthalmoscopic examination should be performed during the first physical examination or within 24 to 48 hours after birth.

Ears. Before 34 weeks, the pinna of the ear is a slightly formed, cartilage-free double thickness of skin. When it is folded, it remains folded. As gestation progresses, the pinna develops more cartilage, resulting in better form, so that it recoils when folded (Figure 5-7). Check ear recoil by folding the ear in half or into a three-corner-hat shape. Consistently folding it the same way helps the care provider develop a baseline for judging maturity. Note the form and cartilage development of the ear. Examine both ears to be sure they are the same and without defects.

Breast Development. Breast development is the result of the growth of glandular tissue related to high maternal estrogen levels and fat deposition. The

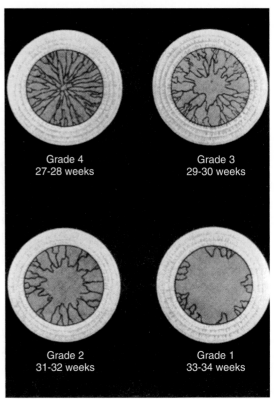

Grade 4
27-28 weeks

Grade 3
29-30 weeks

Grade 2
31-32 weeks

Grade 1
33-34 weeks

FIGURE 5-6 Anterior vascular capsule and gestational age. (From Hittner H, Hirsch NJ, Rudolph AJ: Assessment of gestational age by examination of the anterior vascular capsule of the lens, *J Pediatr* 91:455, 1977.)

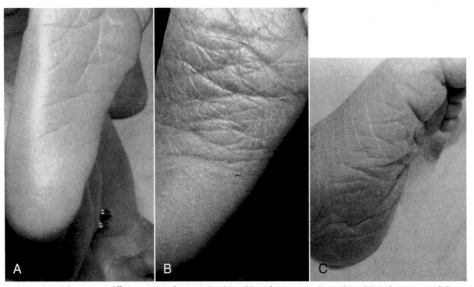

FIGURE 5-5 Sole creases at different gestational ages. **A,** Age 31 to 33 weeks' gestation. **B,** Age 34 to 38 weeks' gestation. **C,** Term.

areola is raised in an infant of 34 weeks' gestation. Note the size, shape, and placement of both breasts. Palpate the breast nodule and determine its size. If the infant is growth restricted, breast size may be less than expected at term.

Genitalia

Male Genitalia. At 28 weeks, the testes begin to descend from the abdomen. By 37 weeks, they are high in the scrotum. By 40 weeks, the testes are completely

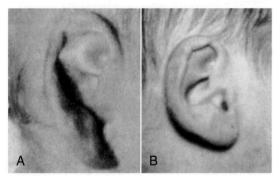

FIGURE 5-7 Ear form and gestational age. **A**, Age 34 to 38 weeks' gestation. **B**, Term.

descended and the scrotum is covered with rugae. As gestation progresses, the scrotum becomes more pendulous (Figure 5-8). Note the presence of rugae on the scrotum and its size in relation to the position of the testes. When examining the baby for descended testes, put the fingers of one hand over the inguinal canal to prevent the testes from ascending into the abdominal cavity and palpate the scrotal sac with the other hand.

Female Genitalia. Early in the female's gestation, the clitoris is prominent with small and widely separated labia. By 40 weeks, the fat deposits have increased in size so that the labia majora completely cover the labia minora (Figure 5-9). Note the labial development in relation to the prominence of the clitoris.

Newborn Classification and Neonatal Mortality and Morbidity Risks. At birth, after establishing fetal maturity and pattern of fetal growth, the next step is to ensure appropriate assignment of a clinical newborn classification, determine neonatal mortality risk, generate a problem list of potential morbidities, and quickly initiate appropriate screening procedures and/or interventions for recognized morbidities.

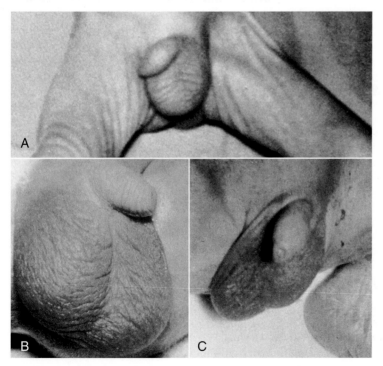

FIGURE 5-8 Male genitalia and gestational age. **A**, Age 28 to 35 weeks' gestation. **B**, Term. **C**, Age 42 or more weeks' gestation.

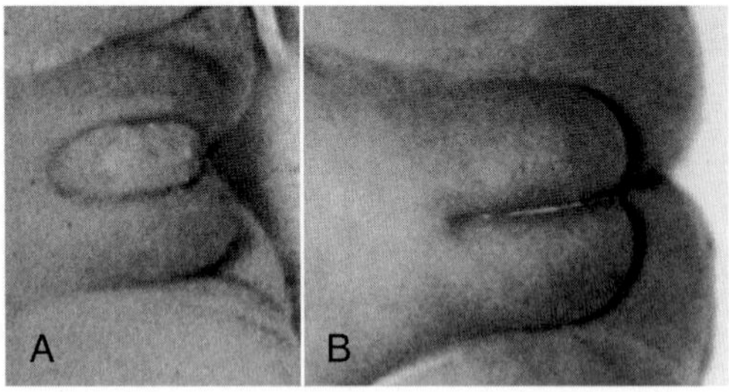

FIGURE 5-9 Female genitalia and gestational age. **A,** Age 30 to 36 weeks' gestation. **B,** Term.

Newborn Classification. The neonatal population can be classified by the use of birth weight, gestational age, fetal growth pattern, and a combination of all of them into the following categories:

By Birth Weight

- Normal birth weight (NBW): 2501 to 3999 g
- Excessive birth weight (EBW): 4000 g and above
- Low birth weight (LBW): 2500 g or less, with the following subcategories: moderate low birth weight (MLBW): 1501 to 2499 g, very low birth weight (VLBW): 1500 g or less, and extremely low birth weight (ELBW): 1000 g or less

By Gestational Age

- Full-term (FT): 37 to 41$^{6}/_{7}$ weeks (259 to 293 days)
- Postterm (PoT): 42 or more weeks (294 or more days)
- Preterm (PT)[43]: Less than 37 weeks (36$^{6}/_{7}$ weeks or less than 259 days), with the following subcategories: late preterm (LPT): 34$^{0}/_{7}$ to 36$^{6}/_{7}$ weeks (238 to 259 days), moderate-severe preterm (MSPT): 28 to 33$^{6}/_{7}$ weeks (196 to 237 days), and extreme preterm (EPT): 27$^{6}/_{7}$ or less weeks (less than 196 days)

By Fetal Growth Pattern. Using the intrauterine growth chart for the 10th and 90th percentiles, newborns can be classified as follows: those below the 10th percentile, *small-for-gestational-age (SGA)* infants; those between the 10th and 90th percentiles, *appropriate-for-gestational-age (AGA)* infants; and those above the 90th percentile, *large-for-gestational-age (LGA)* infants.[12]

By combining gestational age in weeks, birth weight in grams, and intrauterine growth pattern, nine categories of newborns were thus established (see Figure 5-3). This type of classification allows clinicians to anticipate likely problems in the immediate neonatal period and potential morbidities in the long term.

Neonatal Mortality Risk. As the result of significant advances in obstetrics and perinatal-neonatal care during the past 5 decades we have witnessed a remarkable decline in the rate of neonatal mortality (see Chapter 2). Although birth weight is considered to be the best predictor of neonatal survival, with exponential improvement evident with the achievement of optimum birth weight, it is apparent that neonatal mortality risk could be predicted more accurately for any individual infant based on the relation of two factors: birth weight and gestational age.[12,68]

Neonatal mortality risk (NMR), the chance of dying in the neonatal period, can be determined from mortality graphs based on birth weight (BW) and gestational age (GA), such as that shown in Figure 5-10. This figure was constructed based on the Lubchenco Perinatal Database, University of Colorado Hospital, 1980 to 1992. Mortality was calculated for each 100 g/1 week BW/GA block. On the chart, the area of least risk is the FT-AGA infant. Deviations from this area of least risk in relation to either weight or gestational age increase the newborn's mortality risk. Further examination of NMR in Figure 5-10 reveals that two infants with the same birth weight but with different gestational ages may have very different risks for death. For example, infant A may have a birth weight of 2000 g and a gestational age of 33 weeks, and shows an NMR of 2%. Infant B, on the other hand, may also weigh 2000 g but have a gestational age of 39 weeks, and shows an NMR of 0.2%. Infant A thus has a mortality risk 10 times greater than that of infant B, even though they have the same birth weight.

Mortality risk has changed over time because an increasingly physiologic basis of care has been used, coupled with sophisticated professional care, improved technology, new treatment modalities, transport systems, and aggressive management to handle increasingly at-risk populations. Consequently, these neonatal mortality risks need to be reviewed periodically.

Within the National Institutes of Child Health and Human Development (NICHD) Neonatal Research Network, mortality rates for newborns weighing 501 to 1500 g decreased from 23% (1987-1988), to 17% (1993-1994), to 14% (1999-2000). However, within each birth weight category, survival

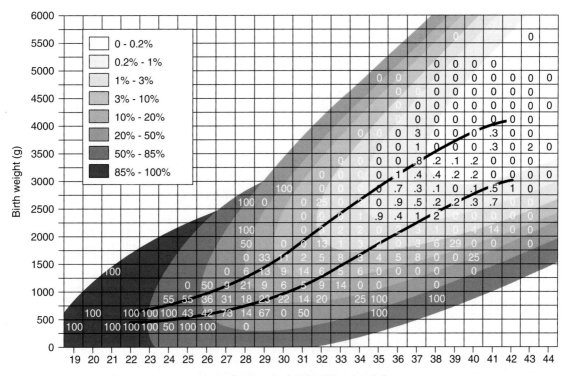

FIGURE 5-10 Neonatal mortality risk by birth weight and gestational age. (From Johnson JL, Merenstein G, Coll J, et al: Colorado intrauterine growth curve, 1980-1992: the new Lubchenco growth curve, *Pediatr Res* 35:274A, 1994.)

free of major morbidity (e.g., chronic lung disease/bronchopulmonary dysplasia, necrotizing enterocolitis, grade 3 or 4 intraventricular hemorrhage) did not change significantly. Because mortality (and morbidity) rates are highest in infants of the lowest birth weights and gestational ages, VLBW and extremely low-birth-weight (ELBW) infants would have better outcomes when they are born in a facility that can provide the appropriate subspecialty care.[16,29,119] These research findings have prompted recommendations that high-risk mothers/infants (e.g., less than 32 weeks of gestational age) be delivered/born in a facility capable of providing the anticipated appropriate level of perinatal/neonatal care.[6]

Neonatal Morbidity Risk. Neonatal morbidity risk (Figure 5-11) is determined by deviations of intrauterine growth and newborn classification. Classification of the newborn assists in identification, observation, screening, and treatment of the

most commonly occurring problems. For every newborn, formulate a problem list based on the morbidities common to the newborn classification. Observe, screen, intervene, and refer as necessary to prevent complications.

SGA/IUGR infants are at increased risk for morbidities (e.g., perinatal depression, hypothermia, hypoglycemia, polycythemia, infection) immediately after birth. There is also an association between size at birth, altered physiologic development, and long-term developmental and health problems (especially heart disease and stroke).[33]

LATE-PRETERM INFANT

In the United States, as a result of shifting distribution of gestational age among spontaneous live, singleton births, 39 weeks has become the most common length of gestation.[37] *Preterm infants are*

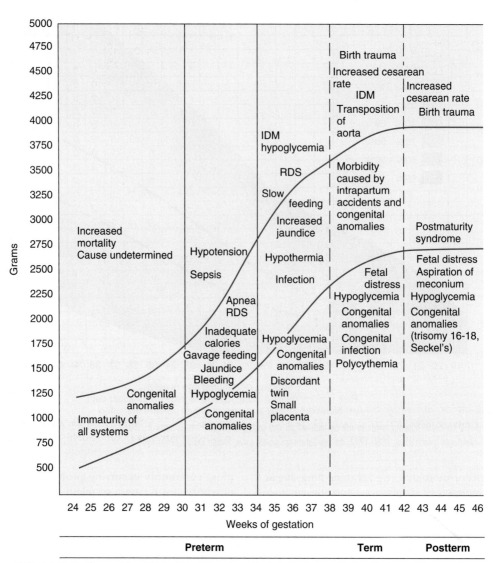

FIGURE 5-11 Specific neonatal morbidity by birth weight and gestational age based on statistics from Newborn and Premature Center at the University of Colorado Medical Center. *IDM,* Infant of diabetic mother; *RDS,* respiratory distress syndrome. (From Lubchenco LO: *The high-risk infant,* Philadelphia, 1976, Saunders.)

infants born before 37 completed weeks of gestation (259th day). *Late-preterm infants* refer to infants born between 34 completed (34⅐ weeks or day 239) and less than 37 completed weeks (36⅐ weeks or day 259).[43] In 2011, the prematurity rate in the United States was 11.7%,[80] and two thirds (8.1%) of these were due to "late-preterm" births. Studies have shown that 70% of all singleton preterm births are 34 to 36 weeks of gestation and

that 36 completed weeks of gestation accounts for 40.1% of all singleton preterm births.[37,81] Because these infants are at increased risk for health and developmental problems, this trend has been considered a growing public health concern.[61]

Historically, infants of 34 to 38 weeks of gestational age have been considered "slightly preterm" or "borderline premature." In the early 1990s, the terminology *near-term* began to be used in the literature. These near-term infants not only were cared for in special care nurseries but also were found in normal newborn nurseries, mother-baby care, and labor/delivery/recovery/postpartum (LDR/LDRP),[51] because they were considered to be "functionally full-term infants."[11]

In 2005 at a National Institutes of Health (NIH) meeting,[94] a proposal was made to use the term *late-preterm* rather than *near-term* to reflect the increased morbidity (and mortality) rates of this group of biologically and physiologically immature neonates.[41] These infants are larger than the usual premature infants, and they are generally "passed off" as mature infants, but they often manifest signs of physiologic immaturity in the neonatal period.

Morbidity and Mortality Outcomes in Late-Preterm Infants

Numerous studies have documented the high incidence of neonatal complications leading to neonatal intensive care unit (NICU) admission (30% to 59%) of late-preterm infants.* In addition, a multicenter study found that 10% of late preterms admitted to mother-baby units required transfer to a higher level of care.[58,84] Table 5-5 shows a list of the most frequently encountered complications in late-preterm infants. These infants have a higher incidence of respiratory complications, such us transient tachypnea of the newborn, respiratory distress syndrome, persistent pulmonary hypertension of the newborn, respiratory failure, and respiratory depression.[32,63,117] In addition they appear to have more episodes of apnea, jaundice (see Chapter 21), temperature regulation problems, hypoglycemia, sepsis, and feeding difficulties than term infants.[11,15,46,50,78] The incidence of these morbidities increases with decreasing gestational age. Some of the respiratory morbidities reported in late-preterm infants are consistent with other studies of elective cesarean section deliveres.[42,57,77]

Recent studies on clinical outcomes in late-preterm infants had 4.4 times the respiratory morbidity and 5.5 times the neonatal infection rate than term infants. They also had more clinical problems, longer lengths of stay, more health care visits with primary providers and specialists, and higher costs compared with full-term newborns.[11,15,42,63,117] In addition, research shows that late-preterm infants have more bronchopulmonary

---

* References 27, 32, 46, 63, 79, 103.

TABLE 5-5	MORBIDITIES IN LATE-PRETERM VERSUS TERM INFANTS			
	WANG et al (2004) FREQUENCY		LEONE et al (2010) FREQUENCY	
MORBIDITY	LATE PRETERM	FULL TERM	LATE PRETERM	FULL TERM
Temperature instability	10%	0%	2.5%	0.6%
Hypoglycemia	15.6%	5.3%	14.3%	0.6%
Respiratory distress	28.9%	5.3%	34.7%	4.6%
Apnea/bradycardia	4.4%	0%		
Jaundice/ hyperbilirubinemia	54.4%	37.9%	47.7%	3.4%
Sepsis evaluation	36.7%	12.6%		
Poor feeding	76%	28.6%		
Intravenous infusions	26.7%	5.3%		

Data from Wang M, Dorer D, Fleming M, et al: Clinical outcomes of near-term infants, *Pediatrics* 114:372, 2004; Leone A, Ersfeld P, Adams M, et al: Neonatal mortality in singleton late preterm infants compared with full-term infants, *Acta Paediatr* 101:e-6, 2012.

dysplasia (BPD)/chronic lung disease (CLD), neurologic complications, poorer family functioning, childhood asthma, and rehospitalizations.[22,72,82,112,115]

Late-preterm infants not only have more morbidities but also have been shown to have *increased mortality risk*. A report from the Institute of Medicine in 2005 points out that whereas the mortality rates for full-term neonates were stable at 2.5 per 100,000 live births, the rate for moderately preterm neonates (32 to 36 weeks of gestation) rose from 8.9 to 9.2 per 100,000 live births from 2001 to 2002.[94] A more recent study compared overall and cause-specific mortality rates between singleton late-preterm and term infants.[112] This study concluded that late-preterm infants have higher mortality rates throughout infancy compared with term infants. Late-preterm infant mortality rates were threefold higher than those of term infants (7.9 versus 2.4 deaths per 1000 live births).[112] In the first month of life, when evaluating deaths in the early (1 to 6 days) and late (7 to 27 days) periods, mortality rates were six and three times higher, respectively, for the late-preterm infant. Postneonatal deaths were twice as high as term infants. During infancy, late-preterm infants were approximately four times more likely than term infants to die. In another study, neonatal mortality rates were significantly higher for late-preterm infants (1.1, 1.5, and 0.5 per 1000 live births at 34, 35, and 36 weeks, respectively) compared with 0.2 per 1000 live births at 39 weeks.[83]

Long-Term Outcomes

Even though it is well known that very preterm infants are at higher risk of psychomotor, behavioral, cognitive, and other developmental disabilities, few studies of long-term outcomes in late-preterm infants have been conducted. A large Swedish population-based study on 32,945 late-preterm infants followed through adulthood found a higher incidence of cerebral palsy (relative risk 2.7), mental retardation (relative risk 1.6), disorders of psychological development, behavior and emotional disturbances, and other major medical disabilities affecting work capacity.[92] Another study comparing learning difficulties among moderately preterm (i.e., 32 to 33 weeks), late-preterm (34 to 36 weeks), and full-term infants found that children born as late preterms scored lower on child assessment tests for reading (but not math) in kindergarten and first grade than full-term born children.[31] When teachers rated these same children, those born late preterm scored lower in reading in kindergarten, first grade, and fifth grade, as well as scoring lower in math assessments in kindergarten and first grade. Children born late preterm also showed an increased need for individualized educational programs.[31,74]

Two recent large reviews[10,92] comparing late-preterm with full-term infants found that the children and adults born late preterm fare worse than full-term born peers in cognitive function, school outcomes, behavior problems, psychiatric disorders, and subtle intellectual and neuropsychological deficits. These findings have been corroborated by recently published studies.[*] These retrospective reports in no way confirm causality. We need to recognize that outcomes are not only the result of physiologic immaturity, but also of the biological determinants of preterm birth interacting with gestational age.[18] Neurodevelopmental follow-up of late-preterm infants has been, until recently, a long neglected area of research. More research, including longitudinal, prospective studies, are needed to fully

---

[*]References 21, 89, 96, 101, 104, 106, 111, 116.

appreciate the impact of late-preterm birth, biologic determinants, and perinatal events on developmental and health outcomes in this population of at-risk infants.[18,102]

Clearly, late-preterm infants are not term infants and need close observation, a high level of suspicion, assessment, and timely intervention by all care providers. Regardless of the geographic location of the late-preterm infant, these immature infants require more nursing time and care than do full-term infants. If the level of care cannot be provided in the infant's current geographic area, these infants should be transferred to a higher-care unit (either within or outside the facility) as soon as possible. Association guidelines for care of late-preterm infants are listed in the Resources for Professionals section at the end of the chapter.

Physical and Neurologic Examination

The purpose of the physical examination is (1) to discover common variations of normal or obvious defects, (2) to quickly initiate intervention or referral for deviations from normal, and (3) to establish a database for serial observations and comparisons. The best data are obtained from the neonate when the physical examination is organized to limit stress, maximize interaction with the examiner, and not overwhelm the newborn. To maximize data and minimize stress, the physical examination should proceed in an orderly fashion from the least stressful to the more stressful aspects of the examination (Box 5-3).

When one appreciates how stressful it is to the newborn to be undressed, it becomes obvious that as much as possible should be done without exposing the infant. Warm hands and instruments are essential, and a warm environment helps. Before touching the infant or removing any covers, observe the face, head, and hands as they appear.

OBSERVATION

Observation of the neonate provides pertinent data without touching him or her. General condition, anomalies, resting posture, and respirations should be observed.

General Condition. The general condition of the infant should be assessed by noting the color, activity, and neonatal state.

BOX 5-3

CRITICAL FINDINGS
PHYSICAL EXAMINATION OF THE NEWBORN

I. Observation Examination

A. General condition
   1. Color
   2. Activity and neonatal state
B. Crying
C. Anomalies
D. Resting posture
E. Respirations

II. Quiet Examination

A. Auscultation
   1. Heart
   2. Lungs
   3. Abdomen
B. Palpation
   1. Fontanels
   2. Abdomen
C. Inspection
   1. Eyes
   2. Blood pressure

III. Head-to-Toe Examination

A. Skin
B. Head
   1. Ears
   2. Nose
   3. Mouth
C. Thorax
   1. Breast
   2. Clavicles
D. Genitalia
E. Rectum
F. Back
G. Extremities
   1. Upper
   2. Lower

Color. The color of the newborn is normally pink. Acrocyanosis, or peripheral cyanosis of the hands and feet, is commonly present in the first 24 hours of life and may be the result of immature circulation or cold stress. Ecchymotic areas, especially on the presenting part, are common; however, they may be confused with cyanosis. To differentiate the two, apply pressure to the area. An ecchymotic area remains blue with pressure, whereas a cyanotic area will blanch.

General cyanosis and central cyanosis of the lips, mouth, and mucous membranes may indicate central nervous system (CNS), heart, or lung disease. Jaundice appearing at birth or within the first 12 hours of life is abnormal. Physiologic jaundice appears after 24 hours, but jaundice may indicate other abnormalities. Pallor at or directly after birth is a sign of circulatory failure, anoxia, edema, or shock. Pallor of anoxia is associated with bradycardia and the pallor of anemia with tachycardia. Plethora, a beef-red color, may indicate polycythemia and is confirmed by hemoglobin and hematocrit determinations. However, lack of plethora does not rule out polycythemia or hyperviscosity.

Activity and Neonatal State. Activity and the neonatal state at the beginning of the examination and appropriate changes throughout the examination should be observed. If the infant is asleep, is it quiet or rapid-eye-movement (REM) sleep? Spontaneous, symmetric movements are normal. Tremors and twitching movements of short duration are normal in relation to states of coldness or startling. Good muscle tone is established with adequate oxygenation soon after birth.

Flaccidity, floppiness, or poor muscle tone should be noted. Spasticity, hyperactivity, opisthotonos, twitching, hypertonicity, tremors, or seizures may be indicative of CNS damage. Asymmetry may result from intrauterine pressure or birth trauma rather than a CNS insult. A lack of crying or evasive behavior in response to the manipulations of a physical examination is abnormal.

Crying. Attempts to calm and console a crying infant during this part of the examination assist in better data collection during the quiet examination. Crying is beneficial in (1) ductal closure and transition from fetal to neonatal cardiorespiratory status, (2) improving pulmonary capacity, (3) maintaining homeostasis, (4) facilitating vocal tract development, and (5) cueing and care-eliciting behavior. Negative effects include (1) changes in cardiovascular (e.g., tachycardia, hypoxia, changes in cerebral blood flow, increases in the risk for brain injury and cardiac dysfunction)[76] and endocrine systems; (2) stress production and energy drainage[76]; and (3) strong, sometimes negative feelings in care providers.

Although uniquely individual, types of cries that reflect the infant's state and contextual basis have been identified as birth, distress call, hunger, pain, spontaneous, and pleasure.[30] At birth, the term neonate has a loud, lusty cry (a signal of robustness and wellness), whereas the preterm's cry may be weak or absent. Observe the infant's ability to quiet himself or herself when crying. High responsivity of the newborn to sustained handling, undressing, and being put down is associated with more infant crying.

A high-pitched cry suggests CNS irritation from increased intracranial pressure, injury, infection, or abnormality. *Weak crying,* no crying, or constant, irritable crying may indicate brain injury, infection, or abnormality. *Hoarse cries* or crowing inspirations result from laryngeal inflammation, injury, vocal cord dysfunction (e.g., paresis/paralysis), or anomalies. *A weak,* groaning cry or expiratory grunt is indicative of respiratory disease.

Anomalies. Obvious bodily malformations such as omphalocele, cleft lip and palate, imperforate anus, syndactyly, polydactyly, spina bifida, or myelomeningocele should be observed and recorded as anomalies. Odd facies or body appearances that are often associated with specific syndromes also should be noted.

Resting Posture. Resting posture should be observed while the infant is quiet and not disturbed. The infant's posture systematically develops according to gestational age: (1) from extension to flexion of the lower extremities, and (2) to flexion of the upper extremities. Asymmetry may result from intrauterine pressure or birth trauma. The infant may take a position of comfort assumed in utero.

Respirations. Respirations should be evaluated while the infant is at rest and before any manipulation. The normal rate is 30 to 60 breaths/min. Count the respiratory rate and rhythm, noticing the infant's use of accessory muscles. Respiration is normally abdominal or diaphragmatic.

After the first hour of life, a respiratory rate of more than 60 breaths/min indicates tachypnea. Tachypnea is the earliest sign of many neonatal respiratory, cardiac, metabolic, and infectious illnesses. Tachypnea, apnea, dyspnea, or cyanosis may indicate cardiorespiratory distress. Labored respirations include retractions, flaring

nares, and expiratory grunt. Maternal epidural analgesia with fentanyl has been shown to cause respiratory depression in neonates because fentanyl freely diffuses from the epidural space to maternal blood, equilibrating within 10 to 30 minutes and freely transporting across the placenta with slightly higher concentrations in the fetal compartment.[71] Neonatal respiratory depression secondary to fentanyl epidural analgesia is more common when mothers receive large amounts of fentanyl during labor; naloxone administration reverses the respiratory depression.[71]

If the infant is swaddled, the observation examination will not be as extensive as is possible when the infant is unclothed in an incubator or under a radiant warmer. If the infant is swaddled, unwrap gently so that observations of the thorax, abdomen, genitalia, and extremities may also be done during this phase of the examination.

Without touching the infant, one can rule out a multitude of conditions. In fact, more than 80% of the newborn examination is made through observation.

Quiet Examination. *Quiet examination* is defined as any part of the examination in which data are best collected from the quiet, cooperative newborn. The heart, lungs, head and neck, scalp and skull, abdomen, eyes, and blood pressure are areas that should be checked during the quiet examination. Using pacifiers, warming hands and stethoscopes, and holding and gently manipulating the infant are ways to avoid overwhelming the baby and to prevent crying.

AUSCULTATION

Heart. Auscultation of the heart, lungs, and abdomen is most effective when the infant is quiet. When the infant is quiet and at rest, auscultate the heart rate, rhythm, and regularity at the apex. The normal rate is 120 to 160 beats/min at a regular rhythm. Sinus dysrhythmia is normal and may be heard. The point of maximal intensity (PMI) of the neonatal heart is lateral to the midclavicular line at the third to fourth interspace. Note the PMI.

A rate of less than 80 beats/min is bradycardia. Newborns with persistent bradycardia may have complete heart block caused by maternal systemic lupus erythematosus (see Chapter 2). A rate greater than 160 beats/min is tachycardia, which may be associated with respiratory problems, anemia, or congestive heart failure when accompanied by cardiomegaly, hepatomegaly, and generalized edema.

Murmurs are noted for loudness, quality, location, and timing. They are best auscultated at the base of the third or fourth interspace. Heart murmurs in the newborn period are common, perhaps as frequent as 10% of the population (see Chapter 24). Note dextrocardia—heart sounds audible on the right side of the chest. Pneumothorax, pneumomediastinum, dextrocardia, and diaphragmatic hernia result in muffled heart sounds or a shift in PMI. To complete the cardiac assessment, careful attention to the femoral pulses is necessary; diminished femoral pulses suggest coarctation of the aorta (see Chapter 24). Often newborns with serious congenital heart disease do not present with clinical signs and symptoms of their anomaly. Use of pulse oximetry to screen all newborns after 24 hours of age and before discharge for critical congenital heart disease is discussed in Chapter 31.

Lungs. Normally, the lungs and chest are resonant after birth and fine rales may be present for the first few hours. Auscultation reveals bronchial breath sounds bilaterally. Air entry should be good, particularly in the midaxilla. A normal respiratory rate is 30 to 60 breaths/min.

Hyperresonance suggests pneumomediastinum, pneumothorax, or diaphragmatic hernia. *Decreased resonance* is a result of decreased aeration—atelectasis, pneumonia, or respiratory distress syndrome. Expiratory grunt suggests difficulty in aeration and oxygenation. Peristaltic sounds heard in the chest may be caused by a diaphragmatic hernia.

Abdomen. Bowel sounds are normally heard shortly after birth.

PALPATION
Palpation of the fontanels and abdomen is best accomplished before the infant begins crying, because guarded muscles and the normally tense fontanels of the crying infant give little useful data.

Scalp and Skull. Temporary deformation of the head is caused by pressures during labor and delivery. The head circumference measurements may be altered so that the occipitofrontal circumference on the first day of life may be smaller than on the second or third. Caput succedaneum is an edematous area over the presenting part of the scalp that extends across suture lines and resolves in 24 to 48 hours. A cephalhematoma is a soft mass of blood in the subperiosteal space on the surface of the skull bone. The blood mass does not extend across suture lines and resolves in 6 to 8 weeks.

Deviating from the normal, skull fractures may be linear or depressed, palpable or nonpalpable. Skull fractures are more common with forceps delivery. *Craniotabes,* softening of the skull bones, is caused by maternal vitamin D deficiency.[121]

The *anterior fontanel,* a diamond-shaped space normally measuring from 1 to 4 cm, may be gently palpated at the junction of the sagittal suture and coronal suture and between the two parietal bones. Normally the anterior fontanel softly pulsates with the infant's pulse, becomes slightly depressed when the infant sits upright and is quiet, and may bulge when the infant cries. Within 24 to 48 hours after birth, the initial molding of the head and overlap of the sutures resolve, resulting in a larger fontanel and in suture lines that should be palpated as depressions.

The *posterior fontanel,* formed at the juncture of the sagittal suture and the lambdoidal suture, is palpated between the occipital and parietal bones. Normally it is triangular shaped and barely admits a fingertip.

A *bulging, tense, or full fontanel* may be associated with increased intracranial pressure caused by birth injury, bleeding, infection, or hydrocephalus. A *depressed fontanel,* a very late sign in the newborn, may indicate dehydration. A *third fontanel,* located along the sagittal suture between the anterior and posterior fontanels, may be a sign of congenital infection or Down syndrome or may be a normal variant.

Sutures are palpable ridges between skull bones. The coronal suture is located between the frontal and two parietal bones. The sagittal suture intersects the two parietal bones, and the lambdoidal suture lies between the occipital and the two parietal bones. With increasing gestational age, the suture edges become firmer and with gentle palpation are felt as hard ridges. Sutures may be open to a varying degree or may be overlapped because of molding. Lack of normal expansion may indicate microcephaly or craniosynostosis. Abnormally rapid expansion indicates hydrocephalus or increased intracranial pressure.

Abdomen. The abdomen will appear slightly scaphoid at birth but will become distended as the bowel fills with air. Gentle palpation of the abdomen for organs or masses reveals that the spleen tip can be felt from the infant's left side and is sometimes 2 to 3 cm below the left costal margin. The liver is palpable 1 to 2 cm below the right costal margin. Superficial veins over the abdominal wall may be prominent.

A markedly scaphoid abdomen coupled with respiratory difficulty may indicate a diaphragmatic hernia. Abdominal distention and lack of bowel sounds may occur because of intestinal obstruction, paralytic ileus, ascites, imperforate anus, meconium plug, peritonitis, omphalocele, Hirschsprung's disease, or necrotizing enterocolitis. The infant should be observed for abdominal wall defects, such as umbilical hernia, omphalocele (a herniation into the base of the umbilical cord), and gastroschisis (a defect of the abdominal wall).

The umbilical cord may also be observed and inspected while the abdomen is being palpated. The diameter of the cord varies, depending on the amount of Wharton's jelly present. Two arteries and one vein are normally present in the umbilical cord. The umbilical cord begins to dry soon after birth, becomes loose from the skin by 4 to 5 days, and falls off by 7 to 10 days. Redness/umbilical erythema, foul odor, or wetness/oozing of the cord may indicate omphalitis. Persistent drainage may indicate a patent urachus, umbilical fistula, or cysts.

INSPECTION

Head and Neck. The head and neck of a newborn make up 25% of the total body surface. The head is usually 2 cm larger than a newborn's chest. Normal head circumference ranges between 32 and 38 cm for a FAGA infant. Note the size, shape, symmetry, and general appearance.

Microcephaly is characterized by a small head size in proportion to body size. *Craniosynostosis* is a small head size caused by early closure of sutures. *Hydrocephalus* is a condition in which an increase in cerebrospinal fluid creates an abnormally large and growing head.

Eyes. Inspection of an infant's eyes is best accomplished when the infant is found in the quiet alert state or when the infant has been aroused to wakefulness during the examination. The eyes cannot be observed while the baby is crying.

Tipping the baby backward and raising him or her slowly or shading the infant's eyes from bright light often causes the eyes to open.

The newborn's eyes open spontaneously, look toward a light source, fix, focus, and follow. Uncoordinated eye movements are common. Subconjunctival or scleral hemorrhages are a common result of the pressures of labor and birth. The size, shape, and structure of the eye should be noted.

The pupils of the normal newborn respond to light by constricting. *Red reflex* is normally present and indicates an intact lens. Tears are not normally produced until 2 months of age. The iris is usually dark blue until 3 to 6 months of age. Doll's eye maneuvers are normally associated with eyes that follow movement of the head, often with a lag and/or nystagmus.

Discharge from the eyes may represent irritation or infection. A lateral upward slope of the eyes with an epicanthal fold may indicate syndromes of mental, physical, or chromosomal aberrations. The absence of red reflex may indicate tumors or congenital cataracts accompanying rubella, galactosemia, or disorders of calcium metabolism. Chorioretinitis is often found in congenital viral diseases such as cytomegalovirus and toxoplasmosis. White speckles on the iris known as *Brushfield's spots* are associated with Down syndrome and developmental delay or are a normal variant. Scleral blueness is associated with osteogenesis imperfecta and scleral yellowness with jaundice. Brain injury may be indicated by a constricted pupil, unilaterally dilated fixed pupil, nystagmus, or strabismus.

Blood Pressure. Blood pressure (BP) with noninvasive Doppler devices is best determined (1) by using the appropriate-size cuff for upper and lower extremities (e.g., using the same size cuff for the leg pressure that was used for the arm pressure results in a falsely elevated leg pressure), (2) by obtaining the measurement when the infant is asleep or before the infant is upset, and (3) by using the mean BP to monitor changes.[36] BP increases in the first 24 hours of life, is higher in more mature infants (e.g., birth weight and gestational age) and in newborns whose mothers smoke,[55] and increases with increasing postnatal age.[35] The BP should be checked in all four extremities to screen for coarctation of the aorta. Because the BP proximal to the area of obstruction is higher than the BP distal to the area of obstruction, BP in the upper extremities is higher (more than 15 mm Hg higher) than in the lower extremities (Figures 5-12 and 5-13).

The only study to evaluate the efficacy of upper and lower extremity BP variations was conducted on 40 healthy neonates.[36] This study showed that with the current Doppler devices, normal neonates may have a wide variation in BPs between limbs. The researchers concluded that a difference of 20 mm Hg is more likely due to random variability than to coarctation and recommended that if weak/absent pulses are present and coarctation is suspected, an echocardiogram is necessary.[36]

Head-to-Toe Examination. The infant's crying will not affect the data to be gathered in the head-to-toe examination.

Skin. As each body part is examined, the skin is also inspected. *Vernix,* a white, cheeselike material that contains quantities of α-tocopherol and surfactant proteins that provide significant protection from infection, normally covers the body of the fetus and decreases with increased gestational age. Discoloration of the vernix occurs with intrauterine distress, postmaturity, hemolytic disease, and breech presentations.

The color of the skin is normally pink. *Mongolian spots* caused by the presence of pigmented cells may cover the sacral-gluteal areas of infants of color (e.g., black, Hispanic, Asian). The degree of generalized pigmentation varies and is less intense in the newborn period than later in life. *Nevus flammeus* may be present at the nape of the neck or on the eyelids.

Note the size, shape, color, and degree of ecchymosis, erythema, petechiae, or hemangiomas. Meconium staining, which occurs in 10% to 20% of newborns, is indicative of prior fetal distress. *Erythema toxicum* appears as a generalized red rash in the first 3 days of life. *Milia* caused by retained sebum are pinpoint white spots on the cheeks, chin, and bridge of the nose.

The normal texture of a neonate's skin is soft. A preterm infant's skin is more translucent than a term infant's skin. Slight desquamation may occur as skin becomes dry. Moderate to severe desquamation occurs in postterm infants with IUGR. Puffy, shiny skin is symptomatic of edema. Localized *edema* of a presenting part is caused by trauma and is only temporary. Edema

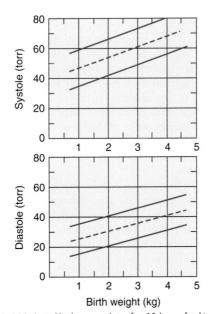

FIGURE 5-12 Aortic blood pressure during first 12 hours after birth. Linear regression *(broken lines)* and 95% confidence limits *(solid lines)* of systolic and diastolic blood pressures on birth weight in healthy newborn infants. (From Versmold HT, Kitterman JA, Phibbs RH, et al: Aortic blood pressure during the first 12 hours of life in infants with birth weight 610 to 4220 grams, *Pediatrics* 67:607, 1981.)

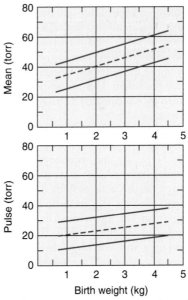

FIGURE 5-13 Mean aortic and pulse pressures during first 12 hours after birth. Linear regression *(broken lines)* and 95% confidence limits *(solid lines)* on birth weight in healthy newborn infants. (From Versmold HT, Kitterman JA, Phibbs RH, et al: Aortic blood pressure during the first 12 hours of life in infants with birth weight 610 to 4220 grams, *Pediatrics* 67:607, 1981.)

should be distinguished from increased subcutaneous fat. *Lanugo* coverage decreases with increasing gestational age.

Tissue turgor is the sensation of fullness derived from the presence of hydrated subcutaneous tissue and intrauterine nutrition. Test the elasticity of the skin by grasping a fold of skin between the thumb and forefinger. When released, the skin should promptly spring back to the surface of the body. A loss of normal skin turgor resulting in peaking of the skin is a late sign of dehydration. A generalized hardness of the skin is a sign of *sclerema* that occurs in debilitated, stressed infants.

Ears. Cartilage development and ear form progress according to gestational age. Observe the external ears for size, shape, and position. The angle of placement of the ears is almost vertical. If the angle of placement is greater than 10 degrees from vertical, it is abnormal. The level of placement is determined by drawing an imaginary line from the outer canthus of the eye to the occiput. If the ear intersects the line, it is placed normally. Slapping hands or other sharp noises will normally elicit a twitching in the eyelid or a complete Moro reflex.

Malformed or malpositioned (low-set or rotated) ears are often associated with renal and chromosomal abnormalities and other congenital anomalies. Abnormalities such as skin tags or sinuses may be associated with renal tract abnormalities or hearing loss. Forceps or difficult deliveries may injure the outer ear. Congenital deafness is suspected if the infant does not respond to noise. It is confirmed by standardized hearing screening tests and follow-up.

Nose. Note the shape and size of the nose. Deformities caused by intrauterine pressure may be temporary. Neonates are obligatory nasal breathers and must have patent nasal passages. Check the patency of the alae nasi by (1) obstructing one nostril, closing the mouth, and observing breathing from the open nostril; (2) placing a stethoscope under the nostrils that will "fog" the diaphragm and auscultate breathing; or (3) passing a soft catheter (if necessary).

Abnormal configuration may be associated with congenital syndromes. Obstructions can be caused by drugs, infections, tumors, nasal discharge, nasal cysts, and mucus. *Choanal atresia,* a membranous or bony obstruction in the nasal passage, may be unilateral or bilateral. Choanal atresia is characterized by the noisy breathing, cyanosis, and apnea of the quiet infant (mouth closed) as opposed to the pink color of the same crying infant (mouth open).

Mouth. The mouth may be examined here or at the end of the examination when the infant is crying loudly with a wide-open mouth. At birth, a normal infant can suck and swallow (this ability develops at 32 to 34 weeks' gestation) and root and gag (this ability develops at 36 weeks' gestation). Elicit each.

Lips and mucous membranes are normally pink. Observe the lips and mucous membranes for pallor and cyanosis. If the infant is well hydrated, the membranes should be moist. Open the mouth to look for anomalies. Palpate the hard and soft palates for a membranous cleft or submucous cleft. *Epithelial pearls* are common along the gum margins and the palate.

Natal teeth may be present and may require removal to prevent aspiration. A large tongue (macroglossia), cleft lip or palate (including submucous cleft), or high-arched palate may be associated with abnormal facies or be an isolated finding. If copious secretions or distress in feeding is present, it is often the result of esophageal atresia or tracheoesophageal fistula.

Thorax. Conformation of the newborn chest is cylindric with an anteroposterior ratio of 1:1. Note the shape, symmetry, position, and development of the thorax. *Asymmetry of the chest* may be caused by diaphragmatic hernia, paralysis of the diaphragm, pneumothorax, emphysema, pulmonary agenesis, or pneumonia. Fullness of the thorax caused by increased anteroposterior diameter occurs with an overexpansion of the lung. Retractions, an inward pull of the soft parts of the chest while inhaling, indicate air-entry interference or pulmonary disease.

Breasts. Breast tissue systematically develops according to gestational age. Enlargement of breasts because of maternal hormones occurs in either sex on the second or third day. Milky secretions may be present. Unilateral redness or firmness indicates infection.

Clavicles. Observe and palpate the area above each clavicle. A fracture of the clavicle is evidenced by a palpable mass, crepitation, tenderness at the fracture site, and limited arm movements on the affected side.

Genitalia. Male and female genitalia systematically develop according to gestational age. *Ambiguous genitalia* result from incomplete or altered differentiation and require urology consultation.

Male Genitalia. Inspect the genitalia for the presence and position of the urethral opening. Palpate the testes either in the inguinal canal or scrotum. The scrotum appears large and pendulous with the presence of descended testes. A tight prepuce may be found. In dark-skinned races, darker pigmentation of the genitalia is normal. *Hypospadias* exists if the urethral opening is on the ventral surface of the penis. *Epispadias* exists if the opening is on the dorsal surface. Inguinal or scrotal swelling, discoloration, palpable masses, and pain/tenderness with palpation may be an inguinal hernia, testicular torsion, trauma, tumor, or *hydrocele*—a collection of fluid in the scrotal sac.

Female Genitalia. Inspect the genitalia for the presence and position of the urethral opening. The introitus is posterior to the clitoris. A vaginal skin tag is a visible hymenal ring.

Edema of the genitalia in both sexes is common in breech deliveries. Note the presence of a hydrocele or hernia. Fecal urethral discharge may indicate rectourethral fistulas.

Rectum. Visualize and check the patency of the anal opening by waiting for meconium passage (it is optional to check patency by gently inserting a soft rubber catheter; do not use rigid objects such as glass rectal thermometers). Observe the anatomy, and feel the muscle tone. Meconium is normally present during the first days of life.

Imperforate anus, irritation, or fissures may be present. Meconium passage before birth suggests fetal intrauterine distress. Failure to pass meconium within 48 hours suggests obstruction. *Meconium ileus* is associated with cystic fibrosis.

Back. Place the infant in a prone position and observe for a flat and straight vertebral column. Separate the buttocks to observe the coccygeal area. To check incurving reflex, stroke one side of the vertebral column. The baby will turn the buttocks toward the side stroked. Deviations from normal include curvature of the vertebral column, pilonidal dimple, pilonidal sinus, spina bifida, or myelomeningocele. A study of spinal congenital dermal sinuses found an increased incidence (greater than 50%) of neurologic deficit, intradural tumors, or tethered cords; recommendations included a prompt radiologic evaluation and neurosurgical consultation so that timely intervention could preserve or improve neurologic function.[3]

Extremities

Upper Extremities. Note the size, shape, and symmetry of the arms and hands. Observe and feel for fractures, paralysis, and dislocations. Count and inspect the fingers. The hands are normally clenched into fists. The infant is capable of adduction, flexion, internal rotation, extension, and symmetry of movement. Note the tone of the muscles. Flexion develops with increasing gestational age.

Simian creases may indicate chromosomal abnormalities that are frequent causes of deformity. *Polydactyly and syndactyly* of the fingers may be found. *Osteogenesis imperfecta* is characterized by multiple fractures and deformities. *Palsies* caused by fractures, dislocations, or injury to the brachial plexus are recognized by limited movement of the extremity. *Fractures* may also be present with edema, palpable crepitus, or the "palpable spongy mass sign" over the clavicle.

Lower Extremities. Note the size, shape, and symmetry of the feet and legs. Note the normal position of flexion (develops according to gestational age) and abduction. Note symmetry of movement, thigh folds, and gluteal folds. A full range of motion is possible, including the "frog position"—a rotation of the thighs with the knees flexed. Observe and feel for fractures, paralysis, and dislocations. Palpate femoral pulses.

Polydactyly and syndactyly of the toes may exist. *Osteogenesis imperfecta,* a rare genetic defect of collagen production that results in brittle bones, manifests as multiple fractures and deformities. Paralysis of both legs is caused by severe trauma or congenital anomaly of the spinal cord. Unilateral or bilateral developmental dysplasia of the hip (e.g., congenital dislocated hip),[62] which is more common in females and breech presentations, causes a hip clunk when the baby's legs are abducted into the frog position. Although soft clicks are common, a sharp click indicates dislocation. Fractures may be present and are characterized by limited movement and edematous, crepitant areas. Chromosomal abnormalities are frequent causes of deformity.

Recoil is a test of flexion development and muscle tone. Recoil appears systematically as flexion first develops in the lower extremities and then in the upper extremities. Extend the legs and then release. Both legs should return promptly to the flexed position in accordance with the gestational age of the infant. Then extend the arms alongside the body. On release, prompt flexion should occur at the elbows.

NEUROLOGIC EXAMINATION[4,5,19,39,60]

The neurologic examination of the newborn is an integral part of the evaluation of the newborn infant. This evaluation often receives little attention and in too many instances the infant is dismissed from the nursery as "normal" when, in fact, little effort was expended to determine the baby's neurologic status. The evaluation and documentation of the development of the nervous system in the normal newborn should be of paramount interest to all the health care clinicians caring for the newborn. Fortunately, for the most part, some portions of the neurologic examination are carried out as a component of the general physical examination of the newborn *(activity, resting posture, symmetry, head size and morphology, rooting reflex, muscle tone, primitive reflexes, tremors and twitching, cry, recoil).* Performing a complete and thorough physical examination of the newly born is paramount.

Clinical, anatomic, and encephalographic studies of the nervous systems in full-term and premature neonates have confirmed the belief that the CNS of the human fetus matures at a fairly constant rate.[39] However, there are recognized limitations and challenges in performing an accurate neurologic evaluation. First, because a newborn is recovering from the stress of birth, the neurologic examination is not reliable until after the infant has successfully completed the transition to extrauterine life. Therefore, the neurologic examination should be performed after the first 12 to 24 hours of life. Second, if the infant was born by cesarean section, or is ill and requiring NICU care, the neurologic examination may not be accurate even after 24 hours. Third, newborns are born at different stages of brain development. Fourth, there are few tests that reflect the status of the cerebrum in the newborn. Nevertheless, in spite of these limitations, it is still possible with a systematic and detailed neurologic examination to obtain enough information to gain a basic understanding of many neurologic problems in the newborn (see Chapter 26).

Assessment of Gestational Age. It is important to remember that neurologic maturity and appropriate developmental milestones correlate with gestational age rather than birth weight. As previously discussed, for an accurate estimation of gestational age most clinicians favor systems that combine neurologic and physical signs of maturation. Each portion of the neurologic examination is objective and easy to perform, relying on muscle tone, posture, reflex movements, and degree of extremity flexion. The most commonly used neurologic signs for gestational age are posture, square window (wrist), arm/leg recoil, popliteal angle, scarf sign, heel to ear maneuver, head lag, ankle dorsiflexion, and ventral suspension.

Assessment of Neurologic Normality and Abnormality. The neurologic examination is most helpful if carried out systematically on an infant during quiet wakefulness between feedings, generally 1 hour before the next meal. The examiner should be especially observant of the general alertness, spontaneous activity, symmetry of posture and spontaneous movements, muscle tone and strength, head control, developmental reflexes, and responses to manipulation and handling.

- *State of alertness:* Alteration in level of consciousness is an extremely important sign in determination of the neurologic status of the newborn. A normal term infant shows a semiflexed posture and smooth spontaneous movements of all extremities. The hyperalert neonate has the appearance of increased vigilance with eyes wide open, often decreased blinking, overreaction to minimal stimulation, and reduced sleeping. Decreased state of alertness could be lethargy, stupor, and coma.
- *Posture:* Observation of posture is one of the first steps in the neurologic examination. Much can be predicted from the position of the limbs at rest. Term infants should have a preponderance of flexor tone during wakefulness and sleep with the normal semiflexed posture of the elbows and ankles. The hand position typically shows a partially closed fist. A tight cortical thumb can be normal, but when it is persistent and obligatory, it suggests a corticospinal abnormality. In prone position the pelvis is elevated by hip and knee flexion. Alterations of expected patterns of posture suggest neurologic abnormalities, which can be focal or generalized.
- *Tone:* Muscle tone is evaluated by resistance to passive movement. Pronounced hypotonia characterizes the premature infant below 29 weeks of gestation, and tone increases in a caudal-rostral direction over the ensuing weeks. There is an orderly progression from a limp "rag doll" at 28 weeks to the flexed "frog legs" posture at 34 weeks and the fully flexed supine posture at term. When evaluating tone in the newborn,

the head should be in the midline position in order to avoid eliciting a tonic neck response, and a comparison should be made between the two sides of the body and between the upper and lower extremities.

- *Neonatal hypotonia:* Term infants with decreased tone will show less flexor posture, less resistance to passive movements, and more head lag. The infant becomes limp and floppy, with little control. The most frequent etiology for hypotonia is generalized depression of the CNS. Other causes include neuromuscular disorders, CNS dysfunction, sepsis, and congenital and genetic disorders.
- *Neonatal hypertonia:* Although decreased tone in the newborn is obvious, at times the determination of increased tone can be more of a problem. Infants with increased tone will show extensor posturing of extremities in supine and prone positions. Extensor posturing of the legs with arms held tightly fisted against the midline points to hypertonicity. The most severe degrees of hypertonia lead to *opisthotonos.* Pronounced hypertonia is usually caused by many of the same conditions that can lead to hypotonia, but usually tends to point to more chronic or subacute conditions. Common etiologies include hypoxic–ischemic encephalopathy (HIE), sepsis and meningitis, congenital structural malformations of the brain, and intraventricular hemorrhage.
- *Developmental reflexes:* The developmental reflexes used to evaluate the newborn are best described as "primitive," because they do not require functional brain above the diencephalon and probably not above the mesencephalon. Many such reflexes have been described; however, it is unlikely that all can be elicited in an infant at any given time. It is better to use six to eight usually present in all newborns and to evaluate them consistently: *Moro's reflex, tonic neck reflex, stepping reflex, Galant reflex (truncal incurvation), palm and plantar grasp reflex,* and *Babinski's reflex.*

Reflexes are complex responses to specific stimulation, probably representing integration of the brainstem and spinal cord level. Asymmetries are always abnormal; these reflexes should never be mandatory or persistent, and a reduction or absence of all developmental reflexes may represent generalized depression of all cerebral activity from any cause such as infection, medications, hypoxemia, or metabolic diseases.

Because the responses vary with the state of alertness of the infant, and the newborn's tolerance for prolonged examination is limited, eliciting a perfect response to each maneuver should not be expected. When the examination is not fully reassuring, repeating selected parts of the examination at a later time may be more helpful in clarifying findings than attempting an extended examination at one time.

Assessment of Neurobehavioral Development

In addition to neurologic examination, the assessment of neurobehavioral development is an important step in the evaluation of the newborn infant. All newborns requiring intensive care, particularly preterm infants, are going to continue their development in extrauterine settings at a time when their brains are growing more rapidly than ever in their life span. Understanding the potential role of illnesses, therapeutic interventions, and NICU environment on their neurobehavioral development is paramount for the provision of quality newborn care during this highly vulnerable phase of brain development.

Caregivers need to become knowledgeable of the tools available for the assessment of the neurobehavioral development and the potential interventions. There are numerous tools for the assessment of neurobehavioral development.[5,17,73] Chapter 13 offers a detailed and comprehensive review of this subject.

THE BRAZELTON SCALE

The Neonatal Behavioral Assessment Scale (NBAS) is a comprehensive behavioral assessment of the newborn.[17] The NBAS psychological scale enables assessment of the infant's individual capabilities for social relationships. Clinical application of the Brazelton scale includes neonatal research and clinical evaluation of newborn infants after illness, prematurity, or maternal medications.

The NBAS focuses on an interactive approach and highly individualized parameters of newborn functioning. Later editions of the NBAS have added supplemental items, which further qualify the behavior of the newborn, particularly of preterm infants.

A modified version of the Brazelton examination is useful in teaching parents about their individual infant's patterns of behavior, temperament, and states. By understanding the uniqueness of their infant, parents may more intelligently assess and interpret their baby's cues for interaction and distance. If the parents know their infant's individual strengths and weaknesses, they will react more realistically to him or her. It is important for the provider to elicit the parents' assessment of their infant's behavior and responsiveness. Unrealistic expectations or incorrect parental perceptions may exist. This is an excellent opportunity for parent teaching, and possibly referral. The NBAS is distinguished from other programs in its use as an intervention with parents and medical staff. Employed in this manner, it is intended to improve and enhance the caregiver's attitude to and interaction with the infant.

The Brazelton examination is usually performed at 2 to 3 days of life, at discharge, or on the follow-up visit at 1 to 2 weeks. This examination assesses the infant's best performance in response to stimulation and handling by the examiner. For research purposes, the scoring technique by a certified examiner is required. For clinical use, knowledge of the specific techniques and interpretations of results is all that is required. Knowledge of the infant's state is necessary (see Chapter 13, Table 13-4). Performing the examination with the parents present provides the opportunity for teaching, parental participation, and observation of their infant's response.

Maternal use of antidepressants and smoking have been shown to alter the newborn's neurobehavioral examination.[91,98] Neonates exposed to selective serotonin reuptake inhibitors late in pregnancy exhibit the following mild and spontaneously resolving behaviors: tremors/tremulousness, restlessness/irritability, abnormal crying, rigidity, fewer state changes, and more active sleep with startles and arousal.[49]

CARE OF THE WELL NEWBORN INFANT

Mother-Infant Bonding and Interventions

FREQUENCY OF ASSESSMENTS

During the transitional period, vital signs should be recorded frequently enough to monitor the infant's condition and provide appropriate care:

- If the infant is distressed (elevated heart rate or respiratory rate, retracting and/or nasal flaring), vital signs may be required every 30 minutes.

- If the baby's vital signs are normal on admission (heart rate 120 to 160 beats/min, respiratory rate 30 to 60 breaths/min, and temperature 36° to 36.5° C), vital signs may be required every 30 to 45 minutes until the infant's condition has remained stable for 2 to 4 hours.
- Vital signs should be recorded at least once every 8 hours.
- Measuring the temperature rectally is *contraindicated* in newborns because of the risk for rectal perforation (see Chapter 6).

Weight, length, and head circumference should be graphed on the appropriate intrauterine growth chart to determine at which percentile the baby falls. Determination of the weight/length ratio (see Figure 5-2) normally increases with fetal age because the fetus becomes heavier for length as term approaches. In intrauterine growth restriction, the weight/length ratio decreases because the rate of growth in weight is affected more than length. Severe and prolonged intrauterine malnutrition may affect head, weight, and length ratios.

PREVENTIVE PRACTICES

Assessment of the infant's gestational age provides a reference point for individualizing care. Whether the infant is term and admitted to the normal newborn nursery or preterm and admitted to the intensive care nursery, attention to care practices that support development and neurologic integrity is essential in preventing iatrogenic disruptions or injury.

In utero, the fetus depends on the mother's physiologic systems to automatically regulate its own. At birth, the neonate's basic physiologic needs are met in new and different ways. Emerging from physiologic dependence into a physiologically independent neonatal state introduces new variables for both mother and baby in the development of their extrauterine relationship. For both term and preterm newborns, the primary developmental task is to reestablish biorhythmic balance by (1) establishing homeostasis through self-regulation of states (e.g., arousal and sleep/wake cycles); (2) processing, storing, and organizing internal and external stimuli; and (3) establishing a reciprocal relationship with primary care providers and the environment.

Although biorhythmic balance is internally determined, caregiving interaction between newborn and parent or caregiver either facilitates or disturbs this transition. After birth, balance is facilitated by contact with familiar surroundings (the mother's body).[47,100,109,110] The mother's sensorimotor (auditory, tactile, visual), thermal, and nutrient stimuli provide regulatory effects on the infant's behavior (activity level, sucking, sleep and wake cycles, stress management, and circadian rhythms) and physiology (endocrine secretion, oxygen consumption, and cardiovascular status).[47,100] Full-term newborns placed on the mother's chest immediately after delivery (within 5 minutes) and longer (more than 60 minutes) display the following stereotypic innate sequence of prefeeding behavior[110,120]:

- Significantly lower salivary cortisol levels and more stable cardiopulmonary function
- No sucking activity in the first 15 minutes
- Rooting and sucking activity begins and reaches maximum intensity at 45 minutes
- First hand-to-mouth movement at 35 minutes
- Spontaneous and unassisted finding of nipple and initiation of breastfeeding at about 55 minutes of age

Within the first 90 minutes after birth, neonates cared for in close body contact with the mother are quiet. However, infants separated from their mothers during this period and cared for in a crib cry and exhibit a *separation distress call* (also seen in several other mammalian species) that ceases at reunion.[30]

Avoidance of Certain Care Practices. Certain care practices (e.g., separation of the mother and infant, gastric suction, noise levels in the newborn nursery) have become "routine" in maternal/child care. These practices are based on few scientific foundations, disrupt maternal and infant regulation and establishment of innate behaviors, may have hidden consequences that surpass human adaptability, and may contribute to behavioral changes that result from violations of an innate agenda.[54,86] For example, gastric suction after birth evokes aversive reflexes (e.g., retching, combative movements, alterations in arterial blood pressure and heart rate, including bradycardia), disrupts development of early feeding behaviors, is unpleasant, and has no advantages in a healthy term infant following a normal pregnancy and normal vaginal delivery.[8,54] Use of maternal analgesia may interfere with the newborn's spontaneous breast-seeking and breastfeeding behavior.

During transition of a term neonate, prone position has been shown to improve oxygenation, decrease heart and respiratory rates, and encourage more favorable behavioral states.[105] In the newborn nursery, the lack of diurnal rhythm in noise levels and care-providing activities disrupts reestablishment of biorhythmic balance. Significant differences in nighttime sleep and wake patterns exist between newborns cared for in the nursery (exposed to more light, noise, crying, and noncontingent care) and newborns rooming with the mother (more quiet sleep and less crying).[67] Term infants exposed to soothing music in the newborn nursery spent less time in high arousal states (i.e., nonalert waking and crying) and had fewer behavioral state changes.[65]

Minimizing Procedural Pain in Newborn Care. Placing full-term and preterm infants skin-to-skin in whole-body contact with their mothers or breastfeeding during heelstick procedures reduces heart rate, crying (by 91%), and grimacing (by 84%).[25,56,64] When possible, breastfeeding throughout the procedure, rather than offering pumped breast milk, offers more comfort because of the synergism between skin-to-skin contact with the mother, sucking, and reception of breast milk by the infant.[2] Either breastfeeding/breastmilk or glucose/sucrose should be used to alleviate a newborn's procedural pain rather than positioning alone or no intervention.[107,108] The proximity and caregiving of the mother provide the term and preterm infants with a barrier against outside stimulation and an ability to increase their threshold to noxious stimuli.[47]

One barrier to using skin-to-skin care and breastfeeding to relieve neonatal pain during invasive procedures such as heelstick and injections is the uncomfortable position of the professional performing the procedure. An ergonomically sound protocol using an adjustable-height stool has been developed and tested in the clinical setting. This approach has resulted in a more comfortable position for the professional and greater use of skin-to-skin care and breastfeeding for neonatal pain relief during procedures.[34]

Nursery Care Practices and Adaptation to Extrauterine Life. Adaptation of full-term neonates is influenced either positively or negatively by nursery care practices (early care and handling). The influence of these practices in the adaptation of preterm or sick neonates may be even greater. Stress-reduction techniques to prevent fluctuations in BP, vital signs, and oxygenation often are not initiated until after the preterm infant has been admitted and stabilized in the NICU. Individualized developmental care (e.g., dimmed lights, decreased noise, gentle handling, contingent stimuli) (see Chapter 13) may be delayed in the presence of urgent expeditious assessment, diagnosis, and life-supporting interventions in the delivery room and on admission to the nursery. Consequently, the physiologic, anatomic, and psychological transition to extrauterine life makes at-risk neonates extremely vulnerable to the stress of resuscitation and initial nursery care.

Minimizing Stress during Respiratory and Circulatory Support. Minimizing stress and conserving energy should accompany establishing and maintaining an airway, adequate oxygenation and ventilation, and circulatory support. An immature preterm infant (under 32 weeks of gestation) (see Chapter 13) who is physiologically unstable may deteriorate if not handled gently and protected from overstimulation. Rapid fluctuations in oxygenation and BP, overwhelming stimuli, too-rapid volume expansion, suction, unrelieved pain, and hypothermia contribute to the incidence of intraventricular hemorrhage that occurs most commonly in the first 24 hours after birth (see Chapters 4, 6, 12, 23, and 26). In preterm infants, "routine" procedures such as bathing[13,114] result in increased heart rate and BP, motor stress behaviors, changes in stability and reorganizational behavior, hypoxia, and increased intracranial pressure (see Chapter 13). Overwhelmed by external stimuli, a neonate's global response to stress may be apnea and bradycardia.

Based on the infant's ability to tolerate an intervention and the benefits of early assessment and intervention, the admission process should be prioritized to (1) provide life-supportive care, (2) conserve energy, and (3) collect data and complete the health care record. Table 5-6 outlines developmental interventions for neonatal admissions and initial nursery care that decrease stress, reduce energy consumption, improve oxygenation and respiratory and heart rates, and prevent iatrogenic stress and injury.

Developmentally supportive care should begin immediately after birth.

KANGAROO CARE

Skin-to-skin "kangaroo" care (KC) benefits both parents and neonates (see Box 13-4). For the neonate, KC improves self-regulation, reduces stress and crying, facilitates breastfeeding, reduces pain, and facilitates neurodevelopment, maturation, and later mental health outcomes.[*] For the mother, KC helps reverse the negative effects of preterm birth and separation; it also increases maternal oxytocin levels, which enhance early bonding and attachment as well as long-term maternal-infant interactions, reduce postpartum depression, increase sensitivity to infant cues, enhance breastfeeding, and contribute to longer breastfeeding.[†]

A meta-analysis of 30 randomized controlled trials (RCTs)[71] showed that early skin-to-skin contact between mothers and their infants resulted in the following significant benefits:

- Better breastfeeding and better glucose levels
- Maintains optimal temperature and less infant crying
- Reduces stress hormones such as cortisol
- Better cardiopulmonary stability and better regulation of BP
- Increased quiet alert state

Kangaroo care not only prevents hypothermia[14] but also is effective in treating hypothermia.[90] KC warms healthy, low-risk, hypothermic preterm infants better (90%) than does incubator care (60%). Few mothers who deliver by cesarean section are offered immediate skin-to-skin contact with their babies after birth in the operating room, although this practice is beginning to occur. If both mother and baby are stable, both remain warm in the operating room during skin-to-skin contact with cardiopulmonary stability, and there is a decrease in maternal anxiety and pain.[100] In an RCT after cesarean section, 34 pairs of mothers and their newborns were randomized to skin-to-skin or routine nursery care within the 2 hours after the mother returned from the operating room.[53] Mean temperatures in both groups were equivalent, but the skin-to-skin care babies attached to the breast earlier, were exclusively or prevalently breastfed at discharge and at 3 months, and mothers were

---

[*]References 20, 48, 52, 69, 87, 88, 97, 100.
[†]References 23, 47, 52, 88, 93, 97.

TABLE 5-6	DEVELOPMENTAL INTERVENTIONS DURING ADMISSION AND INITIAL NURSERY CARE
Oxygenation	Apply noninvasive monitor (see Chapter 7)
	Titrate Fio_2 to maintain saturation at 92%-94% (see Chapters 7 and 8)
	Handle gently, minimally (see Chapters 13 and 23)
	Kangaroo care improves gaseous exchange, especially in preterm infants <1000 g (see Chapter 13)
	Position prone to maximize oxygenation (see Chapter 13 and below)
	Delay or defer bathing (see Chapter 19)
Thermoregulation	Maintain temperature axillary (36.5° to 37.5° C in term infants); skin (36° to 36.5° C in preterm infants) (see Chapter 6)
	Skin-to-skin contact (kangaroo care) provided by mothers or fathers to preterm/term newborns warms better than incubator care[14]
	Prewarm linen, scales, radiant warmer; incubator (see Chapter 6)
	Decrease heat loss with position (i.e., prone, flexion) (see Chapters 6 and 13)
	Use warm water on skin before applying probe, electrodes (see Chapter 19)
	Delay or defer bathing (see Chapter 19) —healthy term infants with axillary temperature >36.8° C can be bathed after 1 hour of age when appropriate care is taken to support thermal stability[114]
	Offer parents opportunity to bathe baby[13,85] (see Chapters 6 and 13)
Nutrition	Screen at-risk and symptomatic infants for hypoglycemia (see Chapter 15)
	Provide fluids and/or calories (orally or intravenously) (see Chapters 14 through 17)
	Decrease energy expenditures by decreasing internal (i.e., hypothermia, hypoxia) and external (i.e., noise, light) stressors (see Chapters 13 and 15)
Pain	Minimize painful stimuli (see Chapters 12 and 13)
	Relieve pain with pharmacologic management (see Chapter 12)
	Provide comfort measures (e.g., pacifier, containment, grasping) (see Chapters 12 and 13)
	Use venipuncture rather than heelstick (see Chapter 12)
	Use sucrose, kangaroo care, or breastfeeding during painful procedures*
Environmental stimuli	*Tactile* (see Chapter 13):
	Handle gently and minimally
	Support and contain in flexion
	Provide rest periods between procedures, handling
	Early (within 5 minutes of birth) and longer (>60 minutes) skin-to-skin care stabilize cardiopulmonary systems and reduce newborn stress after birth[110]
	Visual (see Chapter 13):
	Shield from bright, direct light
	Dim lights as soon as possible
	Cover oxygen hood, face with washcloth
	Cover incubator with blanket or cover
	Auditory (see Chapter 13):
	Talk quietly
	Respond quickly to alarms
	Parents to softly talk to infant
	Keep ill neonates away from crying babies[67]
Position	Promote flexion in side-lying position with blankets, rolls (see Chapter 13)
	Prone (oxygenation better; less apnea; quiet, more restful sleep; decreased caloric expenditure; decreased reflux) (see Chapter 13)
	Swaddle (see Chapter 13)
	Avoid supine if newborn is hypoxic and has an oxygen requirement; otherwise, always position all well, term newborns supine (see Chapter 13)

Continued

TABLE 5-6	DEVELOPMENTAL INTERVENTIONS DURING ADMISSION AND INITIAL NURSERY CARE — cont'd
Assess and interpret newborn cries	Assess avoidance and approach behaviors so that care is individualized (see Chapter 13)
	Support infant strengths and adaptive and coping behaviors (see Chapter 13)
	Modulate environmental and caregiver stimuli based on infant cues (contingent on cues rather than noncontingent stimuli and interaction) (see Chapter 13)
	Teach parents infant cues (see Chapter 13)

*References 25, 56, 64, 69, 107, 108.

highly satisfied with skin-to-skin contact with their babies.[53] Studies involving fathers providing KC for their infants born by cesarean section, compared with infants cared for in cribs and incubators, identified the following outcomes[44,45]:

- Full-term newborns had significantly increased axillary temperatures and blood glucose levels.
- Newborns were more alert, cried less, and were calmer.
- Newborns reached a drowsy state earlier.
- Fathers were able to facilitate and influence their infant's prefeeding behavior.
- Fathers could be primary caregivers during separation of the mother and baby.

Because of this research evidence, the World Health Organization, the American Academy of Breastfeeding Medicine (ABM),[1] the American Academy of Pediatrics (AAP),[8] the Neonatal Resuscitation Program (NRP),[66] and the Centers for Disease Control and Prevention (CDC) recommend use of skin-to-skin (kangaroo care) for the term newborn after birth. The AAP and ABM recommend that full-term neonates should immediately be placed into kangaroo care after birth and remain there until after the first breastfeeding.[8] The CDC and the International Network on Kangaroo Mother Care[97] recommend that the full-term newborn remain in KC throughout the postpartum period as a strategy to facilitate breastfeeding. Even in the LBW infant, continuous KC that is initiated early results in significantly higher proportion of exclusive breastfeeding at 6 months.[93]

SURVEILLANCE FOR POTENTIAL COMPLICATIONS

Complications of common morbidities (see Figure 5-11) are prevented by classification, assessment, and screening of all newborns at birth. These morbidities and their complications are thoroughly discussed in the appropriate chapters. Close monitoring and surveillance of these groups of infants, and long-term follow-up studies, would allow us to establish patterns of potential outcomes for each specific subgroup. For example: Preterm SGA/IUGR infants are at increased risk for mortality, more gross motor and neurologic dysfunction, more cognitive disorders needing special education, but less cerebral palsy compared with AGA infants.

PARENT TEACHING

Transitional care, neonatal assessment, and initial care do not necessarily take place in a nursery in which the newborn and family are isolated from each other. Alternative settings for initial care include birthing rooms, recovery rooms in which family and baby are kept together, the mother's postpartum room, or at a home visit. In fact, keeping the family together not only facilitates bonding but also provides an excellent opportunity for teaching parents about the individuality of their newborn.[85,95]

The assessments of gestational age and physical condition are best performed with the mother and father in attendance so that deviations from normal such as caput, cleft lip, cleft palate, or clubfoot can be explained. Eliciting parental cooperation is important. For example, when the major concern is "Will the procedure hurt?" a response such as "It is routine" will not comfort and reassure well-informed, noninterventionist consumers. Rather, a more physiologically oriented explanation about the condition being screened, why their particular infant is at increased risk, and what interventions are available encourages parental cooperation.

BOX 5-4   PARENT TEACHING[3,29,40-42]

- Every encounter with the parents is a teaching opportunity, so that by the time of discharge, parents are totally competent to care for their infant. Assess each individual family's ability to care for their infant and readiness for discharge.
- Teach parents how to care for the newborn's skin, umbilicus, and circumcision site and the appropriate urination/stooling patterns for newborns.
- Teach parents about the nutritional needs of their newborn, how to breast/bottle feed, and burp their baby. Develop a feeding plan with the parents for the late-preterm infant, and teach parents how and why to adhere to the plan for a late-preterm infant.
- Teach parents how to take an axillary temperature on their newborn and maintain the axillary temperature between 36.5° and 37.4° C (97.7° and 99.3° F) with clothes, blankets, and an appropriate environmental temperature.
- The presence and clinical significance of jaundice are determined before discharge (see Chapter 21), appropriate follow-up care has been determined, and the importance is stressed to parents. Parents are taught how to assess jaundice at home.
- Teach parents the importance of follow-up care, either at a clinic, physician's office, or home visit, within 24 to 48 hours after discharge for late-preterm infants.
- Give parents the newborn immunization record with documentation of what immunizations their infant has received and the importance of follow-up for childhood immunizations.
- Teach parents appropriate safety precautions:
  - Verbal and written information about recognizing signs and symptoms of a "sick"/"ill" infant, how the infant acts, and whom to notify.

- Proper use of car seats including positioning with supports, facing the rear in the backseat, middle of rear seat preferably with an adult seated next to the preterm to enable ongoing observation of the infant during travel.
- Proper positioning supine for sleep: "Back to Sleep." Model "Back to Sleep" by placing babies who are in cribs only on their backs to sleep. *All* care providers (e.g., parents, grandparents, day care providers, babysitters) should sleep babies supine (see Chapter 13).
- Importance of a smoke-free environment because secondhand smoke is associated with an increased risk for developing health problems.
- *NEVER* shake the baby! Babies are shaken by frustrated caregivers when the infant continues to cry. Dangers of shaking infants include blindness, brain damage, developmental delays, seizures, paralysis, and death. (See Resource Materials for Parents at the end of this chapter.) Education of parents about normal sleep and crying patterns, techniques for soothing infants, possible medical causes for crying, and parent self-care advice lowers parental depression and enhances parent confidence in caregiving.
- Information, in writing, about all medications for their infant including name, action, dose, route, side effects, schedule (see Chapter 10).
- Proper swaddling technique: Safe swaddling includes positioning the baby's extremities in slight flexion and abduction; baby should be able to freely move lower extremities. Placing an infant's hips and knees in an extended position with swaddling increases the risk of hip dysplasia and dislocation.[62]
- Teach parents the importance of their own self-care: need for adequate sleep/rest, nutrition/hydration, privacy, stress management, recreation, and sex.

Professional care providers are only temporary caregivers. It is our responsibility to help parents become confident, primary caregivers of their own infants. Actively involving parents in the care and treatment of their newborn further solidifies their position as primary caregivers.[85,95] Encouraging active parental involvement enhances the parents' self-esteem and confidence in their abilities[95]; thus our actions must tell and reassure the parents, "You are able to care for this baby." An RCT comparing the ability of parents to perform the baby's first bath in the mother's room versus a nurse bathing the baby in the admission nursery found no difference in temperature changes irrespective of who bathed the baby or where the bath was given.[85] The newborn heat loss experienced with bathing was significant and returned to normal in 1 hour. Parents in the study wanted the opportunity to bathe their infants and gained

confidence in their parenting skill/ability. With the supervision of the nurse, ensuring an environment to reduce heat loss (e.g., warm, draft-free room, temperature assessment, warm water, use of kangaroo care after the bath) and using the bath as a teaching opportunity, parents can bathe their own infants.

At discharge, performing the physical examination in the room with the parents offers a final opportunity to teach, counsel, and advise them before they take their new baby home. Information about feeding, cord care, bathing, elimination patterns, safety, signs of illness, medications, and the importance of follow-up care is essential for parents of a full-term, healthy newborn (Box 5-4). It is also essential for parents taking home an infant after prolonged hospitalization. In addition, a modified version of the Brazelton examination on all neonates enables parents to become familiar with a newborn's competencies for reacting to and shaping his or her environment and with strategies for parental intervention. Developing written materials for parents about normal newborn care and documenting teaching sessions and return demonstrations ensure that no important information is forgotten. (See Chapter 31 for discharge planning and teaching strategies.)

REFERENCES

For a full list of references, scan the QR code or visit http://booksite.elsevier.com/ 9780323320832.

6

HEAT BALANCE

SANDRA L. GARDNER AND JACINTO A. HERNÁNDEZ

Adaptation to extrauterine life involves the newborn infant in a series of biological adjustments to a totally new set of environmental conditions. Prime among these is the accommodation to a new thermal environment that represents a distinct "cold challenge." Failure to adjust to this cold stress has historically been recognized, particularly in premature and low-birth-weight (LBW) infants, with the development of variable degrees of hypothermia and increased morbidity and mortality rates. At birth, the body temperature of the newborn infant will approximate or slightly exceed that of the mother. Within minutes of birth, however, core temperature begins to fall precipitously, particularly in infants with birth weights less than 1500 g. These infants have a diminished capacity for metabolic heat production, a high surface area to volume ratio, and immature epidermal barrier leading to extraordinarily high evaporative heat losses. Consequently, they are highly vulnerable to the development of hypothermia. Thermal management has become a cornerstone in neonatal intensive care. Earlier studies conducted in term and preterm infants worldwide concluded that maintenance of body temperature through control of the thermal environment is paramount for the reduction of morbidity and mortality risks in LBW infants.[6,54,56,60]

During the past several decades, researchers and clinicians have gained insight into the physiology of thermoregulation and developed the technology to maintain thermal neutrality in the tiniest and sickest neonates.[37,48,51,77,78] Although the staff of modern neonatal intensive care units (NICUs) have the expertise and equipment to avoid or minimize the consequences of inadequate thermoregulation, determining the most appropriate ways of getting the best temperature balance (normothermia) is the subject of ongoing investigation. This chapter discusses the current knowledge of the physiology and pathophysiology of neonatal thermoregulation and techniques used not only to prevent heat loss but also to manage heat balance.

HISTORICAL MILESTONES[18,58,62]

The *first incubator for neonates* was introduced in the early 1830s. Dr. Stephane Tarnier, Chairman of Obstetrics of the University of Paris, first applied the principle of graded incubation (commonly used in chick embryos) in developing a covered incubator chamber that has been widely recognized as the first attempt to systematically provide a warmed environment for premature infants. In 1835 Von Ruehl in St. Petersburg, Russia, introduced an incubator described as a double-walled box that circulated warmed water within the interspace.[58] Tarnier's students, Budin and Auvard, modified Tarnier's incubator by adding a thermometer and regulatory alarms to alert the infant's nurse attendant to either increase or decrease the incubator's prescribed temperature. The care of newborns was delegated to Madame Henry, Midwife-in-Chief, who oversaw the building of a pavilion specifically for the care of these weakling newborns.[72] This pavilion housed 12 incubators in which fragile newborns were warmed over a hot-water reservoir attached to an external source of heat. These were impressive first steps in attempting to control the fragile heat balance of weak preterm infants. Over the next 60 years, in Tarnier's and Budin's clinic, refinements of incubation techniques resulted in an increased survival from 38% to 66% in infants weighing between 1200 and 2000 g.

PURPLE type highlights content that is particularly applicable to clinical settings.

Dr. Tarnier's successor, Dr. Budin, continued this important early practice of neonatology, focusing on the home care of these high-risk babies. Alexandre Lion improved the design of incubators and charged spectators a fee to see them in action, which led to a very popular show at the Berlin Exposition of 1896. An associate of Lion, Martin Couney, brought the incubator shows to the United States, where Dr. Joseph DeLee adopted the technology and opened an "incubator station" in 1900 at the Chicago Lying-in Hospital. Nearly all of the large expositions in America hosted "Incubator Baby Side Shows." These began in 1898 with the Trans-Mississippi Exposition and continued on to the New York World's Fair in 1939.

Dr. Couney's display of incubators at Luna Park on Coney Island and at a second park named *Dreamland* hosted premature babies from New York hospitals that lacked the facilities to care for them. These infants were lined up under heaters in incubators, and they breathed filtered air. At least 8000 babies passed through these incubators, and at least 6000 were saved. Servocontrolled radiant heat in incubators was initially reported by Agate and Silverman in 1963.[58]

Today's *radiant warmer* is an evolution from the original idea of Agate and Silverman. Radiant energy as the sole source of heat from an overhead panel was described in 1969 by Due and Oliver. Widespread use of the warmer in the delivery room was readily accepted and soon led to its use in the NICU. The factors that affect heat loss and heat production were elucidated. As intensive care became more readily available, easy accessibility to the infants became increasingly necessary and the open warmer became more readily used.[38]

Changes in the radiant warmer have included introduction of incubators that are interchangeable with and convert to radiant warmers. The use of humidification in the incubators has also been improved to allow for varying humidification based on the infant's gestational age and weight. These new beds allow the caregiver to rotate the mattress 360 degrees for easy patient access and provide an in-bed scale. In recent years, new approaches to thermal care of the newborn preterm baby have been extensively studied, including* occlusive wrapping, placing on heated mattresses, and skin-to-skin

(kangaroo) care. The role and clinical significance of these approaches will be discussed later.

PHYSIOLOGIC CONSIDERATIONS

Animals that maintain their body temperature within a narrow range through a wide range of environmental temperatures are known as *homeotherms*. Humans, as homeotherms, maintain a "normal" body temperature by balancing the amount of heat lost from the body with the amount of heat generated from within the body. Our ability to cope with changing thermal environments improves physically and physiologically with age. Eventually we are physically able to move to a different place with a more suitable environment or dress more appropriately when the temperature is uncomfortable.

Babies, especially preterm or small-for-gestational-age (SGA) babies, of course cannot physically respond as older children would, and even their physiologic responses are different and limited. Adults lose some thermoregulatory control during rapid-eye-movement sleep. Although newborn infants spend much time in active sleep, their thermoregulatory control is not impaired during this period of active sleep,[48] which indicates the developmental importance of both thermoregulation and active sleep in the maturation of newborn infants.

Neutral Thermal Environment

Physiologic responses to a cold environment include metabolic reactions that consume substrate and oxygen and result in heat production. A neutral thermal temperature is the body temperature at which an individual baby's oxygen consumption is minimized (Figure 6-1). Thus a minimal amount of the baby's energy is expended for heat maintenance, and energy is conserved for other basic functions and for growth. Minimal metabolic activity is possible within a narrow range of temperatures, so temperatures that are too high or too low add stress and increase metabolic rate. Extreme deviations from this range overwhelm the thermoregulatory mechanisms, leading to body temperature imbalances and potentially death.

The goal in controlling a neonate's environment is to minimize energy expended by him or

---

*References 3, 8, 17, 27, 31, 41, 49, 76.

her to maintain a "normal" temperature, thus eliminating thermal stress. This neutral thermal environment is the sum total of factors at which a baby with a normal body temperature has a minimal metabolic rate and therefore minimal oxygen consumption (Figure 6-2). Both traditional indirect calorimetry and the more accurate direct calorimetry are used to study the production and expenditure of heat in newborns. Factors such as ambient air temperature, airflow velocity, relative humidity, and temperature and composition of objects in direct contact with the infant or to which heat may be radiated compose the infant's thermal environment.

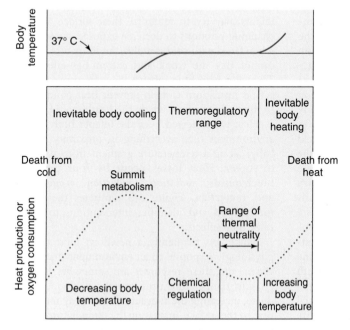

FIGURE 6-1 Temperature versus oxygen consumption. Effect of environmental oxygen consumption and body temperature. (From Klaus M, Fanaroff A: *Care of the high-risk neonate,* ed 2, Philadelphia, 1979, Saunders.)

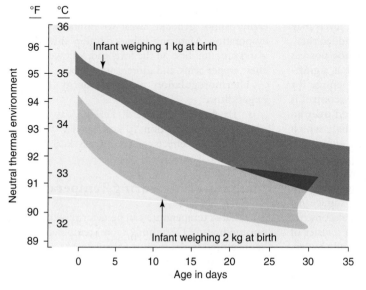

FIGURE 6-2 Neutral thermal environments. Range of temperature to provide neutral environmental conditions for infant lying naked on warm mattress in draft-free surroundings of moderate humidity (50% saturation) when mean radiant temperature is same as air temperature. *Shaded areas* show average neutral temperature range for healthy infant weighing 1 kg *(dark)* or 2 kg *(light)* at birth. Optimal temperature probably approximates to lower limit of neutral range as defined here. Approximately 1° C (1.8° F) should be added to these operative temperatures to derive appropriate neutral air temperature for single-walled incubator when room temperature is less than 27° C (80° F) and more if room temperature is much less. (From Hey EN, Katz G: The optimum thermal environment for naked babies, *Arch Dis Child* 45:328, 1970.)

Maintaining Heat Balance (Heat Production Versus Losses)

When exposed to a cold environment, a neonate senses the reduced skin surface temperature (using sensors in the skin, primarily the face) and senses core body temperature (using sensors along the spinal cord and in the hypothalamus). Information from these various sensors is processed (probably in the posterior hypothalamus), including average temperature, rate of temperature change, and size of the stimulated area. Cold stress results in the initiation of a series of reactions to increase heat production and decrease heat loss. In adults, the most significant involuntary method of heat production is shivering. Neonates rarely shiver and must rely on nonshivering, or chemical, thermogenesis to produce the needed heat. This process is initiated in the hypothalamus and transmitted through the sympathetic nervous system, leading to the release of norepinephrine at the site of brown fat. *Brown fat,* found mostly in the nape of the neck, axillae, and between the scapulae of newborns, is a specialized type of fat. It is unique in that it contains thermogenin, which is the key enzyme regulating nonshivering thermogenesis. Norepinephrine causes the release of free fatty acids, which with thermogenesis undergo combustion in the mitochondria of brown fat cells, releasing heat. Lipoprotein lipase also provides further triglyceride substrate for heat production.

Oxygen and glucose also are consumed during nonshivering thermogenesis. Thus an infant who already has low oxygen or glucose levels may become hypoxemic or hypoglycemic if added thermal stress occurs. Preterm babies do not possess sufficient brown fat stores to mount a significant heat production response to compensate for even minimal cold stress.[22] When servocontrol is used, the thermistor must not be placed over an area of brown fat (such as in the axilla), which may directly heat the overlying skin, causing a decrease in servocontrolled heat output.[2]

Heat generated within the body is transferred by conduction through tissues along a gradient from warmer to cooler areas such as the skin surface. An initial response to a cold environment is to constrict superficial blood vessels to minimize the transfer of heat from the core to the surface of the body. Superficial vasoconstriction, which gives the skin a mottled appearance in response to cold stimulus, results

in a lower skin temperature reading to the thermocontroller and consequently causes an increase in the incubator temperature. The smaller the body size, the less effective vasoconstriction is in conserving heat.

Compared with adults, newborns have a very large surface area to body mass ratio and therefore have a relatively large area exposed to the environment from which heat can be lost. More mature infants may try to minimize their surface area by changing positions to decrease exposed surface area when faced with cold stimulus, but immature infants cannot flex the trunk and extremities effectively. They also have little subcutaneous fat tissue (which acts as insulation) to help prevent heat conduction to the body's surface, where the heat would be lost.

Heat is transferred from the infant's body to the environment (i.e., everything in proximity to the baby) along a temperature gradient from warmest to coolest. Heat losses occur by four principal mechanisms: *radiation, conduction, evaporation,* and *convection.* Figure 6-3 illustrates these four mechanisms and identifies interventions to minimize their effects.

Much less frequently, a newborn must call on physiologic responses to an environment that is too warm, and these responses are somewhat limited. As skin temperature rises, superficial blood vessels dilate, increasing the transfer of core body temperature to the surface. Increasing the temperature gradient between the skin and the environment increases heat loss from the body. When exposed to elevated environmental temperatures, preterm babies generally cannot generate sweat to eliminate heat by evaporation. Maturing babies develop this eccrine gland function first on the forehead, followed by the chest, upper arms, and more caudal areas.

Thermoregulation requires energy (caloric) expenditure:

- Basal metabolic rate: 50 kcal/kg/day
- Thermoregulation: 10 kcal/kg/day
- Thermic effects of feeding: 8 kcal/kg/day[7] (see Chapter 17)

Methods of Measuring Temperature

A neonate's temperature can be determined by various methods.[68] Deep body (core) temperature may be measured in the rectum or esophagus and on the tympanic membrane. Rectal thermistors are thin, flexible probes that must be inserted at least 5 cm

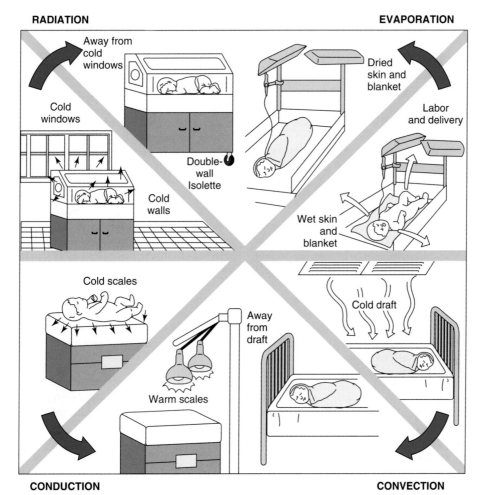

RADIATION

Away from cold windows

Cold windows

Cold walls

Double-wall Isolette

EVAPORATION

Dried skin and blanket

Labor and delivery

Wet skin and blanket

CONDUCTION

Cold scales

Away from draft

Warm scales

CONVECTION

Cold draft

FIGURE 6-3 *Radiation*, or heat loss in the form of electromagnetic photons, occurs from warm skin surfaces to a cooler object not in contact with the newborn (e.g., inside the incubator wall, nursery wall, window). Radiant heat loss is independent of ambient air temperature and is the main source of heat loss because of the infant's large exposed body surface area. *Conduction* is the loss of heat to a cooler object in direct contact with the newborn (e.g., cold scale, unwarmed bed, stethoscope, examiner's hand). *Convection* is the loss of heat to moving air at the skin surface and depends on the air's velocity and temperature. *Evaporation* of water from the skin and mucous membranes also causes heat loss, especially in the delivery room. The thinner stratum corneum layer of skin of very-low-birth-weight infants makes evaporative heat and water loss and fluid management ongoing problems. (Courtesy Lynn Jones, RN.)

to obtain an accurate reading. Insertion to this depth runs the risk for perforation, because the sigmoid colon makes a right-angle turn approximately 3 cm from the anal opening. Esophageal and tympanic readings are difficult to obtain and usually impractical.

Continuous monitoring of abdominal skin temperature with the newborn lying supine is a noninvasive method that has good correlation with rectal temperatures in preterm[21] and very-low-birth-weight (VLBW) preterm infants.[75] *Only* abdominal skin temperature has been shown to be an effective monitor of neutral thermal environment. Box 6-1 clearly illustrates that even a slight change (less than 1° C) in abdominal skin temperatures affects oxygen consumption and basal metabolic rates. Therefore the range of thermal neutrality illustrated in Figure 6-1 is a very narrow range—less than 1° C on either side of abdominal skin temperature of 36.5° C (97.7° F).

> ### BOX 6-1
> ### ALTERATIONS IN OXYGEN CONSUMPTION WITH CHANGES IN ABDOMINAL SKIN TEMPERATURE: RESEARCH BASIS[63,64]
>
> - Abdominal skin temperature of 36.5° C (97.7° F) results in minimal oxygen consumption.
> - Abdominal skin temperature of 35.9° C (96.6° F) results in an increase in oxygen consumption of 10%.
> - Abdominal skin temperature of 37.2° C (98.9° F) results in an increase in oxygen consumption of 6%.

Because of the risks involved, rectal temperatures should not be taken on a routine basis in neonates. Axillary temperatures require disturbing and handling, minimal exposure due to undressing (which may lower temperature), and result in crying and restlessness in some neonates.[23,40] Axillary temperatures are measured by using glass, electronic, or disposable thermometers. The tip of the thermometer should be held firmly in the midaxillary area for at least 3 minutes in preterm infants and 5 minutes in term infants. When taken properly, axillary temperatures provide readings as accurate as rectal and core temperature methods.[25] In term infants, axillary temperatures should be maintained at 36.5° to 37.5° C (97.7° to 99.5° F). For preterm infants, the normal axillary temperature ranges between 36.3° and 36.9° C (97.3° and 98.4° F).[58]

A recent randomized study comparing temperature values from three skin probe positions with digital axillary temperature values was conducted in healthy preterm infants.[61] There was no statistically significant difference in any of the three probe site temperature values or between the probe site values and the digital axillary temperatures.[61] The results of this study are similar to a previous study conducted in healthy full-term infants.[70] Because of the small size of the sample and methodology followed, the results of these studies *cannot* be generalized to all preterm infants, especially those with extremely low birth weight (ELBW). Both researchers recommend consistency in temperature measurement and evaluation of trends and patterns over time, along with evaluation of the entire clinical picture of each individual infant.[61,70]

In search of a quicker, noninvasive, less disruptive mode of temperature taking, the accuracy of noninvasive infrared thermometers in the neonatal population has been evaluated in recent studies in premature[23,40] and in healthy late-preterm and term infants.[30] These studies found the readings between the infrared midforehead and temporal artery and axillary readings to be very comparable. More research with various populations of neonates, in various environments (cribs, incubators, radiant warmers), and using larger numbers of study subjects is necessary.[68]

In critically ill infants, the skin temperature is usually routinely monitored in addition to axillary temperature readings. A skin probe is secured to the right upper quadrant of the abdomen. The temperature probe should not be placed under the axilla or any other position except as recommended by the manufacturer. Because an infant responds to cold stress by vasoconstriction, a drop in skin temperature may be the first sign of hypothermia. The core temperature may not fall until the infant can no longer compensate. The axillary temperature may remain normal (or even be elevated) because of proximity to brown fat stores.

ETIOLOGY OF HEAT IMBALANCES

The ambient temperature range in which a healthy full-term infant maintains a stable core temperature is narrower than the temperature range in which an adult maintains a normal temperature. When measures are taken to provide a neutral thermal environment for the neonate, excessive heat losses or gains are avoided and heat balance is maintained. Recognition of infants at risk for heat imbalance is essential in the prevention of thermal stress.

Premature infants have a limited ability to control body temperature and are extremely susceptible to hypothermia. Factors that contribute to temperature instability include very thin skin, large surface area relative to body mass, limited substrate for heat production, decreased subcutaneous tissue, and an immature nervous system. These infants often have multiple health problems that necessitate frequent interventions by health care providers with consequent disruption of the infant's neutral thermal environment.

A premature infant's very thin skin and larger surface area to body mass ratio allow for increased evaporative heat loss. Term infants can reduce surface area by flexing their extremities onto their trunk, a skill that increases with gestational age. Unable to maintain flexion, a preterm infant lies primarily with extremities extended. Care providers may reduce the surface area by positioning infants in flexion and supporting them with blankets and rolls. The shortened gestation limits lipid supplies, brown fat, and the accumulation of subcutaneous tissue. The immature nervous system delays or mutes the infant's response to thermal stress.

The premature infant is likely to experience other complications (e.g., respiratory distress, sepsis, intraventricular hemorrhage, hypoglycemia) that may increase basal metabolic rate and oxygen consumption, thus interfering with the ability to maintain thermal stability. Numerous procedures and interventions (e.g., medication administration, placement of intravascular catheters, obtaining vital signs) may impede efforts to maintain a neutral thermal environment. Care providers should routinely check the infant's temperature before initiating treatments. If the temperature is low, treatment should be delayed until a more normal temperature is obtained. If interventions are prolonged, temperature should be monitored frequently, an external heat source provided, and the intervention stopped if hypothermia occurs.

Late-preterm infants are predisposed to morbidities because of their developmental immaturity (see Chapter 5). Less adipose tissue for insulation, less brown fat for chemical thermogenesis, more heat loss, and a larger ratio of surface area to weight contribute to problems with heat balance in these infants. Morbidity associated with heat balance in the late-preterm infant is 10% compared with 0% for term infants.[4]

Low-Birth-Weight Newborns

Low-birth-weight (LBW) (less than 2500 g) infants can be divided into two groups: the very-low-birth-weight (VLBW) infant (less than 1500 g) and the extremely low-birth-weight (ELBW) infant (less than 1000 g). Preterms in each of these groups have specific needs for thermoregulation. Heated incubators, radiant warmers, and skin-to-skin care are all methods for maintaining the temperature and promoting weight gain of the VLBW infant. With caregiving, VLBW infants in servocontrolled incubators decrease their abdominal skin temperature with incubator opening in proportion to the type and length of the procedure being done.[20] Infants weighing between 1500 and 1600 g may be weaned to an open crib if all criteria are met.[7,55] (See Figure 6-5 for weaning criteria.)

During the first 12 hours of life, ELBW preterms become hypothermic with procedures such as *intubations, chest x-ray examinations, intravenous (IV) line placement and manipulation, suctioning, repositioning,* and *vital signs.* Like the late-preterm and the LBW infant, ELBW infants have even less brown and subcutaneous fat for maintaining body temperature. Their thin skin also contributes to increased insensible water loss.

SGA infants, like preterm infants, have a large surface area relative to body mass and decreased subcutaneous tissue, brown fat, and glycogen stores, all of which contribute to heat imbalance. Decreased placental blood flow frequently contributes to the small size. The relatively large surface area of an SGA infant increases evaporative and radiant heat loss, whereas limited brown fat stores and subcutaneous tissue contribute to a decreased ability to produce and conserve body heat. Some flexion of the extremities may be present because flexion depends on gestational age and not weight. SGA infants have a higher metabolic rate compared with infants at similar weights who are appropriate for gestational age. This is believed to be caused by the larger brain size relative to body weight. Hypoxia in utero may depress the infant's central nervous system (CNS) and alter the ability to regulate temperature. Increased energy requirements coupled with limited glycogen stores may result in hypoglycemia and limited ability to produce heat. SGA infants may require numerous interventions that disrupt the neutral thermal environment. Care providers should ensure that the infant has a normal and stable temperature before initiation of treatments. If treatments are prolonged, temperature should be monitored frequently, an external heat source provided, and treatments stopped if hypothermia occurs.

Infants with neurologic damage or depression may experience difficulty maintaining a stable temperature. Hypoxia before, during, or after delivery, neurologic defects, and exposure to drugs such as analgesics and anesthetics may depress the infant's neurologic response to thermal stress. Hypoxia decreases the effect of norepinephrine on nonshivering thermogenesis, the main route of thermal regulation in the newborn infant. Hypoxia also may reduce the oxidative capacity of the mitochondria in brown fat and skeletal muscles, which are involved in thermogenesis. Infants who have experienced hypoxia in utero may have increased norepinephrine concentrations, which result in peripheral vasoconstriction. This may cause a delayed metabolic response to cold stress and delayed vasodilation in response to heat stress.

Neurologic defects that affect the hypothalamus also may interfere with heat balance. The hypothalamus coordinates temperature input from various sensors. Drugs such as analgesics and anesthetics cause CNS depression and reduce the infant's ability to respond to thermal stress. Neuromuscular blocking agents inhibit the infant's ability to maintain a flexed position, increasing exposed body surface and heat loss. Care providers must be alert to the effect of drugs on the CNS and the infant's ability to regulate temperature.

Infants with sepsis may have hypothermia or hyperthermia. In a newborn, an elevated temperature may begin as a response to cold stress, with peripheral vasoconstriction and thermogenesis. Heat production continues as the infant attempts to achieve a higher core body temperature. Exogenous and endogenous pyrogens may enhance thermogenesis.

Initially, an infant with sepsis may feel cool to the touch and may have a low body temperature. As fever progresses, temperature may rise and the infant feels warm to the touch. Infants nursed in servocontrolled incubators may not have an elevated temperature. The lower heater output in response to increasing skin temperature (by manual or servocontrol adjustment) may mask a fever by keeping the baby's temperature within normal limits. The care provider should be alert to a sudden decreased need for incubator heat support in a previously stable infant.

Hyperthermia may be iatrogenic, caused by inappropriate control of the neonate's environmental temperature. The most common cause is the inappropriate use of external heat sources. Dehydration also may contribute to hyperthermia. Infants nursed with the use of external heat sources should have their temperatures monitored frequently. Phototherapy, sunlight, and the use of excessive clothing and blankets contribute to overheating. Dehydration may be avoided by early recognition of infants at risk for increased fluid loss. Increased insensible water loss occurs in preterm infants because of increased skin permeability and the use of phototherapy and radiant warmers. Vomiting, diarrhea, gastric suction, and ostomy drainage also increase fluid loss. These infants should receive additional fluids to replace the increased losses (see Chapter 14).

PREVENTION OF HEAT/COLD STRESS

Management of the thermal environment is paramount for newborn well-being. Heat balance is determined by the amount of heat lost to the baby's environment offset by the amount of heat generated by the body plus the amount of heat supplied from outside sources. Because a smaller, more immature, and sicker baby is less able to regulate body temperature, it is crucial that care providers understand the physical and physiologic principles of heat balance and be able to maintain a neutral thermal environment. Two broad categories of interventions foster thermal neutrality[1]: blocking avenues of heat loss, and providing external heat and environmental support to maintain temperature within the normal range of 36.5° to 37.5° C (97.7° to 99.5° F).[6] The theoretical neutral thermal environment necessary for neonates of 1 and 2 kg at a given age is graphed in Figure 6-2. Newborns of less than 800 g are not adequately addressed in currently available tables but should have a starting environmental temperature setting of 36.5° C (97.7° F).

Delivery Room

Attention to the details of these interventions begins in the delivery room, in which the first step is to adjust the ambient delivery room temperature higher than ordinary operating rooms or patient rooms. The air temperature in newborn care areas should be kept at 23.8° to 26.1° C (75° to 79° F), and humidity should be kept at 30% to 60%.[58] Warming the room and placing the resuscitation table away from doors or drafts minimizes convective heat loss. Raising the delivery room temperature to 24° to 26° C, as recommended by the World Health Organization, decreases cold stress in preterm infants less than or equal to 32 weeks of gestation.[33]

The newborn's skin temperature may drop by as much as 0.3° C/min, with core temperature dropping more slowly after delivery. At birth, most heat loss results from evaporation of amniotic fluid from the baby's skin surface. Drying the infant with prewarmed towels and immediately replacing used ones with dry, warm towels minimize evaporative heat loss. Dry towels conduct heat poorly when contacting the neonate's skin. However, cold examiner hands, stethoscopes, scales, and bare mattresses are good heat conductors and can add significant cold stress if not warmed before coming in contact with the newborn.

Hypothermia on admission to the NICU ranges from 31% to 78% in infants less than 1500 g birth weight.[10] The benefit of using *polyethylene plastic bags* and wraps for babies born at 26 to 30 weeks of gestation to preserve body heat and prevent hypothermia at admission has been shown in numerous studies.* This type of warming is ideal for a preterm infant (at birth and the immediate hours following) awaiting transportation to a tertiary care facility or indeed a baby born in a tertiary care facility. The baby is placed on a warm towel (but not dried) and placed under a radiant warming heating device. The baby (excluding his or her head) is placed fully in the polyethylene bag or is wrapped in the polyethylene sheet. The baby should remain under the radiant warmer as the heat, acting through the covering on the baby's moist skin, creates a warm thermal environment. Cutting an appropriate-size hole through the covering over the area of insertion can facilitate the introduction of any catheter or cannula. Polyethylene bags for warmth have been adopted by the Neonatal Resuscitation Program (NRP) (see Chapter 4).

NRP guidelines emphasize how hypothermia may reduce the extent of brain injury after hypoxia and that hyperthermia may worsen the extent of brain injury during reperfusion after hypoxic events. The recommended goal is to maintain normothermia for the infant and avoid iatrogenic hyperthermia in resuscitated newborns (see Chapter 26).

Resuscitation should take place on a preheated radiant warmer so that the adverse consequences of hypothermia are avoided. In an attempt to maintain heat balance, the neonate increases cellular metabolism and oxygen consumption, which increases the risk for hypoxia,

cardiorespiratory problems, and acidosis. Hypoglycemia is also a risk factor, because the infant must consume more glucose for heat production. Other complications include clotting disorders, neurologic problems, hyperbilirubinemia, and even death if the untreated hypothermia progresses.

Because a significant amount of heat is lost through the surface area of the head, with its abundant blood supply and the brain's high heat production, covering the infant's head with some insulating material conserves heat during transfer to the nursery or NICU and afterward. Stockinet material is relatively ineffective for this purpose and provides poor insulation. The best material is thick, maintains its shape with use, and has a high percentage of air volume trapped in the fibers. Knitted wool caps, plastic caps, or Thinsulate material may provide the best results.[12,48,74]

Occlusive plastic wrap alone is not totally effective in preventing hypothermia after birth in the very preterm infant. Several recent studies using plastic wrap and self-heating gel mattresses together to prevent heat loss in preterm infants under 31 weeks' gestation have been conducted.[32,49,59,65,67] These studies have found significant reduction in the incidence of hypothermia with the use of gel mattresses compared with the incidence of hypothermia on admission in very preterm infants who were born before the use of gel mattresses (3.3% vs. 22.6%).[32] Several of these studies have also noticed a higher incidence of hyperthermia on admission.[32,49,67] Three nursing interventions (occlusive wrap, occlusive wrap and chemical mattress, and increasing delivery room temperature) were studied to determine if they normalized admission temperatures in ELBW (less than 1000 g) and LBW (less than 1500 g) preterms.[11,43] Each intervention resulted in a normal admission temperature without the risk of hyperthermia.[11,43] A quality improvement program to reduce hypothermia in preterms less than 35 weeks' gestation after birth used occlusive wrap, a transwarmer mattress, cap, and room temperature between 21° and 23° C.[59a] These interventions resulted in significant increases in delivery room and admission axillary temperatures, no increased hyperthermia, and a reduction of intubation at 24 hours of age.[59a]

There are a variety of ways to maintain thermal neutrality. Accessibility, insensible water loss, servocontrol versus manual control of temperature, and

*References 15, 16, 19, 27, 31, 36, 39, 42, 43, 47, 49, 65, 69, 76.

safety are major considerations when determining the method to use for an individual neonate.

Incubators

Incubators provide a controlled, enclosed environment that is heated convectively with warm air. The temperature in an incubator may be *servocontrolled* to maintain a desired skin temperature or air temperature. As the temperature varies from the desired "set point," proportional control units gradually increase or decrease heat output to maintain a constant temperature (without the wider temperature fluctuations seen with simple on-off controllers). Incubators controlled by abdominal skin servocontrol have been found to reduce neonatal death rates in LBW, and especially in VLBW, neonates.[66] In setting the servocontrolled incubator to the desired skin temperature, the sensor should be attached to the right upper quadrant of the abdomen with insulated temperature patches. The sensor should not be placed over areas of brown fat deposits, because the higher-than-expected temperature information to the controlling unit will result in a lower-than-desired heat output.[2]

Inadvertent cooling may take place if the sensor is covered with clothes or a blanket or if the baby lies on it. Lying prone on the abdominal skin probe results in warmer temperatures than those recorded from probes not entrapped between the skin and mattress, resulting in a cooler incubator than intended.[13] If the sensor becomes disconnected from the skin, unwanted heating may occur because an erroneously low temperature reading causes an unwanted increase in heat output.[66] One also must consider that when an insulated patch is used to cover the thermistor, skin temperature is sensed as being higher than if tape covers the thermistor, resulting in decreased heat output by the warming device. The desired skin temperature used for skin servocontrol is generally 36.0° to 36.5° C (96.8° to 97.7° F).[46] Modern incubators also can be servocontrolled to a desired air temperature. This mode has been shown to provide a more stable thermal environment and less temperature variation compared with skin servocontrol.

Air servocontrol maintains a constant ambient air temperature when other factors such as phototherapy, external radiant heat, unstable room temperature, or direct sunlight are not confounding variables.

Infants who were managed with skin servocontrol had more variable but higher air temperatures and spent more time in a neutral thermal environment. Babies managed with air servocontrol had less variability in air temperatures but more variability in infant body temperature. A review of published trials concluded that VLBW babies whose skin servocontrol is set at 36° C had a lower mortality rate than those managed with air servocontrol at 31.8° C.[66] The question of air versus skin servocontrol or manual control is still debatable for any given situation, and probably neither is the perfect solution for all babies. Figure 6-4 is a research-based algorithm for weaning from servocontrol to air control in an incubator.

Radiant heat loss to cooler incubator walls, especially in single-walled incubators, is a significant source of heat loss. The use of *double-walled*

Criteria for Weaning to Air Control
1. Infant is medically stable and in a condition that permits weaning.
2. Infant requires minimal heat output from servocontrol set at 36.5° to 37° C (97.7° to 98.6° F).
3. Infant is gaining weight adequately: 15 to 20 g/kg/day, based on gestational age and chronologic age.

↓

1. Determine infant's age and weight.
2. Determine appropriate incubator temperature range (see Table 6-1).

↓

Remove the temperature probe and heat-reflecting disk using soap and water or mineral oil.

↓

Obtain the infant's axillary temperature to establish a baseline temperature. Temperature should be at least 36.5° C (97.7° F).

↓

Switch the heat from servocontrol to air control on the incubator and set the incubator control temperature (see Table 6-1).

↓

1. Obtain the infant's axillary temperature every 30 minutes to 1 hour.
2. Increase or decrease the temperature of the air control no more than 0.5 degree per 30 minutes or 1 degree per hour to maintain the infant's temperature.

FIGURE 6-4 Research-based algorithm for weaning from servocontrol to air control mode in an incubator (Courtesy Vivian Brown, RN.)

incubators (with the inner wall warmed to the ambient air temperature inside the incubator) results in less radiant heat loss from the baby. With a skin-set servocontrol temperature, the decreased radiant heat loss (because of warmer incubator walls) is offset by increased convective heat loss (because the ambient air temperature necessary for the desired skin temperature is lower). Consequently, there is no net change in the mean environmental temperature. Double-walled incubators provide less temperature fluctuation when doors are open, thus providing a more stable caregiving environment. Evaporative heat loss is not appreciably different with single- and double-walled incubators. One may increase the humidity in incubators to decrease the infant's metabolic rate only if a neutral thermal environment cannot be achieved by increasing the ambient temperature.

The tiniest neonate has a large evaporative heat loss, and maximum air temperature is limited by the incubator controls, thus making it difficult to reach an air temperature high enough for thermal support. In such cases, hypothermia can be avoided by increasing the ambient humidity within the incubator by using the water reservoir or supplying warmed humidified air into the incubator with respiratory humidifiers. Humidification has been shown to decrease fluid requirements and decrease the incidence of electrolyte imbalances in babies weighing less than 1000 g.[26] Careful attention should be given to preventing bacterial growth in the humidification system (see Chapter 23). Incubator temperatures may also be controlled manually by estimating the appropriate temperature for the baby's age and weight from Table 6-1 and setting the incubator to that temperature.

Regardless of whether one is using skin or air servocontrol or manual temperature adjustments, the baby's temperature and the air temperature must be monitored and recorded regularly. The incubator should be kept away from air conditioning ducts, direct sunlight, and cool windows that may cool or warm the incubator. Room temperature should be kept at 23.8° to 26.1° C (75° to 79° F) and humidity should be kept at 30% to 60%.[5] Seasonal mapping of one NICU showed seasonal variance in humidity level and evaporative temperature, both influences on thermal environment.[71] The researchers recommend periodic assessment of air, evaporative, and radiant temperatures, as well as humidity, in multiroom NICUs.[71] Alarms for both

high and low temperature levels always should be turned on.

The principal disadvantage of maintaining sick newborns in incubators is the limited access to them when extensive procedures are necessary. Incubators also may be perceived by mothers as a barrier between them and their infants and prolong feelings of fear and insecurity, compared with heating methods that provide easier access to the baby. Holding the baby in skin-to-skin (kangaroo care) helps promote bonding and relieves some of maternal and paternal fears (see later). Stable preterm infants dressed in a diaper, shirt, and cap and wrapped in two blankets can also maintain a normal temperature when held close to their parent's body. Keeping the skin probe attached to the infant and plugged into the incubator allows frequent monitoring of the infant's temperature. We also now have an increasing awareness of and concern about the high noise levels within incubators. Such noise poses a potential deleterious effect on the hearing development of preterm infants (see Chapter 13). Improved alarm technology minimizes the risk for inappropriate heating, but malfunctions still occur occasionally. When experienced nurses provide care, infants can be appropriately managed in incubators using any of the three modes of temperature control. Box 6-2 outlines "dos and don'ts" when using an incubator to provide heat and humidity.

Weaning an infant from an incubator to an open crib is an important step in preparing for discharge but may result in an increase in the resting metabolic rate for LBW infants.[22] Indicators that an infant may be successfully weaned include weight of 1600 g or more,[55,79] 5 days of consistent weight gain, an absence of medical complications, and tolerance of enteral feeds. Earlier weaning at lower body weight does not affect weight gain or temperature stability and may result in earlier discharge.[55,79] Weaning may occur over several days and involves dressing the infant in a shirt, hat, and diaper and swaddling with a blanket. The incubator temperature is manually lowered while monitoring the infant's temperature.

Abdominal skin temperature should be 36° to 37° C (96.8° to 98.6° F). Figures 6-5 and 6-6 are research-based algorithms for weaning infants to open cribs. After weaning has been successful, the crib should be placed in a draft-free environment.

TABLE 6-1 NEUTRAL THERMAL ENVIRONMENTAL TEMPERATURES

AGE AND WEIGHT	STARTING TEMPERATURE (° C)	RANGE OF TEMPERATURE (° C)	AGE AND WEIGHT	STARTING TEMPERATURE (° C)	RANGE OF TEMPERATURE (° C)
0-6 hr			**>72-96 hr**		
Under 1200 g	35.0	34.0-35.4	Under 1200 g	34.0	34.0-35.0
1200-1500 g	34.1	33.9-34.4	1200-1500 g	33.5	33.0-34.0
1501-2500 g	33.4	32.8-33.8	1501-2500 g	32.2	31.1-33.2
Over 2500 g	33.9	32.0-33.8	Over 2500 g	31.3	29.8-32.8
(and >36 wk)			(and >36 wk)		
>6-12 hr			**>4-12 days**		
Under 1200 g	35.0	34.0-35.4	Under 1500 g	33.5	33.0-34.0
1200-1500 g	34.0	33.5-34.4	1501-2500 g	32.1	31.0-33.2
1501-2500 g	33.1	32.2-33.8	Over 2500 g		
Over 2500 g	32.8	31.4-33.8	(and >36 wk)		
(and >36 wk)			4-5 days	31.0	29.5-32.6
			5-6 days	30.9	29.4-32.3
>12-24 hr			6-8 days	30.6	29.0-32.2
Under 1200 g	34.0	34.0-35.4	8-10 days	30.3	29.0-31.8
1200-1500 g	33.8	33.3-34.3	10-12 days	30.1	29.0-31.4
1501-2500 g	32.8	31.8-33.8	**>12-14 days**		
Over 2500 g	32.4	31.0-33.7	Under 1500 g	33.5	32.6-34.0
(and >36 wk)			1501-2500 g	32.1	31.0-33.2
>24-36 hr			**>2-3 wk**		
Under 1200 g	34.0	34.0-35.0	Under 1500 g	33.1	32.2-34.0
1200-1500 g	33.6	33.1-34.2	1501-2500 g	31.7	30.5-33.0
1501-2500 g	32.6	31.6-33.6	**>3-4 wk**		
Over 2500 g	32.1	30.7-33.5	Under 1500 g	32.6	31.6-33.6
(and >36 wk)			1501-2500 g	31.4	30.0-32.7
>36-48 hr			**>4-5 wk**		
Under 1200 g	34.0	34.0-35.0	Under 1500 g	32.0	31.2-33.0
1200-1500 g	33.5	33.0-34.1	1501-2500 g	30.9	29.5-32.2
1501-2500 g	32.5	31.4-33.5	**>5-6 wk**		
Over 2500 g	31.9	30.5-33.3	Under 1500 g	31.4	30.6-32.3
(and >36 wk)			1501-2500 g	30.4	29.0-31.8
>48-72 hr					
Under 1200 g	34.0	34.0-35.0			
1200-1500 g	33.5	33.0-34.0			
1501-2500 g	32.3	31.2-33.4			
Over 2500 g	31.7	30.1-33.2			
(and >36 wk)					

From American Academy of Pediatrics and American College of Obstetricians and Gynecologists: *Guidelines for perinatal care,* ed 2, Evanston, Ill, 1988, American Academy of Pediatrics and American College of Obstetricians and Gynecologists. Data from Scopes JW, Ahmed I: Minimal rates of oxygen consumption in sick and premature infants, *Arch Dis Child* 41:407, 1966; Scopes JW, Ahmed I: Range of critical temperatures in sick and premature newborn babies, *Arch Dis Child* 41:417, 1966.

Note: For their table, Scopes and Ahmed had the walls of the incubator 1° to 2° C warmer than the ambient air temperatures. Generally, the smaller infants in each weight group require a temperature in the higher portion of the temperature range. Within each time range, the younger the infant, the higher the temperature required.

BOX 6-2	USE OF AN INCUBATOR
	Dos and Don'ts

Dos

1. Place temperature probes according to manufacturer recommendations.
2. Change the incubator once a month.
3. Use sterile water for humidification.
4. Keep the incubator clean and free of spills.
5. Adequately humidify the incubator according to birth weight and gestational age of the infant.
6. Keep walls locked in place to prevent falls and provide a safe environment for the infant.
7. Clean incubators after each use and between patients with recommended cleaner, by trained staff.
8. Use servocontrol when first placing neonates in an incubator.
9. Follow weaning guidelines when changing from servocontrol to air control, using the weight and age chart (see Table 6-1).
10. Change the temperature probe site as directed by the manufacturer and hospital procedure.
11. Frequently monitor and record the infant's temperature, and observe for changes in clinical condition.

Don'ts

1. *Don't* place the temperature probe in the infant's axilla.[2]
2. Avoid pinching lines/tubes when opening/closing portholes and sides.
3. Avoid placing noisy equipment inside or on top of the incubator.
4. Avoid tapping, hitting, or knocking the incubator when the infant is in the bed.
5. Avoid keeping portholes open except for care and handling.
6. *Avoid* epidermal stripping (see Chapter 19) when applying/changing temperature probe sites.
7. Avoid pulling out lines or extubating the infant when moving/taking him or her out of the incubator.
8. *Don't* wean the servocontrol temperature less than 36.5° C (97.7° F).
9. *Don't* wean the temperature on the air control any faster than 0.5° per 30 minutes or 1° per hour.
10. Avoid cleaning the incubator with alcohol or acetone.
11. Do not keep the incubator in an unlocked position when in use. Do not position the incubator next to an air conditioner duct or in direct sunlight from a window.

Courtesy Vivian Brown, RN.

If an infant cannot maintain his or her temperature in an open crib, he or she is returned to the incubator. An attempt at weaning should be considered again by 48 hours after the initial weaning if all criteria for weaning have been met. The temperature in the neonatal unit should be evaluated, as well as the location of the crib in relation to air conditioner vents or drafts. There may also be other medical reasons (e.g., infection) that the infant cannot maintain his or her temperature in the open crib if all other conditions have been ruled out.[1]

Humidification and Topical Ointments

Many studies and clinical trials have demonstrated the clinical application of the uses of both humidity and topical ointment therapy (see Chapter 19) in preterm infants. The optimal humidity level for the neonate is 50% relative humidity (RH). This is achieved by a variety of methods such as closed humidified incubators and humidity "tents." In the first 2 weeks of life, extremely premature infants may require up to 85% RH. Box 6-3 describes the advantages and disadvantages of using heated, humidified air for ELBW infants while in an incubator.

Radiant Warmers

Radiant warmers provide infrared energy to heat the baby's skin while he or she lies naked on an open bed. The radiant warmer must generate enough energy to offset the tremendous amount of radiant heat lost to the room by a naked baby lying in an open environment. Heat output can be servocontrolled or manually controlled. Because with manual control no feedback from the infant is used, this poses a greater risk for overheating or overcooling. Therefore manual control should not be used routinely except for short periods (e.g., while initiating resuscitation). The servocontrol sensor measuring skin temperature must be protected from the infrared heat source, or the probe will sense a temperature higher than the skin temperature and decrease radiant heat output, leading to cold stress. Conversely, insulating the sensor with an aluminum reflective patch protects the underlying skin from the radiant heat and keeps the protected skin cooler than the surrounding skin. When the skin under the patch is warmed to the desired temperature, the rest of the skin may be overheated. Vasodilation then may increase convective heat loss, resulting in an effective, although precarious, heat balance. Caregivers must use caution to ensure that the

Weaning Criteria
Follow criteria for weaning found in Figure 6-4.

↓

Temperature Regulation
1. Have the infant undressed or dressed in a shirt only.
2. Set the temperature control at 36.5° to 37° C (97.7° to 98.6° F) to maintain a neutral thermal environment (NTE).
3. Keep the temperature probe in contact with the infant's skin to avoid possible overheating of the infant.

↓

Assess
1. Measure and record the infant's axillary temperature every 3 to 4 hours.

↓

Wean
1. Wean to open crib once air temperature of 28° C (82.4° F) has been maintained for 24 hours and infant's temperature remains at 36.5° C (97.7° F) or above.

↓

Insulate
1. Insulate just before moving to an open crib.
2. Dress the infant, and swaddle with one or two blankets.
3. Place a hat on the infant's head.

↓

Reevaluate and Intervene
1. Assess infant's temperature and add extra blankets as needed to maintain normal temperature of 36.5° to 37.5° C (97.7° to 99.5° F).
2. Replace infant into incubator if temperature falls below normal (36.5° C [97.7° F]) in spite of insulation, or if infant is cold stressed.

FIGURE 6-5 Research-based algorithm for servocontrolled weaning from an incubator to an open crib. (Courtesy Vivian Brown, RN.)

Criteria for Beginning to Wean Infant from Incubator
1. 32 weeks postmenstrual age or weighs 1600 g.
2. Medically stable and able to be swaddled.
3. Adequate weight gain, at least 15 to 20 g/kg/day.
4. Tolerating feedings.
5. Ambient temperature is greater than or equal to 32° C (89.6° F) for 24 hours.
6. Infant has normal temperature with a shirt, blanket, and hat during this time.
7. Environmental temperature is 22° to 26° C (72° to 78° F).

↓

Insulate
1. Dress the infant in a hat, shirt, and diaper, and swaddle in one or two blankets.

↓

Thermal Challenge
1. Decrease air temperature by 0.5° to 1° every 4 to 8 hours to maintain a normal axillary temperature. (Larger or more mature infants will wean faster.)

↓

Assess
1. Measure axillary temperature every 3 hours.
2. Wean the air temperature by an additional 0.5° if the axillary temperature is above normal at any time.

↓

Wean
1. Wean to an open crib when air temperature of 28° C has been maintained for 24 hours.
2. Add extra blankets as needed to assist the infant in keeping the axillary temperature at 36.5° to 37.5° C (97.7° to 99.5° F).
3. Stop weaning the infant or place back in the incubator if the temperature falls below 36.5° C (97.7° F) in spite of insulation or if the infant displays signs of cold stress.

FIGURE 6-6 Research-based algorithm for air mode/manual weaning from an incubator. (Courtesy Vivian Brown, RN.)

sensor does not become detached from the skin; otherwise the baby could be exposed to excess heat and become hyperthermic.

Insensible water loss (IWL) for babies cared for under radiant warmers is increased by 40% to 50% compared with losses in incubators. Directly related to the amount of heat necessary from the warmer, this loss also is influenced by other factors (e.g., low RH and convective air currents) on an open bed. Even though transepidermal water loss is increased under radiant warmers, there is evidence that the hydration of the stratum corneum is not affected; therefore the barrier function of the skin remains the same.[46] With very premature infants, severe dehydration may occur if water intake is not increased to replace the inordinate IWL (see Chapter 14). Plexiglas heat shields and polyethylene blankets (plastic wrap) have been used in an attempt to prevent large IWLs. Studies have shown these to be somewhat effective for this purpose; however, the microenvironment created by these blankets undergoes drastic change every time the blanket is removed for procedures or routine nursing care. Even without such blankets, the baby may experience wide swings in heat balance when the infrared heat is blocked from reaching him or her by hands, heads, or drapes during a procedure. These blankets should not be used while the infant is in an incubator, because the purpose is to have the humidity and heat reach the infant.

BOX 6-3	RESEARCH-BASED ADVANTAGES AND DISADVANTAGES OF HEATED HUMIDITY IN THE INCUBATOR OF ELBW INFANTS

Advantages

1. Decreased transepidermal water loss (e.g., insensible water loss [IWL], evaporative water loss, and epidermal heat loss) from the skin of infants less than 31 weeks of gestation. IWL is inversely proportionate to the gestational age of the infant.
2. Increased ability to maintain infant's temperature.
3. Improved maintenance of fluid and electrolyte balance.
4. Improved energy balance—fewer calories expended in temperature maintenance.
5. Improved skin integrity.
6. Possible reduction in the incidence of (1) PDA, (2) IVH (grades III/IV), and (3) BPD because of improved fluid and electrolyte balance.

Disadvantages

1. Increased risk for infection associated with contamination of the humidifier reservoir with bacteria.
2. Moist environment impairs adhesion of equipment (e.g., electrodes, ETT, dressings).
3. Unstable temperatures when procedures are performed and the incubator door is open.

BPD, Bronchopulmonary dysplasia; *ELBW*, extremely low birth weight; *ETT*, endotracheal tube; *IVH*, intraventricular hemorrhage; *PDA*, patent ductus arteriosus.

Both incubators and radiant warmers are effective in maintaining an appropriate thermal balance in sick and preterm infants. Evidence is insufficient to show a clear advantage of one method over the other with the caveat that IWL is significantly higher under radiant warmers.[24] The method chosen should be individualized to the infant and to the situation. Experience, skill, and nurse preference often influence the choice of heating methods. These factors also influence the extent to which incubators are perceived to interfere with the performance of care providers' tasks. Basic principles of care (e.g., keeping bed linens dry to prevent evaporative heat loss) apply to use of both heating methods. Box 6-4 lists advantages and disadvantages of open radiant warmers and incubators for temperature management in premature infants.[46]

Radiant warmers provide easy access for performing procedures—a definite advantage over incubators, in which procedures must be done through portholes. Advances in equipment technology now make it possible to convert a single unit from radiant mode to convection mode without moving the baby from one platform to another. This seems to be an efficient way to provide the improved access needed when a baby's condition changes while maintaining appropriate warming without the potential risks of moving the baby.[29] These hybrid devices improve care of ELBW infants by enhancing

BOX 6-4	ADVANTAGES AND DISADVANTAGES OF OPEN RADIANT WARMER VERSUS INCUBATOR USE FOR PREMATURE INFANTS

Advantages: Open Radiant Warmer

1. Easy access to the infant and larger surface on which to work
2. Useful for initial admission procedures (e.g., intubation, line placement, x-ray examination)
3. Decreased risk for infection without the use of humidity
4. Decreased risk for unplanned extubation and lines being pulled out
5. Better access by parents and staff

Disadvantages: Open Radiant Warmer

1. Increased insensible water loss[24] (without humidification or plastic blanket)
2. Increased stimulation from external noise and light
3. Decreased growth and weight gain patterns
4. Decreased ability to wean the infant slowly from the heat source
5. Better access by parents and staff

Advantages: Incubator

1. Less insensible water loss with use of humidity
2. Acts as a barrier with more difficult access that decreases tactile contact; easier to use minimal stimulation
3. Increased weight gain
4. Heat provided by two methods: convection and conduction
5. Ability to wean temperature control from servocontrol to air control, and from air control to an open crib
6. Ability to cover the incubator to decrease exposure to light

Disadvantages: Incubator

1. Decreased access for treatments, line placements, intubations, and laboratory draws
2. Increased chance of infection with humidity
3. Increased risk for extubation or accidental clamping of lines

BOX 6-5	USE OF OPEN RADIANT WARMER
	Dos and Don'ts

Dos

1. Use the automatic mode (skin probe/servocontrol) for continuous thermal support.
2. Use the manual mode for short-term warming *only;* check the infant's condition and temperature at least every 15 minutes.
3. Place the sensor on the skin surface exposed to the warmer and never beneath the infant. (Follow manufacturer's recommendations.)
4. Check sensor attachments frequently. Poor skin contact causes poor temperature control.
5. Change temperature probe sites according to unit policy and manufacturer's recommendations.
6. Be familiar with the radiant warmer in use as the effectiveness varies among commercial devices.[73]
7. Adjust fluid replacement to compensate for increased insensible water loss.

Don'ts

1. *Don't* forget to switch from manual to servocontrol after weighing the infant. When removing the infant from the radiant warmer, keep the bed on servocontrol and silence the alarm until the infant is returned to the radiant warmer.
2. *Never* use a rectal temperature probe for warmer control. Before normal core temperature is reached, the infant's skin may be burned.
3. *Don't* place anything flammable on top of or under the radiant warmer.
4. *Never* just reset alarms; instead, determine the cause of any alarms.
5. *Never* use your hand to estimate the amount of heat reaching the infant. Set temperature control point at 36.5° C.
6. *Avoid* use of thermal blankets (e.g., bubble wrap); may cause incorrect skin temperature sensing and overheating.

growth velocity, improving electrolyte balance, decreasing fluid intake, and maintaining stable body temperature.[35] Fluid management is easier for infants in incubators because humidity is easily added to the enclosed environment and there are fewer losses from radiation and convection. The large flux of heat exchange between radiant heat source, the baby, and the environment makes wide fluctuations in heat balance more likely when compared with the more easily controlled temperature within an incubator. Many variables influence oxygen consumption using these two heating methods. The metabolic rate and oxygen consumption of infants under radiant warmers are slightly higher than in incubators; however, the clinical significance of this finding is uncertain. Infection rates are comparable between the two methods.[50] Regardless of the type of heat supplied, care must be taken to minimize thermal instability during nursing interventions. Radiant warmers may be able to rewarm a baby faster than an incubator with convective heating after a procedure.[53] Organizing interventions so their frequency and duration limit as much as possible the exposure to a thermally unstable environment can minimize this instability. Box 6-5 outlines dos and don'ts when using a radiant warmer for providing heat.

Other Methods

In the tiniest preterm infants, a conductive heat source (e.g., a heating pad) may also be needed to raise and maintain body temperature. Heated water mattresses provide a neutral thermal environment for less critically ill babies lying in open cribs (making access easier than in closed incubators). This may also provide a feasible and effective means of rewarming hypothermic infants. Heated, water-filled mattresses are most useful in the newborn units of developing countries.

Electric warming mattresses filled with water provide additional moist heat when caring for the infant in surgery, to use for rewarming techniques, or when caring for the LBW or ELBW infant. Manufacturer's recommendations should be followed, and the temperature is usually set at 100° F. Heat is provided by conduction; therefore a linen layer should be placed between the mattress and the infant to avoid skin burns. The temperature of these mattresses should be weaned before weaning any temperature of the open warmer or incubator.

Some portable, disposable, warming mattresses containing a gel that is chemically activated by squeezing may be used for initial stabilization of the infant and for transport. Because heat is provided by conduction, a linen layer is placed between the infant and the mattress surface. The usual temperature for these mattresses is 100° F.

Heel warmers, which are pads that are chemically activated by squeezing, are used to warm the heels of infants before obtaining blood and are especially necessary when obtaining capillary blood gases. The temperature should never exceed 104° F.

Swaddling materials include various types of infant wrappings (e.g., blanket, clothing, foil, or bubble wrap). The use of swaddling materials makes observation of the infant more difficult and blocks heat from overhead radiant warmers. Before one wraps the infant in insulating materials, the infant must be warm, because these merely retain body warmth and do not generate heat.

Oxygen and air delivered to the neonate should be warmed and humidified to minimize convective and evaporative heat loss (see Chapter 23).

Skin-to-skin (kangaroo) care provides a safe and effective alternative method of caring for premature infants. Both appropriate-for-gestational-age (AGA) and SGA infants experience a beneficial warming effect and a stable skin and core temperature when held skin to skin.[45] Mothers exhibit thermal synchrony with the infants so that their body temperature increases or decreases to maintain the infant's thermal neutrality.[9,44] Regardless of the care provider (e.g., father, adoptive parent, grandparent) during skin-to-skin care, heat loss does not occur and temperature rises and can be maintained within acceptable parameters (see Chapter 5). In one study, each mother's skin temperature met the neutral thermal environmental zone of her particular infant. Mothers also preferred this method for holding their infant, compared with the traditional method of wrapping the infant in a blanket and the infant being cradled in the parent's arms. Heat loss may occur during the transfer process from bed to parent. Having a protocol in place that uses one or more staff to help with the transfer and covering the infant with a blanket will reduce the transfer time and subsequent heat loss[45] (see Chapter 13).

Skin-to-skin contact between mother and infant reduces conductive and radiant heat loss and is an excellent way to maintain a neutral thermal condition for the healthy newborn.[52] If the infant remains with the parents for an extended time, temperature should be monitored. In the case of a preterm infant in stable condition, the use of an additional heat source (e.g., a radiant warmer) enables parents to spend more time with their infant before transfer to the NICU. Thermal stability of 26 extremely preterm infants (22 to 26 weeks; 2 to 9 days of age) in early skin-to-skin care has been studied. During skin-to-skin care, extremely preterm infants were able to both maintain and increase their body temperature after the drop that occurred during transfer from the incubator.[34]

Another study analyzing 70 skin-to-skin sessions found lower variation in body temperature in 25 to 28 weeks. gestational age preterms compared with the 29 to 32 weeks' gestational age group at 33 to 36 weeks' post-menstrual age (PMA). These very preterm infants exhibited an advanced maturation of thermoregulation compared with the higher gestational age group.[57]

Bathing is important for removing blood and body fluids from the newborn's skin, to prevent the transmission of infections, and to promote bonding. Sponge bathing is traditionally done in the NICU and newborn nursery and can result in significant heat loss. Immersing the stable infant in a tub of water reduces evaporative heat loss and helps maintain a normal temperature.[14,24]

Transport

The same principles of heat balance that apply to infants in NICUs apply to infants during transport. Infants should have a normal and stable temperature before transport. The infant should be transferred from nursery to transport incubator rapidly to prevent prolonged exposure to an uncontrolled thermal environment. Transport incubators that can provide thermal stability inside the transport vehicle must be used. Oxygen provided during transport also should be warmed and humidified. The infant's temperature should be monitored continuously or at least every 30 minutes. Thin plastic wrap may be useful in decreasing IWL and convective and radiant heat loss. Chemically heated mattresses can also be used to provide a short-term heat source.

After Cesarean Delivery

Most cesarean section (C-section) deliveries are performed using an epidural or spinal anesthesia so the mother is awake and able to hear her infant as soon as he or she is born. Once the baby is assessed after birth, he or she is then placed skin-to-skin on the mother's chest and both are wrapped with a warm blanket. When the infant recovers in the same room as the mother, skin-to-skin contact and bonding are facilitated.[50] If the mother and baby do not recover together in the same room and the mother must return from the operating room, skin-to-skin care is still possible. The father may provide skin-to-skin care and keep the baby warm after C-section until the mother returns to her postpartum room. In a study of elective C-section, 34 pairs of mothers and their newborns were randomized to skin-to-skin or routine nursery care within the 2 hours after the mother returned from the operating room.[28] Mean temperatures in both groups were equivalent, but the skin-to-skin care babies attached to the breast earlier, were exclusively or prevalently breastfed at discharge and 3 months, and mothers were highly satisfied with skin-to-skin contact with their babies[28] (see Chapter 5).

Providing Thermoregulation for the Surgical Patient

The chilled environment of the surgical suite poses extra challenges to the newborn for thermoregulation. Heat losses occur by (1) evaporation during surgery, (2) conduction when placed on cold surfaces, (3) convection with cold drafts around the infant,[66] and (4) radiation of heat from opened body cavities. Coordination between neonatal and surgical staff will be necessary to prevent heat imbalance, as follows:

- Prewarm transport incubator.
- Use portable, disposable mattresses in the incubators and on the operating table.
- Use radiant heat in the operating suite.
- Wrap the infant's extremities in warmed soft cotton material.
- Prewarm all surfaces, as well as all fluids for cleansing and irrigation of body cavities.
- IV fluids should be at room temperature and prewarmed if stored in refrigeration.
- Temperatures should be monitored/documented before, during, and after surgery.

DATA COLLECTION

Anticipation and early recognition of the infant at risk for temperature instability are important in the management and prevention of complications associated with both hypothermia and hyperthermia. The perinatal history and ongoing neonatal evaluation identify events and early risk factors of temperature instability.

History

Events during pregnancy and the early neonatal period may increase an infant's risk for thermal instability. Review of the maternal history should include estimated date of confinement because preterm infants at delivery are at increased risk for hypothermia. Exposure to viral agents (e.g., herpes), as well as vaginal and cervical colonization, increases the risk for acquiring an infection before or during delivery (see Chapter 22). Intrapartal use of analgesics and anesthetics may depress the infant's CNS and mute the thermoregulatory ability.

Fetal stress manifested as fetal decelerations, meconium-stained fluid, or low Apgar scores may suggest an impaired thermoregulatory response. Neonatal interventions that may depress the CNS and thermal response include resuscitation and administration of analgesics, anesthetics, or neuromuscular blocking agents. Invasive procedures (e.g., endotracheal intubations, umbilical catheterization) increase the infant's risk for infection and need for prolonged use of antibiotics. Poor handwashing by care providers also may contribute to infectious nursery outbreaks, such as outbreaks of necrotizing enterocolitis (see Chapters 22 and 28).

Physical Examination: Signs and Symptoms

Physical assessment of the infant should include not only gestational age but also appropriateness of size. Evaluation of the infant's neurologic status (e.g., tone, activity, alertness) may give the caregiver an indication of the extent of neurologic impairment. Hypotonia results in decreased flexion, with an increased exposed surface area and resultant heat loss.

TEMPERATURE DETERMINATIONS

Temperature determinations may need to be made as often as every 30 minutes until thermostability is achieved. After that, temperatures should be recorded every 1 to 3 hours in LBW and preterm infants and every 4 hours in the healthy term infant. Critically ill infants should have continuous monitoring of skin temperature, with axillary determinations every 1 to 2 hours.[5] Documentation should include environmental temperature (e.g., air temperature in the incubator or radiant warmer settings). Measuring the skin and core temperatures simultaneously may help differentiate fever as a result of disease versus environmental overheating. Noting that the baby's servocontrolled skin temperature is relatively stable but that the environmental temperature has dropped also may be indicative of fever as the incubator responds to the high probe reading by cooling the infant's environment.

Laboratory Data

The following may be used to evaluate metabolic derangements associated with thermal instability:

- Arterial blood gases (to assess for hypoxemia and metabolic acidosis)
- Complete blood count (to assess for sepsis)
- Blood glucose level (to assess for hypoglycemia)
- Electrolytes, blood urea nitrogen (BUN), and serum and urine osmolality (to assess hydration, acid–base balance, and renal function)

HYPOTHERMIA

As the infant attempts to conserve heat by vasoconstriction, he or she may be pale, appear mottled, and feel cool to touch, particularly on the extremities. Acrocyanosis and respiratory distress may occur as the infant increases oxygen consumption in an attempt to increase heat production. If hypothermia continues, apnea, bradycardia, and central cyanosis may occur. The hypothermic infant initially may be irritable but may become lethargic as cold stress continues. Other changes that may occur include hypotonia, weak cry, weak suck, increased gastric residuals, abdominal distention, and emesis. Infants generally do not shiver in response to cold stress, but shivering may occur in more mature babies in the presence of severe hypothermia. Chronic hypothermia may result in poor weight gain (Box 6-6).

Treatment and Intervention

To avoid the complications of hypothermia, rewarming of cold infants should begin immediately by providing external heat. However, rewarming too rapidly may further compromise the already cold-stressed infant and result in apnea. Oxygen consumption is minimal when the difference between the skin and the ambient air temperature is less than 1.5° C (2.7° F). Avenues of heat loss should be blocked, temperatures should be monitored, and iatrogenic or pathologic causes should be investigated.

If hypothermia is mild, slow rewarming is preferred. External heat sources should be slightly warmer than the skin temperature and gradually increased until the neutral thermal environmental temperature range is attained. Efforts to block

> **BOX 6-6** **CRITICAL FINDINGS**
> **HYPOTHERMIA**
>
> Critical assessment findings for hypothermia are as follows:
> - Pale, mottled skin that is cool to touch
> - Acrocyanosis
> - Respiratory distress
> - Apnea, bradycardia, central cyanosis
> - Irritability initially
> - Lethargy developing as hypothermia worsens
> - Hypotonia
> - Weak cry and suck
> - Gastric residuals, abdominal distention, emesis
> - Shivering in more mature babies
> - Metabolic acidosis
> - Hypoglycemia

heat loss by convection, radiation, evaporation, and conduction should be initiated. Skin, axillary, and environmental temperatures should be measured and recorded every 30 minutes during the rewarming period. For more extreme hypothermia (i.e., core temperatures less than 35° C [95° F]), more rapid rewarming with radiant heaters (servocontrol 37° C [98.6° F]) or heated water mattresses prevents prolonged metabolic acidosis or hypoglycemia and decreases mortality risk.

Complications

Acute cold stress results in the release of norepinephrine, which causes vasoconstriction to reduce heat loss and initiate thermogenesis. As glycogen stores are depleted and oxygen consumption increases, the infant uses anaerobic metabolism to increase heat production, resulting in lactic acid production (metabolic acidosis). Pulmonary vasoconstriction, accentuated by metabolic acidosis, is associated with hypoxia, decreased surfactant production, and further acidosis (see Chapter 23). Blood flow to vital organs is diminished, and pulmonary hemorrhage and death may occur if hypothermia continues.

Hyperbilirubinemia and kernicterus may occur as nonesterified free fatty acids from brown fat metabolism compete with bilirubin for albumin-binding sites. Acidosis not only decreases the affinity of albumin for bilirubin but also increases the permeability of the blood-brain barrier, allowing bilirubin to enter brain tissue. If hypothermia continues, carbohydrate, protein, and fat supplies will be used for heat production instead of growth.

Close monitoring of the hypothermic infant is essential for early identification and prevention of complications. Evaluation of vital signs, arterial blood gases, and oxygen saturation may give early indication of hypoxia and metabolic acidosis. The infant's skin may be dusky or bright red because failure of dissociation of oxyhemoglobin occurs at low body temperatures. Respirations may be rapid, shallow, and grunting and accompanied by bradycardia. Oxygen and ventilation should be initiated as needed to reduce hypoxia. Sodium bicarbonate may be needed to correct documented metabolic acidosis. Seizures may occur as a result of hypoxia, requiring the administration of anticonvulsants.

Intravenous glucose may be necessary to prevent or correct hypoglycemia. Blood glucose levels should be monitored hourly until stable (see Chapter 15). Blood pressure and urine output should be measured to evaluate hydration and kidney function. An elevated BUN and hyperkalemia may be indicators of decreased renal perfusion and impaired renal function. As fluid is retained, edema of the extremities and face may occur.

Bilirubin should be monitored on a regular basis, and phototherapy may be initiated at a lower-than-usual level to prevent kernicterus. Adequate nutrition to promote growth should be given either intravenously or enterally. While the infant is hypothermic, nipple feedings should be avoided to conserve calories and energy for heat production and growth and to avoid aspiration.

During the rewarming process, the hypothermic infant should be observed for hypotension as vasodilation occurs. Volume expanders may be needed to maintain an adequate blood pressure. Apnea and seizures may occur as a result of hypoxia or decreased cerebral blood flow after vasodilation. Hypothermia as a strategy to minimize adverse outcomes from hypoxic-ischemicencephalopathy continues to be the focus of considerable research to determine safety and efficacy (see Chapter 26).

HYPERTHERMIA

The hyperthermic infant may feel warm to touch, and skin color may be ruddy as the infant attempts to increase heat loss by vasodilation. Sweating may occur in a term infant but generally is not present in infants of less than 36 weeks' gestation. Sweating may first appear on the forehead, followed by the chest, upper arms, and lower body. Hyperthermia is manifested by irritability, lethargy, hypotonia, apnea, a weak or absent cry, or poor feedings. Tachypnea or tachycardia may be seen as the infant attempts to increase heat loss.

Infants with thermal instability should be closely watched for changes in behavior, feeding patterns, and respiratory status. Temperatures should be monitored frequently in any infant exhibiting these symptoms or who feels cool or warm to touch. Early recognition of thermal instability may prevent further consequences and possibly permanent injury or death (Box 6-7).

Treatment and Intervention

The usual approach to treating the hyperthermic infant is to cool by removing external heat sources and by removing anything that blocks heat loss. The most common causes of hyperthermia in intensive care nurseries are iatrogenic. Check the heating controls for proper function and thermistors for proper position. Consider other sources of heat (e.g., direct sunlight, heaters, lights) as possible causes of hyperthermia. Excessive bundling with blankets and a hat and elevated environmental temperature can cause a newborn's body temperature to rise into the febrile range. When evaluating the treatment options in the hyperthermic infant, one should consider removing extra blankets or swaddling materials. Nonenvironmental causes

---

BOX 6-7 | **CRITICAL FINDINGS**
HYPERTHERMIA

Critical assessment findings for hyperthermia are as follows:
- Reddened skin that is warm to touch
- Tachypnea
- Tachycardia
- Irritability, lethargy, hypotonia, weak cry
- Poor feeding
- Apnea
- Sweating in more mature babies
- Dehydration

of hyperthermia (e.g., infection, dehydration, CNS disorders) should be considered. During the cooling process, skin, axillary, and environmental temperatures should be monitored and recorded every 30 minutes.

Complications

Vasodilation to increase heat loss may cause hypotension and dehydration as a result of increased IWL. Seizures and apnea may also occur as a result of high core temperature. Fluid status should be monitored by assessing intake, output, electrolytes, serum and urine osmolality, skin turgor, and mucous membranes. Fluids should be adjusted to account for IWL. Blood pressure should be assessed to detect hypotension, and volume expanders should be administered as needed.

Cardiorespiratory monitoring to detect apnea should be used. Ventilation may be needed if apnea persists or is unresponsive to stimulation. Subtle signs of seizures may include facial grimacing, nystagmus, tremors, apnea, opisthotonos posturing, tongue thrusting, or staring (see Chapter 26).

PARENT TEACHING

While the neonate is in the NICU, parents should be taught the importance of maintaining the newborn's normal body temperature. Temperature should be taken before parents touch the infant through the portholes of the incubator or hold their infant. While the infant is outside the incubator, monitor the skin temperature continuously with a telethermometer. Unwrapping the infant to check the temperature exposes him or her to cold stress. Additional heat sources (e.g., radiant warmer, hat, extra blankets) may be needed while parents hold the infant. Teach parents to monitor their infant's temperature and notify the nurse if it rises or falls (Box 6-8).

Before discharge, teach parents to take an accurate axillary temperature and to notify their physician if it drops below 36° C (96.8° F) or rises above 37.8° C (100° F). A parent should not routinely take a rectal temperature. The temperature should be taken whenever the infant

---

> **BOX 6-8**   **PARENT TEACHING**
> **TEMPERATURE REGULATION**
>
> - Teach parents how to take an axillary temperature on their newborn and maintain the axillary temperature between 36.5° and 37.4° C (97.7° and 99.3° F).[5]
> - Teach parents how to dress their infant with clothes and blankets and use an appropriate environmental temperature to maintain the baby's temperature in the above range.
> - Teach parents appropriate safety precautions, which include verbal and written information about recognizing signs and symptoms of a sick/ill infant, as well as how the infant acts, including temperatures either higher than or, more commonly, lower than the range of 36.5° to 37.4° C (97.7° to 99.3° F).
> - Teach parents to notify their infant's primary health care provider immediately or to take the infant to the nearest emergency department for temperatures out of the above range, especially if the baby's feeding pattern changes.

feels cool or warm to the touch. The nurse should observe the parents taking the infant's axillary temperature before discharge.

The home environment should be kept at a temperature that prevents heat and cold stress. A room temperature that is comfortable for the parent usually is suitable for the infant. The infant should be in clothing appropriate for the room temperature. For example, if the parent requires a sweater to be comfortable, the infant probably also requires a sweater. Parents often overdress the infant or overheat the home, and this may cause hyperthermia. Parents should be given written instructions before discharge on how and when to take an axillary temperature, when to call the physician, and how to maintain a comfortable environment for their infant.

REFERENCES

For a full list of references, scan the QR code or visit http://booksite.elsevier.com/9780323320832.

7

PHYSIOLOGIC MONITORING

WANDA TODD BRADSHAW AND DAVID T. TANAKA

Significant advances in the management of the ill newborn have been made in the past 60 years. The clinical usefulness of the umbilical vein was first demonstrated by Diamond in 1947 to perform an exchange transfusion to prevent kernicterus. Later, James used the umbilical artery for acid-base determination. In most neonatal intensive care units (NICUs), use of these catheters has become the standard of care to assess blood gases, measure arterial and central venous pressures, administer medications and fluids, and obtain laboratory samples. The development of small, indwelling, peripherally inserted central catheters provides a route for administering the aforementioned items and may be used for laboratory sample withdrawal if no other method of obtaining blood is available. Because of the frequency and clinical significance of complications, alternatives to these intravascular routes have been vigorously sought. The development of non-invasive physiologic monitoring devices has been a major step toward this goal. In addition, the use of point-of-care testing for various laboratory values is evolving in neonatal care. This chapter reviews the procedures and advances in physiologic monitoring.

PHYSIOLOGY

Pulmonary Physiology

Gas exchange takes place in the alveoli of the lung. Ventilation is the movement of air into and out of these airspaces. Diffusion is the movement of oxygen (O_2) from the alveolar space into the pulmonary capillary and the movement of carbon dioxide (CO_2) from the pulmonary capillary into the alveolar space for eventual exhalation. Pulmonary perfusion is the flow of blood through the pulmonary capillaries that surround the alveolar spaces. Once oxygen diffuses through the cells lining the alveoli and into the capillaries, it is predominately bound to hemoglobin within the red blood cell. Oxygen content in the arterial blood is the sum of the amount of oxygen dissolved in the plasma and the amount bound to hemoglobin. Approximately 3% of the oxygen content is dissolved in the plasma, with the remaining 97% bound to hemoglobin. PaO_2 is the partial pressure of the oxygen dissolved in arterial plasma. *Fetal hemoglobin* has a higher affinity for oxygen than does adult hemoglobin; therefore, at any given PaO_2, more oxygen is bound to adult hemoglobin (Figure 7-1). Each hemoglobin molecule can carry four oxygen molecules. *Oxygen saturation* (SaO_2) is the percentage of oxygen bound to hemoglobin.

Carbon dioxide content in the arterial blood is the sum of the amount of carbon dioxide in the plasma plus the amount bound to hemoglobin. As hemoglobin gives up oxygen to the tissues it is able to pick up carbon dioxide. Each reduced hemoglobin molecule can carry four carbon dioxide molecules, thus lowering the free hydrogen ion (H^+) concentration. Approximately 10% of the carbon dioxide content is gas dissolved in the plasma (CO_2), 60% is carbonic acid (H_2CO_3), and the remaining 30% is attached to proteins, predominantly hemoglobin. $PaCO_2$ is the partial pressure of carbon dioxide dissolved in arterial blood. It is a measured value that denotes the partial pressure of arterial carbon dioxide. Carbon dioxide values fluctuate as needed to maintain the hydrogen ion

PURPLE type highlights content that is particularly applicable to clinical settings.

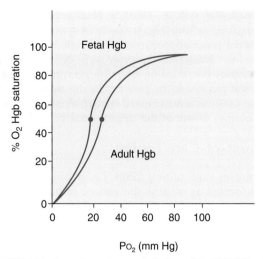

FIGURE 7-1 Oxygen dissociation curves for fetal hemoglobin *(Hgb) (left)* and adult hemoglobin *(right)*.

concentration, or pH, within a normal range. Carbon dioxide combines reversibly with water to yield hydrogen (H^+) and bicarbonate (HCO_3^-) ions. The formula is $CO_2 + H_2O \leftrightarrow H_2CO_3 \leftrightarrow H^+ + HCO_3^-$.

NONINVASIVE MONITORING

Use of noninvasive technologies to monitor *all* neonates in the NICU is the standard of care. Many neonates also require invasive monitoring devices.

Oxygen and Carbon Dioxide

OXYGEN

Noninvasive monitoring of oxygenation can be accomplished by using two monitoring technologies, *pulse oximetry* and *transcutaneous oxygen monitor. Oxygen saturation monitoring* is the most common and widely used method for assessing oxygenation status. Transmission technology relies on a pulsating arterial vascular bed between a dual light source and a photoreceptor. As blood passes between the light source and the photoreceptor, different amounts of red and infrared light are absorbed, depending on the amount of oxyhemoglobin and reduced hemoglobin. With reflectance oximetry, the emitter and receptor are located beside each other. Emitted light is reflected back to the photoreceptor. This method uses the core

body to obtain oxygen saturation and is useful when the patient's peripheral blood flow is diminished. With both methods, the difference in light absorption is electronically processed and displayed by the monitor as the percentage of arterial hemoglobin oxygen saturation expressed as SpO_2. Pulse oximetry probes are easy to apply and require no warm-up period, calibration, or application of heat.

The second method of noninvasive monitoring of oxygenation is *transcutaneous oxygen tension,* which relies on the principle of oxygen diffusing from the skin capillaries through the dermis to the surface of the skin. To measure the oxygen, it is necessary to have adequate perfusion of the site, to intermittently calibrate the sensor, and to heat the skin, which then dilates the local capillaries and arterializes the capillary bed, as well as promotes faster diffusion of the oxygen from the skin.[26]

CARBON DIOXIDE

Carbon dioxide also can be assessed using two different devices, *transcutaneous carbon dioxide* and *end-tidal carbon dioxide* monitors. *Transcutaneous carbon dioxide ($PtcCO_2$)* monitoring works under similar principles as for transcutaneous oxygen monitoring.[24] The probe is a glass pH electrode that detects changes in pH caused by CO_2. Heating of the probe enhances CO_2 diffusion, providing a better correlation between the probe value and the $PaCO_2$ value. The second method used to measure the content of the carbon dioxide in the respiratory gases during the respiratory cycle is *end-tidal carbon dioxide ($PetCO_2$)* monitoring, also called *capnometry.* With capnometry, an infrared light absorption determines the amount of CO_2 present in the sample. Capnography provides a visual graphic curve of $PetCO_2$. The carbon dioxide content varies widely with the phase of the respiratory cycle. During inspiration, there are minimal amounts of carbon dioxide, whereas at the end of expiration, the carbon dioxide values are at their maximum level (Figure 7-2). Until recently, the relatively fast respiratory rate of newborns, combined with the small tidal volumes, resulted in inaccurate values when measured by end-tidal carbon dioxide monitors. Advances in technology have improved the reliability of this monitoring technique for newborn infants.

COMBINED OXYGEN–CARBON DIOXIDE MONITORING

$SpO_2/PtcCO_2$ sensors combining pulse oximetry and transcutaneous carbon dioxide monitoring have

CO_2

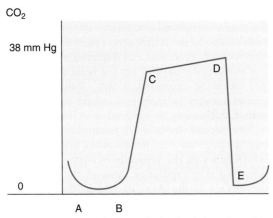

FIGURE 7-2 *Variations in the content of carbon dioxide during phases of the respiratory cycle. A, End of inspiration. B, Beginning of exhalation. C, End of mixed gases washout (dead space and alveolar gases). D, End of expiration of alveolar gases. E, Inspiration.*

been developed. The heated sensor is attached to the patient's ear. It provides rapid SpO_2 values followed by carbon dioxide information within minutes as the site is warmed and arterialized. A single probe, designed to withstand motion artifact and low perfusion states, leads from the patient to the monitor. Because the probe is attached to the ear, its removal for chest radiographs or prone positioning is not necessary. Studies on normal adults, infants, and very-low-birth-weight (VLBW) infants have shown acceptable correlation with both invasive and non-invasive monitoring techniques for oxygen. Carbon dioxide values were less reliable but allowed trending of ventilation status.[25]

Cardiorespiratory Monitoring

The electrical activity of an infant's heart is picked up by chest leads (usually three) placed on the infant and recorded by a cardiorespiratory monitor. The recording is displayed on a visual screen as the infant's electrocardiographic pattern. The infant's respiratory pattern also is recorded, because the chest leads electronically detect movement of his or her chest with each respiration.

Blood Pressure Monitoring

Systolic blood pressure, measured in millimeters of mercury (mm Hg), is the pressure at the height of the arterial pulse and coincides with left ventricular systole. *Diastolic blood pressure,* also measured in mm Hg, is the lowest point of the arterial pulse and coincides with left ventricular diastole. *Mean arterial pressure* is the diastolic pressure plus one third of the pulse pressure. *Central venous pressure* is the pressure in the right atrium and may be approximated by the blood pressure (volume) in any of the large central veins.

Point-of-Care Testing

Point-of-care testing (POCT) involves testing performed at or near the patient rather than in a laboratory. This process has steadily evolved from crude blood glucose determinations to numerous types of monitoring. Currently, whole blood glucose values, transcutaneous bilirubin, fecal occult blood, gastric pH, urine dipstick, activated clotting time, hematocrit, some electrolyte values, and arterial blood gases are part of POCT for the neonatal population.

The indications for using the various techniques for physiologic data collection depend on the infant's clinical situation.

Noninvasive Oxygen and Carbon Dioxide Monitoring

Oxygen monitoring is indicated in infants receiving oxygen for any reason (see Chapter 23). Acute monitoring is used as a part of the management of acute respiratory disorders. Long-term monitoring is used to wean infants with chronic lung disease from oxygen therapy. Noninvasive oxygen monitoring is useful during transport, in emergency situations, and during procedures. However, this method provides no information on hemoglobin level, adequacy of ventilation, and oxygen delivery to the tissues and should be used as one part of total oxygenation and ventilation assessment. Even though oxygen saturation monitoring is used more, less variability in oxygen tension has been demonstrated when transcutaneous oxygen monitoring has been employed.[26]

Carbon dioxide monitoring is useful for verifying that the endotracheal tube is in the trachea (end-tidal CO_2 monitoring) and for the infant with a respiratory disease in which retention of carbon dioxide may become clinically significant (end-tidal CO_2 and transcutaneous CO_2 monitoring).

Cardiorespiratory Monitoring

Cardiorespiratory monitoring should be used in *all* infants who require intensive or intermediate care, as well as in *all* infants at risk for apnea or rhythm disturbances.

Blood Pressure Monitoring

Blood pressure monitoring should be used in the infant requiring surgery, in the acutely ill infant with cardiorespiratory distress, and in any other illness in which hypotension may be a significant contributor to the pathologic state. Central venous pressure should be monitored in infants who may experience an excess or loss of blood volume.

Umbilical Artery Catheters

An umbilical artery catheter (UAC) is placed in those infants requiring frequent arterial blood gas determinations, continuous monitoring of arterial blood pressure, and infusion of parenteral fluids. The practice of medication administration through a UAC varies although there are no published data in the past decade regarding this practice.[21,28] Infants who are candidates for indwelling catheters include critically ill neonates and those with congenital heart disease or disorders that cause respiratory insufficiency (e.g., surfactant deficiency, meconium aspiration syndrome, persistent pulmonary hypertension, diaphragmatic hernia). Although use of an indwelling UAC allows arterial pressure monitoring and accessibility for parenteral infusions, it is generally not used for these indications alone.

Umbilical Vein Catheters

Umbilical vein catheters (UVCs) are useful for exchange transfusions, central venous pressure monitoring, emergency administration of fluids or chemicals in delivery room resuscitation, and administration of parenteral fluids and medications in the NICU, as well as obtaining blood for laboratory analysis. UVCs are being used with increasing frequency for initial management of extremely low-birth-weight (ELBW) infants. Catheters used to cannulate the umbilical vein are

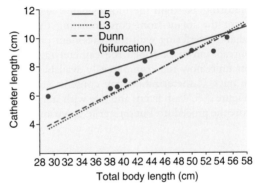

FIGURE 7-3 Graph for distance of catheter insertion from umbilical ring for low placement. (From Rosenfeld W, Biagtan J, Schaeffer H, et al: A new graph for insertion of umbilical artery catheters, *J Pediatr* 96:735, 1980.)

available as both single-lumen and double-lumen items. Double-lumen catheters permit the simultaneous administration of infusates and medications. Use of a UVC reduces the need for peripheral lines when multilumen UVCs are used.

INTERVENTIONS

Invasive Monitoring

Placement of UACs or UVCs and placement of a peripherally inserted central catheter (PICC) are invasive monitoring techniques.

Umbilical Artery Catheter Placement

PROCEDURE

Determine the size and length of the catheter to be inserted. For infants weighing more than 1250 g, use a 5-Fr catheter, and for infants weighing less than 1250 g, use a 3.5-Fr catheter. Figures 7-3 and 7-4 correlate total body length with the length of the catheter to be inserted. Whereas these charts have worked reasonably well in larger preterm and term infants, a newer formula (4 × birth weight in kilograms + 7) resulted in significantly better placement in VLBW infants.[8,14]

Place the infant in a supine position on a radiant heater or in an incubator. Ensure continuous temperature monitoring. Skin temperature should remain between 36° and 37° C (96.8° and 98.6° F). Provide appropriate oxygenation and ventilation. Ensure cardiorespiratory and oxygen saturation monitoring. Restrain the infant's hands and feet to prevent the infant from contaminating the sterile field and interfering with the placement procedure. Don cap and mask. Open the catheterization tray; most units now use commercially available disposable trays. Catheterization tray contents are shown in Figure 7-5. Wash hands and dry with sterile towel before the procedure. Put on sterile gown and gloves.

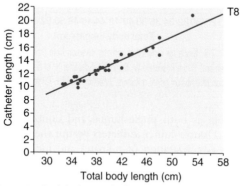

FIGURE 7-4 Graph for distance of catheter insertion from umbilical ring for high placement (T8). (From Rosenfeld W, Estrada R, Jhaveri R, et al: Evaluation of graphs for insertion of umbilical artery catheters below the diaphragm, *J Pediatr* 98:627, 1981.)

Connect the catheter to the stopcock, and flush and fill the entire system, including the catheter, with flush solution. Turn off the stopcock to the catheter to prevent fluid from draining out of the catheter during insertion and securing of the catheter. Cleanse the cord and base of the umbilicus with either povidone-iodine or chlorhexidine with alcohol three times, and allow the site to air-dry.[22] Remove the povidone-iodine with alcohol. For infants weighing less than 1000 g, utilize sterile water. Avoid using an excess of skin disinfectant so the infant is not lying in the solution during the procedure. Any residual skin disinfectant should be washed off the infant carefully after the procedure is completed.

Drape the infant by placing an eye sheet over the umbilicus. An alternative method is to use sterile drapes, as follows:

1. Hold the diagonal corners of one drape, and allow the top half to fold over the bottom half. The result is a V shape.
2. Place the tips of the V on either side of the umbilicus.
3. Repeat with another drape and place on the other side of the umbilicus. The umbilical stump is now visible, yet surrounded by drapes.

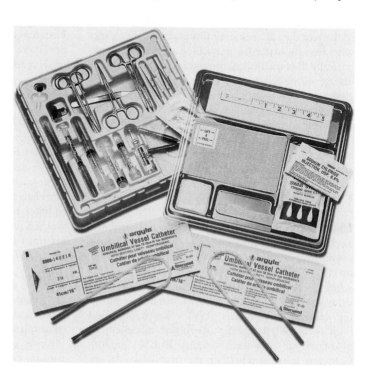

FIGURE 7-5 Argyle umbilical vessel catheter insertion tray. (Courtesy Tyco/Healthcare Kendall-LTP.)

After the UAC is inserted, the drapes can be removed easily without the need to pass the stopcock and catheter through an eyehole of a drape or cut or tear the eyehole drape. Ensure that the infant's head and feet remain visible during the procedure to assess color. A small eye drape with adhesive backing (Steri-Drape) has the advantage of being transparent, so that the infant's color can be seen and temperature can be maintained. Towel drapes may interfere with a radiant heat source used for temperature regulation.

Place an umbilical cord tie (e.g., umbilical cord tape) around the base of the cord to control bleeding. A single overhand knot is preferred because it allows tightening as needed. Using tissue forceps, pick up the cord and cut it with a scalpel about 1 to 1.5 cm above the base. Arterial spasm allows only minimal bleeding. Identify the vessels. There are usually two arteries and one vein. The arteries are small, thick walled, and constricted. The vein is larger, thin walled, and usually gaping open. If the vein is at the 12-o'clock position, the arteries are usually at the 4- and 8-o'clock positions (Figure 7-6).

Stabilize the umbilical stump by grasping the cord between the thumb and index finger or grasping the edge of the stump with a mosquito hemostat. Ensure that the hemostat does not crush the umbilical vessels. With iris forceps, dilate one of the arteries by placing the tips of the forceps in the artery and gently allowing them to spring open. This procedure may need to be repeated several times. In ELBW infants, the artery may be so small that it may be

necessary to initially insert one forcep tip and then both to dilate the artery. While grasping one side of the wall of the dilated artery with small forceps, gently insert the catheter. An alternative method is to insert the catheter between the open prongs of the forceps used to dilate the artery. Instructional aids such as Baby Umb (Medical Plastics Laboratory, Inc., Gatesville, Tex.) and the Umbilical Artery Catheterization Slide-Tape Neonatal Educational Program (Charles R. Drew Postgraduate Medical School, Los Angeles, Calif.) are helpful. As the catheter passes into the artery, resistance may be encountered at several points, as follows:

- At the umbilical cord tie (tape): The tie (tape) may be tied too tightly. Loosen slightly.
- At the point at which the umbilical artery turns downward (caudal) into the abdomen: Steady, gentle pressure is important because forceful pressure may cause the catheter to perforate the artery wall and create a false channel.
- At the point at which the umbilical artery joins the external iliac artery: Once again, steady, gentle pressure is important.

Insert the catheter to the predetermined length. Aspiration on the syringe should provide immediate blood return. Lack of blood return may indicate the following:

- The catheter is not inserted far enough. Insert farther.
- The vessel wall has been perforated or a false channel has been created. If the catheter has pierced the vessel wall, repeat the procedure using the other artery.
- The catheter is kinked. Pull back slightly and then advance.
- The stopcock is turned off. Correct the stopcock position. Return aspirated blood to the infant; then clear the catheter with flush solution.

There are several methods to secure the catheter, including suturing to the umbilical stump, use of an adhesive-type tape after using skin prep to protect the skin, use of a "goalpost" (Figure 7-7), and sterile transparent dressing. The literature denotes these methods but there is no evidence to delineate the most beneficial method. Advantages and disadvantages of each method including skin issues, cost, and ease of use need to be researched.[9]

Connect the stopcock to the intravenous (IV) solution, and set the prescribed infusion rate on

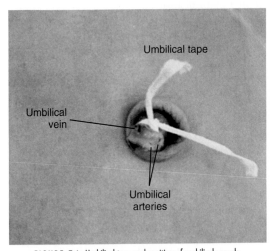

FIGURE 7-6 Umbilical tape and position of umbilical vessels.

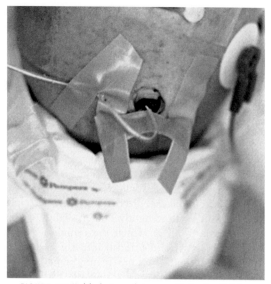

FIGURE 7-7 Umbilical artery catheter secured in "goalpost" design.

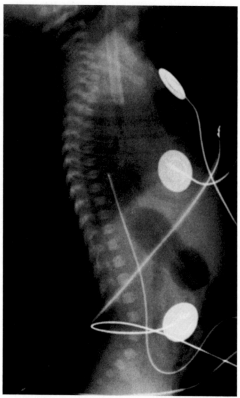

FIGURE 7-8 High catheter demonstrating "leg loop."

the infusion pump. Ensure that no air is in the tubing, stopcock, or catheter. All connections must be secure. Automatic infusion pumps must be used for UACs because arterial pressure must be overcome to permit IV fluid infusion. Determine catheter placement by an x-ray examination (abdominal, chest, or "babygram" depending on placement of the catheter). Figure 7-8 shows how the UAC appears on a lateral x-ray film.

Note that the catheter enters the umbilicus and travels inferiorly before turning superiorly. This "leg loop" is characteristic of an arterial catheter. A UAC follows the aorta and is positioned slightly to the left of the patient's vertebral column. Optimal placement is below the renal arteries and above the aortic bifurcation (L3 to L4) for a *low catheter* and below the left subclavian artery and above the diaphragm (T7 to T9) for a *high catheter*.[17] High catheter placement has fewer complications. Figure 7-9 shows high catheter placement, and Figure 7-10 shows low catheter placement.

If the catheter is too high, measure on the x-ray film the distance from the tip of the catheter to the desired level and pull the catheter back the appropriate distance. Some clinicians multiply this length by 0.8 to account for the magnifying effect of the x-ray film. If the catheter is placed too low, the catheter cannot be advanced but must be

removed and replaced because the external portion of the original catheter is no longer sterile. Remove the umbilical cord tie (tape) or maintain the tie very loosely so as not to obstruct blood flow to the umbilical area.

As a teaching model, the umbilical cord can be used for teaching the procedure of both arterial and venous catheterization. Many of the steps can be effectively carried out using a fresh placenta. Special UACs and monitors are available for continuous PaO_2 or oxygen saturation monitoring.

NURSING CARE AND USE OF UMBILICAL ARTERY CATHETERS

Infants can be positioned on their sides or their backs. The abdominal position may be avoided because accidental slipping, kinking, and removal of the catheter may occur without being immediately apparent. If the abdominal position is used, the catheter should be monitored continuously; ensure pressure alarms are on with parameter settings that would rapidly detect pressure changes.

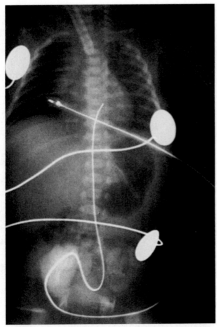

FIGURE 7-9 Umbilical artery catheter in high position (T8).

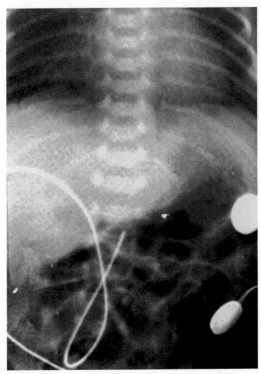

FIGURE 7-10 Umbilical artery catheter in low position (L3).

Care needs to be taken so that the infant is positioned to prevent dislodgement of the catheter. Diapers are effective for preventing the feet and toes from becoming entangled in the catheter. The diaper is folded below the umbilicus. If the infant is receiving phototherapy and thus is not diapered, leg restraints or positioning aids may be indicated. A mitten or positioning aids are useful to prevent hands and fingers from contacting the catheter. Positioning the catheter away from the extremities lessens the chance of accidental dislodgement. Unless using a transparent dressing to secure the UAC, a dressing over the umbilicus is unnecessary. Nontransparent dressings inhibit inspection of the umbilicus and evaluation of the catheter. The IV tubing, connecting tubing, and stopcock should be changed daily. Clots form in the stopcock, so changing it daily prevents the likelihood of embolus formation. Blood backing into the catheter can be caused by the following:

- Increased intraabdominal pressure, commonly caused by vigorous infant crying
- Disconnection of tubing or a loose connection
- Stopcock turned in wrong direction
- Infusion pump malfunction
- A leak in the filter or tubing or a crack in the stopcock

PROCEDURE FOR OBTAINING AN ARTERIAL BLOOD GAS SAMPLE

Drawing blood samples from an umbilical catheter is a sterile procedure. Samples may be obtained for blood gas analysis and to obtain laboratory specimens. Necessary items include a syringe for initially aspirating IV fluid and blood from the catheter, a heparinized blood gas syringe (if a blood gas sample is to be obtained), a syringe for aspirating laboratory samples (if laboratory samples are to be obtained), and a syringe containing flush solution.

The reinfusion method of obtaining blood samples is described. This practice involves returning the "discard" blood and, in theory, minimizes patient blood loss.[3] Remove the stopcock cap and place it down so that sterility will be maintained. Attach the empty aspiration syringe to the stopcock. Turn off the stopcock to the IV solution so that the IV solution stops flowing. Aspirate 1 to 2 ml from the catheter into the dry aspiration syringe (Figure 7-11). The IV fluid is prevented from infusing, and aspiration clears the catheter of

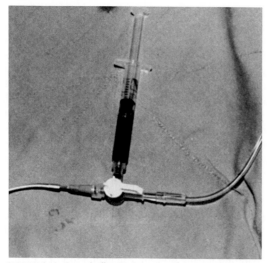

FIGURE 7-11 Stopcock off to IV solution; 1 to 2 ml aspirated into syringe.

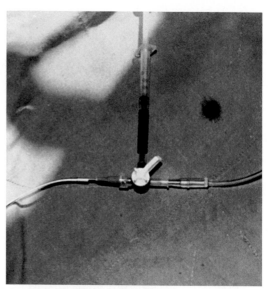

FIGURE 7-13 After blood is aspirated into heparinized 1-ml syringe, stopcock is placed in neutral position before syringe is removed.

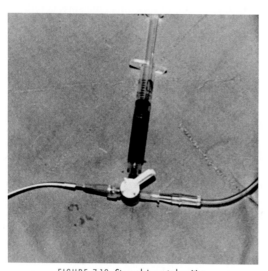

FIGURE 7-12 Stopcock in neutral position.

IV fluid. Turn the stopcock to the neutral position (Figure 7-12), remove the syringe while keeping the tip sterile, and replace it with the heparinized blood gas syringe or laboratory sample syringe. The neutral position of the stopcock prevents contaminating the sample with IV fluid and prevents blood loss from the infant.

CAUTION: Never allow blood to drip from an open stopcock. Attach the sample syringe. Turn the stopcock off to the IV fluid. Using steady, even

pressure, aspirate blood into the laboratory or heparinized blood gas sample syringe. Turn the stopcock to the neutral position, and remove the syringe (Figure 7-13).

For blood gas samples, remove any air from the syringe (because air bubbles in the sample will cause an artificial rise in PaO_2 and a slight fall in $PaCO_2$), cap the end, and chill it to preserve values. Attach the aspiration syringe containing the aspirated blood and IV fluid. Slightly aspirate to remove any air in the stopcock, and then slowly infuse the aspirated blood and IV fluid. Turn the stopcock to the neutral position, and remove the aspiration syringe. Replace the now–empty aspiration syringe that had aspirated blood and IV fluid in it with the syringe filled with flush solution. Turn the stopcock off to the IV fluid. Slightly aspirate to remove any air in the stopcock, and then slowly infuse the flush solution until the catheter is clear. Return the stopcock to the off position, allowing the IV fluid to now infuse. Replace the stopcock cap. Record the amount of blood removed from the infant and the amount of flush solution used to clear the catheter.

To ensure the integrity of all connections, the stopcock and other connections must be visible at all times. Do not place the stopcock and other connections under linen, because this would hamper the immediate detection of an accidental disconnection that would cause severe blood loss in the infant. Immediately remove any air in the tubing or catheter, because air is a potential embolus. It is best removed through the stopcock. If the air has passed the stopcock, it can be aspirated back into a syringe easily.

Obtaining an arterial blood gas specimen from a high UAC is better tolerated in premature infants when the entire procedure is done slowly. Premature and ill term infants have limited cerebral blood flow (CBF) autoregulation. Rapid drops and rises in CBF, especially in the first few days of life, can contribute to neuronal injury and intracranial bleeding. Rapidly obtaining blood samples from a UAC has detrimental hemodynamic effects on CBF. Thus sampling from the UAC should be done slowly.[3]

Umbilical Vein Catheter Placement

PROCEDURE

Determine the size and length of the catheter to be inserted. A 5-Fr catheter is normally used in the UVC placement procedure. The ELBW infant may require a 3.5-Fr catheter. To determine the length of the catheter to be inserted, the distance from the umbilicus to the sternal notch should be measured and multiplied by 0.6. Complete steps for the placement procedure are found under Umbilical Artery Catheter Placement earlier in this chapter. The only difference is that the vein is used instead of the artery. The catheter can be advanced to the desired position easily. The vein is usually gaping open and does not require dilation. The catheter should lie in the inferior vena cava with the UVC above the diaphragm but below the right atrium of the heart. Catheter position must be ensured. Historically, position confirmation was by radiologic examination, using the anteroposterior (AP) and lateral views. Ultrasonography is rapid and determines correct catheter tip placement and prevention of complications such as pericardial effusion and tamponade.[12] UVCs do not have the "leg loop" found on the lateral x-ray film of UACs. An umbilical venous catheter follows the inferior vena cava and is positioned slightly to the right of the patient's vertebral column. The catheter should be secured in the same manner as for an umbilical arterial catheter.

Peripherally Inserted Central Catheter Placement

Peripherally inserted central catheters (PICCs) are silicone or polyurethane products available in a variety of styles including single catheter and needle introducer to a complete insertion kit with instruments, skin disinfectant, and cap, mask, gown, and gloves. Some products provide a stylet and several feature break-away (splittable) needle introducers. PICCs are available in a variety of sizes for the neonatal population from 20 gauge (3 Fr) to 28 gauge (1.2 Fr).

PICCs typically are inserted for the following reasons:
- Infants who require IV access that is expected to be necessary for an extended period
- Infants with limited access
- As a transition from umbilical catheters for infants weighing less than 1000 g
- As a first-line catheter for infants weighing 1000 to 1500 g
- Infants with gastrointestinal anomalies, necrotizing enterocolitis, or gastrointestinal diseases that will require surgical correction

PICCs have long been used to provide highly concentrated parenteral nutrition and hyperosmolar medications.[27] These catheters are relatively easy to insert, affordable, and low maintenance and preclude surgical placement of central venous catheters. Because of extensive dwell time, they significantly reduce or eliminate the need for repeated painful procedures such as peripheral venipunctures, thus improving patient and parent satisfaction.

The nursing care and procedure for drawing blood samples from a UVC are the same as those for a UAC.

PROCEDURE

The insertion sites for PICC lines include the brachial cephalic veins, the axilla, the scalp vessels, and the saphenous veins. This sterile procedure can be performed when the infant is on a radiant warmer or in an incubator. A recent video demonstrating this procedure is available.[19]

For an arm or hand insertion, measure the distance from the insertion site to the axilla and then to 1 cm above the nipple line. If the catheter is to be

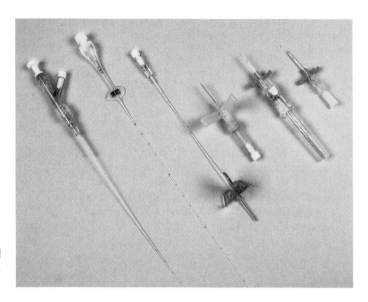

FIGURE 7-14 Peripherally inserted central catheters and introducers. (Courtesy Becton, Dickinson and Company, Franklin Lakes, NJ.)

inserted in the scalp, measure from the insertion site to 1 cm above the nipple line, and for a leg insertion, measure from the insertion site to 1 cm above the umbilicus or to the level of the inferior vena cava.

Determine the size and length of the catheter to be inserted—PICC and introducer: 20 to 28 gauge, varying lengths 20- to 65-cm catheter (Figure 7-14). Recommendations to trim lengthy catheters vary with manufacturer. A recent survey found that 75% of respondents trim catheters. Devices supplied by the catheter manufacturer for catheter trimming result in a precise cut, whereas scissors produced a ragged cut.[27]

A eutectic mixture of lidocaine and prilocaine (various manufacturers) anesthetic cream or a local anesthetic can be used before the procedure is begun (see Chapter 12). Place the infant in a supine position on a radiant heater or in an incubator. Ensure continuous temperature monitoring. Skin temperature should remain between 36° and 37° C (96.8° and 98.6° F). Provide appropriate oxygenation and ventilation. Ensure cardiorespiratory and oxygen saturation monitoring.

Restrain the infant's hands and feet to prevent the infant from contaminating the sterile field and interfering with the placement procedure, or swaddle the infant, with the site to be used exposed. For hand or arm insertion sites, turning the infant's head toward the insertion site will cause a slight occlusion of the jugular vein so that, as the catheter is passed into the subclavian vein, the risk for the catheter advancing upward into the jugular is diminished.

Wear a hat and mask. Open the PICC insertion tray; most units now use commercially available disposable trays. PICC insertion tray contents are shown in Figure 7-15. Open the PICC and introducer (if packaged separately from the PICC insertion tray). Wash hands and dry with sterile towel before the procedure. Put on a sterile gown and gloves. Connect a lipid-compatible T-connector extension tubing to a syringe of flush solution, and fill the entire apparatus.

Grasp the extremity to be used with sterile gauze so that an occlusive dressing can be applied to the distal part of the extremity, thus allowing manipulation of the extremity and precluding contamination of the insertion site by bacteria from distal sites. Cleanse the site with either povidone-iodine or chlorhexidine three times, and allow the site to air-dry. Remove the povidone-iodine with alcohol. For infants weighing less than 1000 g, use sterile water. Avoid using an excess of skin disinfectant so the infant is not lying in the solution during the procedure. Any residual skin disinfectant should be washed off the infant carefully after the procedure is completed. Place sterile drapes under the exposed insertion site. Reglove with new sterile gloves. Place the introducer, catheter either with or without stylet (clinician's choice), syringe, and sterile forceps on the sterile field near the planned insertion site. Insert

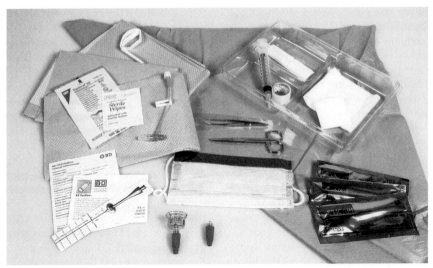

FIGURE 7-15 Disposable tray used for PICC insertion. (Courtesy Becton, Dickinson and Company, Franklin Lakes, NJ.)

the catheter into the introducer, being cautious if a stylet is used not to let the stylet extend beyond the tip of the introducer.

Insert the introducer tip at a flat angle to access the vein. The introducer is *not* advanced into the vein; it is used only as an introducer. At this point, there will probably be no blood return. Once the introducer is in the vein, pick up the catheter with the sterile forceps and gently advance the catheter to the premeasured length. Blood should fill the catheter. If the catheter is not advancing, pull the catheter back beyond the point of the introducer and reattempt to cannulate the vein. Once the catheter is advanced to the premeasured length, remove the stylet if used, and attach an empty sterile syringe. If a break-away cannula is used gently retract the cannula and slowly peel it apart to prevent premature breakage. Blood should be aspirated easily with a syringe. Flush the catheter with 0.5 to 1 ml of flush solution. Secure the catheter using sterile tape or nonfiber adhesive strips at the insertion site. Wrap extra catheter material into a coil above or below the joint to prevent occlusion. Attach the lipid-compatible T-connector extension set, and secure it to the extremity. Dress the insertion site, extra catheter loops, and PICC catheter to T-connector area with a sterile transparent occlusive dressing. Ensure that the dressing does not completely encircle the extremity causing a tourniquet effect. Label the dressing with the gauge and length of the catheter, the line type (PICC), and the initials of the insertion person.

Catheter position must be ensured by AP and lateral x-ray films, ultrasonography, or echocardiography.[12] For PICC lines inserted in the upper extremities, axillae, or scalp vessels, the catheter should lie in the superior vena cava above the right atrium of the heart. Catheters placed in other vessels have a significantly higher rate of thrombus formation and infection. For PICC lines inserted in the lower extremities, the catheter should lie in the inferior vena cava below the right atrium of the heart. Catheter placement in the right atrium can lead to complications of dysrhythmias, pleural effusion, and perforation with cardiac tamponade.[32]

NURSING CARE OF PICCs

Infants should be positioned to prevent dislodgement or kinking of the catheter. Diapers are effective for preventing the feet and toes from becoming entangled in the IV tubing. If the infant is receiving phototherapy and thus is not diapered, leg restraints or positioning aids may be indicated. A mitten or positioning aids are useful to prevent hands and fingers from contacting the catheter dressing and IV tubing. Positioning the catheter away from the extremities lessens the chance of accidental dislodgement. The IV tubing should be changed according to the standard of care. Observe for disconnection of tubing or a loose connection, and ensure an intact and occlusive insertion site dressing.

The occlusive dressing should be changed only when the integrity of the dressing has been lost. A small amount of blood at the insertion site is not a reason to change the occlusive dressing. Maintaining integrity of the occlusive dressing is instrumental in decreasing the risk for infection.

Changing the current dressing is indicated when it is no longer occlusive. The occlusive dressing is changed under sterile conditions. The person performing the dressing change wears a hat, mask, and sterile gloves. Changing the dressing entails removing the transparent film covering the area, cleaning the insertion site with either povidone-iodine solution or chlorhexidine, allowing this to dry, and then cleaning the site with sterile water to remove the preparation agent from the skin. If the nonfiber adhesive tape or strips are no longer adhesive, they are replaced. Dress the insertion site, extra catheter loops, and PICC catheter to the T-connector area with a sterile, clear, occlusive dressing. Ensure that the dressing does not completely encircle the extremity causing a tourniquet effect. Label the dressing with the gauge and length of the catheter, the line type (PICC), and the initials of the insertion person.

Because of the small gauge, PICCs are not routinely used for blood sampling. Clotting of the catheter may rapidly occur. Because the IV tubing does not contain a stopcock, significant blood loss and introduction of air into the venous circulation can occur.

Peripherally Inserted Midline Catheter

In infants not requiring or unable to receive a central catheter (vena cava placement) yet still needing IV access for a few days such as for antibiotic therapy, a peripherally inserted midline catheter (PIMC) can be used. PIMCs are inserted to the midclavicular line. These products are similar to PICCs and are available as single needle introducer and catheter or as complete kits.

Removing Umbilical Artery, Vein, and Peripherally Inserted Central Catheters

When the UAC, UVC, or PICC is no longer needed, it is removed. For UAC catheter removal, make certain the cord tie is snug. Sterile gauze is needed, and a suture removal kit should be available

if the catheter was sutured in place. Turn off the stopcock to the patient and the IV fluid. Withdraw the catheter to 3 cm, and leave it in place for 30 minutes before withdrawing it completely. This procedure works well for infants with respiratory or abdominal issues because it avoids the application of external pressure to the abdomen. Alternatively, withdraw the catheter slowly over several minutes, allowing for the artery to spasm. Pinch the umbilical stump with the sterile gauze for 5 minutes until hemostasis is achieved. Observe the umbilicus for active bleeding or oozing. Observe the lower extremities and buttocks for diminished perfusion secondary to a thrombus or embolus.

The procedure is similar for UVCs, with the exception that the catheter can be slowly withdrawn in one step. Pinch the umbilical stump with the sterile gauze for 5 minutes until hemostasis is achieved. Observe the umbilicus for active bleeding or oozing. Observe the patient for respiratory distress secondary to a pulmonary embolus.

For PICC removal, clamp the catheter, turn off the IV fluid infusion, and withdraw the catheter slowly and steadily. Apply pressure over the insertion site with the sterile gauze for 5 minutes until hemostasis is achieved. Observe the insertion site for active bleeding or oozing. Ensure that the entire catheter was removed.

Oxygen Saturation Monitoring by Pulse Oximetry

Oxygen saturation monitoring by *pulse oximetry* involves placing a small sensor on the infant in such a manner that his or her finger, toe, foot, or wrist comes between the light source and the photoreceptor. The light source emits wavelengths of light in the red and infrared spectrums. The difference between the absorption of the light is picked up by the receptor that is placed directly opposite the light source. The calculation of the ratio of oxyhemoglobin and deoxyhemoglobin is displayed as the percent of oxygen saturation. Key to accuracy of the monitor is that the light source and the receptor must be directly opposite each other over an area in which a pulse can be detected.

Oxygen saturation monitoring provides continuous and instantaneous readout of the oxygen saturation in the infant. In comparison with a blood gas analyzer, which calculates the relative oxygen saturation based on established nomograms, the oxygen saturation monitor measures the actual saturation of the hemoglobin. Calculated values using standard nomograms do not reflect shifts in the affinity of oxygen for hemoglobin based on changes in the patient's temperature, pH, Pco_2, or 2,3-DPG.

An inorganic phosphate produced in red cells; 2,3-DPG binds to the beta chain of reduced haemoglobin (Hb), lowering Hb's affinity for O_2 and by extension, facilitating O_2 release to tissues, causing a "right shift" of the O_2 dissociation curve. 2,3-DPG further shifts the curve to the right by lowering the red cells' pH. When transfused, red cells regain 50% of the 2,3-DPG within 3–8 hours and 100% within 24 hours.

The oxygen saturation monitor relies on adequate perfusion to the site and the ability to detect arterial pulsations; thus if it is placed distal to a blood pressure cuff, the reading will be inaccurate while the cuff is inflated. Newer models of pulse oximetry reduce the artifact that results from motion and low perfusion. These newer models also are indifferent to ambient light, whereas older models were affected by light sources such as phototherapy. Newer neonatal probes have built-in external light source protectors. Pigmentation of the patient's skin may produce artificially high readings, especially at lower oxygen levels.[26]

Oxygen saturation is more indicative of the total oxygen content of the blood than is Pao_2 and is the most sensitive to hypoxemia when it is on the steep part of the oxygen dissociation curve (see Figure 7-1). Keeping the Sao_2 at 90% to 92% keeps the infant in a normoxemic state under most conditions. Oxygen saturation monitoring by pulse oximetry generally is considered reliable and practical for use in infants over a wide range of birth weights and postnatal ages.[1] *Pulse oximetry saturation (SpO₂)* values vary significantly from measured arterial tension values obtained with an arterial blood gas specimen.[26] A contributing factor may be that the calibration of pulse oximeters typically has been performed on healthy adults. A compelling argument for the use of both *pulse oximetry* and *transcutaneous oxygen monitoring* in critically ill infants can be made, because each monitor has its own shortcomings.

Because pulse oximetry monitoring is common in neonatal care and many infants in NICUs require prolonged monitoring, a long-lasting oximeter probe could offer a substantial cost savings. No complications are associated with the use of oxygen saturation monitoring other than the potential for skin trauma caused by adhesive on the probe. Newer probes held in position by gentle elastic pressure have no adhesive touching the infant's skin.

In the asymptomatic newly born infant the incidence of congenital heart anomalies is approximately 1% to 2% of live births, with a quarter of these having critical congenital heart defects (CCHDs). CCHD lesions are ductal dependent or require cardiac catheterization or surgery before 1 year of age, with most requiring intervention within the first month. If not detected early, organ hypoperfusion and hypoxemia occur as the infant continues to transition to adult circulation. Detection of CCHDs before discharge allows medical and surgical interventions that may be lifesaving. The routine screening of all infants after 24 hours of life and before discharge has been recommended by multiple organizations.[6,16] In 2011, the U.S. Department of Health and Human Services (USDHHS) added screening for CCHDs to the Recommended Uniform Screening Panel.[30] The American Academy of Pediatrics endorsed the USDHHS recommendation.[15] Refer to a full discussion in Chapter 31.

Noninvasive Oxygen–Carbon Dioxide Monitoring

END-TIDAL CARBON DIOXIDE MONITORING

End-tidal CO₂ monitors use either sidestream or mainstream analysis. For sidestream analysis, the endotracheal tube has a second narrow lumen that opens at the end of the endotracheal tube. Gases are analyzed from samples taken from the end of the tube. The advantages of this system are that there is no increased dead space in the ventilator circuit and less chance of inspiratory gases contaminating the sample. The disadvantage to this method is that secretions may pool at the tip of the endotracheal tube and occlude the sampling port. The response time to changes in carbon dioxide content is slower than when mainstream analysis is used.

Mainstream analysis of carbon dioxide samples gases in the ventilator circuit. These gases are thought to be reflective of gases at the tip of the endotracheal tube. This method requires a separate chamber attached to the end of the endotracheal tube adapter, thus adding increased dead space and additional weight at the endotracheal tube adapter.

A comparison of sidestream and mainstream analyses of end-tidal CO_2 found that distal values were higher than proximal values and that distal values correlated more closely with $Paco_2$ values.[29] This discrepancy was thought to result from the mixing of end-tidal gases with fresh gases in the ventilator circuit. In an infant with a large alveolar-arterial (A-a) gradient, $Petco_2$ monitoring cannot be relied on for accuracy. In premature infants, it may be useful if the lung disease is mild to moderate; in infants with normal lung function, this method is reliable.[29]

The waveform output of the end-tidal CO_2 monitor can be used clinically if the clinician understands how the waveform corresponds to the exchange of gases in the lung (see Figure 7-2). The waveform has a sharp rise on expiration that reflects the carbon dioxide content of various lung areas. This expiration is followed by a plateau that reflects the cessation of dead space gases and the measurement of alveolar gas. At the end of the plateau is a sharp drop that reflects the inspiration of fresh gases with minimal carbon dioxide content. When using the monitor, the clinician should recognize that a sharp rise indicates compromised exhalation, such as in reactive airway disease. Partially plugged and dislodged endotracheal tubes will change the angle of rise on the capnogram. The plateau phase of the capnogram can be altered by severe hypotension or decreased cardiac output secondary to an altered minute ventilation-perfusion ($\dot{V}/\dot{Q}$) mismatch (as in pulmonary embolus, cardiac arrest, persistent pulmonary hypertension, atelectasis). No waveform or failure of the waveform to change indicates ineffective respiration (dislodged endotracheal tube).

TRANSCUTANEOUS OXYGEN–CARBON DIOXIDE MONITORING

Skin oxygen tension ($TcPo_2$) and carbon dioxide tension ($TcPco_2$) are measured by using one or two electrodes, depending on the model and brand of the monitor. The electrodes, once positioned on the skin, heat the area under the probe and cause certain physiologic changes as discussed. Oxygen and carbon dioxide that diffuse through the heated skin are measured by the electrode, and the value is digitally displayed on the monitor. If intervals between calibration are longer than 4 hours, the readings are subject to drift. The calibration procedures vary with the instruments used. Inherent in

the calibration process is the necessity to change the position of the skin electrode on the infant. Better correlations are found when the instrument is calibrated every 4 hours, the temperature is set correctly, and the infant is well perfused and normothermic. If the temperature of the probe cannot be maintained at 43° to 44° C (109.4° to 111.2° F), a lower temperature should be selected to avoid possible burns. At a lower temperature, the $TcPo_2$ monitor can be used to monitor trends but should not be interpreted as actual Pao_2 values. The range of accuracy of $TcPo_2$ monitors is limited; hypoxia (less than 40 mm Hg) and hyperoxia (greater than 120 mm Hg) may not be accurately reflected.

In an infant with suspected significant right-to-left shunting through a patent ductus arteriosus such as in persistent pulmonary hypertension, two transcutaneous oxygen electrodes can be used: one preductally (right shoulder) and the other postductally (lower abdomen or legs). Significant right-to-left shunting through the patent ductus arteriosus is present when the preductal oxygen tension is significantly higher than the postductal oxygen tension.

The disadvantages of the use of transcutaneous monitoring are that the instrument requires frequent calibration; requires the use of a heated electrode, which may burn the skin, especially in lower-birth-weight infants; requires a 15-minute period after calibration to heat the skin to the correct temperature; and has a 15- to 20-second delay in the readings compared with the patient's real-time values. The advantages are that it is not invasive, does not require the removal of blood for analysis, and displays a continuous readout of skin oxygen–carbon dioxide tensions.

NURSING CARE OF INFANTS WITH NONINVASIVE TRANSCUTANEOUS OXYGEN AND CARBON DIOXIDE MONITORS

The electrode can be placed on any portion of the infant's body as long as good contact between the electrode and the skin is maintained. Uneven areas of skin such as over bones and joints should be avoided because of poor contact between the membrane and the skin surface. The infant should not lie on the electrode. Placing the infant on top of the electrode increases the pressure on the underlying capillaries, thus affecting the flow of blood under the probe and resulting in a drop in $TcPo_2$ values. Because of the heat generated by the electrode

(43° to 44° C [109.4° to 111.2° F]), small red areas resembling first-degree burns are produced on the infant's skin. To minimize trauma to the infant's skin, the electrode should be repositioned every 2 to 4 hours, depending on his or her skin sensitivity. Grouping of nursing interventions has resulted in minimizing the time that the infant receives less-than-optimal oxygenation.

Cardiorespiratory Monitoring

The chest leads are applied in a triangular pattern on the infant's chest. Integrity of the leads must be ensured. Allowing the contact gel to dry or inadvertently dislodging the lead during procedures such as x-ray examination, echocardiography, and lumbar puncture may account for inaccurate tracings. Various components of the electrocardiogram (ECG) pattern may be diagnostically helpful. The QRS complex should be monitored for baseline height and width. A sudden decrease in QRS complex height that is not caused by artifact may be an indication of pneumothorax. The QT interval is helpful in diagnosing hypocalcemia in some infants. Other portions of the strip may be evaluated for electrolyte imbalance and possible cardiac ischemia. Hyperkalemia can induce arrhythmias, including heart block, ventricular tachycardia and fibrillation, and asystole. Initially the ECG will show peaked T waves with a narrow base. As the potassium level rises the P dampens, the PR interval increases, and the QRS widens. Further increases in the potassium value lead to absent P waves, QRS merging with the T wave to form a sine wave, followed by fibrillation, and then asystole.[18]

Humans display variability in vital signs due to the constant adjustments by the sympathetic and parasympathetic nervous systems. Vital sign variability in the healthy infant is maintained near a baseline value. When stressful events such as late-onset sepsis, intraventricular hemorrhage, or severe chronic lung disease are present, there is a corresponding change in vital signs and diminution in variability. Infants developing late-onset infection may exhibit subtle, nonspecific signs in advance of a clinical diagnosis. To aid in detecting heart rate changes that may indicate developing infection, some NICUs now use the HeRO system (Medical Predictive Sciences, Charlottesville, Va.). Heart rate changes over a 5-day period are tracked allowing health care personnel to follow patient trends. Loss of beat-to-beat variability and rising heart rate warrant investigation. As with any instrument, use of this device requires patient assessment and judgment.[11]

Blood Pressure Monitoring

Arterial pressure monitoring may be accomplished via the UAC attached to a transducer and monitor. Central venous pressure monitoring may be carried out in the same manner using the UVC. The same type of transducer may be used for either arterial or venous pressure recording.

Some research has indicated that the predictive value of peripheral blood pressure screening for CCHD is small and that oscillator blood pressure measurements are less accurate than pulse oximetry screening to detect CCHD.[2] This failure to detect CCHD is more pronounced in aortic arch obstructive defects.

Point-of-Care Testing

The Centers for Medicare and Medicaid Services regulates POCT through the Clinical Laboratory Improvement Act (CLIA).[5] Federal regulations require initial education about POCT procedures, as well as annual reassessment of competency. The quality of these tests is imperative to ensure proper diagnosis and treatment, and the CLIA regulations strive to ensure quality testing.

The accuracy of whole blood glucometers compared with laboratory values may vary depending on hypoxia, hematocrit, and elevated triglyceride values. Accuracy also depends on the product that is being measured, because some glucometers measure glucose only, whereas others measure total sugars, including glucose, galactose, maltose, and xylose. In addition, the clinician must remember that an approximately 11% difference exists between plasma glucose (laboratory sample) and whole blood glucose (POCT device). The POCT value should be multiplied by 1.11 to determine a more approximate plasma value.[8] A variance of accuracy also exists with bedside electrolyte assessment devices. Transcutaneous neonatal bilirubin assessments require correlation between the serum bilirubin value and each device, institution, and patient population for which it is used.[7] As neonatal care advances, rapid availability of patient information will become more and more crucial. Expect continuous expansion of POCT.

Event Monitoring

The advancement of physiologic monitors with memory capability has enhanced the ability of the practitioner to review the physiologic status of the infant as measured by multiple physiologic parameters for the past 24 to 48 hours. In many NICUs, the monitor output is integrated into the electronic or computerized chart. This integration allows the care provider to "pull" the data from the monitors into the chart at preselected times, either prospectively or retrospectively. When the monitors are programmed with critical value ranges, any deviation outside these ranges is noted as an "event," which can then be reviewed, tallied, or otherwise annotated. For care providers at the bedside, the challenge is to keep iatrogenic events (e.g., lead removal, excessive activity of the infant, a stopcock turned the wrong direction) minimized such that the infant's record is as valid a reflection of actual physiologic status as possible. Any circumstances noted at the time of the event that may produce false readings should be recorded so that when the infant's record is reviewed, these events can be placed in context of the circumstances at the time.

COMPLICATIONS

UACs act as foreign bodies, causing fibrin deposition and thrombus formation around the catheter. Although most catheters are associated with thrombus formation, it is of clinical significance in fewer than 10% of patients (Box 7-1). A common problem associated with major complications of UACs is ischemic disease resulting from emboli or arterial spasms. In such cases, the catheter should be removed immediately and antithrombin therapy should be considered. Although vasospasm is common, usually it does not require immediate removal of the catheter. Blue discoloration, commonly called "catheter toes," is seen, rather than blanching. Obviously, a hemorrhage may occur when the catheter slips out or when any of the various connections loosen. For reasons such as these, UACs require constant attention. If the lower extremities or buttocks blanch, the catheter should be removed immediately and antithrombin therapy considered. The benefit of antithrombin therapy must be balanced against the increased risk for intracranial hemorrhage.

BOX 7-1

CRITICAL FINDINGS
COMPLICATIONS OF INDWELLING CATHETERS

- UACs
  - Ischemia from thrombi, emboli, or arterial spasms
  - Hemorrhage caused by catheter dislodgement or loose connections
  - Infection
  - Malposition
- UVCs
  - Thrombus formation leading to pulmonary embolization
  - Thrombus formation in portal vessels
  - Hepatic necrosis
  - Intestinal ischemia
  - Hemorrhage caused by catheter dislodgement or loose connections
  - Cardiac complications: dysrhythmias, myocardial perforation, pericardial effusion
  - Infection
- PICC lines
  - Occlusion
  - Clotting
  - Infection
  - Malposition
  - Cardiac complications: dysrhythmias, myocardial perforation, pericardial effusion
  - Breakage and leaking
  - Phlebitis
  - Peripheral edema

PICC, Peripherally inserted central catheter; *UAC*, umbilical artery catheter; *UVC*, umbilical vein catheter.

To prevent bleeding once the catheter is removed, immediately pinch the subumbilical area with sterile gauze for 5 minutes until hemostasis is achieved. Avoid downward abdominal pressure that may compromise respiratory effort. When the color has returned to the affected area and the infant is stable, replacement of the catheter can be considered. If vasospasm occurs in one leg or foot, apply warm wraps (diapers wetted with warm water or chemical heel warmers) to the opposite leg or apply wraps to the upper extremities, thereby producing a reflex vasodilation to the legs. However, inherent in this action is the hazard of obscuring recognition of compromise in that extremity. The wraps should be reheated every 10 to 15 minutes until the spasm has resolved. The skin temperature of the infant must be greater than 36° C (96.8° F) for wraps to be effective.

UVCs may cause thrombus formation. Thrombi can result in pulmonary embolisms. Clots may form in the portal vessels, resulting in portal hypertension. Hepatic necrosis, gut ischemia, and hemorrhage have been associated with UVCs. Other complications include dysrhythmias, myocardial perforation, pericardial effusion, and endocarditis.

PICCs that are placed in central veins have complication rates lower than those placed in noncentral veins. Complications include occlusion, clotting, infection, sepsis, phlebitis, leakage, extravasation, peripheral edema, malposition, catheter migration, cardiac tamponade, and catheter breakage.[32] Bacteremia, always a major concern, will require the removal of the catheter if the blood culture remains positive for more than 24 hours. To prevent central line–associated bloodstream infection (CLABSI), establishment of and strict adherence to a care bundle is beneficial.[4] Bundle items for insertion include a procedure cart with sterile perimeter, skin disinfection, and strict sterile technique. Maintenance items include handwashing, use of gloves, attention to PICC access and fluid tubing changes, and daily CLABSI surveillance. Refer to a full discussion in Chapter 16. Occlusion sometimes may be treated with clot-dissolving agents. Establishment of a PICC team to insert and manage these devices, catheter tip placement in the superior or inferior vena cava, and heparinized solutions have been shown to reduce complications. In an emergent situation evaluate catheter tip placement before administering medications or fluid boluses in case of catheter malposition and cardiac tamponade.

CONTROVERSIES

Clinicians continue to disagree on the optimal placement site for UACs. However, a Cochrane review and subsequent update determined that high UACs resulted in fewer vascular complications than did low UACs and recommended the exclusive use of high placement for UACs.[17] Prophylactic administration of antibiotic agents is not indicated.[22] Use of the UAC for infusion of antibiotic agents, calcium, hyperalimentation solutions, or blood varies, and no definitive studies are available. Blood cultures can be drawn from the UAC for up to 6 hours

---

BOX 7-2	WHAT'S NEXT IN PHYSIOLOGIC MONITORING?

1. Intelligent monitoring systems. Rather than signal when a single parameter exceeds a preset threshold these monitors would integrate multiple data, including patient medications and laboratory results, to provide a more complete view of the patient's status.[1]

2. Telemedicine has demonstrated success in examining and diagnosing retinopathy of prematurity and genetic and neurologic abnormalities. It will now evolve to allow a remote neonatal intensive care unit model where a neonatologist can simultaneously monitor multiple infants continuously—visually and by the integration of multiple data. Virtual rounds as needed, as well as care direction, can occur.[10,31]

---

after insertion. The use of heparin in the infusate has been controversial, because heparin decreases catheter occlusion but not thrombosis.[23] In addition, heparin use in a flush solution alone is not beneficial in preventing catheter occlusion.

Enteral feeding with an umbilical line in place lacks definitive studies; however, this practice is more common than was previously thought. A Cochrane review found that trophic enteral feedings were not detrimental.[20] Select NICUs provided trophic and more substantial enteral feedings with umbilical catheters in place.[13]

Routine monitoring of all infants receiving intermediate or intensive care is the standard of care. Indwelling catheters for blood pressure monitoring have the advantage of continuous readout, but external cuffs are less invasive. There is a continued need for research into the efficacy and safety of umbilical catheters. Box 7-2 cites new research into future possibilities for neonatal physiologic monitoring.

PARENT TEACHING

Important elements of parent teaching are listed in Box 7-3. As with the many other invasive procedures in neonatology, the clinician obtains permission from the parents for umbilical vessel catheterization and PICC placement. This may be the clinician's first contact with the family and thus sets the atmosphere for future contacts. Although parents initially are hesitant about umbilical catheter placement,

<table>
<tr><td>BOX
7-3</td><td>PARENT TEACHING
PHYSIOLOGIC MONITORING</td></tr>
</table>

1. Placement of umbilical lines is invasive. Educate parents about the following:
   - Placement is painless because the umbilical cord contains no nerves.
   - The point of catheter insertion and where the tip of the catheter is located.
   - The umbilical catheter can be used for numerous functions: administering IV fluid, medications, and blood products; monitoring; and obtaining laboratory specimens.
   - Care should be taken when holding or manipulating the infant to prevent catheter dislodgement and blood loss.
   - Holding the infant out of the incubator and wrapped in blankets obscures visualization of the catheter and connections.
2. The NICU environment can be frightening. Educate parents about the following:
   - The baby is being monitored by various methods, including cardiorespiratory, blood pressure, and transcutaneous monitors.
   - The purpose and a short description of each monitor.

generally they are comforted to learn that it will result in a painless way of drawing blood; there are no nerves in the umbilical cord to sense pain. Parents also appreciate that PICC placement will reduce the number of peripheral IV attempts. Before parents visit the infant, providers need to inform parents about the technology that is being used to monitor the infant (i.e., umbilical catheter, transcutaneous monitors, cardiorespiratory monitors, blood pressure monitors), including what the technology is registering. Often parents are confused about where the catheter goes once it enters the umbilicus and the purposes of other monitoring devices.

Parents need to be instructed on how to hold their infant while an umbilical catheter or PICC is in place because manipulating the infant may accidentally dislodge the catheter and result in blood loss and potential infection. When the infant is being held out of the incubator and wrapped in blankets, the integrity of the catheter and connections is not easily evaluated. The parents' vigilance around the technology used on their infant can potentially avoid these incidents.

REFERENCES

For a full list of references, scan the QR code or visit http://booksite.elsevier.com/9780323320832.

8

ACID-BASE HOMEOSTASIS AND OXYGENATION

JAMES S. BARRY, JANE DEACON, CARMEN HERNÁNDEZ, AND M. DOUGLAS JONES, JR.

Accurate interpretation of blood gas values and an understanding of acid-base and oxygenation physiology are essential to proper diagnosis or management of an ill neonate.[8,28,44] The measurement of arterial blood gases allows analysis of two interrelated but separate processes: acid-base homeostasis and oxygen-carrying capacity.[1,27,36] This chapter describes the parameters that designate these processes, their measurements, and the effects of proposed treatment on homeostasis.[1,44] Common abbreviations and their meanings are listed in Box 8-1.

Components of arterial blood gases include (1) measured values (PaO_2, $PaCO_2$, and pH) and (2) calculated values (oxygen saturation, bicarbonate concentration, and base excess). Some analyzer systems also estimate hemoglobin concentration. The pH, $PaCO_2$, base excess, and bicarbonate components are used to assess acid-base homeostasis,[27,36,47] whereas PaO_2, saturation (SaO_2), and hemoglobin concentration[1,8] are used to assess adequacy of oxygen-carrying capacity (Table 8-1).

PHYSIOLOGY

Acid-Base Homeostasis

To review basic chemistry, an acid is a hydrogen ion donor and a base is a hydrogen ion acceptor. The pH refers to the concentration of hydrogen ions [H^+] in a liquid and reflects the acid-base balance in liquid.[47] The quantity of hydrogen ions is minute, approximately 0.0000001 mole/L. Therefore the negative log of the hydrogen ion concentration is used to define pH and create a positive, workable number (pH = 7) (Equation 1). A pH of 7 represents a neutral solution, a pH of less than 7 represents acidity, and a pH greater than 7 represents alkalinity:

$$pH = -\log\left[H^+\right]$$

$$pH = -\log\left[0.0000001\right]$$

$$pH = -\left[-7\right]$$

$$pH = 7$$

Equation 1

The Henderson-Hasselbalch equation describes pH as equal to a constant (pK) plus the logarithm of the ratio of the base-to-acid concentration (Equation 2).[9,31] Thus, if there is an increase in the concentration of hydrogen ions (reflected in the denominator), blood pH value decreases and acidemia results. Conversely, if there is less acid or more base, blood pH increases and alkalemia results.[9]

$$pH = pK + \log\frac{base}{acid}$$

Equation 2

The first step in determining acid-base homeostasis is measurement of pH. Normal human pH is between 7.35 and 7.45. Acidemia and acidosis are often used interchangeably, but strictly speaking, pH of less than 7.35 is acidemia and the process that caused it is acidosis; a pH of greater than 7.45 is alkalemia and the process that caused it is alkalosis.[28] Arterial carbon dioxide ($PaCO_2$) and bicarbonate [HCO_3^-] values represent the two main components of acid-base homeostasis: (1) respiratory contribution ($PaCO_2$) controlled by alveolar ventilation,[1,15,18] and (2) nonrespiratory or metabolic

PURPLE type highlights content that is particularly applicable to clinical settings.

TABLE 8-1

NORMAL (ARTERIAL) BLOOD GAS VALUES

BLOOD GASES	VALUES
pH	7.35-7.45
$Paco_2$	35-45 mm Hg
HCO_3^-	18-26 mEq/L
Base excess	(−5) to (+5)
Pao_2	60-80 mm Hg
O_2 saturation	92%-94%

contribution controlled primarily by renal excretion, retention, or production of $[HCO_3^-]$.[1,25,42] Other factors that affect nonrespiratory components of acid-base balance cause a change in $[HCO_3^-]$; thus $[HCO_3^-]$ is an indicator of the nonrespiratory component.[25,30,42]

RESPIRATORY CONTRIBUTION

Carbon dioxide is produced from cellular metabolism.[1,38] As carbon dioxide is produced, it dissolves in intracellular fluid and can be measured as the partial pressure (P) of the dissolved gas (CO_2). As the pressure of the dissolved gas increases inside the cell, carbon dioxide moves out of the cell into the blood. Blood transports dissolved carbon dioxide (some combined with hemoglobin

as carboxyhemoglobin, most as bicarbonate) to the lung, where the partial pressure in the pulmonary capillary is greater than in the alveoli,[36] causing carbon dioxide to move into the alveoli down a concentration gradient. **Ventilation is the only method of removing carbon dioxide.** The amount of carbon dioxide in the blood is the net result of the body's metabolism (production) and alveolar ventilation (clearance). Because metabolism does not change greatly and CO_2 diffuses easily across membranes, the only clinically important limitation to CO_2 removal is at the lungs. Thus $Paco_2$ reflects alveolar ventilation.[9,15,18,28]

In the red blood cell, the enzyme *carbonic anhydrase* promotes combination of a fraction of dissolved CO_2 with water to form carbonic acid (H_2CO_3), which then dissociates into a hydrogen ion $[H^+]$ and a bicarbonate ion $[HCO_3^-]$[1,38]:

$$CO_2 + H_2O = H_2CO_3 = [H^+] + [HCO_3^-] \quad \text{Equation 3}$$

Therefore, an increase in $Paco_2$ (hypoventilation) causes pH to fall. This is called *respiratory acidosis*.[15] A decrease in $Paco_2$ (hyperventilation) results in less acid formation in the blood and causes pH to rise. This pathophysiologic process is known as *respiratory alkalosis.*

NONRESPIRATORY (METABOLIC) CONTRIBUTION

Nonrespiratory (metabolic) derangements can also disturb acid-base homeostasis. Normal metabolism produces hydrogen ions. Blood pH is maintained within normal limits by renal mechanisms for excreting hydrogen ions. Increased production of $[H^+]$ may occur in conditions such as shock with poor peripheral tissue perfusion or genetically determined aberrations of metabolism.[43] The hydrogen ions produced must be eliminated to avoid a fall in blood pH. Derangements also occur when hydrogen ions are lost (e.g., in gastric fluids) or when bicarbonate is lost (e.g., in diarrheal fluid or ileostomy drainage).[44]

Authorities differ as to the best way to describe nonrespiratory derangements in acid-base status. The traditional approach relies on measurement of pH, Pco_2, and $[HCO_3^-]$. An alternative description is of acid-base status in terms of (1) strong ions (Na^+, K^+, Ca^{2+}, Mg^{2+}, Cl^-), strong because they remain dissociated at normal human blood pH, and (2) weak acids (hemoglobin, albumin, inorganic phosphate), weak because they are partially dissociated at normal human blood pH. Blood pH in this conceptualization is a function of the difference between strong cations and strong anions, the strong ion difference (SID). As an example, the alkalosis associated with loss of gastric fluid would be described exclusively in terms of loss of [Cl⁻] with loss of [H⁺] making no independent contribution to the resulting alkalemia. Advocates maintain that measurement of SID leads to greater understanding of the causes of nonrespiratory and mixed acid-base derangements.[14,20,24,38] Others favor staying with the traditional bicarbonate-centered model.[13,29] The present discussion focuses on the traditional bicarbonate-centered approach. Readers are referred to recent reviews for comparisons of the two methods.[24,29]

A fall in blood [HCO₃⁻] might indicate that bicarbonate, a base and therefore a hydrogen ion acceptor, has been used up by the addition of [H⁺]. As shown in Equation 3, a change in [HCO₃⁻] might also reflect a change in P_{CO_2}. This difficulty is overcome in blood gas analyzers by correcting the P_{CO_2} (graphically) to 40 mm Hg, yielding a "standard bicarbonate" concentration.[38] The standard bicarbonate concentration and the buffering properties of hemoglobin are combined in the concept of base excess (BE). BE is strictly defined as the amount of base or acid that is needed to restore blood to a pH of 7.4 at a normal P_{CO_2} of 40 and temperature of 37° C.[2] A positive value suggests a deficit of fixed (i.e., not volatile as with H_2CO_3) acid or an excess of base; a negative value indicates an excess of fixed acid or a deficit of base.[38] An abnormality of the standard bicarbonate concentration or base excess indicates a process of nonrespiratory (metabolic) alkalosis[25] or nonrespiratory (metabolic) acidosis.[41] Caution is needed because various blood gas analyzers do not calculate base excess in a similar manner and can vary by 3 to 9 mmol/L.[2] Additionally, BE is commonly calculated using assumptions from adult physiology with a normal bicarbonate of 26, which is significantly higher than what would be considered normal for a premature neonate.[33]

In the Henderson-Hasselbalch equation (Equation 2), the pH is equal to a constant, pK, plus the logarithm of the base/acid ratio.[1,28,38] If we substitute [HCO₃⁻] for the base and dissolved CO_2 for the acid,[15,38] multiplying CO_2 by its solubility

coefficient (0.03 mEq/L/mm Hg), the equation becomes the following:

$$pH = pK + \log[HCO_3^- / (P_{CO_2} \times 0.03)] \quad \text{Equation 4}$$

The value of pK is 6.1; normal [HCO₃⁻] is 24 mEq/L, and normal $Paco_2$ is 40 mm Hg.

Substituting, we obtain the following:

$$pH - 6.1 + \log(20/1.2) \quad \text{Equation 5}$$

or

$$pH = 6.1 + 1.3 = 7.4$$

Changes in the 20:1.2 ratio have profound effects on the pH.[1,28] The following are two examples:

1. Hypoventilation of sufficient degree that $Paco_2$ is doubled from 40 to 80 (respiratory acidosis) results in a ratio of 24:2.4, or 10. The logarithm of 10 is 1, and the pH would be 6.1 + 1, or 7.1.
2. If a metabolic acidosis reduced [HCO₃⁻] from 24 mEq/L to 12 mEq/L, the ratio would be 12:1.2 or 10:1, and the pH would be 7.1.

MIXED CONTRIBUTIONS

The two most common reasons for acid-base disturbance in humans are accumulation of carbon dioxide and production of lactic acid through anaerobic metabolism as a consequence of tissue oxygen deprivation. Thus far, these derangements (Figure 8-1) have been discussed as if they happened in isolation, but respiratory and nonrespiratory problems often occur simultaneously depending on pathologic processes in the body. Besides the four single acid-base derangements, there are combined acid-base derangements: (1) respiratory acidosis and metabolic acidosis, (2) respiratory acidosis and metabolic alkalosis, (3) respiratory alkalosis and metabolic acidosis, and (4) respiratory alkalosis and metabolic alkalosis. The combined acidoses or combined alkaloses have a cumulative effect on the pH, whereas an acidosis and alkalosis combination tends to negate the effects of each on the pH value.[27,28,36,47]

COMPENSATION

Acid-base homeostasis maintains pH near the normal range. The body attempts to maintain equilibrium by balancing a pathologic process with

	Respiratory parameter P_{CO_2}	Metabolic parameter HCO_3^-	Cause
Respiratory acidosis	⬆	↑	Hypoventilation
Respiratory alkalosis	⬇	↓	Hyperventilation
Metabolic acidosis	↓	⬇	Add acid or lose base
Metabolic alkalosis	↑	⬆	Add base or lose acid

FIGURE 8-1 Acid-base derangements. *Large arrow* indicates primary process that produces change in pH. *Small arrow* indicates compensatory process.

a physiologic process or predictable buffering response.[9,28,44] Thus, if either the respiratory or nonrespiratory component of the acid-base system is deranged, the other system will compensate to counterbalance the primary process. For example, any respiratory process that leads to retention of carbon dioxide (respiratory acidosis) stimulates a nonrespiratory system, in this case the renal system, to return pH toward normal. Retention of bicarbonate and corresponding excretion of hydrogen ions are the compensatory renal mechanisms that counterbalance respiratory acidosis. Given sufficient time, this may increase blood bicarbonate by as much as 3 to 4 mEq/L for each 10-mm Hg increase in carbon dioxide. Thus a neonate with a chronically increased Pa_{CO_2} and a compensatory rise in bicarbonate may attain a near-normal pH.[28]

Metabolic compensations for deranged respiratory processes can go to remarkable extremes, but respiratory compensations to deranged metabolic processes are limited. Hyperventilation cannot lower the Pa_{CO_2} much below 10 mm Hg in compensation for a metabolic acidosis. Similarly, hypoventilation is limited in compensation for a metabolic alkalosis by the onset of hypoxemia.[44] Hypoxemia stimulates respiratory drive, overriding compensatory hypoventilation, limiting correction of alkalemia.[28]

CORRECTION

Correction of an acid-base disturbance occurs when the health care provider detects the

pathophysiologic process and directs therapy at the primary pathologic process, rather than counterbalancing it with a second pathologic process.

For example, if a respiratory acidosis is present, the clinician assesses the patient to discover the cause of the carbon dioxide retention and directs therapy at improving minute ventilation, the product of respiratory rate and tidal volume, rather than attempting to increase the retention of bicarbonate.

Oxygenation

The remaining components of the blood gas analysis are the P_{O_2}, hemoglobin, and oxygen saturation.[36] Oxygenation is related to but also distinct from ventilation.[9] The two main factors contributing to oxygenation at the tissue level are oxygen delivery and oxygen consumption. Oxygen delivery is the product of the cardiac output and the oxygen-carrying capacity of blood, whereas oxygen consumption is determined by the metabolic needs of the body's tissues. Tissue hypoxia may be caused by many different factors that derange the balance between oxygen delivery and tissue needs. Inability of the lung to oxygenate the blood would decrease oxygen delivery because of arterial hypoxemia. Another cause of tissue hypoxia is interference with blood flow, as in heart failure. The Pa_{O_2} may be normal, but because of heart (pump) failure, oxygenated blood is not delivered in sufficient quantity. Treatment should be directed toward improving cardiac output and tissue perfusion (see Chapter 24). A third cause of tissue hypoxia is decreased blood oxygen–carrying capacity as with anemia. In this instance, the heart and lungs work adequately. PaO_2 is normal but the quantity of hemoglobin available for oxygen transport is insufficient. Finally, tissue hypoxia may result from an abnormally high affinity of hemoglobin for oxygen, which leads to a decrease in tissue oxygen delivery. If oxyhemoglobin affinity is increased, oxygen will not dissociate from hemoglobin unless the venous, and therefore tissue, PO_2 falls to an unusually low level.[12]

Because PaO_2 measures only the partial pressure of oxygen in arterial blood (i.e., measures the amount of dissolved oxygen gas in the blood), it reflects lung function but not tissue oxygenation. Despite this, measurement of PaO_2 together with measurement of hemoglobin and clinical assessment of tissue perfusion is used currently as a surrogate of tissue oxygenation.[9] Two situations merit special comment. First, in a preterm infant whose retinal development is incomplete, high PaO_2 is associated with retinopathy of prematurity, especially at PaO_2 greater than 100 mm Hg (see Chapter 23). Second, in patients with cyanotic congenital heart disease, there is a right-to-left intracardiac shunt. A portion of venous blood goes directly to the left side of the heart, bypassing the lungs. In such patients, the rise in PaO_2 with administration of oxygen is limited. Low PaO_2 in these patients is not related to lung disease, although lung disease may complicate the picture.

Theoretically, in a normal lung with perfectly matched ventilation and perfusion, the alveolar (PAO_2) and the arterial oxygen tension (PaO_2) should be equal. This is not achieved. A difference (gradient) exists between the PAO_2 and the PaO_2. Minor mismatching of ventilation and perfusion leads to a functional intrapulmonary shunt. This creates an alveolar-arterial oxygen gradient (D[A-a]O_2).[9,15] However, a D(A-a)O_2 greater than 20 mm Hg indicates pulmonary disease.[9]

OXYHEMOGLOBIN SATURATION

Oxyhemoglobin saturation is the percentage of hemoglobin that is combined with oxygen. Oxygen binding with hemoglobin increases as the partial pressure of oxygen increases, but not linearly.[9,47] The oxygen dissociation curve is a measure of the affinity that hemoglobin has for oxygen (Figure 8-2).

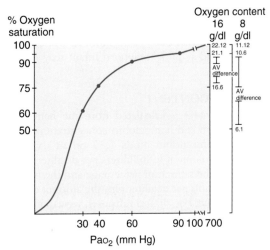

FIGURE 8-2 Oxygen-hemoglobin dissociation curve; the 30-60-90 rule is demonstrated. *Right,* The oxygen content for a hemoglobin concentration of 16 and 8 g/dl is given, demonstrating the effect of anemia on venous saturation and tissue oxygenation.

The "30-60-90 rule" is useful in remembering percent saturation and reconstructing the adult hemoglobin dissociation curve if necessary (see Figure 8-2). At a PaO_2 of 30 mm Hg, the oxygen saturation is 60%; at a PaO_2 of 60 mm Hg, saturation is 90%; and at 90 mm Hg PaO_2, the hemoglobin is 95% saturated. At the normal venous oxygen tension of 40 mm Hg, the oxygen saturation is 75%. Factors that affect this affinity include temperature, pH, and hemoglobin structure. Hypothermia, alkalemia, hypocapnia, and fetal hemoglobin increase the affinity of hemoglobin for oxygen (shift the curve to the left), whereas fever, acidemia, and hypercapnia decrease the affinity of hemoglobin for oxygen (shift the curve to the right).

At a given tissue PO_2, an increased hemoglobin affinity for oxygen leads to less oxygen released at the tissue level, whereas a decreased affinity allows for more oxygen release to the tissues. Alternately, the PO_2 at which the oxygen-binding sites of hemoglobin are 50% saturated (the P_{50}) is low when the hemoglobin affinity is great and higher when the hemoglobin affinity is low.[9] The affinity of fetal hemoglobin for oxygen is higher than adult hemoglobin (see Figure 7-1). The P_{50} of fetal hemoglobin is 19 mm Hg compared with a P_{50} of 27 mm Hg for adult hemoglobin. Approximately 70% of hemoglobin in term infants, and more in preterm infants, consists of fetal hemoglobin.[12] As a result, hemoglobin in a term infant with a Pao_2 of 35 mm Hg will be 80% saturated, and a "pink" newborn infant may have a low Pao_2.

OXYGEN CONTENT

Oxygen content is calculated from the hemoglobin saturation and hemoglobin concentration. One gram of hemoglobin binds 1.39 ml of oxygen. The oxygen content in milliliters per deciliter is the product of the saturation percentage and the hemoglobin in grams per deciliter plus the amount of dissolved oxygen. For clinical purposes, we can neglect the amount of dissolved oxygen in plasma, because it is only 0.003 ml/dl/mm Hg.

Oxygen content becomes critical in anemia, which can decrease tissue oxygenation unless organ blood flow and cardiac output increase to maintain the delivery of oxygen.[9,47] The blood of an infant with a hemoglobin of 8 g/dl will have half the oxygen content compared with that of an infant with a hemoglobin of 16 g/dl at an equivalent oxygen saturation percentage. In Figure 8-2, an infant with 16 g hemoglobin that is 95% saturated (Pao_2 = 90 mm Hg) carries 21.1 ml/dl oxygen, whereas the infant with 8 g hemoglobin carries 10.6 ml/dl oxygen. Tissues require approximately 4 to 5 ml/dl oxygen to maintain aerobic metabolism. With normal cardiac output, venous blood contains 4 to 5 ml/dl oxygen less than the arterial blood. The venous oxygen content in an infant with 16 g hemoglobin would be between 16 and 17 ml/dl, which corresponds to approximately 75% saturation, or a Pvo_2 of 40 mm Hg. However, unless cardiac output increases, the venous oxygen content in an infant with 8 g hemoglobin would be 6.1 ml/dl oxygen. The saturation is 55%, which corresponds to a Po_2 of less than 30.

BLOOD FLOW AND SHUNTS

The product of oxygen content and blood flow returning from the lungs determines the total amount of oxygen in arterial blood if no intracardiac or extracardiac shunting occurs. Total pulmonary blood flow can be divided into the amount of blood in pulmonary capillaries and the amount that is shunted through or around the lungs.

A right-to-left shunt occurs when blood passes from the systemic venous to the systemic arterial circulation. This can occur because of anatomic defects in the heart (e.g., cyanotic congenital heart disease), with a persistently patent ductus arteriosus in the presence of pulmonary arterial pressures that are higher than systemic arterial pressures (pulmonary hypertension), or when pulmonary capillary blood perfuses poorly expanded alveoli (e.g., intrapulmonary shunts). Shunts lower the final arterial oxygen saturation. The usual degree of shunt in a newborn is 15% to 20% of the cardiac output.

Acid–Base and Oxygenation Disorders

Ventilation is defined as the amount of gas leaving the lungs per unit of time (e.g., minute ventilation). Minute ventilation is equal to the product of the tidal volume and respiratory frequency in breaths per minute. Tidal volume comprises (1) gas in the airway and nonperfused alveoli *(physiologic dead space)* and (2) gas in the alveolar space.[9,15] *Alveolar ventilation* is defined as the ratio of CO_2 production by the body to the $Paco_2$. Alveolar ventilation is inversely related to $Paco_2$. When $Paco_2$ doubles, alveolar ventilation is approximately one half of the original value. If the $Paco_2$ triples, alveolar ventilation is approximately one third of the original value, and so forth.[1]

RESPIRATORY ACIDOSIS

When the lungs become less effective at removing carbon dioxide, $Paco_2$ increases and respiratory acidemia ensues. Causes of respiratory acidosis can be separated into pulmonary and nonpulmonary causes.[15] The most common pulmonary cause of respiratory acidosis in term newborns is obstructive lung disease, such as meconium aspiration[47] and transient tachypnea[35] of the newborn. For newborns delivered before 34 weeks of estimated gestational age, surfactant deficiency and immature parenchymal lung and neuromuscular development are the most common reasons for respiratory acidosis. Obstructive lung disease is found in the recovery phase of uncomplicated respiratory distress syndrome and in bronchopulmonary dysplasia.[39] Also included in the pulmonary causes of hypoventilation are conditions that interfere with expansion of the lungs, such as diaphragmatic hernia, phrenic nerve paralysis, or pneumothorax. These limit tidal volume.[15]

A nonpulmonary cause of carbon dioxide retention is poor respiratory effort. Decreased respiratory drive may be secondary to narcosis because of maternal anesthesia before delivery; sepsis; intracranial hemorrhage, including intraventricular hemorrhage; hypothermia; and metabolic disturbances, such as hypoglycemia.[15] Even if respiratory drive is appropriate, newborns may have an inadequate neuromuscular ability to ventilate due to prematurity, degree of illness, and conditions that decrease muscular tone and strength such as those found in certain genetic syndromes (e.g., Prader-Willi syndrome) and maternal conditions (e.g., Graves' disease), and from medication side effects (magnesium sulfate for maternal preeclampsia).

RESPIRATORY ALKALOSIS

In respiratory alkalosis, carbon dioxide clearance is increased and thus $Paco_2$ is below normal.[18] Respiratory alkalosis occurs as a result of hyperventilation, which may be caused by (1) excessive ventilatory support; (2) central nervous system stimulation that increases respiratory drive (e.g., hyperammonemia from a genetic abnormality of the urea cycle)[10]; and (3) hypoxemia, which stimulates respiratory centers through chemoreceptors.[18]

NONRESPIRATORY (METABOLIC) ACIDOSIS

In nonrespiratory (metabolic) acidosis, the metabolic component results from either adding nonvolatile acid (an acid other than carbonic acid) or losing base (bicarbonate).[30,40,44] The underlying mechanisms of metabolic acidosis are (1) loss of base in urine or stool, (2) exogenous acid that is unable to be effectively secreted by the kidneys (high levels of amino acid administration), and (3) abnormal metabolism that leads to an increase in nonvolatile acid levels. Nonvolatile acids originate from lactic acid in circulatory shock and hypoxia, organic acids in inborn errors of metabolism, and ketoacids in diabetic acidosis. Loss of bicarbonate occurs in renal tubular acidosis (inability of the renal tubules to reabsorb bicarbonate appropriately), with stool loss (diarrhea), or through urinary excretion.[42,43,45]

Measurement of the anion gap helps identify the mechanism of metabolic acidosis.[13,16,24,45] The anion gap is variably calculated as the serum sodium concentration minus the serum chloride concentration minus the serum bicarbonate concentration,[28,45] or, alternately, sodium plus potassium

minus chloride minus bicarbonate.★ The upper limit of the normal anion gap with the first method is given as 14 mEq/L[45] and with the second method as 15 mEq/L.[22] Addition of nonvolatile acids is associated with an increased anion gap. Loss of base or excess chloride [Cl^-] is the likely mechanism of acidosis with a normal anion gap.[38,45] An advantage of measuring the anion gap in understanding the effect of excessive chloride administration is clear. Given that there must be balance between blood cations and anions to preserve electroneutrality, [Cl^-] in excess simply displaces [HCO_3^-], resulting in metabolic acidosis.[45] In normal anion gap acidosis, low serum potassium indicates loss of base (e.g., diarrhea) and high serum potassium points to a renal defect (e.g., renal tubular acidosis).[28]

Albumin is a major component of the anion gap. Hypoalbuminemia, common in critically ill neonates and children, may mask the presence of the anions of lactic and organic or other nonvolatile acids.[13,14,16,22,28] A "normal" anion gap in combination with low serum albumin indicates that a nonvolatile acid anion is making up the difference for "absent" anions that albumin would ordinarily provide. Correcting the anion gap for hypoalbuminemia is accomplished by adding 2.5 mEq/L to the anion gap for every g/dl that the concentration of serum albumin is reduced below the normal value of approximately 3.5 g/dl.[13,43]

NONRESPIRATORY (METABOLIC) ALKALOSIS

Nonrespiratory (metabolic) alkalosis is caused by either a loss of acid or an increase of base, principally bicarbonate.[25] Alkalosis occurs when excessive amounts of bicarbonate, acetate, citrate, or lactate are given; metabolism of the later three anions in the liver generates bicarbonate. Loss of acid occurs with gastric fluid removal or prolonged vomiting as can be seen with pyloric stenosis. Acid loss by renal mechanisms can occur through the influence of diuretics, digitalis, or corticosteroids.[18] Urine electrolytes, especially chloride, are useful in the differential diagnosis of metabolic alkaloses. Low urine Cl^- (less than 20 mEq/L) is associated with chloride (saline)–responsive metabolic alkalosis from acid loss (e.g., vomiting, nasogastric suction), whereas high urine Cl^- is associated with chloride

---

★References 9, 14, 16, 20, 22, 38.

(saline)–unresponsive metabolic alkalosis from renal acid loss (e.g., diuretics).[16,28]

OXYGENATION

Inadequate cardiac output, anemia, an increased hemoglobin affinity for oxygen, and hypoxemia (decreased PaO_2) may cause tissue hypoxia. Hypoxemia results from lung disease or cyanotic congenital heart disease. The most common lung abnormality is mismatched ventilation and perfusion.[9] In newborns, there is always some degree of ventilation and perfusion mismatch. Two extreme examples are (1) ventilated and oxygenated alveoli without perfusion (e.g., pulmonary emboli) and (2) perfused but nonventilated alveoli (atelectasis). The former is an example of wasted ventilation, and the latter represents an intrapulmonary shunt. Either extreme is incompatible with life. Clinically relevant degrees of ventilation-perfusion mismatch lie somewhere between those extremes.[9]

Hypoxemia, resulting from ventilation-perfusion mismatch, can be overcome with supplemental inspired oxygen. An increased inspired oxygen concentration will eventually displace nitrogen from even the most poorly ventilated alveoli, and alveolar and then arterial oxygen tension will increase. However, when an extrapulmonary shunt bypasses the lungs PaO_2 does not increase. This is important in that clinicians can differentiate parenchymal lung disease from cyanotic congenital heart disease as a cause of hypoxemia because the latter will not have a significant increase in PaO_2 even with the administration of 100% oxygen.

To perform the *hyperoxia test,* the clinician should place the neonate in 100% oxygen for 10 to 15 minutes and obtain a right radial arterial blood sample. If the PaO_2 rises to more than 150 mm Hg, cyanotic congenital heart disease is very unlikely and lung disease is the most common etiology.

Central hypoventilation from narcosis may cause hypoxemia. As alveolar carbon dioxide rises, PaO_2 falls and PaO_2 decreases. This condition should be clinically evident and should not be confused with lung or congenital heart disease. Other causes of hypoxemia are sufficiently rare in the infant that we need only mention them: decreased inspired oxygen tension, as with increasing altitude, and oxygen diffusion limitation. Diffusion limitation is not usually clinically important in neonatology.

PREVENTION

Prevention of acid-base and oxygenation disturbances and maintenance of acid-base homeostasis require attention to detail. Prevention of premature births or transport of pregnant women who may deliver a high-risk infant to tertiary care centers for treatment can minimize perinatal asphyxia and its consequences.

With respiratory disturbances, immediate assessment and prompt therapy, including supplemental inspired oxygen and assisted ventilation, may help improve oxygenation and respiratory component of acid-base disturbances (see Chapter 23). Careful monitoring of fluid and electrolyte intake and output, minimizing blood loss, and observing for sepsis help the clinician prevent development of nonrespiratory acid-base disturbances (see Chapter 14).

DATA COLLECTION

Monitoring inspired oxygen concentrations and arterial oxygen tension and supplying appropriate concentrations of additional inspired oxygen will prevent hypoxemia (see Chapter 23). Monitoring may be accomplished intermittently through indwelling arterial catheters or continuously by transcutaneous oxygen monitors and pulse oxygen saturation devices (see Chapter 7). Monitoring hemoglobin concentrations and blood loss, with appropriate replacement, helps ensure adequate blood oxygen content.

Reviewing the patient's history, performing a physical examination, and evaluating laboratory data augment each other in the assessment of disturbances in acid-base homeostasis and oxygenation (Box 8-2).

History

An adequate obstetric and perinatal history may warn of potential acid-base and oxygenation disturbances:

- Premature delivery predisposes the infant to shock and respiratory distress.
- Meconium staining may portend respiratory difficulties.
- Prolonged rupture of membranes, maternal diabetes, or abnormal maternal bleeding may be associated with either metabolic or respiratory acid-base disturbances and hypoxemia.

BOX 8-2

EVALUATION OF ACID-BASE DISTURBANCES AND OXYGENATION PROBLEMS IN NEONATES

1. History
   a. Obstetric and perinatal
   b. Neonatal
   c. Family
2. Physical examination
   a. Vital signs
   b. General appearance
   c. Respiratory effort
   d. Pulmonary examination
   e. Cardiac examination
   f. Abdominal examination
   g. Neurologic examination
3. Laboratory
   a. Chest x-ray film
   b. Arterial blood gases
   c. Urinalysis
   d. In selected cases: sepsis evaluation, serum electrolytes, serum albumin, urine electrolytes, and urine osmolality

- A neonatal history of vomiting, diarrhea, or other gastrointestinal disturbances can cause acid-base disturbances.
- The infant's general appearance, feeding habits, and activity level may indicate sepsis or CNS injury, both of which promote acid-base disturbances and hypoxemia.
- Nosocomial infections and pneumonia may significantly influence acid-base and oxygenation disturbances.
- A family history of inherited renal problems such as tubular acidosis may suggest an acid-base disturbance.
- A family history of salt-losing endocrinopathies may produce an acid-base disturbance.

Physical Examination

SIGNS AND SYMPTOMS

Signs of acid-base disturbance vary widely and often go undetected. Hypothermia and low blood pressure should alert caretakers to the possibility of metabolic acidosis. Altered respiratory rate and pattern, grunting respirations, nasal flaring, and chest wall retractions raise the possibility of respiratory acidosis or respiratory compensation for metabolic acidosis. Abnormalities on auscultation of the heart may point to congenital heart disease and resulting acid-base and oxygenation abnormalities. Lethargy, seizures, and abnormal neurologic signs increase concern for acid-base disturbances or hypoxemia.

Laboratory Data

Chest radiograph: A chest x-ray examination may assist in identifying a respiratory or cardiac cause for an acid-base disturbance and hypoxemia.

Urinalysis: The routine urinalysis records urine specific gravity and demonstrates that urine is being produced. Urine electrolytes and pH are helpful in differentiating among the pathophysiologic mechanisms of metabolic derangements.

Arterial blood gases: Interpretation of the arterial blood gases will point to the primary acid-base derangement and may reveal a secondary compensation and define the degree of hypoxemia.[9,27,36,46,47] Presently, methods for monitoring the components of acid-base analysis comprise both invasive and noninvasive techniques. Intermittent arterial punctures or indwelling catheters in various vessels (often the umbilical artery or vein) supply data. However, we can continuously measure transcutaneous Po_2 or O_2 saturation. Monitors can continuously measure expired end-tidal CO_2, which corresponds to the alveolar CO_2. (Alveolar and arterial CO_2 are equivalent unless respirations are excessively rapid.) In addition, skin electrodes are available that measure Pao_2 and $Paco_2$ with varying success (see Chapter 7).

Although the pathophysiologic condition of the acid-base disturbance is determined through the analysis of arterial blood gases, further assessment of the infant is necessary, as follows:

- Respiratory alkalosis or acidosis can be anticipated by obstetric and family history, physical examination, and chest x-ray examination or diagnosed by arterial blood gas analysis.
- Metabolic acidosis often accompanies shock and septicemia. The anion gap and urine electrolytes may provide additional information to delineate causes. Blood pressure measurement, a complete blood cell count, serum and urine electrolytes and pH, serum albumin and glucose determinations, and assessment of intake

and output of fluids are often needed to identify the source of a metabolic acidosis.

- Oxygenation disturbances may be analyzed from the preceding laboratory tests, and, when indicated, electrocardiogram and arterial blood gas response to increased inspired oxygen concentrations are used to evaluate the possibility of congenital heart disease.

Another calculation, the *oxygenation index (OI)*, is used to assess critically ill neonates receiving ventilator therapy. The OI is (FiO_2 × 100 × mean airway pressure) divided by PaO_2 or, simply put, work/result. In some centers, an OI of 25 or greater has been considered an indication for extraordinary ventilatory support, such as inhaled nitric oxide or extracorporeal membrane oxygenation (ECMO).

CORD BLOOD GASES

Providers participating in delivery room stabilization, as well as subsequent care of at-risk newborns, benefit from a thorough understanding of cord gas interpretation, as well as familiarity with the perinatal conditions that may have an adverse effect on fetal outcome. See Table 8-2 for normal cord blood gas values.[49]

When reviewing cord gas values, it is important to note that there is a broader range of normal values than postnatal blood gas values and that the relationship between the venous and arterial norms is the opposite of conventional blood gases.[34] During fetal circulation the umbilical vein transports oxygenated blood from the placenta (acting as the fetal lung) to the fetus. The umbilical arteries transport blood from the fetus back to the placenta for gas exchange. The most useful value is umbilical arterial blood pH because it is indicative of the fetal metabolic condition just before birth and is most strongly associated with perinatal mortality risk and important morbidities.[32]

Umbilical Cord Blood Gas Sampling. Controversy exists as to which perinatal circumstances warrant collection and review of umbilical cord blood gases. The American College of Obstetricians and Gynecologists' Committee on Obstetric Practice updated its opinion statement regarding cord blood gas analysis in 2012.[3] Cord gas collection and review should occur in "circumstances of cesarean delivery for fetal compromise, low 5-minute Apgar score, severe growth restriction, abnormal fetal heart rate tracing, maternal thyroid disease, intrapartum fever, or multiparous gestations."

There are a few points to keep in mind when collecting and analyzing cord blood. After delivery, immediate collection and analysis of cord blood ensures the greatest sampling accuracy. However, samples collected and analyzed within 1 hour at room temperature, or within 6 hours if the samples are refrigerated, maintain valid results.[42] The placenta continues to be metabolically active after delivery and theoretically, if the blood being sampled is in close proximity to the placenta, there may be continued gas exchange, yielding cord gas results that are not truly reflective of the fetal environment.[5]

Cord Blood Gas Interpretation. Asphyxia results when there is interruption of placental-fetal gas exchange and is more specifically defined as metabolic acidemia following birth measured by a pH of less than 7.00 and a base deficit of greater than 12 mmol/L.[34] General causes of intrapartum asphyxia are (1) impaired uteroplacental gas exchange (uteroplacental insufficiency), (2) inadequate umbilical blood flow (cord occlusion), or (3) impaired fetal cardiac output.

General principles of cord blood gas interpretation are as follows:

1. Umbilical venous blood represents uteroplacental status.
2. Umbilical arterial blood represents fetal *and* uteroplacental status.
3. When interpreting an infant's paired cord gases the cord venous gas will *always* have a higher pH, a lower PCO_2, and a higher PO_2 than the umbilical artery cord gas. If these rules of interpretation are not apparent it is likely that the samples were from the same vessel or mislabeled.[7,34]

TABLE 8-2	UMBILICAL VENOUS AND ARTERIAL CORD BLOOD GAS VALUES	
	VENOUS	ARTERIAL
pH	7.25-7.45	7.18-7.38
PCO_2 (mm Hg)	26.8-49.2	32.2-65.8
PO_2 (mm Hg)	17.2-40.8	5.6-30.8
HCO_3^- (mmol/L)	15.8-24.2	17-27
BD (mmol/L)	0-8	0-8

BD, Base deficit.

Uteroplacental Insufficiency. There are multiple perinatal and intrapartum factors that can lead to uteroplacental insufficiency. Some common clinical conditions include maternal hypotension or hypertension, maternal hypoxia, maternal medications, a hyperstimulated contraction pattern, premature placental separation, or a defect in placental development. On many occasions uteroplacental insufficiency is mild in nature and has no lasting effect on neonatal outcome. However, if a critical threshold of uteroplacental insufficiency is reached, the fetus becomes hypoxic. The degree and duration of the hypoxia will determine whether a metabolic acidosis will occur.[19] When intrapartum asphyxia is the result of uteroplacental insufficiency, the umbilical venous and arterial blood gases will *both* reveal derangements in acid-base status. However, due to fetal hypoxia, the arterial gas will demonstrate a lower pH, higher Pco_2, and lower Po_2 than the venous cord sample. On many occasions cord gases reveal a paired respiratory acidosis without a metabolic component, which indicates an acute (less than 30 minutes) event.[7]

Cord Occlusion. Identification of true cord prolapse during labor is enough to raise even the calmest of clinician's heart rates (see Chapter 2). However, there are several less intuitive scenarios leading to functional cord occlusion either by stretching or compression. They include anatomically short cord, breech presentation, occult cord prolapse, shoulder dystocia, nuchal cord, body cord, true knot in the cord, kinking of the cord, cord entanglement between monoamnionic/monochorionic twins, and, following rupture of membranes, any instance in which a fetal body part could intermittently compress the umbilical cord.[34]

The most common cord occlusion scenario is compression of the umbilical vein and at least partial patency of the umbilical arteries. Cord blood gas sampling in this scenario would yield a near-normal venous gas with an arterial sample demonstrating a metabolic and respiratory acidosis to various degrees depending on severity and chronicity of the vessel compression. Overall, the hallmark cord gas findings in cord occlusion are a widened venoarterial pH, Pco_2, and, at times, base deficit differences.

Fetal Circulatory Failure. There are a myriad of causes that can ultimately lead to fetal circulatory failure. Included among these are fetal hemorrhage/anemia, structural heart disease, arrhythmias, cardiomyopathies, extracardiac malformations, and septic shock. For example, in progressive fetal anemia as seen with RH isoimmunization, the fetus compensates for the anemia by increasing cardiac output. As the anemia worsens, oxygenation becomes inadequate to meet cellular metabolism and heart failure occurs. As cardiac output decreases and blood flow slows, there is increased oxygen extraction from the blood and increased production of CO_2. This phenomenon will create widened venoarterial pH, Pco_2, and Po_2. Cord gases following fetal circulatory failure have a similar appearance to gases obtained after cord occlusion.[34]

Pathologic Predictive Value of Cord Blood Gases. Cord blood gas data and analysis are useful for immediate management, but pH alone is poorly predictive of long-term outcomes. Infants that recover quickly with reassuring neurologic examinations tend to have good long-term outcomes regardless of cord blood pH. Although low cord blood pH is clearly associated with poor outcome, association is not cause and effect. The underlying cause of both acidosis and organ damage is tissue hypoxia.[21,26] In contrast, an arterial cord pH less than 7.00 in combination with abnormal clinical signs and symptoms is strongly associated with adverse outcomes.[48] Low and colleagues[31] demonstrated that arterial base deficits of 12 to 16 mmol/L were associated with moderate or severe newborn sequelae in 10% of the neonates studied. That number increased to 40% of neonates once the base deficit reached greater than 16 mmol/L.[31] Conversely, mildly increased base deficits are not usually associated with newborn complications. Although analysis of cord gases can at times be difficult, paired cord blood gases have a role in determining appropriate treatment and guide further evaluation.

TREATMENT

In respiratory acidosis, the pathophysiologic mechanism is decreased alveolar ventilation. Treatment is directed at the underlying cause.[13] Hypoxemia caused by ventilation-perfusion mismatch is treated with increased inspired oxygen concentration. Techniques that may be of benefit to treat respiratory acidosis include continuous positive airway pressure (CPAP), standard ventilation, high-frequency ventilation, ECMO, inhaled nitric oxide,[17] and others (see Chapter 23). Treatment of respiratory alkalosis usually consists of reducing minute ventilation. One of the causes of neonatal central hyperventilation, which requires a high index of suspicion and urgent evaluation and treatment, is hyperammonemia caused by an inborn error of urea cycle metabolism[10] (see Chapter 27).

Asphyxia often leads to a combined respiratory and metabolic acidosis. Ventilation will resolve the respiratory acidosis. Improved oxygen delivery and tissue perfusion usually resolves lactic acidosis without bicarbonate therapy. In narcosis, temporary ventilator support may be necessary. Narcosis may be reversed with administration of naloxone (Narcan) at a dose of 0.1 mg/kg if the possibility of chronic maternal opiate drug abuse has been ruled out. With chronic intrauterine opioid exposure, neonatal Narcan administration may result in acute withdrawal and seizures (see Chapter 4).

With any acidosis and alkalosis, determining the underlying etiology is critical for effective management. If the cause of metabolic acidosis is septicemia, intestinal necrosis, or poor cardiac output severe enough to result in metabolic acidosis, successful treatment of the cause is of far more importance than buffer therapy for acidosis. Historically, sodium bicarbonate has been administered for a neonatal metabolic acidosis. However, controversy exists on the true physiologic benefit from sodium bicarbonate administration.[4,6] Sodium bicarbonate administration may conversely cause harm, especially with a bolus administration because it is a hypertonic solution, which may increase the risk of intraventricular hemorrhage.[30,37] It should not be used if severe lung disease restricts carbon dioxide elimination (see Equation 3).

COMPLICATIONS

Unrecognized or untreated acid-base or oxygenation disturbances may lead to increased mortality rates or morbidity rates in survivors. Complications of the correction of the acid-base and oxygenation disturbance vary according to the disturbance and treatment provided.

One effect of acidosis is CNS depression. In metabolic acidosis, the rate and depth of respiration are increased, whereas in respiratory acidosis, respiration may be labored or depressed. An effect of alkalosis is increased excitability of the CNS and tetany (often of the respiratory muscles).[15,16,25,42]

Treatment of respiratory acidosis by assisted ventilation can produce all of the complications of assisted ventilation, including infection, trauma, oxygen toxicity, sepsis, air leak, and subglottic stenosis (see Chapter 23).

Complications of oxygen therapy include hypoxemia and hyperoxemia. Severe hypoxemia may cause pulmonary vasoconstriction, a change from aerobic to anaerobic metabolism (with eventual metabolic acidosis), bradycardia, hypotonia, or impaired CNS and cardiac function. Prolonged high inspired oxygen concentrations can result in oxygen toxicity, which may be central to significant morbidities such as retinopathy of prematurity and bronchopulmonary dysplasia.[11,23]

Case Scenario Examples

CASE 1

You are caring for a 7-day-old, late preterm (36 weeks) female infant who has poor feeding, sleepiness, decreased urine output, and a new oxygen requirement of 40% Fio_2 on 2 L/min nasal cannula. On examination, she is only mildly responsive to stimulation, has delayed capillary refill of 3 to 4 seconds throughout with poorly palpable peripheral pulses (especially in her lower extremities), respiratory rate in the 80s with labored breathing and clear breath sounds, a cuff-measured blood pressure in her right arm of 65/40, heart rate in the 160s that is regular, and oxygen saturations in the low 90s in right upper extremity. You are concerned about her appearance and order a chest x-ray, complete blood count with differential and platelets, electrolytes, blood culture, urine culture with Gram stain and microanalysis, C-reactive protein, and arterial blood gas. The first result that confirms your concerns is the arterial blood gas: pH 7.03, Pco_2 30, Po_2 55, calculated bicarbonate of 9, base excess minus 16. Serum electrolyte results include sodium of 134, potassium of 5.9, chloride of 95, and bicarbonate of 10. You calculate an anion gap of 35 (134 + 5.9 − 95 − 10). Clinical suspicion is that this newborn has coarctation of the aorta that has become critical on closure of her patent ductus arteriosus, which is confirmed by echocardiogram. The patient receives administration of parenteral prostaglandin, arterial and central venous access, and a cardiology consultation. In patients with metabolic acidosis, it is imperative to identify the cause of the acidosis, which, in this case, was due to decreased oxygen delivery to tissues below the level of the coarctation, resulting in a large anion gap metabolic acidosis from lactic acid production due to anaerobic metabolism.

CASE 2

You attended the delivery of a 32-week, 1.6-kg male infant after preterm labor with rupture of membranes and clear fluid 1 hour before delivery. The mother did not receive betamethasone or antibiotics before delivery. He was delivered vaginally with Apgar scores of 5 and 7 at 1 and 5 minutes, respectively. He presented with poor respiratory effort and responded to drying, stimulation, and positive-pressure ventilation with 30% oxygen after color, and oxygen saturation did not improve with blow-by oxygen. By 5 minutes he was breathing spontaneously with an oxygen saturation measured at 85%. He was admitted to the neonatal intensive care unit and placed in a hood with 50% oxygen. On examination he was grunting with marked retractions, had decreased breath sounds with rales, and had a respiratory rate of 80 with an oxygen saturation of 82%. The rest of the examination was noncontributory. He was placed on CPAP of 5 cm H_2O pressure in 45% Fio_2 and oxygen saturations increased to high 80s. Catheters were placed in the umbilical vein and artery. A chest x-ray revealed low lung volumes, a fine reticulogranular pattern, and prominent air bronchograms. The arterial blood gas results at 2 hours of life were pH 7.13, Pco_2 66, Po_2 51, calculated bicarbonate 14, and base deficit 5. You suspect the infant has respiratory distress syndrome based on symptoms beginning at birth, chest x-ray, and blood gas revealing hypoxemia and, predominantly, a respiratory acidosis. Additional supporting factors include prematurity, lack of antenatal steroids, and examination significant for retractions. Your management includes surfactant replacement therapy and mechanical ventilation in addition to antibiotics and a follow-up blood gas analysis. Respiratory acidosis is a classic finding in respiratory distress syndrome, especially in the preterm population. Treatment goals are aimed at normalizing both oxygenation and ventilation and treating for the possibility of infection.

REFERENCES

For a full list of references, scan the QR code or visit http://booksite.elsevier.com/ 9780323320832.

9

DIAGNOSTIC IMAGING IN THE NEONATE

JOHN D. STRAIN AND JASON P. WEINMAN

Imaging has become an important part of the diagnosis and workup of medical problems of newborns. The ability to use a noninvasive means to diagnose disease, screen for potential pathologic conditions, monitor the effects of therapy, and assist in defining prognosis for counseling has made imaging an essential part of health care. With refinements in diagnostic equipment and capabilities, the role of imaging has expanded significantly in recent years. There are many ways to assess any problem, and the vast potential of the new imaging modalities makes appropriate imaging a constant challenge (Table 9-1). New modalities have been introduced, and advancement in computer technology has added sophistication to established modalities. Nearly 60% of diagnostic imaging involves modalities that were not even available 30 years previously.

There are many excellent reference books and textbooks on neonatal imaging, and specific questions can be addressed most adequately through these resources. This chapter reviews the various imaging modalities available for diagnosis and intervention. A short summary of each imaging modality includes background information, a discussion of image acquisition, and the risks and benefits of each. We have provided a thumbnail description of each modality; however, for clarity, we have taken significant liberty and license in discussing the physics of image acquisition. Each section addresses the most common usage of the modality in neonates, followed by a focused discussion of one or two aspects of image interpretation.

Because there may be more than one appropriate way to evaluate any given problem, it is essential to understand the inherent advantages and limitations of each modality to decide which might be most effective. We have pointed out some of the challenges associated with diagnostic imaging. A focused problem-solving approach with appropriate collaboration and consultation can yield positive results.

RADIOGRAPHY

Background

The 1896 introduction of the roentgenogram was met with great enthusiasm, and x-ray examination quickly became an indispensable diagnostic tool in clinical settings throughout the world. Until 35 years ago, the field of radiology was based almost exclusively on use of the x-ray.

A beam of ionizing radiation from a source (x-ray tube) passes through the patient, and various structures within the body interact to attenuate the x-ray before it is received on the other side. The x-rays pass through the patient and then expose a film, just as light exposes a negative in black-and-white film photography. The film is developed, and the resultant image (radiograph) is a map that corresponds to the transmitted x-ray (that portion of the x-ray not attenuated by absorption or scattered as it passes through the patient). Somewhat analogous to the shadows that result from objects in the sun, the images from x-ray are a shadow of the object being radiographed. (Hence the slang term "shadow doctor" came into use in reference to early radiologists.) Bone attenuates a greater amount of the x-ray (or allows the penetration of fewer x-rays) than lung tissue does, resulting in a film on which the rib is white and the lung is black. In some ways, this can be compared with the different shadows cast by

---

PURPLE type highlights content that is particularly applicable to clinical settings.

TABLE 9-1	COMPARATIVE ANALYSIS OF IMAGING MODALITIES					
IMAGING MODALITY	**IONIZING RADIATION**	**SPATIAL RESOLUTION**	**CONTRAST RESOLUTION**	**COST**	**SEDATION**	**MISCELLANEOUS**
X-ray	Very low	Excellent	Fair	Low	Never	Very fast acquisition eliminates motion
Fluoroscopy	Low	Excellent	Fair	Moderate	Never	Evaluates motion real-time
Ultrasonography	None	Good	Fair	Moderate	Never	Portable; evaluates motion real-time
Computed tomography	Low	Good	Good	Moderate to high	Sometimes	Cross-sectional imaging
Magnetic resonance imaging	None	Good	Excellent	High	Frequent	Multiplanar (i.e., in multiple planes) imaging, flowing blood without contrast
Nuclear medicine	Very low	Poor	Excellent	Moderate to high	Sometimes	Physiologic imaging

the trunk of a tree and by its leaves. With radiography, the spatial resolution is exquisite although the contrast resolution is lacking. One can capture 10 to 20 line pairs per millimeter with film radiography, although only five different densities can be distinguished routinely: air, fat, water (which includes all solid viscera—liver, spleen, kidney, pancreas, and heart), bone, and metal.

More recent developments in x-ray technology include computed radiography (CR) and digital radiography (DR). Although the physics of x-ray generation is essentially the same, the receiver has changed. With CR, a phosphorescent plate replaces film and the latent image is captured digitally. With DR, the image is directly captured in a digital mode. The introduction of these products was driven by the desire to capture, archive, distribute, and display digital images. Almost all medical imaging is now digital, and a *picture archiving and communication system (PACS)* has become an essential component of any imaging department.

Clinical Utility in the Neonatal Intensive Care Setting

Radiography is the simplest and most reliable way to define tube and line position. Radiopaque markers are incorporated into most of these devices. From peripherally inserted central catheters (PICC) to endotracheal, thoracostomy, and feeding tubes,

TABLE 9-2	POSITION OF LINES AND TUBES
LINE/TUBE	**POSITION**
Endotracheal tube	1 cm above the level of the carina
Umbilical artery catheter	Descending aorta between T8 and T10
Umbilical venous catheter	Junction inferior vena cava and right atrium
Central line	Junction superior vena cava and right atrium
PICC line	Junction superior vena cava and right atrium
Nasogastric tube	Antrum of the stomach

PICC, Peripherally inserted central catheter; *T8 and T10,* thoracic vertebrae 8 and 10.

a simple radiograph can help eliminate the complications of suboptimal line or tube placement (Table 9-2). Chest radiographs are most commonly used to evaluate the heart and lungs. Abdominal imaging allows a limited assessment of the solid viscera (the liver, spleen, and kidneys), as well as the bowel gas pattern, useful in evaluating a neonate with a feeding intolerance (Figure 9-1). Bones of the trunk and extremities are assessed easily with plain film radiology.

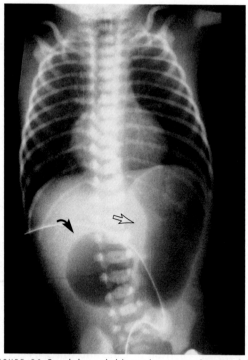

FIGURE 9-1 Frontal chest and abdomen show gaseous distention of the stomach *(open arrow)* and duodenal bulb *(curved arrow)*, the classic double bubble seen in duodenal atresia. Incidental note is made of 13 pairs of ribs in this patient with Down syndrome.

In addition to helping determine a specific diagnosis, imaging is frequently a valuable means for assessing patient response to therapy. For instance, lung compliance and volume, as assessed by x-ray studies, help determine the patient's response to various ventilator rates and pressures; therefore the x-ray findings can be very useful in the selection of the most appropriate ventilator settings.

Focused Discussion: Chest Radiographs

The most common use of x-ray imaging in the neonatal unit is for evaluation of the chest to help define abnormalities that might contribute to respiratory distress. Respiratory distress in newborns can be divided into three categories: conditions that are managed medically, those that are managed surgically, and iatrogenic respiratory distress.

MEDICALLY MANAGED RESPIRATORY DISTRESS

Table 9-3 summarizes plain film diagnosis of respiratory distress in newborns. Use of this approach takes advantage of the fact that only a limited number of changes can be identified radiographically, and a constellation of findings can define a specific group of etiologic factors. A systematic analysis of these various characteristics helps determine a specific group that has a fairly limited differential diagnosis (Box 9-1).

TABLE 9-3	PLAIN FILM DIAGNOSIS OF MEDICALLY MANAGED CAUSES OF RESPIRATORY DISTRESS IN THE NEWBORN (CHIMP DIFFERENTIAL)					
		GESTATIONAL AGE	HEART SIZE	LUNG VOLUME	NATURE OF INFILTRATE	PROGRESSION	ANCILLARY FINDINGS
C	Congenital heart disease		Increased	Normal or increased	Increased pulmonary vascularity or edema	Stable or progressive	Abnormal situs, aortic discordance
H	Hyaline membrane disease*	<36 weeks		Decreased	Diffuse granularity with air bronchograms	Progressive over first 24 hours	No pleural effusions or body wall edema
I	Immature lung	<26 weeks	Normal	Decreased	Diffuse granularity	Progressive	Absent thymus from stress
M	Meconium aspiration	≥39 weeks	Normal	Increased	Streaky and patchy	Stable	Air leak (i.e., pneumothorax)
P	Neonatal pneumonia		Normal or increased		Either diffuse or focal		Pleural effusions and body wall edema

*Idiopathic respiratory distress syndrome (IRDS).

SURGICALLY MANAGED RESPIRATORY DISTRESS

Respiratory conditions that are managed surgically can be subdivided into three groups: (1) those associated with aspiration, such as cleft palate, laryngeal cleft, or tracheoesophageal fistula (TEF); (2) those that compromise functional lung volume, including congenital diaphragmatic hernia (CDH), congenital lobar emphysema (Figure 9-2), pulmonary sequestration, and congenital pulmonary airway malformation (CPAM); and (3) those associated with tracheal or bronchial narrowing, such as a double aortic arch and other vascular rings and slings, congenital tracheal stenosis, and bronchogenic cyst (Box 9-2).

IATROGENIC RESPIRATORY DISTRESS

Most iatrogenic respiratory distress results from either a misplaced catheter or tube or from barotrauma. An endotracheal tube (ETT) can be placed too deep and will preferentially ventilate only a single lung. An ETT may even be inadvertently placed into the esophagus, resulting in inadequate ventilation (Figure 9-3), which is further compromised by

distention of the esophagus and small bowel, limiting lung expansion.

Air leaks are often the result of barotrauma (Figure 9-4). Although barotrauma occurs much less frequently because of the introduction of exogenous surfactant, high-frequency ventilation and nitrous oxide therapy, air leaks continue to be a problem that causes significant concern. Appropriate ventilation management requires timely and accurate diagnosis. One goal in review of a chest

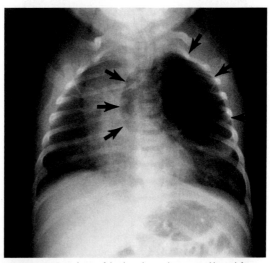

FIGURE 9-2 Frontal view of the chest shows a hyperaerated lucent left upper lobe *(arrows)* associated with mediastinal shift from left to right and is characteristic of congenital lobar emphysema.

BOX 9-1	CHIMP DIFFERENTIAL DIAGNOSIS MODEL

Congenital heart disease
  Transient tachypnea of the newborn (resolves over first 24 hours)
  Extracardiac shunts
Hyaline membrane disease*
  Diffuse atelectasis
Immature lung
  Represents anectasis rather than atelectasis
Meconium aspiration
  Amniotic fluid aspiration
Pneumonia
  Diffuse
    Birth asphyxia
  Focal
    Pulmonary hemorrhage
Bronchopulmonary dysplasia represents the chronic lung disease that may result from any of the causes of respiratory distress.

*The use of exogenous surfactant modifies the picture of hyaline membrane disease (idiopathic respiratory distress syndrome [IRDS]) significantly. The irregular distribution after endotracheal administration causes a much less uniform infiltrate, and the patchy pattern that results has a look similar to that in meconium aspiration, which might be seen in a term or postterm infant.

BOX 9-2	SURGICALLY MANAGED RESPIRATORY DISTRESS

1. Associated with aspiration
   a. Cleft palate
   b. Laryngeal cleft
   c. Tracheoesophageal fistula
2. Compromised functional lung volume involvement
   a. Congenital diaphragmatic hernia
   b. Congenital lobar emphysema
   c. Congenital cystic adenomatoid malformation
3. Cause tracheal or bronchial narrowing
   a. Double aortic arch
   b. Tracheal stenosis
   c. Bronchogenic cyst

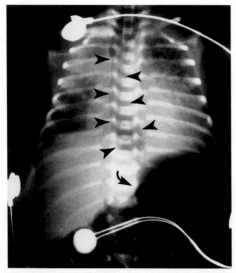

FIGURE 9-3 Frontal chest film. Although the endotracheal tube projects over the midline mediastinum near the thoracic inlet, the dilated esophagus *(arrowheads)* and distended stomach *(arrow)* associated with right upper lobe and left lower lobe atelectasis suggested esophageal intubation, which was diagnosed in this patient.

x-ray film is to define the location of the extra-pulmonary gas. Abnormal extrapulmonary gas can include any one or a combination of the following: pulmonary interstitial emphysema, subcutaneous emphysema, pneumomediastinum, pneumothorax, pneumopericardium, pneumocardia, and portal venous gas.

Focused Discussion: Skeletal Dysplasia

Skeletal dysplasias are a group of bone and cartilage disorders that, although each variety is rare, overall occur in approximately 1 in 5000 births. Today over 450 individual skeletal dysplasias are known and classified by their clinical, radiographic, and genetic findings. The accurate identification and classification of a patient with skeletal dysplasia can have important implications for the patient, with some proving fatal in early life. In patients in whom a complex skeletal dysplasia is suspected, a skeletal survey consisting of anteroposterior (AP) and lateral views of the skull, AP and lateral views of the spine, and AP views of the pelvis and all extremities (with separate AP views of the hands and feet) should be obtained. Although a complete description of the identification and

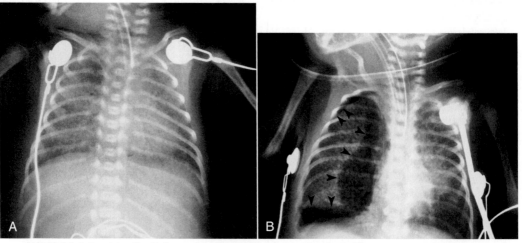

FIGURE 9-4 **A,** Frontal chest film. Hyaline membrane disease in this patient is defined by the diffuse symmetric granular infiltrates with small lung volumes. This patient required intubation, and the endotracheal tube tip projects in satisfactory position. **B,** Follow-up examination in the same patient demonstrates linear lucencies within the right lung resulting from pulmonary interstitial emphysema. A tension pneumothorax *(arrowheads)* is identified on the right with mild mediastinal shift from right to left. The lack of atelectasis on the right is the result of extremely poor lung compliance that accompanies pulmonary interstitial emphysema. The endotracheal tube tip projects in a satisfactory position, but the nasogastric tube is in the midesophagus.

classification of skeletal dysplasias is far beyond the scope of this book, a basic approach to skeletal dysplasias and a few examples will be presented.

The first step in assessing the radiographs in a patient with suspected skeletal dysplasia is to look for disproportion. A disproportionate appearance of the chest, such as a narrowed elongated chest, can be an important early sign of a dysplasia. Other signs include flattening of the vertebral bodies (platyspondyly) with short trunk disproportion, and shortening of the extremities, such as rhizomelia (root or proximal limb shortening), mesomelia (middle limb), or acromelia (distal limb). The next step is to evaluate epiphyseal, metaphyseal, and diaphyseal ossification. Growth of long bones occurs at the ends where the midshaft *(diaphysis)* is contiguous with the distal shaft *(metaphysis)* and separated by a radiolucent cartilaginous plate *(epiphyseal cartilage or physis)* from the distal end *(epiphysis)*. Ossification centers of the distal femur, proximal tibia, calcaneus, and cuboid are often present at birth. With these findings in mind, the patient can often be classified into a group of skeletal dysplasias. With the help of reference books on skeletal dysplasias, such as *"Taybi and Lachman's Radiology of Syndromes, Metabolic Disorders and Skeletal Dysplasias,"* specific findings can lead to a diagnosis.

Achondroplasia is a relatively common dysplasia with 2.8 cases per 100,000 births. Achondroplasia is a disproportionate rhizomelic short-limbed skeletal dwarfism (i.e., the proximal segment [humerus] is shorter than the middle [radius and ulna] and distal [wrist and hand] segments). Patients with achondroplasia also have a disproportionately large head with decreased size of the skull base and narrow foramen magnum. The lower lumbar spine demonstrates narrowing of the distance between the pedicles, which normally widen at the lower lumbar spine and develop kyphosis (posterior angulation) at the thoracolumbar junction. Infants often suffer from respiratory difficulties due to adenoidal hypertrophy, narrow nasal passages, and small thorax. Narrowing of the foramen magnum and cervicomedullary compression can lead to hydrocephalus and neurologic complications.

Thanatophoric dysplasia is also a disproportionate rhizomelic short-limbed dwarfism. Although the radiographic findings are qualitatively similar to achondroplasia, the severity of the manifestations helps differentiate the two. Classic findings in newborns with thanatophoric dysplasia include

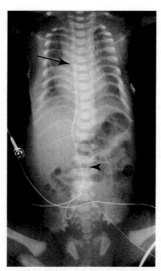

FIGURE 9-5 Anteroposterior film of the chest and abdomen of a patient with asphyxiating thoracic dystrophy (Jeune syndrome) demonstrates short broad ribs with a narrow thorax as well as shortened iliac wings with bony spurs. Also note the malpositioned umbilical venous catheter with its tip in the upper right atrium *(arrow)* and umbilical arterial catheter *(arrowhead)*.

very short bowed femurs with metaphyseal flaring (telephone receiver femurs), narrow thorax, large head with small facial bones and flattened vertebral bodies with notched endplates. Thanatophoric dysplasia is frequently suggested on prenatal ultrasonography by shortened femurs and narrow chest. This dysplasia has important implications in the neonatal intensive care unit (NICU) because infants will die within the first few days of life without respiratory support.

Asphyxiating thoracic dysplasia (Jeune syndrome) presenting symptoms are a long narrow thorax with short horizontal ribs and respiratory difficulties in infancy (Figure 9-5). Shortening of the extremities including the hands and feet, with occasional polydactyly (extra digits), also occurs and can present at birth or later in life. In the pelvis, the iliac wings are shortened in the craniocaudal direction with bony spurs projecting from the acetabula. Complications in asphyxiating thoracic dysplasia in the neonate are primarily respiratory distress due to reduced lung volumes/small chest size. Later in life respiratory infections become a problem and progressive renal disease leading to renal failure may occur. Patients may also develop hepatic fibrosis, pancreatic fibrosis, and retinal degeneration.

FLUOROSCOPY

Background

In fluoroscopy, an x-ray tube similar to that used for plain film radiography is used. The x-ray is generated in the same manner as in plain radiography, but it is received in most cases by a device that is similar to a TV camera or VCR. Fluoroscopy allows real-time evaluation of a patient and can be performed with or without contrast material. Spatial resolution in fluoroscopy is not as good as that in plain film radiography, but it is still excellent. Contrast resolution is about the same: air, fat, water, bone, and contrast are about the only densities that can be separated. Contrast media can be given orally or per rectum, instilled into the urinary bladder, or given intravenously. The contrast attenuates the radiation beam to a variable extent related to physical properties and thickness of the attenuator. Most contrast agents are compounds that use either inert barium or iodine as the attenuator of the radiation beam. The most important characteristic of fluoroscopic imaging is the ability to evaluate motion in real time. This is essential in the evaluation of swallowing function, gastrointestinal (GI) peristalsis, and diaphragmatic motion.

Clinical Utility in the Neonatal Intensive Care Setting

The most common fluoroscopic examinations requested for neonates include the upper GI (UGI) series, the contrast enema, and voiding cystourethrography. The UGI series is useful in the evaluation of swallowing, aspiration, feeding intolerance, vomiting, and abdominal distention with possible bowel obstruction.

A contrast enema can be diagnostic in Hirschsprung's disease (Figure 9-6). It can be both diagnostic and therapeutic in meconium plug syndrome and meconium ileus.

A voiding cystourethrogram is used to evaluate the urinary bladder and the urethra and to look for vesicoureteral reflux (Figure 9-7), which is associated with urinary tract infection. Vesicoureteral reflux is a common cause of hydronephrosis, which is now frequently identified during prenatal ultrasonography. Ureteroceles, periureteral diverticula, and posterior urethral valves all can be associated with hydronephrosis in the neonatal period and demonstrated with cystourethrography.

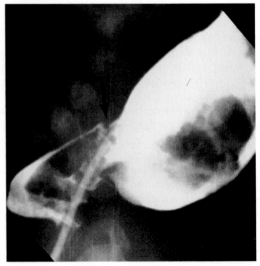

FIGURE 9-6 A lateral film from the early filling phase of a barium enema demonstrates spasm of the distal rectal segment *(short arrow)* with a transition zone to dilated colon *(long arrow)*. These findings are characteristic of colonic Hirschsprung's disease.

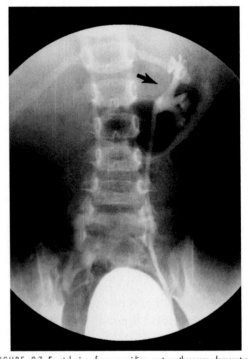

FIGURE 9-7 Frontal view from a voiding cystourethrogram demonstrates grade II vesicoureteral reflux on the left *(arrow)*.

Air works as a fine contrast agent, and the nasal and oral airway, as well as the trachea and proximal bronchus, can be easily evaluated fluoroscopically. Because the diaphragm is immediately adjacent to aerated lungs, diaphragmatic motion and its relationship to inspiratory effort help in the evaluation of phrenic nerve injury and diaphragmatic paralysis. Eventration of the diaphragm also can be evaluated fluoroscopically, but at times can be indistinguishable from diaphragmatic hernia.

Focused Discussion: Upper Gastrointestinal Series

Indications for performing a UGI series include swallowing dysfunction, aspiration, vomiting, choking, and apnea. An appropriately performed UGI series offers a systematic approach to the upper GI tract. Starting with the patient in a left-side-down recumbent position, deglutition is evaluated. Tongue action, transport, nasopharyngeal regurgitation, aspiration, and laryngeal penetration all can be assessed. The right-side-down position better separates the esophagus and the tracheal air column. However, if this position is used initially and the evaluation of the deglutition is prolonged, the stomach may empty, filling the proximal small bowel and obscuring the location of the ligament of Treitz. The left-side-down position allows one to evaluate swallowing without concern that the stomach may empty prematurely. Once deglutition is satisfactorily evaluated, one can concentrate on the esophagus. Vascular rings and slings are evaluated in both the frontal and lateral positions.

Esophageal atresia usually is diagnosed clinically; plain film observation of intraluminal bowel gas defines the most common form, which is associated with a distal tracheoesophageal fistula. Often an enteric tube that coils in the proximal esophageal pouch is the initial radiographic finding in patients with tracheoesophageal fistula. The benefit of a proximal pouch study in esophageal atresia is controversial. There is a small incidence of fistula from the proximal pouch to the trachea; this incidence is independent of the presence or absence of a distal fistula. If the surgical approach to esophageal atresia repair includes direct visualization of the proximal pouch *(esophagoscopy),* the pouch contrast study is superfluous. If, on the other hand, esophagoscopy is not routinely performed, there is some value in evaluating the proximal pouch before surgery. In the absence of esophageal atresia,

the location of the fistula (H type) is at the thoracic inlet. This is higher than the fistula that occurs in the most common form of esophageal atresia, in which the fistula is at the level of the carina.

The caliber of the esophagus is informative, because it is usually dilated in association with significant *gastroesophageal reflux.* Esophageal contour, mucosal detail, and peristalsis are assessed. The configuration of the gastroesophageal junction can indicate gastroesophageal reflux, and rare hiatal hernias can be diagnosed. Gastric emptying is evaluated and gastric peristalsis examined. Because the rotation and fixation of the bowel have important consequences in the newborn period, this is an important part of a complete examination. The duodenal bulb, C-loop, and ligament of Treitz are defined. Both the posteroanterior (PA) and lateral views are essential in localizing the ligament of Treitz. For proximal bowel rotation and fixation to be considered normal, the duodenal-jejunal junction (ligament of Treitz) must be retroperitoneal (and therefore posterior), to the left of the spine, and at the level of the retroperitoneal portion of the second portion of the duodenum (just distal to the duodenal bulb).

The rotation of the proximal bowel may be independent of the rotation of the hindgut. Therefore if the clinical question is malrotation and possible volvulus, the UGI series is the examination of choice. The caliber, contour, and fold pattern of the proximal bowel are evaluated and the transit time observed. This simple, systematic, yet comprehensive approach to a UGI series yields a tremendous amount of information.

ULTRASONOGRAPHY

Background

One of the most prominent mass media introductions of ultrasound (US) technology came when Dr. Robert Ballard located the wreckage of the *Titanic* using US to explore the ocean floor of the North Atlantic. Medical ultrasonography has its roots in sound navigation and ranging (sonar) developed during World War II.

In medical ultrasonography, a transducer (essentially a piezoelectric crystal) converts electrons into mechanical vibration that creates high-frequency sound waves within the body. The same transducer serves as both the transmitter of the sound wave and the receiver of the reflected sound. Within the body, these high-frequency sound waves propagate through the soft tissues until they meet a reflective surface that reflects some of those fluid waves back to the transducer. The percent of the sound beam reflected relates to the difference in the acoustic impedance of the material being evaluated. When the acoustic impedances of materials are similar, as is the case with the abdominal wall musculature (e.g., liver, kidney), most of the sound is transmitted and a small percent reflected at each interface. As the sound wave travels through the abdominal wall to the liver, the abdominal wall–liver interface reflects a portion of the beam and transmits most of the sound through the liver to the liver-kidney interface. The small difference in acoustic impedance between the liver and kidney causes reflection of some of the beam and transmission of most of it to the posterior abdominal wall. This allows the visualization of multiple interfaces that are deeper than the first structure encountered. If the velocity of the sound beam in tissue is known, the distance to the reflective surface can be estimated by measuring the time it takes for the pulse to travel the distance to and from the object imaged.

Most of the tissues in the body have similar acoustic impedances; however, air has extremely low impedance and bone extremely high impedance. This means that there is a big difference in the acoustic impedance between these substances and the organs most commonly imaged. For this reason, both bone and air reflect nearly all of the sound that reaches them. This is why a coupling gel is used on the skin surface to eliminate the air gap between the transducer and the skin. This is also why imaging through the liver gives a good acoustic window to deeper structures but bowel gas obscures imaging lower in the abdomen. For ultrasonographic imaging of the brain in a neonate, the anterior fontanel serves as the acoustic window because the bone of the skull acts as a reflective surface that limits through-transmission of US to deeper structures. The mastoid fontanel serves as a window to the posterior fossa. Bulk fluids within the body, such as urine in the urinary bladder, bile in the gallbladder, or cerebrospinal fluid in the ventricles, have no internal interfaces and therefore are seen as solid black on conventional ultrasonography. Cysts have a sharp posterior wall and have increased through-transmission, because the sound wave penetrates the fluid without any reflections to block transmission of the sound.

Doppler ultrasonography takes advantage of the physical principle that the US reflection from a moving object distorts the wavelength, with the distortion related to the velocity of the object being measured. This is the principle that causes the pitch of a train's whistle to change from high to low as the train passes an observer. It is the same principle police use to monitor the speed of a car and the Judd gun uses to measure the velocity of a pitcher's fastball. In fact, this same principle is responsible for the "red shift" observed by astronomers in determining that we live in an expanding universe. The Doppler evaluation in medical ultrasonography uses the distortion of the wavelength caused by moving red cells to identify flowing blood.

One of the major advantages of US imaging is the lack of ionizing radiation. Although most diagnostic imaging that requires ionizing radiation is of low dose, any radiation exposure is a concern and should be avoided when possible. The portability of ultrasonographic equipment has made it a valuable adjuvant to diagnostic imaging in the neonatal intensive care setting.

Clinical Utility in the Neonatal Intensive Care Setting

Ultrasonography has had a major effect on the evaluation of the neonatal brain. Most of the early work focused on intracranial hemorrhage, which was a common occurrence in preterm neonates. Even though the incidence has decreased, intracranial hemorrhage remains an issue for which US imaging is extremely well suited. Ultrasonographic instrumentation has improved tremendously, and with the addition of color and pulse Doppler technology, great strides have been made in the refinement and sophistication of intracranial imaging. Numerous complex structural abnormalities can be recognized, and screening for developmental abnormalities can largely be accommodated with cranial ultrasonography. Because bone reflects most of the sound-limiting through-transmission, the open fontanel is the window to the brain. As the fontanel closes over time, ultrasonography becomes less and less useful for intracranial imaging. This same limitation affects the utility of ultrasonographic evaluation of the spine as the patient ages.

Renal imaging offers another major role for ultrasonography in the neonatal unit. The kidneys are well visualized ultrasonographically, either through a posterior approach or, more commonly, by using the liver or spleen as soft-tissue acoustic windows to the kidneys. Ultrasonography is an excellent way to evaluate hydronephrosis, which is now frequently picked up on routine prenatal evaluations. Ultrasonography has a role in the evaluation of a jaundiced patient because it is ideal for evaluating cystic structures, such as the gallbladder, and can readily identify dilated biliary ducts. Jaundice caused by biliary obstruction from a choledochal cyst, for instance, can be diagnosed readily ultrasonographically. Because of the reflectivity related to bone and bowel gas, US imaging is much more effective in the upper abdomen, in which the liver and spleen serve as the acoustic windows, or in the pelvis, in which the urinary bladder can function as the window.

Even though ultrasonography is limited by bone, ultrasonographic imaging has a significant role in the evaluation of hips in the neonate. Because the capital femoral epiphysis of the newborn is cartilage, the hip can be well imaged in a neonate. Maternal estrogen causes ligamentous laxity. This changes significantly during the first weeks of life; therefore the accuracy of hip ultrasound examinations improves after the first 3 to 4 weeks of life. Ultrasonography is very good for the detection of developmental dysplasia of the hip and can be used to evaluate the degree of femoral head coverage, the acetabular angle, and any instability of the hip.

Focused Discussion: Cranial Ultrasonography

Ultrasonography is an ideal tool for evaluating the brain in a newborn. In general, an ultrasonographic examination is the first step in the imaging evaluation for any neurologic question. Structural abnormalities, intracranial hemorrhage, sequelae of anoxic or ischemic events, and infection are all well assessed via US imaging. The most common approach is through the anterior fontanel, but additional information can be gained with axial imaging through the squamosa of the temporal bone. The posterior fossa can be evaluated through the posterior lateral fontanel. Familiarity with the normal anatomy is essential. Coronal and parasagittal views are obtained generally. Normal structures can be recognized easily; their absence or deformity is necessary to define developmental abnormalities of the brain. The ventricular size and configuration are

assessed. Characteristic ventricular configurations can define lobar or semilobar holoprosencephaly. In addition, the ventricular configuration can suggest septo-optic dysplasia or agenesis of the corpus callosum. The corpus callosum can be visualized directly; abnormalities of the corpus callosum are associated commonly with *Chiari malformation* and other structural abnormalities of the brain, such as *Dandy-Walker malformation.* Dilation of one or more of the ventricles can be an indication of a pathologic condition. An obstruction of cerebrospinal fluid (CSF) flow in the region of the aqueduct of Sylvius manifests with disparity in ventricular size. The third and lateral ventricles are enlarged, whereas the fourth ventricle remains normal in size. Dilation of one of the lateral ventricles, especially when associated with an area of *porencephaly,* is indicative of an in utero destructive event.

Seizures or apnea may indicate an anoxic or ischemic event in a neonate. Certain structural abnormalities can suggest a specific diagnosis; for instance, periventricular nodules and cortical tubers define tuberous sclerosis. US examination is less sensitive than computed tomography (CT) and magnetic resonance imaging (MRI) in defining subtle areas of gray matter heterotopia or focal pachygyria, examples of developmental abnormalities associated with seizures. US imaging is very sensitive to intracranial hemorrhage, and areas of increased echogenicity can be demonstrated in areas of edema. Intracranial hemorrhage generally is a concern in a premature neonate (Figure 9-8). It is classified into four grades, and each grade generally is associated with a prognosis. Grade I hemorrhage usually has a good outcome, whereas the prognosis with grade IV hemorrhage is frequently poor. Grade I hemorrhage is confined to germinal matrix in the caudothalamic groove. This is the last fetal germinal matrix to mature and is prone to hemorrhage in preterm babies. Grade II intracranial hemorrhage has intraventricular blood. Grade III hemorrhage is associated with ventricular dilation as the intraventricular clot enlarges the lateral ventricles. Grade IV hemorrhage must demonstrate parenchymal extension. It has been hypothesized that grade IV hemorrhage may be the result of venous infarction that occurs from obstruction of the septal veins by the swollen germinal matrix hemorrhage. Periventricular leukomalacia is a consequence of anoxic or ischemic injury to the brain that manifests as increased echogenicity in the

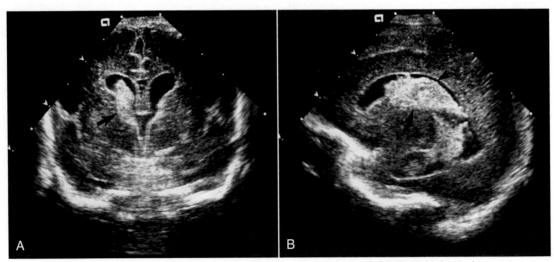

FIGURE 9-8 Coronal **(A)** and parasagittal **(B)** ultrasound images from a cranial ultrasound study demonstrate an echogenic clot *(arrows)* within the dilated right ventricle. The intraventricular clot with ventricular dilation defines a grade III hemorrhage.

deep periventricular white matter of the centrum semiovale. This may progress to cavitation and is then called *cystic leukoencephalomalacia.* Ultrasonographic examination is a very sensitive way to detect this change, which is usually apparent within 2 weeks of birth.

COMPUTED TOMOGRAPHY

Computed tomography (CT) was initially developed in 1972 in Middlesex, England, by EMI. EMI, which stands for Electric and Musical Industries, had been an industrial research company. After signing The Beatles in 1962, the company sold its computer business; however, it kept a researcher named Godfrey Hounsfield and funded his independent research through the revenue generated by the Beatles' success. Hounsfield imagined that he could determine what was inside a box by taking x-rays of the box at all angles. He then worked to build a computer that could reconstruct a slice of an object from the data of these x-rays acquired at various angles. He shared the Nobel Prize in Physiology and Medicine with Allan Cormack, who developed the theoretical mathematics for the invention of CT.

Early CT scanners produced data by acquiring x-ray data in multiple positions in an axial plane moving to a different level between acquiring slices. The initial EMI scanner solved mathematical

equations representing the attenuation of the different x-ray beams, like a giant Sudoku puzzle. The complexity of mathematics involved as well as limitations in computers at the time contributed to the limited speed of the scanner; it took approximately 10 minutes to acquire and reconstruct each slice as well as limited the resolution to an 80×80 matrix. For comparison today's fastest dual-source CT scanners can acquire a slice in about 0.07 second in the fastest scanning mode with a matrix of 1024×1024.

On modern multidetector helical CT scanners, image acquisition takes place as the patient is moved on a mobile table through a rotating gantry containing an x-ray source on the opposite side of the gantry of x-ray detectors. As a ring of data is acquired as the patient is moved through the gantry, the path of image acquisition is in effect a helix, resembling a coil spring, hence the term helical or spiral CT. Multidetector arrays of 4, 8, 16, 64, and even 320 elements allow rapid acquisition of multiple slices in a single rotation of the tube. This renders high-resolution isovoxel data sets (each volume element has the same width, height, and depth). As the data are acquired in a continuous helix in an isovoxel data set, as if peeling an apple from top to bottom in one peel, the data can be reconstructed in any plane as well as rendered in three-dimensional (3D) as you could imagine putting an apple peel back together to look just like an apple. Reconstruction of the acquired data has undergone and continues to undergo revisions. In the most commonly employed method, filtered back projection lines of gray representing the attenuation of the patient are layered on top of each other to create images with different filters applied to accentuate different aspects of the image. This renders a cross-sectional slice that can show all of the structures within that slice. For instance, a slice through the upper abdomen may show the liver, spleen, pancreas, both kidneys, and the spine, each separated by a plane of fat and each with a subtly different density.

New technologies on recently introduced CT scanners include volumetric scanning, dual-source and dual-energy CT scanners, as well as technology designed to reduce dose to patients by limiting the patient's exposure during the scan or allowing for improved reconstruction of scans obtained at lower radiation doses. Volumetric scanning achieved with up to 320 detectors can allow for an area up to 16 cm to be scanned in a single rotation of the scanner gantry. Dual-source, dual-energy scanners can leverage two tubes and two detector arrays, either for increased scanning speed up to 0.07 second per slice with both tubes at the same energy or improved tissue differentiation using different energies. Given the recent attention articles in both the medical literature as well as the lay press have given to radiation effects from CT, there has been a renewed focus on technology to reduce the dose in CT scans. This includes both improving the mechanics of the CT scanners themselves as well as developing more advanced reconstruction algorithms that allow scans obtained at lower doses to obtain excellent image quality.

These recent advances in CT technology have resulted in spectacular images and an explosion in CT utilization. The radiation dose in CT, however, is significantly higher than that in routine radiography. CT now accounts for more than 60% of the radiation exposure from medical imaging in the United States. Trailing this incredible growth in utilization of CT has been greater understanding and concern for the effects of ionizing radiation in medical imaging. Evaluation of the risk associated with the low doses of ionizing radiation used in medical imaging is a complex and evolving topic. The majority of studies estimating risk from low doses of radiation have been based upon models in which survivors of large known doses of radiation, such as from the atomic bombs in Japan, have been followed longitudinally to access the risk of developing cancer. These models assume that by extrapolating the effects of large radiation doses to low doses, the risk for low doses can be assessed in what is called a linear no-threshold model. Although the accuracy and assumptions in this type of model have been questioned, with some investigators claiming that there is in fact no risk nor even benefit to low doses of radiation, more recent studies have suggested that there is a small increased risk of cancer associated with clinical medical imaging. A retrospective cohort study that looked at the incidence of leukemia and brain tumors in pediatric patients who had undergone CT demonstrated an association between the radiation received from CT scans and leukemia and brain tumors. Although there was a significant increase in relative risk suggested in this study, the absolute risk remained low.

Medical research suggests that the radiation dose currently used in diagnostic CT is associated with an increase in the risk for radiation-induced malignancy. Neonates, infants, and children are more susceptible to the effects of radiation than adults. This stems from the fact that, for a given exposure to radiation, the effective dose is greater the smaller the patient as more of the radiation penetrates the patient. Also, longer life expectancy puts younger patients at an increased risk as there is a longer period of time for a radiation-induced complication to develop.

Ionizing Radiation in Perinatal Medicine: The effects of ionizing radiation on the fetus of a pregnant patient is also a complex and important area of concern. Although the general guideline that use of ionizing radiation in patients who are pregnant should be avoided when possible, there still exist indications for which the benefit of performing the examination may outweigh the risk to the fetus. Additionally, on rare occasions a CT may have been performed on a patient who was not known to be pregnant before the examination. Although a comprehensive analysis of risk and radiation exposure of a pregnant patient undergoing CT should be considered in consultation with a medical physicist, general guidelines have been provided by the American College of Radiology in conjunction with the Society for Pediatric Radiology as briefly described in the following paragraphs:

Before conception there has been no documented genetically heritable risk in the human population. *In the first 2 weeks* after conception the only potential risk is felt to be loss of pregnancy. Doses associated with radiographic procedures have not been clearly associated with increased risk, although this is difficult to determine as approximately half of all conceptions are lost in this period, often unbeknown to the woman.

Radiation exposure *between 2 and 15 weeks* postconception has more complex risk implications. In general, radiologic procedures outside of the abdomen and pelvis, including the head, neck, and chest, should result in only a very low dose to the fetus as the only exposure is related to scatter radiation. In a patient who is known to be pregnant, the study should be optimized to even further limit the dose to the fetus. When imaging of the abdomen and pelvis is indicated, or has been performed, consideration of the risk to the fetus takes on greater importance. In centers that carefully manage their CT radiation dose, as do most children's hospitals, the dose to the fetus is thought to be below the level associated with any developmental abnormality. However before counseling takes place, verification of the dose by a qualified medical physicist is recommended. If the dose is determined to be low, the majority of the risk associated with radiation exposure to the fetus is a small increased risk of cancer in later life and termination of pregnancy would not be indicated. Doses associated with increased developmental disorders are uncommon in routine practice and usually occur in circumstances that have important implications to the pregnancy, such as in patients who require complex cardiology or interventional radiology procedures.

The effects of radiation exposure to the *fetus more than 15 weeks* postconception are even smaller, with risk to the developing nervous system occurring only at very high doses, usually beyond what would be typically encountered even with multiple radiology procedures. Therefore, after 2 weeks' gestation, the predominant concern with low-dose diagnostic imaging is the small increase of developing cancer over a lifetime.

Although concern for the deleterious effects of radiation are important, it should always be viewed in the context of the patient as a whole. CT can be a powerful tool in evaluating the pediatric patient. Caution is the key: (1) image only when indicated; (2) limit the scan to the region of concern; and (3) be cognizant of dose and use as low peak kilovoltage (kVp) and milliampere second (mAs) as possible, and use dose-reduction technologies while maintaining diagnostic quality examinations.

Clinical Utility in the Neonatal Intensive Care Setting

Cranial imaging is the most common use of CT in most neonatal intensive care settings. CT adds significant specificity to the abnormalities recognized with ultrasonography. Concern about ionizing radiation and the fact that CT equipment generally is not portable make obtaining a CT more difficult than obtaining a sonogram. CT is more accurate in assessing the nature of extraaxial fluid collections and is very helpful in further defining structural abnormalities of the brain, particularly those associated with abnormal distribution of gray or white matter. It is also very good for evaluating intracranial hemorrhage and infection. Exquisite bone detail defines craniofacial anomalies, choanal atresia and stenosis, and abnormalities of the petrous bone associated with hearing loss. Chest imaging is becoming much more frequent in the NICU. It is used to evaluate abnormalities detected during intrauterine ultrasonographic examination and for potential surgical lesions identified on chest x-ray films. Ultrasonography remains the first-line diagnostic tool for the evaluation of kidneys, liver, and spleen, but when a pathologic condition of the abdomen is a concern and a good acoustic window for US imaging is not available, CT is frequently the examination of choice. CT can be performed with significantly less sedation than that necessary for MRI. CT eliminates many of the artifacts, including those of vascular flow, respiratory motion, and even bowel peristalsis, that limit the utility of MRI. Skeletal lesions are well visualized with CT. Ultrasonography is the method of choice in the evaluation of congenital hip dysplasia, but CT can be very helpful in evaluating the position of the femoral heads after reduction and treatment of congenital hip dysplasia when the patient is immobilized in a plaster cast.

CT can be very helpful in identifying the organ of origin of a specific pathologic condition. This, of course, is the first step in narrowing a differential diagnosis. The addition of intravenous contrast is very useful in defining tumor thrombus in renal arteries and the inferior vena cava, which may affect surgical approach to renal and hepatic neoplasm. The nature of abnormalities seen on CT can frequently lead to a specific diagnosis. Although the spatial resolution of CT is inferior to that of plain film radiography, the contrast resolution is significantly better and CT has taken advantage of this trade-off. The cross-sectional rendition of anatomy, which allows deep structures to be distinguished from one another, is the most significant advantage that CT has over radiography.

Focused Discussion: Intracranial Blood

Noncontrast CT is extremely sensitive and specific for the detection and localization of intracranial blood (Figure 9-9). Blood from acute hemorrhage has a density on noncontrast CT (measured in Hounsfield numbers) higher than any normal structure except bone and calcium. The increased contrast resolution of CT allows the differentiation of gray matter from white matter and lends itself to detailed structural evaluation of the brain. The ventricles are low in density (0 Hounsfield units, equal to water), the white matter more dense, and the gray matter more dense still, followed by blood from acute hemorrhage and, finally, calcium and bone. Blood from acute hemorrhage is visualized as white as soon as a clot is formed, and this high density will slowly decrease over time. For instance, the blood in a subdural hematoma after 2 to 3 weeks will become lower and lower in density until it is indistinguishable from water, which is equal to CSF density in the ventricular system. MRI can differentiate blood from a chronic subdural hematoma for a longer time than CT because

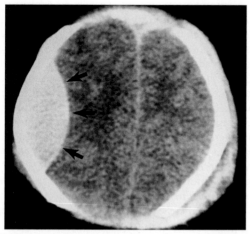

FIGURE 9-9 A single axial image near the vertex demonstrates a high-density lenticular mass *(arrows)* in the extraaxial space over the right cerebral cortex. The lenticular configuration is that of an epidural fluid collection and the high-density characteristic of blood from a chronic hematoma.

the protein within a chronic subdural hematoma modifies the signal on MRI for an extended period. Although all intracranial blood does change density over time, the compartment in which the blood is found affects the rate of change to some extent. Therefore the timing of an event responsible for the blood cannot be precisely determined based on the density alone.

The location of the blood is the next issue. CT is the most accurate imaging method for detection of subarachnoid blood. The presence of subarachnoid blood postpartum is common, even after a relatively nontraumatic birth. Unfortunately, on rare occasions, subarachnoid blood can cause vasospasm of vessels near the skull base, which can result in relative ischemia or hypoperfusion of the peripheral cortex. Areas of edema can be detected by looking for loss of the normal gray-white differentiation or by finding a focal area of brain edema characterized by relatively low density caused by the addition of low-density water to an otherwise normal area of brain.

The shape of a collection of blood is an important variable used in evaluating intracranial hemorrhage. Subarachnoid blood assumes a configuration that follows the arachnoid space. Therefore it is most frequently seen in the suprasellar cistern, the ambient cistern, the sylvian fissure, or the interhemispheric fissure, or layering on the tentorium. The most sensitive locations for identifying subarachnoid blood are in the region of the quadrigeminal plate cistern, the posterior aspect of the third ventricle, and the interpeduncular cistern. Subdural hematomas occur most frequently over the convexities or along the interhemispheric fissure. Those over the convexity can be differentiated from epidural hematomas by their crescentic configuration. This is opposed to the lenticular configuration of an epidural hematoma. The dura is the periosteum of the inner table of the skull; therefore an epidural hematoma is limited by the adhesion of the periosteum to the skull and hence the lenticular configuration. This is also why epidural hematomas are associated most often with higher-pressure arterial bleeding and why subdural hematomas frequently are associated with venous bleeding. Another key to differentiating the compartment is the relationship to cranial sutures. An epidural hematoma will not cross a suture line because of the anatomic limitation of the dura by the suture. A similar limitation by dural attachment at suture lines helps distinguish a cephalohematoma from a caput succedaneum. The direct sagittal imaging of MRI has made us more aware of the high prevalence of subdural blood in the posterior fossa.

MAGNETIC RESONANCE IMAGING

Background

MRI is a modality that images protons or hydrogen ions within the body. Rapid development of magnetic resonance was, in part, because of the transfer of some of the sophisticated reconstruction algorithms used in CT and the computer power developed in other fields, such as 3-D graphics used in cartoon animation, cartography, and seismology. These technologic advances allow tremendous amounts of information to be manipulated quickly enough to make image reconstruction a reality. MRI is essentially hydrogen imaging, and because the human body is 98% water, much hydrogen is available to image.

MRI is performed by placing a patient in a strong magnetic field, which varies slightly from the head to the foot. Each proton acts as a small magnet, and just as the needle on a compass orients itself in one direction when placed next to a magnet, the protons in the body align when placed into the magnetic field of the imaging magnet. This alignment of protons is essential to create an environment that has a net electromagnetic field effect or induces the movement of electrons. Without the alignment of protons by the magnetic field, the random orientation of protons would have no measurable net field effect when stimulated and therefore would create no signal to image.

Once the patient is in the magnet, a radiofrequency (RF) pulse is delivered. In current imaging systems, the pulse wave has a frequency of an FM radio wave. Less than 1 in 1 million hydrogen ions will absorb any energy, and only certain RFs will allow the transfer of energy from the RF pulse to a hydrogen ion.

An analogy of this energy transfer can be seen on a schoolyard playground. Visualize a child on a swing. If you push the swing in rhythm or resonance with the natural frequency of the motion of that swing, then the swing will absorb the energy and the child will swing higher and higher with each push. This natural rate of harmonic motion depends on the length of the rope on the swing and the mass of the swing and the child. If you were to push at a rate that was not synchronous with the swing's natural rhythm, pushing would not allow the energy to assist in propelling the swing higher and higher, and in fact, you would disrupt the normal rhythm of the swing.

In a famous TV commercial for Memorex in the 1970s, the playback of Ella Fitzgerald's voice caused a goblet to break, demonstrating the absorption of resonance frequency by the crystal in the goblet. The absorbed energy caused the goblet to shatter. In MRI, the FMRF energy is used to stimulate hydrogen ions or protons in the body.

Because the field strength of the magnet used for imaging varies slightly from one end of the patient to the other and the resonance frequency depends on the field strength of the magnet, one can selectively stimulate various locations within the patient. By changing the RF slightly, a different specific group of protons is stimulated. Protons stimulated by an RF pulse absorb that energy and move to an unstable higher-energy state. They give up that energy as an RF pulse or "echo" of the pulse they received. The echo is received by an antenna just as with a radio receiver and converted to an image. The signals or echoes received are the result of T1 and T2 relaxation times, which are simply physical parameters that describe the environmental interactions that influence the signal released from a proton. Spin-echo pulse sequences are frequently used sequences in routine MRI.

A spinning top analogy can help to explain the T1 and T2 relaxation times that result in spin-echo imaging. Each hydrogen ion has a dipole moment (a positive pole and a negative pole) and therefore acts like a small magnet within the powerful magnetic field of the imaging magnet. These protons spin or precess with a precessional frequency that is related to the field strength of the magnet. Electromagnetic energy can be transferred to these protons if the energy is delivered at the resonance frequency. Once an RF pulse of resonance frequency is delivered, a certain number of protons (less than 1 in 1 million) absorb this energy and move to a higher-energy state. The T1 relaxation time reflects the time it takes for these excited protons to give up their higher energy and return to baseline.

T2 relaxation times relate to a second parameter of physical interactions. Although the protons are rotating at a frequency proportionate to the magnetic field in which they exist, they are not in phase. In other words, there is no net direction of polarity from all of these spinning magnets. Once the RF pulse perturbs or stimulates these protons, they begin to spin synchronously and therefore create a net magnetic field. This spinning net magnetic field generates an electromagnetic wave that can be picked up by the RF antenna of the imaging system as an "echo" of the original RF pulse delivered. (The principle of a spinning magnet inducing an electromagnetic pulse is the basis for the turbines of hydroelectric generators.)

Because its immediate electromagnetic environment affects each proton differently, these protons will remain synchronous in their precession for a very short period. As they move out of phase or synchrony, the net magnetic field that was created dissipates; therefore the signal received by the RF antenna diminishes. The T2 relaxation time indicates the time it takes the protons to go from a state of synchronous rotation, when maximal signal is created, to random, out-of-phase precession, with zero net magnetic field and hence no signal. The requirement of a net magnetic field to create a signal is used to evaluate flowing blood without the need for contrast. An RF pulse saturates the protons in the field being imaged. The saturated blood within the vessels of that field flow out of the field and are replaced with nonsaturated blood from an adjacent slice. Consequently there is no signal from the vessel containing the blood flowing perpendicular to the slab being imaged.

Diffusion-weighted sequences have proven to be very sensitive in defining neonatal pathology. It is the most sensitive technique in the identification of early anoxic ischemic injury. Diffusion weighting takes advantage of random Brownian motion of molecules in fluid and the restriction of Brownian motion by anatomic barriers or edema. Water within the ventricular system will diffuse homogeneously in all directions (i.e., no restricted diffusion) and will be a low signal on a diffusion-weighted sequence and high signal (white) on an apparent diffusion coefficient map (ADC map). An acute or subacute infarction, for instance, will cause restricted diffusion in the affected region as fluid rushes into cells due to failure of the cells' homeostatic mechanisms, such as ion pumps. The restricted diffusion caused by acute cell death will be a high signal on the diffusion sequence and a low signal on the ADC map. Late findings after infarction will demonstrate facilitated diffusion with a high signal on both the diffusion and ADC map as the infarcted cells burst and therefore no longer

restrict the movement of water molecules. Diffusion tensor imaging measures diffusion in at least six planes simultaneously. From that data, a map of the magnitude and direction of water movement can be generated. The axons within white matter tracts will allow diffusion in the direction of the axon but will restrict diffusion in any direction other than the course of the axon. This allows one to map the white matter tracts and has been studied in relation to developmental abnormalities in brain, the relationship of intracranial neoplasm to white matter tracts, and the plasticity of the developing brain in response to injury.

This is a simplified explanation of the physics necessary for image acquisition. The key is that images are acquired without ionizing radiation, which is particularly attractive in pediatrics. No known harmful effect of either magnetic exposure or RF exposure at levels used in MRI has been observed. However, MRI is still relatively new, and one should be cautious in using fetal and newborn imaging. Energy deposition is a concern, and protocols have been established that limit patient exposure. Another concern is the effect a magnetic field might have on electronic instrumentation, such as pacing devices and metallic surgical clips. The torque on metallic implants can be quite high, but this is rarely of clinical significance. However, the artifact caused by the disturbance of the magnetic field can be significant. The most important and real safety concern is that of the magnetic field attraction of ferromagnetic material. Pens, stethoscopes, or even oxygen canisters can act as projectiles when inadvertently brought too close to a magnetic field. One also should be cautious about the effect that a magnetic field might have on magnetic strips of credit cards and identification badges, but this is more of a nuisance than a safety concern.

The main drawback of current MRI technology is the time it takes to acquire an image. Motion-free imaging is necessary for optimal image quality, and because image acquisition in MRI takes minutes, sedation frequently is necessary. Respiratory and cardiac gating can help for physiologic motion, but even physiologic motion can be problematic.

Focused Discussion: Practical Considerations

The physics of MRI is complex, and variables that influence the signal received are protean (Figure 9-10). These influences variably affect the T1 and

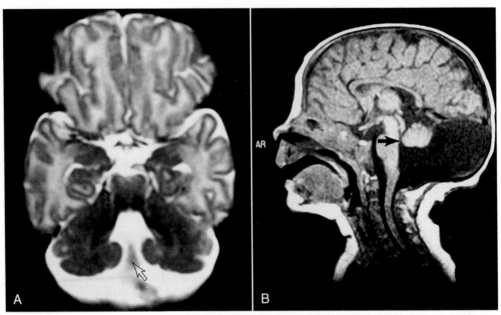

FIGURE 9-10 **A,** Axial T2-weighted image through the posterior fossa demonstrates the high-signal cerebrospinal fluid in the posterior fossa cyst, which communicates with the fourth ventricle more anteriorly *(open arrow).* **B,** Midsagittal T1-weighted image demonstrates a Dandy-Walker variant in this patient. The partial formation of the vermis seen best on the sagittal image defines a Dandy-Walker variant *(black arrow).*

T2 relaxation times in spin-echo imaging. Imaging sequences tend to be called *T1* or *T2 sequences,* depending on which physical parameter has the most influence on the appearance of the image. A simplified approximation of spin-echo imaging helpful for the novice is that in T1-weighted spin-echo sequences fluid is black, and in T2-weighted imaging fluid is white. Most pathologic conditions are characterized either by the distortion of the normal anatomy or by edema, which is manifested by increased fluid in an otherwise normal structure or within the particular lesion. Therefore if one looks for a fluid collection (e.g., CSF in the ventricles of the brain, such as CSF in the subdural space around the cord; orbital fluid of the aqueous humor; or fluid in the heart or urinary bladder), one usually can determine whether the imaging sequence is T1 weighted, in which the fluid appears black, or T2 weighted, in which the fluid appears white. On T1-weighted sequences, a pathologic condition is seen as a black or lower signal, because a pathologic state is associated with increased water in the area of abnormality. In T2-weighted sequences, the pathologic lesion tends to be white.

Focused Discussion: Fetal MRI

Historically, ultrasonography has been the most effective and informative imaging modality in fetal medicine. However, as the field of maternal fetal medicine evolves, fetal MRI is becoming an essential part of the imaging armamentarium (Figure 9-11). The explosion in fetal MRI is the result of advanced instrumentation, imaging sequence development, and finally imaging expertise. The newer equipment and modified sequences shorten acquisition time and therefore minimize artifact, which yields better quality images.

Ultrasonography continues to offer the advantage of availability, portability, and real time acquisition. MRI, like US, is performed without ionizing radiation. Although fetal US continues to be the screening modality of choice, MRI as an adjuvant modality can clarify US findings. Literature also has demonstrated that fetal MRI can identify additional abnormalities not seen by fetal ultrasonography, particularly in the central nervous and genitourinary systems. A fetal MRI examination takes much longer to perform than an US study and, in general, the imaging is not real-time. However, MRI offers

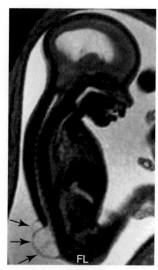

FIGURE 9-11 Saggital T2-weighted fetal MRI demonstrates a defect within the lumbosacral spine with associated cystic structure consistent with a lumbosacral myelomeningocele. The associated findings of a small posterior image, with dilatation of the lateral ventricles consistent with a Chiari II malformation are also partially visible.

a number of advantages. Tissue characterization with MRI is superior to that of US. This is particularly helpful when evaluating the fetus for developmental anomalies of the central nervous system. Cerebral sulcation, cortical and white matter development, and ventricular size and configuration can be readily displayed with fetal MRI. MRI can clarify spinal abnormalities suggested by screening US. MRI is an essential part of the Management of Myelomeningocele Study (MOMS Trial) comparing the results of prenatal versus postnatal repair of myelomeningocele. Another important role of fetal MRI relates to imaging of airway and lungs. Valuable information concerning the degree, location and nature of bronchial obstruction can have significant effect on EXIT (Ex Utero Intrapartum Treatment) procedures to deal with complex anatomy that could result in fatal airway compromise after birth.

NUCLEAR SCINTIGRAPHY

Nuclear scintigraphy is the most physiologic of the tools commonly used in neonatal imaging. A pharmaceutical is tagged with a radiotracer, which is a radioactive isotope that can be detected by a nuclear medicine camera. The pharmaceutical may be injected intravenously, given orally, or delivered directly into the urinary bladder. The pharmaceutical is distributed in the body based on the parent compound to which the radioisotope is chelated or bound. The patient then is imaged using a detector that maps the distribution of the tagged isotope in the body.

The radiation dose in scintigraphy is small. With the doses used for diagnostic purposes, there is no risk to the individual or anyone who is in immediate contact with the patient. The pharmaceutical agents have both a biologic half-life that is related to the natural elimination of the parent compound from the body and a radioactive half-life that is determined by the isotope used to label the pharmaceutical. The spatial resolution is poor, but contrast resolution is exquisite, because the radiopharmaceutical is distributed so specifically within the body.

Clinical Utility in the Neonatal Intensive Care Setting

Three common investigations for which nuclear medicine is well suited are renal scintigraphy, hepatobiliary imaging, and splenic imaging. In patients with the syndrome defined by vertebral, anal, cardiac, tracheal, esophageal, renal, and limb (VACTERL) anomalies, renal scans can be helpful in determining the number and location of the kidneys. Renal scintigraphy can be used to quantify relative renal function. Scintigraphy is a functional way to evaluate the degree of obstruction in hydronephrosis. Nuclear cystography has a very low radiation dose; therefore it is a good method for following vesicoureteral reflux. Fluoroscopic cystography usually is performed for the initial evaluation because the excellent spatial resolution can assist in defining anatomic abnormalities that may be responsible for reflux (e.g., that might be missed with the poor spatial resolution of nuclear imaging).

Hepatobiliary imaging can assist in the evaluation of the jaundiced patient. The radiopharmaceutical is extracted from the blood pool by the liver and excreted like bile, allowing one to determine transit time and flow of the bile from the liver into the gallbladder, through the common bile duct, and into the duodenum. Hepatobiliary imaging can help diagnose neonatal hepatitis, in which there is limited clearance of the pharmaceutical agent from the blood by the liver; therefore the liver shows little activity compared with the background. In biliary atresia, the clearance or extraction of the radiopharmaceutical agent from the blood is closer to normal, but the isotope never leaves the liver and therefore no activity is seen in the duodenum and small bowel, even on delayed images. A choledochal cyst accumulates radiotracer and is diagnosed by an intense area of focal activity and a dilated biliary system more proximally.

Splenic imaging can be performed with technetium sulfur colloid, which is taken up in the Kupffer cells in the liver and spleen. Alternatively, radiolabeling of red blood cells can be used for splenic images because damaged cells are sequestered in the spleen. Splenic imaging frequently is helpful in patients with complex congenital heart disease and situs abnormalities to diagnose asplenia or polysplenia.

Focused Discussion: Renal Scintigraphy

The radiopharmaceutical choices for renal imaging are either cortical agents that bind in the renal cortex, filtered agents that transit the cortex and then are excreted into the collecting system, or a combination of both cortical and filtered agents. Cortical agents are useful in defining size, number, location, and relative function of the kidneys (when there are two kidneys). The US characteristics of multicystic dysplastic kidney (MDK) usually are diagnostic; however, renal scintigraphy (Figure 9-12) occasionally can help differentiate the hydronephrotic form of MDK from severe ureteropelvic junction (UPJ) obstruction. A combination agent, such as mercaptoacetyltriglycine (MAG3), is useful in the evaluation of hydronephrosis, because one can determine the relative function of each kidney and evaluate the degree of obstruction. Addition of the furosemide (Lasix) washout study augments the evaluation of hydronephrosis by rendering a washout curve that is indicative of the severity of obstruction. In evaluating hydronephrosis, generally it is helpful to place a catheter in the urinary bladder to prevent possible vesicoureteral reflux from confounding examination results. Although all of these tests can be performed in the newborn period, the concentrating ability of the newborn kidney is marginal. Therefore the tests often are reserved until the patient is 3 to 6 months of age to improve their accuracy and prognostic capability.

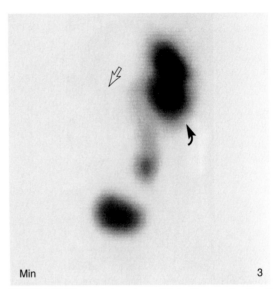

Min   3

FIGURE 9-12 This posterior image from a diethylenetriaminepentaacetic acid (DTPA) renal scan demonstrates the collecting system, ureter, and urinary bladder associated with the functioning right kidney *(black arrow)*. The multicystic dysplastic kidney on the left shows no functional renal tissue *(open arrow)*.

POSITRON EMISSION TOMOGRAPHY

Background

The radiation dose required for positron emission tomography (PET) is significant, and the utilization in neonates and young infants to this point has been limited. Nonetheless, the recent growth and interest in PET requires a section if for no other reason than for completeness.

The concept of PET was initially put forth in the early 1950s. Medical positron emission tomography was first attempted in the mid-1970s. The physics of PET involves introduction of a positron emitting radiopharmaceutical combined with a biologically active substance. These short half-life radiopharmaceuticals require a cyclotron to produce and are therefore less available than the technician chelate pharmaceuticals most commonly used in routine nuclear scintigraphy. A positron is a particle with the opposite charge of an electron that travels only a very short distance within the body until it hits an electron. The collision of the positron with an electron results in two annihilation electrons (gamma rays) of the specific energy 511 keV being emitted in opposite directions at equal velocity. The location in space of the point source of the electrons can be calculated from the fractional difference in the time it takes for the electron to reach the detector. The positron-emitting tracer attached to a metabolically active substance is introduced into the body intravenously, and the radiotracer is distributed throughout the body with the active metabolite. After 30 to 60 minutes of redistribution within the body, a scintillation scanning device detects the nearly coincident paired gamma rays. In the body, bones and other attenuators block some of the electrons from reaching the detector. Therefore a means of identifying the blockers is needed.

Computed tomography happens to be a very efficient means of locating bones and other blockers but has the added benefit of rendering anatomic images. This allows for more precise localization of signal and its relationship to internal structures. Because of the ability to acquire both anatomic and metabolic information simultaneously, the combination of PET and CT (PET/CT) has been responsible for the rapid growth of PET in recent years. Not only can one identify regions of high metabolic activity, but also the location can be more precisely correlated with the internal anatomy with significant improvement in diagnostic accuracy. In humans, the most common pharmaceutical used is fluorodeoxyglucose (FDG), which is a glucose analog. FDG is distributed like glucose throughout the body. Regions of abnormal metabolic activity can be identified and, with CT, localized to a specific structure in the body. A metabolically active tumor, for instance, would demonstrate a focus of increased activity in a PET image. For example, if it were localized in the anterior mediastinum, it would be consistent with the diagnosis of lymphoma.

Clinical Utility in the Neonatal Intensive Care Setting

The relatively high radiation dose associated with PET has limited its use, but it has been effectively utilized in staging neonatal neoplasm. The role PET will play in the evaluation of hypoxic ischemic injury and the evaluation of neonatal seizures is yet to be determined.

INTERVENTIONAL RADIOLOGY

Intervention is one of the newest but most rapidly growing subspecialty areas in medical imaging. Interventional radiology has assumed an important role as a minimally invasive way to treat disease. Imaging is used to direct the surgical approach. From a practical standpoint, there are four major areas of radiology intervention: (1) vascular access, (2) tissue sampling for minimally invasive diagnosis of neoplasm or infection, (3) catheter or needle drainage of fluid collections or abscesses, and (4) directed delivery of cells, chemotherapy, or embolic material, which may be used to diminish flow in a vascular lesion.

Any of the imaging modalities may be used to guide the intervention, but the most commonly used are fluoroscopy, ultrasonography, and CT.

Clinical Utility in the Neonatal Intensive Care Setting

Vascular access is the most commonly requested radiologic intervention in most pediatric institutions. Ultrasonography or fluoroscopy can be used to visualize veins for venous access.

Most *tissue sampling* is performed to diagnose neoplasm. In general, a needle can be placed into an area of abnormal tissue and either a fine-needle aspirate is obtained or, in solid tumors, a core needle biopsy may be performed. The advantage of a core needle biopsy is that the tissue obtained is frequently of volume sufficient to complete many of the biologic studies necessary in the preoperative evaluation of the neoplasm. This can be particularly helpful in patients in whom a neoplasm, once defined, can be pretreated before definitive surgical resection is performed.

Cysts or abscesses can be drained, obviating the need for an open surgical procedure and thus minimizing morbidity and shortening recovery time.

A *gastrostomy or gastrojejunostomy tube* also can be placed in a minimally invasive manner, rather than a more invasive standard surgical procedure. This can be an ideal approach for placement of a temporary feeding tube.

Directed delivery of chemotherapy has been used in neonatal units for the treatment of hepatoblastoma. Chemotherapy can be directed through the hepatic artery into the involved lobe and the tumor reduced in size before excision. The technique allows a previously nonresectable tumor to be resected.

Another example of directed delivery is the *embolization* of hepatic hemangioendothelioma. Hemangioendothelioma is an infrequent cause of congestive heart failure resulting from an extracardiac shunt in the neonatal period. It is possible to embolize the benign neoplasm, thereby diminishing the shunt and correcting the heart's failure. Vein of Galen malformation is another extracardiac vascular shunt that frequently predisposes the patient to high-flow cardiac failure. A significant spectrum of disease is related to vein of Galen malformations, and the success of embolization is highly dependent on the degree of vascular insufficiency related to the steal associated with a high-flow lesion. In patients who present early and in florid heart failure, the outcomes are predictably less positive than in patients who present later with an abnormality discovered during a routine physical examination, in which an intracranial bruit might be identified.

Finally, directed delivery for cell implantation and genetic engineering shows great promise. These areas are early in their development, but the ability to direct a catheter to a specific organ for cell implantation or genetic engineering will clearly have a role in future applications of interventional radiology.

Focused Discussion: Vascular Access

The availability of ultrasonographic equipment can allow placement of peripherally inserted central catheters (PICCs) or central venous catheters in vessels as small as 2 mm. With US imaging, the vessel is visualized directly. Fluoroscopic guidance requires limited venography through a peripheral intravenous (IV) line. Indirect visualization of the venous system is possible because intravascular contrast defines the vascular lumen. After visualization with either ultrasonography or fluoroscopy, a 21-gauge needle is placed into the selected vessel. Once good blood return confirms the intraluminal position of the needle tip, a 0.18-wire is passed through the needle. The needle is removed, and the tract is dilated. Next, a peel-away sheath is placed over the wire. The catheter is sized and then passed through the peel-away sheath. The location of the catheter tip is confirmed fluoroscopically.

PICTURE ARCHIVING AND COMMUNICATION SYSTEMS

The widespread use of picture archiving and communication systems (PACSs) has had a significant effect on diagnostic imaging and medicine

---

BOX 9-3   PICTURE ARCHIVING AND COMMUNICATION SYSTEM

- Acquires, displays, distributes, and archives patient images
- Displays digital images on computer monitors (soft copy)
- Enables manipulation of images to enhance visualization
- Provides brightness, contrast, magnification
- Makes simultaneous viewing at multiple sites possible
- Improves efficiency and accelerates results reporting
- Enhances decision support, which improves patient management

---

throughout the United States and the world. Simply put, a PACS is the process of image acquisition, display, distribution, and archive as it relates to radiology (Box 9-3). A PACS allows images obtained by CT, MRI, ultrasonography, nuclear imaging, and plain radiography to be obtained and distributed to any location for simultaneous access by any number of caregivers and specialists. Examination images can be distributed via a local network within a hospital, over a regional network to a group of providers, or over the Internet for viewing anywhere in the world. Systems have been developed that offer resources never before possible with film. Archives are protected for patient privacy and safety.

For a number of years, CT, MRI, and ultrasound images have been acquired digitally or, at a minimum, were handled digitally after an analog-to-digital conversion. Before computerized radiography (CR) and digital radiography (DR), x-ray images obtained in a conventional manner could be converted into a digital format by scanning the image in a laser scanner. Fluoroscopic and x-ray images now can be captured digitally with CR or DR and thereby become immediately available for "soft copy reading." *Soft copy reading* is the term used to describe reading from a computer monitor as opposed to viewing a radiograph at a view box, known as *hard copy reading.* CR is very similar to conventional radiography except that it replaces film with a phosphorescent imaging plate that transfers the latent image into a digital format when developed. DR provides for direct conversion of the x-ray into an electronic digital format that requires no processing of the imaging plate.

The subtleties of CR and DR acquisition are beyond the scope of this chapter. Suffice it to say that the flexibility provided by digital imaging is incredible. The contrast and brightness (window and level) can be adjusted to optimize visualization of selected images or even portions of an image. These parameters can be changed when viewing an image to enhance a particular structure or finding. The window and level can be changed when viewing a chest x-ray image, for example, to accentuate the lung, bones, a central catheter, an endotracheal tube, or a gastrostomy button. Images can be magnified, rotated, inverted (black to white and white to black), and even screened by sophisticated computer programs to improve detection of pathology. Radiology reports can be transcribed with voice recognition software, allowing the radiologist to edit and sign a report within minutes of acquisition. The reports then are associated with images from the examination. It is now common to have images and interpretations available on a computer monitor in the NICU by the time the patient returns from radiology. Reports and images then are assimilated into the patient's electronic medical record. The PACS is a powerful tool that improves medical management by translating bits of data into clinically relevant information. It enhances medical care and decision support by making images and interpretations available simultaneously in numerous locations in a fraction of the time previously necessary.

FAMILY EDUCATION AND INVOLVEMENT

The caregiver can have a positive effect on imaging by helping educate the parent. When the parents understand the procedure and know what to expect, they can be very helpful. Not only is the imaging made optimal but also the experience of the parent and patient is improved. An informed parent can effectively assist in the imaging process when included in the treatment plan.

An optimal study requires motion-free imaging. Even with fluoroscopy and ultrasonography in which motion is being recorded, the actual acquisition of the image must be motion free. With x-ray and CT studies, shortening the acquisition time accomplishes that. Respiratory motion can be limited by taking the image at the end of inspiration. Some modalities cannot acquire the image data fast enough to eliminate motion. These examinations frequently require sedation. The most common modalities to require sedation are MRI, nuclear scintigraphy, and CT.

Sedation protocols vary from institution to institution, but certain aspects of sedation are universal. The patient must be given nothing by mouth (NPO) for a period of time before sedation. It is simply unsafe to sedate a patient who has eaten recently. Failure to keep a patient NPO is one of the most common reasons that a scheduled examination has to be canceled and rescheduled. Parents generally are informed of the need for sedation and asked for consent (verbal or written). The choice of sedation depends on many factors. These include the length of the examination, the fragility of the patient, and the experience and training of the individual responsible for sedation. The route of administration also is variable and includes IV, intramuscular (IM), oral (PO), rectal, and inhalation. The sedated patient is monitored throughout the procedure and recovery. Recovery can occur in the imaging suite, a recovery area, or newborn center, but the patient must be monitored until fully recovered.

Some unique aspects of newborn care require special attention in the imaging suite that might not be as important in older patients. These important issues are of even more concern in the sedated patient. Thermoregulation is always of concern in the neonate. Imaging suites frequently are cold. Maintaining body heat is especially problematic in studies that require prolonged imaging times and in those in which the patient could get wet, such as cystography and fluoroscopic GI procedures. Blankets and heat lamps can mitigate the problem, but one must anticipate the issue.

Fluid administration also can be problematic in the neonate. Newborns need dextrose in their IV lines, especially if they are not feeding. Keep IV lines open and functioning. Most IV pumps are not compatible with MRI, and many cause interference that degrades image quality. However, it is not appropriate to suspend fluid administration for the duration of the study. The issue should be anticipated and addressed in a timely fashion.

Care of a critical newborn in the imaging suite can be challenging. It requires cooperation between the NICU staff (nursing and medical) and the imaging staff. Parental education enables the parents to participate in the care of their newborn and has a positive effect on the care the newborn will experience.

Numerous imaging alternatives are available for the evaluation of any patient condition. The best imaging choice varies depending on local expertise and availability. A clear understanding of the differential diagnosis, along with a thoughtful and specific analysis of the clinical question, is essential for optimal imaging consultation. The clinician should consider the pros and cons of each modality and consult with a radiologist if there is any uncertainty as to the best method of imaging.

REFERENCES

For a full list of references, scan the QR code or visit http://booksite.elsevier.com/9780323320832.

10 | PHARMACOLOGY IN NEONATAL CARE

MARY MILLER-BELL, CHARLES MICHAEL COTTEN, AND DEANNE BUSCHBACH

Optimal pharmacotherapy delivers the maximum intended beneficial effect with the minimum toxicity. Determining the optimal pharmacotherapy for neonates is problematic in that much of the data have been extrapolated from research in adults, children, and laboratory animals. Neonates show dramatic differences in the way they respond to drugs compared with older children and adults and within the neonatal population.[22,28] Gestational age, chronologic age, and disease state alter a neonate's ability to metabolize medications and affect response to the drug.[28,44]

This chapter discusses pharmacology as it relates to the neonate and illustrates how rational medication decisions can be made for neonatal intensive care unit (NICU) patients. The chapter also includes discussions on strategies to avoid medication errors, strategies for drug delivery, information on how therapeutic hypothermia affects pharmacokinetics, and a summary of recent pharmacokinetic studies in NICU patients.

PHYSIOLOGY

Pharmacodynamics and Pharmacokinetics

The drug-receptor theory states that the amount and duration of a drug's availability to a receptor determine its effectiveness. *Pharmacokinetics* describes what the body does to the drug (concentration/time), which then determines how much drug is available to the receptors and for how long (Figure 10-1).[20,46] *Pharmacodynamics* describes what the drug (or its active metabolite, such as caffeine for theophylline or morphine-3 and morphine-6 glucuronide for morphine) does to the body at certain concentrations (effect/concentration). The drug's effectiveness also depends on receptor availability, affinity of the drug for the receptor, and cellular function in response to the drug-receptor interaction.

Antagonist drugs block a receptor's cellular and physiologic activity (e.g., naloxone), whereas *agonist* drugs elicit the receptor's action (e.g., cardiovascular agents such as dopamine and epinephrine). Some drugs act with receptors to increase or decrease gene expression (e.g., antenatal steroids), whereas others affect cell membrane permeability. Some drugs, such as methylxanthines, increase or decrease the amount or activity of "second messenger" molecules within cells. Antibiotics and antiviral agents act through some of these mechanisms to reduce the viability of pathogenic organisms by changing vital characteristics and functions. Readers should note that most drugs have more than one effect, so although the desired therapeutic effect may occur, the drug's other effects can limit its usefulness. *Side effects,* which can vary from minor to prohibitive, occur within the therapeutic range of concentration. *Toxic effects* result from drug overdose or serum concentrations higher than the recommended therapeutic range.

Individual infants may have *idiosyncratic responses* to medications, as well as expected responses. Infants who are low-sensitivity responders exhibit a drug response less than that expected for a usual dose, whereas infants who are extreme-sensitivity responders exceed the expected response for a given dose and drug level. Unpredictable adverse reactions differ from expected responses. Patients may become

---

PURPLE type highlights content that is particularly applicable to clinical settings.

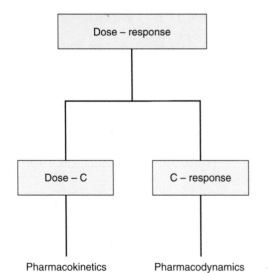

FIGURE 10-1 Variability in dose–response relationship can be the result of differences in pharmacokinetics or pharmacodynamics. *C,* Drug concentration (plasma or serum).

tolerant to a given drug dosage, as is commonly seen with opiates. *Tachyphylaxis,* a rapid decrease in drug response without a dosage change, may be related to limited receptors or other intracellular mechanisms.[6,17]

Developmental differences in number and function of receptors and intracellular mechanisms are critical to estimating drug actions.[46] An example of developmental effect on pharmacodynamics is the diminished sensitivity of the cardiovascular system to digitalis in the youngest patients; the receptor number increases with age. Changes in alpha- and beta-adrenergic receptors also occur with gestational and chronologic age and must be considered in determining dosage with pressors and inotropes.[29]

A clinician bases drug choice and dosage regimen largely on the likelihood of achieving the desired therapeutic response with minimal toxic effects in "average" patients. We target a concentration of drug in the body compartment where we want the desired effect. *Plasma concentration* provides a surrogate for effect when the relationship between concentration (C) and effect has been demonstrated in similar patients. The *minimum effective concentration (MEC)* is that at which 50% of patients exhibit the desired response (Table 10-1). The *maximum safe concentration (MSC)* is that at which 50% of patients exhibit a toxic response (Figure 10-2).

TABLE 10-1	ABBREVIATIONS	
ABBREVIATION	ABBREVIATION DEFINED	UNIT OF MEASUREMENT
C	Drug concentration (plasma or serum)	mg/L
Css	Steady state concentration (average)	mg/L
MEC	Minimum effective concentration	mg/L
MSC	Maximum safe concentration	mg/L
F	Extent of drug availability (0–1): how much active drug gets to the systemic circulation	Unitless
Vd	Volume of distribution: relates to loading dose	L/kg
Cl	Clearance: relates to maintenance dose	L/kg/hr
$t_{1/2}$	Drug elimination half-life: relates to the time course of changes in drug concentration	Hours

L, Liter = 1000 milliliters; *mg,* milligram = 1000 micrograms.

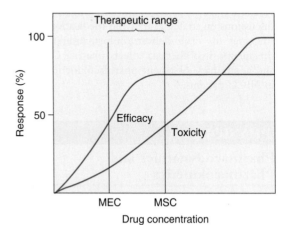

FIGURE 10-2 Percentage of patients with desired and toxic responses as a function of drug concentration. Therapeutic range is bounded by minimum effective and maximum safe concentrations. *MEC,* Minimum effective concentration; *MSC,* maximum safe concentration.

To elicit the desired therapeutic effect, the drug must be delivered to the receptor and remain available for an appropriate amount of time.[52] If a clinician aims to continue the therapy beyond a single dose, then plasma concentration at "steady state" (Css) is targeted, somewhere between the MEC and the MSC, where most patients exhibit the desired effect and few suffer toxic effects. With ideal maintenance therapy, drug input equals drug elimination. The variability around the Css depends on dose, dosage interval, and drug disposition. Even before NICU clinicians consider the changes in drug metabolism over time when prescribing maintenance therapy, clinicians should anticipate the need to modify dosages because there is a 10-fold variation in weight range for NICU patients (0.5 to 5 kg), and in the first 3 to 4 postnatal months in term newborns, when weight doubles, while in prematures the rate is even faster.[52]

The target Css is influenced by the amount of drug bound to plasma protein. In a newborn, free unconjugated bilirubin can displace numerous medicines of lower protein affinity, including ampicillin, penicillin, phenobarbital, and phenytoin,[47] while other medicines can displace unconjugated bilirubin, increasing unconjugated bilirubin's serum concentration and its potential for toxicity, as noted with ceftriaxone, ibuprofen, benzyl alcohol, and sulfisoxazole.[1,5] Intravenous (IV) lipid infusions also can affect protein binding of both bilirubin and some medicines, such as nafcillin and ceftriaxone. The drug concentration measured in most available assays is usually the total, both protein-bound and free; therefore the available concentration at the receptor usually is somewhat less than the total serum concentration. This changes over time for NICU patients; as bilirubin production changes, plasma proteins change in amount and biologic properties. The lower affinity of fetal albumin to weak acids, and the presence of bilirubin displacing a drug from binding albumin can lead to higher levels of freely circulating active drugs (protein binding of ampicillin, phenytoin, and phenobarbital in neonates is about half of that noted in adults).[22,46]

As an example of variation between neonatal and adult pharmacokinetics, we offer the example of theophylline, which has been used to treat apnea of prematurity. The reported therapeutic range for bronchodilation for theophylline in adults is 10 to 20 mcg/ml. In neonates, the effective range to treat apnea of prematurity has been 4 to 12 mcg/ml.[52] Theophylline is reported to be 8% bound to plasma protein at a total concentration of 8 mcg/ml in newborns, compared with 40% bound in adults. A total theophylline concentration of 10 mcg/ml in an adult represents 3 mcg/ml free theophylline available to receptors, whereas in a neonate, a total circulating level of theophylline of 4.7 mcg/ml provides the same 3 mcg/ml of free theophylline. In addition to the direct effects of theophylline itself, metabolism of theophylline in neonates leads to measurable free caffeine. Decreased bound theophylline in neonates could explain why therapeutic effect is achieved (and toxicities noticed) with lower total serum concentration in neonates.

DOSE–CONCENTRATION-TIME CONSIDERATIONS RELATED TO AGE

In the NICU, doses and intervals must be adjusted based on changes in the dose–concentration and the concentration–response relationships. This enables a more accurate and precise response to changes in dose–concentration effects, especially total concentrations, but as with the theophylline case, we must watch for clinical effects and estimate other factors' influences to estimate the free concentration's effectiveness and the receptor and cellular responsiveness. As noted earlier, pharmacokinetics describes the delivery and removal of the drug to and from the body. Four processes can describe a drug's disposition: drug entry (absorption), distribution, biotransformation (metabolism), and elimination. Doses and dose intervals are expressed mathematically by pharmacokinetic disposition parameters related to distribution, biotransformation, and elimination, such as clearance, volume of distribution, and half-life. Potential causes of changes in dose–concentration relationships unique to newborns are described for the pharmacokinetic processes that follow.

Absorption

The process of *absorption* defines the rate and amount of drug that enters the bloodstream. In the NICU, drugs are given by intravenous injection (100% bioavailability) and by means other than directly into the bloodstream, including inhalation, intranasally, intrarectally, topically, intramuscularly, and subcutaneously. When extravascular administration methods are used, the drug must overcome physical, chemical, mechanical, and biologic variables to enter the circulation. When considering extravascular administration, clinicians must keep in mind the clinical and developmental stage of the patient. For example, extreme preterm infants, transdermal absorption is much more efficient than in term infants with thicker stratum corneum and adipose tissue, but intestinal absorption in the extremely preterm infant may be less, given slow transit time and delayed gastric emptying.[22,46]

The parameter *F* indicates the percentage of dispensed drug available in the systemic circulation, with *F = 1* indicating the drug is 100% available. We lack systematic studies of absorption in sick newborns, and differences in absorptive processes are expected but remain unmeasured generally. Some differences in newborns that potentially affect bioavailability include developmental changes in surface area and permeability of gastrointestinal (GI) mucosa, age-dependent changes in acid secretion in the stomach (higher pH than in older children and adults in the first postnatal days), changes in gastric emptying time and total GI transit time, and the characteristics of GI flora. Drugs such as ranitidine and metoclopramide also affect absorption of other medications by altering gastric and intestinal pH and gastric emptying time and intestinal motility (faster transit time = less absorption).[46]

"First-pass" pharmacokinetics: First-pass elimination takes place when a drug is eliminated between its site of administration and the site of sampling for measurement of drug concentration. The liver is usually assumed to be the major site of first-pass metabolism of a drug administered orally, but other potential sites are the gastrointestinal tract, blood, vascular endothelium, and lungs.[39] Different drugs are absorbed at different rates, and different formulations of the same medication may be protected from first-pass metabolism.[21] The first-pass phenomenon is why many drugs (e.g., furosemide, propranolol, theophylline, morphine) need a larger oral than intravenous dose.

Distribution

Medications rely on blood flow and drug solubility for distribution to their sites of action. The *volume of distribution* for a drug is a parameter that relates total amount of drug distributed throughout the body to the serum or plasma concentration.[6]

It is an attempt to quantify the space in which the drug can go. Strictly defined, it is the hypothetical volume of body fluid necessary to dissolve the total amount of drug as found in the serum. *Volume of distribution* must be used to estimate the amount of a loading dose or a change in plasma concentration with any bolus dose:

$$\text{Loading dose} \times F \text{ (the absorption parameter)}$$
$$= \text{Change in concentration } (\Delta C)$$
$$\times Vd \text{ (volume of distribution)}$$

Or, put another way:

$$\Delta C = F \times \text{Loading dose}/Vd$$

Volume of distribution usually is expressed as a function of body weight, with units of volume per kilogram. Major factors that affect distribution volume are plasma protein binding and body composition.[12,18,29] Changes in body composition happen throughout fetal and newborn life. Total body water decreases with increasing age: 85% in the smallest, most preterm infants; 70% in term infants; and 55% in most adults. Total body water may increase with such conditions as the syndrome of inappropriate antidiuretic hormone (SIADH) excretion, which increases total body water. Extracellular water composes about half this amount in a healthy term neonate. Large water-soluble molecules reach this compartment. Intravascular water composes about 10% of the body weight; protein-bound medications stay in this small compartment. Water-soluble drugs such as penicillins, aminoglycosides, and cephalosporins are distributed in a greater volume in smaller, more preterm infants than in older infants in whom total body water is a lower percentage of overall body weight—therefore they require a higher loading dose per kilogram, if total body water was the only determinant of volume of distribution.[32,46]

Plasma protein amounts and binding capacities also differ with gestational and chronologic age. Protein binding is decreased in newborns, because lower amounts of albumin are available, and fetal albumin has less capacity to bind some drugs. Acidic drugs such as ampicillin, phenytoin, and phenobarbital bind less well, thus increasing the free (available to receptor) fraction of the drug, with resultant increase in effect. Changes in pH also can affect a drug's affinity for albumin. Fat content varies with gestational age and degree of illness; increased fat content increases the volume of distribution, leading to a large volume of distribution for lipophilic medications such as propofol and fentanyl.[22,46]

As described previously, the interaction of circulating unconjugated bilirubin and protein-bound drugs is particularly concerning in neonates. Several anionic compounds bind to albumin and can displace bilirubin, increasing free bilirubin, thus increasing its potential for toxicity. Bilirubin has a higher affinity for albumin than some other medications; it may displace them from albumin, increasing the medication's availability and potential to reach toxic levels.[1,5]

Biotransformation

Biotransformation, or *drug metabolism,* occurs most commonly in the liver. Phase I metabolism describes the nonsynthetic metabolism of medications. Phase II, usually conjugation, or the addition of a substance to a medication, is synthetic metabolism. Oxidation, conjugation, glucuronidation, and hepatic blood flow change with gestational and chronologic age, diseased states, and use of certain medications. For example, oxidation and glucuronidation are decreased in newborns. Drugs such as acetaminophen, phenobarbital, and phenytoin, which require oxidation for elimination, remain available longer and may be transformed to other active metabolites (the neonatal liver metabolizes theophylline to caffeine), or the drug may remain at significant free concentrations for a prolonged period. The possibility of prolonged peak concentrations of available drug or active metabolites for many pharmaceuticals mandates careful monitoring of drug levels and clinical conditions to titrate dose intervals. To further the potential for confusion and trouble, and further the argument for careful assessment of levels and clinical signs of effectiveness and toxicity, a decrease in plasma protein binding (or any other change in volume of distribution) may increase the hepatic clearance of a drug.

Clearance (Elimination)

Drug clearance or *elimination* occurs by excretion of unaltered drug or biotransformation to

an inactive metabolite. Most drug elimination pathways can become saturated if the dose is high enough and dose intervals are too frequent. Most drugs in use in the NICU have therapeutic doses less than those necessary to saturate the elimination system. When clearance mechanisms are not saturated, the Css in plasma is proportional to the dose rate. Clearance equals the rate of drug elimination divided by the drug concentration.[21] Just as volume of distribution relates to loading dose and initial concentration, clearance relates to a maintenance dose that keeps a drug's concentration at steady state. So for an ideal drug maintained at steady-state concentration:

$$(\text{Dose/dose interval}) \times F = Cl \ (\text{clearance}) \times Css$$

Stated another way:

$$Cl = F \times \text{Dose}/(\text{dose interval} \times Css)$$

Or, to tailor the dose for a desired steady-state concentration:

$$\text{Dose rate} = (Cl \times Css)/F$$

The appropriate dose rate can be calculated if the clinician can specify the desired steady-state plasma concentration and knows the clearance and bioavailability of a drug (from peak and trough levels in a particular patient).

For example, clearance of theophylline in preterm infants is reported to be 0.017 L/kg/hr. If the desired Css = 8 mg/L, assuming F = 1, particularly if the dose is to be given intravenously:

$$\text{Dose rate} = (Cl \times Css)/F = (0.017 \times 8/1 = \\ 0.136 \text{ mg/kg/hr or } 1.1 \text{ mg/kg q 8 hr}$$

RENAL EXCRETION

The kidney is the primary route of excretion for many drugs commonly used in the NICU. The kidney clears drugs through glomerular filtration and tubular secretion. Examples of medications eliminated through the kidney are aminoglycosides, digoxin, diuretics, and penicillins. Doses and dose intervals of drugs that have renal excretion must change with age and disease state. The glomerular filtration rate or GFR (i.e., the amount of blood filtered by the kidney in a unit of time) is low at birth and gradually increases over the first weeks. In preterm infants, the GFR starts even lower than in term infants, with a somewhat significant increase occurring at 34 weeks after conception. Tubular secretion also matures with increasing gestational age and depends on tubular function. In adults, aminoglycosides may be dispensed based on creatinine clearance, but in neonates less than 1 week old, serum creatinine may reflect maternal levels, as well as renal impairment. Acidosis and a history of hypoxia or ischemia also may modify an infant's renal function, slowing excretion and altering pharmacokinetics. Again, measuring levels in cases of suspected renal impairment, whether from suspicious history or laboratory values, is important to determining an appropriate dosage strategy.

Half-Life

A drug's *"half-life"* ($t_{1/2}$) is the time necessary for the drug level to decline by 50%. Half-life is related to both volume of distribution (V) and clearance (Cl), so that:

$$t_{1/2} = 0.7 \times V/Cl$$

The $t_{1/2}$ is used to predict and interpret the time course of changes in plasma drug concentrations. For example, the time to steady state is 4 to 5 half-lives. The half-life is useful in selecting dose intervals. This concept is illustrated in Figure 10-3.

Loading doses help expedite reaching desired therapeutic concentrations, especially for drugs with long half-lives, in which a desired effect is needed immediately. For drugs with one-compartment distribution that stay in the circulation and are not stored in cells or tissue, the loading dose may be given as a simple single dose. Drugs that are fat soluble or stored intracellularly are more difficult to assess, and therapeutic levels must be included in the loading dose assessment.

$$LD \text{ (loading dose)} = (Vd \times Concentration)/F$$

If the volume of distribution for caffeine in preterm infants is 0.8 L/kg and 20 mg/L is the desired concentration, and *F* for an intravenous dose is assumed to be *1,* a loading dose can be calculated.

$$\begin{aligned} LD &= (Vd \times C)/F = 0.8 \text{ L/kg} \times 20 \text{ mg/L} \\ &= 16 \text{ mg of caffeine/kg} \end{aligned}$$

Pharmacogenetics and Pharmacogenomics

In the 30,000-plus known genes, there are over 4 million "common" variants (occurring in more than 1% of the population), many of which directly affect the function of the coded protein. In addition to multiple factors like age, gender, disease, and concurrent medications, a patient's genetic code can cause variation in the response to a particular

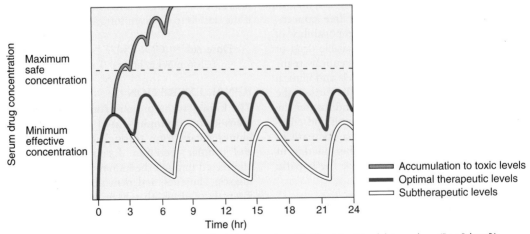

FIGURE 10-3 Effect on serum drug concentration of multiple dosage along with different time intervals between doses. (From Roberts RJ: *Drug therapy in infants,* Philadelphia, 1984, WB Saunders.)

drug. Once a drug is administered, it is absorbed and distributed to its site of action, then interacts with targets, and is finally metabolized and excreted. The enzymes and other compounds involved in each of these processes are subject to genetic variation that leads to variation in function. *Pharmacogenetics* is the study of the role of inheritance in the individual variation in drug response. *Pharmacogenomics* is the study of the influence of multiple genes, and their interaction with the each other and the environment, on drug effects.[7,41,46]

More than 40 years ago, the first description of a genetically caused variation in drug metabolism focused on the enzyme responsible for hydrolysis of succinylcholine. One in 3500 people are homozygous for the gene encoding an atypical form of the enzyme *butyrylcholinesterase,* which is quite slow to hydrolyze the succinylcholine, a condition leading to prolonged muscle paralysis. Concurrently, an enzyme responsible for N-acetylation, another form of drug metabolism, was found to have a common genetic variant, such that some patients are fast metabolizers of drugs such as hydralazine while others are slow metabolizers.

The cytochrome P-450 enzymes are important in phase I drug metabolism. Researchers have extensively studied one in particular, CYP-450 2D6, which is responsible for metabolism of many drugs. About 5% to 10% of the adult Caucasian population has genetic variants of the enzyme, leading to decreased activity, and higher and more prolonged active drug levels.

Recently, a genetic variant in mitochondrial DNA, the A1555G mutation gene, has been linked to risk of hearing loss associated with aminoglycoside toxicity. The risk-additive variant's frequency in the general population is estimated between 1% and 3%, but among deaf subjects tested, concurrence of deafness with aminoglycoside treatment associated with this mutation is quite common. This could lead to future testing before use of aminoglycosides. It is unknown whether tight control of aminoglycoside levels would reduce risk of hearing loss. No recommendations can be made until more extensive, population-based studies are done. Such studies must include accounting for drug levels and duration and genotypes in assessment of risk of hearing loss.[33]

In addition to genetic variation in drug metabolism, genetic polymorphisms of drug targets, including adrenergic and dopamine receptors, enzymes like acetylcholinesterase are likely to have effects on response to drugs targeting these proteins such as bronchodilators, pressors, and inotropes, and angiotensin-converting enzyme (ACE) inhibitors such as enalapril and captopril.

The study of pharmacogenetics and pharmacogenomics is new, especially to neonatology, in which so little is currently known about pharmacokinetics and pharmacodynamics of commonly used medications. The genetic revolution that has come with completion of the sequencing of the entire human genome is on its way to reaching neonatology with the availability of rapid analysis of large population-based samples for thousands of genes and their variants, and how they relate to drug response. In the future, these studies will lead to improved understanding of individual variation in drug response, which should allow development of strategies to individualize care and help avoid complications resulting from heretofore-unaccounted-for genetic variations. The challenge will be to understand how the multiple genes and environmental factors interact in fragile infants to alter risk of disease and adverse drug responses.

DATA COLLECTION

Clinicians should be aware of a medication's desired effects, side effects, and toxicities. They should also know when these are expected to occur and should monitor for these effects. Whether a dose effect occurs or not should be noted. Dose–plasma concentration results should be recorded when therapeutic drug monitoring is done. If the drug's serum concentration relates to clinical response, the blood concentration should be followed in addition to clinical signs. To optimally use drug serum levels, the expected blood concentration is calculated from the dosage history, and patient variables that may affect pharmacokinetics with the timing of blood samples are considered. A comparison of expected values with measured values allows rational adjustment of future dosage.[7] Potential explanations for differences between measured and expected concentrations are listed in Box 10-1.

Even if predictable pharmacokinetic and pharmacodynamic changes are taken into account, other factors may influence a drug's effect. Clinical end points must be followed and recorded and dosage regimens adjusted accordingly. One example is the monitoring of renal function with

B O X 10-1	POTENTIAL EXPLANATIONS FOR DISCREPANCIES BETWEEN MEASURED AND EXPECTED DRUG CONCENTRATIONS

- Inadequate compliance
- Inadequate medication delivery
- Inappropriate timing of samples
- Laboratory error
- Revision in initial estimates of necessary pK required

pK, Pharmacokinetics.

indomethacin dosage: If clinical signs of renal dysfunction are noted, the drug is not administered. A pharmacist should be included in the caregiving team to clarify dose and disposition parameters for individual patients with their various conditions.

If a suboptimal clinical response is noted in conjunction with a subtherapeutic plasma concentration, revised estimates of clearance should be adjusted with one or two available plasma concentrations. If a single level is drawn after absorption and distribution is complete or near steady state, then the maintenance dose formula can be rearranged to calculate the revised clearance. The common-sense approach suggests that if a patient has half the expected concentration of a drug, then perhaps the clearance is twice the initial estimate. If the patient has twice the expected concentration, the clearance likely is half the initial estimate. However, this technique is misleading if steady state has not been reached. If a drug's level is higher than expected and higher than what is considered safe, or if toxicity is noted, the drug should be discontinued until the concentration decays to the appropriate target. If two concentrations are available after absorption and distribution, half-life is determined by plotting the concentrations on semilog paper. The revised clearance is calculated by rearranging the half-life formula:

$$\text{Clearance} = 0.7 \times \text{Vd}/t_{1/2}$$

Once the clearance and desired steady state are known, a new dose rate can be calculated:

$$\text{Dose rate} = (\text{Cl} \times \text{Css}_{\text{desired}})/\text{F}$$

Examples

The following examples illustrate the need to pay close attention to issues of drug delivery and clinical effects. The following examples are for caffeine citrate in neonates. The half-life of caffeine citrate in neonates is 3 to 4 days, the *Vd* is *0.8 to 0.9 L/kg* and clearance is *0.008 L/kg/hr*.

EXAMPLE 1: A 15-day-old, 1-kg preterm infant receives oral caffeine for apnea of prematurity. After the loading dose of 20 mg/kg, the infant has received 5 mg every 24 hours for 5 days. At 8 AM on the fifth day, 4 hours after the last dose, the baby's heart rate is more than 180 beats/min, but apnea has not been a problem. Clinical and laboratory evaluation of tachycardia includes consideration of caffeine toxicity. A blood sample for caffeine is sent to the laboratory. To estimate the concentration of caffeine, use the following formula:

Necessary data:

Total body weight: 1 kg
Vd = 0.8 L/kg = 0.8 L in this patient
Cl = 0.008 L/kg/hr = 0.008 L/hr in this patient
$t_{1/2} = 0.7 \times \text{Vd}/\text{Cl} = 0.7 \times 0.8 \text{ L}/(0.008 \text{ L/hr}) = 70 \text{ hr}$
Time to steady state (Tss) = $4t_{1/2}$ = 280 hr
  Assume F = 1, maximum safe concentration (MSC)
      = 30 mg/L, minimum effective
         concentration (MEC)
      = 20 mg/L

Therefore:

$$\text{Css} = \text{F} \times \text{Dose}/(\text{Dose interval} \times \text{Cl})$$
$$= 1 \times 5 \text{ mg}/(24 \text{ hr} \times 0.008 \text{ L/hr})$$
$$= 26 \text{ mg/L}$$

The Css was estimated using average Vd and Cl values reported in similar infants, adjusted for this infant's weight. If this infant has diminished clearance relative to "average," toxicity may result from the standard dose. Toxicity may not have been noted until day 5 because of the estimated time to steady state (Tss) of 115 hours.

EXAMPLE 2: At 4 AM, 24 hours after the last dose, when the next dose is due, caffeine concentration of 27 mg/L is reported. This is higher than the therapeutic range for caffeine in neonates and is most likely the result of decreased clearance. Using this concentration, estimate the time when the concentration will decline to 20 mg/L and determine a 24-hour dosage schedule to maintain that concentration. The 4 AM dose is held, and the tachycardia resolves 24 hours later.

Clearance revised = F × Dose/(Interval × Css)
= 1 × 5 mg/(24 hr × 27 mg/L) = 0.008 L/hr

Revised $t_{1/2}$ = 0.7 × Vd/Cl$_{revised}$
= 0.7 × 0.7 L / 0.008 L/hr = 70 hr

Therefore the concentration 70 hours later should be one half of the measured 27 mg/L, or about 13.5 mg/L. To maintain a concentration of 20 mg/L:

Dose = (Interval × Cl$_{revised}$ × Css)/F
= (24 hr × 0.008 L / hr × 20 mg / L)/1
= 3.8 mg caffeine PO q 24 hr

EXAMPLE 3: Before the new oral regimen is initiated, another blood specimen is drawn 70 hours after the first and is found to be 14 mg/L. Because tachycardia has resolved, an oral regimen based on the last two levels is begun to maintain a caffeine concentration of 20 mg/L. Estimate the necessary maintenance dose: The concentration fell 50%, from 27 to 13.5 mg/L in 70 hours, which confirmed our original estimate of half-life.

DRUG CATEGORIES

Antimicrobial Agents

Antimicrobial agents inhibit growth or kill microorganisms; they include antibacterial, antiviral, and antifungal agents. *Bacteriostatic* agents limit growth, allowing host defenses to control spread; this will not reliably eliminate a pathogen. *Bactericidal* agents kill the pathogen. Bactericidal agents at low concentrations may be bacteriostatic. *Minimum inhibitory concentration (MIC)* is the lowest concentration of an antimicrobial that stops the spread of an organism in laboratory culture media. This cannot be directly measured in an infected neonate and depends on tissue concentration and number of bacteria present. *Minimum bactericidal concentration (MBC)* is the lowest concentration of antimicrobial that reduces microbial number in laboratory media by 99.9%. Pathogens can develop *resistance* to antimicrobials by changing their cellular structures or producing enzymes that reduce antimicrobial activity.

For effective antimicrobial action, the drug must reach an adequate concentration in the infected tissue. The ideal concentration elicits maximum effect on the pathogen with minimum effects on the patient. Selection criteria for antimicrobials include the microorganism's sensitivity, the availability of the drug to the target tissue (some antibiotics do not cross the blood-brain barrier), bioactivity of the antimicrobial in the target tissue, the known MIC and MBC relative to side- and toxic-effect levels for the medication, and the infant's biologic state—that is, whether the systems of absorbance and elimination are working adequately for effective and safe drug delivery and removal. When the use of antimicrobial agents is planned in a seriously ill infant, as with other drugs, greater consideration must be given to clinical status than to the gestational or chronologic age.

In particular, the pharmacokinetics of antifungal drugs in preterm neonates has begun to be studied. Guidance of dosage based on these more recent studies in the neonatal population has been reviewed recently.[27] Of note, one cited study suggests that a loading dose (25 mg/kg) followed with maintenance achieved the therapeutic target more rapidly than traditional dosage that starts with and continues a single maintenance dose.[38] More pharmacokinetic studies of commonly used antimicrobials are under way.

Diuretics

Diuretics are used in the NICU to remove excessive extracellular fluid. Diuretics commonly cause a loss of electrolytes along with water. Response to any diuretic depends on renal function and the drug's ability to reach its target in adequate amounts. Most diuretics work within the tubule, but any drug that increases GFR can increase water loss. Drugs that increase cardiac output without decreasing renal perfusion, and others that specifically increase renal blood flow, also cause diuresis.

In infants, renal tubular function improves with increasing chronologic and gestational age. Because of poor absorption and response to aldosterone (especially in extremely preterm infants), electrolyte losses can be clinically significant with the addition of a loop diuretic such as furosemide or bumetanide. The ongoing losses may lead to hypochloremic metabolic alkalosis and less response to the diuretic.

Delivery of diuretics to the kidney loop increases with increasing chronologic and gestational age. Most diuretics rely on secretion from the proximal tubule and filtration through the glomerulus to reach their site of action. Both these functions improve with age. Enteral absorption of some diuretics is limited, so clinical effectiveness and electrolyte stability must be monitored closely to help determine safe and effective dosage regimens. The kidney also is responsible for diuretic excretion, again through tubular secretion and glomerular filtration. Because these functions are age dependent, the clinician must ensure that clearance time is adequate to avoid toxic levels.

Cardiovascular Drugs

Medicines used to improve cardiovascular function include digitalis and the sympathomimetic amines, which include drugs such as dopamine, dobutamine, and epinephrine. *Antiarrhythmics,* including digoxin, act to control the electrical conduction within the myocardium.

The sympathomimetic amines bind to β and G receptors; the number and availability of receptors determine response. β_1 receptor response leads to constriction of vascular smooth muscle. β_2 receptors cause decrease in GI motility. Stimulation of the G1 receptor stimulates cardiac contractility, and G2 response includes vascular and bronchial smooth muscle relaxation. The response in any individual, and in any individual's specific organ system, depends on the relative amount of these receptors. Receptor numbers and their linked response elements within cells vary with gestation and clinical condition, and response must be monitored to aid in dosage decisions. Prolonged administration of sympathomimetic amines can lead to decreased response—an example of tachyphylaxis.

Antihypertensive agents occasionally are used in neonates for essential hypertension and occasionally to decrease afterload in neonatal patients with heart failure. These include volume reducers such as diuretics, inhibitors of physiologic regulators of blood pressure like enalapril, and drugs that decrease vascular resistance through β and G receptors.

The pathophysiology of neonatal disease should direct the choice of cardiovascular agent. Extremely close monitoring of physiologic effects helps determine safety and efficacy of therapy. Monitoring must include very frequent, if not continuous, monitoring of blood pressure, heart rate, perfusion, and oxygen saturation (preductal and postductal in some cases). Because other drugs are often given as a neonate receives cardiovascular medicines, thorough knowledge of possible drug interactions is mandatory. Absorption of cardiovascular drugs is unpredictable. The sympathomimetic amines must be given by the intravenous route unless used in an emergency situation when endotracheal (ET) administration of epinephrine is indicated. Once dosed, the drug must be delivered to the target organ system. Infants in shock may not have the circulatory wherewithal to deliver the medication to elicit the desired therapeutic response. Because of the variability in β and G receptor development and distribution, undesired side effects in various organ systems may accompany desired responses. Rapid metabolism of the sympathomimetic amines demands continuous IV infusion, and infiltration of IV fluids may lead to significant tissue damage. Along with the physiologic effects, these IV lines must be carefully monitored.[28,43]

Central and Peripheral Nervous System Drugs

Nervous system drugs include analgesics, which decrease pain sensations; *anesthetics,* which control pain peripherally or in the central nervous system (CNS); *sedatives/hypnotics* including barbiturates (phenobarbital) and nonbarbiturates (chloral hydrate, lorazepam), which do not control pain and can control some seizures; and *antiepileptic* agents, which are designed to control seizures (phenytoin, fosphenytoin). These drugs are associated with problems of addiction, tolerance, dependence, and withdrawal.

Addiction is a complex lifestyle change that involves drug-seeking behavior, which is not applicable to neonates. Tolerance occurs with many drug types. *Tolerance* exists when increasing doses and serum concentrations of a medicine are necessary to achieve a desired effect. A patient is *dependent* on a medication when regular drug administration is necessary for physical well-being. *Withdrawal* is a collection of physiologic and behavioral signs attributed to the absence of a medication in a dependent individual. Withdrawal has been identified for many medications, but it has been classified and described, along with weaning protocols, for opiate analgesics[10] (see Chapter 11).

The mechanism of most CNS medications is not clearly known. Again, careful monitoring of therapeutic effects relative to dose, duration, and serum concentrations is extremely important. Significant respiratory depression can occur with most CNS medications, so appropriate resuscitation equipment must be available. Variations in hepatic metabolism and volume of distribution are important in the ongoing assessment of dose response. Some medications are highly fat bound and are slowly released into the circulatory system, causing prolonged effects, both therapeutic and undesired (e.g., respiratory depression, poor gastric motility, and abnormal neurologic function such as feeding difficulties).

If therapeutic hypothermia is used for infants with hypoxic-ischemic encephalopathy (HIE), evidence suggests that opiates accumulate in the circulation in excess of the accumulation in similar infants with HIE who are not cooled. Therefore, when using opiates in cooled infants with HIE, opiate levels are likely to be higher than expected for a given dose and expectations for neurologic examination must be modified given accumulation of high levels and delayed expectations.[41]

Pharmacokinetics During Hypothermia

In recent years, therapeutic hypothermia has become the usual approach in intensive care nurseries for term newborns with neonatal hypoxic-ischemic encephalopathy (HIE).[44] Neonatal HIE is often accompanied by metabolic acidemia in the first postnatal hours to days, along with kidney and liver injury. Hypothermia entails lowering the core body temperature below 34° C for the first 72 postnatal hours, followed by gradual rewarming.[44] This complex combination of end organ injury and cooling below the usual physiologic core body temperature influences pharmacokinetics of commonly used medications in the NICU.[53]

Antiepileptics, opiates, and antibiotics are among the more commonly used medications for infants with HIE. In adults, the systemic clearance of cytochrome P-450 metabolized drugs is decreased between approximately 7% and 22% per degree Celsius below 37° C during cooling. Several studies have assessed specific medications often used for term neonates with HIE. Phenobarbital (PB) administered to newborns under whole body hypothermia results in higher plasma concentrations and longer half-lives than expected in normothermic newborns. In the report on phenobarbital pharmacokinetics for neonates cooled for HIE, Cmax, Cmin, and Cavg, were higher, and half-lives longer, than reported in normothermic newborns in earlier studies. Clinicians using PB to treat seizures in such newborns should be aware of the risks of elevated serum PB concentrations with doses of 40 mg/kg or higher.[11] In the Total Body Hypothermia Study (TOBY), one center measured and reported morphine pharmacokinetics on the infants enrolled in the study.[41] All of the infants were treated with a continuous infusion of morphinehydrochloride, with the rate adjusted according to clinical status. Serum morphine concentrations reached a steady state after 24 hours in normothermic infants with HIE but continued to increase throughout the assessment period in the hypothermia group. The authors concluded that infants with HIE have reduced morphine clearance and elevated serum morphine concentrations when morphine infusion rates are based on the clinical state. Potentially toxic serum concentrations of morphine are more likely with the combination of HIE, moderate hypothermia, and infusion rates greater than 10 microg/kg per hour, than with HIE not treated with hypothermia.[41] In a study of 29 infants treated with hypothermia for HIE, gentamicin clearance was decreased in neonates with HIE treated with hypothermia compared with previous reports in nonasphyxiated normothermic full-term neonates. At a 36-hour dosage interval, a dose of 4 to 5 mg/kg was predicted to achieve target gentamicin peak and trough concentrations in more than 90% of neonates.[15] In a subsequent study, this group demonstrated that a gentamicin dosage strategy of 5 mg/kg every 36 hours in neonates with HIE receiving therapeutic hypothermia improved achievement of target trough concentration less than 2 mg l(−1) compared with every 24-hour dosage, while still providing high peak concentration exposure.[14]

From these few examples, the effect of hypothermia on the pharmacokinetics of important drugs in a very vulnerable population is evident.[8] An ongoing, multicenter study in the Netherlands is investigating how therapeutic hypothermia influences the pharmacokinetic and pharmacodynamic time profiles of analgesics, sedatives, antibiotics, and antiepileptic drugs in infants with HIE.[8]

PREVENTION OF THERAPEUTIC MISHAPS

More individuals die each year in the United States from medical error than from traffic accidents. Many medical errors are medication errors.[25] Even after making a correct choice of medication, one must pay attention to the appropriate dose and interval based on factors that affect a drug's pharmacokinetics and pharmacodynamics. Drug delivery must be ensured: This includes appropriate dose calculations, appropriately written and read orders, and appropriate mixing with diluents, as well as attention to drug interactions, incompatibilities, contraindications, and drug delivery systems. In addition, effects of therapy at the chosen dose and systematic monitoring for therapeutic and toxic effects must be included in NICU care when medications are used.

Human error may occur, and it is in the highest-acuity hospital areas, such as intensive care units and emergency departments, that the majority of medication errors have been described. In a review of medication errors in a large general hospital, pediatric medication errors occurred at a higher rate (5.89 errors per 1000 patients) than in the emergency department and medicine, surgery, and obstetric and gynecology units, with dosage calculation errors being the most common problem.[25] The authors suggested initiatives designed to prevent, detect, and avert problems associated with major error factors. In addition to calculation errors, problems included lack of information and accessibility to information on drug therapy such as pharmacokinetic and drug interaction information, appreciation of patient characteristics that alter drug therapy, and confusing drug nomenclature.[1,2,12,25] In another review of hospital errors involving dosage equations,[28] antibiotics were the principal drug class involved. Errors in the equations used to calculate doses for all drug classes accounted for 29.5% of the errors.

Completing the "six rights" of medication administration (Box 10-2) in the NICU is complicated by the small doses and dosage adjustments based on infant weight or surface area.

BOX 10-2 THE "SIX RIGHTS" OF DRUG ADMINISTRATION

Right drug
Right patient
Right route
Right dose
Right time
Right response

Investigators estimate that 8% of drug doses calculated and administered by competent NICU nurses are at least 10 times greater or less than the ordered dose.[43] Another error risk arises from the fact that many drugs must be diluted, because they are ordered in amounts that are not commercially available. The rate of drug entry, or absorption, also varies, depending on route of administration. Calculations can be difficult and must be double-checked. Examples should be available readily to those responsible for calculating doses. Other suggestions include the use of standardized drug preparations and dosage, as well as standardized nomenclature or computer/digital order entry, with alerts for unusual doses. To avoid errors with emergency "code" medications, the doses of emergency medications should be calculated on admission, along with appropriate infusion rates (Figure 10-4). The calculated doses for the most commonly administered medications should be posted at the bedside; these should be updated routinely with the passage of days and weight changes (as the pharmacokinetics and pharmacodynamics change).

The *Rule of Six* was developed originally for use with vasopressor agents in code situations, and its use has extended beyond that. The rule, which allows nurses to estimate a pediatric dose by using a factor of 6, is prone to error. Standardized drug concentrations are less error prone and safer for patients than the *Rule of Six*.[34] Because of medication errors, The Joint Commission (TJC) has required the use of standardized intravenous drug concentrations for pediatric patients prescribed medications for which the *Rule of Six* was routinely used. Another error avoidance strategy, not mandated by TJC but strongly recommended, is to integrate a clinical pharmacist into patient care rounds with

NEONATAL RESUSCITATION MEDICATIONS

Name: _____ Weight: _____ Suction depth: _____

Date of birth: _____ ET tube size:_____

Drug	Strength	Dose	Route	Amount to administer
Epinephrine	1:10,000	0.1 mL/kg	IV, ET	_____
Atropine	0.1 mg/mL	0.1 mL/kg	IV	_____
Volume expanders		10 mL/kg	IV	_____

Signature of preparer

FIGURE 10-4 *Calculations for neonatal resuscitation medications. Other drugs and dosages could be added.* ET, *Endotracheal;* IV, *intravenous.*

physicians and nurses, particularly in intensive care and oncology, to provide more direct patient care and consultation rather than the traditional role of drug preparation and dispensing. Pharmacist interventions can reduce medication errors and adverse drug events.[48] In addition, designing the ordering system to reduce complexity and provide rule-based order screening and double-checking of calculations and developing effective information delivery may be more effective than traditional education or process-improvement efforts that target interventions after an error occurs.[10,16]

The American Academy of Pediatrics has published further recommendations for reducing medication errors for pediatric patients.[4] These include some hospital-wide actions, including the establishment of a clearly defined system for drug ordering, dispensing, and administration, with review of the original drug order before dispensing and administration. Confirmation of patient weight, drug dosage, and strength are also recommended.[28] Avoiding the use of the terminal zero to the right of the decimal point (e.g., writing 5 instead of 5.0), and using a zero to the left of a dose less than 1 (e.g., using 0.1 rather than .1) will help reduce medication errors. Avoid abbreviations of drug names (e.g., MS may mean either morphine

sulfate or magnesium sulfate), spell out dosage units rather than using abbreviations (e.g., units rather than U, or mcg for microgram rather than μg), and use generic medication names rather than trade names. Avoid verbal orders whenever possible.[34] See Table 10-2 for other interventions to reduce medication errors. For pediatric nurses, recommendations include:

- Familiarizing oneself with the medication ordering and use system
- Verifying drug orders before administration
- Confirming patient identity before each dose
- Verifying calculations with a second individual
- Verifying any unusually large volumes or dosage units for a single patient dose
- Verifying verbal orders by "reading back" the complete order to the prescriber
- Listening to the patient, parent, or other caregiver
- Asking questions as to whether a drug should be administered
- Maintaining familiarity with the operation of administration devices and the potential for errors with such devices

TABLE 10-2 INTERVENTIONS TO REDUCE MEDICATION ERRORS

STRATEGY	EXAMPLES
Develop a neonatal and pediatric formulary	Neonatal/pediatric dilutions of pediatric formulary for gentamicin, hydrocortisone, magnesium sulfate
Develop age-specific dosage guidelines	All medications commonly used to treat neonatal and pediatric patients
Develop protocols and procedures	Fluid management, skin care, insulin
Support nonpunitive error reporting	Medication incident reports
Provide up-to-date references	Neonatal and pediatric drug dosage handbooks

METHODS OF ADMINISTRATION

Once a clinician orders a medication and the drug and dose are found to be appropriate for that particular infant, the nurse's challenge is to administer the medication correctly. The following section addresses methods that help improve accuracy of drug delivery.

Oral Administration

It must be noted that all oral medications should be prepared and administered using only oral syringes and oral orogastric (OG) or nasogastric (NG) tubing. These oral syringes and tubing do not allow oral medications to be given inadvertently through an IV.[48] Variations in oral bioavailability and unanticipated and unmeasurable loss of the drug complicates administering oral medications to newborns. Loss of medication occurs when infants regurgitate or require gastric suctioning and lose residual fluid that may include medication. If an infant is receiving OG or NG feedings, medication should be placed into the center of the barrel of a syringe containing a small portion of the feeding. Medication may adhere to the plastic and decrease the amount of medicine delivered. The nurse must document drug administration attempts and any possible loss of drug, with an estimate of the amount lost. For infants receiving oral medications, documenting the color of the emesis or residual material helps determine presence of medications that have distinctive color.

If an infant is bottle-fed, the nurse may put the medication in the full bottle. However, if the infant fails to take the whole volume, he or she has not received the full dose. One option is to finish the volume with gavage feeding. Another option is to gently introduce very small portions of a dose into the cheek pouch and wait for the infant to swallow. Another method is to put 5 to 10 ml of a feeding, with the medication, in a small bottle and let the infant take that amount, then continue with the remainder of the feeding. Medication also may be placed into a nipple with a small volume of formula and then offered to the infant. For breastfeeding infants, medication may be administered into the mouth as described previously, with or without a small volume of expressed breast milk. As with all dosage of medicines, it is imperative to record doses and volume and characteristics of any residual material or emesis.

Intramuscular Injection

A newborn infant has relatively little muscle mass to receive injections. When intramuscular (IM) injections are necessary, as with vitamin K, the anterior thigh is the site of choice. Comfort measures should be given before and after injection (see Chapter 12). Clean the site with your hospital-approved antiseptic solution. Insert a 22- to 25-gauge needle into the muscle, and, for most medications, draw back on the syringe to ensure safe needle placement (unless specifically contraindicated), then inject the medication. For an infant weighing less than 1500 g, the volume injected into one leg should not exceed 0.5 ml. The final step is to document the administration.

Intravenous Administration

IV medication can be given by push or pump infusion. Rarely is retrograde injection used because it is no longer recommended to administer IV medications to neonates.[6] Although drugs directly enter the bloodstream, the time necessary to complete drug delivery to receptors is a function of dosage volume, IV flow rate, and injection site (depending on particular IV methods).[52] Failure to recognize these potential time lags could result in inappropriate expectations of the timing of physiologic responses and peak and trough concentrations. The use of microbore IV tubing will facilitate rapid drug delivery because the volume of the fluid in the tubing is reduced. An example of a pediatric syringe infusion preparation and delivery chart for common neonatal drugs may be useful to the reader.[34] Certain drugs should never be administered into the umbilical vein or artery, and drug incompatibilities should be recognized before setting up multiple drug dosage through the same IV line. Careful monitoring for infiltrates and knowledge of drug-specific treatment for this complication are essential to safe IV drug administration. Continuous IV infusion of pressors is common in the NICU, and because of their rapid clearance and physiologic importance, these infusions should never be interrupted or given by bolus without orders. Because of the sudden influx of potent medication, flushes to clear lines with continuous infusions of sympathomimetic amines should be avoided.

PUSH INJECTION

IV push medications must be mixed in appropriate volumes, delivered through appropriately sized syringes, and followed with an appropriate flush solution: heparin with normal saline solution (NS), 10% or 5% dextrose, and water ($D_{10}W$ or D_5W). If numerous flushes are given, care must be taken with the osmolality of the flush solution.

To administer an IV push injection, prepare the IV port closest to the patient. Administer a small volume of appropriate flush solution, and then administer the medication over 1 to 2 minutes. Slow pushes are ordered sometimes, but the rate should be specified by the ordering medical care provider. A postmedication flush is given at the same rate as the medication to clear the line of remaining medication. IV push administration of many medications used in the NICU is

contraindicated because of the possibility of immediate adverse reactions associated with rapid bolus injections. Opiates and sedatives should be given with great care and constant attention to respiratory and cardiovascular parameters. Check a pharmacology reference if there is any uncertainty.

ANTEGRADE INJECTION

Antegrade injection is the introduction of medication into an entry port along the course of the IV tubing. The flow of maintenance fluid carries the medication to the patient at its rate. Because infusion rates in neonates are characteristically low, significant delays in drug delivery result. If rapid infusion is necessary, as with emergency resuscitation medications, more rapid infusion rates are necessary. This can lead to a significant medication error if, after drug delivery, the IV rate is not returned to baseline.

PUMP INFUSION

To avoid delay of drug delivery, two methods of pump infusion using a mechanical infusion device allow control of drug amount and delivery rate. These devices consist of a pump that can be set to deliver a specific volume over a specific time, a syringe or other container that holds the medication or fluid to be delivered, and connecting tubing to connect the pump to a port for drug delivery. Because pumps vary by manufacturer and some may be used in a variety of ways, each NICU should have a policy to ensure that each staff member carries out pump infusions in the same manner. If different care providers start and end an infusion, the method used must be communicated.

Method 1. An exact ordered amount of medication is drawn into a syringe and diluted if necessary to provide the volume necessary for pump operation. This drug plus diluent fluid is flushed through the tubing, and the syringe is placed in the pump. After the pump finishes the infusion, some medication remains in the tubing and syringe hub. This medication needs to be flushed into the IV line with a flush solution to deliver the entire ordered dose.

Method 2. Medication is drawn into the syringe through the connecting tubing until the desired volume is in the syringe. The syringe then is placed on the pump and a volume carrying the ordered amount of drug is infused. The tubing and syringe hub need not be flushed, because the infant has already received the entire ordered dose.

OTHER CONSIDERATIONS

Health care providers must remain attuned to additional concerns when administering IV medications. Medications may require filters or protection from light sources, or have significant specific gravity osmolarity. A 0.22-mcg filter may provide "cold sterilization" (i.e., remove particulate matter and bacterial contamination). Some medications cannot be administered through a filter, because the filter removes the active ingredient. Medications with a specific gravity less than that of the IV fluid have a tendency to accumulate at high points in the IV tubing, whereas those with a higher specific gravity settle into low tubing loops, in both cases resulting in delayed and inaccurate drug delivery.

ACCESS VIA PERIPHERALLY INSERTED CATHETERS (PICCs) OR PERIPHERAL INTRAVENOUS LINES (PIVs)

PICCs have been used in the neonatal world for more than 30 years. Their use has decreased mortality and morbidity. They have proven to be a reliable safe method to deliver medications and high osmolar fluids.[36] Training in PICC placement is accomplished through specialized courses that adhere to strict sterile techniques. Two methods of PICC placement include the traditional method using breakaway needle/peel-away plastic or an advanced method where the catheter is threaded over the needle.[37]

How to Get Intravenous Access: Inserting Peripheral Intravenous Lines (PIVs). PIVs may be placed by the bedside nurse without the specific training course that is needed to place a PICC. Common sites for IV placement in neonates include the hands, feet, arms, legs, or scalp veins. A transilluminator or ultrasound machine[20] may help locate vessels in extremities. Some transilluminators have a high-intensity light source. Use care not to cause burns.

Equipment
- Catheters with needles of appropriate size for the vessel
- Tape
- Antiseptic
- Gauze
- Syringe with flush solution

- Tourniquet
- Arm or leg board
- Restraints (as necessary)
- Gloves
- Nonpharmacologic comfort measures (see Chapter 12)

Procedure. Always use comfort measures with any potentially painful procedure. Use of local anesthetic or other analgesia also should be considered in addition to the comfort measure (see Chapter 12). Assemble equipment at the bedside. Provide adequate temperature support. Prepare your securing tape/dressing. Select a vessel after confirming it is not an artery. Determine the direction of flow; veins fill toward the heart, arteries away from the heart.

Stabilize the infant enough to avoid movement that prevents line placement. Some care providers place a leg or arm board before the catheter is placed; others secure the limb after the catheter is in position. Some providers prefer to flush the needle/catheter before beginning the procedure. The syringe should be removed before the attempt if this method is used. Place a tourniquet around the extremity, taking care to not pinch the skin. (Some caregivers prefer not to use a tourniquet and with practice may achieve success equal to that of caregivers using one.) Clean the site with antiseptic solution and follow manufacturer instructions for drying time. After gloving, insert the needle catheter into the vessel using hand and fingers to anchor the skin surrounding the vessel. Insert at an acute angle and in the direction of blood flow. Observe for blood return or flashback into the tubing or cannula of the catheter. Some vessels do not provide blood return; babies in hemodynamic shock also may not have blood return. If the needle is thought to be in the vessel but no blood return is seen, then a small amount of flushing solution may be injected. If the needle is not in the vessel, the tissue will swell. If it blanches, the vessel is most likely an artery. If blood return is seen, inject flushing solution to clear the needle; remove the needle and gently advance the catheter.

Place a short piece of tape across or small piece of transparent dressing across the catheter to secure it. Cross a longer piece of tape around the back of the catheter and cross the ends across the front of the catheter. Check for proper position by disconnecting the IV from the syringe to note blood return or by infusing a small amount of flushing solution. If necessary use gauze behind the needle for support. Secure the IV in place by using another long piece of tape or additional transparent dressing. Leave adequate access to skin close to the IV site to allow monitoring for changes in color or edema that indicate complications such as infiltrates, phlebitis, or hematomas.

If the medication is to be administered intermittently and the line is not otherwise used, it may be "heparin-locked" and flushed every shift, or per unit protocol with your unit's standard heparin solution. Heparin solutions are available in several concentrations. It is good unit practice to standardize the volume and container type for each concentration, and individualize how each concentration-specific container looks and where they are kept. Controversy exists over the use of heparin versus normal saline (NS) for flushing lines.

Teaching Model. Models for teaching IV insertion with various needles and catheters vary from the highly sophisticated (and expensive) computerized human patient simulator to the "low-tech" and inexpensive human placenta. The current gold standard in teaching IV insertion is simulation. The simulator allows this common but technically difficult procedure to be practiced repeatedly in a safe environment.[51] The computerized human patient simulator is currently available in three models: adult, pediatric, and neonatal. The simulator allows lines to be inserted in vessels; then bar-coded syringes of "drugs" can be administered through the lines, and the simulator will respond with the appropriate physiologic response, which may include changes in blood pressure, heart rhythms, respiratory effort, and changes in pupil dilation. Less advanced techniques include various models of neonate-sized manikins with visible "vessels" in the scalp, arms, legs, and feet.

The fetal side of a human placenta is an inexpensive and easy-to-use model. The needed supplies and procedure follow:

Supplies
- Placenta
- Assorted needles and catheters
- Syringes with flush solution
- Gloves
- Tape

Procedure. Place the placenta fetal side up on drapes. Remove the fetal membranes, exposing the rich network of vessels. After gloving, insert IV needles with catheters into the larger vessels first, then into smaller vessels with improving technique. Tortuous or branching vessels can be used for various

---

B O X 10-3	CRITICAL ASSESSMENT
	INTRAVENOUS EXTRAVASATION

- Check all indwelling lines hourly for signs of extravasation.
- Look for phlebitis, edema, burns, adequacy of perfusion to site, hardness of tissue, or inflammation at needle site.
- For scalp veins, check dependent side of head for trauma.

---

methods. Once catheters are in position, practice securing with various taping methods.

COMPLICATIONS OF INTRAVENOUS THERAPY

Complications include phlebitis, infiltration, hematomas, chemical burns, compartment syndrome, and emboli.[28] Long-term complications include disfigurement, contractions, and the need for surgical repair or amputation. Frequent *(at least hourly)* assessment of IV sites helps reduce, but does not absolutely prevent, all IV complications (Box 10-3). Swelling or discoloration of the extremity or skin at the needle tip is a sign of trouble, and the line should be removed. In the scalp, infiltration may be difficult to assess, because swelling occurs not only at the IV site, but also on the dependent side of the head. Scalp edema on the dependent side or a swollen eye is an indicator of scalp vein infiltration.

Footdrop[12] and *compartment syndrome,* in which nerves and vessels are damaged by swelling of tissue within a limited space, have been associated with positioning a foot board along the lateral aspect of the fibula, with or without an IV infiltration. The use of rolled washcloths as foot boards or extensive padding of IV boards with cotton or gauze may prevent excessive pressure. Unnoticed infiltrations may result in significant tissue loss. Warm soaks are *contraindicated* because, when warmed, extravasated fluid may exacerbate the burn, maceration, and necrosis. In addition, heat increases oxygen demand in already compromised tissues.

Elevating the infiltrated area increases venous and lymphatic drainage helping to decrease the edema. Hyaluronidase[35] destroys extracellular barriers, allowing rapid diffusion and absorption of the extravasated fluid. For vasoconstrictive substances that extravasate, local use of vasodilators like phentolamine can aid in reperfusion. Table 10-3 lists treatment approaches for extravasation.

TABLE 10-3   TREATMENT APPROACH FOR EXTRAVASATION

DRUG SUPPLIED	DOSAGE/ADMINISTRATION	COMMENTS
Hyaluronidase (Amphadase) 150 units (ml)	1 ml (150 units) given as 4 or 5 intradermal 0.2-ml injections with a 25-gauge needle around the periphery of the IV extravasation site	Use with extravasation of hyperosmolar or extreme pH drugs. Administer within 1 hr of event. Not for use with vasoactive drugs.
Phentolamine (Regitine) 5 mg/ml in 1-ml vial	0.5 mg/ml given as 4 or 5 intradermal 0.2-ml injections with a 25-gauge needle around the periphery of the IV extravasation site	Prepare a dilution. Use with vasoactive drugs. May be given up to 12 hr after an event.

Modified from Roberts RJ: Intravenous administration of medication in pediatric patients: problems and solutions, *Pediatr Clin North Am* 28:23, 1981.

BOX 10-4   PARENT TEACHING
INDWELLING LINES FOR PARENTS

Talk with parent about indwelling lines. Discuss the following:
- Type of line, purpose, and any limitations on holding, handling, or feeding the infant
- Pain control measures for the placement of lines
- Need for restarting lines
- At discharge: The name of the medications, the dosages, purpose, routes, and any potential side effects
- At discharge: Medication administration and what to do if the infant does not receive the full dose of medication

---

PARENT TEACHING

IV lines in newborns may frighten the child's parents, especially scalp vein lines (Box 10-4). Without information, parents may mistakenly believe the fluid or a needle is going directly into their baby's brain. It is helpful to reassure the parents that a needle, the fluid, and possibly medications, are going into large veins. Also, reminders that, although an infant has an IV line in place, parents may still touch, hold, and feed their child can help parents to cope with interventions.

Parents should be made aware that pain assessment and control are part of the caregiver's ongoing efforts, and both are addressed during IV placement and maintenance. They should be told that a newborn's venous fragility, combined with the types of solutions used, make restarting IV lines and multiple sticks per line relatively commonplace. The potential for infiltration also should be addressed, and parents should be included in the effort to monitor the appearance of IV sites (see Chapter 12).

As for an infant's medications, the parents should be made aware of treatment choices in the NICU. They need not know the details of medication dosage but should be made aware of significant medications in their child's treatment regimen. At discharge, parents must know the names of their child's medications, their actions and the dose, frequency of administration, and side effects, as well as where to obtain refills for each drug. Some of the medications given for infants are not readily available at some of the smaller pharmacies. Caregivers must teach parents to administer prescribed medicines, and the parents must demonstrate their ability to safely and reliably give their child the recommended doses. The parents should receive written drug information instructions, which may be developed by the unit for their families or may be commercially available. Instructions must include actions, dose amounts, routes of administration, dosage schedule, and potential side effects.

REFERENCES

For a full list of references, scan the QR code or visit http://booksite.elsevier.com/ 9780323320832.

11 DRUG WITHDRAWAL IN THE NEONATE

SUSAN M. WEINER AND LORETTA P. FINNEGAN

The epidemic of maternal substance abuse over the past 40 years has continued to escalate at an alarming rate, most recently with the rise of prescription opiate abuse.[17] The extent of drug use during pregnancy is often underestimated, as are the effects on the fetus and neonate. According to the National Survey on Drug Use and Health (Substance Abuse and Mental Health Services Administration),[90] an estimated 5.9% of pregnant women (aged 15 to 44 years) reported using illicit drugs in any given month with data averaged across 2011 to 2012. An average of 10.8% of pregnant women reported current alcohol use with 2.7% reporting binge drinking and 0.3% reporting heavy drinking. These rates have dropped over the past 6 years. The prevalence of cigarette use among pregnant women did not change significantly during the same period (18% in 2002–2003 and 15.9% in 2011–2012) in women of the same age.[75] Patrick et al., in a 2012 article in the *Journal of the American Medical Association,* discuss health care expenditures and point out that of the approximately 4 million births per year in the United States, neonatal abstinence syndrome (NAS) is diagnosed at a rate of 3.9 of 1000 hospital births per year.[73] Infants with NAS were 19% more likely to have low birth weight, and their length of stay was approximately 13 days longer than non-NAS infants (16 vs. 3 days).[72] Data also showed that 8% of black pregnant women reported using an illicit drug in the past month, compared with 4.4% of white women and 3% of Hispanic women.[75]

The National Institute of Drug Abuse funded the 2007 Monitoring the Future study, which showed that 0.8% of 8th graders, 0.8% of 10th graders, and 0.9% of 12th graders had abused heroin at least once in the year before being surveyed.[65] As health care providers, we must recognize these data as a snapshot of affected young people who are future parents. The sequelae of both licit and illicit substance abuse by the mother during pregnancy must be recognized and addressed to provide optimal medical care of the neonate. Stereotypic biases should not interfere with the diagnosis or treatment. Drug dependence in pregnancy crosses all socioeconomic and racial barriers. Therefore, health care providers should not rule out drug exposure in any neonate who is exhibiting symptoms at birth related to withdrawal from or exposure to illicit or prescribed drugs.

Opioid addiction in the mother during pregnancy has been studied in detail for decades in terms of its effects on the woman, the fetus, and the developing child.[*] An *opioid* is defined as any natural or synthetic drug that has pharmacologic properties similar to those of opium.[28,30,40] An opiate is derived from opium or contains opium. Because time, circumstances, and knowledge have changed, other factors now should be considered in treating neonates. Diagnostic data can no longer be gathered on the assumption that one drug or substance was used. Polydrug use (the concurrent use of three or more drugs) is now the norm and not the exception. Polydrug use also can be the combination of illicit substances with those that are legal or found over the counter. The effect on the fetus and neonate is not necessarily minimized by the legality of the substance. Patterns of abuse, purity of the illicit drug, and sometimes potent or

---

[*]References 19–21, 24, 26, 29, 30, 40, 46, 57, 59.

PURPLE type highlights content that is particularly applicable to clinical settings.

poisonous additions to them also may cause catastrophic sequelae in newborns. According to a July 2013 report from the Centers for Disease Control and Prevention, abuse of prescription pain killers by pregnant women caused NAS cases to rise almost 300% in the United States between 2000 to 2009.[12]

Iatrogenic physical dependence has been documented in infants given intravenous fentanyl or morphine to maintain continuous analgesia and/or sedation during extracorporeal membrane oxygenation (ECMO) and mechanical ventilation.[93] The signs of withdrawal are much like those reported in infants born to opioid-dependent mothers. Fifty to 84% of neonates removed from fentanyl within a 24-hour period exhibited withdrawal symptoms, and 48% exhibited signs and symptoms with morphine withdrawal.[93] Regardless of the agent(s) used for sedation, once the decision is made to start weaning the medication, careful observation of the infant is crucial to monitor for signs and symptoms of withdrawal.[10,93] A review of the literature points out the importance of initiatives for adequate analgesia in neonates, the development of formal policies concerning intensive care sedation, and the treatment of the withdrawal[3,10,92,93] (see Chapter 12).

In a Cochrane Database Review of opiate treatment for newborn withdrawal, Osborn et al. discuss the use of the Lipsitz Tool (1975), the Finnegan Scoring System (1975), and the Neonatal Withdrawal Inventory by Zahorodny (1998) for the documentation of manifestations of withdrawal by various institutions.[66,70] The literature cites various pharmacologic agents that have been used to alleviate the symptoms of opioid withdrawal with methadone, buprenorphine, and oral morphine sulfate.* Advances in neonatology have continued to broaden the period of viability as many more premature infants are surviving. What appears to be decreased severity of abstinence in preterm infants may be related to developmental immaturity of the central nervous system (CNS) or to differences in total drug exposure. This proves to be a problem in evaluating the severity of abstinence signs in a smaller preterm infant because scoring tools were developed largely for use with term or near-term infants.[3,30,40,63]

This chapter presents current information about treatment issues surrounding drug-exposed neonates, with the main focus on opioid withdrawal. The effects of other substances such as stimulants, hallucinogens, selective serotonin reuptake inhibitors (SSRIs), tricyclic antidepressants, nonopioid CNS depressants, tobacco, methamphetamines, and alcohol are addressed when symptoms deviate from those of NAS.

PHYSIOLOGY

Because of their low molecular weight and lipid solubility, all drugs of abuse reach the fetal circulation by crossing the placenta, causing direct toxic effects on the fetus.†

Although certain drugs may produce specific effects, many abused drugs produce similar manifestations of fetal and neonatal disease. In addition, the effects of legal drugs such as tobacco, caffeine, and alcohol may confound simple drug–effect relationships.[3,5,9] A hostile intrauterine environment may also be caused by adverse effects of the mother's drug addiction and must be considered when diagnosing the neonate's problems. Examples of factors that could affect neonatal outcome include lifestyle, homelessness, physical or sexual abuse, prostitution, poverty, poor or no prenatal care, polydrug abuse, intravenous drug abuse, binge and withdrawal cycles, anorexia, poor maternal nutrition, pica, dehydration, alcoholism, sexually transmitted diseases, dental abscesses, preexisting medical conditions requiring pharmacologic therapy, human immunodeficiency virus (HIV)–positive status or acquired immunodeficiency syndrome (AIDS), and hepatitis B and hepatitis C.‡

Opioid Substances

When drugs such as heroin, methadone, morphine, buprenorphine, and meperidine cross the placenta, the fetus may become passively dependent. Morphine, the major metabolite of heroin, methadone, as well as buprenorphine and its metabolite have been identified and measured in amniotic fluid, cord blood, breast milk,[1,32,35] neonatal urine, and meconium.[20,40,51,64] Nonopioid CNS depressants (e.g., benzodiazepines, barbiturates) and the other opiates/opioids (e.g., codeine, hydrocodone, oxycodone,

---

*References 22, 30, 49, 62, 66, 70.

† References 4, 5, 11, 16, 20, 22, 24–26, 29, 43, 52.

‡ References 3, 16, 20, 22, 47, 68.

hydromorphone, pentazocine, propoxyphene) all have been identified in neonatal urine and meconium.[22,101] Ethanol and its primary metabolite, acetaldehyde, have been identified in placental tissue and amniotic fluid.[15,87,89]

Human and animal studies have shown that use of opioids during pregnancy directly affects fetal growth. Heroin is associated with intrauterine growth restriction (IUGR), with only a slight reduction in gestational length, although the mechanism through which heroin inhibits growth is not known.[21] Early speculation reported that maternal opiate (heroin) use during pregnancy accelerated fetal lung maturity, but this has not been borne out when formally studied, and no plausible mechanism through which heroin exposure resulted in this has been elucidated—even the associated growth restriction and chronic stress.[38] Older studies comparing methadone-exposed with nonexposed infants have found that methadone-exposed infants had lower birth weights. However, infants born to methadone-maintained women have been reported to have higher birth weights than those born to women using heroin. Decreased head circumference has been an inconsistent finding with these babies. Schempf conducted a meta-analysis looking at illicit drug use and neonatal outcomes and found birth weights of newborns born to mothers using heroin were lower than those of newborns whose mothers used methadone alone and those of newborns whose mothers used both heroin and methadone during their pregnancy.[79] A mean reduction of 483 g in birth weight and a relative risk for low birth weight were associated with any opiate use during pregnancy.[79] Heroin, methadone, and buprenorphine have not been associated with congenital malformations or any specific dysmorphic syndrome in offspring.

Methadone maintenance has been an accepted treatment strategy for opioid dependence for more than 40 years. In the past few years, buprenorphine has been extensively researched for treatment of maternal addiction and NAS by medical professionals in the United States and Europe.★

Neonatal withdrawal from psychoactive substances that the fetus is exposed to occurs in varying degrees. Because most opiates/opioids are short acting and not stored by the fetus in appreciable amounts, neonatal abstinence is usually

★References 14, 33, 40, 43, 46, 48, 49.

apparent within the first 24 to 72 hours of life.[29] The onset of clinical NAS symptoms depends on which opiates/opioids the pregnant women used.[19,29] For example, with heroin, NAS may occur in the first 24 hours, whereas with methadone, it may not develop until after 48 hours.[20] Symptoms of NAS in heroin-exposed infants occur earlier than in infants of methadone-maintained mothers because of heroin's shorter half-life.[29] Compared with methadone, a lower incidence of NAS has been reported in buprenorphine-exposed neonates, and it has been suggested that it is because of the limited placental transfer of this drug, thereby limiting fetal exposure and development of dependency.[39,42,52] The Maternal Opioid Treatment: Human Experimental Research (MOTHER) Study showed that neonates of buprenorphine-maintained mothers required less pharmacologic treatment of their withdrawal and had shorter lengths of hospital stay.[46,48,49]

Nonopioid Substances

COCAINE

Although still controversial, the neonatal effects of maternal cocaine use, especially on fetal growth, is more consistently observed.[79] Researchers hypothesize that cocaine reduces fetal growth through maternal vasoconstriction, reduced uteroplacental transfer, and direct effect on fetal metabolism interfering with fat deposition.[79] Cocaine crosses the placenta by simple diffusion. This occurs because of its high lipid solubility, low molecular weight, and low ionization at physiologic pH. In addition, the low level of plasma esterases in the fetus and the relatively low pH of fetal blood (cocaine is a weak base) enhance the accumulation of cocaine in fetal compartments.[41,64] Taking advantage of the fact that cocaine and its metabolite *benzoylecgonine (BE)* accumulate and can be detected months after exposure in maternal and neonatal hair, an analytic test for cocaine and BE was developed by Garcia-Bournissen et al. These investigators looked at the characteristics of maternal and neonatal hair cocaine as biomarkers of fetal exposure.[34] They found that cocaine in hair and BE concentrations were not normally distributed, and they did not observe a correlation between maternal hair cocaine concentration and the baby-to-mother cocaine ratio, which ruled out a dose-dependent mechanism.[34,41,64,101] However, the positive correlation between cocaine concentrations in maternal and neonates' hair corroborates previous reports showing transplacental transfer of cocaine.[34,41,64,101] Cocaine has a significant vasoconstrictive property, which decreases blood flow to the placenta and fetus, contributing to fetal growth restriction and hypoxia.[34]

Accumulated evidence from well-designed prospective investigations done in the past few years have revealed less severe sequelae in the majority of infants exposed to cocaine than originally anticipated.[6] Unlike opioids, which may produce NAS and neurobehavioral deficits, cocaine exposure appears to be associated with significant but subtle decrements in neurobehavioral, cognitive, and decreased language function.[6]

Maternal cocaine abuse has been shown to produce infants of lower birth weight and birth length and infants who were significantly more likely to require medical support or resuscitation.[31] The most important central action of cocaine is its stimulation of the central nervous system by inhibiting the reuptake of norepinephrine, serotonin, and dopamine. In the neonatal period, cocaine, unlike opiates, does not produce an abstinence syndrome.

As part of the Maternal Lifestyle Study, Bada et al. used multivariate regression models with more than 11,000 mother–infant dyads to try to estimate the effects of cocaine exposure on intrauterine growth and to investigate when fetal growth deviation would manifest itself in the woman's gestation.[4] After controlling for confounders, at 40 weeks' gestation, cocaine exposure was estimated to be associated with decreases of 151 g in birth weight, 0.71 cm in length, and 0.43 cm in head circumference. Investigators concluded that in utero cocaine exposure was associated with growth deceleration that becomes more pronounced as gestation advances.[4]

ALCOHOL

Alcohol is the most common teratogen that fetuses are exposed to in Western societies, and unlike other teratogens, ethanol has no receptor but affects cellular activity.[84] In both recent prospective and retrospective studies of animals and mammals, ethanol has been shown to cause multiple problems during gastrulation and organogenesis that includes cellular growth, differentiation, and migration.[84,96] These cellular effects can be seen with both ethanol and acetaldehyde and are instrumental in inducing fetal malformations.

Early exposure to alcohol, whose effects are globally referred to as fetal alcohol spectrum disorders (FASD) are well-known causes of mental retardation.[96] FASD is an umbrella term describing the range of effects that can occur in an individual who was prenatally exposed to alcohol. These effects may include physical, mental, behavioral, and/or learning disabilities with lifelong implications. FASD is not a diagnostic term. It refers to specific conditions, such as fetal alcohol syndrome (FAS), alcohol-related neurodevelopmental disorder (ARND), and alcohol-related birth defects (ARBD).[85,89] Recent research documenting deleterious outcomes for children prenatally exposed to even small amounts of alcohol (0.5 drink per day) has led to a realization that a threshold has not been adequately identified. Current research has also found a genomic effect that is different in all individuals.[84] When ethanol exposure is held constant, genetic factors modulate the risk for cardiac, craniofacial, skeletal, and central nervous system defects in the developing fetus.[84] In light of these facts, health care professionals should counsel all women not to drink any alcohol while pregnant.[74,75]

When women consume cocaine and alcohol together, they compound the danger. Researchers have found that the human liver combines cocaine and alcohol to produce a unique metabolite, cocaethylene, which intensifies cocaine's euphoric effects. Cocaethylene is associated with a greater risk for sudden death than cocaine alone.[67] Discussions in the 1990s surrounding the use of cocaine and alcohol together suggested that cocaethylene was reported to be 10 times more potent than cocaine alone and more toxic to the growing fetus. The authors have not been able to find this in current literature.

AMPHETAMINES

Amphetamines and methamphetamines known as crystal, ice, or crank are abused by pregnant women in many geographic areas in the United States with the same frequency as cocaine. Like cocaine and "crack," the amphetamines are potent stimulants, and effects on the fetus and neonate are similar; also like cocaine, the preponderance of available data would suggest little or no effect of amphetamine on organogenesis.[26,39] Early research has shown how in utero amphetamine exposure can lead to congenital brain lesions, including hemorrhage, infarction, or cavitary lesions. Investigators also described the sites of these lesions as frontal lobes, basal ganglia, posterior fossa, or generalized atrophy; the effects of the lesions are not exhibited until the child is older. In the neonatal period, neurologic abnormalities including decreased arousal, poor state control, difficulty with habituation, tremors, hyperactive neonatal reflexes, abnormal cry, increased stress, drowsiness, poor feeding, and seizures have been reported.[26,83] Outcome effects of prenatal exposure to amphetamines have yet to be isolated from the effects of alcohol and nicotine, the two drugs most often used with the methamphetamines.[67]

A review of the most recent literature documents lack of prenatal care as the hallmark of maternal cocaine and amphetamine use with an increase in maternal morbidity and mortality as its consequence.[40,80,87,88] The use of these stimulants is reported to be toxic to the fetal brain, and there may be an increase in sudden infant death syndrome (SIDS). Stimulants (amphetamines and cocaine) have been found in breast milk in extremely high levels, and may produce an acute neurotoxic syndrome with hypertonia, tremors, apnea, and seizures.⋆

MARIJUANA

Marijuana, one of the most popular illicit drugs used by pregnant women,[30] has been studied for many years. de Moraes et al., in a prospective cross-sectional study that included full-term infants born to adolescent mothers who used marijuana, found that marijuana exposure was detected in both the mother's and the infant's hair and that the exposure during pregnancy altered the neurobehavioral performance of the term newborns when assessed with the neonatal intensive care unit (NICU) Network Neurobehavioral Scale (NNNS).[16,40] Other recent studies have highlighted the long-term effects of marijuana use in pregnancy on the neonate and child. These studies showed that prenatal marijuana use was "significantly related to increased hyperactivity, impulsivity, inattention symptoms, and delinquency" as the child grew older.[67]

INHALANTS

No well-controlled, prospective studies have been done on maternal inhalant use—often substances of abuse in poor and underprivileged communities

and groups because they are widely available, legal, and relatively inexpensive. Organic solvents are chemical compounds used to dissolve substances, and although their chemical structures widely differ, they share some common features: low molecular weight, lipophilia, and volatility at room temperature.[60,81] Inhalants are classified into four groups: volatile solvents, aerosols, gases, and nitrites.[60,61,81]

Inhalants may produce a variety of rapid neuropsychiatric effects with euphoria or drowsiness occurring within seconds to minutes. Case reports and follow-up studies of children of inhalant/solvent–abusing mothers are available. Inhalant/solvent–abusing mothers give birth to babies who are small for gestational age (SGA) and who have developmental delays, craniofacial deformities, and an alcohol-like withdrawal syndrome.

ANTIDEPRESSANT USE IN PREGNANT WOMEN AND NAS OCCURRENCE

Another area of concern is the psychopharmacology employed in the complex care needs of pregnant women with coexisting mental health diagnoses.[40] It has been estimated that up to 70% of pregnant women experience some symptoms of depression, with 10% to 16% of pregnant women meeting diagnostic criteria for a major depressive disorder.[94] The typical or atypical antipsychotic drugs and lithium all pass the blood–placenta barrier, with significant difference among compounds.[76] Continuing treatment throughout the pregnancy may be necessary to prevent relapse, and the pharmacologic treatment for depressive disorders may be either the tricyclic antidepressants (TCAs) or the SSRIs. A prospective study done by Kallen showed that both maternal TCA and SSRI use significantly increased the risk for neonatal respiratory distress, hypoglycemia, neonatal convulsions, and the occurrence of NAS.[40,53,54] Table 11-1 gives the signs and symptoms of withdrawal from TCAs and SSRIs.

Lithium. Lithium, often used for bipolar disorders, should be avoided during the first trimester of pregnancy. The placenta provides no protection to the developing fetus, and neonatal lithium toxicity is exhibited as hypotonia, cyanosis, lethargy, jaundice, hypothermia, poor sucking, poor respiratory effort, poor Moro reflex, reversible inhibition of thyroid function, and diabetes insipidus.[66]

⋆References 4, 34, 38, 40, 41, 78, 83.

TABLE 11-1 NEONATAL SSRI AND TCA EXPOSURE SYMPTOMS

	CNS, SLEEP, ENERGY		GI SYSTEM		MOTOR		SOMATIC		RESPIRATORY/CARDIO	
	SSRI	TCA	SSRI	TCA	SSRI	TCA	SSRI	TCA	SSRI	TCA
Somnolence	X	X								
Irritability	X	X								
Convulsions	X	X								
Abnormal cry patterns	X									
Aberrant stool			X							
Poor suck/may need tube feedings			X	X						
Agitation					X	X				
Tremors, jitteriness, shivering					X	X				
Decreased tone					X	X				
Increased tone, rigidity, apathy					X	X				
Temperature instability							X	X		
Hypoglycemia							X			
Tachypnea									X	X
Dyspnea, respiratory distress									X	X
Dysrhythmias, unstable B/P, cyanosis									X	X

Modified from ter Horst PG, Jansman FG, van Lingen RA, et al: Pharmacological aspects of neonatal antidepressant withdrawal, *Obstet Gynecol Surv* 63(4):267, 2008.
B/P, Blood pressure; *CNS*, central nervous system; *GI*, gastrointestinal; *SSRI*, selective serotonin reuptake inhibitor; *TCA*, tricyclic antidepressant.

ETIOLOGY OF NEONATAL ABSTINENCE SYNDROME

NAS is occurring in two ways: (1) by the passive exposure to opiates/opioids in utero as a consequence of maternal addiction to heroin, methadone, and other narcotic analgesics or to treatment of opiate/opioid addiction with methadone or buprenorphine; and (2) iatrogenically, by the administration of opiates/opioids such as fentanyl, morphine, and methadone to the neonate for analgesia and sedation. Infants exposed in utero and born to heroin-, methadone-, or buprenorphine-dependent mothers have a high incidence of NAS (60% to 90%).[23] Less potent opioids or opioid-like agents have also been implicated in the development of NAS. (Box 11-1 gives a complete list.) Neonatal abstinence is described as a generalized disorder characterized by CNS hyperirritability, gastrointestinal dysfunction, respiratory distress, and autonomic dysfunction manifesting as vague symptoms such as yawning, hiccups, sneezing, mottled skin color, and fever.* When narcotics cross the placenta, equilibrium is established between maternal and fetal circulations. Before birth, the drug is cleared from the infant's circulation primarily by the mother's excretory and metabolic mechanisms.[28,30,40]

In reviewing current literature, there are studies being done that may add to what we know about the causes and severity of the neonate's NAS. Some studies are outside the realm of NAS occurrence due to drug exposure alone. Here are two examples of studies being done with future implications:

- Jansson et al. studied the change in vagal tone of 50 pregnant women on methadone

---

*References 19, 24, 30, 40, 56, 57.

BOX 11-1 DRUGS ASSOCIATED WITH NEONATAL ABSTINENCE SYNDROME

Opioids
- Heroin
- Fentanyl
- Methadone/buprenorphine
- Morphine
- Meperidine (Demerol)

Less Potent Opioids and Opioid-like Agents
- Propoxyphene hydrochloride
- Codeine
- Pentazocine (Talwin)

Nonopioid Central Nervous System Depressants
- Tranquilizers and sedatives
- Bromides
- Chlordiazepoxide (Librium)
- Desipramine (Pertofrane, Norpramin)
- Diazepam (Valium)
- Ethchlorvynol (Placidyl)
- Glutethimide (Doriden)
- Hydroxyzine HCl (Atarax)
- Oxazepam (Serax)
- Alcohol
- Inhalant solvent abuse

BOX 11-2 FACTORS INFLUENCING THE ONSET OF PASSIVELY ACQUIRED NEONATAL ABSTINENCE SYNDROME

- Drugs used by the mother
- Both the timing and the dose of the drugs before delivery
- Character of labor
- Type of analgesia and/or anesthesia given during labor
- Maturity, nutritional status, and the presence of intrinsic disease in the neonate
- Possible gene variations of the *OPRM1* gene or *COMT* gene (currently under investigation)

BOX 11-3 FACTORS INFLUENCING THE ONSET OF IATROGENIC NEONATAL ABSTINENCE SYNDROME

- Prolonged opiate sedation for mechanical ventilation
- Duration of opioid analgesia use during extracorporeal membrane oxygenation
- Type of opiate used
- Maturity and presence of intrinsic disease in the neonate

maintenance therapy. The study defined vagal tone as an indicator of autonomic control and concluded that NAS severity was associated with the change in the maternal vagal tone due to taking methadone.[44]

- Wachman et al. conducted a multicenter cohort study on the association of *OPRMI* and *COMT* single nucleotide polymorphisms on NAS, the infant's length of stay, and need for pharmacologic treatment. This study concluded that infants with the *OPRMI* gene had a length of stay 8.5 days less than those without the variation and a better chance of not needing pharmacologic treatment. Neonates with the *COMT* gene variation were in he hospital 10.8 fewer days and had less treatment.[98]

The onset of withdrawal symptoms varies from minutes or hours after birth to 2 weeks of age, but the majority of symptoms appear within 72 hours. Many factors influence the onset of NAS (Boxes 11-2 and 11-3).

Once the umbilical cord has been cut, the neonate is no longer exposed to the drug, and monitoring of symptoms of withdrawal should commence. Because heroin is not stored in appreciable amounts by the fetus, signs of heroin withdrawal usually are apparent shortly after delivery and generally within 24 to 48 hours. However, methadone is stored in the fetal lung, liver, and spleen, facilitating the slow decline of methadone levels, but the rate of metabolic disposition varies for each infant, making the age at onset of NAS unpredictable.

Buprenorphine

Buprenorphine and methadone both act on the μ-opioid receptor; however, each has a unique pharmacology.[46] Whereas methadone has approximately 90% oral bioavailability, buprenorphine has approximately 50% oral bioavailability. This is because methadone is a full μ-agonist and buprenorphine is a partial μ-agonist and κ-agonist. Buprenorphine has higher receptor affinity[14] and a longer duration of action than methadone.[46]

The MOTHER Study, an eight-site, international, double-blind, double-dummy, flexible-dosing trial compared buprenorphine and methadone in a comprehensive care environment, enrolling 175 opioid-dependent pregnant women, of whom 131 delivered while on the study.[46,48] Among the women who completed the study, there were no significant differences between the buprenorphine and methadone groups with respect to any baseline characteristics.[48] There also were no significant differences between the groups in primary outcomes (i.e., percentage of neonates requiring NAS treatment, peak NAS scores, and head circumference).[46,48] However, there were significant differences in two primary outcome measures: (1) the total amount of morphine needed for NAS treatment (mean dose 1.1 mg vs. 10.4 mg) and (2) the length of hospital stay (4.1 days vs. 9.9 days). On average, the buprenorphine-exposed neonates required 89% less morphine and spent 43% less time in the hospital than those exposed to methadone.[48]

Withdrawal may be mild, transient, and delayed in onset, or it may increase stepwise in severity. Symptoms may be present intermittently or follow a biphasic course characterized by acute NAS signs, followed by improvement and then the onset of a subacute withdrawal reaction.[21,24,26,30,40] Withdrawal seems to be more severe in infants whose mothers have taken large amounts of drugs for an extended period. In general, the closer to delivery a mother takes the drug, the more severe the symptoms and the greater the delay in onset.

Usually the origin of NAS lies in the abnormal intrauterine environment. A series of steps appear to be necessary for the onset of NAS and thus the recovery of the infant. The growth and ongoing survival of the fetus are threatened by the continuing or episodic transfer of addictive substances from the maternal to the fetal circulation. During this time, the fetus goes through a biochemical adaptation to the abnormal element. At delivery, abrupt removal of the drug is the catalyst needed to start the onset of symptoms. The newborn continues to metabolize and excrete the substance, so that withdrawal signs occur when critically low tissue levels have been reached. Recovery from NAS is gradual and occurs as the infant's metabolism is reorganized to adjust to the absence of the offending drug.[25,26,30,40]

Studies of the relationship between maternal dose of methadone and severity of NAS have yielded

---

BOX 11-4 EFFECT OF MATERNAL METHADONE MAINTENANCE ON MOTHER AND CHILD

- Reduces illegal opiate use as well as use of other drugs, diminishing the risk for hepatitis, HIV/AIDS, and other sexually transmitted diseases
- Helps remove the opiate-dependent woman from the drug-seeking environment
- Eliminates illegal behavior, including prostitution
- Prevents fluctuation of the maternal drug level that may occur throughout the day
- Decreases mortality and severe maternal morbidity
- Permits a more stable intrauterine environment for the fetus, decreasing chances of hypoxia; *increases birth weight*
- Increases retention in substance abuse treatment
- Stabilized mothers on methadone more likely to retain custody of their children
- Children can be monitored by methadone clinic staff
- Provides opportunity for parenting education and other life skills
- No association between neonatal abstinence syndrome severity and the following:
  - Maternal methadone dose
  - Trimester of methadone initiation
  - Duration and amount of methadone exposure
  - Duration of maternal drug use before pregnancy

Modified from Pregnant, Substance-Using Women (TIP2) BKD127 Guideline 4, Substance Abuse and Mental Health Services Administration, U.S. Department of Health and Human Services.

---

inconsistent results: 50% of the studies find a relationship, whereas 50% find no relationship.[8,23,30,40,82] Use of adequate maternal methadone for therapeutic effect may decrease concomitant drug use and fetal risk; there is no compelling evidence to reduce maternal dosing to avoid NAS.[23] Box 11-4 outlines the effect of maternal methadone maintenance on mother and newborn.

PREVENTION

Neonatal drug withdrawal is preventable if women do not use dependence-producing substances, licit or illicit, during pregnancy. Through intense educational efforts, the desirability and availability of drugs may be thwarted. Unfortunately, the psychosocial and socioeconomic milieu of modern society continues to propagate dysfunctional families, victimization of women, and an intergenerational cycle of substance abuse.

Therefore, our goals must be to provide prenatal care for the pregnant drug-dependent woman and her fetus to diminish or eliminate the sequelae of passive addiction. The medical community is challenged to become more astute in its assessment and intervention for the problems of drug-dependent parturients. More treatment is necessary for these women and their neonates through inpatient residential care and outpatient interdisciplinary clinics that focus on the elimination, as well as the consequences, of addiction.

Birchley, in addressing iatrogenic NAS, discusses the need for guidelines for effective weaning of neonates from opiate analgesics and sedatives are becoming more established.[10] Investigators encourage dose reductions of 10% to 20% per day. For the prevention of iatrogenic NAS, discussions in recent literature include limiting total doses of fentanyl during ECMO therapy by administering morphine boluses or using continuous morphine infusions to replace fentanyl, substituting enteral methadone for morphine, or using sublingual buprenorphine.[56,62]

DIAGNOSIS

History

A comprehensive prenatal medical and drug history, especially with respect to polydrug abuse, is of prime importance. All pregnant patients who are substance abusers, regardless of the drug used, are considered high risk because of the effects of the drug, as well as complications arising from concomitant infections and lifestyle.[29] Fear of referral to child welfare agencies or the legal system in recent years has prompted women to conceal their drug abuse and/or pregnancy. This fear and denial may prevent the pregnant woman from seeking prenatal care. Thus, she may appear in the emergency department of the hospital either in crisis or ready to deliver. In this instance, a prenatal history is absent, making neonatal assessment more difficult.

Signs and Symptoms of Neonatal Abstinence Syndrome

At birth, most infants exposed to opioids appear physically and behaviorally normal with symptoms of withdrawal beginning shortly after birth and up

---

BOX 11-5	**CRITICAL FINDINGS**
	NEONATAL ABSTINENCE SYNDROME[20,21,29]

- Signs and symptoms of neonatal abstinence syndrome may not be exhibited for up to 72 hours.
- Most common signs and symptoms of neonatal abstinence syndrome are central nervous system hyperirritability, gastrointestinal dysfunction, respiratory distress, and autonomic instability.
- The closer to delivery a mother takes the drug, the more severe the symptoms and the greater the delay in onset.
- Acute signs and symptoms that may persist for several weeks:
  - Restlessness
  - Tremors (disturbed at first to undisturbed)
  - High-pitched cry
  - Increased muscle tone
  - Irritability and inconsolability
  - Increased deep tendon reflexes
  - Exaggerated Moro reflex
  - Seizures in approximately 1% to 2% of heroin-exposed neonates and approximately 7% of methadone-exposed neonates
- Subacute signs and symptoms that may persist for 4 to 6 months:
  - Irritability
  - Sleep pattern disturbance
  - Hyperactivity
  - Feeding problems
  - Hypertonia

---

to 2 weeks of age, but the majority are exhibited within 72 hours.[20,26,30,40] Acute symptoms may persist for several weeks, whereas subacute symptoms (e.g., irritability, sleep problems, hyperactivity, feeding problems, hypertonia) may persist for 4 to 6 months.[11]

The most common signs and symptoms of NAS are those of CNS hyperirritability, gastrointestinal dysfunction, respiratory distress, and autonomic instability (Box 11-5). A NAS scoring system is recommended and discussed on p. 211; however, for the convenience of referencing, the signs and symptoms discussed here are in the order in which they appear on the assessment sheet shown in Figure 11-2 (neonatal abstinence score sheet).

Initially, the infants appear only to be restless. Tremors develop, which are mild and occur only when the infants are disturbed, but these progress to the point at which they occur spontaneously without any external stimulation of the infant. Disturbed and undisturbed tremors and hyperactive Moro reflex, excessive irritability, and failure to thrive have been observed significantly more frequently in methadone-exposed neonates.[48] A high-pitched cry, increased muscle tone, and further irritability to the point of inconsolability develop. When examined, the infant tends to have increased deep tendon reflexes and an exaggerated Moro reflex.* Buprenorphine-exposed infants had higher frequency of nasal stuffiness, sneezing, and loose stools.[48–50]

One of the most serious but rare consequences of neonatal narcotic abstinence is the development of seizures. The relationship between maternal methadone dosage and the frequency or severity of the seizures has not been established. In addition, no significant differences were found between neonates with seizures and those without seizures in birth weight, gestational age, occurrence of their withdrawal symptoms, day of onset of withdrawal symptoms, or the need for specific pharmacologic treatment.[20,29] The mean age at seizure onset was 10 days. Generalized motor seizures, or myoclonic jerks, are the principal seizure manifestation, although in some infants the seizure manifestation can be complex. Seizures may occur even while the infant is being treated for NAS. The short-term prognosis for abstinence-associated seizures is favorable compared with the prognosis after seizures associated with other causes. Finnegan and Kaltenbach suggested that this observed improvement in neurologic function may be based on the replenishment of neurotransmitters after transient depletion in the neonatal period.[25]

Infants with NAS frequently exhibit respiratory distress symptoms such as rhinorrhea, a stuffy nose, tachypnea, nasal flaring, chest retractions, intermittent cyanosis, and apnea. These symptoms may increase in severity when the infant regurgitates, aspirates, or develops aspiration pneumonia.

There is some evidence of transient abnormality of lung compliance and tidal volume in infants born to methadone- or heroin-abusing mothers, as well as tachypnea in NAS, suggesting that opioids may alter the fetal development of the respiratory system. Infants with acute heroin withdrawal have shown increased respiratory rates associated with hypocapnia and an increase in blood pH during the first week of life. The observed

respiratory alkalosis was thought to have a beneficial role in the binding of indirect serum bilirubin to albumin and possibly in the prevention of respiratory distress syndrome, which is rarely observed in infants of opioid-abusing mothers. However, alkalosis can decrease the levels of ionized calcium and lead to tetany.[27]

The risk for SIDS should be considered when the neonate has an especially difficult course of NAS, when the mother supplemented her methadone with other substances (stimulants such as cocaine or amphetamine, nicotine), and when a combination of therapeutic agents is used for treatment. The rate of SIDS in these infants has been demonstrated to be 5 to 10 times over that in the general population. Research reports that the risk for SIDS is increased in opiate-exposed infants and varies from 2.5% to 4%.[42] Wingkun and other investigators studied carbon dioxide sensitivity in infants of substance-abusing mothers and found that these infants have abnormal sleep ventilatory patterns and "an impaired repertoire" of protective responses to hypoxia and hypercapnia during sleep cycles.[100] Infants undergoing withdrawal from narcotics have disturbed sleep patterns and exhibit excessive spontaneous generalized sweating. Other autonomic nervous system signs include yawning, elevation of temperature, sneezing, and skin mottling. The rooting reflex is exaggerated. It is not surprising, then, that these infants frequently suck their fists or thumbs; yet when fed, their suck and swallow reflexes are uncoordinated and ineffectual. Therefore they tend to regurgitate or vomit in a projectile manner. The infant also may develop loose stools and is susceptible to dehydration and electrolyte imbalance.[3,24,29,30,40]

These symptoms are exhibited as a result of exposure to opioids, as well as to nonopioid CNS depressants. However, with nonopioid CNS depressant exposure, symptoms tend to begin at a later age, with malnourishment at birth an unusual feature. Because barbiturate withdrawal may not develop until an infant has been discharged from the nursery, it may not be treated unless suspicion has been aroused by the mother's symptoms or actions. Furthermore, there is a greater risk for seizure activity in neonates withdrawing from barbiturates than in those withdrawing from opioids.[3,23,25,29,40]

Symptoms exhibited by stimulant-exposed newborns differ significantly from those associated with maternal opiate use, unless the mother was using cocaine or amphetamines along with

---

*References 20, 29, 30, 40, 66, 74, 79, 97.

the opiates. Recent literature describes cocaine-exposed infants as tremulous, irritable, lethargic, unable to respond appropriately to stimuli, and having abnormal state control and cry patterns.[3,4,40,41,79] Also described are abnormalities in orientation, motor ability, state regulation, muscular hypertonia, and abnormal reflexes. Infants may show symptoms of lethargy intermittently with irritability, poor sucking patterns, and sleep disturbances. When cocaine has been the primary drug of abuse, most clinicians have not seen symptoms severe enough to treat the infant pharmacologically.[27,29] Most would refer to the symptoms associated with cocaine not as withdrawal but, instead, as a manifestation of toxicity.

Laboratory Data

Before initiating medication for treatment of NAS, one must rule out common neonatal metabolic alterations that can mimic or compound withdrawal, such as hypocalcemia, hypomagnesemia, hypoglycemia, and hypothermia. Serum glucose and calcium tests may be indicated. If the mother has had no prenatal care, it would be prudent to thoroughly assess the infant at birth, including testing for occult disease, sepsis, and intracranial bleeding. A urine test for toxicology should also be obtained. Meconium testing, although expensive and not readily available in all institutions, appears to be more accurate and can detect a longer period of drug exposure.[101] Recent studies support meconium drug analysis, because the test is noninvasive, highly accurate, and can detect prior drug use over a 20-week period.[62,91]

TREATMENT AND INTERVENTION

Gaalema et al. studied the differences in the profile of NAS in methadone versus buprenorphine-exposed neonates. Among treated neonates, methadone-exposed infants required treatment significantly earlier than buprenorphine-exposed infants (i.e., 35 hours vs. 59 hours, respectively). Overall, methadone-exposed neonates had more severe NAS.[33]

To determine whether an infant will need pharmacologic treatment for withdrawal, appropriate assessment of symptoms is essential. Because only 50% to 60% of exposed infants have symptoms significant enough to require medication, an assessment tool is helpful.

We have used a *scoring system* to monitor the neonate in a *comprehensive and objective* way. With this score, one can assess the onset, progression, and resolution of symptoms. The score is used also to monitor the infant's clinical response to pharmacotherapy for the control of NAS symptoms. Titration of therapeutic agents is thus based on the degree of withdrawal symptoms that correspond to a specific score (Figure 11-1). Although a number of scores have been used in both clinical and research settings, in our experience, the 21-item Finnegan neonatal abstinence score has remained useful. The nurse is vital in the assessment of withdrawal symptoms because he or she will administer and record the score and any other activities that may affect the infant's progress. Therefore, it is essential that interrater reliability be developed among all nurses responsible for the infant.

The ***Finnegan abstinence scoring sheet*** uses a weighted scoring of 21 actual items most commonly observed in an opioid-exposed neonate.[24-27,40] Scoring includes the following: (1) a score of 1 for tremors regardless of which of the four varieties noted, (2) 1 for the Moro reflex, (3) 1 for stooling, (4) 1 for crying, and (5) 1 for regurgitation/projectile vomiting. Signs and symptoms are recorded as single entities or in several categories if they occur in varying degrees of severity. Each symptom, with its associated degree of severity, has been assigned a score. Higher scores are assigned to symptoms found in infants with more severe withdrawal. The total score is determined by adding the scores assigned to each symptom observed throughout the entire scoring interval. The scoring system is dynamic rather than static; all of the signs and symptoms observed during the 4-hour intervals at which infant symptoms are monitored are point-totaled for that interval. Infants are assessed 2 hours after birth and every 4 hours afterward.

If medication is not warranted, the infant is scored for the first 4 days of life at the prescribed intervals. If the symptoms are severe enough to require medication, the infant is scored at 2- or 4-hour intervals, depending on whether the score is 8 or less or 8 or higher, as described previously, throughout the duration of the therapy. Once medication is discontinued, if there is no

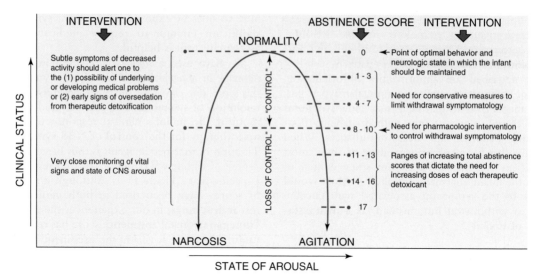

FIGURE 11-1 **Management of the neonatal abstinence syndrome.** *CNS,* **Central nervous system.** (From Finnegan LP: Neonatal abstinence syndrome. In Nelson N, editor: *Current therapy in neonatal-perinatal medicine,* ed 2, Ontario, 1990, Decker.)

resurgence of the total score to 8 or higher after 3 days, scoring may be discontinued. However, if there is a resurgence of symptoms with scores consistently equaling 8 or higher, scoring should be continued for a minimum of 4 days after discontinuation of medication to ensure that the infant is not discharged prematurely, with the consequent development of symptoms at home.

The Lipsitz Tool, also known as the Neonatal Drug Withdrawal Scoring System, was recommended in the 1998 American Academy of Pediatrics (AAP) statement on neonatal drug withdrawal.[13] However, the Finnegan Neonatal Scoring Tool is the predominant tool used in the United States.[30,40]

Figure 11-2 shows the NAS scoring system. Symptoms are listed on the left, scores to the right. Times of each evaluation are listed at the top, and the total score is listed for each evaluation. A new sheet should be started at the beginning of each day. A "Comments" column has been provided for nursing and medical staff to record important notes about the infant's progress.

The first score should be recorded approximately 2 hours after the neonate's admission to the nursery. This score reflects all infant behaviors from admission to that first point in time when the scoring interval is complete. The times designating the end of the scoring intervals (whether every 2 or 4 hours) have been left blank to permit the nursing

staff to choose the most appropriate times for scoring intervals in relation to effective planning and implementation of nursing care.

Salient points to consider in using the scoring system are as follows:

- All infants should be scored at 4-hour intervals unless high scores indicate a need for more frequent scoring.
- All symptoms exhibited during the entire scoring interval, not just a single point in time, should be included.
- The infant should be awakened to elicit reflexes and specified behavior, but if the infant is awakened to be scored, one should not score him or her for diminished sleep after feeding. Sleeping should never be recorded for a scoring interval except when the infant has been unable to sleep for an extended period: more than 12 to 18 hours. If the infant is crying, he or she must be quieted before assessing muscle tone, respiratory rate, and the Moro reflex.
- Respirations are counted for 1 full minute.
- The infant is scored if prolonged crying is exhibited, even though it may not be high pitched in quality.
- Temperatures should be taken (mild pyrexia is an early sign indicating heat production by increased muscle tone and tremors).

NEONATAL ABSTINENCE SCORE

Date: _____   Weight: _____

System	Signs and Symptoms	Score	Time AM ... PM	Comments
Central nervous system disturbances	Excessive high-pitched cry	2		
	Continuous high-pitched cry	3		
	Sleeps <1 hour after feeding	3		
	Sleeps <2 hours after feeding	2		
	Sleeps <3 hours after feeding	1		
	Hyperactive Moro reflex	2		
	Markedly hyperactive Moro reflex	3		
	Mild tremors when disturbed	1		
	Moderate - severe tremors disturbed	2		
	Mild tremors when undisturbed	3		
	Moderate - severe tremors undisturbed	4		
	Increased muscle tone	2		
	Excoriation (specific area)	1		
	Myoclonic jerks	3		
	Generalized convulsions	5		
Metabolic/vasomotor/ respiratory disturbances	Sweating	1		
	Fever <101° F (37.2° - 38.2° C)	1		
	Fever 38.4° C and higher	2		
	Frequent yawning (>3 - 4 times/interval)	1		
	Mottling	1		
	Nasal stuffiness	1		
	Sneezing (>3 - 4 times/interval)	1		
	Nasal flaring	2		
	Respiratory rate >60/min	1		
	Respiratory rate >60/min with retractions	2		
Gastrointestinal disturbances	Excessive sucking	1		
	Poor feeding	2		
	Regurgitation	2		
	Projectile vomiting	3		
	Loose stools	2		
	Watery stools	3		
	TOTAL SCORE			
	Initials of Scorer			

FIGURE 11-2 **Neonatal abstinence score sheet. Check sign or symptom observed at various time intervals and add scores for total at each evaluation.** (Modified from Finnegan LP, Kaltenbach K: The assessment and management of neonatal abstinence syndrome. In Hoekelman RA, Nelson N, editors: *Primary pediatric care*, ed 3, St Louis, 1992, Mosby.)

- If the infant is sweating solely because of conservative nursing measures (e.g., swaddling), a point should not be given. **Medication is not indicated if consecutive total scores or the average of any three consecutive scores continues to be 7 or less during the first 4 days of life.**

The total scores dictate the specific dose of medication, such as morphine, methadone, or phenobarbital, and all subsequent doses are determined by and titrated against the total score. In the phenobarbital loading dose approach, an initial dose of 20 mg/kg is administered in an attempt to achieve an expected therapeutic serum level with a single dose. Current recommendations are an opiate. Phenobarbital is used only in resistant polydrug exposures.

The need for medication is indicated when the total score is 8 or higher for three consecutive scorings (e.g., 9, 8, 10) or when the average of any three consecutive scores is 8 or higher (e.g., 9, 7, 9). Once an infant's score is 8 or higher, the scoring interval automatically becomes 2 hours, so that the infant exhibits symptoms that are out of control for no longer than 4 to 6 hours before therapy is initiated. If subsequent 2-hour scores continue to be 7 or less for 24 hours, 4-hour scoring intervals may be resumed.

If the infant's total score is 12 or higher for two consecutive intervals or the average of any two consecutive scores is 12 or higher, therapy should be initiated at the appropriate dosage for that score before more than 4 hours elapse.

The longer the delay in initiating an appropriate medication dose, the greater the risk for increased infant morbidity. *Comfort measures* used for the infant should include the following[11]:

- Swaddling
- Offering a pacifier for nonnutritive, excessive sucking. (A new study used a pacifier connected to a recorder that played a song sung by the infant's mother.[13] This device improved oral feeding skills in preterm infants, including those with brain injury. Larger studies will be conducted and these devices may be used with NAS infants in the future.)
- Aspirating nasal secretions when needed
- Changing the diaper frequently; exposing hyperemic buttocks in severe cases for air-drying
- Providing soft sheets or sheepskin to decrease excoriations
- Positioning on right side-lying to reduce aspiration if vomiting or regurgitation is a problem
- Protecting the infant from face scratching by using mitten cuffs on the undershirt or tying a rubber band to the end of the shirt sleeves
- Considering demand feedings if weight-change patterns are an issue
- Modifying the infant's environment (noise and light control). (For severe cases, some literature recommends self-activated nonoscillating waterbeds as a useful adjunct to supportive care of narcotic-exposed neonates.)

Table 11-2 describes the symptoms of withdrawal and appropriate nursing interventions.

The pharmacologic agents of choice in the United States and United Kingdom for treatment of withdrawal include morphine or methadone. Paregoric is no longer used because it contains variable concentrations of other opioids and toxic ingredients such as camphor. The AAP has recommended methadone, and data are available concerning its safety and efficacy.[30] However, Finnegan cautions methadone use for NAS because of its long-acting properties.[30]

Table 11-3 outlines drug treatment for NAS. Any infant who exhibits a precipitous drop in a total score of 8 points or higher should be monitored for vital signs immediately. It is important to determine whether any underlying medical problems are developing, such as sepsis, meningitis, hypocalcemia, or hypoglycemia. Detection of underlying medical problems may be difficult, because poorly controlled abstinence may mimic and/or disguise many common neonatal conditions.

An infant may become increasingly depressed by a medication that is not used specifically for withdrawal. This situation may be seen in the infant's gradual development of depression and simultaneous poorly controlled withdrawal, requiring reevaluation for appropriateness of the medication (Box 11-6).

The efficacy of the medication always must be assessed. Two common situations indicate the need for reassessment: (1) CNS depression and (2) failure to achieve "control" despite aggressive pharmacologic intervention and/or near-toxic serum levels of the agents. In these situations, the following measures are indicated:

- Evaluate the infant for metabolic derangements, sepsis, and CNS disturbances to detect an occult problem compounding the clinical picture. Evaluate laboratory data, including serum calcium, electrolytes, glucose determinations, and blood cultures.
- Review maternal drug history along with both maternal and infant urine toxicology results to ensure appropriate medication.
- If a single medication is ineffective, consider a combination of therapeutic agents. Phenobarbital may be used in conjunction with an opiate in cases of *maternal* polydrug abuse.

Breastfeeding the NAS Infant

Both methadone and buprenorphine are found in breast milk. Methadone appears in low levels so that the mean daily methadone ingestion for an infant is 0.05 mg/day.[23] Buprenorphine is excreted into breast milk approximately 2 hours after maternal ingestion. The concentrations of buprenorphine and norbuprenorphine in breast milk are highly variable because of differences in breast milk protein and fat. However, neither concentrations of buprenorphine and norbuprenorphine were found to exceed plasma concentrations.[46]

One study comparing breastfeeding rates and the relationship between breastfeeding and NAS in buprenorphine-exposed neonates found the following[46]:

- 76% or (65 of 85 participants) in the study chose to breastfeed.
- 66% were still breastfeeding at 6 to 8 weeks' postpartum.

TABLE 11-2	CREATING A SUPPORTIVE ENVIRONMENT FOR THE DRUG-EXPOSED NEONATE	

INFANT BEHAVIOR	OBSERVATIONS	INTERVENTIONS
High-pitched cry	Note onset. Note length of time the cry persists: Is it continuous? Is it high pitched and piercing as though infant were in pain? Observe infant for other causes of abnormal crying patterns (e.g., meningitis, intracranial bleed, pain): Is anterior fontanel full or bulging? Are cranial sutures widely separated? Is head circumference increased? Does infant stare without blinking; exhibit tongue darting? Is cry aggravated or alleviated when infant is picked up?	Soothe infant by swaddling, holding firmly and close to your body; soft-pack baby carrier; smooth, slow rocking. Nonnutritive sucking. Decrease feeding intervals or implement a demand-feeding schedule. Reduce environmental stimuli (noise, light). Use waterbeds, lambskin.
Inability to sleep	Note how long infant sleeps after feeding. Note general sleep–wake patterns. If drug therapy has been initiated, note changes in sleep patterns, ability to rest, and any decreased activity indicative of drug overdose.	Decrease environmental stimuli (noise, light). Swaddle or use soft-pack baby carrier. Feed small amounts at frequent intervals. Use waterbeds, lambskin. Organize care to minimize handling.
Frantic sucking of fists	Note onset and amount of fist sucking. Observe for blisters on fingertips and knuckles. If blistering occurs, observe sites for signs of infection.	Use infant shirts with sewn-in sleeves for mitts to prevent skin trauma. Offer pacifier for nonnutritive sucking. Keep skin area clean; use aseptic technique.
Yawning	Note onset and frequency.	None.
Sneezing	Observe onset and frequency.	Aspirate nasopharynx as needed.
Nasal stuffiness	Note severity of nasal stuffiness and determine whether it hinders breathing and feeding; if mucus is excessive, consider possibility of other underlying problems, such as esophageal atresia, tracheoesophageal fistula, and congenital syphilis.	Allow more time for feeding with rest between sucking. Aspirate trachea if tracheal mucus is increased. Check rate and character of respirations frequently. Use cardiorespiratory monitor with alarms set.
Poor feeding	Note sucking pattern: Is infant uncoordinated in attempt to suck, swallow, and breathe? Observe for other possible causes of poor feeding (e.g., sepsis, hypoglycemia, immaturity, bowel obstruction, pyloric stenosis).	Weigh daily. Decrease environmental stimuli. Feed small amounts at close intervals. Wrap securely. Maintain fluid and caloric intake required for infant's weight. Consider demand feedings. Use alternative feeding methods (e.g., gavage). Avoid rocking; may be helpful for some babies. Avoid talking or eye contact during feeding.

Continued

TABLE
11–2   **CREATING A SUPPORTIVE ENVIRONMENT FOR THE DRUG-EXPOSED NEONATE**—cont'd

INFANT BEHAVIOR	OBSERVATIONS	INTERVENTIONS

Regurgitation	Note when regurgitation or vomiting occurs: Is there a precipitating factor (e.g., medication, handling, manipulation, position)?
	Observe for signs of dehydration:
	    Specific gravity >1.015
	    Urinary output <1 ml/kg/hr
	    Dry mucous membranes
	    Marked weight loss
	    Poor skin turgor
	    Sunken anterior fontanel
	Note time, color, consistency, and quantity of vomitus or stool.
	When stools are loose, estimate amount of water loss with stools.
	Note whether vomiting is forceful (projectile) or not.
	Observe for electrolyte imbalance.
		Measure intake and output closely, and correlate with infant's general condition, progress, and therapy.
		Offer supplementary fluids if signs of dehydration appear
		Weigh frequently if weight loss, vomiting, and diarrhea persist.
		Maintain IV at prescribed rate.
		Maintain infant in side-lying position.
		Head of bed may be elevated.
		Give skin care to prevent excoriation of neck folds, buttocks, and perineum.
		Change diaper frequently; expose hyperemic buttocks for air-drying.
		Consider barrier dressings on knees, elbows, etc.

Hyperactive Moro reflex	Is reflex moderately or markedly exaggerated? If drug therapy has been started, is Moro reflex diminished or absent? Is there asymmetry of the reflex? Asymmetry may indicate underlying pathophysiology (Erb's palsy, fractured clavicle, intracranial hemorrhage).	None

Hypertonicity	Note degree (mild, moderate, or severe) of increased muscle tone by:
	    Attempting to straighten arms and legs and recording degree of resistance
	    Picking infant up by hands and noting body rigidity with degree of head lag (a withdrawing infant often exhibits trunk rigidity and holds the head on a plane with the body for a prolonged time)
	    Raising infant by arms and letting baby stand (a withdrawing neonate exhibits marked leg rigidity and can support body weight for considerable periods)
	Correlate mother's obstetric history and delivery with infant's condition; observe baby for other pathophysiology—hypocalcemia, hypoglycemia, meningitis, asphyxia, and intracranial hemorrhage.
	Observe for reddened areas over heels, occiput, sacrum, and knees.
	Observe temperature frequently; increased activity may cause hyperthermia.
		Change infant's position often because prolonged or marked rigidity predisposes the infant to develop pressure areas.
		Use sheepskin to reduce pressure and for relaxation and comfort.
		Decrease environmental temperature if infant's temperature is >37.6° C (99.7° F).

TABLE 11-2 CREATING A SUPPORTIVE ENVIRONMENT FOR THE DRUG-EXPOSED NEONATE — cont'd

INFANT BEHAVIOR	OBSERVATIONS	INTERVENTIONS
Tremors, convulsions	Note whether tremors occur when infant is disturbed or undisturbed. Note location of tremors: Upper extremities Lower extremities Generalized Note whether degree of tremors is mild, moderate, or severe. Observe skin over nose, elbows, fingers, toes, knees, and heels for excoriation. Observe face for scratches. Observe for underlying pathology mentioned in the "Hypertonicity" section. Check temperature often for hyperthermia. Observe for seizures; if they occur, note onset, length, origin, body involvement, type (tonic, clonic, or both), eye deviation, and infant's color.	Change position frequently to prevent excoriation. Give frequent skin care (cleansing, ointment, and exposure to air and/or a heat lamp). Use sheepskin. Observe excoriations for healing, worsening, and infection. Decrease environmental temperature if infant exhibits hyperthermia. If infant convulses, maintain patent airway and prevent self-trauma. If infant is apneic after seizure, stimulate appropriately and be prepared to resuscitate. Decrease environmental stimuli. Organize nursing care to decrease handling. Support movements during caregiving. Swaddle as much as possible during caregiving.

Modified from Finnegan LP, MacNew BA: Care of the addicted infant, *Am J Nurs* 74:685, 1974.

TABLE 11-3 DRUGS USED FOR NEONATAL ABSTINENCE SYNDROME

DRUG	DOSAGE	COMMENTS
Tincture of Opium (1 ml is added to 24 ml sterile water) Final concentration equal to 0.4 mg morphine sulfate Contains variable concentrations of other opioids, camphor, anise oil, alcohol and benzoic acid[41]	Starting dose is 0.4 mg PO in 6–8 divided doses. Dose should be increased by 0.04 mg/kg/day or 0.1 ml as needed as frequently as every 4 hours until control is achieved. Weaning: decrease infant's dose by 10% daily, or as tolerated until daily dose is 0.2 mg/kg/day; then discontinue.	Control is evidenced by an NAS average score <8, rhythmic feeding/sleep cycles, optimal weight gain, same opium dose for 72 hours, pharmacologic weaning. Continue to score for NAS. Scores must remain <8.
Oral Morphine First choice of U.S. clinicians	Initial dose: 0.04 mg/kg every 3–4 hours Increment: 0.04 mg/kg/dose Maximum dose: 0.2 mg/kg/dose[41] Use a 0.4 mg/ml dilution: 1 ml of the 4 mg/ml injectable solution added to 9 ml preservative-free normal saline solution. Protect from light; stable for 7 days, refrigerated.	Advantages: Diminishes bowel motility and loose stools; 20%–40% bioavailability when administered orally; lower doses and shorter dosing interval are associated with shorter hospital stays in infants with NAS resulting from maternal methadone treatment. Disadvantages: Respiratory depressant, hypotension, delayed gastric emptying, ileus, urine retention.

Continued

TABLE 11-3	DRUGS USED FOR NEONATAL ABSTINENCE SYNDROME—cont'd	
DRUG	**DOSAGE**	**COMMENTS**
Phenobarbital Only useful if polydrug use occurs	Loading dose: 20 mg/kg to achieve an expected therapeutic level in a single dose. If score is ≥8, give 10 mg/kg every 12 hours until control or signs of toxicity appear. Maintenance dose (once under control): 2–6 mg/kg/day for 3–4 days. Decrease dose to 3 mg/kg/day. Discontinue: serum levels <15 mcg/ml.	Daily serum levels can be obtained. Advantages: Drug of choice for polydrug use; especially effective in controlling irritability and insomnia; controls symptoms in 50% of infants. Disadvantages: Does not prevent loose stools. Infant should be in a nursery where he or she can be monitored closely.
Oral Methadone[40]	Initial dose: 0.05–0.1 mg/kg every 6 hours Increment: 0.05 mg/kg/dose Maximum dose: to effect	Many practitioners do not wish to use methadone as a first-line drug for NAS because of its long half-life. However, many articles written from the United Kingdom and United States have compared it to oral morphine.[40]
Oral Clonidine[40]	Initial dose: 0.5–1 mcg/kg every 6 hours Increment: not studied Maximum dose: 1 mcg/kg every 3 hours	Alpha-2-adrenergic receptor agonist that has been used in combination with an opioid or other drug in older children and adults to reduce withdrawal symptoms. Via a negative feedback mechanism, clonidine reduces CNS sympathetic outflow and palliates symptoms of autonomic overactivity, such as tachycardia, hypertension, diaphoresis, restlessness, and diarrhea. Cessation of clonidine treatment can result in a rebound of autonomic activity. Reported experience with clonidine as a primary or adjunctive treatment of NAS is limited but promising.[40]

CNS, Central nervous system; *NAS,* neonatal abstinence syndrome; *PO,* by mouth.

BOX 11-6	COMPLICATIONS OF EXCESSIVE PHARMACOLOGIC TREATMENT

- Diminished or absent reflexes: Moro, sucking, swallowing, Galant, Perez, tonic neck, corneal, grasp (palmar, plantar)
- Truncal (central) or circumoral cyanosis or persistent mottling not associated with ambient temperature decreases
- Decreased muscle tone with passive resistance to extension of extremities, or decreased neck or trunk tone
- Altered state of arousal (e.g., obtunded, comatose)
- Diminished response to painful stimuli
- Failure of visual following
- Hypothermia
- Altered respirations: irregular (periodic breathing in full-term infants), shallow (decreased air entry), decreased respiratory rate (<20/min), apnea
- Cardiac alterations: irregular rate, distant heart sounds with weak peripheral pulses, heart rate of 80 to 100 beats/min, poor peripheral perfusion (pale, gray, mottled skin), cardiac arrest

- NAS was less severe with the breastfeeding group (mean peak NAS scores of 8.83 vs. 9.65 on the Finnegan scoring system).
- Breastfed infants were less likely to require pharmacologic treatment (23.1% vs. 30%) than infants who were not breastfed.

The Norwegian National Cohort Study of 124 women treated with either methadone or buprenorphine found that 77% of the women chose to breastfeed. Methadone-exposed infants had a lower incidence of NAS requiring pharmacologic treatment (53% vs. 80%). Breastfed infants exposed to both methadone and buprenorphine needed less medication for a shorter period of time.[58] In summary, the limited published research (barring other complications and contraindications, such as HIV-positive mother) support current guidelines that recommend breastfeeding for mother stabilized on either methadone or buprenorphine[2,46] (see Chapter 18).

PARENT TEACHING

It is important for primary caretakers to understand that infants exposed to narcotics through maternal addiction have been found to be more irritable and less cuddly, exhibit more tremors, and have increased tone (Box 11-7). These infants are also less responsive to visual stimulation and are less likely to maintain an alert state. Some symptoms of withdrawal may persist for 2 to 6 months, and the nurse should discuss this possibility with the caregivers well before discharge so that they may begin building the skills they will need under the watchful eye of supportive staff. The infant may continue to feed poorly and regurgitate, yet vigorously suck fists and hands. Mothers frequently misread this continued, exaggerated rooting reflex as hunger and therefore may overfeed the infant. Loose stools may continue.

These infants may have hyperacusis or are easily disturbed by normal household sounds and do not sleep well. They sweat more than other infants and, when crying, continue to have a high-pitched cry. They may have poor tolerance of being held or to abrupt changes in position. This, along with hypertonia, may continue, and the mother may interpret this as a sign of rejection. Nursing support, including thorough descriptions of the potential symptoms and their management and the fact that they are time limited, is vital if maternal–infant attachment is to occur and potential neglect and abuse are to be avoided.

In recent studies, drug-dependent mothers and their infants were assessed for patterns of interaction. Both drug-dependent mothers and their newborns demonstrated poor performance on a measure of social engagement. The drug-dependent mothers demonstrated significantly less positive affect and greater detachment, and the drug-exposed infants presented fewer behaviors promoting social involvement. Drug-exposed infants and their mothers experience a difficult early period during which both are less available, less likely to initiate, and less responsive to social involvement.[87] Therefore, parents of the drug-exposed infant may need assistance in recognizing important symptoms that signal problems and cues necessary for caregiving.

All drugs of abuse pass through the breast milk. However, breastfeeding in the methadone-maintained mother need not be discouraged, because it does not appear to shorten or worsen the course of withdrawal.[23,41] In contrast, women using stimulants and other drugs, as well as those who are infected

BOX 11-7	PARENT TEACHING CARING FOR AN INFANT EXPOSED TO OPIOIDS

Some symptoms may persist for 2 to 6 months.

- Infants exposed to narcotics in utero are more irritable, less cuddly, and tremulous and have increased tone: Parent(s) may interpret these behaviors as signs of rejection; infant may not want to be held or cuddled as other babies.
- Less responsive to visual stimulation
- Less likely to maintain a quiet-alert state: Let parent know symptoms are time limited.
- Poor feeding habits: Continue to regurgitate yet show vigorous sucking of fists or pacifier: Constant sucking and exaggerated rooting reflex may lead to overfeeding the infant.
- Continuation of loose stools: Important to stress good diaper hygiene to prevent infection from excoriated skin.
- Infants easily disturbed by sounds: Parent may decrease stimuli in house.
- Sweat more than other newborns: Dress infant appropriately to avoid overheating.
- High-pitched cry: Not easily consoled, parents need someone to share infant care and give them some rest from an irritable infant to prevent neglect or abuse.
- Hypertonia
- Less eye-to-eye contact, which decreases social interaction.

with HIV, should not be encouraged to breastfeed because of the potential toxic and negative effects on the neonate. Finally, secondary crack smoke, crystal methamphetamine smoke, marijuana smoke, and tobacco smoke can be detrimental to the health of the newborn; therefore, parents should be warned of the consequences of using these substances around their infant.

Although much has been learned over the past several decades from research in the field of perinatal substance abuse, continued evidence-based studies are essential if we are going to determine the intricacies of neonatal abstinence syndrome and the overall immediate and long-term effects of in utero substance exposure.

REFERENCES

For a full list of references, scan the QR code or visit http://booksite.elsevier.com/9780323320832.

PAIN AND PAIN RELIEF

SANDRA L. GARDNER, MARY ENZMAN HINES, AND RITA AGARWAL

Pain is a complex phenomenon, the nature of which is, at best, elusive in the neonate. Extremely fragile premature infants experience multiple painful procedures (e.g., heel sticks, intravenous sticks, intubation, lumbar punctures, introduction of chest tubes, placement of nasogastric tubes) during their stay in the neonatal intensive care unit (NICU). The number of exposures to these procedural events varies from 0 to 53 a day, and approximately 30% of these neonates fail to receive analgesia.[17,206] Rationalization for inadequate treatment of pain has resulted in unnecessary suffering for these fragile infants. Research has shown that the "unchecked release of stress hormones by untreated pain may exacerbate injury, prevent wound healing, lead to infection, prolong hospitalization, and even [lead] to death."[263] These fragile neonates are simply too sick to *not* have their pain treated. Health care professionals are responsible for influencing positive change in clinical practice about neonatal pain.[3,7-11,171,257,317]

Several decades ago, neonates did not receive analgesia and/or anesthesia agents for surgery because of the controversy as to whether they feel pain and whether they are physiologically stable enough to tolerate the effects of these drugs. The rationale for withholding analgesia and/or anesthesia agents included the following beliefs:

- Neonates have an immature central nervous system (CNS) with nonmyelinated pain fibers and are thus incapable of perceiving pain.
- Neonates have no memory of pain.
- Pain is a highly subjective experience that is difficult to objectively assess in nonverbal neonates.

- Anesthetics and analgesics are dangerous when administered to neonates, and neonates are safer if they are not medicated.

There is increasing evidence from more than 30 years of research that neonates, including preterm infants, have a CNS that is much more mature than previously thought.[7,25,95] Pain pathways are myelinated in the fetus during the second and third trimesters and are completely myelinated by 30 to 37 weeks' gestation. Even thinly myelinated or nonmyelinated fibers carry pain stimuli. Incomplete myelination implies only a slower transmission, which is offset in the neonate by the shorter distance the impulse must travel.[25]

Even though pain is not expressed verbally in semiconscious patients, nonverbal adults (e.g., intubated, mute), or infants, this does not negate their experience of pain. In response to the question of whether the neonate's responses are reflexive or express a perception of pain, research has focused on measuring the infant's pain experience. The infant's capacity for memory is far greater than was previously thought,[7,16,17] and a neuropsychologic complex of altered pain threshold and pain-related behavior has been identified.*

Concern has been expressed that giving potent medications to an already critically ill infant might be dangerous. Local and systemic drugs now available, as well as new techniques and devices for monitoring, enable all neonates to be safely anesthetized and provide safe and effective analgesia while maintaining a stable condition.[25]

Neonates exhibit (1) physiologic, (2) hormonal, (3) metabolic, and (4) behavioral responses to invasive procedures that are similar to, but more

---

*References 6, 97, 132, 228, 229, 245, 258, 294, 295, 300.

PURPLE type highlights content that is particularly applicable to clinical settings.

intense than, adult responses.[12,14,18,25,72] Exposure to multiple painful procedures may increase the vulnerability of preterm infants to gross neurologic damage (intraventricular hemorrhage, periventricular leukomalacia).[13,15,17,48,126] Pain relief benefits the neonate by decreasing physiologic instability, hormonal and metabolic stress, and the behavioral reactions accompanying painful procedures.*

The Committee on Fetus and Newborn of the American Academy of Pediatrics (AAP) has recommended the administration of local or systemic drugs for anesthesia or analgesia to neonates undergoing surgical procedures.[8] The committee further states that any decision to withhold these drugs should not be based solely on the infant's age or perceived degree of cortical maturity but should be based on the same criteria used in older patients.[8,18] The AAP, in the latest version of the guidelines, cites that prolonged exposure to untreated pain increases morbidity and alters subsequent behavioral and physiologic responses to pain.[9] National associations have promulgated standard-of-care guidelines or position statements about neonatal pain management.[3,7-11,257,317] The focus of these documents is on the proactive assessment and management of pain in the neonate. The National Association of Neonatal Nurses (NANN) guidelines outline the following recommendations[317]:

- Parents should be informed of pain relief as an important part of the neonate's health care plan and should be encouraged to actively participate in their neonate's assessment and management of pain.
- *Every* institution must mandate clinical practice guidelines that ensure access and safe administration of pain control to the neonate. Institutions also should develop guidelines for assessing and monitoring pain management practices that include parental input with the goal of measuring the adequacy of pain relief and control in the neonate.
- Institutions should support interdisciplinary research and ongoing education that includes a description of neonatal pain, accurate pain assessment, interventions to improve patient care and reduce morbidity, as well as guidelines ensuring adequate administration of analgesics and sedatives for the neonate.

A national study of experienced, highly educated neonatal nurses who were members of NANN was recently published.[72] Only 50% of the surveyed nurses felt knowledgeable about pain, some disagreed about the neonate's capacity to feel pain or that there were long-term consequences of unrelieved pain. Other findings of the survey include the following: (1) 81% use a pain assessment tool; only 65% thought the tool was appropriate for neonates, and 60% thought it was an accurate measure; (2) 83% felt confident in use of pharmacologic interventions; (3) 79% felt confident in use of nonpharmacologic interventions.[72] Only 44% of the respondents reported that neonatal pain was well managed, and only 43% thought that their pain protocols were evidence-based. Barriers to relief of neonatal pain were identified as (1) professional (both nurses and doctors) resistance to change (44%), (2) lack of knowledge (23%), (3) fear of side effects of pain medications and incorrect evaluation of pain symptoms (15%), (4) time-delay from pain assessment to receipt of medications (13%), and (5) lack of trust in the assessment tool (13%).[72] One hundred and forty-seven of the total 237 respondents identified strategies to improve pain management: (1) education about pain (45%), (2) reading and using research (15%), and (3) more interdisciplinary communication.[72]

All neonatal health care providers have an ethical and legal obligation to practice the standard of care* in assessing and intervening to relieve the neonate's pain, as well as to reevaluate the safety and efficacy of the pharmacologic and comfort interventions used to treat pain.[18,100,145,209,237]

PHYSIOLOGY AND PATHOPHYSIOLOGY

"Pain is an unpleasant sensory and emotional experience associated with actual or potential tissue damage, or described in terms of such damage."[158] The neonate's expression of pain does not fit the self-report aspect of this definition, which often results in the health care provider's failure to recognize and treat pain. Because self-report is absent in the preverbal neonate, nonverbal behavioral information needs to be assessed and used to determine the treatment options for neonates. The definition

---

*References 12, 13, 25, 26, 132, 228, 323.

*References 3, 7–11, 18, 100, 171, 177, 257.

of pain has been amended. "The inability to communicate in no way negates the possibility that an individual is experiencing pain, and is in need of appropriate pain-relieving treatment."[158] Although we cannot assess the emotional experience associated with pain in these babies, the necessary sensory pathways are now better understood. Neonates have a developing, incompletely myelinated nervous system at birth; however, all the components of the nociceptive (pain) pathways are present.[96,138] As background for an understanding of neonatal responses and their differences from adult responses, the basic mechanisms of adult pain transmission are presented in Figure 12-1.

Types of pain experienced by the neonate have been identified as (1) *physiologic,* caused by tissue injury; (2) *inflammatory,* caused by inflammation of tissues, (3) *neuropathic,* caused by nerve inflammation/damage; and (4) *visceral,* caused by distention, inflammation, and contraction of viscera.[20,21] Sources of neonatal pain are either acute, established, or chronic/prolonged.[20,21] Chronic pain in the neonate has not yet been defined, but a recent Delphi survey found that it is persistent and recurring pain associated with inadequate pain management and that *every* newborn in an NICU is at risk for developing a chronic pain state.[106,313] Pain in the neonate can and should be viewed as an *adverse event.*[200]

NEUROANATOMY

Peripheral Nervous System

Peripheral nerves can be classified into three broad categories based on fiber diameter and velocity (Table 12-1). Pain receptors (nociceptors) are the A-delta fibers (A-δ) and C fibers that are widely spread in the superficial layers of the skin, periosteum, fascia, peritoneum, joints, muscle, pleura, dura, and tooth pulp. Most visceral tissues have fewer nociceptors, and these transmit to the spinal cord through the sympathetic, parasympathetic, and splanchnic nerves. Tissue damage and inflammation cause the release of arachidonic acid and

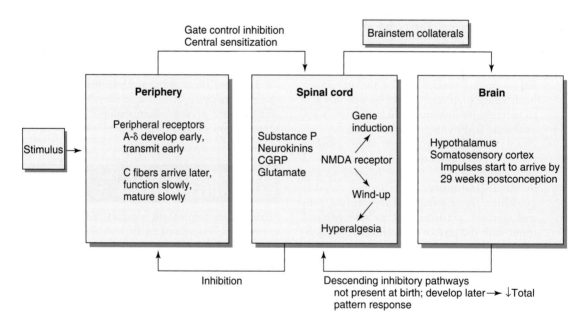

FIGURE 12-1 Schematic representation of transmission of noxious stimuli from the periphery to the brain. CGRP, Calcitonin gene–related peptide; NMDA, N-methyl-D-aspartate.

other chemicals that can sensitize nerve endings and cause vasodilation and plasma extravasation. This causes pain, swelling, and hyperalgesia.[84]

A-δ fibers are myelinated and therefore capable of fast impulse conduction. These nerves are responsible for "fast" or "first" pain. They are also known as *high-threshold mechanoreceptors (HTMs)* because they respond to strong pressure or tissue injury. The C fibers (polymodal nociceptors) are unmyelinated, conduct impulses more slowly, and are the main nociceptors for transmitting chemical, thermal, and mechanical noxious stimuli to the spinal cord.[214] The A-δ fibers develop ahead of the C fibers in the skin and the spinal cord. A-δ fibers are involved in the cutaneous flexion reflex. This reflex is exaggerated in the preterm. Thresholds to mechanical skin stimulation (which may or may not be perceived as pain in a newborn) are lower and responses last longer. Complete myelination occurs during the second and third trimesters. Lack of myelination had been thought to indicate the inability of a neonate to perceive pain; however, incomplete myelination leads only to slower conduction, which is offset by the shorter distances traversed in the infant.[25,138]

Reflex responses to somatic stimuli begin at 7.5 weeks postconceptual age (PCA) in the perioral skin and continue to develop in the palms of the hands before finally reaching the hind limbs by 13 to 14 weeks. Peripheral pain receptors are in place throughout the body by 20 weeks' gestation.[280] It is likely that both A-δ fibers (touching) and A-δ fibers (pinching) transmit painful stimuli in the human fetus. In rat pups, the C fibers reach the spinal cord but do not start to stimulate dorsal horn cells until the end of the first postnatal week. They subsequently continue to mature for several weeks. This slow maturation in rats may be caused by low levels of neuropeptides such as substance P (SP), neurotransmitters, or immature receptor sites. These changes in rat pups appear to correlate with the third trimester and the early neonatal period in humans.[96]

Spinal Cord

The pain transmission system begins with the peripheral pain receptors (nociceptors). Once a noxious stimulus is detected by the nociceptors, the signal is transmitted via the primary afferents to the dorsal root ganglia and from there to the dorsal horn of the spinal cord.[64] Neurotransmitters and their receptors amplify or attenuate the signal in the dorsal horn before sending the signal to the brain.

Excitatory neurotransmitters such as SP and other neurokinins are increased after acute inflammation and may be necessary for the transmission of painful stimuli to the brain.[163] Glutamate and aspartate are amino acids that appear to be involved in central hypersensitivity and wind-up.[24] *Wind-up* is a phenomenon in which repetition of the same noxious stimulus leads to an exaggerated response. This response continues even after the noxious stimulus ceases. Wind-up also may be responsible for converting a low-level, pain-related activity to a high-level, pain-related activity.[84,300] The preterm experiences increased stress and activity in the nociceptive pathways after prolonged periods of exposure to painful stimuli. After prolonged exposure, the preterm exhibits

TABLE 12-1	CLASSIFICATION AND CHARACTERISTICS OF PERIPHERAL NERVES	
NAME/CHARACTERISTICS	**FUNCTION**
A-alpha (A-α) d: 10–20 μ v: 70–120 m/sec myelinated	Innervate skeletal muscle
A-beta (A-β) d: 12–20 μ v: 30–70 m/sec myelinated	Light touch or pressure may be involved in peripheral sensitization and allodynia; in the premature and newborn infant, may be involved in the transmission of noxious stimuli
A-gamma (A-γ) d: 3–6 μ v: 15–30 m/sec myelinated	Muscle tone
A-delta (A-δ) d: 2–5 μ v: 12–30 m/sec myelinated	Fast, well-localized pain; high threshold mechanoreceptors
B d: 3 μ v: 3–15 m/sec myelinated	Preganglionic autonomic fibers may be involved in sensory or sympathetic coupling
C d: 0.4–1.2 μ v: 0.5–2 m/sec unmyelinated	Slow pain, touch, temperature, postganglionic sympathetic fibers, polymodal nociceptors

d, Nerve diameter; *v,* nerve velocity.

similar pain responses when exposed to other caregiving activities (e.g., handling, suctioning the endotracheal tube, positioning).[91]

An additional factor in the development of hypersensitivity (e.g., decreased pain threshold) and hyperalgesia is the presence of nociceptive-specific receptors,[138] which respond only to pain. In the presence of peripheral inflammation, the threshold of these receptors is decreased so that they are capable of responding to other nonnoxious stimuli.[84] For example, an infant whose heel has been repeatedly stuck for blood samples may demonstrate pain behavior, even when the heel is merely touched. Many of these responses can be blocked by low doses of opioids. However, once these responses are established, a 10-fold increased dose of opioids may be necessary to reverse them.[97,323]

The spinal cord also contains inhibitory neurotransmitters (γ-aminobutyric acid [GABA], glycine), which are activated by descending neural pathways (from the brain to the spinal cord) and decrease the intensity of pain transmission. This results in modulation of pain transmission from the spinal cord to the cortex. Descending inhibition is necessary to modulate the pain response and yet allow for specific pain responses (e.g., withdrawal from a needle stick). Delayed maturation of the descending inhibitory fibers results in a *higher pain threshold* in the upper extremities and lower in the lower extremities, resulting in more pain sensitivity in the lower extremities.[20] Lack of inhibition produces exaggerated, generalized, but definite, responses to pain such as body wriggling, facial grimacing, and excessive crying. These pathways, in contrast to the excitatory ones, are not fully developed at birth in "rat pups and probably in preterm infants[138]; therefore, the neonatal spinal cord is more excitable.[96] The pain transmission system of the premature infant (<36 weeks) is more developed than the pain modulation system; therefore preterm infants are *more* sensitive to pain than are term or older infants.[138,280]

Neurotransmitters in the developing nervous system may be expressed early but are not necessarily located in areas normally found in an adult. This is particularly true of SP and glutamate, which may contribute to the unorganized responses noted with pain stimuli in the newborn (e.g., the whole body moves when an intravenous [IV] line is started).

Brain

Much less is known about the development of the pathways to the higher brain centers, such as the hypothalamus and cortex. Once again, there is evidence of immaturity of the inhibitory pathways.[96] Development in the human cortex continues for many years after birth. Contrary to previous beliefs that newborns do not feel pain, it appears that, in fact, cutaneous responses are exaggerated and occur at much lower thresholds and reflex muscle contractions last longer in newborns than in mature individuals. Using real-time near-infrared spectroscopy (NIRS) in 18 preterm infants (25–45 weeks postmenstrual age [PMA]), an increase in cerebral oxygenation over the somatosensory cortex was measured in response to heel stick blood draws[277] and in response to venipuncture in another study.[36] From these findings, researchers concluded that pain is transmitted to the cerebral cortex of preterm infants from 25 weeks' PMA.[277] Other recent research has found that low biobehavioral responsiveness to pain at 32 weeks' PCA is associated with poorer quality of motor function at 8 months' PCA; therefore pain reactivity in the NICU may be a marker of neuromotor development in later infancy.[133] In summary, the newborn's nervous system, although still developing, is fully capable of transmitting, perceiving, responding to, and probably remembering noxious stimuli.

PHYSIOLOGIC RESPONSES

Acute pain in adults is associated with increased sympathetic stimulation, heart rate, respiratory rate, blood pressure, cardiac output, myocardial oxygen consumption, peripheral resistance, anxiety, emotional distress, and hormonal imbalance and greater morbidity and mortality. Numerous studies have shown that both premature and full-term infants express the same physiologic responses to pain and noxious stimuli (e.g., intubation) as adults do (Box 12-1).[8,25,72,325] Infants undergoing circumcision without the use of pain medication demonstrated higher pain scores, increased irritability after the procedure, an altered sleep-wake state, and abnormal feeding patterns for up to 22 hours. These responses can

BOX 12-1	CRITICAL FINDINGS
	NEONATAL PAIN RESPONSE*

Physiologic

- Increase in
  - Heart rate
  - Blood pressure (also fluctuations)
  - Intracranial pressure/cerebral blood flow,[203] which leads to higher risk for intraventricular hemorrhage
  - Respiratory rate
  - Mean airway pressure
  - Muscle tension
  - Carbon dioxide ($\uparrow TcP_{CO_2}$; P_{CO_2})
  - Pulmonary vascular tone
  - Oxygen consumption
- Decrease in
  - Depth of respiration (shallow)
  - Oxygenation ($\downarrow P_{O_2}$; Sa_{O_2}), which leads to apnea or bradycardia
  - Vagal tone and peripheral blood flow
  - Cerebral oxygenation with vigorous crying
- Pallor or flushing
- Diaphoresis or palmar sweating
- Dilated pupils
- Nausea, vomiting, gagging, and hiccoughing

Behavioral

- Vocalizations
  - Crying (higher pitched, tense, and harsh)
  - Inaudible crying
  - Whimpering
  - Moaning
- Facial expressions
  - Grimacing
  - Furrowing or bulging of the brow
  - Quivering chin
  - Eye squeeze
  - Nasal flaring
  - Curling/curving of the tongue
  - Facial twitching
  - Lips open and pursed

- Body movements
  - General diffuse body activity (flexing/extending extremities; extending legs; finger splay, fisting, hand on face)
  - Limb withdrawal, swiping, thrashing
- Changes in tone
  - Hypertonicity, rigidity, fist clenching
  - Hypotonicity, flaccidity
- Touch aversion
- States
  - Sleep-wake cycle changes, wakefulness
  - Activity level changes: increased fussiness, irritability, listlessness, lethargy
  - Feeding difficulties
  - More difficult to comfort, soothe, quiet
  - Disruption of interactive ability with parents

Hormonal/Catabolic Stress Response

- Increase in
  - Plasma rennin activity
  - Catecholamine levels (epinephrine and norepinephrine)
  - Cortisol levels (serum and hair)
  - Nitrogen excretion/protein catabolism
  - Release of
    - Growth hormone
    - Glucagons
    - Aldosterone
  - Serum levels of
    - Glucose
    - Lactate
    - Pyruvate
    - Ketones
    - Nonesterified fatty acids
- Decrease in
  - Insulin secretion
  - Prolactin
  - Immune responses

*References 12, 13, 25, 72, 73, 116, 130, 134, 136, 145, 169, 220, 227, 284, 291, 318, 321.

be attenuated or blocked with the appropriate use of analgesics.[252] Despite research on infants' pain response to circumcision and recommendations to use anesthetics or analgesics during circumcision, a survey in a large academic medical center showed that only 30% of infants being circumcised by obstetricians received any pain relief, and there was no documentation of discussion with parents about pain management.[182]

Pain reactivity varies by prior experience with pain.[72,265,295] Studies on pain reactivity in very-low-birth-weight (VLBW) infants at 32 weeks' PCA found that younger gestational ages (GAs) and increased numbers of invasive procedures at birth resulted in a "dampening" of normal pain reactions (e.g., delayed or fewer facial changes; lower pain scale scores)[72,90,170] and cortisol response.[128] These infants had higher baseline heart rates, which may have indicated that they were in a perpetual state of stress or pain. A longitudinal comparison of 81 preterm infants' pain responses to repeated heel sticks found that both a higher severity of illness and number of previous heel sticks lowered pain scores.[90] Previous exposure to morphine was associated with a "normalization" of responses to painful stimuli. More recent studies of the pain response in extremely low-birth-weight (ELBW) preterms (<27 weeks' GA) found (1) similar responses to older infants but also "dampened" responses[112,113,325] and (2) lower cortisol levels representing down-regulation of the hypothalamic-pituitary-adrenal axis that is not counteracted by morphine use.[128] Two other studies have compared the biobehavioral pain responses of ELBW infants with term controls. The studies found that (1) at 4 months' corrected age, behavioral and cardiac autonomic responses were similar, with less parasympathetic withdrawal and more sustained sympathetic response during recovery in the ELBW group[228] and (2) at 8 months' corrected age, behavioral response was similar to that in term infants but less sustained (i.e., faster dampening); baseline heart rate was significantly higher in ELBW neonates.[132] The number of previous painful experiences in the NICU was significantly related to subsequent pain reactivity in the ELBW infants, and those ELBW infants exposed to higher doses of morphine had heart rate recovery more similar to that of the term infants.[132] Higher numbers of invasive procedures are significantly associated with brain structure alterations, specifically reduced white matter and subcortical gray matter maturation in preterm infants.[48]

ETIOLOGY

Invasive Procedures

Pain is produced with any invasive procedure (Box 12-2).[18,137,273] Two studies of the first 14 days in the NICU found (1) an average of 196 procedures per neonate with 14 invasive procedures per day per infant[273] and (2) a median of 115 procedures

per neonate with 16 invasive procedures per day per infant.[59] In the most recent study, treatment for painful procedures included the following[59]:
1. Pharmacologic-only therapy (2.1%)
2. Nonpharmacologic-only therapy (18.2%)
3. Combination therapy (both No. 1 and No. 2) (20.8%)
4. No specific analgesia (79.2%)
5. Concurrent analgesia/anesthesia for other purposes (34.2%)

Another study examining the use of analgesics for "minor" procedures in NICUs and pediatric intensive care units (PICUs) found that analgesics were rarely used for the placement of IV catheters, suprapubic bladder aspiration, urinary bladder catheterization, venipuncture, arterial line placement, lumbar puncture, and paracentesis in NICUs. Analgesics were used approximately 60% of the time in NICUs for the placement of chest tubes, central lines, and bone marrow aspiration.[37] By contrast, analgesics were used in the majority of patients in PICUs undergoing arterial line placement, lumbar puncture, and paracentesis and in more than 90% of chest tube insertions, central line placements, and bone marrow aspirations. Possible reasons for these differences were that (1) neonates were more often critically ill and the use of analgesics may have prolonged the procedure or exacerbated the infants' medical problems, (2) the use of neuromuscular blocking agents prevented the physical response to pain, and (3) not all infants respond to pain by crying loudly, withdrawing, or otherwise "protesting." A study of painful procedures in NICUs found that 239 patients were subjected to 2134 invasive procedures in 1 week and an analgesic was administered in only 0.8% of these procedures.[167] More recent studies have found that only one third of the neonates received an analgesic for painful procedures,[273] no pain guidelines were present in 25% of surveyed NICUs, and the majority of these NICUs had no guideline for pain relief for routine invasive procedures.[210] Health care providers underestimate the pain caused by procedures,[86] and even when they believe that most NICU procedures are painful, relief is provided only 33% of the time.[273] A study of neonates at increased risk for neurologic impairment found that these infants had the highest number of invasive procedures but received the least amount of analgesic on the first day of life.[285] These studies indicate that considerable work is needed to educate practitioners about the safety, efficacy, and benefits of

BOX
12-2 **SELECTED COMMON CAUSES OF PAIN IN NEONATES**

Invasive Procedures	Surgical Procedures	Others
Intravenous cannulation	Central line placement	Clavicle, rib fracture
Venipuncture	PDA ligation	Extremity fracture
Heel stick	TEF repair	Chest pain
Intramuscular injection	Gastroschisis repair	Central pain syndrome (i.e., pain derived from
Arterial line, blood gas	Omphalocele repair	CNS damage)
Umbilical catheterization	CDH repair	Spasticity
Chest tube insertion or removal	Inguinal hernia repair	Abdominal pain resulting from short gut syndrome,
Bone marrow aspiration	Cardiac surgery	multiple abdominal surgeries
Lumbar puncture	Circumcision	Necrotizing enterocolitis
Paracentesis	Broviac catheter insertion or removal	Bowel obstruction
Endotracheal intubation/removal	ECMO catheter insertion or removal	Prolonged and/or improper positioning
Endotracheal or nasal[217] suction		Position changes
Mechanical ventilation		NG tube placement
NCPAP		Flushing lines
Bladder catheterization		Dressing changes
Suprapubic aspiration		Eye examination for ROP
Ventricular tap		IV administration of medications
Endoscopy		Addition/withdrawal of fluid from umbilical catheter
Bronchoscopy		Transient mechanical birth trauma (e.g., cephalic
PICC line insertion/removal		hematoma, molding, bruising, forceps marks,
Cutdown (arterial/venous) for access		petechiae)
		Cryo/laser surgery for ROP
		Chest physiotherapy
		Changing tape/suture removal
		Therapeutic hypothermia[146]

Data from Anand KJ and the International Evidence-Based Group for Neonatal Pain: Consensus statement for the prevention and management of pain in the newborn, *Arch Pediatr Adolesc Med* 155:173, 2001; Barker D, Rutter N: Exposure to invasive procedures in neonatal intensive care unit admissions, *Arch Dis Child Fetal Neonatal Educ* 72:F47, 1995; Bauchner H, May A, Coates E: Use of analgesic agents for invasive medical procedures in pediatric and neonatal intensive care units, *J Pediatr* 4:647, 1992; Belda S, Pallas C, Dela Cruz J, et al: Screening for retinopathy of prematurity: is it painful? *Biol Neonate* 86:195, 2004; Evans JC, Vogelpohl DG, Bourguignon CM, et al: Pain behaviors in LBW infants accompany some "nonpainful" caregiving procedures, *Neonatal Netw* 16:33, 1997.
CDH, Congenital diaphragmatic hernia; *CNS*, central nervous system; *ECMO*, extracorporeal membrane oxygenation; *IV*, intravenous; *NCPAP*, Nasal continuous positive airway pressure; *NG*, nasogastric; *PDA*, patent ductus arteriosus; *PICC*, peripherally inserted central catheter; *ROP*, retinopathy of prematurity; *TEF*, tracheoesophageal fistula.

appropriate pain management in neonates. Use of "better practices" strategies, clinical practice guidelines, and proven quality improvement methods has resulted in better pain management for neonates in the NICU.*

Endotracheal intubation is associated with hypoxia, bradycardia, catabolism, increased intracranial pressure, increased systemic and pulmonary hypertension, and release of stress hormones.[183] Recent research has shown that use of premedication for elective, nonurgent intubations is safer and more effective than awake intubations (see the Endotracheal Intubation section in Chapter 23). Unmedicated endotracheal intubation in the neonate should be reserved for emergency resuscitation in the delivery room.[183]

No consensus exists about pain relief in the mechanically ventilated neonate.[140,174,211] Benefits of pain management in the ventilated neonate

---

*References 82, 88, 185, 186, 191, 244, 270.

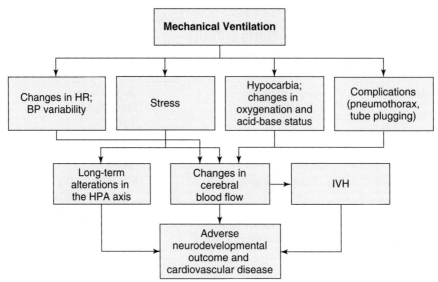

FIGURE 12-2 Potential mechanisms leading to adverse effects from mechanical ventilation in preterm neonates. *BP,* Blood pressure; *HPA,* hypothalamic-pituitary-adrenal; *HR,* heart rate; *IVH,* intraventricular hemorrhage. (Modified from Hall RW, Boyle E, Young T: Do ventilated neonates require pain management? *Semin Perinatol* 31:289, 2007.)

include (1) improved ventilator synchrony, (2) improved pulmonary function, (3) less neuroendocrine (cortisol, beta-endorphins, catecholamine) response, (4) better oxygenation, and (5) potentially ameliorated adverse effects (Figure 12-2) of mechanical ventilation in the preterm.[32,140,211] Two approaches to pain management in ventilated neonates are commonly used: (1) preemptive, continuous opioid infusion and (2) as-needed (prn) intermittent bolus administration of opioids.[29,79,174,212] The NOPAIN pilot study found poor neurologic outcomes in only 4% of the ventilated preterms receiving continuous morphine sulfate (MS) for pain compared with 24% in the placebo group and 32% in the midazolam group.[23] In this study the MS-treated preterms were the only group with significantly lower pain scores.[23]

The NEOPAIN double-blind randomized controlled trial (RCT), conducted in 12 American and 4 European NICUs, studied whether preemptive morphine analgesia would decrease early neurologic injury in 898 ventilated preterms less than 32 weeks' gestation.[24] There was a higher incidence of severe intraventricular hemorrhage (IVH) in the morphine-treated group of 27 to 29 weeks' gestation, possibly due to higher MS infusion rates or less MS clearance in hypotensive infants.[24] Further analysis of cohorts from the NEOPAIN study have found

(1) significantly longer ventilation in MS-treated preterms, as well as more air leaks and supplemental oxygen use in preterms who received additional intermittent boluses of MS[42]; (2) MS delays the start of and the full attainment of enteral feedings but does not increase gastrointestinal (GI) complications,[213] (3) both preemptive and additional MS and lower GA are associated with hypotension[141]; (4) IVH (i.e., any and severe) and death are associated with preexisting hypotension, but morphine therapy did not contribute to these outcomes[141]; and (5) although MS infusions cause hypotension, they can safely be used for most preterm neonates.[141] Use MS cautiously for 23- to 26-week preterms and those with preexisting hypotension.[141] Another randomized, double-blind, placebo-controlled trial of morphine infusion for ventilated preterms showed that (1) the analgesic effect was similar between the treated and placebo group, (2) routine morphine infusion decreased the incidence of IVH but did not influence poor neurologic outcome, (3) the routine use of MS infusions is not supported by the lack of analgesic effect and the absence of any beneficial effect, and (4) the long-term effects of MS on the neurologic outcomes of preterm infants need study.[274]

Studies have also compared fentanyl with morphine and fentanyl with sufentanil for analgesia during mechanical ventilation in neonates.[260,264] Fentanyl was equianalgesic with morphine, sufentanil equianalgesic to fentanyl, and sufentanil did not reduce the weaning period for ventilated (term) infants.[260,264] Continuous fentanyl infusion (plus open-label PRN boluses of fentanyl) for very preterm ventilated infants has been shown to reduce acute, but not prolonged, pain with more side effects (longer ventilation and delayed meconium passage) than use of PRN fentanyl boluses alone.[29] Morphine, fentanyl, and sufentanil reduce the pain and stress of preterms being mechanically ventilated but may prolong the duration of ventilation.[29,32] Only two studies have investigated the effect of fentanyl analgesia on acute brain outcomes, and there was no difference in the incidence of IVH, PVL, or mortality.[184,260]

Dexmedetomidine hydrochloride, an α-adrenergic receptor agonist, provides analgesia, anesthesia, and sedation for mechanically ventilated neonates.[211,230] Advantages include (1) less adjunctive sedation needed, compared with fentanyl; (2) minimal effect on blood pressure, heart and respiratory rates, oxygen saturation, and gastric motility; and (3) its safety and effectiveness for short-term pain relief during invasive procedures in ventilated and nonventilated neonates.[211,230] Only one study of the effect of dexmedetomidine on brain injury has been conducted. In a comparison of dexmedetomidine versus fentanyl used for sedation in mechanically ventilated preterms, there was no difference in the incidence of severe IVH or PVL between the two groups.[305] An RCT of the safety and efficacy of dexmedetomidine hydrochloride and the short- and long-term neurologic outcomes are needed.[68,90]

Although use of analgesia in ventilated infants is recommended,[9,18] a meta-analysis concludes there is insufficient evidence for "routine use" of opioids during mechanical ventilation.[40] The meta-analysis states that opioids should be selectively used for individual neonates based on clinical judgment and pain assessment.[40] Long-term neurologic outcomes of MS analgesia for ventilated preterms are being studied. A recent pilot study of 5- to 7-year-olds from the NEOPAIN cohort of ventilated preterms, who had received preemptive MS, found them to be 7% smaller in head circumference, 4% less in body weight, slower and completed fewer (27%) short-memory tasks, and had more social problems, specifically with creating and maintaining friendships.[94] This same cohort was again studied at 8 to 9 years of age and found to have significantly better executive function as evaluated by parents and teachers.[81] The method of pharmacologic pain relief, the appropriate drug to use, the use of preemptive or bolus, based on pain scores, and minimizing long-term adverse outcomes remain clinical and research challenges.

Surgery

Painful stimuli, surgery, and traumatic injuries have been shown in adults to trigger the "stress response," which causes the release of a variety of hormones, including epinephrine, norepinephrine, corticosteroids, glucagon, and growth hormones. These hormones prepare the body for a *fight-or-flight response* and cause, among other things, an increase in heart rate, respiratory rate, glucose production, and muscle and fat breakdown. This response allows the body to deal with an insult in the short term. If the insult continues or is untreated, the ongoing catabolic stress response may become deleterious to the body's well-being by promoting more tissue breakdown and preventing growth and tissue repair. During the period of rapid brain growth and development, the immature brain of the preterm infant has heightened vulnerability to pain. The first study to link cumulative neonatal pain stress to alteration in brain function in extremely low gestation (≤28 weeks) preterms has recently been published. This study found an association between cumulative neonatal pain-related stress and alteration in cortical function resulting in visual-perceptual difficulties at school age in this vulnerable population.[87]

Both premature and full-term infants have a decreased stress response with the use of appropriate analgesia both during and immediately after surgery.* Physiologic indicators (e.g., heart/respiratory rate, blood pressure) of postoperative pain may be unreliable or confounded by illness severity and use of analgesics and neuromuscular blocking agents.[52,98]

Use of adequate operative anesthesia[8,9] and postoperative analgesia is mandatory, even if its use might prolong postoperative ventilatory support.

A special example of untreated operative pain is newborn circumcision. In addition to the previously mentioned short-term effects of not treating the pain associated with circumcision, male infants who have undergone circumcision without analgesia

---

*References 11, 13, 18, 23, 25, 26.

have an increased pain response to vaccination at 4 to 6 months of age.[294,296] When these infants were pretreated for their immunizations with a topical anesthetic, their pain response was lessened.[296] Another study of 14- and 45-month-old children who had major surgery with appropriate analgesia (in their first 3 months of life) found that their biobehavioral pain response to immunizations was not altered compared with a matched group of toddlers who had not had surgery.[240] However, prolonged exposure to early hospitalization did contribute to an altered pain response (in areas of prior tissue damage) that "recovered" over time.[240,241] Although early painful memories may not be consciously recalled, experiences of pain are "remembered" by the developing nervous system.[15,16,28,241] Newborns have a much greater capacity for memory than was previously thought.

Other Causes

Rib, clavicular, and extremity fractures are not uncommon and should be considered in the presence of prolonged crying and failure to move the affected extremity.

Bronchopulmonary dysplasia (BPD) is a common problem in infants who were premature and may cause chest pain, a syndrome known to occur in some older patients with chronic lung disease. Neurologic dysfunction can leave patients with ongoing pain from central pain syndrome or excessive spasticity. One study showed that 27% of former ELBW infants who were now teenagers had neurosensory impairment, and 9% reported moderate or severe pain.[261]

PREVENTION

Prevention of pain in the neonate and preterm infant begins with a proactive plan of care aimed at preventing the pain cycle. The key approaches in this plan include (1) anticipation, (2) comprehensive and ongoing assessment of the variables; (3) distinguishing agitation and irritability from pain expressions and responses of the preterm infant; (4) ongoing communication among health care providers, using input from the parents; (5) advocating and implementing timely and effective treatment for irritability, agitation, and pain (e.g., pharmacologic and comfort measures); (6) reducing the number of painful procedures[59,85,221,315]; and (7) ongoing

reevaluation of this proactive plan of care.[3] Different types of common procedures in the NICU can be anticipated to be painful. *Diagnostic procedures* include arterial puncture, heel stick, lumbar puncture, and retinopathy of prematurity (ROP) examination. *Therapeutic procedures* include tracheal intubation and extubation, tracheal suctioning, chest tube insertion, mechanical ventilation, suture removal, therapeutic hypothermia,[146] and removal of adhesive tape. Some of the *common surgical procedures* are circumcision, patent ductus arteriosus ligation, insertion of central venous catheters, and laser therapy for ROP. Anticipation and prevention of pain during such procedures can markedly affect the success of the procedure and the condition of the infant. Preventing, reducing, and relieving neonatal pain constitute an essential health care provider goal to maintain the sick neonate's behavioral, physiologic, and biochemical homeostasis.[18]

Individualized behavioral and developmental care is another important area in preventing stress and sensory overload, which often contribute to an ongoing pain cycle.[78,275] These approaches help prevent disorganization in the neonate. Several studies have shown that clustering care, a common practice in the NICU (see Chapter 13), actually results in an increase in behavioral responses and cortisol secretion for preterms of younger GAs when exposed to a painful procedure.[147,148,151] To facilitate stability and self-regulation before and during an invasive painful procedure, (1) do not cluster care and provide a period of rest before the procedure, (2) assess the infant's state and facilitate a change to an alert state, (3) contain extremities (see Chapter 13), (4) provide a pacifier and an opportunity to grasp (a finger, hand, or blanket), and (5) use another person (e.g., parent, caregiver) to support, contain, and observe for stress. After the procedure, provide support, comfort, and slow withdrawal so that the infant remains calm.

The suffering of neonates can be avoided. Needless suffering is prevented by an established plan of care for assessment, management, and evaluation of pain and attempts to relieve pain. Neonates depend on the skilled observations, assessments, and interventions of care providers for *prompt, safe* and *effective* relief. A cooperative effort among health care providers and the parents in the form of pain management teams[207] and well-established pain protocols[82] prevents unnecessary suffering of both neonates and their families.[177] Controlling environmental stimuli (e.g., dimming lights, controlling noise level, speaking softly, performing rounds outside of the unit), although often difficult in the NICU, is crucial for decreasing stress and preventing unnecessary agitation. Use of an individualized, developmentally appropriate plan of care reduces the need for sedation in severely ill, VLBW neonates.[12,275] Quieting techniques are also a useful way to help control pain response in the neonate; these include nonnutritive sucking, containment interventions, and rocking (see Chapter 13).

DATA COLLECTION

History

Neonates experiencing procedural, surgical, and/or chronic pain must be provided measures to alleviate pain. Neonatal irritability and agitation (Box 12-3) secondary to chronic conditions (e.g., BPD, necrotizing enterocolitis, short bowel syndrome, neurologic deficits) and/or environmental overstimulation also may require a combination of environmental interventions and sedation.[9]

Signs and Symptoms

Assessment of pain in neonates is often challenging because they cannot verbalize their subjective experience.[17] The four objectives in the assessment of pain are (1) detecting the presence of pain, (2) assessing its effect, (3) providing pain-relieving interventions, and (4) evaluating the effectiveness of interventions.[73] Guidelines for the assessment of pain are listed in Box 12-4. Expression of pain through behavior is one of the neonate's only means of communicating about pain. Behavioral

---

BOX 12-3

CRITICAL FINDINGS

INDICATORS OF IRRITABILITY AND AGITATION

Physiologic
- Increase in
  - Heart rate and blood pressure only with activity
  - Oxygenation (↑TcPco$_2$; Po$_2$; Sao$_2$)
  - Respiratory rate and effort
- Decrease in
  - Oxygenation (↓Po$_2$; Sao$_2$) after prolonged agitation
  - Heart rate (bradycardia)
  - Respirations (apnea)
- Alterations in skin color: cyanosis, mottling, duskiness, pallor
- Diaphoresis
- Vomiting
- Poor pattern of weight gain

Behavioral
- Vocalizations
  - Whining cry
  - Intense, urgent cry
  - High-pitched cry
  - Resumes fussiness when consolation ceases

- Facial expressions
  - Frowning
  - Worried facies
  - Gaze aversion
  - Closes eyes to tune out
- Body movements
  - Random movements of head and body
  - Hypertonic, rigid posturing; arching; hyperextended neck
  - Flailing, thrashing, frantic activity of extremities during fuss or cry
  - Decreased activity
  - Tremulousness
- States
  - Hyperalert—easily aroused from sleep; startles easily
  - Rapid and frequent state changes to fuss or cry
  - Sleep-wake cycles unpredictable
  - Feeding difficulties
  - Difficult to console, soothe
  - High level of persistence
  - Needs environmental structure to fall asleep; takes a long time to fall asleep
  - Ineffective in self-consoling; requires vestibular stimulation or body containment to console; responds inconsistently to consolation
- Noncuddly

Modified from Broome ME, Tanzillo H: Differentiating between pain and agitation in premature neonates, *J Perinat Neonat Nurs* 4:53, 1990; Burdeau G, Kleiber C: Clinical indicators of infant irritability, *Neonat Netw* 9:23, 1991; Franck LS: A national survey of the assessment and treatment of pain and agitation in the NICU, *J Obstet Gynecol Neonat Nurs* 16:387, 1987.

Modified from Anand KJ and the International Evidence-Based Group for Neonatal Pain: Consensus statement for the prevention and management of pain in the newborn, *Arch Pediatr Adolesc Med* 155:173, 2001; Prince W, Horns K, Latta T, et al: Treatment of neonatal pain without a gold standard: the case for caregiving interventions and sucrose administration, *Neonatal Netw* 23:33, 2004.

cues may include diffuse or localized motor activity, facial grimacing, crying, agitation, and change in level of activity (see Box 12-3). Female infants, both preterm and term, show more facial expressions of pain compared with male infants.[136] In an analysis of the responses of 149 infants to a painful event, facial actions were found 40% of the time to account for pain indicators in vulnerable neonates.[281]

Assessment of pain in the neonate is complicated by the infant's level of neural development and maturation.* Infants of younger GAs have limited autonomic and self-regulatory abilities. Developmental immaturity also results in disorganized, ineffective responses to stimuli and makes it more difficult for these immature preterm infants to communicate pain.[111] Fewer facial changes related to painful stimuli have been observed in young preterm infants.[111,113] However, crying, change in arousal state, and facial grimacing have been found to be the most robust pain behaviors.[325] Another study showed a change in facial expression with heel lance in preterms as young as 25 weeks' gestation.[278]

*References 111, 134, 148, 170, 220, 248, 325.

However, in this study, preterms less than 32 weeks' PMA took a significantly longer time to change their facial expression than did older infants.[278]

A more immature, fragile neonate may manifest alterations in sleep-wake cycles and habituate to the overwhelming stimuli of the NICU (see Chapter 13) and thus cannot exhibit any response to pain. Illness severity as an influence on pain response has shown contradictory findings in research studies. Some studies show altered pain response in more severely ill neonates, whereas others show no alteration in the most severely ill.[72,90,283]

Behavioral expressions of pain by the neonate are further hampered by intubation, use of restraints, and neuromuscular blockers.[227] Similarly, chronically ill infants who have been exposed to repeated painful procedures have difficulty generating a pain response and exhibit a "dampened" pain response.[73,112,113,128] Recent research shows that several body movements (e.g., fisting, flexing/extending extremities, finger splay, hand on the face) commonly assessed in the Newborn Individualized Care and Assessment Program (NIDCAP) developmental care program (see Chapter 13) are associated with acute pain response in preterms[220] (see Box 12-1). Preterm infants who have experienced more invasive procedures, who are lower in GA at birth, and who have spent more days on ventilators have a diminished behavioral and cardiac autonomic pain response to acute pain at 32 weeks' PCA.[111,126,129] Another study indicates that both term and preterm neonates who undergo handling and immobilization may exhibit exaggerated behavioral and physiologic response to later painful procedures.[140] Other studies have demonstrated no difference in biobehavioral response to pain in preterm infants with neurologic injury.[226,278,325]

Physiologic parameters also may indicate pain (e.g., increased heart and respiratory rates, elevated blood pressure, desaturation, apnea, palmar sweating). These symptoms are the result of sympathetic nervous system activation (see Box 12-1). One study found that some physiologic responses to pain (e.g., facial activity and state) moderately correlated to heart rate changes, whereas other behavioral expressions (e.g., finger splay) did not correlate with any autonomic changes.[219] However, in the same study, specific measures of cardiac autonomic modulation did not correlate with behavioral change, suggesting that cardiac alterations are influenced by a multitude of factors[227] and may be independent measures of pain

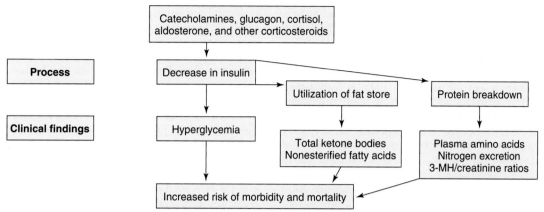

FIGURE 12-3 Hormonal response to pain in infants. *3-MH*, 3-methylhistidine. (From Johnston C, Stevens B: Pain in infants. In Watt-Watson J, Donovan M, editors: *Pain management: nursing perspective,* St Louis, 1992, Mosby.)

in the preterm.[219] A more recent study found higher physiologic reactivity (i.e., heart rate changes) in male preterm infants but the evidence was insufficient to confirm a gender difference in pain responsivity.[307] Some preterm infants respond to pain with more behavioral changes, whereas others respond with more physiologic changes.[284] In the first week of life, all infants of different GAs (e.g., <28–36 weeks) can differentiate between mild and more invasive procedures.[246] At 36 weeks, these same infants exhibited differing physiologic pain responses based on their GA at birth. (e.g., infants born closer to term had lower increases in heart rate than those born at a younger GA).[111,246,325]

When pain is repetitive or persists for hours or days, there is a *decompensatory* response, resulting in hormonal and metabolic alterations (Figure 12-3; see also Box 12-1). The fight-or-flight mechanism of the sympathetic nervous system can no longer compensate, so an adaptation syndrome begins with a return to baseline physiologic parameters. The return of the heart rate, respirations, and blood pressure to baseline parameters makes assessment of the infant's pain more difficult and does not mean that the infant has "adjusted" to or is no longer experiencing pain.[52]

The lack of an expression of pain through physiologic and behavioral responses also does not mean that the neonate is not experiencing pain.[158] Pain responses may be delayed, cumulative, or absent. In the preterm infant, sustained elevations in vital signs and decreased oxygenation confirm the persistence of physiologic alterations after painful stimuli.[283] Critically ill neonates and immature preterm infants may be so weak and overwhelmed that they have completely exhausted their energy and cannot respond.[131] The incidence of crying in response to painful or noxious stimuli is less than 50% in the preterm infant.[283] Depending on GA, a preterm infant's behavioral responses to pain are similar to those of the term infant.[15,131,283] A prospective cohort study comparing full-term infants (e.g., of diabetic mothers who were exposed to repeated heel sticks in the first 1–2 days of life) showed that these infants learned by conditioning to anticipate pain after their heel was swabbed with alcohol and exhibited a more intense pain response to a later venipuncture than infants who had not been exposed to repeated painful procedures.[300]

Pain responses of the neonate are also influenced by the number and timing of painful procedures, the technique used, and the degree of professional expertise.[9,73,300] Lack of a response to a painful stimulus occurs more frequently in younger newborns (both GA and PCA) who are asleep and who have recently undergone another painful procedure.[170,227,246] Pain scores may be lowered in preterms with higher severity of illness and higher number of previous invasive procedures,[121] whereas there is a larger heart rate response to repeated pain.[243] Use of mechanical lancets rather than manual lancets results in less behavioral and physiologic distress, fewer repeat punctures, and less bruising.[90,312]

Venipuncture has been shown to be associated with less pain in the neonate than heel stick,[231,268] and a new blood glucose device using the forearm has been found to be less painful for term infants than heel sticks.[262]

Assessment of neonatal pain is influenced by the attitudes and beliefs of care providers; amount of time spent observing for and having knowledge of pain responses; discrepancy between attitudes and practice, knowledge, and education of parents and professionals about pain; prioritization of pain recognition and relief in the NICU; interdisciplinary communication and collaboration; and the social community.* If professionals (1) deny that newborns experience pain, (2) become desensitized to newborns' pain experience, (3) rationalize reasons for not assessing or treating pain, and (4) do not take responsibility for inflicting pain, there can be no improvement in neonatal pain management.[17,189,209]

Numerous other social factors influencing pain recognition and relief include the following: (1) appearance, behavior, and responsiveness of a sick neonate that varies markedly from the usual expectations about newborns; (2) lack of knowledge about analgesia and belief that pain is secondary in importance to the focus on survival; and (3) lack of knowledge about the effect on morbidity, mortality, and long-term consequences.[18,209]

Researchers have examined the beliefs and management techniques of 374 clinicians (both physicians and nurses) about procedural pain in newborn infants. Although the majority of clinicians believe that infants experience pain in the same or greater degree than adults, 9 of 12 commonly performed bedside procedures (e.g., intubation, chest tube insertion, arterial or venous catheter insertion, heel sticks) were rated as "moderately to very painful." Neither pharmacologic nor comfort measures were frequently used.[246] More recent surveys and studies of professional attitudes have found the following: (1) assessment for neonatal pain is based on instinct rather than tested pain tools,[4,53,244] (2) there is inadequate staff knowledge and lack of evidence-based guidelines,[4,53] (3) there is difficulty translating knowledge to clinical practice,[4,189] and (4) nurse-physician collaboration is a strong predictor of evidence-based procedural pain control.[18,189,209] A recent qualitative study revealed NICU staff attitudes concerning neonatal pain. Pain causes unnecessary suffering and staff members

realized how multiple and repeated procedures result in long-term consequences from previous pain experiences. Second, health care providers realized how approaches to pain relief are based on feeling rather than facts. Furthermore, while comforting the neonate and when suffering is detected, health care providers have doubts and concerns about the use and side effects of drugs for pain relief. Lastly, staff members felt that the parent's presence and caretaking in the NICU had the potential to decrease the neonate's response to painful stimuli.[105] Despite more than 30 years of research into pain and pain control in neonates, "clinical use of pain-control measures in neonates undergoing invasive procedures remains sporadic and suboptimal."[27]

IRRITABILITY AND AGITATION

Differentiation between pain and irritability or agitation is a challenge (Figure 12-4). Agitation is a behavioral symptom of many problems, including environmental overstimulation, respiratory insufficiency, neurologic irritability, and pain. Factors influencing chronic irritability and agitation in neonates in the NICU are shown in Figure 12-5. Causes of agitation other than pain should be eliminated before pain management and/or sedation is initiated. Assessment of environmental stimuli should be a routine part of the neonate's care. The neonate may associate certain stimuli with unpleasant events over time, and repeated exposure (e.g., ventilator alarms, placement of heel warmer, the odor of an alcohol wipe) may trigger agitation. Although these stimuli are inevitable, identifying, avoiding, or limiting them will help prevent anticipatory decompensation in these fragile infants.[316]

Strategies to prevent and intervene with irritable or agitated infants include the following:
- Avoid negative labels and ascribing psychological intentionality to the infant's behavior.
- Minimize caregivers and provide consistency in care by staff and family.
- Determine whether there is a "locus of pain" (e.g., pain-related irritability).
- Determine whether physiologic instability (e.g., needs suction/position change; hypoxemia) is the cause or the result of irritable behaviors.
- Use developmental care (see Chapter 13).
- Use sedatives judiciously.[316]
- Use of individualized, developmental care significantly reduces the need for sedatives in VLBW infants.[316]

---

*References 18, 86, 103, 137, 142, 173, 189, 209, 232, 244, 282.

Agitation
Rule out respiratory cause, increase support
Calming occurs
Agitation continues
Look for pain source, provide analgesia
Agitation continues
Calming occurs
Assess environment, reduce stimulation
Agitation continues
Calming occurs
Provide sedation

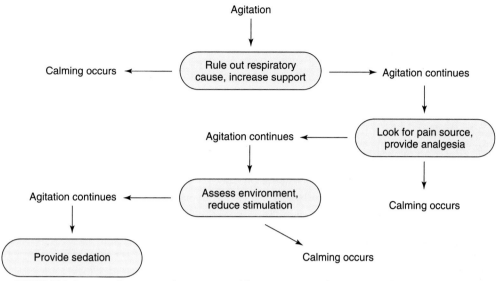

FIGURE 12-4 Decision tree for assessing and managing pain and/or agitation. (From Gordin P: Assessing and managing agitation in the critically ill infant, *Matern Child Nurs* 15:26, 1990.)

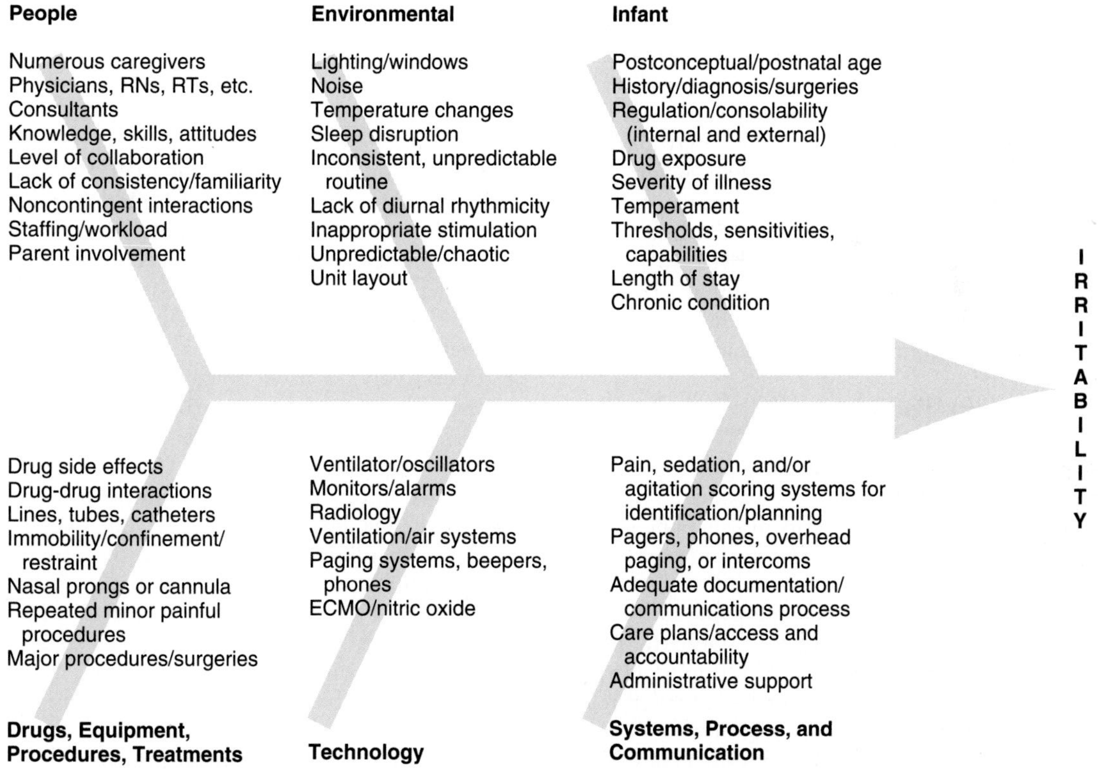

People
Numerous caregivers
Physicians, RNs, RTs, etc.
Consultants
Knowledge, skills, attitudes
Level of collaboration
Lack of consistency/familiarity
Noncontingent interactions
Staffing/workload
Parent involvement
Environmental
Lighting/windows
Noise
Temperature changes
Sleep disruption
Inconsistent, unpredictable routine
Lack of diurnal rhythmicity
Inappropriate stimulation
Unpredictable/chaotic
Unit layout
Infant
Postconceptual/postnatal age
History/diagnosis/surgeries
Regulation/consolability (internal and external)
Drug exposure
Severity of illness
Temperament
Thresholds, sensitivities, capabilities
Length of stay
Chronic condition
IRRITABILITY
Drug side effects
Drug-drug interactions
Lines, tubes, catheters
Immobility/confinement/ restraint
Nasal prongs or cannula
Repeated minor painful procedures
Major procedures/surgeries
Drugs, Equipment, Procedures, Treatments
Ventilator/oscillators
Monitors/alarms
Radiology
Ventilation/air systems
Paging systems, beepers, phones
ECMO/nitric oxide
Technology
Pain, sedation, and/or agitation scoring systems for identification/planning
Pagers, phones, overhead paging, or intercoms
Adequate documentation/ communications process
Care plans/access and accountability
Administrative support
Systems, Process, and Communication

FIGURE 12-5 Fishbone diagram of factors influencing irritability. *ECMO,* Extracorporeal membrane oxygenation; *RNs,* registered nurses; *RT,* respiratory therapist. (From Walden M, Carrier C: Sleeping beauties: the impact of sedation on neonatal development, *J Obstet Gynecol Neonatal Nurs* 32:393, 2003.)

TABLE 12-2 CRIES: NEONATAL POSTOPERATIVE PAIN ASSESSMENT SCORE

	SCORING CRITERIA FOR EACH ASSESSMENT			
	0	1	2	INFANT'S SCORE
Crying	No	High pitched	Inconsolable	_____
Requires O$_2$ for saturation greater than 95%	No	<30%	>30%	_____
Increased vital signs*	HR and BP within 10% of preoperative value	HR or BP 11%–20% higher than preoperative value	HR or BP 21% or more above preoperative value	_____
Expression	None	Grimace	Grimace/grunt	_____
Sleepless	No	Wakes at frequent intervals	Constantly awake	_____
			TOTAL SCORE†	_____

From Krechel SW, Bildner J: Neonatal pain assessment tool developed at University of Missouri-Columbia.
BP, Blood pressure; *HR*, heart rate.
*BP should be done last.
†Add scores for all assessments to calculate total score.

Pain-related irritability must be treated by alleviating pain with the use of opioids and comfort measures. Use of sedatives *alone* for pain-related irritability suppresses behavioral expression of pain, has no analgesic effects, and may *increase* pain. Sedatives should be used only when pain has been ruled out as the source of the irritability or agitation. Although no research documents the safety or efficacy of combining sedatives and analgesics for the treatment of neonatal pain, sedatives are used with opioids to wean infants who have developed tolerance from prolonged opioid therapy.[316]

Assessment Tools

To quantify and objectify a neonate's pain experience and to facilitate health care professionals' recognition of the presence and severity of pain in neonates, research has developed 40 infant pain measurement tools.[74] The Joint Commission requires the selection and use of a valid, reliable pain assessment tool; however, there is no "gold standard" neonatal pain assessment tool.[19,74,171] Pain tools have been developed for research purposes; limited reliability and validity have been established for clinical practice,[74,282] especially in the critically ill newborn or the extremely premature infant. Clinical utility— the ability of users to obtain needed information to

plan, implement, and evaluate interventions or services of pain tools—is beginning to be studied.

The most commonly used pain assessment tools in clinical practice are the CRIES; Neonatal Postoperative Pain Assessment Score; Premature Infant Pain Profile (PIPP); and Neonatal Pain, Agitation, and Sedation Scale (N-PASS). All of these pain tools (except the N-PASS) assess only acute, not chronic/prolonged, pain.[21] The CRIES assessment tool (Table 12-2), developed to measure physiologic and behavioral pain responses of term babies postoperatively, is used hourly with vital sign assessment. CRIES uses a scoring system similar to the Apgar score: A score of 4 or higher indicates pain and requires intervention. CRIES requires the calculation of a percentage of change from the infant's baseline physiologic values and relies on continuous cardiorespiratory monitoring. Validity and reliability to measure postoperative pain and pain relief after administration of an analgesic have been established,[180] whereas use of CRIES to measure procedural pain has not been validated.

The PIPP (Table 12-3) is a multidimensional (physiologic and behavioral) assessment tool intended for use within clinical practice.[284] The PIPP is a seven-item, four-point scale; its maximum score depends on the infant's GA and behavioral

TABLE 12-3 **PREMATURE INFANT PAIN PROFILE (PIPP)**

Infant Study Number: _____

Date/Time: _____

Event: _____

PROCESS	INDICATOR	0	1	2	3	SCORE
Chart	Gestational age	36 wk and more	32–35 wk, 6 days	28–31 wk, 6 days	Less than 28 wk	
Observe infant 15 sec	Behavioral state	Active/awake; eyes open; facial movements	Quiet/awake; eyes closed; no facial movement	Active/asleep; eyes closed; facial movement	Quiet/asleep; eyes closed; no facial movements	
Observe baseline heart rate oxygen saturation						
Observe infant 30 sec	Heart rate (max)	0–4 beats/min increase	5–14 beats/min increase	5–24 beats/min increase	25 beats/min or more increase	
	Oxygen saturation (min)	0%–2.4% decrease	2.5%–4.9% decrease	5.0%–7.4% decrease	7.5% or more decrease	
	Brow bulge	None 0%–9% of time	Minimum 10%–39% of time	Moderate 40%–69% of time	Maximum 70% of time or more	
	Eye squeeze	None 0%–9% of time	Minimum 10%–39% of time	Moderate 40%–69% of time	Maximum 70% of time or more	
	Nasolabial	None 0%–9% of time	Minimum 10%–39% of time	Moderate 40%–69% of time	Maximum 70% of time or more	

Scoring method for the PIPP:
1. Familiarize yourself with each indicator and how it is to be scored by looking at the measure.
2. Score gestational age (from the chart) before you begin.
3. Score behavioral state by observing the infant for 15 seconds immediately before the event.
4. Record baseline heart rate and oxygen saturation.
5. Observe the infant for 30 seconds immediately after the event. You will have to look back and forth from the monitor to the infant's face. Score physiologic and facial action changes seen during that time and record immediately after the observation period.
6. Calculate the final score.
From Stevens B, Johnston C, Petroshen P, et al: Premature Infant Pain Profile: development and initial validation, *Clin J Pain* 12:13, 1996.

state of the premature at baseline. The PIPP has been validated with both full-term and preterm neonates and can distinguish between procedural and postoperative pain and nonpain (e.g., noxious) events. The revised PIPP (PIPP-R) has recently been validated in full-term neonates and preterms greater than 26 weeks' GA, is easy to use, and higher pain scores require effective interventions.[114] Lower pain scores in the PIPP-R indicate that pain intervention strategy is efficacious.[114] The PIPP has not been validated for assessment of the efficacy of analgesia nor for its usefulness in the assessment of continuous pain.

The N-PASS (Table 12-4) is an easily used clinical scale to assess, document, and manage pain and sedation.[156,157] NICU infants being mechanically ventilated or in the immediate postoperative period were assessed with the N-PASS before and after pharmacologic intervention. N-PASS measures acute, prolonged and chronic pain.[73] N-PASS is a reliable and valid assessment

TABLE 12-4 NEONATAL PAIN, AGITATION, AND SEDATION SCALE (N-PASS)

ASSESSMENT CRITERIA	SEDATION		SEDATION/PAIN	PAIN/AGITATION	
	−2	−1	0/0	+1	+2
Crying Irritability	No cry with painful stimuli	Moans or cries minimally with painful stimuli	No sedation/No pain signs	Irritable or crying at intervals Consolable	High-pitched or silent, continuous cry Inconsolable
Behavior state	No arousal to any stimuli No spontaneous movement	Arouses minimally to stimuli Little spontaneous movement	No sedation/No pain signs	Restless, squirming Awakens frequently	Arching, kicking Constantly awake or Arouses minimally/no movement (not sedated)
Facial expression	Mouth is lax No expression	Minimal expression with stimuli	No sedation/No pain signs	Any pain expression intermittent	Any pain expression continual
Extremities Tone	No grasp reflex Flaccid tone	Weak grasp reflex ↓ muscle tone	No sedation/No pain signs	Intermittent clenching toes, fists, or finger splay Body is not tense	Continual clenched toes, fists, or finger splay Body is tense
Vital signs: HR, RR, BP, SaO_2	No variability with stimuli Hypoventilation or apnea	<10% variability from baseline with stimuli	No sedation/No pain signs	↑↓ 10%–20% from baseline SaO_2 76%–85% with stimulation, quick recovery	↑↓ >20% from baseline SaO_2 ≤75% with stimulation, slow recovery Out of sync with vent

ASSESSMENT OF SEDATION

- Sedation is scored in addition to pain for each behavioral and physiologic criterion to assess the infant's response to stimuli.
- Sedation does not need to be assessed/scored with every pain assessment/score.
- Sedation is scored 0 → −2 for each behavioral and physiologic criterion, then summed and noted as a negative score (0 → −10).
- A score of 0 is given if the infant has no signs of sedation, does not underreact.
- Desired levels of sedation vary according to the situation:
  - "Deep sedation" → goal score of −10 to −5
  - "Light sedation" → goal score of −5 to −2
- Deep sedation is not recommended unless an infant is receiving ventilatory support, related to the high potential for hypoventilation and apnea.
- A negative score without the administration of opioids/sedatives may indicate the following:
  - The premature infant's response to prolonged or persistent pain/stress
  - Neurologic depression, sepsis, or other pathology

ASSESSMENT OF PAIN/AGITATION

- Pain assessment is the fifth vital sign. Assessment for pain should be included in every vital sign assessment.
- Pain is scored from 0 → +2 for each behavioral and physiologic criterion and then summed:
  - Points are added to the premature infant's pain score based on his or her gestational age to compensate for his or her limited ability to behaviorally communicate pain.
  - Total pain score is documented as a positive number (0 → +11).
- Treatment/interventions are indicated for scores >3.
  - Interventions for known pain/painful stimuli are indicated before the score reaches 3.
- The goal of pain treatment/intervention is a score ≤3.
- More frequent pain assessment indications:
  - Indwelling tubes or lines that may cause pain, especially with movement (e.g., chest tubes) → at least every 2–4 hours
  - Receiving analgesics and/or sedatives → at least every 2–4 hours
  - 30–60 minutes after an analgesic is given for pain behaviors to assess response to medication
  - Postoperative → at least every 2 hours for 24–48 hours and then every 4 hours until off medications

Continued

PARALYSIS/NEUROMUSCULAR BLOCKADE

- It is impossible to behaviorally evaluate a paralyzed infant for pain.
- Increases in heart rate and blood pressure at rest or with stimulation may be the only indicator of a need for more analgesia.
- Analgesics should be administered continuously by drip or around-the-clock dosing.
  - Higher, more frequent doses may be required if the infant is postoperative, has a chest tube, or has other pathology (e.g., NEC) that would normally cause pain.

SCORING CRITERIA

Crying/Irritability

−2 → No response to painful stimuli:
  - No cry with needle sticks
  - No reaction to ETT or nares suctioning
  - No response to caregiving
−1 → Moans, sighs, or cries (audible or silent) minimally to painful stimuli (e.g., needle sticks, ETT, or nares suctioning, caregiving)
0 → No sedation signs or No pain/agitation signs
+1 → Infant is irritable/crying at intervals but can be consoled
  - If intubated, intermittent silent cry
+2 → Any of the following:
  - Cry is high pitched
  - Infant cries inconsolably
  - If intubated, silent continuous cry

Behavior/State

−2 → Does not arouse or react to any stimuli:
  - Eyes continually shut or open
  - No spontaneous movement
−1 → Little spontaneous movement; arouses briefly and/or minimally to any stimuli:
  - Opens eyes briefly
  - Reacts to suctioning
  - Withdraws to pain
0 → No sedation signs or No pain/agitation signs
+1 → Any of the following:
  - Restless, squirming
  - Awakens frequently/easily with minimal or no stimuli
+2 → Any of the following:
  - Kicking
  - Arching
  - Constantly awake
  - No movement or minimal arousal with stimulation (not sedated, inappropriate for gestational age or clinical situation)

TABLE
12–4   NEONATAL PAIN, AGITATION, AND SEDATION SCALE (N-PASS) — cont'd

Facial Expression

−2 → Any of the following:
- Mouth is lax
- Drooling
- No facial expression at rest or with stimuli

−1 → Minimal facial expression with stimuli

0 → No sedation signs or No pain/agitation signs

+1 → Any pain face expression observed intermittently

+2 → Any pain face expression is continual

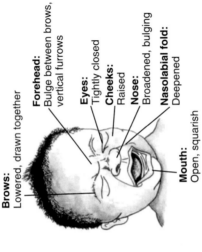

Brows:
Lowered, drawn together

Forehead:
Bulge between brows,
vertical furrows

Eyes:
Tightly closed

Cheeks:
Raised

Nose:
Broadened, bulging

Nasolabial fold:
Deepened

Mouth:
Open, squarish

**Facial expression of physical distress and
pain in the infant**

Extremities/Tone

−2 → Any of the following:
- No palmar or plantar grasp can be elicited
- Flaccid tone

−1 → Any of the following:
- Weak palmar or plantar grasp can be elicited
- Decreased tone

0 → No sedation signs or No pain/agitation signs

+1 → Intermittent (<30 seconds' duration) observation of toes and/or hands as clenched or fingers splayed
- Body is *not* tense

+2 → Any of the following:
- Frequent (≥30 seconds' duration) observation of toes and/or hands as clenched or fingers splayed
- Body is tense and stiff

Vital Signs: HR, BP, RR, and O₂ Saturations

−2 → Any of the following:
- No variability in vital signs with stimuli
- Hypoventilation
- Apnea
- Ventilated infant—no spontaneous respiratory effort

−1 → Vital signs show little variability with stimuli—less than 10% from baseline

0 → No sedation signs or No pain/agitation signs

+1 → Any of the following:
- HR, RR, and/or BP are 10%–20% above baseline
- With care/stimuli, infant desaturates minimally to moderately (Sₐ0₂ 76%–85%) and recovers quickly (within 2 minutes)

+2 → Any of the following:
- HR, RR, and/or BP are >20% above baseline
- With care/stimuli, infant desaturates severely (Sₐ0₂ <75%) and recovers slowly (>2 minutes)
- Out of sync/fighting ventilator

TABLE 12-5 NEONATAL FACIAL CODING SYSTEM

ACTION	DESCRIPTION
Brow bulge	Bulging, creasing, and vertical furrows above and between brows occurring as a result of the lowering and drawing together of the eyebrows
Eye squeeze	Identified by the squeezing or bulging of the eyelids; bulging of the fatty pads about the infant's eyes is pronounced
Nasolabial furrow	Primarily manifested by the pulling upward and deepening of the nasolabial furrow (a line or wrinkle that begins adjacent to the nostril wings and runs downward and outward beyond the lip corners)
Open lips	Any separation of the lips
Stretch mouth (vertical)	Characterized by a tautness of the lip corners coupled with a pronounced downward pull on the jaw; seen when an already wide-open mouth is opened a fraction further by an extra pull at the jaw
Stretch mouth (horizontal)	Appears as a distinct horizontal pull at the corners of the mouth
Lip purse	Lips appear as if an "oo" sound is being pronounced
Taut tongue	Characterized by a raised, cupped tongue with sharp tense edges; the first occurrence of taut tongue usually is easy to see, often occurring with a wide-open mouth; after this first occurrence, the mouth may close slightly; taut tongue is still scorable on the basis of the still visible tongue edges
Chin quiver	An obvious high-frequency up-down motion of the lower jaw

Data from Grunau RVE, Craig KD: Pain expression in neonates: facial action and cry, *Pain* 28:399, 1987; Grunau R, Craig K: Facial activity as a measure of neonatal pain expression. In Tyler DC, Krane EJ, editors, *Advances in pain, research and therapy*, vol 15, New York, 1990, Raven.

tool for pain/agitation and sedation in postoperative and/or ventilated neonates (0–100 days of age) at 23 or more weeks' gestation.[156,157]

The Neonatal Facial Coding System (Table 12-5) is an assessment tool based on nine facial expressions of term newborns in four sleep-wake states while experiencing the discomfort of heel rub and the pain of heel lance. Quiet, awake neonates demonstrate the most facial activity, whereas those in quiet sleep demonstrate the least.[130,134] Facial activity also increases with GA, so both infant state and GA must be considered when using this scale. Because this tool is sensitive to changes in pain intensity, it is also useful for evaluating the effectiveness of interventions. There is recent evidence of reliable clinical use of this tool in term and preterm infants and for postoperative pain assessment; however, it is time-consuming, unidimensional, and requires experienced coders.[131]

The Neonatal Infant Pain Scale (NIPS) (Table 12-6) is a behavioral assessment tool for preterm and term neonates responding to a needle puncture. NIPS scores reveal an increase in behavioral response during the procedures and a decline in response scores after the procedure (Figure 12-6).

Thus, NIPS provides a measurement of intensity of infant responses to a painful procedure during and after the event.[190] NIPS scores have been correlated with GA and Apgar scores. NIPS provides an objective measure of pain-relieving interventions and their effectiveness.[190] NIPS is objective and nonintrusive and assesses only behavioral response to pain; compared with other pain scales, it has been found to be easy and quick to use.[190] Flow sheets also have been designed to facilitate the documentation of pain scores and behaviors.[190]

The National Practice Guidelines provides a list of assessment questions to ask when assessing pain management in the neonate (Box 12-5). Lack of validated assessment tools may leave health care providers wondering if behaviors are indicators or responses to pain. The Acute Pain Management Guideline suggests that "if care providers are unsure whether a behavior indicates pain, and if there is reason to suspect pain, an analgesic trial can be diagnostic, as well as therapeutic."[3]

Assessment of pain and delivery of effective pain-relieving interventions in daily clinical practice must *not* be delayed while adequate, objective assessment tools are developed.[72,283]

TABLE 12-6	NEONATAL INFANT PAIN SCALE (NIPS) OPERATIONAL DEFINITIONS

FACIAL EXPRESSION	
0 — Relaxed muscles	Restful face, neutral expression
1 — Grimace	Tight facial muscles; furrowed brow, chin, jaw (negative facial expression — nose, mouth, and brow)

CRY	
0 — No cry	Quiet, not crying
1 — Whimper	Mild moaning, intermittent
2 — Vigorous cry	Loud scream; rising, shrill, continuous (*Note:* Silent cry may be scored if baby is intubated as evidenced by obvious mouth and facial movement)

BREATHING PATTERNS	
0 — Relaxed	Usual pattern for this infant
1 — Change in breathing	Indrawing, irregular, faster than usual; gagging; breath holding

ARMS	
0 — Relaxed/restrained	No muscular rigidity; occasional random movements of arms
1 — Flexed/extended	Tense, straight arms; rigid and/or rapid extension, flexion

LEGS	
0 — Relaxed/restrained	No muscular rigidity; occasional random leg movement
1 — Flexed/extended	Tense, straight legs; rigid and/or rapid extension, flexion

STATE OF AROUSAL	
0 — Sleeping/awake	Quiet, peaceful sleeping or alert and settled
1 — Fussy	Alert, restless, and thrashing

From Lawrence J, Alcock D, McGrath P, et al: Children's Hospital of Eastern Ontario, 1993.

The usefulness of pain scores was recently assessed in 196 ventilated premature infant patient-days.[255] Although only 2% of pain scores suggested the presence of pain and only 0.1% of the pain scores resulted in analgesic use, these ventilated infants were obviously exposed to multiple pain-related procedures. In this study, regular reassessment and assignment of a pain score was poorly correlated with exposure to painful procedures.[255] All health care providers must use their highly developed assessment skills, along with input from the parents, to gather information about infant behavioral, physiologic, and hormonal or catabolic stress responses before, during, and after painful stimuli.[73] These same assessment skills enable care providers and parents to evaluate the effectiveness of pharmacologic and comfort interventions and institute more and/or different interventions as necessary to relieve pain and suffering.

Laboratory Data

Hormonal and metabolic changes are listed in Box 12-1. Serum glucose levels and reagent test strips monitor for hyperglycemia, which may result in increased serum osmolality and increase the risk for IVH. Glucosuria, ketonuria, and proteinuria

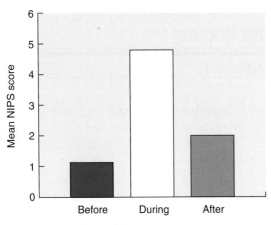

FIGURE 12-6 Mean Neonatal Infant Pain Scale (NIPS) scores over time in 22 infants. (From Lawrence J, Alcock D, McGrath P, et al: The development of a tool to assess neonatal pain, *Neonat Netw* 12:62, 1993.)

BOX 12-5 CRITICAL QUESTIONS TO ASK ABOUT PAIN MANAGEMENT IN NEONATES

- Is the infant being adequately assessed at appropriate intervals?
- Are analgesics ordered for prevention and relief of pain?
- Is the analgesic strong enough for the pain expected or the pain being experienced?
- Is the timing of the drug administration appropriate for the pain expected or being experienced?
- Is the route of administration appropriate (preferably oral or intravenous) for the infant?
- Is the infant adequately monitored for side effects?
- Are side effects appropriately managed?
- Has the analgesic regimen provided adequate comfort and satisfaction from the family's perspective?

Questions to Consider About Nonpharmacologic Strategies
- Is the strategy appropriate for the infant's developmental level, condition, and type of pain?
- Is the timing of the strategy sufficient to optimize its effects?
- Is the strategy adequately effective in preventing or alleviating the infant's pain?
- Is the family satisfied with the strategy for prevention or relief of pain?

From Acute Pain Management Guideline Panel: *Acute pain management: operative or medical procedures and trauma—clinical practice guideline* (AHCPR Pub No 92-0032), Rockville, Md, 1992, Agency for Health Care Policy and Research, Public Health Service, U.S. Department of Health and Human Services.

---

result in elevated specific gravity. Metabolic acidosis may result from increased serum levels of lactate, pyruvate, ketones, and nonesterified fatty acids. These data also may be indicative of other serious neonatal problems (e.g., sepsis, acute tubular necrosis).

In the search of more objective measures of pain assessment, use of heart rate variability (HRV), skin conductance (SC) measurements, and brain-oriented techniques such as near-infrared spectroscopy (NIRS), electroencephalography (EEG), and magnetic resonance imaging (MRI) are being investigated. Although HRV is a reliable measure of the neonate's response to acute and prolonged pain,[93,113] lack of availability of monitoring devices may preclude its use clinically.[72] SC, which measures stress-induced sweating in the palms and soles of the feet, has shown conflicting results in research, especially in preterm infants.[155,222,289,308] It requires further investigation in the preterm infant before it will be ready for clinical use.[309]

Current and future research is focused on brain-oriented approaches (e.g., NIRS, EEG, and MRI) instead of pain assessment tools. Painful stimuli cause hemodynamic changes in the brains of preterm and term infants.[36,250,276,277] As early as 25 weeks' gestation, preterm infants have increased oxygenated hemoglobin in response to a heel stick.[277] Cerebral changes are dependent on GA and sleep-wake state; less robust changes are seen in the younger GA and while asleep compared with the awake infant.[277] The first study to assess the correlation between cortical hemodynamic activity (by NIRS) during a heel stick in 25- to 43-week PMA neonates and the PIPP score found significant correlation between the NIRS and the pain score.[276] Use of the NIRS remains clinically challenging due to multiple factors (i.e., movement, external stimuli, birth weight, medications, ventilator settings, infection, PDA) that alter results.[149,150]

EEG changes in the frontal lobes of the brain during noxious and painful stimuli have been researched in preterm and full-term infants. Developmental maturation in response to touch and pain has been found in the neonate: (1) before 35 weeks' gestation nonspecific neuronal bursts to both touch and pain were the dominant response and (2) after 35 to 37 weeks' gestation specific responses to touch versus pain were present.[92] MRI has documented procedural, pain-related stress to alterations in brain maturation in preterm infants in an NICU[48] and altered brain metabolites in full-term asphyxiated neonates.[31] Research into use of

EEG and MRI, especially technical challenges such as movement artifact, for pain assessment is in its infancy.[72,149,150,202]

Future assessment of neonatal pain may combine validated and reliable tools as well as laboratory data collected at the point-of-care. One such study used a multimodal approach to measure pain: (1) electromyography (EMG), EEG, and NIRS; (2) video-recording of behavioral responses; and (3) autonomic responses (i.e., heart and respiratory rates, oxygen saturation with pulse oximetry and cardiovascular activity with ECG.[326] In more than 100 test occasions this multimodal system is precise, accurate, and 100% sensitive and specific in detecting touch versus a heel stick.[326]

TREATMENT

The neonate relies on the skilled observations, assessment, and interventions of care providers for prompt, safe, and effective relief of pain. Pain management is an interactive, relationship-based process that comprises the (1) environment of pain management, (2) preparation of the newborn for a procedure, (3) pain relief during a procedure, and (4) restoring safety and security to the infant after a procedure.[38,137] Barriers in providing adequate analgesia in these patients include an unfamiliarity with medication doses and with regional techniques and concern over increased drug sensitivity in neonates. Because routine care can be irritating to newborns, differentiating between agitation, which may respond well to comfort measures, and pain, which will not, is mandatory. Opioids are the mainstay of pharmacologic treatment; however, other useful medications and techniques may be used for pain relief.[9] Guidelines for managing pain in the neonate are listed in Box 12-6. Table 12-7 and Table 12-8 present evidence-based pain management strategies for commonly performed painful procedures and surgical interventions.

Pharmacologic Measures

Absorption, metabolism, distribution, and clearance of drugs in the neonate differ from those in the older child and adult (see Chapter 10). These differences are summarized in Table 12-9.

BOX 12-6	GUIDELINES FOR PAIN MANAGEMENT IN THE NEONATE

- Use strategies to prevent pain (e.g., avoid recurrent painful stimuli).
- Use developmental care and environmental interventions to reduce noxious stimuli and stress in the NICU (see Chapter 13).
- Use comfort measures (e.g., sucrose, nonnutritive sucking, containment with swaddling or facilitated tucking).
- Sucrose administration recommendations:
  - Preterm infants: 0.1 to 0.4 ml; dipping a pacifier into sucrose results in 0.1-ml intake
  - Term infants: 2 ml
  - Administer 2 minutes before a painful procedure
  - Analgesic effect lasts about 5 minutes
- Use pharmacologic therapy for preemptive analgesia (see Table 12-10).
- Use pharmacologic therapy for ongoing pain.
- Use of a combination of pain interventions (e.g., sucking, containment, medication) may have an additive or synergistic clinical effect[195]

Modified from Anand KJ and the International Evidence-Based Group for Neonatal Pain: Consensus statement for the prevention and management of pain in the newborn, *Arch Pediatr Adolesc Med* 155:173, 2001; Prince W, Horns K, Latta T, et al: Treatment of neonatal pain without a gold standard: the case for caregiving interventions and sucrose administration, *Neonatal Netw* 23:33, 2004.

OPIOIDS AND BENZODIAZEPINES

Opioids have their primary effect on the μ-receptor in the brain and spinal cord. High-affinity μ-receptors are associated with analgesia, and low-affinity μ-receptors are associated with respiratory depression. There may be fewer high-affinity μ-receptors in the newborn that are less sensitive to the analgesic effects of opioids. Higher initial doses of opioids may therefore be necessary for effect, which may in turn increase the risk for respiratory depression. A randomized, double-blind study of postoperative (e.g., thoracic or abdominal surgery) pain relief in full-term newborns receiving either continuous or intermittent morphine found an age-related difference in morphine requirements and metabolism.[45,46] Younger infants (e.g., 7 days or younger) needed less morphine postoperatively (e.g., loading dose [50 mcg/kg], continuous dose [5–10 mcg/kg/hr], and need for additional "breakthrough" doses) than neonates older than 7 days (e.g., loading dose [100 mcg/kg] and continuous dose [10 mcg/kg/hr]). This study also found that neonates being mechanically

TABLE 12-7								
NURSE-DIRECTED/PERFORMED PROCEDURES AND EVIDENCE-BASED NEONATAL PAIN RELIEF *								

NURSING CARE STRATEGIES	SKIN-TO-SKIN/ KANGAROO CARE	BREAST-FEEDING	ORAL: NONNUTRITIVE SUCKING OR SUCROSE PACIFIER	TACTILE: SWADDLING/ CONTAINMENT/ FACILITATED TUCKING/ HOLDING AND ROCKING	MEDICATIONS: TOPICAL: EMLA CREAM, AMETHOCAINE GEL	REGIONAL INFILTRATION WITH LIDOCAINE	OPIOIDS	NONOPIOID ANALGESIA OR GENERAL ANESTHESIA
Heel lance	X	X	X	X				
Venipuncture			X	X	X		X	
Arterial stick			X	X	X	X		
Gavage tube insertion	X	X	X	X				
IM injection			X	X	X			
ETT or nasal suction	X†		X	X				
Catheterization of bladder	X‡	X‡	X	X				Nonopioid analgesia‡
Dressing changes/ tape removal/ suture removal	X†	X†	X	X				Nonopioid analgesia‡

Adapted from Gardner SL: *Clinical practice tool: nurse-directed/performed procedures and nurse assisted procedures: evidence-based neonatal pain relief,* 2008. Used with permission.
ETT, Endotracheal tube; *IM,* intramuscular injection.
*Using a combination of nonpharmacologic, comfort strategies potentiates their pain relieving effects as does combining comfort measures and pharmacologic measures.
†If already kangaroo caring.
‡Postprocedure.

ventilated had slower morphine metabolism and clearance.[45] A retrospective analysis of the postoperative use of morphine in 82 full-term neonates after thoracic and/or abdominal surgery[89] found that both dosage and duration of infusion prolonged mechanical ventilation. After extubation, no apnea or hypotension was associated with morphine use.

Decreased protein binding, drug metabolism, and drug clearance may contribute to higher plasma and CNS concentrations and prolonged drug effect. Effective drug doses and metabolism by the individual neonate depend on weight, GA, postnatal age, genetic variation, and the corresponding pharmacokinetics and pharmacodynamics, which may change in the first days of life.[293,305,210] All doses must be titrated to the individual neonate's needs and current clinical circumstances.[305]

All the opioids have similar mechanisms of action; however, there are a few important differences in side effects (Table 12-10). Morphine is the most commonly used opioid and may cause hypotension in dehydrated patients or when used in high doses; it provides more sedation than fentanyl. Recent research on the blood pressure effects of morphine administration showed (1) no hypotensive effects on ventilated newborns[259] or on preterms[310] given analgesic doses[16] and (2) occurrence of hypotensive effects with loading and higher dosages.[24,310] However, morphine should be used with caution in preterms of 23 to 26 weeks' gestation and those with preexisting hypotension.[141] For acute procedural pain (e.g., heel stick), a loading dose of morphine followed by continuous IV infusion does not provide adequate analgesia for invasive procedures in ventilated preterms.[58]

TABLE 12-8 NURSE-ASSISTED PROCEDURES AND EVIDENCE-BASED NEONATAL PAIN RELIEF*

NURSING CARE STRATEGIES	SKIN-TO-SKIN/ KANGAROO CARE	BREAST-FEEDING	ORAL: NONNUTRITIVE SUCKING OR SUCROSE PACIFIER	TACTILE: SWADDLING/ CONTAINMENT/ FACILITATED TUCKING/ HOLDING AND ROCKING	MEDICATIONS: TOPICAL: EMLA CREAM, AMETHOCAINE GEL	REGIONAL INFILTRATION WITH LIDOCAINE	OPIOIDS	NONOPIOID ANALGESIA OR GENERAL ANESTHESIA
PICC line insertion/removal			X	X	X	X	X	
Taps: lumbar; suprapubic; ventricular; paracentesis; bone marrow			X		X	X	X	
Line placement/removal: (CVP; Broviac; ECMO; arterial/venous cutdowns			X	X	X	X	X	Consider general anesthesia Nonopioid analgesia†
Chest tube insertion/removal			X	X		X	X†	Nonopioid analgesia†
ETT intubation; NCPAP; ventilation	X‡		X‡	X			X	Nonopioid analgesia†
Circumcision			X		X	X		Nonopioid analgesia†
Scopes: endoscopy/bronchoscopy			X (preprocedure)	X			X	Nonopioid analgesia†
Eye examination for ROP	X†	X†	X†	X†			X	Nonopioid analgesia†
Any surgical procedure: PDA ligation; TEF/gastroschisis repair/omphalocele/CDH/inguinal hernia/CHD repair/shunt placement			X†	X†			X†	Nonopioid analgesia†

*Using a combination of nonpharmacologic, comfort strategies potentiates their pain relieving effects as does combining comfort measures and pharmacologic measures.
†Postprocedure.
‡With NCPAP/ventilation.

CDH, Congenital diaphragmatic hernia; CHD, congenital heart disease; CVP, central venous pressure; ECMO, extracorporeal membrane oxygenator; ETT, endotracheal tube; PDA, patent ductus arteriosus; PICC, peripherally inserted central catheter; ROP, retinopathy of prematurity; TEF, tracheoesophageal fistula.

Adapted from: Gardner SL: Clinical practice tool: nurse assisted procedures: evidence-based neonatal pain relief, 2008. Used with permission.

TABLE 12-9 PHARMACOLOGIC DIFFERENCES BETWEEN NEWBORNS AND ADULTS

DIFFERENCES	CAUSE	EFFECTS
Altered gastric activity	Presence of alkaline amniotic fluids at birth Immature gastric mucosa Consumption of alkaline milk	Variable drug absorption
Decreased gastric emptying time		Increased absorption of some drugs
Decreased protein binding	Lower levels of albumin, α-acid glycoprotein Increased competition for binding sites by endogenous substances (bilirubin)	Increased levels of free drug (opioids, local anesthetics)
Increased volume of distribution	Larger volume of body water in the newborn	Larger initial dose may be needed for effect (e.g., neuromuscular blocking agents, local anesthetics)
Decreased drug metabolism	Immature liver enzyme systems	Prolonged effect of some medications (e.g., morphine, fentanyl, neuromuscular blockers)
Decreased drug clearance	Immature renal system and decreased glomerular filtration rate	Prolonged effect of some medications (morphine)

From Rovee-Collier C, Hayne H: Reactivation of infant memory: implications for cognitive development, *Adv Child Dev* 10:185, 1987.

TABLE 12-10 ANALGESICS, SEDATIVES, AND REVERSAL AGENTS FOR THE NEONATE

DRUG	DOSAGE	COMMENTS
OPIOIDS		
Morphine	0.05–0.1 mg/kg/dose q 4–6 hr PRN IV, IM, or Sub-Q Continuous IV infusion: 10–15 mcg/kg/hr (up to 30–40 mcg/kg for ventilator therapy and major surgery)[231] Mean onset of action: 5 min Peak effect: 15 min Duration: 4–5 hr	CNS and respiratory depressant; bronchospasms; peripheral vasodilation with hypovolemic infants; hypotension, decreases gastric/intestinal motility; intestinal obstruction; risk for NEC; increases intracranial pressure; seizures; urinary retention. Easily reversed with naloxone; slower onset but longer duration than for fentanyl; withdrawal symptoms may occur. Ceiling effect (after reaching a therapeutic level, higher doses result in more adverse rather than analgesic effects) reached by using doses up to 0.5 mg/kg.[20] Sleep-wake cycling, measured by EEG, resumed soon after surgery in neonates ≥32 weeks' gestation who received high doses of morphine and midazolam.[233] Does not alter the physiologic response to ETT suctioning[22] As premedication for ETT intubation: use only if other opioids not available; must wait at least 5 minutes for onset of action[183]
Fentanyl (Sublimaze)	0.3–2 mcg/kg/dose q 1–2 hr PRN IV or Sub-Q Continuous IV infusion: 0.3–5 mcg/kg/hr Onset of action: 2–3 min Peak effect: 3–4 min Duration: 30–60 min	Same as for morphine. Eighty to 100 times more potent than morphine. Rapid onset of action; decreases motor activity; does not increase intracranial pressure in the absence of respiratory depression. Easily reversed with naloxone; short duration of action; may cause bradycardia, hypotension, apnea, seizures, or rigidity if given too rapidly; hypothermia. Less hypotension, urinary retention, GI motility effects than with morphine.[260] Withdrawal symptoms occur with prolonged use (>5 days). Drug of choice for premedication for ETT intubation.[183]

T A B L E 12-10	ANALGESICS, SEDATIVES, AND REVERSAL AGENTS FOR THE NEONATE—cont'd	
DRUG	**DOSAGE**	**COMMENTS**
OPIOIDS—cont'd		
Sufentanil citrate (Sufenta)	0.5–1 mcg/kg/dose q 30 min to 1 hr Peak effect: 5–6 min Duration: 30 min	Ten times more potent than fentanyl; has a quicker onset and shorter duration of action than fentanyl. Use with caution in neonates with intraventricular hemorrhage, hepatic or renal impairment, or pulmonary disease. Same side effects as for fentanyl. Bolus and continuous infusion affects electroencephalogram (EEG) results in very/extremely low-birth-weight infants; use of sufentanil must be considered in EEG interpretation.[306]
Remifentanil	1–3 mcg/kg/dose IV Repeat in 2–3 minutes PRN Onset of action: almost immediate Duration: 3–10 min	Same as for fentanyl. Easily reversed with naloxone. Short duration of action. Limited experience in neonates.[183,187,239] Premedication for ETT intubation: acceptable analgesic
Meperidine (Demerol)		*Not* recommended in preterm or term infants. The active metabolite normeperidine accumulates in tissues and causes CNS stimulation (e.g., tremors, muscle twitching, hyperactive reflexes, dilated pupils) and also lowers the seizure threshold level.[9]
NONOPIOIDS		
Acetaminophen (Tylenol)	Oral loading dose: 20–25 mg/kg PO; then 12–15 mg/kg PO q 8 hr	May cause hepatotoxicity in overdose. Potentiates effects of opioids but alone does *not* relieve surgical pain or heel lance pain. Do not use in patients with G6PD deficiency.
Ibuprofen (Advil, Motrin)	4–10 mg/kg/dose q 6–8 hr PO	Gastric irritant—administer with or after feeding; use with caution in neonates with necrotizing enterocolitis, impaired renal function, hypertension, or compromised cardiac function.
LOCAL ANESTHETICS		
Lidocaine	0.5%–1% solution (to avoid systemic toxicity, volume should be less than 0.5 ml/kg of 1% lidocaine solution—5 mg/kg)	Local infiltration anesthesia for invasive procedures; use solution *without epinephrine* to avoid vasoconstriction. Use topical creams (EMLA/amethocaine) before needle insertion; warm solution to body temperature; inject slowly to reduce the pain of injection.[193]
Bupivacaine Levobupivacaine Ropivacaine	2.5 mg/kg one-time epidural dose Continuous IV infusion: 0.2 mg/kg/hr (maximum dose)	Monitor for CNS (e.g., seizures, irritability) and cardiotoxic (e.g., ventricular dysrhythmias) side effects. Monitor catheter integrity. Epidural infusion is titrated to effect but *must not* exceed maximum dose. Levobupivacaine and ropivacaine are less cardiotoxic than bupivacaine.
EMLA (lidocaine and prilocaine)	2.5–5 g to site for at least 60 min Peak effect: 2–3 hr Duration: 1–2 hr after removal	Vasoconstriction at the site. Site must be covered with water-impermeable dressing (e.g., Tegaderm). Single doses have not been shown to cause methemoglobinemia in preterm or term neonates.[298] Does not relieve pain of heel lance.[9] The possibility of toxicity is increased when EMLA is applied to (1) open skin and (2) a larger area than recommended by manufacturer.[235] Cannot be used on abraded skin or mucous membranes.

Continued

TABLE 12-10	ANALGESICS, SEDATIVES, AND REVERSAL AGENTS FOR THE NEONATE — cont'd	
LOCAL ANESTHETICS — cont'd		
Amethocaine gel* (4%) (liposome-encapsulated tetracaine) (Ametrope)	1.5 g to site for 30 min to 1 hr	Site must be covered with water-impermeable dressing (e.g., Tegaderm). Vasodilation at the site — mild transient (≈20 min) erythema or blanching.[161,193,229,297] Case report of ELBW preterm developing a clinically significant cardiac arrhythmia after topical use for PICC insertion[205]
Liposomal lidocaine (4%) cream	Onset of action: 20–30 min	Available in United States without a prescription. Does not cause methemoglobinemia; can be applied without an occlusive dressing, and has fewer vasoactive effects.
SEDATIVE-HYPNOTICS		
Barbiturates		Do *not* provide pain relief; help reduce agitation precipitated by painful events. Frequently produce hyperalgesia and increased reaction to painful stimuli; contraindicated for neonates who have pain and also require sedation.
Phenobarbital	Loading: 10–20 mg/kg IV to maximum 40 mg/kg Maintenance: 5–7 mg/kg in two divided doses beginning 12 hr after last loading dose	Prolonged sedation possible once therapeutic levels achieved (20–25 mg/ml); depresses CNS — motor and respiratory; slow onset of action; little or no pain relief; not easily reversed; withdrawal symptoms may occur; incompatible with other drugs in solution.
NONBARBITURATES		
Dexmedetomidine HCl (Precedex)	Bolus for procedural sedation: 1–3 mcg/kg Slow IV infusion: Loading dose: 0.5 mcg/kg over 10 minutes Continuous IV infusion: Maintenance dose: 0.25–0.6 mcg/kg/hr Distribution half-life: 6 min Elimination half-life: 2 hr	Sedative, analgesic and all anesthetic properties for mechanically ventilated preterms and invasive procedures in ventilated and nonventilated neonates Minimal effect on blood pressure, heart and respiratory rates, oxygen saturation, and gastric motility.[211,230] Wean slowly to avoid withdrawal symptoms. Adverse reactions: hypo/hypertension, tachycardia, hypoxia, acidosis, elevation in temperature and blood sugar, anemia, and oliguria
Chloral hydrate	25–75 mg/kg/dose q 6 hr PRN, PO, or PR Onset: 10–15 min Duration: 2–4 hr	Gastric irritant — administer with or after feeding; paradoxical excitement; prolonged use associated with direct hyperbilirubinemia[188]; not to be used for analgesia; respiratory depressant; in repeated doses to premature infants — adverse effects — CNS depression, dysrhythmias, and renal failure.[117] For occasional procedural sedation, although not recommended. Recovery from chloral hydrate accompanied by a "hangover."
Benzodiazepines		Do *not* provide pain relief. Produce sedation, muscle relaxation, amnesia, anxiolysis, and anticonvulsant effects.
Diazepam (Valium)	0.02–0.3 mg/kg IV, IM, or PO q 6–8 hr	Do *not* dilute injection; venous sclerosing; may displace bilirubin and result in kernicterus; respiratory depression; hypotension; may cause agitation; induces sleep; relaxes muscles; withdrawal symptoms may occur; no analgesic effect; this drug should be used with caution in the neonate because of its long half-life, long-acting metabolites, and preservative (benzyl alcohol).[9]
Lorazepam (Ativan)	0.05–0.1 mg/kg/dose (give over ≥3 min) q 4–8 hr	Respiratory depressant, partial airway obstruction, drowsiness; respiratory depression potentiated when opioids or barbiturates also being given; infuse slowly to avoid apnea, bradycardia, and hypotension. Rhythmic myoclonic jerking in preterms.

TABLE 12-10	ANALGESICS, SEDATIVES, AND REVERSAL AGENTS FOR THE NEONATE—cont'd

NONBARBITURATES—cont'd		
Midazolam (Versed)	0.05–0.15 mg/kg/dose IV (give over ≥5 min) q 2–4 hr PRN Continuous IV infusion: <32 wk: 0.03 mg/kg/hr or 0.5 mcg/kg/min >32 wk: 0.06 mg/kg/hr or 1 mcg/kg/min PO: 0.25 mg/kg/dose of oral syrup Onset: IV—1–2 min; PO—15–30 min Duration: 1 hr after single IV dose For procedural sedation: Give 0.05 mg/kg IV and repeat ×1 PRN for procedure	Same as for lorazepam; continuous IV infusion enables precise titration until sedative effect is obtained; calms agitated infant on ventilator. Rapid bolus delivery and/or use with fentanyl is associated with (1) myoclonus—rhythmic twitching of all extremities that ceases with discontinuation of drug and does not return, and (2) respiratory depression and hypotension—caution use in hypotensive and hypovolemic neonates.[160,201] A systematic review shows (1) increased incidence of adverse neurologic outcomes (e.g., grade 3–4 IVH; PVL, altered CBF); (2) longer duration of NICU stay with midazolam use; and (3) conclusion that there is insufficient evidence to support IV midazolam use as a sedative for neonates in NICU.[224]

REVERSAL AGENTS		
Naloxone (Narcan)	1–10 mcg/kg	Reverses effects of opioids (both side effects and analgesia).
Flumazenil (Mazicon) 10 mcg/kg	10 mcg/kg	Reverses the effects of benzodiazepines (e.g., midazolam, diazepam, lorazepam).

CBF, Cerebral blood flow; *CNS*, central nervous system; *EMLA*, eutectic mixture of lidocaine and prilocaine; *ETT*, endotracheal tube; *G6PD*, glucose-6-phosphate dehydrogenase; *GI*, gastrointestinal; *IM*, intramuscular; *IV*, intravenous; *IVH*, intraventricular hemorrhage; *NEC*, necrotizing enterocolitis; *NICU*, neonatal intensive care unit; *PO*, per os; *PR*, per rectum; *PRN*, as needed; *PVL*, periventricular leukomalacia; *Sub-Q*, subcutaneous.
*Not yet approved by the Food and Drug Administration for use in the United States.

Fentanyl is the preferred drug in many NICUs because of its cardiovascular stability and its ability to decrease pulmonary vascular resistance. It can, however, cause chest wall rigidity and decreased lung compliance if administered too quickly. Neuromuscular blocking agents or slow administration of the drug will prevent this problem. Fentanyl also is commonly used in patients on extracorporeal membrane oxygenation (ECMO) to provide sedation and analgesia and to prevent increases in pulmonary vascular resistance and pressure.[194] Fentanyl is used also for artificial ventilation, persistent pulmonary hypertension of the newborn (PPHN), diaphragmatic hernia, and postoperative pain.[305] Because of its rapid onset and short duration, fentanyl relieves procedural pain.[305] Sufentanil is 10 times more potent than fentanyl and significantly more expensive. It is shorter acting and can have even greater effects on lung and chest wall compliance. Hydromorphone and methadone have also been used particularly in the postoperative period.

Administering drugs by as-needed (PRN) schedule results in peaks and valleys of pain relief and increases in side effects. Because an analgesic is most effective if given before the peak of pain (wind-up), continuous infusions or regular administration can help prevent undue neonatal suffering.[9,293]

Benzodiazepines are commonly used in the NICU for sedation. Midazolam (Versed) has been used increasingly to provide sedation in mechanically ventilated neonates. A meta-analysis of the research on midazolam concluded that there are significant adverse effects and no clinical benefit to the use of midazolam; there is insufficient evidence to justify the use of midazolam for ventilated neonates in the NICU (see Table 12-10).[32,224] Benzodiazepines potentiate the effects of opiates.[280] Therefore, when they are used in combination (e.g., fentanyl and midazolam), lower doses of each medication may be used to gain the same effect as would be attained if either one was used separately. There is increasing concern regarding the neurotoxicity of midazolam[196] (see Table 12-10). It is important to note that although benzodiazepines provide sedation, they have no analgesic effect.[280]

The long-term effects of analgesic use on the developing brain are poorly understood because of a paucity of data on neurodevelopmental outcomes. Several researchers have found a protective effect of analgesic use on neurodevelopmental outcomes, perhaps because of decreased fluctuation in blood pressure, cerebral blood flow, oxygenation, respiratory synchrony with ventilation, and stress hormones.[15,23,28,184,203]

More recent studies on the long-term neurologic effects of morphine analgesia in ventilated preterm infants caution against the lack of protective effects and have documented: (1) an increase in severe IVH,[24] (2) a decrease in the incidence of IVH that did not influence poor neurologic outcomes,[274] and (3) subtle neurobehavioral differences in preterm infants exposed to morphine analgesia.[251]

LOCAL ANESTHETICS

Local anesthetics have a variety of uses and provide analgesia by preventing the transmission of noxious stimuli at either the peripheral receptor site or the spinal cord. Bupivacaine, ropivacaine, and lidocaine are the most commonly used local anesthetics (see Table 12-10). A recent study showed that bupivacaine confers better analgesia for neonatal circumcision than that achieved with lidocaine.[288]

Bupivacaine is longer acting but more cardiotoxic than lidocaine. Both are more toxic in neonates than in adults because of increased organ sensitivity and free fraction of drug. The cardiovascular toxicity may be enhanced if epinephrine-containing local anesthetics are used. The long-acting local anesthetics *levobupivacaine* (available in Europe) and *ropivacaine* are as effective as bupivacaine but less cardiotoxic.[324] Procainamide is used as a continuous infusion in many centers because of its' rapid ester metabolism and decreased toxicity.

Regional Technique. Regional techniques provide adequate analgesia, thus reducing the need for higher doses of opioids (Table 12-11). Advantages include the following[83]:
- Stress responses are significantly decreased.
- Normal respiratory patterns return more quickly.
- The need for postoperative ventilation may be avoided or shortened.

TABLE 12-11	TYPES OF REGIONAL BLOCKADE *Potential Uses*	
BLOCK	**POTENTIAL USES**	**COMPLICATIONS**
Spinal	In place of general anesthesia for surgery below the umbilicus; decreased incidence of postoperative apnea	Inability to access space; incomplete block or inadequate duration of anesthesia
Caudal/epidural	Intraoperative and postoperative analgesia for thoracic, abdominal, perineal, and lower extremity surgery	Inadequate block; local or opioid-related toxicity; nerve damage, paralysis
Dorsal penile nerve/ring block	Circumcision, analgesia for any penile surgery	Hematoma formation; end-organ damage if epinephrine-containing solutions are used
Intercostal nerve block	Rib fractures, thoracic surgery	Pneumothorax; local anesthetic toxicity (highest rate of absorption)

- Intestinal motility recovers more quickly.
- Morbidity decreases, particularly with the use of epidural blocks.

Dorsal Penile Nerve/Ring Block.[179] Dorsal penile nerve block is extremely easy to perform with a high degree of success that can provide surgical anesthesia for circumcision.[179] The block is performed by injecting 1% lidocaine 3 to 5 mm below the skin at the 2 o'clock and 10 o'clock positions on the dorsum of the penis (Figure 12-7). In a full-term neonate, 0.5 ml/side is used, and 0.2 ml/kg/side is used in premature infants. An alternative technique less likely to cause hematoma is to inject a subcutaneous ring of 0.5% or 1% lidocaine around the base of the penis. All solutions should be without epinephrine, and a "wait time" of 5 to 8 minutes is necessary to achieve adequate anesthesia.[192]

A study of pain responses to circumcision using dorsal penile nerve block/ring block, topical ELA-Max, and 24% oral sucrose solution found that infants receiving a combination of dorsal block/sucrose or ring block/sucrose had lower pain scores than those with use of ring block or sucrose alone.[252,256] Infants receiving topical ELA-Max had pain scores that were not significantly different from those in the infants

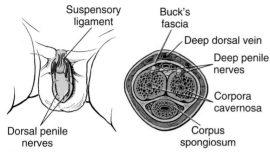

FIGURE 12-7 *Anatomic landmarks for placement of a dorsal penile nerve block. (From McClain B, Anand KS: Neonatal pain management. In Deshpande J, Tobias J, editors:* The pediatric pain handbook, *St Louis, 1996, Mosby.)*

receiving dorsal penile or ring block. Both dorsal and ring nerve blocks resulted in similar pain scores. As a result of this nursing research, the institutional policy was changed so that newborn circumcision is performed only with the use of analgesic and not oral sucrose alone.

Liposomal lidocaine was compared with a eutectic mixture of lidocaine and prilocaine (EMLA) and dorsal penile block in a study of 54 full-term infants being circumcised; liposomal lidocaine was found to be a safe and effective topical anesthetic.[192] A video study found that the dorsal penile nerve block was significantly more effective for pain relief during circumcision than use of topical EMLA cream.[108] A recent meta-analysis of 14 studies of infant circumcision found that pain was dramatically decreased with the combined use of dorsal penile block, acetaminophen, oral sucrose, and topical analgesic cream.[39] Addition of liposomal lidocaine to sucrose did not further decrease the pain of venipuncture in healthy term newborns.[303]

Epidural Block. The epidural space is an area surrounding the dura of the spinal cord. This space can be accessed from the caudal, lumbar, or thoracic region. An epidural block is performed by a skilled pediatric anesthesiologist, often with the patient under general anesthesia.[208] A small catheter can be left in the space, or a one-time dose of medication can be given. Local anesthetics act by anesthetizing either the local nerve roots or the spinal tracts at the level of the spinal cord where they are placed. The most commonly used medications in neonates are the local anesthetics *procainamide, ropivacaine,* or *bupivacaine.* They are often used in combination with low doses of opioids and/or clonidine, which have both local and systemic action. The major advantages of these techniques include their ability to provide continuous pain relief and the potential to minimize respiratory depression, facilitate extubation, and hasten recovery.

Eutectic Mixture of Local Anesthetic and Infiltration. Eutectic mixture of local anesthetic (EMLA) is a local anesthetic cream that anesthetizes the skin and has been used for a variety of procedures (e.g., lumbar puncture, venipuncture).[154,321] A study of EMLA, applied 60 to 90 minutes before lumbar puncture, showed a significant decrease in pain response during needle insertion and withdrawal but not during positioning/handling of the newborn.[175] EMLA has been used for analgesia with circumcisions in newborns and has been shown to be efficacious.[321] However, its analgesic properties are not as effective as those of dorsal penile blocks in relieving postoperative circumcision pain.*

A meta-analysis of the efficacy of EMLA for a variety of procedures in neonates found that EMLA diminishes pain during circumcision, venipuncture, arterial puncture, and placement of a peripheral/central IV line.[298,321] For maximum effectiveness, EMLA should be applied and left on for at least 1 to 2 hours before starting an invasive procedure. Unfortunately, EMLA does not appear to alleviate pain resulting from heel sticks.[99,298,321] Infiltration of local anesthetic can also help decrease pain for such procedures as placement of percutaneous central lines, removal of Broviac catheters, and circumcision. Methemoglobinemia does not appear to be a problem when single daily doses of 0.5 g EMLA are left in place for 60 minutes,[298] but studies are ongoing to address this issue.

Amethocaine gel (lysosome-encapsulated tetracaine) is a topical local anesthetic preparation that provides more effective superficial analgesia than EMLA in adults. Amethocaine has demonstrated similar efficacy to EMLA when appropriate application times are used and has a more rapid onset and longer duration of action than EMLA.[229] Studies have documented its effectiveness in neonates as follows:

- It relieves pain during venipuncture,[161,197] IV insertion, and injections of vitamin K.[269]
- It does not relieve pain from heel sticks[238] or peripherally inserted central catheter (PICC) insertion, unless combined with morphine use.[297]

---

*References 43, 137, 145, 153, 179, 223, 252, 287, 299, 321.

- It relieves circumcision pain.[321]
- It does not cause methemoglobinemia.
- It is effective within 30 to 40 minutes of application.

OTHER MEDICATIONS

Acetaminophen and nonsteroidal antiinflammatory drugs (NSAIDs) can be helpful in providing analgesia for mild to moderate pain (see Table 12-10). These medications are more effective when administered on a regular schedule, augment the effects of opioids, and may be delayed in effect because of the rate of gastric emptying.[30,310] Acetaminophen given 2 hours before circumcision does not reduce pain during the procedure but is effective in postoperative pain relief; repeated doses every 4 to 6 hours for the first 24 hours after circumcision are recommended. The analgesic effects of IV NSAIDs have not been studied in preterms, and the adverse effects of prolonged NSAID use may lead to renal, circulatory, hepatic, gastrointestinal, and hematologic complications.[21,27] Although use of acetaminophen as a prophylactic for febrile response to immunizations is effective, there is a significantly lower antibody response to vaccine antigen when acetaminophen is used.[247]

Sedatives can help decrease agitation and improve comfort but do *not* by themselves provide analgesia. Use of developmental care significantly reduces the need of VLBW infants for sedative drugs.[316] Sedatives are appropriate to induce sleep for diagnostic procedures (e.g., computed tomography [CT] scan, magnetic resonance imaging [MRI]), to calm chronically irritable infants whose physiologic stability or ventilatory status is compromised by agitation, and for pain-related agitation.[23,316] Sedatives have potential toxicities, effect behavioral changes, and affect consciousness, which deprive neonates of their ability to communicate and interact with their parents, caregivers, and the environment.[317] Furthermore, the short-term and long-term effects of frequent or continuous use of sedatives on the developing brain are unknown.

Comfort Measures

Comfort measures alone do not relieve pain; however, their use reduces agitation, which indirectly reduces pain by promoting behavioral organization, relaxation, general comfort, and sleep.[9,195] Although comfort measures may prevent the intensification of pain (e.g., guarding an abdominal incision by positioning is less painful than four-point restraint), they may not relieve moderate to severe pain. Comfort measures are helpful but inadequate by themselves, considering the intensity of the noxious stimuli causing moderate to severe pain.[9,77]

Provision of comfort measures (i.e., nonpharmacologic interventions) for neonatal pain is an evidence-based nursing practice that should be initiated by neonatal nurses and parents.[107] As partners in care, parents should be encouraged and facilitated to engage in providing comfort measures for their infants having painful procedures.[54] Nonnutritive sucking, kangaroo care, facilitated tucking, rocking, and holding have been found to be the nonpharmacologic interventions that offer the most comfort during a painful intervention.[65,234] Who better than parents to provide these interventions? Research shows the efficacy of parental involvement. Initiation of skin-to-skin contact,[123] taste, and suckling was described in full-term infants receiving heel sticks for genetic screens, who experienced less crying (91%) and grimacing (84%) when being held and breastfed by their mothers.[60,122] Numerous studies show that very preterm, healthy preterm, and term newborns (between 28 and 36 weeks' PMA) receiving heel sticks experienced diminished behavioral and physiologic pain response, less crying, and quicker recovery when being held skin-to-skin (e.g., kangaroo care) by their mothers for 15 to 30 minutes before and during the procedure.* If the preterm infant's mother is not available, does provision of skin-to-skin care by the father or an unrelated woman result in lower pain responses? This question has been researched in two published studies with the following results: (1) fathers were marginally less effective than mothers in decreasing their preterm infant's pain response[166]; (2) unrelated females had a small, although not negligible, decrease in their ability to relieve infant pain, and fathers are more acceptable to the baby's mother than an unrelated female to provide this intimate care.[164] Animal studies show that the short-term and long-term effects of repeated pain are ameliorated by the presence and ministrations of the

---

*References 62, 65, 71, 74, 123, 168, 178, 199, 225, 234.

mother[318]; perhaps the presence of the human mother or parent provides the same protection for the human neonate.[38,54]

One barrier to using skin-to-skin care and breastfeeding to relieve neonatal pain during invasive procedures such as heel stick and injections is the uncomfortable position of the professional performing the procedure. An ergonomically sound protocol using an adjustable height stool has been developed and tested in the clinical setting.[72] This protocol has resulted in a more comfortable position for the professional and more use of skin-to-skin care and breastfeeding for neonatal pain relief during the procedure.[73]

Developmental care not only prevents pain but also decreases behavioral and physiologic pain scores in preterm infants.[63,90,275] A recent study of a simple diaper change in VLBW preterms showed less physiologic response (e.g., alteration in heart rate, hypoxia, bradycardia, desaturation events) and less pain response (measured with two pain scales) when developmental care was used before and during the procedure.[275] In this study, developmental supports such as opportunities for grasping, hand swaddling, decreasing light and noise, nonnutritive sucking, and body support and containment were used.

NONNUTRITIVE SUCKING

Nonnutritive sucking (NNS; e.g., the infant's own fingers or hands or a pacifier) soothes by reducing the infant's level of arousal and duration of cry while promoting the quiet alert state.[55] NNS is effective in reducing pain in preterm infants during heel stick, circumcision, and immunizations and during retinopathy of prematurity (ROP) screening eye examinations.[47] The effect of NNS is immediate, but the effect ceases immediately on cessation of sucking/removal of the pacifier. Combining NNS and sucrose before and during painful procedures provides a synergistic effect on pain relief for both term and preterm neonates.[44,57,223,287]

ORAL SUCROSE/GLUCOSE

Distressed infants offered oral sucrose calmed quickly, stayed calm longer, and spent more time in a quiet alert state than did infants offered only a pacifier.[44] Sucking soothes, reduces heart and metabolic rates, induces hand-to-mouth behavior, and elevates the pain threshold through opioid and nonopioid systems.[44] Administration

of sucrose (into the mouth) within 2 to 3 minutes before an invasive procedure (e.g., heel stick/venipuncture; bladder catheterization; eye examinations for ROP; insertion of gavage tube; arterial stick) has been shown to decrease crying duration, heart rate, facial activity, and electroencephalogram (EEG) changes associated with pain in full-term and preterm infants.*

In these studies, the amount (0.05–2 ml) and concentrations (24%–50%) of sucrose varied, but even the smallest dose administered once to preterm infants of 26 to 34 weeks' gestation reduced pain behaviors.[41,287] The small doses of concentrated sucrose solution used to treat neonatal pain have not been shown to cause hyperglycemia in preterm infants.[49]

When sucrose is paired with developmental interventions such as rocking, carrying,[119] NNS,[76,111] prone positioning, or parental holding,[69,115,137] sucrose is more effective in decreasing behavioral pain responses. A recent RCT study of the combination of NNS, oral sucrose, and facilitated tucking during heel stick in preterms found reduced arousal during the procedure, less crying and fussing, and better sleep than routine care alone.[195] Use of oral sucrose alone has been shown to result in higher pain scores than use of any other form of analgesia during circumcision; sucrose is an adjunct to pain control during circumcision and should not be the only analgesic used for this operative procedure.[252] In a systematic meta-analysis of 21 studies of sucrose use for analgesia, sucrose was found to be safe, effective, and cost-effective for single painful procedures (e.g., heel stick/venipuncture).[287] Addition of liposomal lidocaine to sucrose in one study did not further decrease the pain of venipuncture in healthy term newborns.[303] Despite being aware that sucrose relieves pain, only 10% of surveyed NICUs used sucrose before a heel stick, and only 11% used sucrose before venipuncture.[124] Another survey showed only 33% of responding NICUs using sucrose before routine painful procedures.[210] A more recent survey of NICUs in eight European countries found poor compliance with pain management guidelines for heel stick and other invasive procedures.[198]

An RCT of 2 ml of 25% oral sucrose solution given to healthy preterms (e.g., <37 weeks' GA)

---

*References 41, 43, 95, 104, 137, 159, 181, 215, 216, 254, 266, 287, 301.

2 minutes before a venipuncture significantly decreased heart rate and crying during the venipuncture.[2] The safety and efficacy of "routine use" (e.g., use for every invasive procedure in the first week of life; administered a maximum of three times, 2 minutes apart) of sucrose (0.1 ml of 24% solution) in preterms less than 31 weeks' PCA were studied in a randomized controlled trial.[169] In the group of preterms receiving sucrose, the higher number of doses of sucrose predicted poorer neurobehavioral development (e.g., scores on motor development, vigor, alertness, and orientation at 36 weeks; lower motor development and vigor at 40 weeks) and poorer physiologic outcomes.[169] Other studies have found that repeated sucrose use is safe (no side effects) and effective for pain relief from repeated procedural pain in the NICU.[109,286]

The benefits of sucrose for pain relief have been shown to provide comfort to the infant during subsequent caregiving activities.[302] Two hundred and forty neonates were randomized to a placebo or sucrose-treated group for all needle procedures. After the painful procedure, those infants receiving sucrose reacted to a diaper change with lower pain scores than the infants receiving only a placebo. The comforting benefits of sucrose remained even after the painful procedure was complete.[302]

The Academy of Breastfeeding Medicine states that "when available breastfeeding should be the first choice to alleviate procedural pain in neonates."[1] When possible, breastfeeding throughout the procedure, rather than pumped breast milk, offers more comfort because of the synergism between skin-to-skin contact with the mother, sucking, and reception of breast milk by the infant.[1] An RCT comparing breast milk with sucrose for pain relief in 71 late preterm infants (born at 32–37 weeks' PMA) undergoing heel lance was conducted in the Netherlands.[271] Using the PIPP assessment scale, there was no significant difference in pain scores between the preterms receiving breast milk (directly breastfed or bottle-fed) and those receiving sucrose. Salivary cortisol levels from birth to 1 year of age are 40% higher in breastfed infants compared with formula-fed infants.[63] The analgesic effect of breast milk may be due to these higher cortisol levels.[56] Concerns about breastfeeding as a comfort measure during painful procedures have been raised. To explore these concerns a study of 57 preterms

(30–36 weeks' GA) were randomized to be breast-fed or given a soother during a blood collection procedure.[150] Preterms with mature breastfeeding skills had lower pain scores during the procedure, all breastfed infants had lower pain scores after the procedure, and use of breastfeeding as a comfort measure did not interfere with the acquisition of breastfeeding skills.[150]

Several studies have compared use of glucose versus sucrose for pain relief, with conflicting results. A comparison of oral glucose versus sucrose showed that glucose solution (e.g., 33%–50%) was more effective in reducing pain response in term newborns having heel sticks.[135] Another study found that 30% sucrose solution was more effective in reducing crying time than 10% to 30% glucose solutions.[159] When oral glucose (30% solution) was given to full-term newborns undergoing venipuncture compared with (1) EMLA cream[121] and (2) subcutaneous injections,[57] the infants treated with glucose had significantly lower pain scores. Oral glucose and facilitated tucking by parents was found to be more effective and preferred over the use of opioids in preterm infants receiving heel sticks and pharyngeal suction.[35] Future studies of glucose and sucrose for pain relief should examine (1) the most effective method of administration, (2) the optimal dose and solution strength, (3) the effectiveness when paired with other behavioral and pharmacologic interventions, (4) the long-term effects of repeated administration, and (5) the use in the VLBW infant (e.g., at risk for necrotizing enterocolitis, nil per os [NPO] status, unstable; ventilated).[41,111,169,287]

TACTILE INTERVENTIONS

A reassuring human presence (of parents or caregivers) during painful procedures for all neonates in the NICU is *mandatory*.[38] Body containment of extremities in a flexed position (e.g., holding, swaddling, nesting; providing an opportunity to grasp a finger or pacifier) decreases gross motor movements that contribute to the infant's increased level of arousal, reduces physiologic and behavioral stress, facilitates energy conservation in the preterm infant, and lowers pain scores.[55,66,304] Improper body position contributes to discomfort and pain. An RCT combining five tactile interventions (i.e., swaddling, side/stomach lying, shushing, swinging, and sucking) for infant immunizations resulted in less crying time and lower pain scores;

these outcomes were greater than those obtained with sucrose alone.[144]

Facilitated tucking—gentle containment of flexed extremities in the midline on the trunk while side-lying or supine—during a painful procedure (e.g., heel stick) results in lower heart rate, shorter crying time, less sleep disruption, and fewer sleep-state changes.[77] A study of facilitated tucking (provided by parents for endotracheal tube suctioning) showed that participation by parents was a safe, effective pain-management strategy that provided parents with an active role in their infant's pain care and was also preferred by parents.[34] A more recent study by the same researchers found lower pain scores with oral glucose and facilitated tucking by parents during heel stick and pharyngeal suction in very preterm infants.[35] Facilitated tucking was perceived positively by mothers who were either internally motivated to provide it or were externally motivated by nurses who suggested their involvement.[33] However, two other studies of facilitated tucking[115] and facilitated tucking and oral sucrose[69] found that using facilitated tucking alone was less effective in pain management.

Use of a 2-minute massage of the ipsilateral leg before heel stick in preterm infants was safe and resulted in a decreased pain response (decreased pain score and heart rate) compared with nonmassaged preterms.[162] Massage of the arms and hands of infants for 2 minutes prior to an invasive procedure such as heel stick or other needle stick has been shown to reduce pain scores.[66]

Motoric boundaries (e.g., containment of extremities) assist a preterm infant to maintain a more secure, controlled response and facilitate self-regulation. Therapeutic interventions include the use of positions that support flexion and restraint in physiologic position, periodic release of restraint and exercise of extremities, gentle change in body position, and positioning to guard operative sites. Along with comfort measures, minimizing stimulation in the NICU environment enables a neonate who is agitated or in pain to use internal and external resources in organizing his or her behavior and develop self-soothing strategies (see Chapter 13). Individualizing care and handling to the infant's likes and dislikes and listing these at the bedside help maintain consistency of care and build trust in these developing neonates.

Picking up, holding, and rocking provide tactile soothing, vestibular stimulation, and the calming effect of rhythmic, repetitive movement. Use of massage, rocking, and water mattresses provides tactile, vestibular, and kinesthetic stimuli that modify and accelerate behavioral, state control, and decreased stress behaviors (see Chapter 13).

AUDITORY INTERVENTIONS

Four small studies of the use of music therapy to relieve the stress and pain of procedures evaluated physiologic and behavioral responses in a total of 75 infants.[5] In two studies, intubated preterms were exposed to music/no music during routine suctioning. Positive results in the music-exposed preterms included (1) improved oxygen saturation, (2) heart rates between 120 to 160 beats per minute for a longer period of time, (3) more time in sleep state, and (4) quicker recovery time after suctioning.[50,67] Two other studies exposed irritable, agitated, infants in a naturally occurring inconsolable crying episode to music and measured their responses. Again positive results of music therapy included (1) improved oxygen saturations, (2) better respiratory and heart rates, (3) state change to drowsy or quiet alert, and (4) fewer crying episodes.[70,176] Additional data from well-designed studies are required before use of music therapy for preterms during painful, stressful conditions can be recommended.[5]

COMPLEMENTARY HEALING MODALITIES

Complementary healing (e.g., therapeutic touch [TT], acupressure, acupuncture, Reiki) is gaining increasing interest among neonatal health care providers. Little research exists, but clinical reports have depicted the benefits of pain relief with integration of these modalities. A study conducted with registered nurses (RNs) who provided TT to preterm infants (25–37 weeks' gestation) revealed that the infants' responses to TT included (1) decreased heart and respiratory rates; (2) enhanced restful periods; (3) improved sucking, swallowing, and breathing; and (4) a greater ability to interact with the environment.[143] Two more recent studies of the use of TT with a painful procedure have been conducted. In the first study, 10 preterm infants (34–40 weeks' conceptual age) received TT during a low-intensity sensory punctuate stimuli and responded with an increase in cerebral oxygenation.[152] The researchers concluded that TT may have a protective effect on the autoregulation of cerebral blood flow in the preterm infant during a painful stimuli.[152] Another randomized study of the effects of TT before and after procedural pain (heel lance) found no comforting effect for 27 preterm infants less than 30 weeks' GA.[165] These researchers recommended use of other tactile interventions for pain relief.

Acupuncture and acupressure may be safely used to treat pain, agitation, and drug withdrawal in the neonate.[118] A retrospective review of 10 hospitalized infants exposed to acupuncture found a decrease in the use of sedative and analgesics for agitation, successful weaning from ventilators and transitioning to oral intake after oral aversion without adverse effects.[110] Additional research in this area is needed to validate the use of these modalities for pain management.[110]

Activation of cutaneous sensory nerves with a transcutaneous electrical nerve stimulation (TENS) unit and application of thermal (topical skin refrigerant) blocks transmission of peripheral pain impulses from procedural pain. Low-frequency, monotonous sounds (e.g., heartbeat, vacuums) quiet the infant and increase behavioral organization. Use of music (see Chapter 13) and recordings of family voices soothe term and preterm infants, resulting in fewer state changes, less time in the arousal state, and increased behavioral organization. However, during circumcision, music (with or without a pacifier) is not an effective distraction or soothing strategy for relief of the pain of the procedure. Another recent study showed that preterm infants presented with a familiar odor during venipuncture exhibited significantly less crying and grimacing, compared with the preterms presented with an unfamiliar odor or no odor.[120]

END-OF-LIFE CARE

When the decision is made to terminate or not begin aggressive medical intervention, the neonate receives end-of-life care, also known as comfort care or palliative care (see Chapter 32). Neonates who receive end-of-life care are at the threshold of viability, have multiple congenital anomalies that are incompatible with life, or are not responding to NICU interventions (e.g., deterioration in condition despite medical efforts).[242,253]

End-of-life care should combine comfort measures, pharmacologic management, developmental care (see Chapter 13),[291] and spiritual and psychosocial support for the neonate and family (see Chapters 29 and 30).[61,64,242,290,291] The family is provided a quiet, private, homelike area in which to touch, hold, and interact with their terminally ill neonate. Use of skin-to-skin care (kangaroo care); soft, soothing music; dimmed lighting; infant massage; holding; and rocking provides both a comforting environment for the infant and family, as well as parenting and comforting opportunities.[65,291] Parents, siblings, and extended family members remain with their infant during and after death. Clergy may be present for family support and may perform a religious service, such as baptism or blessing.

For comfort care, all invasive procedures, including measurement of vital signs, monitors, machines, and artificial feeding, are discontinued. The infant, cleaned and wrapped in a warm blanket, is held by the family. Intravenous access may remain in place for administration of pain medications or sedatives. Medication is administered in sufficient doses to provide comfort, relieve pain, and ensure that the infant does not suffer at the end of his or her life.

In the only study that documents use of analgesia for dying infants whose life support is withdrawn or withheld, 165 deaths in a university-based NICU were reviewed.[236] Opioid analgesia was administered to 84% of infants when life support was withdrawn or withheld. Infants with major congenital anomalies (93%) and necrotizing enterocolitis (100%) were more likely to receive opioids than were ELBW infants (66%–83%). Overall, opioid analgesia was administered to at least 65% of infants. Reasons for life support discontinuation also influenced administration of opioids: (1) futility of treatment (84% medicated), (2) severe lifelong impairment (85% medicated), and (3) suffering caused by treatment (100% medicated). The median dose of opioids was within the usual pharmacologic range in 64% and greater in 36%. Of the infants receiving a higher dose, 94% had previously been receiving an analgesic and may have needed a higher dose as a result of tolerance. The median time until death from the discontinuation of life support was 18 minutes for those who received the standard dose and 20 minutes for those who received the higher dose.

A survey of hospital staff providing pediatric palliative care found that 50% of physicians and 30% of nurses reported feeling inexperienced in pain management.[75] Providers also shared how personally distressing it is to witness a child's suffering, especially when pain relief was possible but not available or delivered. In the same study, families also described their anguish in watching their child experience and suffer any amount of pain and discomfort. Unlike the health care providers, families thought that everything had been done to alleviate their child's pain. Another recent study found that insufficient education in pain and palliative care of pediatric care providers was a barrier to use of palliative care in children.[80]

COMPLICATIONS

A neonate's complex behavioral response to pain has both short-term and long-term ramifications (Box 12-7).

These behavioral changes may disrupt parent-infant interaction and attachment, adaptation to the postnatal environment, feeding behaviors and growth.[25,314] An alteration in brain development and maldevelopment of sensory systems can occur when distorted or inappropriate sensory input occurs during a critical period in development.* Because of a neonate's memory, painful experiences increase the infant's sensitivity to subsequent medical encounters.† These initial experiences may affect the development of attitudes, fears, anxiety, conflicts, wishes, expectations, and patterns of interactions with others.[97,204]

Younger infants are more susceptible to long-term consequences (see Box 12-4) because there is heightened sensitivity at earlier developmental stages.‡ In the most immature preterm infants, lower pain thresholds and the lack of inhibitory controls influence hypersensitivity.[125] When tissue injury occurs early in development, increased pain sensitivity develops both at the site of the damage (primary hyperalgesia) and in the surrounding skin (secondary hyperalgesia) because of hyperinnervation at the site.[125,241] The lower pain threshold of the more preterm infant is also influenced by repeated exposures.[125] The consequences of this altered excitability include

*References 14–16, 23, 28, 48, 97, 138, 139, 245, 249, 258, 313, 319.
†References 14, 132, 139, 228, 240, 245, 258, 279, 295, 298, 300.
‡References 48, 138, 139, 249, 313, 314.

BOX 12-7	LONG-TERM CONSEQUENCES OF REPETITIVE PAIN*

- Less physiologic stability (e.g., alterations in heart and/or respiratory rates and blood pressure)
- Less postnatal growth (less weight gain and lower head circumference) in very preterm infants[314]
- Alterations in basal cortisol levels in extremely low gestational age preterms at 8 and 18 months that suggests a "resetting" of the endocrine stress systems with potential for negative implications for neurodevelopment and later health
- Alterations in cerebral blood flow,[203] increasing the risk for intraventricular hemorrhage and periventricular leukomalacia
- Inappropriate sensory input (pain) disrupts neural activity, and chronic activation of neuroendocrine system results in abnormal brain development
- Hyperinnervation (e.g., neural reorganization in the periphery and the spinal cord) associated with increased pain behaviors such as allodynia and hypersensitivity
- Altered pain responsiveness:
  - Heightened responsiveness to pain (hyperalgesia)/lower pain threshold
  - Decreased responsiveness to pain (associated with more exposure to painful experiences) in the NICU and later in infancy and childhood
  - Reduced tolerance to pain in adolescence (after being born extremely preterm, with most painful experiences and most doses of morphine), but pain response that closely resembled control group, born at term[311]
- Neurodevelopmental and behavioral sequelae of prematurity (see Chapter 31)
- Alteration of parent-infant interactions and relationships; temperament and pain expression

*References 14–23, 28, 31, 48, 97, 125–127, 132, 138, 139, 204, 228, 240, 246, 258, 279, 294–298, 300, 318, 319.

---

(1) perceiving nonnoxious tactile stimuli as noxious,[5] depending on the number of invasive procedures in the previous 24 hours[129]; (2) systemic responses of chronic pain and discomfort; (3) associating earlier pain with decreased behavioral responses to pain; (4) variable physiologic responses[125]; and (5) lower tenderness thresholds and more tender points in adolescence.[51,311] Ongoing studies demonstrate the importance of infant and family factors (Figure 12-8) in ameliorating developmental alterations initiated by early and repeated pain exposures.[125,313] NICUs with a higher

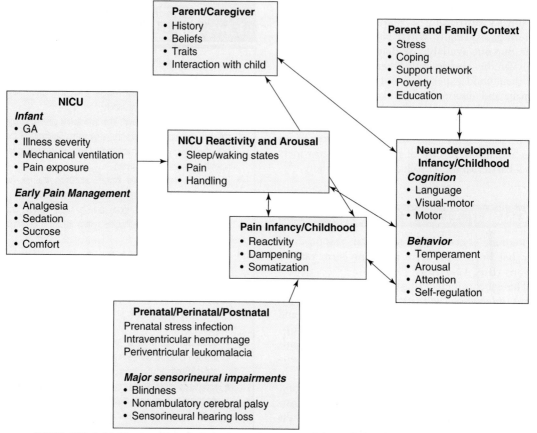

FIGURE 12-8 Model of long-term effects of pain showing complex, interactive, bidirectional relationships among multiple biologic and environmental factors. *GA,* Gestational age; *NICU,* neonatal intensive care unit. (From Grunau R: Early pain in preterm infants: a model of long-term effects, *Clin Perinatol* 29:376, 2002.)

level of infant pain management are associated with better neurobehavioral performance (i.e., better attention and arousal, less lethargy, and better reflexes as measured by the NNNS scale) in very preterm infants.[218] Studies to evaluate the long-term effects of pharmacologic and comfort interventions are also needed.[125,212,313]

As mentioned, unanesthetized surgery and/or unrelieved pain causes suffering that might itself be a risk to life.[25] Maintaining metabolic homeostasis by the appropriate use of anesthetics and analgesics improves postoperative outcome by preventing (1) protein wasting, (2) electrolyte imbalance, (3) impaired immune function, (4) sepsis, (5) metabolic acidosis, (6) pulmonary and cardiac insufficiency, (7) hypermetabolic state, and (8) death.[12,26,83,116] Increasing evidence confirms that exposure to prolonged, severe, or untreated pain increases morbidity and alters brain development and subsequent behavioral and physiologic responses to pain.*

Opioid analgesics may produce respiratory depression severe enough to require mechanical ventilation. Naloxone (0.1 mg/kg IV or intramuscular [IM]) is the specific antidote for opioid overdose (see Table 12-10). Lower doses of naloxone (0.001–0.01 mg/kg IV or IM) can be used for moderate respiratory depression. Complete opioid reversal with 0.1 mg/kg naloxone increases agitation and stress response in neonates with ongoing pain. Subsequently, it is more difficult to manage the neonate's pain until the effects of

_____

*References 9, 11, 15, 16, 18, 25, 52, 97, 126, 204, 311, 314.

the naloxone wear off. Lower doses of naloxone should be used and the dose titrated to prevent this outcome. An ampule of neonatal naloxone should always be immediately available with the appropriate dose precalculated on the infant's emergency card. Flumazenil is a specific antagonist for the benzodiazepines and should be used to treat respiratory depression (see Table 12-10). Respiratory depression may produce hypoxemia, so a pulse oximeter should be standard equipment along with cardiorespiratory monitoring.[9,293] All equipment for assisted ventilation should be at the bedside.[9]

An overdose of local anesthetics can cause seizures, ventricular tachycardia, bradycardia, and cardiovascular collapse. Toxic doses for neonates should be carefully calculated, and lower doses should be administered. Benzodiazepines or phenobarbital can be used to treat refractive seizures; cardiopulmonary resuscitation (CPR) and defibrillation may be necessary to treat the cardiovascular complications. Administration of intralipids 20% in a dose of 1 to 2 mg/kg/day is a specific antidote for cardiac toxicity from local anesthetics. Patients who are receiving epidural analgesia for postoperative pain control should be monitored for signs of potential CNS toxicity (e.g., irritability, jitteriness, twitching, myoclonic jerking). If an opioid is being administered with the local anesthetic infusion, then respiratory depression is also a possibility and patients should be monitored as described. Clonidine in the epidural infusion can lead to hypotension and decreased heart rate. Other extremely rare complications of epidurals are nerve injury and/or paralysis.

Hematoma formation can occur (1.2%) with the placement of a dorsal penile nerve block. Using a ring block usually avoids this problem. Epinephrine-containing solutions must *never* be used, because this can lead to compromise of the blood supply to the penis and severe tissue damage.

Tolerance and Withdrawal

Tolerance is the need for escalating doses of drug to achieve the same effect. Tolerance (1) occurs sooner with the use of synthetic opioids (e.g., fentanyl) than with naturally occurring opioids (e.g., morphine); (2) is related to the duration of use—the longer the use (>5 days),[21] the more likely tolerance is to develop (use for less than 72 hours usually is not associated with tolerance); (3) develops more rapidly with continuous infusions versus intermittent therapy; (4) may develop more rapidly in preterm neonates than in term neonates; and (5) occurs more often in males than in females.[20,292,293,310]

Physical dependence is the state in which continued drug is needed to prevent the signs of withdrawal.[310] Withdrawal arises when discontinuing the drug causes symptoms such as irritability, diarrhea, tachycardia, hypertension, insomnia, restlessness, diaphoresis, or palmar sweating and muscle twitches. Addiction occurs when there is psychological, as well as physical, dependence and is associated with active drug-seeking behavior and use (abuse) of the drugs for nonmedical conditions. Infants are incapable of this level of cognition and therefore cannot become addicted to analgesics and sedatives.[118,280] Tolerance, dependence, and withdrawal can occur with opioids and benzodiazepines. Medications should not be restricted because of fear of addiction. Family members should be made aware of this.

Critically ill infants sometimes need long-term infusions of opioids or benzodiazepines to provide analgesia and sedation. ECMO and prolonged mechanical ventilation are two examples of this situation. Use of fentanyl for more than 5 to 7 days can lead to tolerance and withdrawal (also known as *opioid abstinence syndrome;* see Chapter 11). Tapering doses to wean neonates off opioids will depend on the duration of the medication's use and the infant's response to the changes. For short-term use, decrease opioid dose by 25% to 50% of the drug dose per day, so that the drug is discontinued within 2 to 3 days. For longer opioid use, decrease doses by no more than 10% to 20% every 1 to 3 days. Infusion regimens can be changed to intermittent administration before the drug is discontinued.[293] Oral forms of opioids should be used whenever possible. Shorter-acting medications such as fentanyl and midazolam can be switched to methadone and lorazepam, which have the advantage of being longer acting and being available in an oral form. Addition of oral clonidine 1.5 to 3 mcg/kg two times daily (BID) can help alleviate withdrawal symptoms. The dose of clonidine can be titrated up to 5 to 10 mcg/kg BID as tolerated. The side effects of clonidine include bradycardia, hypotension, and sedation. In addition, minimal handling and a quiet, darkened environment help decrease external stimuli. A pacifier, swaddling, and holding are effective comfort measures.

PARENT TEACHING

Mothers of neonates in the NICU report dissatisfaction with pain management, worry about their infant's pain and pain management, and want to participate in comforting their distressed infants.[98,102,300] A multicenter international study is the first to provide a comprehensive description of parental concerns, distress, information needs, and involvement in care of their infant in pain.[98] Both mothers and fathers from 11 NICUs participated in completing questionnaires: (1) both parents reported a moderate degree of stress, (2) stress responses were slightly higher for mothers, (3) mothers' stress was related to the sights and sounds of the NICU and their inability to perform their maternal role, and (4) mothers reported higher anxiety levels. Specific parental concerns about pain included (1) effects of pain on the infant, (2) immediate medical problems caused by pain, and (3) long-term effects of pain. Parents reported few worries about the effects of pain medications. Parents rated their infant's worst pain as moderate to severe and had expected there to be less pain and that their infant would receive a high degree of pain relief. A more recent study showed that pain management was a priority concern for parents and that seeing their babies in pain and being unable to protect them from pain was very stressful.[172] An RCT to increase parental involvement in pain management for their NICU infants was conducted to evaluate reduction in parental stress and postdischarge parenting ability.[101] Although NICU-related stress was not reduced, parents who received information about pain and comforting techniques were better prepared to be active participants in their infant's pain care and have more positive views about their parenting role after discharge.[101]

Parents in two studies received primarily verbal information (i.e., 81%[102] and 58%[99]) rather than any written (4%)[99] information about pain and pain relief. Nurses (41%) more commonly than physicians (28%) provided information about pain to parents.[99] Although parents usually were satisfied with the pain information they received, 30% indicated that they wished they had received more information about infant pain.[99] Fifty percent of parents reported that they were shown how to recognize if their infant was in pain and how to provide comfort.[102] In the more recent study, 18% of parents were shown how to assess pain in their infant, and 55% were shown how to comfort the infant.[99]

In the multicenter study, 57% of parents reported that they would prefer to be with their infant during procedures.[102] Yet most parents had never (52%) or not often (24%) been asked about their preference. Parents who would have preferred to be absent during procedures reported higher stress levels, anxiety, and current worry about pain for their infant than did parents who preferred to be present. Eighty-seven percent of parents stated that they wanted greater involvement in their infant's pain care. Generally, the parents in this survey reported a high level of satisfaction with their infant's pain care.[99]

Parental stress was related to (1) their estimation of infant pain, (2) their worries about infant pain, and (3) their degree of satisfaction about information about infant pain care.[99] The influences of these factors on the degree of parental stress were "strikingly consistent" among the diverse NICUs in the study. More research is needed to determine whether (1) more parental information, involvement, and satisfaction with pain care reduces parental stress; (2) greater parental involvement in pain care improves parent-infant attachment, interaction, competence, and confidence after discharge; (3) culturally and socially diverse families respond similarly; and (4) barriers exist to providing more parental information and facilitating more involvement.[99]

The lack of information (Box 12-8) and passive involvement of parents in pain care for their infant[99,272] should be addressed in the NICU. Parents are excellent observers of their infant and often recognize when the infant is experiencing pain even before the care provider does.[20] The health care provider loses credibility and parental trust when he or she does not acknowledge and effectively treat the infant's pain.[209] Listening to parents' concerns about their infant's pain, including the parents' report of their assessment, communicating the plan of care about analgesia or sedation, and offering the rationale behind the medication decision making help the parents

---

BOX 12-8

PARENT TEACHING

PAIN IN NEWBORNS

- The body that is in pain is "stressful" to the infant.
- The body that is in pain cannot grow, cannot heal, and may not survive.
- Newborn infants, both full-term and preterm, feel pain in the NICU. Remember that pain (and repeated pain) may have long-term consequences.
- Newborns in the NICU deserve to have their pain assessed, adequately treated with medications and comfort measures, and reevaluated to determine whether the therapies have relieved their pain.
- Newborn infants, both full-term and preterm, DO NOT become "addicted" to medications that are used for pain relief, although they may develop tolerance and withdrawal, which can be managed by the health care provider.
- Comforting distressed infants and children is basic to the maternal/paternal role.
- No research or reports have documented a newborn forming a negative association with the mother/parent while she or he was providing comfort during a painful event.
- Research shows that skin-to-skin contact with mother before, during, and after a painful procedure decreases the pain response in preterm and full-term infants.[123]
- Breastfeeding full-term and preterm newborns before, during, and after a painful procedure markedly decreases their pain response (e.g., crying, grimacing, less tachycardia).[122,267]

---

become active participants in the management of their infant's pain.

Parents of medically fragile infants have identified specific sources of stress in the NICU: (1) parental role alterations, especially inability to comfort the infant, and (2) infant appearance and behavior, especially pain and difficulty breathing. The most common fear expressed by parents is that their infant will experience undue pain while being cared for in the NICU. Three years after their infant's NICU experience, mothers can still recall the pain and procedures that their infants endured.[322] The care provider's sensitivity to the neonate's pain and advocating for pain relief are comforting for parents.[98,209,320] Teaching parents to report their assessments and encouraging parents to comfort their infants will help them in the attachment process and foster a trusting relationship with the health care team. Comfort measures are ideally provided by parents, who may then actively participate in their infant's pain relief.[38,78,101]

REFERENCES

For a full list of references, scan the QR code or visit http://booksite.elsevier.com/9780323320832.

13 THE NEONATE AND THE ENVIRONMENT
Impact on Development

SANDRA L. GARDNER, EDWARD GOLDSON, AND JACINTO A. HERNÁNDEZ

For centuries the newborn baby has been considered a *tabula rasa*—a blank slate on which parents and the world "write" to create the individual. In the first half of the 20th century, research emphasized the contributions of the environment in shaping the infant and child. Only recently has the individuality of the infant been recognized as a powerful shaper of the caregiver, the care given, and thus the environment.

This chapter explores the psychosocioemotional development of term and preterm neonates. Infant development is a reflection of the dynamic relationship between endowment and environment. Understanding the dynamic relationship between endowment and environment is enhanced by a review of the principles of development in Box 13-1. First, the developmental tasks of infancy are presented, along with the influences of endowment and environment on mastery. Home and family life, in which most infants are raised, is then contrasted with the experiences of babies in the neonatal intensive care unit (NICU). Intervention strategies to normalize the NICU environment also are presented, along with strategies for parent teaching. The developmental and social outcomes of infants exposed to the NICU are then presented.

DEVELOPMENTAL TASKS OF THE NEONATE AND INFANT

Neonates begin extrauterine life able to attend with their sensory capabilities, communicate with their environment through a complex repertoire of behaviors, and store remembrances. Infancy (birth to 12 months) is the time of further development and maturation of these capabilities through self-mastery and adaptation to the extrauterine environment.

Biorhythmic Balance: The Primary Developmental Task of Newborns

In utero, the fetus depends on the mother's physiologic systems to regulate its own systems. At birth, the neonate's basic physiologic needs (i.e., feeding, elimination, cleaning, heat balance, stroking, communicating) are met in new and different ways. The process of emerging from a physiologically dependent state as a fetus into a physiologically independent neonate introduces new variables for both mother and infant in the development of their extrauterine relationship.

The primary task of newborns is to establish independent biorhythmic balance by stabilizing the function of sleep-wake cycles, respiratory and heart rates, blood chemistry levels, metabolic processes, and eating patterns. Biorhythmic balance is the establishment of innate, cyclic recurrence of biologic functions. Although biorhythmic balance is internally determined, caregiving interaction between newborn and parent or caregiver either facilitates or disturbs this transition.[254] After birth, this balance is facilitated by contact with familiar surroundings (the mother's body) (see Chapter 5).

When immediate recontact between the neonate and the mother is not possible (e.g., when the mother refuses or is ill) or when the neonate is preterm or sick and requires immediate emergency medical intervention or transport, the primary "mothering" role is temporarily transferred to professional (medical and nursing) care providers. Interactional dynamics

PURPLE type highlights content that is particularly applicable to clinical settings.

BOX 13-1 PRINCIPLES OF DEVELOPMENT

- Development is a continuous process of increasing complexity from conception to maturation (i.e., development also occurs in utero).
- Growth (i.e., number and size of cells) and development are influenced by genetic traits and environmental experiences.
- Development occurs in an orderly sequence, largely determined by readiness or maturation.
- The sequence of development is the same in all children; the rate of development is individual.
- Development is cephalocaudad (head→foot), centripetal (from the outside toward the center) and from gross to specific (e.g., peripheral→central→lateralization).
- The first 5 years are marked by a rapid period of growth of all body systems. During this time, behavior patterns are developed and are greatly influenced by the environment.
- Environmental stimulation influences conceptual development and has an effect on cognitive function.
- Learning occurs when behavioral change does not result solely from maturation; learning is facilitated by reinforcement of the behavior through experience.
- Development of the infant occurs within the framework of interaction with a caregiver and the family.
- Equifinality postulates multiple paths to the same developmental outcome: complex developmental patterns rather than simple development milestones.

Modified from Barnard K, Erikson M: *Teaching children with developmental problems,* ed 2, St Louis, 1976, Mosby; Illingworth RS: *The development of the infant and the young child,* ed 5, Edinburgh, 1972, Churchill-Livingstone.

necessary for reestablishing biorhythmic balance and fostering the psychosocioemotional development of the newborn also are transferred into the NICU.

Just as in a home or family setting, the infant's personality and behavioral development are affected by the nature and dynamics of the stimuli and relationships encountered with the staff in a nursery or NICU setting. The level of function or dysfunction in the biorhythmic balance affects the neonate's long-range outcomes and is interwoven with the development of a sense of self and a basic trust.

Sense of Self

In utero, the fetus has continuous tactile-kinesthetic stimulation that contributes to the development and maturation of the central nervous system (CNS)

and establishes kinesthesis as the most natural pathway for growth and development. The interaction between infants and the extrauterine environment also is kinesthetic. However, tactile contact and vestibular stimulation are also essential for (1) the development of a physical identity (body image), (2) organization and sorting of stimuli, (3) coordination of sensorimotor skills, (4) a psychologic and social sense of self, (5) normal neurophysiologic development (mental and cognitive abilities), and (6) emotional stability and temperament.[40]

Daily caregiving and interactions such as feeding, diapering, holding, and playing with the parent or caregiver provide infants with reciprocal stimuli for further developing their identity. Through the manner in which the infant is handled, he or she receives messages about how the caregiver feels about him or her.

Response cues given by an infant affect the caregiver's response to and interaction with the infant.[9,40] As the infant quiets in response to caregiving, the parent is positively reinforced to continue nurturing and soothing behavior. Withdrawal, irritability, or continuous crying is perceived by the caregiver as rejection or inadequacy and may result in parental frustration, depression, withdrawal, and decreased interaction. Repeated exposure to the caregiver's style and nonverbal messages thus enables the infant to adapt to these patterns of caregiving. The self of the infant is formed through interaction with people and objects within the environment.

Because the nature (amount and type) of the kinesthetic interaction between infants and caregivers influences how infants develop and mature, a lack of appropriate stimulation can have long-term negative consequences. Stimulus deprivation results in impairment or retardation of, or deviancy in, skill development for productive living. The degree or extent of impairment depends on the severity of the restrictions and limitations encountered.[40,304] Institutionally reared infants who had minimal contact and no social interaction with their caregivers displayed significant developmental delays.[266] The effect of kinesthetic deprivation was seen in the minimal expression of social skills (e.g., cooing, babbling, crying), minimal interest in objects in the environment, increased self-stimulation (rocking), touch aversion, flat or withdrawn affect, and retarded mental and motor development. Environmental deprivation may also affect the physical growth of the infant. Montagu[225] stated that infants can overcome mental and nutritional deprivation as long as they are not deprived of tactile stimulation.

The Psychosocial Task: Trust versus Mistrust[96]

Trust versus mistrust in self and the environment is solidified during infancy.[9] The response of the environment from the moment of birth is the means through which neonates continue to develop trust in themselves and decide on the reliability of their new environment. Two major factors influence the development of trust versus mistrust: (1) the infant's ability to communicate needs to the environment and (2) the reliability and contingency of the responding environment.

In the course of routine caregiving, an infant associates the caregiver with either comfort and trust or lack of need satisfaction and mistrust. The infant cries to communicate a need (e.g., "I'm hungry"; "I'm wet"). The caregiver responds to the infant and meets the need—the infant is fed; the diaper is changed. Thus, the newborn learns to communicate when the need arises again, because the environment or caregiver has responded and will respond. This *contingent response* of the caregiver to the infant's need is the necessary reinforcement for the development of trust in self, others, and ultimately humankind. As a result, the infant develops a sense of mastery over his or her world and a sense that it is okay to experience needs and that they will be met.

Caregiving that ignores or delays needs gratification is *noncontingent* to the infant's cues for care. Need meeting that is externally defined by the caregiver's agenda (e.g., feeding schedule, rigid or inflexible routines, medical or nursing procedures in the NICU) discourages the infant from being aware of and experiencing needs and communicating them. Such infants eventually detach themselves (emotionally and kinesthetically) from the sensation of their needs, thus no longer experiencing or communicating them.[41]

As a result, these infants conclude that they and their needs (which they perceive as one and the same) are not important and that they have no effect on their environment. They do not cultivate their sense of self or their own existence, physically (where their boundaries end and another's begin) or psychologically (their identity, which exists independent of another).

Survival depends on the caregiver's meeting the newborn's needs. Need meeting is either contingent on the infant's cues or noncontingent on an external agenda. The degree of the mother's emotional investment and connectedness with the newborn will determine the nature and quality of the caregiving. Likewise, the temperament and responsiveness of the infant will affect the mother's feelings of competence, success, and emotional connectedness to her infant.[41] This relationship facilitates the ongoing development of a good sense of self (e.g., esteem, confidence, emotional security) and mastery of the world. Caregivers who do not perceive infants as individuals do not respond to their "need cry" or interact with them during caregiving. This style fosters the development of mistrusting, suspicious, helpless, emotionally insecure, and isolated children and adults.

ENDOWMENT

Infants possess innateness and individuality. Primitive reflex behaviors, higher cognitive abilities, temperament, and sensorimotor competencies are the endowment of the individual infant. Individual variation and use of these endowments are influenced by the environment of the newborn.

Even before conception, the genetic endowment of the parents and preceding generations affects the fetus or newborn. Everything that the individual will inherit from his or her parents is determined at the moment of conception. Of the vast number of possible combinations of chromosomes, chance determines which characteristics the individual receives. Thus each individual, except monozygotic twins, is genetically and biologically different from every other person. Either a faulty gene (e.g., sickle cell anemia) or an altered number of chromosomes (e.g., Down syndrome) is responsible for inherited defects (see Chapter 27).

Although after the moment of conception, hereditary endowment can never be changed, it is influenced by the intrauterine environment. Some birth defects are caused by teratogens or poisons—any environmental agent (e.g., drugs, virus, chemical, pollutant) that interferes with normal fetal development. An individual's potential for growth and development is strongly influenced by his or her genetic endowment. As Montagu[225] stated, "Genetic endowment determines what we can do—environment what we do do."

The exact influence of genetics for most psychologic traits is unknown. Introverted (timid, shy, withdrawn) and extroverted (active, friendly, outgoing) personality types may be partially genetically controlled. The degree to which intelligence is inherited is currently unknown, although the intelligence of children is most often similar to parental intelligence (i.e., intelligence is more similar between child and biologic mother than between child and adoptive mother).

Freedman[115] studied newborns of many ethnic groups to determine whether there were any similarities in disposition within the group or differences from other ethnic groups. He found that Chinese American newborns were more adaptable, less irritable, and easier to console than Caucasian American newborns. Maneuvers such as the Moro and covering the face with a cloth elicited different responses, depending on the newborn's ethnic origin.

The same environmental stimuli elicit different behavioral responses, which are individual and genetically influenced. These genetically influenced behaviors are also influenced by environment—both internal and external. Thus, an individual may be more vulnerable to or more resilient in a specific environment. Therefore, we are totally endowment and totally environment (100% endowment + 100% environment = an individual).[115]

Temperament

Parents often notice behavioral differences in their children from the first day. These differences are obvious in motor activity, irritability, and passivity. Some infants are quiet and placid, others are irritable and easily upset, and others are somewhere in between (Table 13-1). These temperamental qualities enable the following three basic types of infants to be identified:

- The "easy" child, who is seen as regular, pleasant, and easy to care for and love
- The "difficult" child, who is difficult to rear and reacts with protest and withdrawal to strange events or people
- The "slow to warm" child, who reacts with withdrawal or passivity to new events

Neurologic Development

Brain growth of the fetus and newborn occurs in two stages.[80]

STAGE I

Stage I is from 10 to 18 weeks of pregnancy. The number of nerve cells that the individual has develops during this period. Any environmental

perturbation (e.g., maternal malnutrition, medications, infections) that affects brain growth during this stage also may affect neonatal behavioral responses.

STAGE II

Stage II is from 20 weeks' gestation to 2 years of age. This period marks a brain growth spurt and is the most vulnerable period of growth of the dendrites of the human cortex.

The maturity of an infant is reflected in his or her behavior. Infants of a younger gestational age have less mature responses than infants of an older gestational age. A neurologic assessment of the newborn includes evaluation of (1) newborn reflexes, (2) neonatal states, (3) psychosocial interaction, and (4) sensory capabilities. The neonate is born with behaviors that are unlearned, instinctual, and of an adaptive and survival nature. They reflect the state of the nervous system and the level of neonatal maturation (Table 13-2). Serial testing of reflex behavior gives more reliable data than one observation. Observations indicative of major deviations include asymmetry—total absence or no response on one side or in upper versus lower extremities.

Psychologic Interaction and Neonatal States

For years, newborn behavior was thought to occur only on a reflexive, instinctual level. Through the work of Brazelton[43] and others, newborns have been shown to have the ability to interact with and shape their environment. With the Neonatal Behavioral Assessment Scale (NBAS),[43] care providers can observe and score the interactive behavior of newborns. The NBAS enables assessment of the infant's individual capabilities for social relationships rated on the infant's best performance. Six categories of abilities are considered in evaluating an infant's performance: habituation, orientation to auditory and visual stimuli, motor maturity, state changes, self-quieting ability, and social behaviors.

Response decrement (i.e., *habituation*) is the protective mechanism through which a fetus or infant decreases responsivity to external stimuli. Habituation represents the cerebral behavior of memory—the fetus or infant stores the memory

TABLE 13-1	CRITICAL FINDINGS BEHAVIORAL CATEGORIES DESCRIPTIVE OF INDIVIDUAL TEMPERAMENT

TEMPERAMENTAL QUALITY	RATING
Activity level	*Low*—Decreased movement when dressed or during sleep *High*—Increased movement when asleep; increased wiggling and activity when diaper changed
Rhythmicity	*Regular*—Establishes own feeding; sleep and bowel movement patterns are fairly predictable *Irregular*—Amounts of sleep, feeding variable; "no 2 days are alike"; no pattern established
Approach and withdrawal	*Positive*—Eagerly tries new foods, interested in new surroundings and people *Negative*—Rejects new foods, new toys, and new environments; apprehensive, cries with new people
Adaptability	*Adaptive*—Little resistance to first bath; may enjoy bath *Nonadaptive*—Startles easily; resists diapering, bathing, and other manipulating
Quality of mood	*Positive*—Pleasant, easygoing disposition; easy to comfort; smiles *Negative*—Fussy; cries easily and is not easily comforted by external stimuli; unable to comfort self easily
Intensity of mood	*Mild*—No crying when wet; frets instead of crying when hungry *Intense*—Vigorously cries; rejects food
Sensory threshold (intensity of stimulus necessary to elicit a response)	*High*—Not startled or interested by noise or other stimuli *Low*—Noise, activity, or other stimuli enough to interrupt infant's behavior
Distractibility	*Distractible*—Rocking, pacifier, toy, voice, music decrease fussing *Nondistractible*—No stimuli decrease distress until need is met—food; stop changing diaper; bath over
Attention span and persistence	*Short*—Cries when awakened but stops immediately, mild objection if needs are not immediately met *Long*—Repeatedly rejects substitutions for perceived needs (no pacifier until diaper is changed; no water if milk is wanted)

Data from Thomas A, Chess S: *Temperament and development,* New York, 1977, Brunner-Mazel.

of the stimulus and, with repeated presentation, learns not to respond.[232] Infants who are able to habituate are not interested in nonnovel repetition in the environment and protect themselves from overstimulation.

Infants who become "bored" with their toys have habituated to them—infants like variety. *Dishabituation* represents increasing attention to a new stimulus (e.g., new mobile, toy, face) after habituation to an old stimulus. The fetus or infant thus "recognizes" the novelty of the new stimulus and chooses to respond.

An infant who is unable to habituate will continue to react vigorously to the same stimuli. Compared with term infants, preterm infants are more reactive (e.g., less able to control their level of excitation) and less able to self-regulate (e.g., modulate reactivity, reflected in habituation rate and self-soothing abilities).[90] Very-low-birth-weight (VLBW) infants are less able to (1) modulate attention, (2) take brief breaks from

processing information, and (3) habituate to stimuli.[90] Thus the preterm is less able to deal with multiple sources of stimuli and thus is easily overstimulated.[5]

Neonates are able to imitate the facial and manual gestures of adults.[221] Infants as young as 12 days imitate gestures such as mouth opening and tongue protrusion. Because a neonate has never seen his or her own face, this innate ability to match behaviors to those of another is a remarkable use of the cerebral cortex. Imitation may operate as a positive feedback mechanism to caregivers; thus it is significant in parent-infant reciprocity and represents early learning behaviors.

Learning, a function of the cerebral cortex, occurs with habituation and imitation. Early cognitive development is important to later learning and future cognitive function. Learning occurs in the context of experience and influences structural maturation; there is marked CNS development during the first 2 years of life.[43,80]

TABLE 13-2	CRITICAL FINDINGS
	NEONATAL REFLEX BEHAVIORS

BEHAVIOR	BEGINS (IN UTERO) (wk)	INTEGRATES
	PROTECTION	
Moro reflex	28	At 6–8 mo to allow sitting and protective extension of the hands
Palmar grasp	28	At 5–6 mo to allow voluntary grasping of objects
Plantar grasp	28	At 7–8 mo with foot rubbing on objects; complete at 8–9 mo for standing and walking
Babinski reflex	28	Same as for plantar grasp
Tonic neck reflex	35	At 4 mo, so rolling over and reaching or grasping may occur
Gag* reflex	36	Protects against aspiration — does not disappear
Blink reflex	25	Does not disappear
Crossed extension	28	Disappears around 2 mo of age
	SURVIVAL	
Rooting*	28	At 3 mo; decreased response if baby is sleepy or satiated
Sucking*	26–28	Not yet synchronized with swallowing
Swallowing*	12	32–34 wk, stronger synchronization with sucking; perfect by 34–37 wk

*Although isolated components of feeding behaviors are all present before 28 weeks' gestational age, they are not effectively coordinated for oral feedings before 32 to 34 weeks' gestational age.[123,219,291] Coordination of respiration with sucking and swallowing during bottle feeding is consistently achieved by infants more than 37 weeks' postconceptual age.[47]

State of consciousness influences the reactions of a newborn to internal and external stimuli. The infant's state at the time of observation must be considered in interpretation of the findings (Table 13-3).

Clinical application of the NBAS includes evaluation of infant capabilities after illness, prematurity, or maternal medications. The most important application of the NBAS is in anticipatory guidance for parents. Demonstration of parts of the examination for parents enables them to become familiar with their infant's individual patterns of behavior, temperament, and states.

Circadian Rhythm

Circadian rhythms are cyclic variations in function that occur daily at about the same time. Humans cycle their bodily functions (e.g., temperature, hormonal changes, blood pressure, urine volume, sleep-wake cycles) in a 24-hour period.[273,274] These daily fluctuations are innately controlled by the individual's "biologic clock" in the suprachiasmatic nuclei (SCN) in the anterior hypothalamus. The SCN are located at the base of the third ventricle, above the optic chiasm.[228] The circadian pacemaker must be reset daily by the relay of photic (light) information from the retina to the SCN, along the direct pathway from the retinohypothalamic tract (RHT) to the SCN.[273] During the 18th week of prenatal life, the SCN form and continue maturation after birth. In utero, the fetus expresses endogenous circadian rhythms (in heart/respiratory rates and steroid secretion) that are influenced by the mother.[273] The RHT has been identified in human newborns of 36 weeks' gestation; SCN are functionally innervated by the retina at stages equivalent to 25 weeks after conception in human infants.[273]

In infants, the development of circadian rhythm is influenced by genetic factors, gender, brain maturation, and the environment.[273-275,328] There are individual differences in the development of circadian rhythms, in both preterm and full-term infants.[272-275,328] These circadian rhythms in the neonate are influenced by feeding, environmental lighting, interactions with mother, and chronologic/postconceptual age.[272-275,327,328] Intrauterine growth

TABLE 13-3	CRITICAL FINDINGS
	NEWBORN STATES AND CONSIDERATIONS FOR CAREGIVING

NEWBORN STATE	COMMENTS
SLEEP STATES	
Deep sleep (non–rapid-eye-movement [REM] or quiet sleep): Slow state changes Regular breathing Eyes closed; no eye movements No spontaneous activity except startles and jerky movements Startles with some delay and suppresses rapidly Lowest oxygen consumption	Infant is difficult if not impossible to arouse. Infant will not breastfeed or bottle feed in this state, even after vigorous stimulation. Infant is unable to respond to environment, which is frustrating for caregivers. Term infants may exhibit a "slow" heart rate (80–90 beats/min), which may trigger heart rate alarms and result in unnecessary stimulation by NICU staff. At birth, preterm infants have altered states of consciousness. Early dominant states are light sleep, quiet, and active alert. "Protective apathy" enables the preterm to remain inactive, unresponsive, and in a sleep state to conserve energy, grow, and maintain physiologic homeostasis.[273] As maturation occurs, there is an increase in quiet alert.
Light sleep (REM or active sleep): Low activity level Random movements and startles Respirations irregular and abdominal Intermittent sucking movements Eyes closed, REM Higher oxygen consumption	Full-term infants begin and end sleep in active sleep; preterm infants are more responsive (than term infants) to stimuli in active sleep. Infant may cry or fuss briefly in this state and be awakened to feed before truly awake and ready to eat. Lower and more variable oxygenation states.
AWAKE STATES	
Drowsy or semidozing: Eyelids fluttering Eyes open or closed (dazed) Mild startles (intermittent) Delayed response to sensory stimuli Smooth state change after stimulation Fussing may or may not be present Respirations are more rapid and shallow	Infants may awaken further or return to sleep (if left alone). Quietly talking and looking at the infant or offering a pacifier or an inanimate object to see and listen to may arouse the infant to the quiet, alert state. Less mature infants (30 weeks) demonstrate a more drowsy than quiet alert state than more mature infants (36 weeks).
Quiet alert, with bright look: Focuses attention on source of stimulation Impinging stimuli may break through; may have some delay in response Minimal motor activity	Immediately after birth, term newborns exhibit a period of quiet alert, which is their first opportunity to "take in" their parents and the extrauterine environment. Dimmed lights, quiet talking, and stroking optimize this time for parents. Best state for learning to occur, because infant focuses all of attention on visual, auditory, tactile, and sucking stimuli; best state for interaction with parents — infant is maximally able to attend and reciprocally respond to parents.
Active alert — eyes open: Considerable motor activity — thrusting movements of extremities; spontaneous startles Reacts to external stimuli with increase in movements and startles (discrete reactions difficult to differentiate because of general higher activity level) Respirations irregular May or may not be fussy	Infant has decreased threshold (increased sensitivity) to internal (hunger, fatigue) and external (wet, noise, handling) stimuli. Infant may quiet self, may escalate to crying, or with consolation by caregiver, may become quiet alert or go to sleep. Infant is unable to maximally attend to caregiver or environment because of increased motor activity and increased sensitivity to stimuli.
Crying — intense and difficult to disrupt with external stimuli Respirations rapid, shallow, and irregular	Crying is the infant's response to unpleasant internal or external stimulation — infant's tolerance limits have been reached (and exceeded). Infant may be able to quiet self with hand-to-mouth behaviors; talking may quiet a crying infant; holding, rocking, or putting infant upright on caregiver's shoulder may quiet infant.

Data from Blackburn S: *JOGN Nurse* 12(suppl 3):76S–86S, 1983; and Brazelton TB: *Neonatal behavioral assessment scale*, ed 2, Philadelphia, 1984, International Medical Publishers/Lippincott.

influences the development of circadian rhythms; in one study, more appropriate-for-gestational-age (AGA) than small-for-gestational-age (SGA) infants developed body temperature and heart rate rhythms.[124] More mature infants (i.e., greater postconceptual age) of 35 to 37 weeks' gestation have a higher amplitude on body temperature rhythm compared with infants of 32 to 34 weeks' gestation.[124] Infant biorhythms have been studied in the areas of temperature, heart and respiratory rates, blood pressure, sleep-wake cycles, rest-activity patterns, endocrine secretion, and feeding frequency.[124,273–275,327]

SLEEP CYCLES AND PATTERNS

Active (or light) sleep is characterized by rapid eye movements (REM), whereas quiet (or deep) sleep has no rapid eye movements (i.e., non-REM sleep; see Table 13-3). At 29 to 30 weeks' gestation, sleep differentiates into REM and non-REM sleep.[129] At birth and for the first few weeks of life, term newborns generally distribute sleep over a 24-hour period and sleep from 16 to 19 hours a day. As sleep begins, a term infant enters active, rather than quiet, sleep and spends more time in active sleep than does an adult.[84]

Active sleep durations vary from 10 to 45 minutes, whereas quiet sleep lasts about 20 minutes.[84] An infant's sleep cycle is 50 to 60 minutes, compared with an adult's 90- to 100-minute cycle. Although day-night rhythms are difficult to detect in the neonatal period, some infants exhibit such rhythms as early as 1 week of age.[273,274]

Maturation of infant sleep is characterized by (1) increased organization of sleep states, (2) decrease in total sleep time, (3) increase in quiet sleep, (4) decrease in active sleep, and (5) increase in active and quiet waking.[84] Arousability from sleep is altered by gestational and postnatal age. In term infants, arousal thresholds are significantly elevated in quiet sleep compared with active sleep (at 2–3 weeks and at 2–3 months of age), so that spontaneous arousal is greater in active (REM) than in quiet (non-REM) sleep.

Infants have their own "clock" for sleep-wake, hunger, and feeding or fussy times. This clock often does not coincide with the family's rhythms and may cause disruption and conflict. Sleep-wake states reflect the underlying status of the neurologic system. The infant's maturity at birth greatly affects his or her rhythms and development of normal circadian rhythm. Early relationships with caregivers provide the organization and stabilization necessary for sleep regulation, as well as other biologic functions.[327]

In preterm infants, active and quiet sleep cycles are less organized and of shorter duration (a sleep cycle is about 30–40 minutes) than in term infants.[83] Active sleep is "lighter" than quiet sleep—there is more response to stimuli in active sleep.[83] Quiet sleep is a more controlled state and occurs more frequently in term infants than in premature infants. Quiet sleep does not become significant in the preterm until approximately 36 weeks' gestation. Hence, a third sleep state, *transitional sleep,* has been identified for premature infants.[248] This state is characterized by quiet sleep with periods of closed eyes, regular or periodic respirations, no body movements, and no REM. Before 36 weeks' gestation, a preterm infant's predominant sleep state is transitional sleep. As the preterm infant matures, he or she spends progressively less time in transitional sleep, has more quiet than active sleep, and has more awake, alert time. However, a preterm of 40 weeks' postconceptual age does not have sleep patterns that are as organized as those of a term newborn.[248] Spontaneous arousal from sleep is greater in active sleep compared with quiet sleep. Long-term follow-up studies fail to show a difference in sleep distribution between preterm and term infants when corrected for age.[295] Both preterm and full-term infants who are exposed to an appropriate light intensity at home develop day-night rhythmicity by 44 and 48 weeks' postconceptual age, respectively.[274,275,295]

As day and night rhythms in sleep-wake cycles develop, diurnal rhythm in hormone production also develops: (1) melatonin production is detectable at 12 weeks of age; and (2) variations in cortisol levels appear between 3 and 6 months of age.[273] Sleep disruption may interfere with growth and development by altering neuronal maturation, cortex development, and growth hormone secretion.[4,49] Human growth hormone has a rhythmic pattern associated with sleep-wake cycles. The highest peaks of growth hormone in infants occur during REM (active) sleep. A fetus (29–32 weeks' gestation) spends 80% of the time in utero in REM sleep; a term newborn's sleep is 50% REM sleep.[83,84] Because growth hormone secretion depends on the regular recurrence of sleep, any disturbance of the sleep-wake cycle results in irregular spikes of growth hormone during a 24-hour period.

Sleep disruption, especially of REM sleep, also interferes with healthy visual development.[129]

Although infant circadian rhythms are synchronous with those of the mother, desynchronous rhythms at birth may occur.[248,273] An infant whose cycles are discrepant from his or her family's may be perceived as "difficult." Gradually, through caregiving, parents teach the infant synchronization with family rhythms.[327] By 9 months of age, most term infants develop day-night fluctuations that are similar to adult patterns.

Sensory Capabilities

At birth, a neonate's senses are developed and functioning. Sensory development proceeds in a specific order: tactile/vestibular, olfactory/gustatory, and auditory/visual. Stimuli (e.g., type, timing) to one sense affect the development of other senses. Sensory enhancement or deprivation of a later-developing sensory system (e.g., vision) could either accelerate or decelerate the development of behavior mediated by earlier-developing sensory systems (e.g., tactile and olfactory).[308] Through the neonate's sensory perception, learning occurs by (1) habituating to some stimuli while attending to other stimuli, (2) discriminating between related and unrelated sensory events, and (3) integrating multisensory stimuli. As the neonate takes in the sensory information, he or she associates features of the environment that occur together (e.g., sound, smell, sight, touch of "mother" or "father"), demonstrating complex and intermodal abilities for handling the sensory input from the environment.

TACTILE/KINESTHETIC

Touch is the major method of communication for neonates and infants. Touch is the first sense to develop (at about 7.5 weeks' gestational age) and the last sense to fade. In utero, a fetus's existence has been primarily one of movement—floating within the amniotic fluid and experiencing rhythmic maternal movements. The senses of touch, temperature, and pressure are all well developed, and receptors lie in the newborn's skin. Pleasant touch is associated with a slowing of the heart rate, a decrease in physiologic arousal, and increased engagement.[100] Even preterms as young as 28 weeks' gestation tactilely memorize the shape of an object by manipulating it in their hands and discriminate between objects.[201] The sensitivity to touch is especially well developed

in the face, around the lips (root reflex), and in the hands (grasp reflex). Because newborns are nonverbal, they pick up messages through the manner in which they are held and handled—by the adult's "body language." Infants are often barometers for adult feelings; if the adult is tired and irritable, the infant knows and may respond with irritability and crying.

Infants love to be held, rocked, and carried; note the soothing effects on a crying infant. Adults do not spoil infants by providing these important stimuli. Increased carrying of infants contributes to less crying at 6 weeks of age.[29] In response to being held, infants adjust their body posture to the body of the caregiver. Adults describe an infant as "cuddly" (assumes a comfortable, relaxed curl; snuggles to adult body; and attempts to root or suck) or "noncuddly" (sprawls; tenses or stiffens; and pushes away). The most comforting position for a crying infant is upright on an adult's shoulder.[164] Responsiveness to tactile stimulation has been found to be greater in female than in male neonates.[164]

HEARING

The fetus in utero has heard the voices of mother, father, and siblings beginning in the second trimester of pregnancy, at about 27 weeks of pregnancy.[228,229,308] These voices are "familiar" to newborns, so they "know" and have learned their family and are able to differentiate them from the voices of strangers.[71,72,228,229,232] Neonates prefer their mother's voice and the maternal language that they heard in utero.[229] Studies have suggested that fetuses and neonates exhibit memory.[71,72,229,232] Newborns who had been read a particular story while in utero responded to the story reread to them after birth with a recognition and attentiveness that was not exhibited in response to unfamiliar stories.[71,72] A more recent study presented fetuses with music five times per week and measured their brain activity at birth and at 4 months of age. Brain activity at birth and at 4 months of age was much stronger when the neonates and infants heard the "familiar" music they had listened to in utero.[249] The ability to hear the outside world, particularly the spoken word, is a prerequisite to further verbal language development.[228,229]

Fetal responses to sound include increases in breathing, body movements, fetal heart rate, cerebral blood flow, and glucose use and changes in behavior states, as well as recognizing and habituating to familiar sounds.[232] Neonates with an intact CNS are able to orient and respond to the auditory environment. In response to a sound, the neonate will demonstrate the following:

- Change in motor activity (eye blink, decrease in activity, limb movements, head turn)
- Change in heart rate (if the infant is quiet, the heart rate increases with stimuli; if the infant is crying, the heart rate decreases with stimuli) and/or change in respiration (increase in rate, decrease in amplitude, or decrease in respiratory cycle rate)
- Smile
- Startle or grimace
- Alert or arouse
- Cry or cease to cry
- Stop sucking

The response to sound depends on the sound's quality. The intensity of intrauterine noise is approximately 85 dB. When frequency and pitch are low, the infant is soothed and distress is decreased; high frequency and pitch alert and distress the infant and disturb sleep.

Frequencies less than 4000 Hz (the range of human speech is 500–3000 Hz) produce the most newborn response. Infants are maximally reactive to the human voice in typical speech patterns (rather than disconnected syllables). Infants prefer the high-pitched (e.g., female) voice over the low-pitched (e.g., male) voice.

Experience with sound improves an infant's behavioral responses to sound. Stimuli presented for 5 to 15 seconds elicit the best reaction. Stimuli lasting longer than several minutes are less effective because the term infant habituates to the sound and ceases responding. The ability to habituate to sound is indicative of an intact CNS.[232] Full-term newborns habituate to sound better and faster than do preterm infants. Infants exhibit startle behavior if the stimulus rapidly reaches maximal loudness. Infant state is important in evaluation of response to auditory stimuli; light sleep is the optimal state. Infants quiet and soothe in response to rhythmic sounds (rather than dysrhythmic ones). Neonates move their bodies in rhythmic synchrony *(entrainment)* with the spoken word.

VISION

Eye development begins 22 days after conception. The eyelids fuse at about 10 weeks' gestation and remain fused until about 26 weeks' gestation. Eyelid opening is a function of maturity—more mature neonates open their eyes more than younger gestation neonates. At birth, photoreceptors are already developed, but maturation is not complete for several months. The fetus can distinguish light from dark and recoils from a bright light shone at the mother's abdomen. Even at term birth, the visual system is immature; significant development occurs over the next 6 months to a year. The ability to fix, follow, and alert is indicative of an intact CNS.[223]

At birth, infants can see an object within 8 to 10 inches of the face (visual acuity of 20/140).[102] Within seconds after birth, the neonate can recognize his or her mother's face—the voice that he has heard for the last trimester of pregnancy comes from the face he now sees! The cradled-in-the-arms position of feeding is the exact distance from the adult's face that the newborn can see. In response to an interesting visual stimulus, neonates stop sucking to look, alert, and attend to the object; horizontally scan the object; and fix and follow a moving object in a 90-degree arc.

Infants prefer the human face as a visual stimulus, prefer a patterned over a nonpatterned stimulus and attend longer to larger patterns with more complex patterns and angles.[102] Infants prefer black and white because of the greater contrast and will focus on the outside of a figure where the contrast is the greatest[223]; color discrimination occurs around 2 to 3 months.[129] Newborns are sensitive to bright light and will tightly close their eyes in its presence. They prefer moderate, diffuse lighting. Newborns exposed to cycled light (e.g., day-night changes) open their eyes more than those exposed to continuous bright light. Presentation of visual stimuli enables development of the neural pattern for vision. During the infant's first year of life, visual investigation of the environment is a primary mode of learning.

SMELL AND TASTE

In utero, the fetus learns his mother's scent by exposure to amniotic fluid.[308] The fetus increases its amniotic fluid consumption when saccharin is added to the fluid and decreases consumption with the injection of distasteful substances. Taste may be a way the fetus monitors the intrauterine environment. Olfaction is well developed at full term and preterm birth.[202] Olfactory cues guide the full-term newborn to the maternal nipple. Flavors and smells in the mother's diet are present in amniotic fluid and in mother's breast milk so that infants show a preference for these familiar flavors and smells at birth and later in infancy.[308,326,330]

At 5 days of age, a neonate can differentiate his or her mother's breast pad and demonstrates a preference for the smell over that of a "stranger"; full-term newborns stop crying and increase their mouthing behaviors when exposed to their mother's odor.[309] The infant's response to pleasant odors is to arouse and suck. After several presentations of the stimulus, the infant will habituate to the odor. Infants withdraw from unpleasant odors such as vinegar and ammonia. They are also able to differentiate tastes, preferring sweet solutions[326,330] and refusing, by turning the head away, bitter, acid, and sour substances. Intrauterine growth restricted (IUGR) 1-day-old newborns have been shown to strongly prefer a sweet solution (24% sucrose) that is inversely related to their degree of IUGR.[21] Asphyxiated infants demonstrate a loss of olfaction that parallels the suppression of brainstem reflexes and activities.

COMMUNICATION SKILLS

A neonate's ability to communicate is a naturally endowed survival skill. Crying is an infant's language to communicate needs.[192] Crying also may be a response to the environment: noisy, cold, overstimulating, multiple caregiving, or lack of synchrony. Because the cry brings someone to meet the need, the infant soon learns that the caregiver gives attention and the world is a trustworthy place. The more responsive the caregiver is to the infant's crying, and thus the infant's needs, the less crying behavior is necessary.[29,192] Learning occurs as the infant associates comfort with the caregiver. The temperament of the individual infant and his or her ability to habituate to disturbing stimuli influence the amount of crying behavior. Tension in the caregiver or the environment is communicated nonverbally to the infant and may potentiate or contribute to the infant's crying.

The amount and tone of the newborn's cry are influenced by birth weight, gestational age, and the events of birth. Types of cries include birth cry, hunger cry, pain cry, and pleasure cry.[59,60] Infants separated from their mothers in the first 90 minutes after birth exhibit a "separation distress call" (also seen in other mammal species) that ceases at reunion.[59,60] The newborn's cry physiologically affects the mother: her breasts change and prepare to nurse. Neonates possess a repertoire of self-quieting behaviors when in a fussy

state: (1) hand-to-mouth efforts, (2) sucking on fist or tongue, and (3) use of visual or auditory stimuli from the environment.[43]

After birth, crying develops a diurnal pattern: term infants cry more during the day than at night. Persistent crying (>3 hours a day) is more likely in breastfed babies, whereas early-evening crying is more likely by formula-fed infants. Postnatal age is a significant predictor of crying. Crying decreases with increasing chronologic age.[316] The neonatal cry may be a signal of robustness or wellness, a signal of pain, or diagnostic of existing conditions or trauma. CNS insult often results in a high-pitched, shrill cry.

A smiling infant is a joy to the caregiver. Smiling may be either spontaneous (from birth) or a response to the social human face (at 4–12 weeks of life). A smile is most easily elicited by the stimulus of a moving, smiling human face. The ability to smile begins before 40 weeks in a preterm infant, as observed during REM sleep. The social implications of the smile include positive feedback to the caregiver that the infant is happy and contented, which results in parental feelings of adequacy and competence.

ENVIRONMENT

Prenatal Environment

In utero, the fetus depends totally on the mother's emotional and physical health and well-being for his or her own. Through the mother the fetus receives nurturance, housing, and stimulation to develop the body, the sensory organs, and the rudiments of personality and temperament.

Conditions present at birth may not be congenital but, rather, the result of the effect of uterine environmental conditions on development. Maternal-fetal programming, known as the *Barker hypothesis,*[26] postulates that the maternal prenatal environment influences the developing fetal brain and also the long-term permanent effects on health and susceptibility to disease.[44,233]

Intrapartal Environment

Birth is a major transition from physiologic dependence to physiologic independence. At term, a neonate's physiologic systems are developed, sensory organs function, and the foundation of personality and temperament is established. Birth is disorienting and disruptive. The amount of disruption depends on the degree of trauma incurred during the labor and birth processes. Not having a social support system compounds the stress, often escalating it beyond the mother's tolerance and coping skills. Anxious and fearful women have longer labors and more delivery complications than women who are confident about themselves and their infants.[286] The shift toward family-centered birth enables mothers to receive support from their families, be an active participant in the birth process, and have immediate contact with their newborns (see Chapter 29)

A neonate also is influenced by medications and the events of labor and birth (see Chapter 2). Maternal medications for analgesia and anesthesia affect neonatal behaviors, resulting in decreased sucking ability, lethargy, and decreased habituation. They also give less feedback to their parents than do unmedicated infants. The parents may feel rejected, tend to stimulate the infant less, and thus begin a pattern of suboptimal interaction.

Postnatal Environment

Home and family are the primary media through which newborns (1) reestablish their biorhythmic balance, (2) stabilize themselves in the extrauterine world, (3) develop a sense of self and mastery in the world, and (4) become socialized as human beings. Socialization teaches the adaptive psychosocial skills necessary for survival and functioning in society. Cultural and family values, behavioral expression, and ways of meeting social and emotional needs are learned within the family. Thus, the home and family environment is considered to be a "socializing" environment for human development.

CAREGIVER FACTORS
The dyadic relationship continues postpartum between the caregiver and the infant—the behavior of one reinforces the behavior of the other. The infant's physical and emotional needs are satisfied by caregivers. The infant's response to the caregiver depends on how the infant perceives and receives ministrations; this response affects the level of emotional satisfaction the caregiver receives from the interaction. Parental expectations have a major effect on their perceptions and their behavior and ultimately affect the child's development. Parents must work out the discrepancy between the wished-for and the actual child, especially if the

infant is preterm or ill or has an anomaly. How attached the parents are to the infant influences their relationship with and ability to care for their infant (see Chapter 29). If the pregnancy has failed to produce a normal, healthy infant, the parents must grieve the loss of their expectations. Parents have problems attaching to and caring for the infant until they have completed their grief work (see Chapter 30).

A caregiver and an infant have a reciprocal interaction when their cycles and signals are synchronized with each other. The biorhythmic cycle of the newborn has been in synchrony with one person (mother) in utero, and the infant is accustomed to her cycles and rhythms for developing adaptive behavior. Consistent, sensitive maternal caregiving enables a newborn to regulate his or her rhythms to those of the mother and begin adapting to the postnatal environment.[293,303] From her, they expand their adaptation to the family and the larger world of society.

Experience in relating to infants influences the caregiver's efficiency in interpretation of and sensitivity to infant cues. Multiparous women have more sensitivity to infant cues than do primiparous mothers. Mothers with little or no experience exhibit more difficulty in quieting a crying infant. The competence of parents may be improved through acquisition of knowledge about infants, so that the quality of interaction between parent and infant is enhanced. Better informed first-time mothers may result in significant differences in sensitivity to infant cues and social and emotional growth fostering behaviors in early (first 24 hours) mother-infant interaction.[341] In addition to experience, maternal hormones, oxytocin and estrogen, enable mothers to retain and respond to their infant's vocal cues.[25,306]

Consistency and sensitivity in maternal responses[303] is especially important as the infant continues to learn the accepted patterns of cues from the caregiver. Cared for by one or two people, an infant is able to develop synchrony with and expectations of the parents. Single caregiving improves establishment of biorhythms for sleep-wake cycles, feeding, and visual attentiveness. Consistent cues soon elicit a consistency of response from the infant. Consistency and promptness of maternal (and other caregivers) response results in less infant crying during the first year of life. A predictable and responsive environment enables the infant to progress to varied types of communication (not just crying). Care by parents provides for mutual cueing and mastery of the environment through interaction. Inconsistent cues distress and confuse the infant. Multiple caregivers, who may not be knowledgeable about a particular infant, may confuse the infant, increase distress with feeding, cause irritability, and upset visual attention.

Regardless of how stable or unstable, consistent or inconsistent it is, family life has a rhythm, synchronicity, and predictability of its own. Through interaction with parents and siblings, infants further develop their ability to form relationships. From these primary relationships, the foundation and format for other relationships are established. The quality of subsequent relationships depends on the quality of the relationship experienced within the primary family from birth throughout infancy.[125]

NEONATAL FACTORS

The neonate is not a passive recipient of the environment of the family but, rather, is an active participant in shaping that environment. Infants send cues about their ability and readiness for interpersonal interactions. In their first 4 months of life, infants' interactions with persons differ from their interactions with inanimate objects. The excitement generated by interpersonal interaction is seen in an infant's arm and leg movements, bodily movement toward the other person, smiling, vocalizing, and increased visual attention. Because of the infant's immaturity, he or she is unable to maintain a continuous interaction. Maternal or care provider sensitivity[303] to the attention-withdrawal cycle of interaction enables the adult to modulate his or her behavior in synchrony with the infant's cues. Successful interaction with an infant includes reading the infant's cues, responding appropriately, and not overwhelming the infant with too much stimulation (thus overstepping the infant's tolerance for interaction). Overwhelming the infant results in withdrawal for progressively longer periods to protect himself or herself from overstimulating and insensitive others.

Attachment of the newborn to the mother/parent functions to keep the infant in proximity for caregiving and promotes brain and emotional development.[308] Just as the parent has expectations, the infant also has physiologic and emotional needs that require care. Relief from the discomforts of hunger, cold, sleeplessness, and boredom enables the infant to respond positively to the care provider.

Care-eliciting behaviors are those neonatal cues used to signal the caregiver that attention is needed. Crying, visual following, and smiling are care-eliciting behaviors. Newborn responses to care include quieting, suckling, clinging and cuddling, looking, smiling, and vocalizing. These social interactions positively reward the care provider and encourage and promote continued care. Infant characteristics that modify maternal attitudes include (1) a healthy or sickly infant; (2) an attractive, pretty infant or an infant with obvious congenital anomaly; (3) a premature infant; (4) a calm and contented or a fussy and irritable infant; and (5) an infant responsive to or rejecting of maternal care. A maternal or care provider ability to soothe the infant reinforces a feeling of success (or failure) in his or her feelings of competence.

The infant's gender also affects the cues and the caregiver's response. Male infants exhibit more startles, more muscle activity, and more physical strength. In response, caregivers hold them more as a means of soothing.[164] Females exhibit more tactile and oral sensitivity, more smiling, and more responsivity to sweet taste. As a result, girls are more often soothed by talking, eye-to-eye contact, and a pacifier.[164]

The infant's level of neurophysiologic development influences the appropriateness of maternal and caregiving behaviors. The neurologically mature term infant who has already mastered autonomic, motoric, and state regulation is able to actively elicit and respond to caregiving behaviors.[43] Because of the immaturity of the CNS, a preterm infant lags behind a term infant in care eliciting and responsivity to the care provider[215,338] (Box 13-2). Because a young preterm infant's priority is mere survival, interaction with the environment and care providers will occur at the expense of physiologic stability.[325] Although overwhelming the term infant results in withdrawal from interaction, overwhelming the preterm infant results first in a real threat to physiologic survival and then to withdrawal from interaction.

The ability of an infant to be a social partner and to respond in a social interaction is developmentally determined and influenced by the infant's physical condition. The response of preterm infants (weight <1500 g) to social stimulation (e.g., talking and talking combined with touching) develops over time: (1) at 29 to 32 weeks' gestation, respond with distress (e.g., eye closing) to all forms of social stimuli; (2) at approximately 33 weeks' gestation, begin to respond with increased attention

CRITICAL FINDINGS
STAGES AND CHARACTERISTICS OF BEHAVIORAL ORGANIZATION IN PRETERM INFANTS

ALS & BRAZELTON*

Physiologic homeostasis — stabilizing and integrating temperature control, cardiorespiratory function, digestion, and elimination. Characteristics: become pale, dusky, cyanotic; heart and respiratory rates change — all symptoms of disorganization of autonomic nervous system.

Motor development may infringe on physiologic homeostasis resulting in defensive strategies (e.g., vomiting, color change, apnea, bradycardia). State development becomes less diffuse and encompasses full range: sleep, awake, crying. States and state changes may affect physiologic or motor stability.

Alert state is well differentiated from other states; may interfere with physiologic or motor stability.

GORSKI†

"In-turning" — physiologic stage of mere survival characterized by autonomic nervous system responses to stimuli (rapid color changes caused by swings in heart and respiratory rates); no or limited direct response; inability to arouse self spontaneously; jerky movements; asleep (and protecting the central nervous system from sensory overload) 97% of the time. Preterms (<32 weeks) are easily physiologically overwhelmed by stimuli.

"Coming out" — first active response to environment may be seen as early as 34–35 weeks (provided some physiologic stability has been achieved). Characteristics: remains pink with stimuli, has directed response for short periods, arouses spontaneously and maintains arousal after stimulus ceases; if interaction begins in alert state: maintains quiet alert for 5–10 min, tracks animate or inanimate stimuli, spends 10%–15% of time in alert state with predictable interaction patterns.

"Reciprocity" — active interaction and reciprocity with environment at 36–40 weeks. Characteristics: directs response, arouses and consoles self, maintains alertness, interacts with animate/inanimate objects, copes with external stress.

*Data from Als H, Brazelton TB: A new model of assessing the behavioral organization in preterm and full-term infants: two case studies, *J Am Acad Child Psychiatry* 20:239, 1981.
†Modified from Gorski PA: Stages of behavioral organization in the high-risk neonate: theoretical and clinical considerations, *Semin Perinatol* 3:61, 1979.

to talking; they remain distressed with combined stimuli; and (3) at approximately 35 to 36 weeks' gestation, pay more attention to talking; more distress at combined stimuli is seen in high-risk infants (e.g., preterms <1500 g) and better habituation seen in healthier infants.[89] Sicker preterm infants have a more difficult time attending to and modulating their response to social interactions than do healthier preterm infants.[88–90,338] Although VLBW preterm infants respond to talking with increased attention and eye opening, the addition of touch results in increased eye closing and facial grimacing.[77] Sicker infants demonstrate the same pattern of response but in a more exaggerated way that reflects their increased reactivity and decreased ability for self-regulation.[88,90,325]

Because preterm infants are not as neurologically mature as term infants, the NBAS has little value with this population. A behavioral assessment scale for preterm infants, the Assessment of Preterm Infant's Behavior (APIB), has been developed that evaluates the preterm infant's behavioral organization along five subsystems of functioning: autonomic, motor, state, attentional-interactive, and self-regulatory.[11] This examination delineates

the quality and duration of the preterm infant's response, the difficulty in eliciting the response, and the effort and cost to the preterm infant of achieving and maintaining a response. Because it, too, is an interactive test, the nature and amount of organization provided by the care provider is an indication of the preterm infant's lack of integrative skill. As the preterm infant matures and advances in development of organization, he or she is more able to interact with the environment (animate and inanimate). However, it must be remembered that this maturation process is "uneven"; as the preterm infant advances in one area of development, he or she may become, at least temporarily, more vulnerable in other areas.[125]

Another examination, the Neonatal Intensive Care Unit Network Neurobehavioral Scale (NNNS), assesses neurologic integrity and behavioral factors of high-risk infants (e.g., preterms, drug-exposed infants) by evaluating neurobehavioral organization, neurologic reflexes, motor development, muscle tone (active/passive), and signs of (drug) withdrawal and stress.[324] The NNNS differs from the NBAS in that the NNNS (1) was developed for at-risk populations, not for the normal newborn; (2) is more structured and standardized than the NBAS; and (3) gives results more reflective of infant capabilities rather than infant-examiner interaction.[324] The NNNS is performed on medically stable infants, between more than 30 weeks' gestation and 46 to 48 weeks' postconceptual age, for research purposes and for clinical practice.[324] Clinical applications include the following[324]:

- Evaluates the infant's personality and temperament as capacities for state regulation of arousal, response to stimuli, self-soothing, and tolerance of handling
- Documents the physiologic and behavioral manifestations of drug withdrawal or stressors in the environment
- Documents the capacity to habituate, orient to stimuli, and respond to handling, as well as muscle tone and quality of movement
- Evaluates infants withdrawing from in utero drug exposure and those being weaned from analgesia in the NICU
- Determines when the infant is ready for discharge
- Is used as a teaching and care-planning tool when the examination includes parents and other care providers
- Is a tool that bridges the assessment from early gestation/neonatal period to 2 months corrected age when other tools are unreliable

INTERVENTIONS

Life in a special care nursery is characterized by sensory deprivation of normal stimuli that the preterm infant would have experienced in the womb and that term infants would experience at home with their families. However, the NICU is also an environment of sensory bombardment—constant noise, light, and tactile stimulation; intrusive, invasive procedures; upset of sleep-wake cycles; and multiple caregivers. Rather than too much or too little stimulation, infants in the NICU receive an inappropriate pattern of stimulation (e.g., non-contingent, nonreciprocal, painful [rather than pleasant], and multiple stimuli).[6,125,127] Because the immature CNS of the premature infant cannot tolerate these stimuli, the easily overstimulated preterm infant protects himself or herself by physiologic and interactional defensive maneuvers that are maladaptive.

Inappropriate patterns of stimuli that stress the preterm infant in the NICU environment influence brain structure and function during a critical period of brain development.[308] The first study to examine a relationship between stressors in the NICU and alterations in brain development was published in 2011. This prospective cohort study used the Neonatal Infant Stressor Scale (NISS)[238] to measure daily exposure to stressors of preterms (<30 weeks' gestation) for the first 14 and 28 days of life and from admission to the NICU until term equivalent postmenstrual age (PMA) or discharge.[298] Magnetic resonance imaging (MRI) examinations were performed at term equivalent age (about 36–44 weeks' PMA) and the association between exposure to stressors and abnormal brain development was then calculated. The most immature, sickest preterms were exposed to the highest number of stressors and procedures, particularly in the first 14 days of life. Higher exposure to stressors was associated with decreased brain size in the frontal and parietal sections.[298] Increased stress was also associated with altered microstructure in the temporal lobes, especially the right lobe, that resulted in less mature, poorly developed connections between the temporal lobes.[298] A combination of destructive and developmental mechanisms contribute to the encephalopathy of prematurity.[333] White matter injury to the developing brain is recognized as the cause of common motor, behavioral, and cognitive problems in surviving premature infants[91] (see Chapter 31).

A recent study by the same investigators found altered neurobehaviors at term equivalent in a prospective study of preterm infants (<30 weeks' estimated gestational age).[258] Using the NNNS, differences in neurobehavior were examined between preterm infants at term and full-term controls, between 34 weeks' PMA and full-term equivalent and relationship of neurobehavior to perinatal exposures (such as days of intubation, postnatal steroids, oxygen use after 36 weeks' corrected age).[258] At term equivalent, preterm infants exhibited a broad range of altered behaviors (Box 13-3). Studied preterms between 34 weeks' PMA and term equivalent also exhibited behavioral and motor changes that were not influenced by any of the measured perinatal exposures. At 34 weeks' PMA, preterms with significant cerebral injury had increased excitability compared with non–brain-injured preterms.[258] The researchers concluded that the neurobehavioral changes occurring before

BOX 13-3	ALTERED NEUROBEHAVIOR IN PRETERM INFANTS IN NICU

Preterms (at Term Equivalent) Compared With Full-Term Infants

- Poorer orientation
- Lower ability to tolerate handling
- Lower ability to self-regulate
- Poorer reflexes
- Increased stress
- More excitability
- Altered muscle tone—hypotonic or hypertonic

Preterm Infants From 34 Weeks' Premenstrual Age to Term Equivalent

- Changes in motor function:
  - Declining quality of movement
  - Increasing hypertonia
  - Decreasing hypotonia
- Changes in behavior:
  - Increasing arousal
  - Increasing excitability
  - Decreasing lethargy

Adapted from Pineda RG, Tjoung TH, Vavasseur C, et al: Patterns of altered neurobehavior in preterm infants within the neonatal intensive care unit, *J Pediatr* 162: 470, 2013.

term may present a rich opportunity in the NICU for interventions to ameliorate developmental disadvantages evident in the studied preterms by term equivalent age.

Altered neurodevelopmental outcomes and resulting altered neurobehavior may also affect the infant's ability to attach to parents. A recent study involving very preterm/VLBW infants, full-term infants, and their mothers examined the security of the infant's attachment to the mother at 18 months of age.[346] A majority of the full-term (72%) and the very preterm (61%) were securely attached. However, more very preterm infants (32%) had disorganized attachment than the full-term infants (17%). Researchers concluded that neurodevelopmental problems in the very preterm infants altered their ability in social relationship with their mothers.

Research has shown medical, developmental, and cost benefits to low-birth-weight (LBW) infants from individualized behavioral and environmental care in the NICU (Box 13-4). The most effective interventions (1) follow the Newborn Individualized Developmental Care

and Assessment Program (NIDCAP),[*] (2) are contingent on the infant's responses, (3) balance protection from sensory overload with provision of enough stimulation to promote emerging capabilities, and (4) involve the parents.[6,10]

The first randomized controlled trial (RCT) of individualized developmental care (NIDCAP)[10] for VLBW (inborn and transported) infants conducted in three diverse NICUs showed improvement in medical well-being and neurobehavioral and family function.[10] Neurobehavioral benefits included better autonomic or motor system regulation and self-regulation and reduced need for facilitation.[10] Given the diversity of the NICU settings and populations, the biggest differences in beneficial outcomes were appreciated in the most challenged settings (e.g., NICUs initially using the least developmental care, families with multiple social and cultural vulnerability, the sickest infants).[10]

Another RCT studied the effectiveness of NIDCAP initiated within 72 hours of NICU admission in 30 preterms (28–33 weeks' gestational age [GA]) on brain structure and function.[6] The group of preterms receiving NIDCAP showed significantly better neurobehavioral functioning at 2 weeks' and 9 months' corrected age on mental and psychomotor development than that of the control group. Changes in the brain on MRI included a more mature brain fiber structure between brain regions (e.g., frontal to occipital; frontal to parietal) than is consistent with enhanced neurobehavioral functioning. The study's conclusion is that the quality of early experiences (e.g., before term) significantly alters brain structure and function.[6] Several more recent RCTs of NIDCAP show improved health and neurodevelopmental outcomes, shorter length of stay, less chronic lung disease (CLD) for VLBW preterms and severe intrauterine growth restricted (IUGR) preterm infants at 2 weeks' corrected age, 9 months corrected age, and at 8 years.[†] Higher quality of developmental care in the NICU is associated with better neurobehavioral performance (i.e., better attention and self-regulation, less excitability and hypotonicity, and lower stress scores.[227]

Preterm infants are not the only infants at risk from the stress of overstimulation in the NICU. Acutely ill infants and chronically ill infants with prolonged hospitalization also experience stress.

---

[*]References 7, 8, 10, 207, 208, 255.
[†]References 7, 8, 199, 207, 208, 243, 255.

BOX 13-4 OUTCOMES OF INDIVIDUALIZED DEVELOPMENTAL INTERVENTION IN THE NICU*

Physiologic Benefits	Developmental Benefits	Cost Savings
Decrease in:	Improvement in:	Shorter length of stay
Incidence of IVH or pneumothorax and severity	Behavioral organization of autonomic, motor, attention	Earlier discharge at younger age
of BPD, ROP, NEC	modulation, and self-regulatory abilities	Decrease in hospital charges
Ventilator/CPAP use	Interactive capability of infant with staff and parents	
Need for supplemental oxygen	Quality of parent-infant interaction (perception of preterm	
Need for gavage feedings/IV nutrition	as better regulated, more autonomous, and more	
Number of apneic episodes	gratifying; enhanced competence in parental role)	
Need for sedation/analgesia	Less parental personal stress	
Increase in:	Feelings of closeness with preterm	
Daily weight gain; head growth/length	Cognitive function/IQ	
Stability of cardiorespiratory function	Development of feeding skills (earlier full oral feedings)	
Sleep states/sleep duration	Fewer behavioral problems and attentional difficulties	
Significant electrophysiologic differences in frontal, tempo-	Continuation of maternal ability to read and respond to	
ral, central, occipital, and parietal lobes of the brain	infant behavioral cues/appreciation of the infant	

BPD, Bronchopulmonary dysplasia; *CPAP*, continuous positive airway pressure; *IQ*, intelligence quotient; *IV*, intravenous; *IVH*, intraventricular hemorrhage; *NEC*, necrotizing enterocolitis; *NICU*, neonatal intensive care unit; *ROP*, retinopathy of prematurity.
*References 6–8, 10, 111, 162, 199, 207, 208, 227, 255.

A term infant with persistent pulmonary hypertension (see Chapter 23) is particularly vulnerable to repeated handling, procedures, and interventions that decrease PaO_2. Thus, these infants are managed on a minimal intervention regimen: care is organized, coordinated, and individualized to decrease noxious stimuli and physical manipulations. The chronically ill infant with bronchopulmonary dysplasia (BPD) has been shown to improve when behavioral or environmental changes were initiated.

The ultimate goal of intervention strategies in the NICU is to facilitate and promote infant growth and development and thus task mastery.[254] During rapid stages of brain development, neuroprotection of the preterm and sick term infant's brain in the NICU by providing an environment that nurtures brain growth and minimizes brain injury is essential.[39,46,190] In the NICU, these goals are achieved by the following:

- Altering the environmental and caregiving stressors that interfere with physiologic stability
- Promoting individual neurobehavioral organization and maturation by identifying and facilitating stable behaviors and reducing stressful behaviors

- Conserving energy
- Teaching parents to interpret infant behavior
- Promoting infant-parent interaction and caregiving

Core measures for evidence-based developmental care have been identified: (1) protected sleep; (2) pain and stress assessment and management; (3) developmental activities of daily living, such as positioning, feeding, and nonnutritive sucking (NNS); (4) family-centered care; and (5) a healing environment.[66]

Establishing biorhythmic balance and physiologic homeostasis is necessary for survival and is enhanced by a sensitive, responsive NICU environment. An unresponsive environment may so stress the preterm infant that apnea, bradycardia, and other physiologic instabilities severely compromise and prolong recovery.[125,177,254,325] For the hospitalized infant, development of the sense of self and trust is undermined by noncontingent stimulation that prevents establishing a sense of competence and control of the environment.[127] When the ventilated infant experiences hunger or is wet, he or she cannot signal the care provider with a cry because of the tube. Thus, the infant experiences a need but cannot signal and bring care and relief. The infant soon learns that he or she is not in control of the situation.

BOX 13-5	CRITICAL FINDINGS
	CLASSIC SIGNS OF "HOSPITALITIS"

Asocial Behavior

- Gaze aversion—fleeting glances at caregiver with inability to maintain eye contact
- Flat affect—social unresponsiveness (little fixing and following; little smiling) to caregiver
- Little or no quiet alert state—infant abruptly changes state and often is described as "either asleep or awake and crying" (crying is only "awake" state); out-of-control crying

Touch Aversion*

- Becomes hypotonic or hypertonic with caregiving or attempts at socialization
- Fights, flails, and resists being cared for or held
- Aversive responses (see Table 13-4) to caregiving or holding

Feeding Difficulties

- Have multiple origins, including delayed onset of oral feedings; touch aversion around mouth secondary to invasive procedures; multiple caregivers; feeding on schedule, rather than demand
- Rumination syndrome—voluntary regurgitation, a form of self-comfort and gratification when environment is not nurturing or gratifying

Failure to Thrive

- Poor or no weight gain despite adequate caloric intake
- Develops mental delays (language, motor, social, emotional)

*Infant associates human touch with pain.

Similarly another intubated infant may be quietly asleep and not experiencing a need; however, it is "care time," so the nurse moves, wakes, changes, and generally disturbs the infant. This infant also soon learns about not being in control of the situation.

Hospitalized infants, especially those with prolonged stays, may exhibit the classic signs of institutionalized infants or infants suffering from maternal deprivation (Box 13-5).[304] It is the goal of "environmental neonatology"[127] to prevent this maladaptive behavior by altering the NICU to be more developmentally appropriate and responsive to infants. Normalizing the environment begins with an assessment of the stimulation to which the individual infant is exposed. The type (i.e., noxious versus pleasant; contingent versus noncontingent), amount, and timing of stimulation should be noted. To decrease noxious stimuli, no infant should have "routine" care (e.g., all infants are suctioned every 2 hours; all infants have a glucose test every 4 hours).[125] Care should be individualized by asking these questions: "Why are we doing this procedure?" and "Is this procedure necessary for this infant's care?" Overstimulation in the NICU occurs when 81% to 94% of all contacts are medical or nursing procedures, an average of 40 to 132 of which are performed per day.[97] The frequency, pattern, and trends of caregiver encounters and disturbance have not changed over the past 20 years,[19,50,254] although caregivers grossly underestimate the amount of handling to which NICU infants are exposed. Nurses,

who are best able to control overstimulation, provide the majority of handling, sleep disruption, excessive disturbance, and noncontingent interaction to these fragile infants (number of contacts ranging from 79 to 164 times, evenly distributed over a 24-hour period).[19] Painful, invasive procedures that are not vital to the individual infant are stress-producing events that should be eliminated (see Chapter 12).

Rest may be the most important environmental change.[144,254] Sleep disruption is stressful to preterm and sick term neonates in the NICU and alters weight gain, visual development, state regulation, cortical growth, and physiologic stability.[49,129] In a study of ventilated extremely LBW (ELBW) infants, the relationship between hypoxemia and state revealed that sleep disruption with its accompanying motor activity was associated with hypoxemia more often than when these infants were in active/quiet sleep.[177] Recommendations of this study include (1) using strategies (e.g., clustering care, kangaroo care [KC]) to promote sleep in ventilated infants and (2) sleep cycling analogous to in utero patterns (e.g., more quiet sleep) to improve ventilatory stability, decrease hypoxemia, and improve oxygenation.[177] Quiet sleep for preterm infants is enhanced by (1) no caregiving; (2) social interaction, especially with the parents in skin-to-skin care; (3) NNS; and (4) lateral positioning.[184] Conversely, quiet sleep is disrupted with routine and intrusive care.[184] Individualized developmental care promotes sleep.[4]

TABLE 13-4	CRITICAL FINDINGS
	SELF-REGULATORY VERSUS STRESS BEHAVIORS

ORGANIZATION	DISORGANIZATION
	PHYSIOLOGIC
Cardiorespiratory: stable heart and/or respiratory rate; regular, slow respirations	Cardiorespiratory: increase or decrease in respiratory rate; irregular respirations; apnea; gasping; bradycardia; blood pressure instability; sneezing, hiccoughs, coughing, sighing
Color: pink, stable	Color: mottling, duskiness; cyanosis—central or generalized; pallor or plethora
Gastrointestinal: tolerates feedings	Gastrointestinal: abdominal distention; spitting up; vomiting; gagging; stooling
	BEHAVIORAL
Body movements smooth and synchronous: consistent tone of all body parts; arms and legs flexed with smooth movements	Tremors, jittery and jerking movements; hypotonia or hypertonia (flaccid trunk, extremities; movements arching, flailing, extended extremities; finger splays, fisting)
States: well-defined sleep-wake	Unable to modulate states: sudden state changes; more active than quiet sleep; awake states with gaze aversion, frowning, grimacing, staring, irritability, wide-eyed "help me" look
Self-quieting behaviors: hand-to-mouth, hand or foot clasping, finger folding or grasping, sucking, foot or leg bracing	Limited use of self-quieting behaviors (may need assistance from caregiver)
Attentive behaviors: alert gaze; fixes and follows visual stimuli; ceases to suck or slows suck rate, turns toward auditory stimuli, smiles; imitates; opens mouth, extends tongue; vocalizes: coos, babbles, habituates to stimuli	May demonstrate any of the foregoing stress signals when attempting to interact with one or more modes of stimuli (e.g., rocking, talking) simultaneously in environment (either animate or inanimate)

Data from Als H, Brazelton TB: A new model of assessing the behavioral organization in preterm and full-term infants: two case studies, *J Am Acad Child Psychiatry* 20:239, 1981; Gorski PA: Stages of behavioral organization in the high-risk neonate: theoretical and clinical considerations, *Semin Perinatol* 3:61, 1979.

Although rest periods are necessary for normal growth and development and optimal immune function,[277] care continues to be evenly distributed over 24 hours without adequate periods of undisturbed rest.[4,254] Rest periods of less than 60 minutes are ineffective and insufficient for the preterm to complete a normal sleep cycle.[254] The length of rest periods in most NICUs has not changed (Table 13-5), and institution of a rest period (even only 1 hour in length) does not necessarily decrease the amount of disturbance.[147]

A fetus in utero and a term infant at home relate to a minimum of caregivers and thus need to learn one or only a few sets of cues. Consistency of caregivers is essential for an infant's developmental agenda. Multiple caregivers in the NICU confuse the infant by providing many care-related cues for the infant to learn—many techniques of handling and many emotional, nonverbal messages to decode. *Primary nursing* minimizes the number of care providers, because the primary nurse and one or two associates always (or as much as possible) care for the infant; assess, revise, and write the care plan; and coordinate care.[190] *Primary nursing* also adds consistency and continuity for parents and satisfaction for nurses.[190]

The infant's state or level of arousal provides an appropriate context for caregiving. Some infants exhibit a low threshold for stimuli; they are easily overwhelmed and fatigued. Others with a higher threshold are quieter, more difficult to arouse, initiate less, and thus receive less interaction.[11] Organizing care to be reciprocal to the infant's state reinforces the infant's competence in signaling a need (sense of self) and having it met (sense of trust and mastery). As the infant matures, feeding on demand rather than on a schedule not only teaches this valuable lesson but also increases absorption and use of caloric intake.[125,213,296] If the infant is asleep, ask: "Should we do this now? Would another time be better?" In some centers, physicians make an appointment with the nurse to examine the infant at a time that is optimal for the infant.

TABLE 13-5	REST PERIODS FOR NICU INFANTS: RESEARCH BASIS

AUTHOR, YEAR	LENGTH OF REST PERIOD
Korones, 1976[165]	Range of mean rest periods 5.6–19.2 min
Duxbury, 1984[87]	Average time of 30.2 min
Evans, 1994[97]	Time between handling: 1–38.45 min in first nursery 1–60 min in second nursery
Appleton, 1997[19]	2–59 min

NICU, Neonatal intensive care unit.

Because preterm infants exhibit short duration of state cycles until around 38 weeks, they have decreased tolerance for stimuli. The smaller, sicker, and less mature the infant, the less he or she is able to handle stimuli. Some preterm infants tolerate all care done at once and long periods of rest; others do not and need care spread out to decrease overstimulation and decompensation. *Clustering of care*—performance of several procedures together in a short period of time—may result in more physiologic alterations (changes in cardiorespiratory stability, changes in blood pressure, increased cortisol levels, and heightened pain responses) than a single care-taking event or the actual length of the handling episode.[146] Studies show increased and prolonged behavioral motor responses and increased cortisol levels indicative of stress during clustered care; clustered care is especially stressful for preterms less than 28 weeks' gestational age.[145] Clustering care may not ensure long rest periods, because 50% of all rest periods in several NICUs were shorter than 10 minutes (see Table 13-5).[97] If the practice of clustering care, with its prolonged disturbance of the preterm infant, results in alterations of vital signs, oxygen saturation, and infant stress and fatigue, then care should be individualized and provided to minimize physiologic and behavioral disturbances.[136,146,177,254] A study of medically stable preterms found that after nursing interventions, these infants generally sleep—either from satiety or from the significant energy expenditure associated with caregiving.[310]

Even "preterm growers" may be unable to tolerate more than one stimulus at a time—they feed best if visual, auditory, and social stimuli are not provided until after the feeding. As the infant matures and is able to tolerate integrated experience, multimodal stimuli are provided.[340] Studies of multimodal stimuli (e.g., auditory, tactile, vestibular, visual) provided to preterms demonstrate (1) increased alertness, (2) earlier discharge, (3) faster progression to full oral feedings, (4) improved organization of behavioral states, (5) stable respiratory rate and oxygen saturation, and (6) a significant decrease in resting heart rate.[340,341]

Alterations in the individual infant's daily schedule are made to accommodate a more flexible or structured schedule—whichever is better for the infant.[127] Assessing the infant before, during, and after an interaction or intervention guides the care provider in adapting care and the environment to the individual infant (Table 13-6).

An organized infant is able to interact with the environment without disrupting his or her physiologic and behavioral functioning.[11] When a disorganized preterm interacts with the environment, signs of physiologic and behavioral stress may occur (see Table 13-4), in which case the interaction should cease.[136,164] The potential effects of stress and trauma to fragile preterm infants have not only short-term but also long-term effects on their outcomes.[257,298] An intubated preterm infant cared for in a NICU with a strict suction "routine" every 2 hours responds with profound cyanosis, lowered $TcPo_2$ and pulse oxygenation, and bradycardia and requires bagging after every suction (with no secretions obtained), an obviously unnecessary and stressful intervention. In a less rigid, more individualized care setting, that same infant may signal the need for suction by becoming restless, by a decrease in oxygenation, or by heart rate changes (tachycardia or bradycardia). Suctioning improves the infant's condition—the infant lies quietly and has improved oxygenation, and the heart pattern stabilizes. This infant has signaled his or her need, and the care providers have read the cues and responded with a stabilizing intervention—the infant has not been stressed by an unnecessary procedure.

Knowledgeable professionals are able to role model for and teach parents how to relate to their premature infant.[162] Parents are taught to recognize and use infant states to maximize appropriate interaction.[162,178] The drowsy premature infant may be unable to engage in eye-to-eye

TABLE 13-6 PARAMETERS FOR ASSESSING INTERACTION AND INTERVENTION WITH NEONATES

TIME FRAME	ASSESSMENT
	BEFORE
Gather baseline data **before** touching the infant	Gestational age and postconceptual age
	Diagnosis
	Level of physiologic homeostasis:
	Previous vital signs
	Oxygenation state — continuous pulse oximetry or transcutaneous monitor
	Neonatal state:
	Sleep — deep, light, drowsy
	Awake — quiet, active alert, crying
	Self-regulatory versus stress behaviors (see the Critical Findings in Table 13-4)
	DURING
Gently and as unobtrusively as possible assess physiologic and behavioral signs during intervention	Level of (current) physiologic homeostasis — vital signs and changes:
	Observation (without touching infant) — color, posture, general appearance, respiratory rate, temperature (skin, incubator), blood pressure (transducer), oxygenation (from continuous monitor)
	Quiet (with minimal disturbance) — auscultate heart, lungs, and abdomen; axillary temperature, blood pressure (cuff); head-to-toe assessment; oxygenation (saturation decreases with distressful, disturbing stimuli)
	Neonatal state change:
	Sleep — deep, light, drowsy
	Awake — quiet alert, active alert, crying
	Self-regulatory versus stress behaviors (see Table 13-4)
	AFTER
Assess physiologic and behavioral signs after intervention (delayed reactions may occur minutes after care)	Level of physiologic homeostasis
	Vital signs — Returned to baseline values? More stable or less stable than baseline values?
	Neonatal state change — Return to baseline state? To a higher state? Unable to be consoled? More consolable left alone?

contact with the parents or be able to sustain it for too short (for the parents) a period. Waiting until the infant is more awake to initiate eye contact is more rewarding for the parent and less stressful for the infant. Role model for parents that their infant is an individual and, although premature, can signal for more or less stimulation (see Table 13-4).

A preterm infant who is lightly touched may startle, jerk, or withdraw from parental touch. In response, the parent suddenly and sadly pulls his or her hand away and is reticent to touch the infant again. Intervention includes helping parents read cues and learn appropriate responses to their infant. Teach parents how to recognize a stressed infant and how to intervene. At the same time, be sure to acknowledge the parents' knowledge of the infant and support them. Above all, do not patronize. Professionals have much to learn from parents, who are "professionals" in their own right. The prime rule of relating to infants is this: The infant leads; the adult follows.

Feeding a premature infant may be difficult because the infant "goes to sleep" during feedings. The usual parental ministrations of talking to the infant, soothing with touch, or holding upright on the shoulder may not work with a fussy, irritable preterm infant.

The preterm infant's behavior may be so disorganized, unpredictable, or misunderstood by the parents that an appropriate response is not possible.[5,125] Thus, parents often become exhausted, bewildered, and frustrated in their encounters with their preterm infant's behavioral response to their care as rejecting and unloving: "My baby doesn't like me." Teach parents that their infant's disorganization with stimuli is related to prematurity (i.e., an immature CNS) and not to parent ministrations. Reassure them that as the premature infant grows and evidences maturational changes, he or she will be able to tolerate more stimulation and will be more responsive to their care.

Just as parent-infant interaction is responsible for normal development of the term infant, parent-infant interaction is crucial in the development of at-risk infants. Many parents of premature infants have been observed making heroic efforts, over long periods, to interact with their less alert, active, and responsive infants.[88,125,215] Parenting the preterm has been described as "more work and less fun." "Setting parents up to succeed" involves placing parents in situations in which they will experience positive feedback from their infants. Suggesting and role-modeling intervention strategies show parents what and how to play and interact with their infants. Parent participation in intervention strategies is ensured by stressing how important it is to infant development, that professionals are too busy to provide all the necessary interventions, and that parents are in a unique position to provide developmental care in the hospital and at home after discharge. Parents, with help from professionals, are the ideal planners and providers of developmentally appropriate intervention strategies[293] (see Table 13-1).

A rooming-in setting for parents and their at-risk newborns is the best environment for cues to be learned and care given according to these cues. Unlimited and unrestricted contact of parents and newborns should be the policy in every normal, medium-risk, and high-risk nursery (see Box 29-2). Providing a single-room NICU, a family room, bonding room, or apartment in which parents and their soon-to-be-discharged newborn can room-in helps the transition from hospital to home care. Rooming-in before discharge gives mothers and fathers an opportunity to assume full responsibility for their infant's care, tests the reality of caregiving, helps them learn caregiving activities and their infant's behavior patterns, and confirms their readiness for independent parenting and the infant's readiness for discharge.

Intervention Strategies

Because infants experience their environment through sensory processes, intervention strategies are based on tactile/kinesthetic, auditory, visual, olfactory/gustatory, and communication skills. Interventions must be individualized according to the infant's state, sensory threshold, physiologic homeostasis, and stability or stress cues.[97,146,177]

CIRCADIAN RHYTHMS

In utero, the states of the fetus are regulated by the sleep-wake cycles of the mother. In the NICU, multiple intrusions disrupt regulation.[273–275] How this affects an infant is not fully known, although limited energy may be drained, the infant may be subjected to further stress,[5,127] neurodevelopment altered, and outcomes of therapeutic interventions may not be optimized. To minimize interruptions and excessive handling, infants should not be awakened when asleep; if they must be awakened for care, it should be during active sleep by talking softly and stroking gently.[4,83] Appointments for examinations should be made before feeding to decrease unnecessary disturbance of sleep but with enough rest time (if needed) before actual feeding.

Adequate numbers of caregiving encounters—physical assessment, vital signs, diaper or linen change, and procedures—must be balanced against constant manipulations.[125] Because essentially all NICU (levels II and III) infants are continuously monitored, "laying on of hands" every 1 to 2 hours is often unnecessary. Thorough physical assessment and vital sign recording every 4 hours is easily alternated with recordings from the monitors every 4 hours. Thus, the infant is evaluated every 2 hours but not disturbed that often. An acutely ill infant may need closer observation, but alternating "hands-on" with monitor readings accomplishes the goal without overwhelming an infant with few reserves.

Sleep-wake patterns are influenced by feeding method,[316] temperature, position, CNS maturation, birth weight, caregiving practices, and environmental effects (e.g., ambient light, noise).[273–275,327] Sleep-wake patterns in breastfed and bottle-fed infants differ. Full-term breastfed infants awaken more and sleep less during the night.[117]

Day-night cycles are facilitated by afternoon nap time and nighttime in which the dimming of lights or covering of incubators and cribs with blankets and quieting of NICU noise enable infants to sleep. Deep, quiet sleep is facilitated by quiet and dark, soft music or nature sounds, gentle stroking of the head, and self-regulated tasks (self-sought proximity of infant to "breathing bear").[315] Maintaining daily nap-time and nighttime hours helps infants reset their diurnal rhythms and become accustomed to sleeping in dim light and a quiet environment. Among convalescing preterm infants (<34 weeks' gestational age), four standard rest periods per day resulted in (1) increased daily weight gain, (2) increased sleep, (3) less-active states during nap time, (4) decreased occurrences of apnea, and (5) by 3 weeks, less quiet waking time and longer uninterrupted sleep episodes.[144,322] Uninterrupted sleep and diurnal rhythmicity also are associated with improved state organization in VLBW infants, as well as less fussing and crying.[131,274,275]

TACTILE AND KINESTHETIC INTERVENTION

Because the sense of touch is highly developed in utero, even a very immature preterm has acute tactile sensitivity. For newborns, human touch is the most important tactile stimulation. Not all touch is equal, however, nor is it responded to equally by term or preterm infants who are well, critically ill, or recovering from illness. One study has shown the effect of the vulnerability of LBW infants in their response to the nurturing touch of their mothers. Nurturing maternal touch was associated with a secure attachment in robust infants; in highly vulnerable, sick LBW infants, this same nurturing touch was associated with a less secure attachment.[338] Any type of tactile stimulation is composed of six factors: duration, location, action, intensity, frequency, and sensation. Tactile sensation both arouses and quiets. Gentle but firm handling quiets infants because they feel more secure; light, uncertain touch often results in agitation and withdrawal. Handling for routine care (e.g., vital signs, changing the diaper or position, venipuncture for blood draws or placement of IV lines, feeding, heel sticks, suction, and physical or neurologic examinations) can result in hypoxia, increased intracranial pressure, episodes of apnea/bradycardia, agitation, elevated pain scores for VLBW preterms, and increased or decreased heart rate and blood pressure.*

Handling. How a neonate is handled during care affects his or her physiologic and behavioral response. Use of body containment during suction decreases the physiologic and behavioral responses to this stressful procedure.[313] Comparing preterm responses to swaddled and unswaddled weighing, unswaddled infants exhibit more physiologic distress, more motor disorganization, poorer self-regulation, and more need for caregiver facilitation than when they were swaddled for weighing.[236] Transferring preterm infants from the incubator to the parent for holding or KC is stressful. One study evaluated physiologic disorganization in preterms according to the method of transfer from the incubator for KC (nurse picking up the baby and transferring to the parent versus the parent picking the baby up directly from the incubator).[239] Both transfer methods resulted in increased physiologic and motor disorganization (i.e., oxygen desaturation, tachycardia, cyanosis/pallor, hypotonia, decreased self-regulation, and increased need for caregiver facilitation to maintain physiologic stability during transfer). In both methods of transfer (which lasted 6–9 minutes), the ventilator was disconnected (for 5 seconds). Both the infant's desaturation readings and tachycardia recovered to baseline levels faster with the parent transfer.[239]

Excessive handling of preterm, VLBW, or sick neonates results in significant physiologic consequences, such as blood pressure changes, alterations in cerebral blood flow, hypoxia, and other stress behaviors.[188] One study of ventilated VLBW infants found an average of 53 handling episodes, for an average length of 3 minutes over a 24-hour period.[50] These infants had pain scores significantly higher after than before handling despite the reason for the handling (i.e., invasive/noninvasive or social/nonsocial).[50] A particularly vulnerable group of preterm infants, those with periventricular leukomalacia (PVL), react to handling and multisensory stimulation (e.g., auditory, tactile, visual, vestibular) with an increase in heart rate above their already higher resting heart rate.[290] These CNS-injured preterms require close observation and monitoring during handling, stressful procedures, and interventions.[341]

---

*References 50, 68, 69, 98, 188, 252, 310.

A total body position change is not considered a painful procedure, but in LBW preterm infants with endotracheal tubes and umbilical artery catheters, the handling necessary to change the infant's position elicits pain behaviors.[99] Nonpainful tactile stimulation (e.g., routine nursery handling) of preterm infants has been shown to produce equal or higher levels of physiologic stress activation than does a painful stimulus (e.g., heel stick).[50,140] In the same study, the relatively low behavioral activation during "routine handling" led the researchers to conclude that this tactile stimulus was not unpleasant to the infants, even though it produced a high level of physiologic stress response.

In the NICU, infants who are repeatedly subjected to painful, intrusive procedures develop touch aversion—the association of human touch with pain. Tactile vulnerability has also been found in infants who require multiple postnatal medical interventions, who are exposed to illicit drugs in utero, and whose mothers had their own predisposition regarding being touched (a genetic component?).[337] These infants cry uncontrollably, squirm away, flail arms and legs, and recoil when touched, knowing that pain will soon follow. An infant who has received ventilatory therapy may have touch aversion around the mouth: the infant is averse to facial stroking and rooting, has a hypersensitive gag reflex, and refuses to nipple feed. Painful procedures should be minimized to those absolutely (medically) indicated—no infant should be subjected to "routine" painful procedures. During those necessary procedures, it is essential to provide body containment, comfort measures (e.g., a pacifier), and adequate pain relief (see Chapter 12).

Touch. Touch that is not related to caregiving (i.e., social contact) should be provided by parents and professionals when the preterm infant is aware, alert, and receptive. When parents touch their babies, the amount and types of touch vary widely—most frequently, holding, stroking, rubbing, or placing a finger in the infant's hand. Preterm infants respond individually and physiologically to their parents' touch; there is more variation in heart rate and oxygen saturation levels compared with baseline values. These variations depend on gestational age, infant state, and the amount of handling before parent handling.[135] Less touching by the nurse within the 2 hours before parental holding results in less mean decrease in heart rate during parental holding.[135] Parents provide more positive touch (kissing and stroking); preterm infants are more likely to smile and sleep for their parents compared with responses after a nurse's touch. In animal studies, increased parental touching in infancy results in changes in brain structure, decreased levels of stress hormones, and better ability to survive a stressful environment.[218,335] Perhaps parental touch of preterm humans enables them to withstand the stress of illness and the NICU environment.

Nonpainful touch such as stroking (the head, trunk, or hands) during care may calm, soothe, and prevent touch aversion. Stroking of physiologically stable preterm infants has been associated with increased activity and alertness, a faster regaining of birth weight, more rapid weight gain, less crying and apnea, enhanced developmental status, and better social scores.[134,136] In another study, systematic stroking of ventilated preterms resulted in no adverse effects on oxygenation and respiratory or heart rates.[75] However, in preterm infants (26–30 weeks' gestation) who are not physiologically stable, stroking results in decreased oxygen saturation, signs of behavioral stress (e.g., grasping, grunting, gaze aversion), and more avoidance cues (e.g., grimacing, yawning, fussing or crying, tongue protrusion). Other behavioral and physiologic effects include heart rate and blood pressure changes, changes in respiratory rate and rhythm, increase in avoidance signals (e.g., increased startle reflex, agitation, crying), increase in activity and movement, and decreased visual responsivity.[69,135,188,239]

If the preterm infant becomes agitated with stroking, a hand firmly placed on the head and lower back, buttocks, or abdomen often quiets.[65,134] Hand placement without stroking does not decrease oxygen saturation or alter heart rate and has a soothing effect (i.e., decreases active sleep, increases quiet sleep, decreases respiratory and heart rates, decreases motor activity and behavioral distress) on small preterm infants.[136,137,149,224] Handle gently to avoid stressful reactions (e.g., flailing, arching, oxygen desaturation) and enable the infant to become calm and rest between caregiving. Parents should be taught and encouraged to provide their preterm with "gentle human touch"[134,224] in the form of supportive containment with their hands, use of gradual and rhythmic action, observation of infant responses (see Table 13-4), and modification, alteration, or cessation of touch when necessary.[134,136]

Therapeutic touch (TT), a complementary therapy of balancing and increasing energy to promote healing, does not require physical contact as hands are suspended over the body. A randomized double blind study of the use of TT on 10 physiologically fragile, very preterm infants showed no adverse effects (i.e., oxygen desaturations or apnea).[343] Clearly more research is indicated.[300]

Massage. The touching and stroking of massage stimulate nerve pathways and aid myelinization by increasing hypothalamic activity and production of the growth hormone *somatotropin*. In animal studies, touch deprivation decreases growth hormone secretion, which results in undergrowth of all organ systems; a return to normal secretion occurs with tactile stimulation.[288] Massage affects the maturation of the brain's electrical activity and simulates intrauterine development as observed in term infants.[132] A growth gene that responds to tactile stimulation has been discovered; this suggests a genetic origin for the touch-growth relationship.[106] Because touch stimulation of the inside of a neonate's mouth increases the release of gastrointestinal food absorption hormones (i.e., gastrin, insulin), it is postulated that the tactile stimulation of massage leads to a similar hormone release. Assays of glucose and insulin levels in heel-stick samples of preterm infants suggest that massaged infants show increased levels of insulin.[106]

Research on massage therapy with preterm infants has been conducted on medically stable, growing infants (i.e., preterm growers). Despite positive outcomes of massage research in Table 13-7 and its cost-effectiveness in decreasing length of stay, only 38% of NICUs practice massage on their stable preterm infants.[108,336] Massage therapy provides social touch rather than painful touch, prevents or treats touch aversion, and should be taught to and provided by parents in the hospital and at home.[217] Confidence in parenting skills and tactile communication between parents and infant is encouraged when parents massage their infant. Because massage has not been studied in acutely ill preterm infants, its use should be confined to preterm growers.[106,331] Chronically ill infants (e.g., babies with BPD or congenital heart disease) may exhibit physiologic and behavioral disorganization with massage, so the risk-benefit ratio must be assessed carefully. The M Technique, used for fragile infants who do not tolerate conventional massage, is a

gentle, structured stroking technique that reduces stress and anxiety. Outcomes of those exposed to the M technique included (1) lower heart rate, (2) increased oxygen saturations, (3) increase in quiet sleep, and (4) fewer behavioral distress cues.[300]

Varying sensations and touch patterns keep infants interested in stroking and massaging. As a preterm infant matures and is able to tolerate variety, he or she should be introduced to different textures (e.g., lambskins, stuffed toys, cotton, satin). Baby clothes provide various textures, decrease heat loss (especially hats), and make the infant more attractive ("He looks like a real baby!"; "She looks like a girl because her shaved head is covered!").

Holding. When the infant is preterm or a sick term baby, holding him or her, an essential step of parent attachment, is disrupted. Some NICUs promote parental holding as soon as possible, whereas others have specific protocols about weight criteria and extubation before parents are able to hold their infant.[113] A national survey on holding policies found (1) written protocols for conventional holding (26%) and for KC (40%), (2) for extubated infants: 73% offered KC, 99% conventional holding, and (3) for holders of extubated babies: mothers 73% KC, fathers 68% KC, and 99% conventional holding for both parents.[113] Potential benefits of enhanced parent-infant interaction and attachment,[163] closeness of parents to their infant, increased lactation, and improved parental self-esteem are factors that influence staff to facilitate holding.[113]

A recent prospective cohort study of parental presence and holding in the NICU found significant neurobehavioral benefits for preterm infants less than or equal to 30 weeks' gestation.[271] Early parenting (i.e., holding) in the NICU resulted in lower arousal and excitability, better quality of movement, less stress and less hypertonic muscle tone, thus a developmental advantage.[271] Another recent study conducted in an urban NICU with low levels of parental presence and holding compared the neurodevelopmental outcomes of preterm infants (<30 weeks' gestation) cared for in single-family rooms versus open ward NICU rooms.[257] The study outcome showed that at age 2 years, children cared for in the private rooms had lower language acquisition, more externalizing behaviors, and a trend toward lower motor scores than those in open wards. The researchers were surprised by their findings and remarked on the relative

TABLE 13-7	BENEFITS OF MASSAGE WITH PRETERM INFANTS: RESEARCH BASIS

STUDY	RESULTS
Three times/day massage of preterms with physiologic and biochemical measurements[287]	21% increase in daily weight gain Discharged 5 days earlier Superior performance on habituation Fewer stress behaviors (mouthing, grimacing, clenched fists) Increase in catecholamine secretion in neonatal period (analogous to the normal developmental increase after birth) Increase in vagal activity
10 healthy preterm "growers": 3 times/day massage for 15 min in a randomized sequence of 5 days of massage and 5 days without massage[171]	Energy expenditure significantly lower after 5 days of massage than after 5 days without massage in metabolically and thermally stable preterms Decreased energy expenditure may contribute to enhanced growth caused by massage
Massaged for 15 min three times/day for 5 days: 68 preterms (mean GA = 30 wk) with either light- or moderate-pressure massage[107] 80 preterms randomized to moderate-pressure massage or standard care[76] 72 preterms randomized to massage or control therapy[77] Massaged or exercise for 10 min 3 times/day for 5 days[78]: 30 preterms randomized to moderate-pressure massage *or* passive flexion and extension of limbs 21 preterm infants (8 males and 13 females)[301]	Fewer stress behaviors and less activity from first to last day of the study Moderate-pressure group: significantly more daily weight gain; more relaxed, less aroused than light-pressure group Increase in vagal activity and gastric motility, which may contribute to greater weight gain in massaged preterms Greater increase in body temperature in massage versus control preterms (even though incubator portholes were open for the massage but not for the control group) Greater weight gain in both massage and exercise groups due to different mechanisms: • Massage increased vagal tone • Exercise increased calorie consumption Massaged male infants had improved autonomic nervous system function during caregiving and sleep compared with nonmassaged male preterms. There was no difference in heart rate variability between massaged and nonmassaged female preterm infants.[301]
	MOTHER MASSAGE
104 VLBW infants (≥750 to ≤1500 g; ≤32 wk GA) randomized to control or standard care with maternal massage 4 times/day of face and limbs with passive limb exercises[222]	Significantly lower incidence of late-onset sepsis Discharged from the hospital 7 days earlier Improved neurodevelopmental outcomes at 2 years CA with massage[265]
66 stable preterm infants (32 massaged by their mother; 34 control group)[1]	Lower pain scores after massage with heelstick and at discharge; higher cognitive scores at 12 months' CA compared with control group. No difference in weight gain, LOS, breastfeeding duration, and motor skills between two groups.
Medically stable preterms (33–37 wk GA; BW 1500–1999g) randomly assigned to massage group or massage with sunflower oil by their mothers 3 times/day for 14 consecutive days[101]	Oil massage group: mean weight at 1 month and 2 months of age significantly greater than body massage alone group

BW, Birth weight; *CA,* corrected age; *GA,* gestational age; *LOS,* length of stay; *NICU,* neonatal intensive care unit; *VLBW,* very low birth weight.

sensory deprivation of the preterms in private rooms whose parents were not often present and handling their infants. Long periods of sensory deprivation—lack of parental presence, holding, and auditory stimuli—may be as detrimental as the sensory overload of a noisy, open NICU.[257] A qualitative study of factors affecting parental presence found that active involvement in the care of their extremely preterm infants, including skin-to-skin holding, increased their motivation to be present and their feelings of control.[139] Factors discouraging parental presence included excessive noise and light levels in the NICU and dismissive staff attitudes.[139] Communicating to parents the

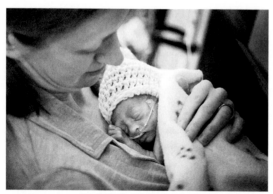

FIGURE 13-1   Kangaroo care.

importance of their presence and their care for their baby, as well as providing a welcoming, nurturing, and comfortable place for parents is the responsibility of all the NICU staff, especially nurses.

KC (Figure 13-1), skin-to-skin contact between parents and infant by placing the infant in a vertical position between the maternal or paternal breasts, benefits both parents and neonates (Box 13-6). KC for the healthy preterm has been used in the delivery room, in the transitional period (see Chapter 5), for adoptive parents, and for transport. National surveys of holding/KC have been conducted and have found that KC is practiced more commonly in subspecialty (level III) than in specialty (level II) care NICUs.[95,113]

KC is well tolerated in the first week of life by preterm infants with current or resolving neonatal illness. KC of preterm infants for even 1 hour has been shown to provide benefits: significant decrease in heart and respiratory rates, increased temperature and oxygen saturations, especially in SGA and female preterms.[38] A RCT of healthy preterms (33–35 weeks' GA) found that KC for 3 hours improved breathing patterns and resulted in no apnea or bradycardia or periodic breathing or temperature instability.[191] KC improves gas exchange in preterm infants of less than 1800 g. The smallest infants (<1000 g) remained more clinically stable (i.e., smallest increase in heart rate, highest decrease in respiratory rate and increase in oxygen saturation, no hypothermia) compared with infants larger than 1000 g.[112]

When KC is compared with conventional cuddling care (i.e., mother holding her swaddled, clothed infant), there is no difference in maintenance of vital signs, oxygenation, parental stress/expectation, or breastfeeding.[276] A randomized study of three holding methods

(i.e., KC, cuddled, and a no restrictions method) in preterms between 32 to 35 weeks' gestation concluded that both KC and cuddled holding by parents may provide equal developmental benefits in the form of early behavioral organization to preterm infants.[237] All infants being held either conventionally or by KC should be continuously monitored for vital signs and oxygen saturation.[191]

Parental holding is often (17%–33%) limited or not supported by nurses and physicians.[35,113] Parents identify both the hospital staff and the environment of the NICU as barriers and supportive of KC.[35,179] A recent phenomenologic study found that NICU nurses attempt to balance the developmental needs of infants with parental readiness to participate in skin-to-skin care.[170] A second phenomenologic study found that information, communication, consistency, and support from staff to parents along with knowledgeable staff assisted in parents performing and having positive experiences with KC.[179] Barriers to holding infants include (1) infant safety concerns (e.g., accidental extubation, loss of arterial/venous lines, vital sign or oxygenation instability) and (2) reluctance of professionals and families to initiate or participate in KC (e.g., adding to workload, difficulty providing care, lack of experience, used for babies who are not developmentally ready, belief that technology is better than KC).[95,113] More than 60% of NICUs responding to one survey stated that low birth weight and gestational age were not contraindications for KC; many NICUs did not permit KC for babies on high-frequency oscillator ventilation (HFOV) or vasopressors.[95]

"Risky populations" for KC include infants who are intubated (Figure 13-2), have arterial/venous lines and chest tubes, are on pressors to maintain blood pressure, and are on HFOV. One of the national surveys found that 64% of NICUs offered conventional holding to parents of intubated infants and 45% offered KC of intubated infants; the second survey found that 60% of NICU nurse managers thought that intubated infants should not receive KC.[95,113] In a recent study, 43 intubated, hemodynamically stable preterms less than 1500 g were assessed for 90 minutes (15 minutes of transfer; 60 minutes of KC; 15 minutes of transfer) and found to have stable heart rates, oxygen saturations, axillary temperatures, and mean arterial blood pressures.[22] The researchers concluded that KC was safe for these ventilated preterms under their study conditions.

On the basis of a 3-year study in five NICUs of mechanically ventilated infants receiving KC,

BOX 13-6   BENEFITS OF KANGAROO CARE/SKIN-TO-SKIN CONTACT*

Parental

- Activates maternal/paternal processes of search for meaning and mastery of the experience of premature birth
- Increases maternal/paternal self-confidence, competence, and self-esteem
- Enhances parent-infant attachment
- Initiates and maintains maternal/paternal behavior
- Positively affects mother's mood/behavior; less maternal depression; calming (decrease in salivary cortisol levels)[32,237]
- Positive and personally beneficial experience
- Positively affects parental identity and knowledge of infant[279]
- Increases confidence in meeting infant's needs
- More frequent visiting
- Parental eagerness for infant's discharge
- Long term:
  - More consistent/contingent maternal/paternal responses at 15 months of age
  - More sensitive, less intrusive, more reciprocal interactions from 6 months to 2 years from both mothers and fathers
  - More affectionate touch, more adaptive to infant signals, and infants more alert during interactions at 3 to 6 months
  - Less maternal/paternal separation anxiety at 6 months
  - Improved family cohesiveness

Neonatal

- Thermal synchrony: mother's body temperature rises and falls to maintain infant in neutral state (see Chapter 6)
  - Higher body temperature resulting from advanced maturation of thermoregulation
- Cardiopulmonary:
  - Adequate or improved oxygenation
  - Fewer/no episodes of periodic breathing, apnea, and bradycardia
  - Lower heart rate/stable respiratory rate
  - Higher vagal tone: indicative of quicker maturation of the autonomic nervous system
- Breastfeeding:
  - Increased milk supply
  - Increased incidence and length (even in very-low-birth-weight preterms)[110]
- Behavioral:
  - Increased alert activity
  - Increased deep sleep

- Improved self-regulation: sleep-wake cycles, arousal, sustained exploration
- Better emotional regulation and arousal modulation for interaction and rest
- Decreased stress response: decrease in beta-endorphin and cortisol levels
- Decreased or no crying[98,99]
- Increased *en face* positioning
- Better orientation and habituation
- Less pain response to painful procedure in both preterm and term infants (see Chapter 12)
- Accelerated brain maturation
- Earlier discharge:
  - Increased weight gain
  - No increased infection/fewer infections; decreased severity of infection and mortality
  - Out of incubator earlier
- Decrease in mortality of infants with birth weight <2000 g.
- Regulatory interaction:
  - Behavioral
  - Sucking
  - Neurochemical
  - Metabolic
  - Sleep-wake cycles/improved sleep organization[195]
  - Cardiovascular
  - Endocrine
  - Immune
  - Circadian
- Long-term:
  - Increased length and head circumference at 9 months and 1 year of age
  - Less crying at 6 months of age
  - Higher psychomotor scales at 6 months and higher mental scales at 6 months to 2 years
  - Enhanced mental and psychomotor development at 1 year
  - Better self-regulation, less frustration and better able to calm themselves at 1 year of age
  - Improved cerebral motor pathways and synaptic efficacy at adolescence
  - Enhanced cognitive development and executive functioning from 6 months to 10 years. By 10 years of age: attenuated stress response, improved autonomic functioning, organized sleep, and better cognitive and behavioral control

*Data compiled from references: 45, 48, 51, 63, 103, 112, 121, 133, 174, 191, 193, 216, 220, 240-242, 246, 278, 279, 289, 290.

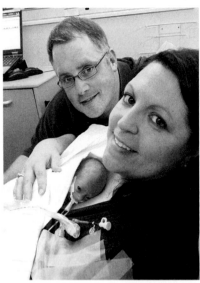

FIGURE 13-2 Kangaroo care of awake, alert, intubated, and ventilated premature infant.

BOX 13-7	SELECTION CRITERIA FOR KANGAROO CARE WITH VENTILATED INFANTS

- Birth weight >600 g; ≥30 weeks' GA
- Ventilator for at least 24 hr before first kangaroo care
- SIMV: <35 breaths/min; FIO_2 <0.50 (50%)
- Stable vital signs (TPR, B/P) and oxygen saturation
- Stable blood gases, bilirubin level
- No signs/symptoms of sepsis
- Not receiving vasopressors; no chest tube
- Lines (Broviac, umbilical, arterial, IVs) well secured

Modified from Ludington-Hoe S, Morgan K, Abouelfrettoh A: A clinical guideline for implementation of kangaroo care with premature infants of 30 or more weeks' postmenstrual age, *Adv Neonatal Care* 8:S3, 2008.
B/P, Blood pressure; *FIO_2*, fraction of inspired oxygen; *GA*, gestational age; *IV*, intravenous; *SIMV*, synchronous intermittent mandatory ventilation; *TPR*, temperature, pulse, respiration.

selection criteria (Box 13-7) and a safe protocol (Box 13-8) for KC in this population have been developed.[193,196] During this study, no adverse physiologic or behavioral events or accidental extubations occurred. None of these babies was agitated, and all slept and tolerated KC well. Previously reported parental perceptions of KC with ventilated babies include the following:

- Ambivalence toward KC: yearning to hold the infant yet being apprehensive about it

- The necessity of a supportive environment
- The special quality of parent-infant interaction: intense connectedness and active parenting

Perhaps these parental concerns, as well as staff concerns, may be overcome with careful selection of infants, education about KC, a consistent procedure for transfer, increase in confidence of the staff assisting parents in KC, and a clinical guideline for implementing KC.[141,193,196,240,241] Parents and staff need education about KC, and staff can offer KC to parents instead of waiting for parents to request this intervention.* Recommendations about KC include the following:

- It is an important therapeutic intervention for healthy preterms (gestational age ≥34 weeks) and their mothers in a modern, well-equipped NICU[191,339] as recommended by the World Health Organization.[348]
- It is a simple, safe, cost-effective intervention that reduces severe infant morbidity without serious side effects, and more well-designed randomized controlled trials are needed.[63]
- Parents need education, a trusting relationship, individualized support, and consistent information and communication from health care providers to be comfortable with KC.[179,235]
- Nursing staff members need education about the benefits of KC, as well as confidence and competence in skills to transfer and evaluate families and infants during KC.[141]
- Well-written NICU protocols for KC should contain criteria for initiation, positioning, transfer to/from KC, care practices while in KC, provision of privacy, parental role, and interventions for neonatal instability.[179,240,241]
- Written information for parents about the benefits of KC, expectations of parents during KC, preparing for KC (i.e., eat, go to the bathroom, bring a drink) assist parents and provide consistent, complete information to all families.[179]

One should also note that fathers can also participate in KC without endangering the infant. Aside from the positive effects on the baby, paternal KC enhances the engagement and attachment of the father, helps fathers attain their paternal role, adapt to the crisis of preterm birth, and includes the father in the infant's care.[35,179,314] The Hug Your Baby (HUG) program improves fathers'

---

*References 18, 45, 79, 95, 141, 179, 191.

BOX 13-8

PROTOCOL FOR KANGAROO CARE WITH VENTILATED INFANTS

In Preparation for Transfer

1. Record baseline vital signs, oxygen saturation, and ventilator settings. Secure and maintain continuous monitoring of these parameters during kangaroo care (KC) to determine infant's tolerance of KC.
2. Place infant supine on a clean blanket (folded in fourths) with assistance of second person, and note changes in vital signs, saturations, or ventilator settings.
3. Auscultate chest and evaluate breath sounds, suction endotracheal tube, and change diaper.
4. Drain water from ventilator tubings to decrease resistance, maintain airflow, and prevent retrograde water flow toward infant when moved or positioned lower than or at the level of the ventilator.
5. Assess infant's responses: Wait 15 minutes to enable physiologic adaptation (e.g., return of baseline vital signs/oxygenation for 3 minutes). If still unstable at 15 minutes, the infant is probably not stable enough for KC at this time.
6. Position the reclining chair near the ventilator, making sure there is ample tubing length.
7. Two or three staff members will assist the parent in transfer of the infant:
   - One person gathers lines to one side of the infant.
   - One person transfers and secures the ventilator tubing.
   - One person assists the parent.

Transfer Procedure

1. After a staff member disconnects the endotracheal tube (ETT) from the ventilator, the parent slides his or her hands under the blanket and infant, lifts both, and places the infant prone against his or her chest in one movement. Reconnect the ventilator tubing, and let the infant stabilize. (If the infant was not placed on a clean blanket or it was soiled before transfer, the parent can lift the baby and a clean blanket is placed over the infant when he or she is prone on the parent's chest.)
2. Disconnect ventilator tubing from ETT and move parent backward toward recliner, having him or her sit down when he or she feels the edge of the

chair against the calves of the legs. Reconnect the ETT to the ventilator tubing.
3. Assist the parent in being comfortable by raising the footrest, position the infant in a flexed position with head and neck in a neutral position to avoid ETT movement (e.g., downward into the bronchi with head flexion or possible extubation with head extension) and/or obstructive apnea with head flexion or extension if the infant is on nasal continuous positive airway pressure.
4. Secure the ventilator tubing by draping it over the parent's shoulder. *Do not tape the tubing to the blanket, parent clothing, etc.*
5. If using ISC temperature control (on the radiant warmer/incubator), turn to air control, set temperature at 33° C while the baby is receiving KC, and monitor the infant's skin temperature from the temperature gauge on the radiant warmer/incubator. (There is then no need to uncover or cold stress the infant to take a temperature.)
6. Maintain continuous electronic monitoring throughout KC; check both the infant's and/or parent's condition every 10 minutes during KC.
7. If the infant's condition remains stable, facilitate KC for a minimum of 1 hour.

Transfer after Kangaroo Care

1. Slowly place the recliner in an upright position, and assist parent to move forward to the front edge of the chair.
2. One staff member handles the lines, and another disconnects the ETT from the ventilator lines.
3. Assist the parent to stand, reconnect the ETT to the ventilator tubing, and let the infant stabilize.
4. In one movement, disconnect the ventilator tubing and place the infant in the radiant warmer/incubator.
5. Reconnect the ventilator tubing to the ETT, stabilize, and secure all lines inside the radiant warmer/incubator.
6. Document KC, length of session, and how the infant and parent tolerated KC.

ISC, Infant servocontrol.
Modified from Ludington-Hoe S, Ferreira C, Swinth J: Safe criteria and procedure for kangaroo care with intubated preterm infants, *J Obstet Gynecol Neonat Nurs* 32:586, 2003; Ludington-Hoe S, Morgan K, Abouelfrettoh A: A clinical guideline for implementation of kangaroo care with premature infants of 30 or more weeks' postmenstrual age, *Adv Neonatal Care* 8:S3, 2008.

understanding of their preterm infant behaviors, lowers paternal stress, and improves paternal confidence.[156]

Bathing. There is a lack of evidence of the safety and efficacy of sponge bathing preterm babies in the NICU on a daily or every-other-day schedule.[114] Sponge bathing critically ill infants (28–34 weeks' gestational age) results in significant increases in behavior state and activity levels

(i.e., motor stress behavior, stability, reorganization), increase in stress cue frequency, increase or decrease in heart rate, decrease in oxygen saturation preterm, and need for enhanced temperature support.[252,312] These detrimental effects caused by handling were exhibited most frequently by neonates of younger gestational ages. Because sponge bathing of critically ill preterm infants clearly increases physiologic risk and provides no clear benefits, the procedure of routine bathing of these infants is unnecessary and not recommended.[253] Frequency of sponge bathing can be reduced to every 4 days without increasing skin flora colony counts or colonization with pathogens.[114]

Waiting to bathe these infants until they are physiologically stable with introduction of the bath as a "recovery milestone" for parents to complete is a more developmentally and physiologically appropriate practice.[93,253] In one study, late preterm infants (LPI) who were tub bathed experienced less hypothermia and were significantly warmer at 10 minutes and 30 minutes after bathing compared with LPIs who were sponge bathed.[189] Parents may tub bathe the premature grower, and this may provide a soothing, relaxing, tension-relieving experience of multiple textures (i.e., water, water temperature, soap, washcloth).

A study of the effects of tub bathing on preterm infants (done by nurses) found disruption of sleep and an increase in stress behaviors; the study recommended considering the effects of "routine" nursing procedures and modifying handling of the preterm to promote recovery, growth, and development and to decrease stress.[182] It is evident that more supportive behaviors by the nurse (i.e., position support and containment) enhanced the preterm infant's self-regulation during bathing.[183]

Swaddled bathing (i.e., swaddled in a flexed, midline position in a blanket while bathing) provides containment and helps the infant self-regulate. Benefits of swaddled bathing are listed in Box 13-9. A protocol for swaddled bathing is available with best results occurring with an initial water temperature of 100° to 101° F and a bath length of 8 minutes.[267]

Self-Consoling. Consoling hand-to-mouth behaviors are observed more frequently during caregiving (by nurses, rather than parents) and before and after feeding (especially in gavage-fed infants). Hand-to-midline behaviors are encouraged by cradling the infant for feedings (for both bottle and gavage feedings if the infant tolerates it) with both arms in the midline. If a premature infant needs an oxygen hood, using one large enough so that the infant's whole upper body will fit inside encourages hand-to-mouth quieting (Figure 13-3). VLBW preterm infants whose whole body was not inside the oxygen hood have been videotaped expending energy in persistent attempts (30–40 minutes) to self-console and reduce stress by trying to get their hands to their mouths.

> **BOX 13-9** **BENEFITS OF SWADDLED BATHING**[104,267]
>
> - Decrease in physiologic and motor stress
> - Better energy conservation
> - Improvement in state control
> - Less crying and agitation
> - Fewer stress cues
> - Less temperature instability

Use arm restraints only when necessary, and immobilize the extremity in a physiologic position. Release and exercise the restrained extremity with each caregiving encounter. Avoid restraining both arms so that one is free for hand-to-mouth behaviors. If both must be restrained (e.g., the infant pulls out the orogastric tube), give the infant a pacifier.

Positioning. Preterm infants display motor development that is different from that of term infants.[226,285] A continuous assessment of muscle tone, response to positioning and handling, oral-motor function, and response to sensory stimuli provides data for individualizing intervention. The goal of intervention is to provide opportunities for normal development and organization of the sensory systems, detect early developmental problems, and educate parents about stimulation, handling, and positioning. Although some studies have shown that specific positioning for premature infants does not significantly affect development, others have shown that a developmental approach to care of VLBW infants greatly reduces the long-term, negative effects of prematurity.[81,231]

Preterm infants usually have less developed physiologic flexion in the limbs, trunk, and pelvis compared with term newborns (Table 13-8). Even at 40 weeks' postconceptual age, preterm infants have less flexion than their full-term counterparts have. For preterm infants, long periods of immobilization without a positioning device on a firm mattress with the influences of gravity result in a number of abnormal characteristics: (1) increased neck extension with a right-sided head preference, (2) shoulder retraction and abduction (reduces forward rotation and ability to reach midline), (3) increased trunk extension with "arching" of the neck and back, (4) frog-leg position: hips abducted and externally rotated, and (5) ankle and feet eversion

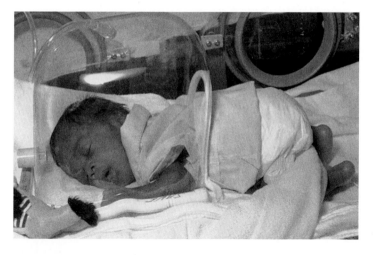

FIGURE 13-3 Preterm infant in oxygen hood that is large enough to accommodate upper body to facilitate hand-to-mouth behavior. Note sling that helps maintain flexion without frog-leg position.

TABLE 13-8	DEVELOPMENT OF TONE*	

GESTATIONAL AGE (wk)	DEVELOPMENT
28	Completely hypotonic and lacks all physiologic flexion
32	Hips and knees begin to show some flexion while arms remain extended
34	Flexor tone apparent in legs
36	Loose flexion of arms and legs evident and grasp reflex present
40	Develops tone in utero and develops flexed position in intrauterine space; after birth, reflex activity and central nervous system maturity help term infant unfold and extend; term infant holds all four limbs in flexed position

From Anderson J, Auster-Liebhaber J: *Phys Occup Ther Pediatr* 4(1): 1984; Dubowitz LM, Dubowitz V, Goldberg C: *J Pediatr* 77:1, 1970; Palisano R, Short M: *Phys Occup Ther Pediatr* 4(4):43, 1984.

*Muscle tone develops in caudocephalic and centripetal (distal to proximal) directions and interacts with simultaneous cephalocaudal development of movement to help affect posture. Although knowledge of normal development before term helps detect signs of abnormality, variability of ±2 weeks' gestational age must be considered.[85]

(Figure 13-4).[226,325] These characteristics interfere with development of eye-hand coordination, head control in prone/sitting, crawling/walking, cognitive development, and equilibrium.[285] Box 13-10 lists the reasons for proper positioning in the NICU.

To prevent overstretching of the joints, facilitate development of flexor tone, and prevent deformities, the infant should be provided with a variety of positions. Goals of proper positioning include (1) optimize alignment (e.g., neutral neck/trunk and foot positions), semiflexed, midline extremity posture, (2) support posture and movement within containment boundaries (avoid producing a barrier of immobilization), (3) modify positioning and handling to support behavioral state regulation of sleep-wake states, and (4) provide positions that encourage controlled, individual exposure to stimuli while monitoring for signs of behavioral stress from overstimulation and adjust stimuli accordingly. A physical therapist can be helpful in facilitating these positions.

Side-lying is used to improve visual awareness of hands, encourage hands-to-midline movement, and discourage the frog-leg position. In this position, the infant can bring the hands to the mouth for sucking and self-comforting. Side-lying is best maintained with swaddling or commercial positioning devices rather than single blanket rolls (Figure 13-5). Position extremities so that the bottom arm is in a comfortable position and the upper shoulder and hip are slightly forward of the weight-bearing lower hip or shoulder, provide a small roll (e.g., folded cloth diaper or washcloth or small bean-stuffed toy), and bundle for security but not so that the upper extremity compromises chest expansion. Alternating sides reduces head molding and may prevent atelectasis of the dependent lung. The head and trunk should be maintained in neutral alignment (e.g., the head and trunk are in the same vertical plane). The left lateral position has been

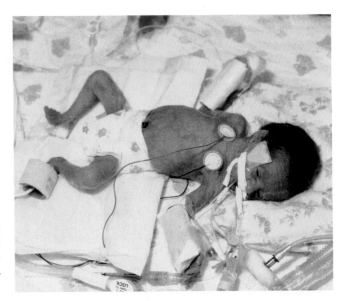

FIGURE 13-4 Premature infant hypotonic resting posture exhibiting the W configuration of arms, frog-leg position of the legs, abducted hips, externally rotated ankles, everted feet, and asymmetric head position. This position promotes positional deformities and developmental gaps and delays. (From Hunter J: The neonatal intensive care unit. In Case-Smith J, editor: *Occupational therapy for children*, ed 4, St Louis, 2001, Mosby.)

BOX 13-10   REASONS FOR PROPER POSITIONING

1. Inhibits or shortens dystonic phase while infant remains in fetal position during postnatal period
2. Facilitates hand-to-midline and midline orientation[85]
3. Stimulates visual exploration of environment (through head to midline)
4. Facilitates development of head control (making feeding easier and helping respiratory problems)[85]
5. Helps balance flexors and extensors to facilitate symmetric posture[81,226,231,285]
6. Helps develop antigravity movement
7. Enhances comfort and decreases stress
8. Has an organizing effect that facilitates development of flexor tone[85]
9. Promotes normal and prevents abnormal development[81,85,285]
10. Helps enhance development of motor skills, reflexes, and postural tone[81,231,285]

From Pelletier-Sehnar JM, Palmeri A: High-risk infants. In Pratt PN, Allen AS, editors: *Occupational therapy for children*, ed 2, St Louis, 1989, Mosby.

shown to improve oxygenation, lung mechanics, and breathing patterns in preterm infants, similar to the benefits of prone positioning.[128] Left lateral position reduces gastroesophageal reflux, whereas right lateral position reduces gastric residuals.[92]

To accommodate their ventilators, umbilical catheters, and other devices, acutely ill preterm infants may be positioned supine; the preterm neonate's head should be in the midline. Positioning VLBW infants supine with their heads turned to either side causes mechanical obstruction of cerebral venous return and alters cerebral blood flow, which may contribute to the development of intraventricular hemorrhage (IVH).[250] Cerebral (and mesenteric) tissue oxygenation was recently measured in clinically stable VLBW infants in two supine positions (i.e., with head tilted up 30 degrees and lying flat) and prone (lying flat).[74] Regardless of position these stable VLBW infants were able to maintain stable cerebral and mesenteric tissue oxygenation, both before and after feeding.[74]

Supine positioning does not promote flexion and may be stressful to acutely ill infants. Earlier studies found an increase in apnea, bradycardia, and periodic breathing in supine positioning, although a more recent study of 22 preterm infants with apnea and bradycardia found no significant difference in the incidence of clinically significant events between supine and prone positioning.[158] Placed supine, infants exhibit more startle behaviors, agitation, motor disorganization, calorie expenditure, and sleep disturbance from environmental stimuli.

Prolonged supine positioning is associated with the hypertonic "arched" position (hyperextension

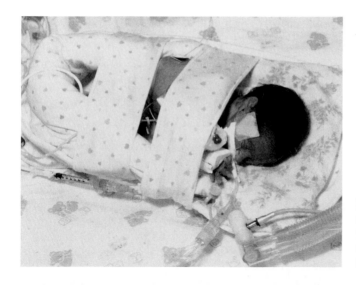

FIGURE 13-5 Small preterm infant in side-lying position supported in flexion and with a midline orientation of the extremities. (From Hunter J: The neonatal intensive care unit. In Case-Smith J, editor: *Occupational therapy for children,* ed 4, St Louis, 2001, Mosby.)

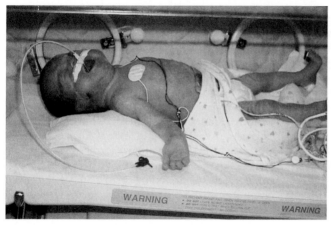

FIGURE 13-6 Supine positioning without positioning supports results in motor disorganization, agitation, arching posture, and burning of significant calories. (From Hunter J: The neonatal intensive care unit. In Case-Smith J, editor: *Occupational therapy for children,* ed 4, St Louis, 2001, Mosby.)

of head, neck, and shoulder girdle) of many chronically ventilated infants (Figure 13-6); use of a gel or water pillow under the infant's head and neck (e.g., to the nipple level to prevent neck flexion; used as a mattress under the head or body of a VLBW infant) provides comfort and maintains neutral alignment.

Supine positioning should promote as much flexion as possible. Use of a positioning device of foam with the middle cut out and sloping under the scapulae is another method of obtaining supine flexion. Use of hip support results in less lower extremity abduction and external rotation than in infants without such hip support. Pillows filled with polystyrene beads (i.e., preterm bean bags) require skill for optimal positioning and close infant monitoring but are useful in providing positioning for very small premature infants (1000–1500 g).

Body containment increases the infant's feeling of security, promotes quieting and self-control, enhances physiologic stability, promotes energy conservation, reduces physiologic and behavioral stress, and enables stress to be better endured.[313] Without positional supports, many premature infants "travel" (no matter how many times they are returned) to the sides or bottom of their incubator. Parents and professionals are inclined to move the uncomfortable-looking infant back to the middle of a "boundary-less" world. Infants should be left where they feel safe and comfortable; if they become uncomfortable, they will let you know. Providing boundaries (e.g., blanket rolls, positioning

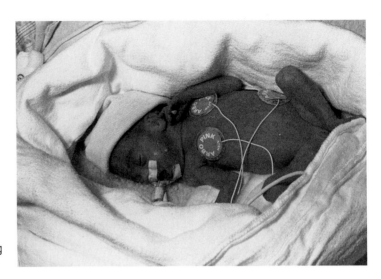

FIGURE 13-7 Very small premature infant resting quietly in a "nest" of pads and blankets.

devices) stops this migration and the expenditure of precious calories that could go to growth.

Small, acutely ill premature infants who are positioned supine are often extremely agitated, thrashing arms and legs, tachycardic, and expending precious energy and calories. Instead of needing medications, these infants often are calmed by providing a nest of blankets or a commercial nesting device (which simulates the boundaries and security of the uterus). This artificial womb must be closely surrounding the infant to promote flexion, security, and quiet rest (Figure 13-7). If agitation recurs, a limb (usually a leg) has extended outside the infant's secure boundary; flexing and returning it to the "womb" quiets the infant.[11]

Body containment maneuvers such as swaddling, holding onto a finger or hand, and crossing the infant's arms in the midline and holding them securely help with self-regulation during feeding, procedures, or other stressful manipulations.[65] Safe swaddling includes positioning the baby's extremities in slight flexion and abduction. Placing an infant's hips and knees in an extended position with swaddling increases the risk of hip dysplasia and dislocation.[150] Because being wrapped in a blanket with extremities flexed simulates in utero position, swaddling (1) improves flexed posture and flexor muscle tone, (2) facilitates behavioral responses, and (3) improves the development of primitive reflexes. Picking up the preterm infant from a supine position often produces startles, apnea, or head hyperextension. A better technique is

to roll the infant prone, which flexes the head, and then flex the limbs onto the trunk and pick up the infant. If the infant has difficulty breathing in prone position, swaddle or contain the extremities before picking up the infant.

Prone positioning encourages the infant to work on using neck extension and promotes flexion of the extremities. Position devices for prone include a small hip roll or sling to assist in maintaining flexion; use of gel/water pillows for head support; and secure lower boundary for foot bracing. Use of a rolled cloth or gel pillow placed under the infant (from top of the head to the umbilicus) (1) provides elevation of the body to promote extremity flexion without placing excessive pressure on the knees and elbows, (2) enables the shoulders to round forward over the top of the roll, and (3) enables the legs to flex over the bottom edge of the roll. Prone (versus supine) positioning has numerous benefits and is the position of choice for many NICU infants (Box 13-11). A study showed that sleeping in the prone position did not improve oxygenation in preterms 32 weeks' PMA or older for infants without respiratory problems. The study concluded that preterms older than 32 weeks' PMA and without respiratory difficulties should be placed supine and monitoring continued to ensure adequate oxygen saturation. Prone positioning of highly agitated, fretful narcotic-withdrawing neonates showed that they experienced less distress (i.e., lower withdrawal scores and lower caloric intake) than supine-lying infants.[200] Use of a sheepskin or lambskin helps to further facilitate flexion and prevents skin abrasion, especially on the knees.

Sleep Position. The most recent American Academy of Pediatrics (AAP) position paper on infant sleep states that healthy infants should be placed *only* in the supine position for sleep beginning immediately after birth.[17] Side-lying for sleep is not endorsed because the infant may spontaneously roll from side-lying to prone.[17] Overheating sleeping infants; use of soft sleeping surfaces, stuffed toys, and positioning devices[55]; and inappropriate sleep environments (e.g., waterbeds, pillows, bed railings, bed sharing[52,62,323]) should all be avoided in healthy infants.[17] The National Infant Sleep Position study, conducted from 1993 to 2010, found an increase in bed sharing especially among black and Hispanic mothers throughout the study period.[62] Use of a pacifier for sleep and sleeping in proximity (same room) to parents is also recommended.[17]

Use of side-lying and prone positioning, as well as containment with soft bedding for physiologically compromised term and preterm infants, is safe and appropriate in a NICU setting. Parents may question these practices; therefore, their physiologic base and rationale should be explained. Parents should be taught that when their baby is medically stable, by 32 weeks' PMA,[17] he or she will be physiologically and developmentally mature enough to tolerate supine sleep position in preparation for discharge.[118,181] Many of the beneficial effects of prone positioning listed in Box 13-11 are no longer necessary[181] and become detrimental in increasing the risk for sudden infant death syndrome (SIDS) in the stable, mature preterm infant.

Since the "Back to Sleep" campaign, the rate of SIDS has decreased by 53%.[17] VLBW infants (<1500 g), the group at highest risk for SIDS, have been found in one study to be more likely to sleep prone after discharge than larger LBW infants.[330a] Reasons cited by mothers included (1) infant's preference and (2) advice from professionals (NICU doctors, nurses) who may remain uncomfortable recommending supine sleep in this population[118,181,330a] despite the AAP recommendations and the research that supports them[17] (Table 13-9).

Implementing Back to Sleep principles in the NICU remains a problem and influences parental behavior. One study found that only 50% of NICU nurses place preterm infants supine during

---

BOX 13-11 EFFECTS OF PRONE POSITIONING

1. Decreases heart rate variability
2. Improves oxygenation by 15% to 25%[24,31,128]
   a. Increased TcP_{O_2} values
   b. Increased Pa_{O_2} values
   c. Decreased apnea, bradycardia, and periodic breathing
   d. Increased peripheral oxygenation and decreases cerebral blood flow[30]
3. Improves lung mechanics and lung volumes[128]
   a. Increased lung compliance
   b. Increased tidal volume
4. Decreases energy expenditure[126]
   a. Increased quiet sleep; higher arousal threshold[152]
   b. Decreased awake time; more sleep time[56,152]
   c. Decreased caloric expenditure (median difference supine vs. prone: + 3.1 kcal/kg/day)
   d. Decreased heat loss[56]
   e. Less crying[56]
   f. Lower levels of activity[56]
5. Decreases (by 50%) gastric residuals in the first 30 minutes after feeding[57]
6. Decreases gastroesophageal reflux[92]

---

transition to an open crib and more than 20% never place preterms supine or do so only 1 to 2 days before discharge.[130] A recent project to increase NICU compliance with supine positioning for sleep used staff and parent education, an algorithm, crib card, audit tool, and postdischarge telephone survey.[118] Compliance with the principles of Back to Sleep resulted in (1) supine positioning increased from 39% to 83%, (2) firm sleeping surface increased from 5% to 96%, (3) removal of soft objects improved from 45% to 75%, and (4) continuation of parental provision of a safe sleep environment improved from 23% to 82%.[118]

In term infants, supine sleep position may delay some motor milestones by 1 month but does not delay walking. Increased amounts of time in supervised prone play ("tummy time") encourages earlier motor milestone attainment in supine sleepers and helps prevent head molding.[173] Head molding (i.e., bilateral flattening of the head and elongation of the face) is a significant problem in preterm infants; it results from flattening of the skull as the baby lies against the firm incubator mattress.[173] To parents, this

TABLE 13-9 SLEEP POSITION AS A RISK FACTOR FOR SUDDEN INFANT DEATH SYNDROME (SIDS): RESEARCH BASIS

SUPINE	PRONE
Preterm infants at 36–38 wk PCA[126] No significant difference in sleep organization based on body position. More awakenings in supine vs. prone position. Standard deviations of heart rate increase during quiet sleep in supine position; low frequency and high frequency of heart rate higher in supine vs. prone position in both active and quiet sleep states. More sleep transitions, a lower arousal threshold, and higher heart rate variability while sleeping supine contribute to decreased vulnerability to SIDS	Prone position reduces spontaneous arousals from sleep in term infants,[157,245,272] which may be related to a decrease in cerebral oxygenation in prone sleeping.[347] First quiet sleep after feedings significantly longer, fewer number of awakenings, and decrease in overall heart rate variability in prone vs. supine.[126,272] Preceding characteristics of prone sleep constitute a higher arousal threshold, and thus increased vulnerability to SIDS in prone position.[245,272,347] Decreased baroreflex sensitivity, which increases vulnerability to hypotensive events.[349]
Full-term (n = 10) infants in prone/supine sleep positions given 0.4 ml water; instillation into the mouth resulted in airway protective responses of swallowing (95%) and arousal (54%).[153]	Sixty-two healthy, growing low BW infants (26–37 wk GA; 750–1600 g BW); sleeping position—a shift of EEG activity toward slower frequency, which may be related to mechanisms associated with a decrease in behavioral arousal in prone position.[272,283]
Swallow rate rapid in supine position in response to small infusions of fluid, whereas respiratory rate remains largely unaffected. When supine, term infants can coordinate rapid swallowing while maintaining breathing.	A significant decrease in swallowing and breathing in active sleep in prone vs. supine position; airway protection is compromised in prone sleeping position during active sleep in healthy term infants exposed to minute pharyngeal fluid.
Full-term (n = 3240) ≥37 wk GA evaluated in the first 24 hr of life for frequency/severity of spitting up incidents while asleep[311]: • 96.6% did not spit up during sleep. • 130 episodes of spitting up while sleeping supine (55% required no intervention; 37% brief bulb suction; 6% gentle stimulation; 2% wall suction). • <4% spit up while sleeping supine, and none required significant intervention or experienced serious sequelae.	Six episodes of spitting up while infants side-lying (66.7% no intervention; 33.3% bulb suction).

BW, Birth weight; *GA,* gestational age; *EEG,* electroencephalogram; *PCA,* postconceptual age.

head flattening is concerning, and they may find the infant less cute and desirable than a term infant with a rounded head. To prevent head molding, preterm infants are often placed on waterbeds, water pillows, air mattresses, or eggcrate-type mattresses, with variable results. Preterm infants (<32 weeks' gestation with birth weight <1500 g) who are turned every 3 hours, repositioned in one of six positions, and never placed in the same position twice in 8 hours had significantly rounder head shapes from 9 to 13 weeks of life compared with infants repositioned according to a standard NICU procedure.[142]

Kinesthetic. A combination of vestibular and tactile stimulation increases quieting behaviors, decreases apneic and bradycardic episodes, entrains respirations, increases visual and auditory fixation, and increases brain growth.[164,166] Waterbeds provide contingent stimuli because they move in response to the infant's movement; oscillating waterbeds provide rhythmic motion. Kinesthetic stimulation is provided by rocking chairs, hammocks, baby swings, and baby carriers, the effects of which have not been investigated. In Brazil, a combination tactile/kinesthetic stimulation program enrolling 16 clinically stable preterm infants less than 2500 g was conducted and compared with a control group of 16 preterms.[105] Outcomes of the preterms receiving the tactile/kinesthetic program included (1) higher daily weight gain, (2) predominance of self-regulated behaviors (i.e., regular respirations, balanced tone, state of alertness, range of postures, coordinated movements, hand-to-mouth movement control, suction, grip and support), and (3) a trend toward shorter length of stay.[105]

Upright positioning in a car seat or infant seat encourages symmetry and spatial orientation. Soft rolls or foam padding maintains flexion; a rolled blanket in a horseshoe configuration around the infant's head and shoulders prevents lateral slouching. Carrying quiets the infant, provides sensory communication with the caregiver, changes the infant's environment, and provides visual, auditory, and tactile stimuli. A nasal cannula (see Chapter 23) and portable tank enable mobility for an infant receiving oxygen.

Rather than standardized protocols, tactile interventions must be individualized by assessing each infant's physiologic and behavioral responses before, during, and after touch (see Table 13-6). While an infant is acutely ill, tactile intervention should include minimal handling, containment, and gentle touch (without stroking). As the infant matures and becomes physiologically stable, stroking, rocking, and holding are integrated based on the individual infant's tolerance and preferences. In healthy preterm infants, a program of range-of-motion exercises with passive resistance is associated with an increase in weight gain and growth, bone mineral content and density, and muscle mass and a decreased risk for osteopenia.[13,185,332]

Cobedding. Cobedding, the practice of placing medically stable twins and higher-order multiples together in the same open warmer, incubator, or crib, was initiated after the observed stress response in separated siblings. The practice of cobedding spread based on anecdotal information, because there is limited research to support or refute its use. Few differences between cobedded and non-cobedded infants have been demonstrated. Limitations of the research on cobedding include small sample size, short follow-up periods, lack of randomization, and blinding of evaluators.

Infection, safety, and parents continuing the practice after discharge are major concerns of cobedding. To date, increased infection rates in cobedded infants have not been reported. Infection concerns are addressed by good hand washing and color-coding of equipment. Other safety concerns include proper identification for medication administration and medical emergencies and maintenance of temperature stability for all cobedded infants.[12] Because parents continue care practices at home that they have witnessed and become accustomed to in the hospital, the possibility of continuing cobedding at home (and the lack of evidence as to its safety) must be considered.[118]

The National Association of Neonatal Nurses (NANN) recommends that a decision to cobed be made with input from parents, involve education of staff and parents about potential benefits/risks, the experimental nature of the practice, and the development of a clinical evaluation protocol to collect data on risks and benefits.[234] The AAP recommends separate sleep areas in the hospital and at home.[17] Both NANN[234] and the AAP[17] have concluded that neither the safety or benefit of cobedding has been established by current research and that parents should be instructed to follow established safe sleeping practices at home.[17]

AUDITORY INTERVENTION

The NICU is a noisy environment that has no diurnal rhythm or predictability; it is as noisy at night as in the daytime (Table 13-10).[70,127,206] An infant in the NICU is exposed to an onslaught of noise 24 hours a day for days, weeks, or months. At follow-up, preterm infants exhibit a lower threshold for sound and a reduced responsiveness to auditory stimulation.[28] Assisted ventilation, severe asphyxia, drug therapies, and possibly acoustic insult account for the increased risk (i.e., in up to 10%–12% of LBW infants) for sensorineural hearing loss in NICU infants (regardless of gestational age).[16,228,351] Moderate to severe conductive hearing loss also occurs in 42% of VLBW infants. Conductive hearing loss is attributed to endotracheal intubation, poor eustachian tube function, increased otitis media, and CLD in preterm infants.

The first goal in auditory intervention is to assess the current level of noise in the NICU and decrease the noise decibel level wherever possible.[167,206] The noise environment of an individual infant depends on the ambient sounds in the nursery, the type of incubator and support equipment, and the baby's own behavior (i.e., quiet or crying). Noise measurement protocols must sample multiple noise sources and sites.[206] Some NICUs have

TABLE
13-10 **NOISE LEVELS IN THE NICU**

LEVEL (dB)	COMMENTS
48–69	Humidifiers and nebulizers
50–60	Normal speaking voice
50–73.5*†	Incubator (motor noise)
53	Median noise level on conventional ventilator
55–88	Bradycardia alarm
58–85‡	Noise in NICU (talking, equipment alarms, telephones, radio)
59	Median noise level on high-frequency oscillator
65–80†	Life support equipment (ventilator; intravenous pumps)
66–76	Sink on/off
67	Incubator alarm
70	Background noise mean level should not exceed
85§	Noise level at which hearing damage is possible for adult; (?) neonatal effects
90	Peak sound intensity in the NICU not to exceed
90§	Adult exposure for 8 hours requires protective device and hearing conservation program
92.8†	Opening incubator porthole
84–108	Placing a plastic bottle of formula on top of incubator
96–117†	Placing a glass bottle of formula on top of incubator
70–116†	Closing one or both cabinet doors
80–124†	Closing one or both portholes
120	Threshold for pain
130–140†	Banging incubator to stimulate apneic premature infant
160–165§	Recommendations for peak, single noise level not to exceed to prevent (adult) hearing loss; (?) neonatal effects

Data from Thomas KA, Uran A: How the NICU environment sounds to a preterm infant: update, *MCN Am J Matern Child Nurs* 32:250, 2007.

NICU, Neonatal intensive care unit.

*Modern incubators generate less than 60 dB; exceeds hourly recommendation of 50 dBA (see Table 13-11).

†Measures from inside the incubator.

‡Noise levels do not vary from morning to night.

§Occupational Safety and Health Administration (OSHA) standard. (No safety standards for neonates have been established.)

BOX
13-12 **EFFECTS OF LOUD NOISE**[138,169,284,334,344]

- Increase in stress behaviors:
  - State lability
  - Arousal state
  - Avoidance behaviors—more fussy, more startles, etc. (see Table 13-4)
  - Sympathetic nervous system arousal measured by noninvasive skin conductance, which was higher in male preterms
- Decrease in approach behaviors (see Table 13-4)
- Cardiorespiratory changes:
  - Increased heart rate
  - Increased respiratory rate
  - Increased apnea or bradycardia
  - Increased hypoxemia (decreased pulse oximeter)
  - Increased peripheral and arterial vasoconstriction:
    - Increased systemic blood pressure
    - Increased intracranial pressure
  - Increased sensory neural hearing loss
  - Abnormal auditory development and processing
  - Prevents habituation
- Alters development of sleep-wake cycles:
  - Disturbs sleep; interrupts light sleep
  - Increases wakefulness and agitation
- Increased risk for intraventricular hemorrhage:
  - Increase in cerebral blood flow
  - No change in cerebral oxygenation when peak sound levels increased by 5 dB for short duration; cerebral oxygenation at higher sound levels for longer durations unknown[94]

installed decimeters that present a flashing or blinking light when the noise level exceeds a preset level (about 50–65 dB). Sources of noise include heating, ventilation, and air conditioner flow units (noise levels may decrease by 2.5–10.5 dB when these units are turned off). The greatest contributor to loud noise in the NICU is talking and conversation by the staff. Noise levels vary with location, time of day, and day of week within the NICU; therefore various locations or various times and days should be measured.[70,167,206]

Increased environmental noise levels are a stressor to all infants in the NICU—preterm infants, as well as ill term infants (e.g., infants with persistent pulmonary hypertension of the newborn or drug withdrawal; Box 13-12). The sudden, high-pitched, shrill, dysrhythmic noise of equipment alarms alerts the care provider, but it also results in infants manifesting an extreme hypersensitivity to sound (as a learned conditioned response). CNS-injured preterms are particularly vulnerable to sound stress in the NICU, are less able to habituate to NICU noise, and respond with exaggerated and prolonged physiologic responses (e.g., alterations in respiratory rate, bradycardia, desaturations). Noise is stressful not only to the infants but also to parents and care providers in the NICU.[139] Three years after their NICU experience, mothers recall the noise level in the NICU as a stressor. NICU noise is stressful to care providers and has the potential to damage hearing; cause physiologic responses (e.g., increase blood pressure, alter immune response, increase stress hormone secretion, disturb sleep); cause fatigue, irritability, and "burnout"; interfere with communication with coworkers and parents; alter concentration; and increase errors.[317]

Although the AAP recommends that noise levels be less than 45 dB,[64] most NICUs' noise levels range between 38 and 90 dB, with higher noise bursts (see Table 13-10).[70,138,167,206] To protect sleep, support stable vital signs, and improve speech intelligibility, recommended standards for noise criteria have been established. Recent noise studies in NICUs have found the following★:

- Noise levels are still louder than recommended.
- Environmental changes to reduce noise must be monitored because they may increase rather than decrease noise.
- Nurses perceived their own NICU as "pretty quiet" when, in fact, noise levels were above recommendations.
- Noise levels have not significantly decreased in the NICU.
- Single-room NICUs attenuate noise, but equipment noise is not decreased in single-room units

Table 13-11 presents specific noise criteria and their rationale. Parents and care providers must be involved in planning, developing, and being educated about quieter NICUs.[138,167,307]

Strategies to minimize external auditory stimuli include quieting alarms with suction (and remembering to reset them); not taking a shift report over or allowing medical rounds near the infant's incubator; having noisy equipment repaired immediately; emptying sloshing water in ventilator or nebulizer tubing; maintaining cardiac monitors in a quiet state

---

★References 70, 138, 167, 186, 206, 329.

TABLE 13-11	RATIONALE FOR SPECIFIC NOISE CRITERIA[64]
NOISE CRITERION	**RATIONALE**
Hourly Leq (equivalent sound level) of 45 dB in infant room; 50 dB in staff work areas	Preserves sleep for healthy term infants most of the time
Hourly L_{10} of 50 dB in infant room; 55 dB in staff work areas (sound levels may exceed 55 dB only 10% of the time or a total of 6 min/hr)	Preserves sleep for infants; enables caregivers to speak at normal conversational levels and be clearly understood 12 feet away, approximately 90% of the time
L_{max} of 65 dB in infant room; not to exceed 70 dB in staff work areas (maximum decibel sound level ≤1 sec in duration—transient bursts of noise)	Minimizes rousing babies and causing startle responses

with alarms on (decreasing the sound of alarms by 50%); and purchasing quieter equipment (e.g., plastic instead of metal trash containers; quieter incubators). Choosing heated humidifiers (48 dB) rather than nebulizers (69 dB) and keeping the containers full of water, rather than low, decrease noise from respiratory equipment. Nursery design changes[64] include smaller cubicles rather than one large room, soundproofing materials, lights for phones and alarm systems, and minimizing equipment noise. Placing a blanket on top of the incubator or using an incubator cover muffles the noise of equipment placement; gentle, considerate (to the infant) placement of equipment on or in the incubator muffles sound; and closing portholes and drawers gently decrease the structural noises of caregiving. Prohibiting placement of equipment (e.g., clipboards, stethoscopes, formula bottles) on top of the incubator prevents such noises. Two studies of the effects of earmuffs for noise reduction for NICU neonates found the following: (1) reduction in heart and respiratory rates and oxygen requirements[2] and (2) increase in quiet sleep in neonates wearing earmuffs (87.5%) compared with 29.4% without earmuffs.[86] However, another study combining eye goggles and earmuffs found that preterm infants with these devices had higher stress responses, measured by higher heart rates.[3]

Tapping (by parents or siblings) or banging (by medical, nursing, or ancillary personnel) on the incubator Plexiglas should *never* be permitted. This (along with a brisk startle reflex from the infant) is an opportunity to teach about the noise levels generated by such activity. Infants should be kept in incubators as long as necessary to maintain heat balance. Older incubators do *not* protect the infant from noise. A well-managed NICU environment may be much quieter than the continuous noise of an incubator. Noise in modern incubators varies according to the model. Sound sources within an incubator include its motor, infant sounds, equipment sounds inside the incubator, equipment sounds transmitted from outside the incubator, and ambient nursing noise (e.g., personnel, phones). Modern incubator walls attenuate impulse noises from the NICU and may decrease the infant's noise exposure. Inside modern incubators, motor noise does not exceed 60 dB, but this level exceeds the more recent recommendation of 50 dB. However, impulse noises from the incubator (i.e., doors, latches) are louder on the inside of the incubator (see Table 13-10). Prolonged stays in an incubator not only expose the infant to repeated caregiving noises but also mean there will be a dearth of kinesthetic stimulation (e.g., carrying, holding, rocking, swinging, sitting upright in an infant seat) and socially relevant speech patterns. Both the internal noise generated by the incubator and how well the incubator attenuates external noise should be considered in incubator purchases.

Noise levels in the NICU may interfere with development of other sensory systems and delay the development of hearing and language. Radios have been banned in most NICUs. Day-night cycles (nap time, nighttime) when auditory stimulation is decreased should be established in the NICU. Institution of a quiet time or rest period—through reduction of (1) noise from talking, equipment, telephones, and so on; (2) light by dimming overhead light; and (3) procedures to only emergency treatment—has resulted in enhanced infant sleep (34%–85%), less crying (14%–2.4%), and less parental and caregiver stress.[307] At discharge, NICU infants often will not sleep in a quiet room. Softly playing a radio facilitates sleep, and the infant gradually is weaned from it. Signs such as "Quiet . . . baby sleeping" or "Do not disturb, I'm asleep (talk to my nurse)" ensure undisturbed sleep *if* they are heeded.

The "in-turning" premature infant (see Box 13-2) of less than 34 weeks' gestation probably receives enough auditory input from the NICU. Auditory enhancement at this stage is probably overstimulation. Just as high-frequency sounds arouse, low-frequency ones, such as the heartbeat, respiratory sounds, and vacuum cleaners, quiet and facilitate sleep.[83] One study showed less behavioral response and less salivary cortisol release by infants who were presented with a heartbeat sound or white noise (both at 85 dB) during and after heel stick.

Although music has been shown to soothe full-term babies, the use of music with preterm infants has not been as well studied. Presentation of in utero sounds and a female voice to agitated, intubated preterm infants has resulted in improved oxygen saturation and behavioral states. A recent RCT of the effects of live music replicating womb sounds was conducted at multiple sites with preterms (≥32 weeks' gestation).[187] Music therapists chose lullabies identified by parents as important to their cultural heritage and that were within the parents' vocal range; parents were taught to entrain their singing to their infant's respiratory rate and activity. Outcomes included (1) lower heart rates during lullabies and music with a rhythm, (2) increased caloric intake and sucking behavior with parent-selected lullabies, and (3) decreased parental stress.[187]

A meta-analysis of music therapy showed benefits to preterm infants including improved oxygen saturations, increased weight gain, decrease in hospitalization, an increase (over time) in tolerance for stimuli, reinforcement of NNS, and increase in the rate of feeding at 34 to 36 weeks in poor feeders.[305] This meta-analysis showed more benefits of live music and benefits for the use of music early in the NICU stay (for birth weights <1000 g and <28 weeks' gestation). Music therapy in the NICU is used for pacification, reinforcement of sucking, and as a basis for multimodal stimulation.[305] Both neonatal nurses and parents believe that music in the NICU decreases stress, improves sleep, and reduces pain and crying.[260,261]

Although the use of recordings of music or family voices has been advocated and widely practiced, some investigators have recommended that such recordings not be used. Among the reasons cited against their use are that their benefits and long-term consequences have not been established, their use places a nonresponsive machine between a caring person and the preterm infant, and recordings may replace exposure of the preterm to the contingent human voice. However, if used with preterm infants, auditory stimuli should be (1) kept at a reasonable distance from the infant's ear (never use earphones), whether placed inside or outside the incubator; (2) played at levels below 55 dBA; (3) played for brief periods; and (4) used if the infant is soothed and discontinued if the infant becomes stressed, restless, or agitated. However, because preterm infants cannot habituate to sound as well as term babies can, they may be unable to tolerate any added sound and may become exhausted by such stimuli.

The human voice is the most preferred sound. The preterm in an incubator may be isolated from important exposure to his or her mother's voice that would have occurred over months in utero. Parental talking to their preterm infant in the NICU has been shown to be a strong predictor of infant vocalizations at 32 weeks and conversational turns (i.e., infant coos and parent gives a vocal response) at 32 and 36 weeks.[53] This study found that preterms begin vocalizing at 32 weeks and that the rate increases over time. When parents are present in the NICU, preterm vocalizations increased by as much as 129%, particularly at 32 weeks.[53] Another study of maternal talking and singing found greater oxygen saturation levels, fewer negative critical events, and a prevalence of calm alert state in the preterms who were reconnected to their mother's voice while in the NICU.[109] An exploratory study of VLBW preterms (16 exposed to biologic maternal sounds [BMS] matched with 16 exposed to usual NICU sounds) was conducted to measure weight gain.[352] VLBW infants exposed to BMS (maternal voice and heartbeat) gained more weight and had a higher growth velocity compared with the control group.[352] While in the NICU, parents reading to their newborns resulted in parental feelings of closeness to their infants, developing a sense of control, intimacy, and normalcy.[172]

Teach parents the neonate's preference for high-pitched voices speaking in typical speech patterns (not baby talk). While in the NICU parents can talk to the baby about their day, essentially conversing with the baby, and listening for responses. Parental talking to the baby in the NICU is associated with higher scores on language and cognition at 7 and 18 months corrected age.[54] The degree of attenuation of the higher frequency of mother's voice by the lower frequency of incubator noise, the incubator walls, and the ambient noise of the NICU has not been measured. Role model and teach parents to gently talk to the infant

while touching and giving care. Teach parents to talk to their infant while presenting their faces in the infant's range of vision. Watch for infant tolerance, and increase or decrease talk time to avoid overload. For older infants, imitate the infant's coos and babbles; this reinforces and encourages vocalizations.

For a neonate, hearing is more important than vision for attachment and bonding to the parents. Within seconds after birth, newborns are able to discriminate and prefer their mother's face. They have connected her familiar voice with her unfamiliar face. A high index of suspicion about hearing loss is warranted if caregivers do not observe normal responses to sound stimulation. Hearing screening by high-risk factors alone identifies only about 50% of newborns with significant hearing loss; therefore, universal newborn hearing screening is the standard of care.[14,16]

VISUAL INTERVENTION

The NICU is lit with bright, cool-white fluorescent lights 24 hours a day. Light levels vary between and within various NICUs. Early studies showed light levels in the low range, from 34 to 100 lux at night and 184 to 1000 lux during the day; more recent studies report light levels ranging from low levels of 1 to 25 foot-candles (ftc) to high levels of 235 ftc.[297] The amount of light to which the preterm infant is exposed is influenced by (1) location in the NICU, (2) seasonal or climactic variations, (3) use of phototherapy, (4) ophthalmoscopic examinations (e.g., at birth and for retinopathy of prematurity [ROP] follow-up), (5) use of procedure lights,[244] and (6) infant-related factors (e.g., maturity and amount of eye opening, head position, or eye shielding). Ambient light levels in the NICU should be adjustable through a range of 10 to 600 lux (approximately 1–60 ftc) at every bedside.[64] Other light recommendations for newly built NICUs are outlined in Table 13-12.

Although decreased light levels and response to bright light have not been shown to reduce the incidence of ROP, ophthalmic sequelae of preterm birth are common.[129] (See Chapter 31 for a discussion of ROP.) There are three broad categories of ophthalmic sequelae: (1) decreased visual function, (2) strabismus, and (3) decreased eye size (arrested growth) and abnormal refractive state (increased myopia). In addition, there is abundant animal, child, and adult research documenting negative biochemical and physical effects (e.g.,

TABLE 13-12 LIGHT RECOMMENDATIONS IN THE NICU[64]

ILLUMINATION LEVEL	PURPOSE
High levels: 60–100 foot-candles (ftc)	Evaluate and assess skin color and perfusion.
Lower levels: 10–20 ftc	Safe and adequate because of concerns over retinal/ocular damage from continuous exposure to high levels (60–100 ftc).
Nighttime levels: 0–5 ftc	Diurnal variation in light levels.
Procedure light: 100–150 ftc	Available at every bedside to temporarily increase lighting for infant assessment/procedure without increasing light exposure to all other babies. Prevent light from reaching infant's eyes.
Support areas	For charting, medication preparation, etc., should provide adequate and separate light to accommodate sleeping babies and working health care providers. Lighting should be located to avoid any infant's direct line of sight to the fixture.
Daylight	One source visible from care areas for its psychologic benefit for staff and families.

NICU, Neonatal intensive care unit.

BOX 13-13 EFFECTS OF CYCLED LIGHT*

- Behavior:
  - Decreases movement or motor activity
  - Increases motor coordination
  - Increases sleep time
  - Decreases fussing and crying
  - More eye opening
- Cardiorespiratory changes:
  - Decreases heart rate
  - Decreases respiratory rate
- Feeding behavior:
  - Quicker progression to oral feedings
  - Feeds more efficiently and in less time
  - Increased weight gain and better growth
- Circadian rhythm development:
  - Melatonin level
  - Temperature
  - Heart rate
  - Rest and activity patterns
- Decreased cortisol levels
- Decreased incidence and severity of retinopathy of prematurity
- Decreased parental and/or care provider stress
- Decreased infant handling and noise levels

*References 42, 131, 230, 274, 275.

change in endocrine function, increased hypocalcemia, cell transformations, immature gonadal development, chromosome breakage).[127] Exposure to bright lights in the NICU is associated with the following[127,244]:

- Decreased oxygenation
- Increased incidence of retinopathy
- Altered vital signs
- Alteration in state organization (i.e., altered sleep patterns, poorer circadian rhythms)
- Skin changes (e.g., tanning, rashes)
- Alteration of nutrients in total parenteral nutrition (TPN) solution, formula, and breast milk

Rapid increase in the intensity of ambient light causes a decrease in oxygen saturation in younger, immature preterm infants; slower increasing of light levels enables easier adaptation.[244]

The first goal in visual intervention is to assess the current level of light and decrease it wherever possible. A very immature preterm infant is accustomed to the muted light of the uterus (light filtered through the abdominal and uterine walls) and has fused eyelids (if the infant is less than 26 weeks' gestational age). Draping blankets on top of the incubator or using a handmade or commercial incubator cover[176] decreases the light at the infant's level during rest but allows immediate maximal illumination when the cover is pulled back. Using adjustable lighting at each infant's bedside enables every infant to have more or less light, depending on the care and rest circumstances of the individual infant. Because infants are continuously monitored, not all infants need to be subjected to maximal illumination at all times.[127]

Cycled light, dimming the lights in day-night cycles, is associated with positive effects (Box 13-13). Randomized controlled studies show that the circadian clock of the preterm infant is entrained by cycled light.[129] Preterm infants exposed to low-level cycled light for 2 weeks before discharge showed night/day rest-activity patterns within the first week after discharge. Preterms exposed to

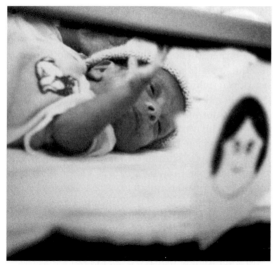

FIGURE 13-8 Premature infant fixing the gaze on a black-and-white face.

low-level uncycled light were delayed in their development of day-night differences in activity and rest till 3 weeks after discharge.[273–275]

Visual attentiveness is correlated with birth weight and gestational age: the more mature the infant, the more the infant is able to fix and follow. An infant at 28 weeks' gestation fixes and follows but may become apneic, behaviorally disorganized, and stressed as a result. Visual stimulation is very tiring and taxing (increases the heart rate) for the immature infant: those of less than 34 weeks' gestation probably receive enough stimulation from the NICU environment. Premature visual stimulation also may interfere with auditory neurosensory development. When these infants reach the "coming-out stage" (see Box 13-2), they may signal their readiness for visually enhancing activities.

Infants receiving phototherapy are deprived of visual sensory stimuli because of their protective eye pads. These should be removed during care and feeding and interaction with parents and professionals. Interesting visual stimuli include inanimate objects (e.g., toys, black-and-white faces and patterns, pictures of family members, artwork from siblings, mobiles) and animate objects (e.g., faces of parents, siblings, professionals; Figure 13-8). Infants prefer the human face as a visual stimulus, especially the talking face, which stimulates both visual and auditory pathways. Parents often need to be encouraged that, rather than toys, their infant prefers to watch and listen to their faces and voices.

Teach parents the abilities of the infant and appropriate methods of visual stimulation:

- Place mobiles, pictures, and faces of high contrast (i.e., black and white) within the visual range of the newborn: 8 to 12 inches for term infants, a little closer for preterm infants.
- Quiet alert is the best state for visual encounters after feedings, if awake; swaddle the infant to quiet, or unwrap the infant to arouse; hold infant upright.
- Place the infant on the abdomen (called "Tummy Time") with objects of various sizes and shapes within visual range.
- Change toys and visual stimuli. Infants become bored with the same thing.
- When the preterm infant tolerates multiple stimuli, hold him or her in *en face* position (see Chapter 29) to feed, talk to, and rock. Whether the infant is nipple or gavage fed, alternate sides so the infant sees both sides of the care provider's face (especially important if the preterm infant exhibits the common preference for right-sided head turning).
- Place the infant at varied heights (in a baby carrier, crib, swing, infant seat, on the floor) so the infant sees the world from various angles.
- Place the infant so that he or she can bring the hands to midline and see his or her hands and fingers and eventually reach for toys.

Infants who exhibit gaze aversion should not be "pursued" by the face of the parent or professional, because this only potentiates the time "spent away" with their gaze to protect themselves from overload. Gaze aversion, flat facial affect, and absence of a smile may cast doubt on the ability of these infants to see, because there is no eye "language" or caregiver feedback of preference, recognition, and delight. These infants do see, but they fix only fleetingly. Minimizing the number of care providers is crucial for these babies so that they deal with as few caregiver cues, styles, and ways of being handled as possible. Most important, the caregiver must be sensitive and responsive to the infant's negative and positive cues.

SMELL AND TASTE INTERVENTION

Newborns, including preterms, can detect, discriminate, respond (e.g., facial expression, change in respirations, apnea), learn, and remember olfactory stimuli.[202,330] The neonate's well-developed sense of smell is not stimulated in the NICU with pleasant odors. A high-risk infant is stimulated by the smell of forgotten alcohol, skin prep, or povidone-iodine (Betadine) pads inside the incubator and the unpleasant taste or smell of oral medications.[202] Because a premature infant cannot respond by crying or moving away, the infant responds to noxious smells by a decrease in respiratory rate, transient apnea, or an increase in heart rate.[202] Removal of noxious odors from the incubator is as critical as removal of sharp instruments after a procedure. Alcohol vapors from alcohol-based hand rubs that had not completely dried before touching the preterm was cited as the most common unpleasant smell to which the infants were exposed.[168] Other unpleasant odors included cleaning solutions, detergents, soaps and skin care products, and wipes such as alcohol or adhesive removers.

Enhancing the olfactory environment includes having parents hold the infant or sit close if the infant cannot yet be held. The smell of the mother's breast milk is especially pleasant and elicits more suckling than the smell of formula.[34,330] Olfactory stimulation of sucking in preterm infants increases with increasing postnatal age.[34] Placing a drop of human milk on the infant's lips with a cotton ball or gauze sponge helps the infant recognize the mother's smell and associate that smell with food and feeding when the infant is able to nipple feed.[73]

Nonnutritive suckling (during gavage and between feedings) is associated with better oxygenation; quieter, more restful behavior; increased readiness for nipple feedings because of a more alert state; fewer gavage feedings; acceleration of the sucking reflex; better weight gain; accelerated transition to full oral feedings; no alteration in breastfeeding success; decreased tension; and increased insulin and gastrin secretion that may stimulate digestion and storage of nutrients.[33,116,124,256,350]

However, meta-analyses of NNS studies have found no consistency in these benefits but rather a decreased length of hospital stay, efficacy in pain relief, and no adverse effects (see Chapter 12).[259] Sucking on a pacifier satisfies the infant's sucking needs and may facilitate early learning that satiety and sucking are associated. However, nutritive and nonnutritive suckling are not alike (see Chapter 18); the fact that an infant vigorously sucks on a pacifier does not mean the infant will be able to suckle nutritively, because the expressive and swallow phases

have not been present in nonnutritive suckling and coordination of suck, swallow, and breathing has not been necessary. This is confusing to most parents and many professionals and should be clarified for them.

High-risk infants often undergo prolonged periods during which a nil per os (NPO) status has been ordered, and during these times, their sensation of hunger is not relieved. Although pacifiers are soothing, these infants may learn that sucking and satiety are not related. NICU infants also experience many aversive stimuli around and within the mouth (e.g., oral intubation, oral and endotracheal tube suction, intermittent gavage) that result in touch aversion of the mouth and a hypersensitive gag reflex. Feeding difficulties may result from the following:

- Severity of illness[155,210,281]
- Neurologic damage (e.g., IVH)
- Structural abnormalities (e.g., cleft palate or submucous cleft, recessed chin)
- Prematurity: the infant is too neurologically immature and tires easily with "work" of feeding
- Aversive feeder (acquired or developmental: sucking defect; psychologic: "hospitalitis," rumination) and aversive feeding experiences[46,293] that alter brain structure[298,301]
- A combination of these types[280]

Neural maturation (34–35 weeks' gestation) is the developmental guideline for initiation of oral feedings (see Table 13-2),[46,123,213,296] although some infants are ready at an earlier age (30–34 weeks' gestation) (see Box 13-2). Maturation of feeding skills occurs because of developmental changes in the CNS, coupled with experiential learning.* So intimately interrelated are these indicators that maturity depends on experience and experience depends on maturity; therefore, the more opportunities to nipple feed, the more improved the preterm neonate's feeding performance. However, preterm infants may exhibit periods of apnea and tachypnea with bottle feeding, because consistent coordination of breathing with sucking and swallowing does not occur until 37 weeks' gestation (see Table 13-2).

The research basis for determining readiness for initiation of oral feedings is discussed in Chapter 18 and in Box 13-2. *Cue-based or infant-driven feedings* are individualized feedings initiated and

---

*References 46, 120, 143, 148, 151, 209, 213, 219, 256, 293, 294, 296, 321.

discontinued based on the infant's cues of readiness to feed and satiety, rather than on time or volume of feeding.[160,161,293,294] Research supports the efficacy of cue-based feedings in (1) initiating feeding[155]; (2) earlier achievement of full oral feedings[82,160,293]; (3) enhancing the quality, rather than the quantity, of feeding; and (4) providing a safe, pleasurable experience for the infant and parents.[46,280,320]

Coregulated feeds, the ability of parents to know their infant's cues and read and respond dynamically to changing needs of the infant, focuses on the feeding relationship, rather than the volume consumed.[320] Parents learn from professional care providers how to individualize every feeding encounter by (1) respecting infant cues, (2) seeing their infant as an active partner, (3) evaluating readiness to feed, (4) adjusting feeding to be contingent with the infant's breathing rhythm and other physiologic cues, (5) using proper positioning, and (6) decreasing physical and environmental stimuli that interfere with feeding.[282,293,320] These strategies enable a safe, learning experience for both parents and their infant, a pleasant feeding experience, and lay the foundation for positive feeding outcomes and improved neurodevelopment.[293,320] There is no one approach for feeding preterms; strategies in Box 13-14 are individualized to each infant and parent.

Feeding difficulties at the beginning of life often lead to eating problems in infancy and later in life.[280,282,293] Severe behavioral eating difficulties are associated with prematurity, low birth weight, CNS injury, distress during feeding in the first 6 months of life, and regular or frequent vomiting. Feeding difficulties are stressful to all family members, complicate parenting and strain the parent-infant bond.[198,280,282,293]

Because criteria for discharge include full oral feedings with adequate weight gain, transition to full oral feedings is a topic of ongoing research. Longer transition time to full oral feedings is significantly influenced by (1) apnea, (2) birth weight or gestational age, (3) younger age at first oral feeding, (4) BPD/CLD, (5) number of days being tube fed/receiving ventilatory therapy, and (6) desaturations of oxygen with feeding.* Shorter transition time to complete oral feeding is associated with (1) greater weight and (2) older postconceptual age at initiation of nipple feeding,[47,219] (3) use of oral stimulation (e.g.,

stroking, NNS, NNS with lullabies, NNS with mother's voice),† (4) use of oral colostrum,[119] and (5) a semidemand or demand-feeding protocol.[160,209–211,213]

A randomized study of early introduction of oral (bottle) feeding (e.g., within 48 hours of full tube feeding) found the following[296]:

- Transition time to all oral feedings was significantly shorter.
- Oral feeding was introduced 2.6 weeks earlier.
- Total oral feeding was achieved at earlier postmenstrual age (e.g., 54% of 33 weeks' postmenstrual age infants versus 12.5% of control group).
- Weight gain and discharge weights were similar for both groups.
- Episodes of feeding-related bradycardia and desaturations were similar for both groups.
- Discharge was 10 days earlier for the earlier fed infants.

These researchers postulate that feeding opportunities in young infants provide them with practice and experiential opportunities to develop their oral motor skills and coordination of suck-swallow-breathe.[148,296]

For infants with BPD/CLD, the more days receiving positive-pressure ventilation and supplemental oxygen, the older (in postconceptual age) the infant when he or she is first fully nipple fed. For these infants, transition time to full nipple feeding may be lengthened because of the increased work of breathing, the precedence of breathing (at an increased rate) over feeding, and changes in heart rate variability.[67,214] However, a randomized study found that infants with BPD/CLD fed by an individualized, semidemand method (using the infant's behavioral cues and cardiorespiratory state to determine frequency, length, and method) achieved nipple feeding earlier (5.9 days) compared with control infants (12.3 days).[210]

The goals of intervention include (1) a safe feeding (i.e., diminished risk for aspiration), (2) a functional feeding (i.e., adequate caloric intake for optimal growth and with minimal energy expenditure), and (3) a pleasant, social interactive experience for the infant and parents or caregivers.[155,263,293,321]

The use of individualized developmental care may assist VLBW and preterm infants with

---

*References 116, 151, 209, 213, 219, 296, 342.

†References 20, 58, 116, 211, 294, 350.

BOX 13-14 STRATEGIES TO FACILITATE ORAL FEEDING

1. Minimize noxious stimuli to the mouth.
   a. Suction only as needed (not routinely).
   b. Consider indwelling gastric tube rather than intermittent gavage (e.g., an infant fed every 2 hours would have a gavage tube passed 12 times a day).
   c. Pass intermittent gavage tube down mouth through hole in pacifier nipple; if infant has hypersensitive gag, passing smaller tube down nose stimulates gag reflex less than passing tube down mouth.
   d. Perioral and intraoral stimulation techniques[20,23,37,116,180]:
      i. These techniques are only more aversive, rather than therapeutic, on babies with touch aversion at mouth area; individualizing therapy is important
      ii. When performing oral exercises, do so with care—do not stimulate aversion reflexes (e.g., gag reflex).
      iii. Use of a new motorized pulsating pacifier results in faster emergence of NNS and increase in proportion of oral nutrition.[27]
2. Enhance pleasant stimuli to mouth (first experiences with suckling have lasting neurobehavioral effects).[46,111,282]
   a. Have infant smell or taste breast milk; use colostrum/human milk for oral care[119]
   b. Provide nonnutritive suckling[143] and NNS with lullabies[350] or with mother's voice[58] while tube feeding[282]
   c. Facilitate hand-to-mouth behaviors.
   d. Use nipple with proper flow rate.[120,122,204,292] If flow rate is too fast, increased flow stimulates anxiety and/or gag reflex and causes bradycardia—promotes incoordination. If flow rate is too slow, fatigue and frustration are increased and may result in inadequate consumption/growth failure.
   e. Perioral and intraoral stimulation—facilitates development of normal sucking behaviors.[20,116,180]
   f. Use Lact-Aid nursing supplementer (see Chapter 18):
      i. Never frustrate infant with dry breast.
      ii. Positive reinforcement for infant to nurse.
      iii. Calorically and energy efficient method.
      iv. Oral therapy—teaches infant proper nutritive suckle.
   g. For infants with difficulty in coordination of respiration with suck or swallow (prevents stress of apnea and hypoxia and enhances pleasure of feeding experience) (see Chapter 18)[67,318,319]:
      i. Assess feeding pattern (e.g., continuous or intermittent suck), pulse oximeter, muscle tone, breathing pattern, heart rate.[321]
      ii. Remove nipple from mouth to enable infant to breathe (pace feeding).[175]
      iii. Begin breastfeeding before bottle feeding (see Chapter 18 Critical Findings: Readiness for Initiation of Oral Feedings: Research Basis on p. XXX).

   iv. Use of orthodontic nipple results in physiologic stability and more effective feeding behavior in some infants
   v. Use of soft-walled bottle system improves oxygenation and coordination and is more like breastfeeding than rigid-walled bottle[122]
3. Positioning: use proper position to facilitate swallow and improve suction—symmetric positioning with predominance of flexion.[321]
   a. Hold with feedings (even gavage) as much as possible.
   b. Consistent caregivers—parents, primary nurses, foster grandparents.
   c. Kangaroo care before feeding improves alertness; does not tire infant and should not be avoided before feeding; promotes breastfeeding.[63,282]
   d. Swaddle[293,321,345]:
      i. Decreases startles
      ii. Optimizes postural stability and control
      iii. Infant may become too warm and sleepy.
   e. Facilitate swallowing:
      i. Position with chin tucked.
      ii. If breastfeeding, turn infant's whole body toward mother so head and trunk are in alignment (infant is not trying to swallow with head turned to one side).
      iii. Upright position with neck, shoulders, and back supported—slows gravitational flow of formula from nipple (as when infant is in semireclined position); restricted milk flow (e.g., milk flows only with active sucking, not with gravity) beneficial (e.g., more efficient; more volume obtained).
      iv. Head-elevated, side-lying position results in more physiologic stability (fewer and less severe bradycardia; slower, more relaxed breathing) for bottle feeding[293]
      v. Cuddling, semireclined position increases flow of formula by gravity—may be too fast, regardless of nipple chosen; results in increased gags, choking, and bradycardia.
      vi. Prone with neck extended (slightly): Keeps tongue forward and airway unobstructed.
      vii. Good for aversive feeder who chokes.
      viii. Gentle, upward pressure under chin (chin support) or at base of tongue facilitates swallowing, because it mimics upward thrust of tongue with swallowing.
   f. Improve formation of suction:
      i. Semireclining (>45-degree angle) on lap of caregiver—frees both hands to work with infant on oral control.
      ii. Cupping both cheeks (check support)[143] with fingers of free hand (i.e., hand not holding bottle) improves lip closure, suction formation, minimizes fluid loss, stabilizes the jaw, and organizes deglutition.[37,143,345]
      iii. Gentle tugging at nipple (as if to take it out of mouth) may smooth and strengthen suck; avoid prodding infant to suck[293]

Continued

BOX 13-14	STRATEGIES TO FACILITATE ORAL FEEDING—cont'd

4. Timing
   a. Do not allow infant to cry to exhaustion before feeding—infant will be too tired to eat.
   b. Keep external stimuli to a minimum in immature preterm infants (<34 weeks) for optimal intake and weight gain.[292,320]
   c. If or when satiated, infant will not suck:
      i. Feed on demand/semidemand or when alert[210-213] (demand feeding reinforces sleep-wake cycle) and the development of self-regulation.[211,264]
      ii. If feeding on schedule, note whether infant gives cue of hunger: fussiness and crying, hand-to-mouth behaviors or rooting, hiccups. Infants as young as 32 to 33 weeks can provide cues

so that feeding can be individualized.[209,213,281,282,293]
   iii. If feeding on schedule, space time and see whether infant exhibits cues of hunger (as described earlier).
   iv. First, nipple what infant is able to feed; then tube feed (presence of an indwelling nasogastric tube may result in compromised respirations, oxygen desaturation, and bradycardia in the VLBW infant).[296]
   d. Try to nipple feed for no longer than 20 to 30 minutes (infant becomes too tired and uses up energy and calories to feed instead of to grow).[281]
   e. Infants of advanced age (around 6 months) may be unable to nipple if they have never had the opportunity. It may be more developmentally appropriate to cup feed or spoon-feed infant because normal infants begin cup drinking between 6 and 8 months of age.

NNS, Nonnutritive sucking; *VLBW,* very low birth weight.

BPD/CLD in obtaining and maintaining an optimal condition for progression to oral feedings. Use of skin-to-skin KC improves weight gain, supports and promotes breastfeeding, and shortens length of stay (see Box 13-6). Because KC improves alertness and does not tire the infant, it can be used as a strategy to facilitate oral feeding (see Boxes 13-6 and 13-14). The use of developmental care enables VLBW preterm infants to initiate the first oral feeding and have the last gavage feeding at an earlier age compared with VLBW infants not receiving developmental care. Preterm infants successfully completing oral feeding spent significantly more time in awake states than did preterm infants who were unsuccessful in their feeding.

Using developmental principles, health care providers are able to facilitate both the preterm infant and parents in effective feeding experiences.[281,293] A self-regulating preterm infant shows these signs of stability during feeding: (1) smooth, regular respirations (no or minimal increase in respiratory rate or effort); (2) consistent postural control—flexed, hands near face, maintains muscle tone, calm/organized behavior; (3) maintains optimal color; (4) quiet, alert state, focuses on feeding; and (5) coordinates suck-swallow-breathe.[292,321] Coordination of feeding is facilitated by (1) imposing breaks/pacing (e.g., removing the nipple from the mouth; tipping the bottle so that the nipple is empty but remains in the infant's mouth), (2) limiting bolus size (limiting the number of sucks

before a swallow results in smaller bolus size) by limiting the number of successive sucks before the infant becomes stressed, and (3) slowing the flow rate (e.g., using low-flow-rate nipples,[204] upright positioning to decrease hydrostatic pressure and gravitational flow).[292]

Signs of stress during nipple feeding, their significance, and appropriate interventions are listed in the Critical Findings in Table 13-13. Even preterm infants who are near discharge still have oxygen desaturations when fed by their mothers; the incidence is decreased in infants receiving supplemental oxygen, beginning a feeding with a higher baseline oxygen saturation, and in those of an older postconceptual age.[318,321] Parents must be taught how to interpret their infant's cues of stability and stress so that they can modify their behavior and learn to intervene to help their infant safely and successfully feed.[269,293,320] Skills parents need for effective feeding include (1) following the infant's lead about readiness to feed—preterms are able to root and open their mouths to the stimulus of a nipple; (2) assessing breathing cues, providing adequate rest (see Table 13-13), and not interrupting by "jiggling" or moving the nipple to stimulate sucking; and (3) recognizing that noisy swallowing and drooling indicate dysfunction[293,320] (see Table 13-13). Strategies that parents consider helpful in mastery of these skills are (1) being included in decision making about feeding and its success, (2) observing a nurse feed their baby, and (3) having a nurse spend time with

TABLE 13-13	**CRITICAL FINDINGS**	
	STRESS DURING NIPPLE FEEDINGS	

SIGN	SIGNIFICANCE	INTERVENTION
Color change Pallor, dusky, gray, central cyanosis—perioral/periorbital	Oxygen desaturation[168] Feeding too rapidly with brief, shallow breaths Low hematocrit level Breath-holding	Assess baseline color before feeding Assess bottle-feeding delivery system: soft-walled system significantly improves oxygen saturation, coordination of suck/swallow/breathe, and more like breast feeding compared with rigid-walled feeding bottle[12] Periodic removal of nipple to facilitate deep breathing Monitor changes in color during feeding Use pulse oximeter during feeding to maintain saturation ≥92%[318,319]
Changes in state of alertness	Quiet alert state optimal for successful feeding Increased infant focus on feeding Increased organization of oropharyngeal muscle movements	Offer preterm opportunity to suck on pacifier before feeding—encourages awake/alert behavior[319]
	Increasing drowsiness, falls asleep: Respiratory fatigue resulting from rapid feeding, desaturation, increased respiratory rate, and/or work of breathing Fatigue resulting from behavior/energy expenditure (e.g., crying; bathing) before feeding	Pulse oximeter monitoring during feeding—give and/or adjust oxygen to maintain saturations ≥92% during nippling efforts Unwrap if sleepy
	Fussiness/restlessness—resulting from oxygen desaturation (e.g., hypoxia) because of the work of breathing (WOB) and nippling; disorganized behavioral state	Periodic rest periods and pace energy expenditure with nipple feeding Swaddle/rock if fussy
Breathing	Increased respiratory effort resulting from work/exercise of feeding,[203,318] especially in the infant with CLD/BPD[67]	
1. Respiratory fatigue: Falls asleep, ceases feeding before adequate volume obtained	WOB before feeding is increased further with effort of feeding Infants with poor endurance may be unable to feed or may demonstrate poor weight gain despite acceptable intake	Pulse oximeter monitoring with feeding to ensure adequate oxygenation; give oxygen PRN to keep saturation ≥92% Provide chin/cheek support (see Table 13-12) that decreases energy expenditure, enhances state organization and sucking activity
2. Tachypnea Respiratory rate >60/min	WOB increases with feeding; respiratory rate increased with work of feeding Increased incoordination of suck-swallow-breathe with feeding; predisposes to aspiration Increased risk for aspiration if gasping for breath	Brief and/or frequent breaks in feeding to enable deep breaths and reorganize breathing patterns[319]
3. Nasal flaring	Attempts to increase oxygen intake because of hypoxia or increased WOB	Pulse oximeter; supply adequate oxygen Brief breaks to reorganize breathing
Nasal blanching	Distress of breathing/hypoxia Incoordination of suck-swallow-breathe with possible aspiration if flaring/blanching occur	
4. Chin tugging/head bobbing/"catch-up" breathing/grunting	Attempting to increase air entry because of "air hunger"/hypoxia/WOB/decreased tidal volume Incoordination of suck-swallow-breathe; increased risk for aspiration	As for signs 1 through 3

Continued

	CRITICAL FINDINGS—cont'd	
TABLE 13-13	**STRESS DURING NIPPLE FEEDINGS**	

SIGN	SIGNIFICANCE	INTERVENTION
5. Crowing sounds— high-pitched stridorous noise on inspiration	Incoordination of opening/closing of vocal cords that increases the risk for aspiration into the trachea[345]	As for signs 1 through 3
Swallowing	Primary swallow dysfunction predisposes to aspiration,[293] swallowing may be evaluated by videofluoroscopy	
1. Drooling	Loss of bolus control because of: Inability of tongue to collect and hold fluid that is flowing too fast Rapid respiratory rate, excessive WOB that shortens time for swallowing to occur; so that only part of bolus is swallowed	Give fewer sucks in a row, followed by brief break (pacing) so that bolus is smaller and easier to completely swallow[175]
2. Gulping	Use of prolonged sucking pattern or long sucking bursts (especially at the beginning of feeding) without deep breathing at the appropriate intervals Results in oxygen desaturation, bradycardia, apnea resulting from suppression of respiration Increases incoordination of suck-swallow-breathe and stimulates pharyngeal stretch receptors, resulting in vagally stimulated apnea	Give brief breaks (pacing) to assist the infant in slowing down the feeding[175]
3. Gurgling sounds in the pharynx (breathing sounds are wet/noisy)[293]	Fluid collecting in the throat, pharynx, or supraglottic space above vocal cords Noisy respirations caused by breathing through fluid in hypopharynx because bolus is too large or flow is too fast	Brief break from feeding to enable extra swallow/ dry swallow to clear fluid from throat
4. Swallowing (several times) in succession	Deliberate swallows in succession to clear bolus (that is too large/flow is too fast) from pharynx Breathing is delayed with successive swallowing and may result in apnea/bradycardia[205]	Break from feeding to clear throat and regain control of respiration
5. Coughing, choking, gagging, spitting up	Fluid has entered (or nearly entered) the airway.[168] Changes in color, heart rate, respiratory rate suggest swallowing problems Occurrence toward end of feeding suggests gastroesophageal reflux; frequent or intense spitting up also may indicate reflux	Usually can be prevented by close attention and intervention to previous signs of feeding difficulty Breaks from feeding to clear airway, regain control of respiration and state organization Ability to cough enables infant to clear airway Inability to cough, color change, hypotonia, bradycardia, and apnea are symptoms of airway obstruction that may require suction and cardiopulmonary resuscitation Change nipple and/or bottle system

BPD, Bronchopulmonary dysplasia; *CLD,* chronic lung disease; *PRN,* as needed; *WOB,* work of breathing
Modified from Shaker C: Nipple feeding preterm infants: an individualized, developmentally supportive approach, *Neonatal Netw* 18:15, 1999.

them while they are feeding their baby to give them feedback, ideas, and tips about feeding.[269,293,320] For parents, learning to feed their infant is viewed as a significant symbol of parenting, as an opportunity to read and react to infant cues, and as a coregulator of feeding.[269,293,320]

A feeding plan, developed with parents,[282,293,320] must be individualized for each infant and posted at the bedside (Box 13-15 and the Case Study). All care providers must adhere to the plan for consistency and continuity of stimuli and to promote infant learning.[293] Evidence-based approaches to nipple feeding

1. *Sit upright.* This decreases the flow of formula from the bottle and thus decreases:
   a. His gag reflex, which causes the bradycardia.
   b. His anxiety, which is caused by a bolus of formula in his mouth.
2. *Use a blue nipple.* This is the shortest nipple and decreases stimulation of his hypersensitive gag reflex, which causes his bradycardia. (All other nipples stimulated him to gag.)
3. *Gently push up under his chin when he gets a mouthful of formula.* This pushes his tongue upward against his palate, the same way the tongue moves during swallowing. (READER: Swallow and note your tongue motion.) He becomes frightened (i.e., eyes wide open and fearful; increased respiratory rate; arching and struggling) when he has a mouthful of formula, because he is used to sucking only on a dry pacifier and having nothing to swallow. His fear raises his heart rate, respiratory rate, and gag reflex, which causes bradycardia.
4. *Talk to him.* Softly and gently, tell him he can swallow and praise him when he does.
5. *Nipple.* Have him do this as much as possible (he will only get better with practice) and supplement feeding with the indwelling nasogastric tube (no more intermittent tube passage).

CASE STUDY

Tommy was a 28-week preterm infant with severe RDS, prolonged ventilation, and now BPD. He is now 38 weeks' postconceptual age, receiving hood and nasal cannula oxygen and trying to learn to nipple feed. In the morning report, the night nurse says that Tommy "has bradycardia with tube passage so that 24 hours ago he had a cardiorespiratory arrest that required resuscitation. He also has bradycardia and tachypnea with bottle-feeding."

Tommy's nurse evaluated his initial attempts to bottle-feed (after waiting for him to demand) and wrote the care plan (Box 13-15) after feeding him 45 ml in 20 minutes without tachypnea, cyanosis, or bradycardia.

BPD, Bronchopulmonary dysplasia; *RDS*, respiratory distress syndrome.

(for NICU preterms and sick term infants) have been developed that integrate contingent, developmental principles with more nurse autonomy and multidisciplinary collaboration and support.* The Early Feeding Skills (EFS) Assessment checklist has been developed to assess a preterm infant's readiness for oral feeding, oral feeding skill, and ability to maintain physiologic stability and tolerance of oral feeding.[321] The Premature Infant Oral Motor Intervention (PIOMI) is an evidence-based, validated intervention that facilitates the development of oral feeding skills, improves oral feeding, shortens length of stay, and lowers costs.[180] The Supporting Oral Feeding in Fragile Infants (SOFFI) method contains an algorithm to assist nurses in decision making, using specific evidence-based strategies and interpreting behavioral cues for bottle feeding preterm, sick, and fragile infants.[281] SOFFI is recommended to be used in conjunction with the National Association of Neonatal Nurses Guideline for Practice: *Infant directed oral feeding for premature and critically ill hospitalized infants.*[282]

---

*References 60, 209, 213, 262, 294.

CRYING OR SMILING INTERVENTION

Crying is the infant's innate care–eliciting behavior, a signal that he or she needs attention. The energy expenditure of a crying infant is increased by 7.5% compared with the resting state.[268] Immediate response decreases the infant's physiologic stress, increases the infant's trust in the environment, and enhances the sense of self and of control over the world.[192] The infant's need to escalate to "out-of-control" crying is decreased with immediate response, so that infants are easier to soothe. Consoling the crying infant also helps the infant change states so he or she is able to attend to and interact with the environment.

Term infants vocalize, cry, and look at their caregiver more than do preterm and ill infants.[88,127] Although preterm infants are more irritable than full-term infants, preterm infants cry less throughout the day than do full-term infants. NICU infants exhibit fewer care-eliciting behaviors (some preterm infants in one study never cried, vocalized, or looked at their caregiver).[127] Preterm infants thus are less responsive to the caregivers (both parents and professionals), who receive less positive feedback from the infant and hence are less rewarded. In one study, those NICU infants who were able to cue the care provider (cry, look, vocalize) were consistently responded to 80% to 100% of the time.[127]

Intubated infants who cannot produce an audible cry signal their needs by agitation, heart rate changes, and changes in oxygenation. Preterm infants (<32 weeks' gestation) may recover better from agitation when left alone, because active consolation is overstimulating. How caregivers attempt to soothe a crying infant while giving NICU care includes (1) no response to cries (58.1% of the time), (2) response by talking (29.2% of the time), (3) response by social touching (5.5% of the time), and (4) response by talk and social touching (7.2% of the time).[127]

Parents and staff should use graduated interventions in quieting a crying infant by the following:

- Soothing with gentle, high-pitched talking (loud enough that the infant can hear it above his or her crying)
- Placing the palm of the hand across the infant's chest or holding arms on chest with the palm of the care provider's hand
- Swaddling with blankets to decrease self-upsetting startles
- Picking up infant, holding (upright is the most soothing position), and rocking
- Placing the infant skin-to-skin on the parent's chest
- Offering a pacifier

Most stimulation in the NICU is procedural. The lack of social stimulation in the NICU not only affects the infant but also teaches parents that their infant is too weak for, too fragile for, uninterested in, or incapable of social interaction. Again, social stimulation must be paced according to the stage of development and stability of the infant[90] (see the Critical Findings in Box 13-2). Enhancing the infant's social environment includes presenting the smiling, moving, talking care provider's face to the alert infant; touching and stroking; and soothing and consoling the distressed infant.

In many busy NICUs, parents and a foster grandparent program provide this sensory integrated social experience. If the infant has been transported to a referral center, parents may live some distance away and be unable to visit daily. A chronically ill 4- to 5-month-old infant who begins to recognize the foster grandmother may smile, relax, and feed better for her and is often fussier and more irritable on her day off. A foster grandparent program benefits both infants and seniors—the infant receives love and socialization, and the senior "has a reason to get up in the morning."

If possible, parents should be encouraged to perform the "firsts" with their infant (e.g., first nipple feeding, first bath, first time out of the incubator). Because parents are not always present, they will miss some important milestones for their infant (e.g., extubation). Many NICUs have developed baby diaries (or calendars) and/or use videotaping in which the nurses, physicians, and foster grandparents write or record important information about the infant's day (as if the infant were the author). The text is accompanied by self-developing pictures with humorous captions (e.g., "Look at me. I've got my tube out!"). Staff members are very creative in relating "what's been happening," so that the parents have not only a verbal report (that, over time, may be forgotten) but also a keepsake of NICU progress.

The pursuit of "humane,"[159] relationship-based[9,10] developmental care continues with redesign of NICU environments,[64] including single-room care, as well as changing the attitudes and care practices among health care providers. Single (family) room care has been shown to be associated with (1) increased developmental and family-centered care, (2) increased parental participation in their infant's care (i.e., more skin-to-skin care, visits), (3) increased parental satisfaction and reduced stress, and (4) improved neonatal outcomes (i.e., better attention, less stress, hypertonicity and lethargy due to developmental care; less pain and stress due to parental care).[244a] However, a comparison study of single-family NICU rooms versus open-ward NICU was conducted in an urban NICU with low levels of parental visiting and holding and found poorer outcomes at 2 years—rather than the room configuration, the presence and care-by-parents influences improved outcomes.[257]

Creating an integrated, relationship-based, family-centered, developmental care philosophy requires the following:

- A commitment by individual care providers to alter practice for the benefit of neonates and families and to integrate family-centered developmental care into their individual practice
- Relationship building with neonates, families, and colleagues
- The use of effective change strategies within the institution's organizational climate
- Implementing the guidelines of national professional organizations[15,64] to satisfy ethical, legal, and professional standards of care
- Changing health care providers' knowledge base, which requires multidisciplinary educational opportunities (e.g., orientation, in-service, continuing education, consultation) and written resource materials[5]

Developmental care can no longer be considered "nice, but optional," especially with the evidence that not only brain function but also actual brain structure are positively affected by the early experiences of family-centered developmental care in the NICU.[6–8,207,208,227]

REFERENCES

For a full list of references, scan the QR code or visit http://booksite.elsevier.com/9780323320832.

14 FLUID AND ELECTROLYTE MANAGEMENT

MICHAEL NYP, JESSICA L. BRUNKHORST, DAPHNE REAVEY, AND EUGENIA K. PALLOTTO

Advances in the management of specific neonatal disorders have contributed to a remarkable decline in morbidity and mortality rates in newborns. Fluid and electrolyte therapy, nutritional support, thermal regulation, and maintenance of oxygenation remain central features of modern, supportive neonatal intensive care. Fluid and nutrition data have accumulated over time, but opportunities remain for increasing knowledge in order to optimize clinical management and long-term outcomes. For example, it is clear that the restrictive fluid policies of the 1950s were misguided efforts that caused hyperosmolarity, hyperbilirubinemia, and hypoglycemia. On the other hand, the degree to which initial fluid, electrolyte, and glucose administration should be "liberalized" remains uncertain—particularly in very-low-birth-weight (VLBW) infants (infants with birth weights less than 1500 g).[1,14,19] Many high-morbidity outcomes such as patent ductus arteriosus (PDA), necrotizing enterocolitis (NEC), bronchopulmonary dysplasia (BPD), intraventricular hemorrhage, and hyperglycemia in VLBW infants are associated with larger volumes of fluid, electrolyte, and glucose administration.[1] At best, clinicians make approximations for therapy in many clinical situations, which is why good measures of fluid and electrolyte requirements are needed. Infants requiring neonatal intensive care commonly receive parenteral fluids, often for prolonged periods of time. The fluid requirements of both premature and term infants vary based on the underlying diagnosis and therapies used to treat these disease processes.

This chapter discusses implementation of the following fundamental principles: (1) rapidly assessing the infant's initial condition; (2) developing a short-term, time-oriented management plan; (3) initiating therapy; (4) monitoring the infant; and (5) modifying the plan based on clinical and biochemical data.

PHYSIOLOGY

Neonates show physiologic differences when compared (on a per-kilogram basis) with older children and adults: (1) their basic metabolic rate is greater, even double; (2) their fluid requirements are four to five times higher; (3) their sodium excretion is only 10% that of older children and adults; and (4) their glomerular filtration rate is 5 to 10 times less than that of adults.[14] The subdivisions of total body mass (TBM) are illustrated in Figure 14-1. Total body water (TBW) as a percentage of TBM demonstrates a curvilinear decline with increasing gestational age (Figure 14-2). During the early fetal period, the fetus's TBW is 95% of total weight and decreases to 80% at 8 months' gestation and then to 75% at term.[14] Intracellular fluid (ICF) and extracellular fluid (ECF) as percentages of TBM change in opposite directions as gestational age advances, ECF decreases, and ICF increases with growth.[9]

These physiologic and body composition phenomena highlight the importance of accurately calculating fluids and electrolytes for small infants,

---

PURPLE type highlights content that is particularly applicable to clinical settings.

especially those less than 1500 g. The ability of infants, especially those premature, to remove free water and/or remove a solute load is impaired. Caregivers should independently calculate all requirements and compare calculations with standard guidelines. Intravenous (IV) fluid should be administered by a special infusion pump that can regulate fluid with precision of at least 0.01 ml/hr. Intake should be measured hourly and all output measured. The balance of intake versus output should be assessed at least every 8 to 12 hours using a standard format (Figure 14-3).

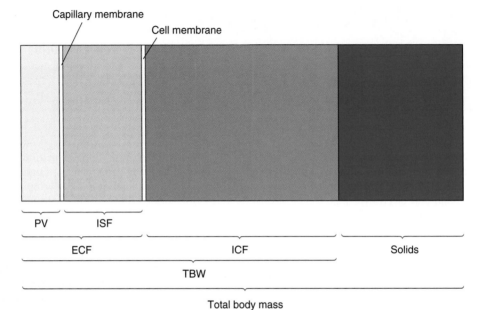

FIGURE 14-1 *Major subdivisions of total body mass. ECF, Extracellular fluid; ICF, intracellular fluid; ISF, interstitial fluid; PV, plasma volume; TBW, total body water. (From Winters RW, editor: The body fluids in pediatrics, Boston, 1973, Little, Brown.)*

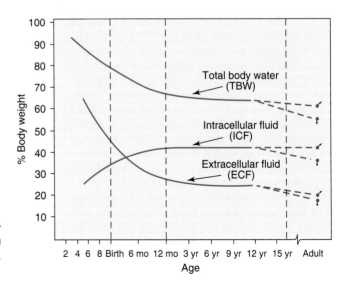

FIGURE 14-2 *Effects of age on TBW, ICF, and ECF. Note curvilinear changes that are maximal during perinatal period. (From Winters RW, editor: The body fluids in pediatrics, Boston, 1973, Little, Brown.)*

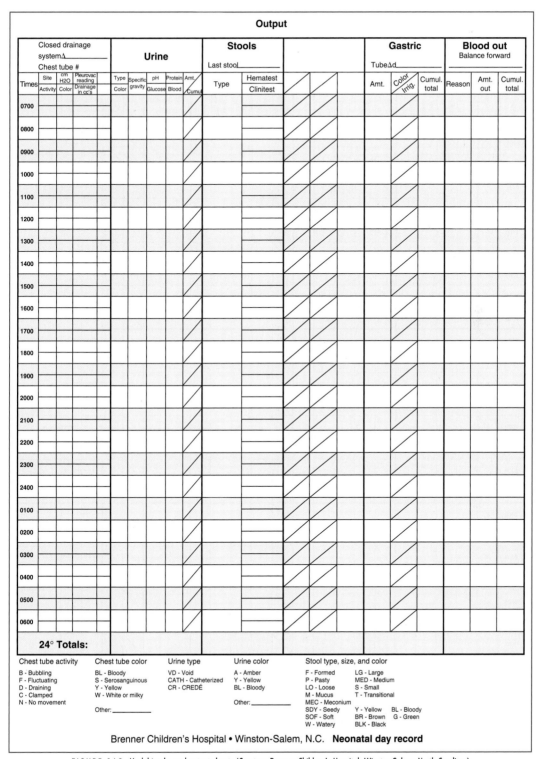

FIGURE 14-3 Model intake and output sheet. (Courtesy Brenner Children's Hospital, Winston-Salem, North Carolina.)

Continued

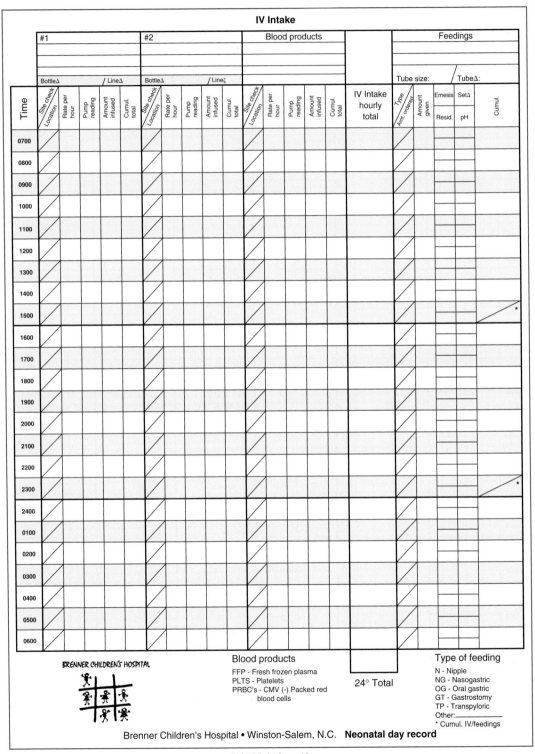

FIGURE 14-3, cont'd

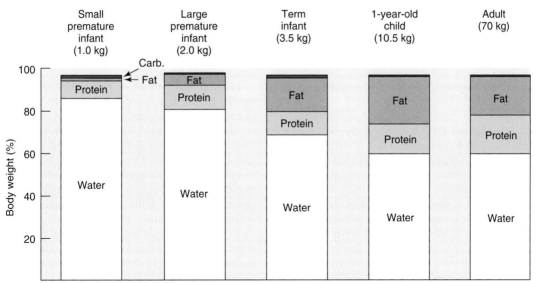

FIGURE 14-4 Effects of gestational age on body composition compared with older children and adults. (From Heird WC, Driscoll JM Jr, Schullinger JN, et al: Intravenous alimentation in pediatric patients, *J Pediatr* 80:351, 1972.)

Once clinical signs of fluid overload or deficit occur, it may be difficult to regain balance. Fluid balance should be managed prospectively; consistent assessments and laboratory evaluations should be a part of every initial care plan.

The effect of gestational age on body composition is striking (Figure 14-4). Because gestational age is a determinant of the percentage and distribution of TBW, accurate assessment is important. In utero, fetal fluid and electrolyte balance occurs through feto-placental exchange. Changes in the distribution and percent of body water will be influenced by intrauterine growth, maternal fluid balance, maternal medications, maternal health conditions, and placental blood flow. For example, a preterm infant born to a mother receiving magnesium sulfate may have elevated serum magnesium levels at birth, which may remain elevated up to 3 to 5 days following birth. Small-for-gestational-age (SGA) infants have reduced amounts of fat, and their TBW (as a percentage of TBM) increases. Conversely, large-for-gestational-age (LGA) infants with an increased amount of body fat have a lower percentage of TBW.

The initial (first 3 to 5 days of life) weight loss of healthy term (up to 5% to 10% of TBM) and preterm (up to 10% to 15% of TBM) infants should be considered a normal physiologic loss of fluid. This loss is from the interstitial fluid (ISF).

It is not a pathologic catabolism of body tissues but a result of the maturation of specific regulators of fluid and electrolytes. One such example, vasopressin (antidiuretic hormone), is secreted during the early stages of labor. This hormonal secretion contributes to renal maturation and has a limited antidiuresis effect at birth.[23]

After birth, contraction of the ECF compartment occurs, followed by natriuresis, diuresis, and weight loss.[9,14] This weight loss is then regained over 7 to 10 days as muscle and fat. Preterm neonates often demonstrate relative oliguria during the first 24 to 48 hours. Disease processes, such as asphyxia, pneumonia, and respiratory distress syndrome (RDS), increase vasopressin release; thus the fluid and electrolyte transition during the first few days of birth may be altered in these conditions.[20,38,50] Neonates with RDS will also have delayed postnatal contraction of the ECF compartment, further delaying diuresis. Onset of the diuresis, during the first few days of life, usually coincides with the initial stages of recovery from RDS.[24]

Despite the period of natriuresis after birth, infants usually do not require additional sodium during the first 24 to 48 hours of life. It is normal to have an initial negative sodium balance, but later it is necessary to retain sodium for appropriate growth; additional sodium supplementation may be required.[24]

A review of maternal history and the intrapartum course may be helpful in calculating the infant's fluid and electrolyte requirements. For example, if the mother received large amounts of electrolyte-free fluids in the intrapartum period, the neonate may be hyponatremic and have an expanded ECF space at birth.[30,56]

Extracellular fluid comprises both intravascular fluid (plasma) and ISF. The electrolyte composition of ISF and plasma is similar, but it is strikingly different from ICF (Figure 14-5). Sodium is the major cation in ECF (both ISF and plasma) and is easily measured. Potassium, the major cation in ICF, on the other hand, cannot be measured readily because ICF is not easily accessible. Because 90% of the total body potassium is intracellular, low levels of plasma potassium are assumed to reflect low total body potassium.

Maintaining appropriate fluid and electrolyte balance may be difficult due to the immaturity of the neonatal renal system: (1) inability to dilute urine secondary to lower glomerular filtration rate (GFR) and (2) inability to concentrate urine secondary to renal tubular immaturity. The neonatal GFR, a measure of renal function, is low in utero but increases rapidly within a few hours after delivery as renal blood flow increases. This increased GFR is a result of increasing cardiac output and increasing glomerular permeability.[24]

GFR is independent of gestational age. It rises rapidly during the first 6 weeks of life, increasing more slowly during infancy, and reaches adult values by 12 months of age. A VLBW infant in satisfactory condition at 6 weeks should have a similar GFR to that of term infants. The formation of nephrons is complete at 34 to 35 weeks' gestation, whereas maturation of the nephrons continues beyond 40 weeks' gestation.[14,19] The GFR can be compromised in critically ill neonates.

In addition to fluid balance, the renal tubules are responsible for mineral and electrolyte excretion and reabsorption. Renal tubular function is influenced by gestational age.[24] Therefore urine sodium losses are a function of gestational age and sodium intake. Preterm infants with immature tubular function have a limited ability to excrete sodium and are more likely to experience electrolyte imbalance. Urine sodium excretion increases slowly during the

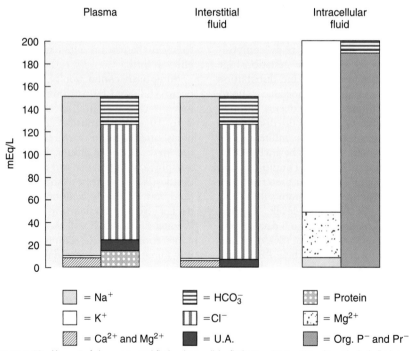

FIGURE 14-5 "Gamblegram" of plasma interstitial fluid and intracellular fluid. (From Winters RW, editor: *The body fluids in pediatrics*, Boston, 1973, Little, Brown.)

first 2 years of life. If increased amounts of sodium are provided to more mature infants, they are able to respond by increasing urine sodium excretion in an attempt to normalize serum sodium.

The use of the urinary fractional excretion of sodium (FENa) [FENa = (Urine sodium × Plasma Cr)/(Urine Cr × Plasma sodium)] is an important tool in assessing sodium balance, but must be interpreted cautiously, especially shortly after birth, due to the immaturity of renal tubular function. When using FENa to diagnose the etiology of hyponatremia, a value greater than 3% reflects an intrinsic renal problem, whereas a value less than 2.5% reflects a prerenal problem (e.g., volume depletion); both values are higher than that expected for an adult.[16] A falsely elevated FENa may be present when excessive sodium is lost in the urine due to prematurity or with diuretic use.[27,59]

The ability to excrete potassium is impaired at birth, especially in low-birth-weight infants, thus increasing their risk of hyperkalemia, particularly when given a potassium load before establishing stable renal function. Calcium reabsorption is also reduced with immaturity and results in higher urinary levels of calcium; thus early use of loop diuretics may lead to an increased risk of renal stones.[28]

The capacity to concentrate urine in VLBW infants appears limited but can be influenced by gestational age and nutrient intake. The immature concentrating ability (maximum of approximately 600 mOsm/L) (Figure 14-6) coupled with an inability to rapidly excrete an acute water or sodium load results in a narrow margin of safety when prescribing fluid and electrolytes, especially in the VLBW infant.[1,14,19]

In general, urea is the major component of urine osmolality (and hence specific gravity). When total parenteral nutrition is provided, urine specific gravity may rise because of a low renal threshold for glucose and amino acids. The renal protein and glucose threshold increases with increasing gestation.

Neonatal urinary acidification is limited and the threshold for bicarbonate excretion is reduced, leading to both decreased bicarbonate retention and acid excretion. Both physiologic and pathologic factors can contribute to this urinary alkalinization. Acidemia develops in premature infants due to this limited capacity for hydrogen ion excretion, whereas if this is present in more mature infants they may have acute illnesses, such as bicarbonate-losing tubular necrosis or a urinary tract infection. The ability to distinguish acidemia occurring from an acute illness versus a developmentally impaired urinary acidification system is important for proper treatment. The anion gap [serum Na^+/(serum Cl^- + serum bicarbonate)] is a useful tool in this assessment. The normal anion gap typically is less than 8. A widened anion gap is suggestive of increased production of organic acid, in particular lactic acid (a pathologic condition), whereas a normal

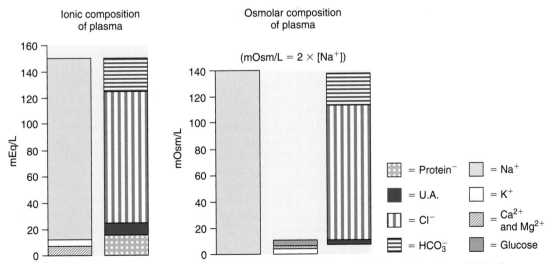

FIGURE 14-6 Ionic and osmolar composition of plasma. (From Winters RW, editor: *The body fluids in pediatrics*, Boston, 1973, Little, Brown.)

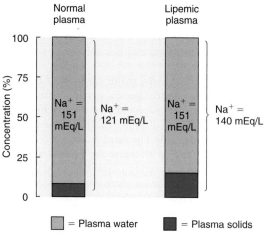

FIGURE 14-7 Effects of hyperlipidemia on plasma water and plasma sodium concentration. (From Winters RW, editor: *The body fluids in pediatrics,* Boston, 1973, Little, Brown.)

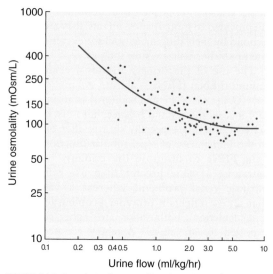

FIGURE 14-8 Normal urine flow rates. (From Jones MD, Gresham EL, Battaglia FC: Urinary flow rate and urea excretion rates in newborn infants, *Biol Neonate* 21:322, 1972.)

or narrow gap suggests bicarbonate loss due to the lowered threshold for bicarbonate excretion in the neonate. Further details are available in Chapter 8.

Hormones, including antidiuretic hormone, aldosterone, atrial natriuretic factor, and parathyroid hormone, are involved in regulating the neonatal fluid and electrolyte balance, yet the specific roles are not well defined. Most hormonal effects occur by modifying renal function through either changes in GFR or renal tubular permeability. For example, the increased osmolality that occurs in dehydration is a trigger for antidiuretic hormone release leading to changes in the permeability of the distal tubule and collecting duct. This change results in more water reabsorption and thus more concentrated urine.

Osmolality can be satisfactorily estimated in many clinical settings by the following formula (Figure 14-7):

$$(\text{Osmolality} = (2\,[\text{Na}^+] + \text{Glucose (mg/dl)} \div 18) + (\text{BUN (mg/dl)} \div 2.8)$$

Osmotic forces are responsible for apparently low plasma electrolyte concentrations in some common clinical settings. For example, in hyperglycemia, the plasma sodium concentration reported by the laboratory is usually low but the total effective osmolality may be normal.

An analogous situation exists for the less frequent condition of hyperlipidemia, in which low laboratory plasma sodium values are reported with a normal osmolality (Figure 14-8). Low laboratory values for plasma sodium (pseudohyponatremia) occur because the increase in plasma solids (lipids) causes a lower plasma water content resulting in water displacement and hence a lower sodium concentration per liter of whole plasma.

Osmotic forces largely determine shifts in the internal redistribution of water in hydration disturbances. An example of changes in osmolality occurs in preterm infants who undergo insensible water loss because of skin immaturity, decreased body fat, and a large surface-to-volume ratio leading to increased evaporation. This water loss from the interstitial space results in a hyperosmolar extracellular compartment exhibited by hypernatremia and occasionally hyperkalemia and hyperglycemia.[9,14]

Another key concept in fluid and electrolyte balance involves insensible water losses (IWLs) that occur via pulmonary and cutaneous routes and are influenced by the factors listed in Table 14-1. However, IWL varies greatly depending on gestational age and birth weight (Table 14-2). The neonate's environment also can affect the fluid balance. Radiant warmer usage decreases the neonate's radiant heat loss but can increase IWL by

T A B L E 14-1	EXAMPLES OF OSMOTIC FORCE		
	mM	N	mOsm
NaCl	1	2	2
Glucose	1	1	1
CaCl$_2$	1	3	3

T A B L E 14-2	FACTORS THAT INFLUENCE INSENSIBLE WATER LOSS (IWL)
DECREASE IWL	INCREASE IWL
Heat shield or double-walled incubators	Inversely related to gestational age and weight
Plastic blankets	Respiratory distress
Clothes	Ambient temperature above thermoneutral
High relative humidity (ambient ventilator gas)	Fever
	Radiant warmer
Emollient use	Phototherapy
	Activity

50% to 200%, resulting in hypernatremic dehydration.[36] Incubators reduce radiant heat loss via their double-walled Plexiglas design.

Modern incubators provide sterile humidity (80% or greater) and are very effective in decreasing IWL by reducing evaporative heat loss. Internal incubator humidification was discontinued in the 1970s when it was associated with *Pseudomonas* infections.[37] Presumably, the nature of *Pseudomonas* promoted its stability and growth in the water humidification reservoirs. However, present humidification designs provide for direct heating of water in an external reservoir to a temperature that kills most organisms. The water is transformed into vapor, rather than mist, and carried in a gaseous state by the incubator's convective air flow, thus reducing the possibility of airborne bacterial transfer.[37]

Because added environmental humidity reduces transcutaneous evaporative water loss, a preterm infant managed in humidity needs less fluid than those managed without humidity to achieve the same water balance. A relative humidity of 80% can reduce water loss to one tenth of the water loss of a preterm infant

receiving care in 50% humidity.[36] This reduction in evaporative water loss affects the management of fluid requirements and the electrolyte balance in premature infants. For infants with birth weight less than 1000 g, the use of humidity at 60% to 80% results in lower fluid intake and fewer episodes of hypernatremia in the first week of life. A decreased risk of severe BPD has also been reported in extremely low-birth-weight (ELBW) infants cared for in humidified incubators.[32] Despite these improvements, the optimal level and duration of humidification have yet to be determined.

The ability to provide the proper fluid and electrolyte balance is determined by assessing initial fluid status, renal function, and estimated insensible fluid losses. Frequent assessment of fluid balance remains essential in preventing fluid deficit or overload that can be difficult to correct once it has occurred.

ETIOLOGY

The causes of common electrolyte problems and common clinical syndromes are discussed under Treatment later in this chapter.

PREVENTION

Prevention of fluid and electrolyte imbalance in neonates begins with knowing how to calculate fluid and electrolyte requirements correctly. The estimated metabolic rate forms the reference base for all calculations. The metabolic rate (and hence oxygen consumption) normally increases steadily over the first weeks of life, so changes in water and electrolyte requirements should be anticipated.

If the daily caloric requirement is approximately 100 *kcal/kg/day,* the physiologic basis of metabolic rate may be used to calculate needs; however, most institutions determine an infant's daily fluid need on a *milliliters per kilogram (ml/kg)* basis, which is modified by factors that influence IWL and is usually adjusted depending on body weight, clinical composition, serum chemistry results, and urine volume and composition (Figure 14-9; see also Table 14-2).

Preterm infants have lower metabolic rates than those of term infants.[6] SGA infants may have higher metabolic rates than those of preterm infants of similar weight,[5,9] which may be

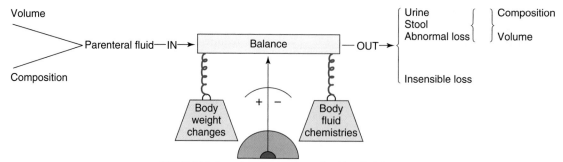

FIGURE 14-9 Basic scheme for monitoring and modifying fluid therapy.

because of their relatively large brain/body mass ratio. Infants with congenital heart disease,[40] as well as infants in the immediate postoperative period,[43] also have higher metabolic rates compared with appropriate-for-gestational-age (AGA) infants. Both SGA and preterm infants, especially VLBW infants, should be expected to require more frequent assessment and modification of requirements.

Preterm infants, however, are subject to other problems that may diminish the influence of this metabolic rate when calculating fluid needs. SGA infants may require less water per kilogram than either preterm or term AGA infants due to their increased extracellular volume.[41] Input should be recorded every hour. Output should be recorded hourly on critically ill infants but may be recorded every 4 to 6 hours on infants who require minimal stimulation. The smallest infants require frequent fluid balance monitoring, so if output is unusually large, intake can be adjusted immediately. If fluid intake lags behind losses, critically ill infants may develop hypernatremia and may not tolerate "catching up." Continuous monitoring is necessary to ensure that fluid is administered in appropriate amounts. Current infusion pumps can accurately infuse volumes of 0.01 ml/hr and must be used for the smallest, sickest infants.

Requirements for fluid and electrolytes are divided into maintenance and deficit needs. *Maintenance* indicates the infant remains in a zero balance state and can be subdivided into (1) normal loss, which consists of water and electrolyte loss through stool, urine, and insensible (lung and skin) routes; and (2) abnormal or increased losses, such as gastrointestinal/diarrhea, ostomy, and chest tube drainage.

All diapers should be preweighed using a gram scale and marked with dry/tare weight.

After each stool or void, the diaper is reweighed; the difference equals the amount of loss. For example, if the dry weight is 20 g and the wet weight is 26 g, the difference is 6 g, or 6 ml of stool or urine. All losses should be calculated to the nearest milliliter.

The term *deficit* refers to previously incurred losses. These should be uncommon in the newborn but can occur when there are unrecognized losses such as "third space" or interstitial losses with NEC (see later discussion). In older neonates, deficits may occur with disorders that have an insidious or delayed onset, such as renal tubular dysfunction or nonvirilizing congenital adrenal hyperplasia.

Deficits are best estimated by body weight comparisons. Weight loss greater than 10% to 15% in 1 week should be considered excessive, although in VLBW infants it can be difficult to maintain within 10% to 15% of birth weight during the first week of life.[60] Infants who are SGA have less weight loss compared with AGA infants[61] in the first 10 days after birth. Growth charts assist with calculations of weight loss and/or gain and help consider the normal physiologic weight loss that occurs during the first several days after birth when calculating an infant's fluid needs.

The initial choice of parenteral solution depends on the weight and postnatal age of the infant (Table 14-3). Also important is whether the infant is in an incubator with a heated humidified environment or under a radiant warmer without a plastic blanket or heat shield. Uncovered VLBW infants under radiant warmers demonstrate IWLs of up to 170 ml/kg/day,[24] and thus use of radiant warmers should be avoided if possible. Maintenance of water and glucose needs in larger infants on the first day of life can usually be met by a 10% glucose solution infused at 60 to

TABLE 14-3	GUIDELINES FOR FLUID (ml/kg/day) AND SOLUTE PROVISION BY PATIENT WEIGHT AND DAYS OF AGE				
WEIGHT (g)	**RANGES OF WATER LOSS**		**DAY 1***	**DAYS 2-3***	**DAYS 4-7***
Less than 1250	IWL[†]	40-170			
	Urine	50-100			
	Stool	5-10			
	TOTAL	95-280	120	140	150-175
1250-1750	IWL[†]	20-50			
	Urine	50-100			
	Stool	5-10			
	TOTAL	75-160	90	110	130-140
More than 1750	IWL[†]	15-40			
	Urine	50-100			
	Stool	5-10			
	TOTAL	70-150	80	90	100-200

Increment for phototherapy: 20-30 ml/kg/day if patient is in open warmer and has radiant phototherapy. No adjustment if baby is in humidified environment and/or has fiberoptic phototherapy source.
Increment for radiant warmer: 20-30 ml/kg/day.
Maintenance solutes: glucose: 7-12 g/kg/day (4-8 g/kg in VLBW infants)
  Na: 1-4 mEq/kg/day (2-8 mEq/kg/day in VLBW infants)
  K: 1-4 mEq/kg/day
  Cl: 1-4 mEq/kg/day
  Ca: 1 mEq/kg/day

*Adjustment based on a urine flow rate of 2 to 5 ml/kg/hr and a stable weight.
[†]May be reduced by 30% if the infant is on a ventilator.
IWL, Insensible water loss; *VLBW,* very-low-birth-weight.

80 ml/kg/day, which provides an acceptable glucose infusion of about 4.2 to 5.5 mg/kg/min. The infusion rate can be gradually increased over 4 to 5 days to 120 to 140 ml/kg/day using principles of monitoring discussed later in this chapter.[4]

All sick infants require IV access for fluid administration. Placement of an IV line is the most common procedure in the neonatal intensive care unit (NICU).[45] The IV equipment should include (1) a needle or catheter, (2) connecting tubing, and (3) an infusion pump.

Electrolytes such as sodium and potassium are usually omitted the first and second day of life and then added as the salt of acetate, chloride, or phosphate in amounts of 1 to 4 mEq/kg/day. Mildly acidotic and VLBW infants may be given their sodium requirements as sodium acetate.[4] Potassium should never

be added to IV fluid until urine flow and renal function have been assessed. The initial requirement for calcium is 1 mEq/Kg/day (20 mg/kg/day), but rises to a maintenance requirement of 3 to 4 mEq/kg/day (about 60 to 80 mg/kg/day) of elemental calcium preferably given as calcium gluconate (about 600 to 800 mg/kg/day).[55] This maintenance is most important in VLBW infants and those who are severely ill. Careful observation of peripheral IV sites with infusion of IV fluids containing calcium is critical due to the risk of tissue necrosis associated with infiltration.[31]

Factors that influence IWL must be identified early and maintenance needs adjusted appropriately to prevent problems with water and electrolyte balance. Humidified incubators significantly decrease the IWL of ELBW infants. They require less fluid intake, have lower percentage of weight loss, and have fewer episodes of hypernatremia than infants cared for in a nonhumidified incubator.[32] Management of VLBW infants presents special, complex problems, and continued research is needed. The following observations may be helpful:

- Total fluid requirements should typically start at 100 to 120 ml/kg/day at birth although some authors suggest as low as 80 ml/kg/day[11,42,57] and often need to be increased by 20 to 40 ml/kg/day over days 2 to 6 of life, typically plateauing at 150 to 160 ml/kg/day. Higher fluid requirements may be necessary for VLBW infants managed on a radiant warmer or in nonhumidified incubation. Careful restriction of fluids, without allowing dehydration, has been shown to decrease the risk of PDA and NEC.[8] A lower risk of BPD has also been associated with early appropriate weight loss in ELBW infants.[32,61] Careful restriction of fluids allows for the normal contraction of extracellular fluid and appropriate weight loss while maintaining physiologic needs.[8,42]
- Cumulative weight loss plateaus at 10% to 15% of birth weight by postnatal day 3 to 5.
- Sodium requirements (including medications) are 2 to 3 mEq/kg/day after 24 to 48 hours of age and may reach a maximum of 4 to 5 mEq/kg/day during the first few weeks of life.[16]
- Maintaining normal serum glucose concentrations (50 to 150 mg/dl) in VLBW infants may initially require relatively less glucose than that of term or near-term infants because their own endogenous glucose production may not be effectively suppressed. However, in order to preserve endogenous stores of glucose (e.g., glycogen) in clinical practice, the preterm infant may need up to 8 to 9 mg/kg/min of glucose, whereas the term infant requires about 6 mg/kg/min.[17] In VLBW infants, a gradual increase in the glucose infusion rate to 11 to 12 mg/kg/min by the end of the first week of life is usually well tolerated.[4] The glucose concentration of the fluids administered may need to be changed, sometimes frequently, to maintain an appropriate serum glucose concentration. With the larger initial fluid requirements of very tiny babies, lower glucose concentrations, sometimes down to

D_5W (5 mg% or 5 mg/dl) in IV fluids are often prescribed for ELBW infants as the initial fluid. As anticipated, infants weighing less than 1000 g are the most difficult to manage without inducing excessive weight loss, hypernatremia, or hyperglycemia, especially those stabilized under radiant warmers. They may have greatly increased IWL with fluid requirements in the range of 175 to 200 ml/kg/day or greater. By the end of the first week of life, as the epithelium cornifies, their daily requirements decrease to 120 to 150 ml/kg/day. When enteral caloric intake is low (fewer than 50 kcal/kg/day), neonates will require administration of IV fluids, which should be provided as parenteral nutrition[39] containing glucose, amino acids, lipids, vitamins, and micronutrients in order to support growth (see Chapter 17).

DATA COLLECTION

Parenteral therapy should be based on the following principles: (1) assess the patient's clinical status for maintenance needs, factors that modify IWL, and confounding medical or surgical disorders; (2) calculate short-term (12 to 24 hours) fluid and electrolyte needs; (3) initiate therapy at the proper site and infusion rate; and (4) monitor and adjust the fluid infusion rate and content based on clinical and biochemical data.

History

Factors influencing IWL (see Table 14-2) include gestational age, birth weight, and postnatal age. When the patient's condition changes, it is important to detail the change to evaluate the potential effect of the new condition on fluid and electrolyte balance and requirements. Thus NEC may be associated with an acute need for additional volume expansion–type fluids because of "third space losses," whereas with acute renal failure, anuria should prompt clinical reassessment and usually indicates the need for reducing daily fluid administration.

Signs and Symptoms

Weight, urine output (Box 14-1), and serum sodium concentration (Box 14-2) are the best overall clinical guides to assess whether therapy is

BOX 14-1 **DATA COLLECTION**

CLINICAL EVALUATION OF FLUID AND ELECTROLYTE STATUS

- Serial weight (sometimes two to three times per day)
- Heart rate
- Blood pressure
- Skin perfusion
- Urine output
- Other drainage (ostomies, gastric, chest tubes)

BOX 14-2 **DATA COLLECTION**

LABORATORY EVALUATION OF FLUID AND ELECTROLYTE STATUS

Essential values are included in this box. Other measurements are routinely made but are less valuable in the rapid determination of fluid status and complications of imbalances.

- *Sodium* (most sensitive indicator of water loss in excess of electrolytes, as is insensible water loss)
- *Potassium* (may rise with decreased kidney perfusion and acidosis)
- *Hematocrit* (will rise with extracellular fluid contraction)
- *BUN* (relatively insensitive indicator of dehydration in neonate)
- *Creatinine* (will rise slowly with renal failure)
- *Total CO$_2$* (low level indicates acidosis, either because of bicarbonate loss or metabolic acidosis from poor tissue perfusion and anaerobic metabolism)

adequate. Weight is the most sensitive index of IWL and must be accurately determined at least every 24 hours. Accurate daily weights in VLBW infants require special nursing efforts and may be facilitated with electronic bed scales.

Urine output should be 2 to 5 ml/kg/hr with a specific gravity of 1.005 to 1.012.[22] Blood pressure and peripheral perfusion may be used to reflect changes in vascular volume and cardiac output. Normal capillary refill is typically less than 3 seconds and is more reliable when tested on the forehead or sternum. However, its sensitivity and specificity have been questioned in infants and should be interpreted with caution as a sign of adequate hydration. Blood pressure and heart rate should be evaluated in conjunction with capillary refill time.

Loss of skin turgor is a late and variable sign and usually is not helpful in assessing therapy, but vital signs (heart rate, respiratory rate, and temperature) provide useful signs about metabolic rate and stress. However, temperature may be affected by many external factors. Drainage volume and content from ostomies, chest tubes, nasogastric tubes, and other sites should be quantitated accurately. Fluid samples can be submitted for laboratory analysis to improve the accuracy of the replacement fluids. The amounts of drainage represent maintenance requirements that must be added to the calculation of baseline daily maintenance needs (abnormal + normal = total maintenance).

Laboratory Data

Tests for concentrations of electrolytes (Na$^+$, K$^+$, Cl$^-$, Ca^{2+}), red blood cells (hematocrit), glucose, blood urea nitrogen (BUN) or creatinine, and acid-base status should be performed serially (see Box 14-2). Occasionally, serum osmolality and protein concentrations are helpful in assessing the neonate's condition. The anion gap may be calculated from the difference of the positive and negative ions, sodium, chloride, and bicarbonate: $[Na]^+ - ([Cl^-] + [HCO3^-])$.

Urine volume must be recorded with every void. Measuring urine osmolality and glucose and electrolyte concentrations helps clarify fluid and electrolyte balance when amounts of glucose, protein, or other solutes appear in the urine. In a preterm infant, especially a VLBW infant, an elevated urine pH may signal bicarbonate loss due to renal function immaturity.[48]

All drainage must be collected and measured, with the concentration of solutes determined (see Box 14-2). Accumulations over 4 to 6 hours are preferable to a single "spot" collection, which may be misleading. Occasionally, determining trace electrolyte elements, hematocrit, and protein content of urine or drainage can be crucial to management. However, there are no "normal" values for urine electrolyte concentrations because they must be interpreted with respect to the infant's clinical diagnosis, medications, and the serum electrolyte concentrations.

Electronic health records allow for real-time evaluation of fluid balance. Data can be downloaded directly from IV pumps or entered manually on an hourly basis. The practitioner can review actual intake and output (see Figure 14-3), evaluate total fluid balance, and quickly make adjustments, if needed, to ensure optimal fluid balance in the neonate. Graphs are also available to provide further detail and trend changes over time.

TREATMENT

Techniques of IV Therapy

In modern neonatal intensive care, peripherally inserted central venous catheters (PICCs) have become an invaluable tool. Placement permits long-term administration of IV fluids, avoiding multiple painful procedures for peripheral IV placement and the need for surgical placement of a long-term central catheter. This is particularly valuable for ELBW infants for whom the time to establish full enteral feedings may be prolonged. This technique is also helpful for long-term parenteral nutrition. Complications of long-term indwelling central catheters include infection, thrombosis, phlebitis, infiltration, effusion, occlusion, and catheter breakage.[62] The risk for infection significantly increases after the PICC has been in place for longer than 2 weeks[35]; therefore, these catheters should be discontinued as soon as enteral nutrition is adequately established. Thrombosis is more likely to occur when the flow rate of IV fluids is extremely low (less than 1 ml/hr). Although the use of heparin in PICC-line fluids has been shown to prolong patency of the line, it does not decrease the incidence of thrombosis.[46] Infiltration usually occurs at the site of the catheter tip. This includes infiltration into the mediastinum, pleural space, or pericardium, depending on the location of the tip of the catheter (see Chapter 7).

Peripheral insertion of central venous catheters can be accomplished readily but requires clinical training and experience. Insertion sites include the saphenous, antecubital, axillary, basilic, cephalic, popliteal, posterior auricular, and external jugular veins.[47] Avoidance of upper extremity PICCs in infants with single-ventricle cardiac anatomy is recommended to prevent thrombosis or occlusion of upper extremity veins required in the eventual Fontan procedure.[2] The catheter is advanced so the tip is in the superior or inferior vena cava; suboptimal positioning is associated with increased risk of complications.[13,29] The position of the catheter tip must be confirmed radiographically. Confirmation by lateral radiograph is recommended with saphenous insertion due to a risk of inadvertent placement in spinal vessels.[49] Cannulation of the subclavian vein of VLBW infants requires insertion by a pediatric surgeon. Venesection or cutdown of peripheral or central vessels can be performed with appropriate training.

Midline catheters can be used for infants who will require more than a few days of IV fluid administration. Midline catheters are longer than peripheral IVs and are inserted deeper into the vein where blood flow is greater but remain outside of central vessels. Because of their placement, midline catheters can only be used to provide fluids appropriate for peripheral access. The length of duration is an advantage of midlines compared with peripheral IV lines; catheters can last 1 to 2 weeks with some reports of midlines lasting up to 3 months.[34]

Peripheral venous access continues to be a valuable approach to IV therapy when short-term vascular access is needed. The advent of extremely small catheter and introducer sets has permitted prolonged use of a single peripheral infusion site. "Butterfly" infusion sets are rarely used for IV access.

A rubber band is an effective tourniquet for the extremity of a small infant. Attention must be paid to antiseptic technique when acquiring venous access. Before puncturing the skin, prepare materials for placement. It is important to recognize the significant risk for infiltration and skin necrosis with a peripherally inserted IV line. Calcium-containing solutions in parenteral nutrition present an additional risk, particularly for skin damage. Prevention of such extravasation injuries is paramount because few treatment options are available. Although the needle or catheter must be taped in place, the tape should allow for adequate visualization of the site. The fluid administered should be recorded at least every hour, and the site should be observed for signs of infiltration. Although traditionally, splints/padded boards have been used to decrease movement and increase catheter duration, there are no studies to support the practice in neonates.[15] If splints/padded boards are used to stabilize an IV line, it should be taped in a manner that allows visual inspection of the insertion site. The most common complication of IV therapy is infiltration, with rates as high as 70%.[63] If extravasation occurs, the infusion should be stopped immediately and the IV catheter removed. The affected extremity should then be elevated to limit swelling.[18] Hyaluronidase is an enzyme that degrades hyaluronic acid, a constituent of the normal interstitial barrier, which increases the distribution and absorption of locally injected substances.[7] By facilitating more rapid absorption of potentially damaging fluid, tissue necrosis may be lessened. A plastic surgery consultation should be considered when tissue necrosis is anticipated.

Umbilical vessel catheterization should be limited to several days' duration until a central catheter can be placed (see Chapter 7).

It is important to provide pain relief during the placement of peripheral IVs, midlines, and/or PICC lines. Methods that have been shown to decrease pain during venipuncture in infants include oral sucrose,[52] swaddling, nonnutritive sucking, breastfeeding, kangaroo care, and topical anesthetics.[3] The use of sucrose has been found to be superior compared with topical lidocaine in infants[54] (see Chapter 12).

The combination of pharmacologic and non-pharmacologic pain management modalities is recommended, but additional research is needed. When undergoing venipuncture the use of topical lidocaine and sucrose was found to be superior compared with sucrose alone in preterm infants,[10] but not in term infants.[54] Intravenous morphine and the combination of morphine and topical tetracaine reduces the pain associated with peripheral central line placement in ventilated neonates; however, use of morphine also increases the need for respiratory support,[53] so it should be used with caution. At minimum, nonpharmacologic pain treatments should be used for all venipuncture procedures in neonates.

Common Problems

In NICUs, virtually all patients initially receive IV fluid therapy. Therefore conventional rules of pediatric fluid therapy that estimate losses and project deficit replacement may not be appropriate. Weight, urine output and concentration, and the concentration of various solutes in serum and other body fluids are usually known. The correct diagnosis usually rests on clinical and laboratory measurements (not estimates). Attempts should be made to identify the etiology of the deficit or excess while these conditions are being corrected.

HYPOCALCEMIA (INFANTS WITH TOTAL SERUM CALCIUM LESS THAN 7 mg/dl)

Hypocalcemia is a common finding in critically ill babies. Clinical findings may correlate poorly with biochemical data (total or ionized calcium). Jitteriness, irritability, and twitching are common, but nonspecific, initial signs. Both serum calcium and glucose should be measured. Hypocalcemia is often a clinical concern in infants of diabetic mothers and in infants with asphyxia, prematurity, and delayed nutrition. Risk for "early" hypocalcemia within 72 hours of birth is minimized by supplementing IV fluids with 35 or more mg/kg/day of elemental calcium or initiating parenteral nutrition with 60 or more mg/kg/day for preterm infants.[9] Alternatively, early neonatal hypocalcemia may be prevented with oral calcium supplementation of 80 mg/kg/day of elemental calcium gluconate[9] (100 mg of calcium gluconate = 9.3 mg of elemental calcium).

It should be noted that a normal physiologic neonatal calcium nadir occurs at around 48 hours of neonatal life.[25] At birth, when the infant is disconnected from the maternal calcium supply, calcium levels begin to fall and parathyroid hormone secretion is stimulated. The parathyroid gland's response is somewhat insufficient, leading to a calcium nadir within the first 2 days of life. During this nadir, ionized calcium typically remains within the normal adult range, but undergoes a substantial decline from fetal levels.[25] Early administration of calcium to the neonate may interfere with the anticipated natural history of calcium homeostasis. Treatment during this physiologic nadir, in term infants, is often not necessary unless the infant has confirmed low ionized calcium level. This would be typically associated with other medical concerns such as hypoxic-ischemic encephalopathy or in infants of diabetic mothers.

Confirmation of low serum calcium values with an ionized calcium level is necessary, because the albumin level, acid-base balance, and other factors could affect serum calcium levels. Attempts to rapidly correct hypocalcemia, using bolus infusions and slow infusions over 2 to 3 minutes, are not as successful and may induce dysrhythmias, compared with more gradual attempts to correct hypocalcemia. Either repeated slow infusions every 6 hours or a continuous infusion is best. Additional calcium should be given intravenously as 100 to 200 mg/kg/dose of calcium gluconate over 4 to 6 hours if seizures or biochemical abnormality persists. "Late" hypocalcemia, occurring at more than 7 days of age, usually has a specific cause such as malabsorption, hypomagnesemia, hypoparathyroidism, long-term diuretic therapy, or rickets and should be evaluated in detail.

Care should be taken when administering IV calcium: (1) the infant should receive cardiac monitoring to detect bradycardia; (2) calcium administration should be discontinued immediately if bradycardia occurs; and (3) the peripheral IV site should be checked for patency before and during administration because of the potential for skin necrosis, sloughing, and dystrophic calcification caused by infiltrated calcium.

HYPERCALCEMIA (INFANTS WITH SERUM CALCIUM MORE THAN 11 mg/dl)

Hypercalcemia is typically asymptomatic but may present with nonspecific symptoms in the infant. Symptoms can include poor feeding, emesis, lethargy, irritability, polyuria, and constipation. Both serum and ionized calcium should be measured along with phosphate and alkaline phosphatase. The most common presentation of hypercalcemia is iatrogenic in the setting of excessive vitamin D or calcium supplementation or in response to inadequate phosphorus supplementation during the administration of parenteral nutrition. Hypercalcemia may also be seen secondary to maternal hypoparathyroidism or increased maternal vitamin D intake. Neonatal disease such as hyperparathyroidism, hyperthyroidism, Williams syndrome, and hypophosphatasia can also present with hypercalcemia. Drug-induced hypercalcemia can occur with thiazide diuretics.[12]

Initial management is often directed at adjusting the calcium-phosphorus ratio in parenteral nutrition solutions. Hypercalemia in the setting of inadequate phosphorus supplementation results from increased bone reabsorption of calcium and therefore treatment should be aimed at providing appropriate phosphorus supplementation as opposed to decreasing calcium. If hypercalcemia is severe, furosemide can be given to facilitate calcium excretion in the urine. Electrolytes must be monitored carefully, as well as the infant's volume status, with careful avoidance of dehydration. Normal saline can be given if there is concern for dehydration. Hydrocortisone can also be used to decrease intestinal calcium absorption. If the etiology of hypercalcemia is not apparent, further evaluation with additional laboratory studies, such as parathyroid hormone, 1,25-dihydroxy-vitamin D, 25-OH-vitamin D, urine calcium, and urine phosphate should be considered.[12]

HYPERNATREMIA (INFANTS WITH SERUM SODIUM MORE THAN 150 mEq/L)

Clinical signs of hypernatremia are rare, except for late-occurring seizures. The most common causes of hypernatremia are (1) dehydration, usually caused by too little "free water" administration; (2) injudicious use of sodium-containing solution, such as sodium bicarbonate bolus infusion and sodium-containing medications; and (3) congenital or acquired reduction in antidiuretic hormone resulting in excess loss of "free water," diabetes insipidus. Intracranial bleeding correlates strongly with hypernatremia.[36] Management should be directed toward prevention, and infants with hypernatremia should have serum sodium reduced slowly to prevent seizures. Infants who experience hypernatremic dehydration often appear better hydrated than they are because hypernatremia shifts fluid into the intravascular space.

HYPONATREMIA (INFANTS WITH SERUM SODIUM LESS THAN 130 mEq/L)

Hyponatremia is usually asymptomatic because it develops chronically rather than as an acute imbalance; however, a late clinical sign is seizure. The most common causes include (1) excess hydration as a result of administration of electrolyte-free solutions; (2) renal loss of sodium in neonates receiving diuretic therapy, especially in VLBW infants; and (3) the syndrome of inappropriate antidiuretic hormone secretion (SIADH) that is suspected when decreased serum sodium and decreased urine output occur. This syndrome is associated with central nervous system and lung pathologic conditions. Clinical criteria include (1) low serum sodium, (2) continued inappropriately high urine sodium loss, (3) urine osmolality greater than plasma, and (4) normal adrenal and renal function. Management is by volume restriction until diuresis follows, and treatment is directed toward resolving the etiology.

In the case of sodium deficit as primary etiology, one can compute the amount of sodium required to correct a deficit using the following formula:

$$\text{Necessary sodium} = (\text{Sodium desired} - \text{Sodium observed}) \times 0.6 \times \text{Weight (in kilograms)}$$

The target goal amount and the replacement rate given are a matter of clinical judgment based on underlying diagnosis and treatments for individual patient situations. In practice, often the clinician prescribes a percentage of the calculated deficit, repeats the serum measurement, and modifies the IV solution.

HYPERKALEMIA (INFANTS WITH SERUM POTASSIUM MORE THAN 7 mEq/L)

Causes of hyperkalemia include (1) acidosis with or without tissue destruction, (2) renal failure (water overload may limit management), (3) adrenal insufficiency (relatively uncommon), and (4) iatrogenic secondary to inappropriate potassium administration. Nonoliguric hyperkalemia may be seen in ELBW infants; even in the absence of potassium intake, it tends to occur more frequently in infants at a younger gestational age who did not receive antenatal steroids. Other electrolyte imbalances, such as elevated phosphate, can also predispose ELBW infants to nonoliguric hyperkalemia. If potassium levels are low at birth, the infant is less likely to develop nonoliguric hyperkalemia. Careful monitoring for electrolyte disturbances must occur in this population.[33,58]

Table 14-4 outlines clinical signs and electrocardiogram (ECG) changes that may be seen in hyperkalemia. Management is directed toward resolving the causes and nonspecific treatment, depending on the severity of the hyperkalemia and the associated clinical signs:

- Stop all potassium administration.
- Evaluate total and ionized calcium.
- If hypocalcemia is present, infuse 100 to 200 mg/kg of calcium gluconate to lower the cell membrane threshold. This is transient therapy but may be lifesaving.
- Infuse sodium bicarbonate 1 to 2 mEq/kg, slowly over 30 minutes or longer. This is also transient therapy designed to promote intracellular sodium and hydrogen exchange for potassium. It is particularly useful when the hyperkalemia is associated with acidosis.

However, if hyperkalemia is associated with acute renal failure, the relatively large volume of fluid required to deliver the sodium bicarbonate may be concerning.

- Administer 1 g/kg cation exchange resin (sodium polystyrene sulfonate [Kayexalate]) as an oral or rectal solution. Little experience has been reported in neonates, and technical problems of retention can be substantial. Furthermore, this may not be an option if the infant is on nothing-by-mouth status or has an injured gastrointestinal tract. When this resin is used, sodium in the resin is exchanged for serum potassium, which may result in hypernatremia. Therefore, careful attention must be paid to serum electrolyte concentrations.
- An insulin infusion given simultaneously with a dextrose infusion can help shift potassium to the intracellular space. There are several challenges to this form of therapy. First, the actual dose of insulin administered to the patient varies unpredictably because the insulin adsorbs to plastic IV tubing. Second, significant hypoglycemia and seizures may occur. Serum glucose concentration must be monitored frequently and the glucose infusion adjusted accordingly.
- Perform peritoneal dialysis. With neonatal hyperkalemic peritoneal dialysis, sodium bicarbonate frequently must be added to dialysate to prevent acidosis. Peritoneal dialysis is a complicated procedure in neonates, involving catheter placement and dialysis monitoring. It may be technically impossible in VLBW babies and difficult or impossible when there is injured bowel, as with NEC.

HYPOKALEMIA (INFANTS WITH SERUM POTASSIUM LESS THAN 3.5 mEq/L)

About 90% of the body's total potassium is intracellular. Low serum potassium always implies significant intracellular depletion; most potassium is intracellular, and total body potassium can be low even with normal serum levels. Management is directed toward the cause. The most common causes of hypokalemia are (1) increased gastrointestinal losses from an ostomy or nasogastric tube and (2) renal losses from diuretic therapy. Diuretic-induced hypokalemia can be treated with supplemental potassium chloride. Caution is needed, particularly if sending the patient home on this medication,

TABLE 14-4	HYPERKALEMIA (INFANTS WITH MORE THAN 7 mEq/L SERUM POTASSIUM)	
CLINICAL SIGNS	**ELECTROCARDIOGRAM CHANGES**
Muscular weakness	Short QT interval
Cardiac dysrhythmias	Widening QRS
Ileus	Sine wave QRS/T

because incorrect dosing can have serious consequences. Caution must also be used in providing supplementation if the patient is treated with potassium-sparing medications such as spironolactone or captopril.

Clinical signs of hypokalemia are related to muscular weakness and cardiac dysrhythmias. Ileus may also occur. Electrocardiographic changes include decreased T waves and ST depression.

Common Clinical Syndromes

RESPIRATORY DISTRESS SYNDROME

Before the widespread use of surfactant, pulmonary function in RDS tended to improve following a period of brisk diuresis on the third or fourth day of life. It was hypothesized that increased endogenous surfactant production led to improved pulmonary capillary integrity and lymphatic drainage. As a result, hypotonic interstitial lung fluid was reabsorbed back into circulation and a delayed physiologic diuresis occurred. Although antenatal corticosteroids and routine use of exogenous surfactant have altered the natural history of RDS, the preterm infant remains at risk for a more severe course should excessive fluid overload occur. Daily fluid intake should be monitored closely and restricted to allow for the natural contraction of extracellular volume to occur.

Because of the observation of improved lung function associated with diuresis, furosemide and other diuretics have been suggested for the treatment of RDS. Although short-lived improvements in lung function were seen, no long-term effects on morbidity or mortality rates were shown.[21] Use of diuretics shortly after birth could also lead to hypotension and compromised peripheral perfusion, as well as electrolyte disturbances. Aggressive use of diuretics is not indicated in the setting of RDS.

PATENT DUCTUS ARTERIOSUS

Excessive fluid overload can increase the risk of PDA in premature infants. Treatment of a PDA with nonsteroidal antiinflammatory drugs can lead to renal vasoconstriction with a resultant decrease in renal blood flow and glomerular filtration rate. Therefore, it is not uncommon to see an increase in serum creatinine, oliguria, and hyponatremia during PDA treatment. Nonsteroidal antiinflammatory drugs should be given in the lowest effective dose and concomitant administration of other

nephrotoxic drugs should be minimized. Once the drug effect diminishes, accumulated free water should be excreted rapidly, especially if the ductus has closed and cardiovascular status has improved. Fluid status and electrolytes must be monitored closely before, during, and after PDA treatment.

BRONCHOPULMONARY DYSPLASIA

Infants with BPD typically have increased metabolic needs and require higher caloric intake. However, volume overload can potentiate worsening of pulmonary disease.[21] It becomes a delicate balance to provide adequate nutrition while avoiding excess volume. Diuretics are often used in this population, creating an additional set of complications, as discussed previously. Electrolytes must be monitored closely, and diuretic dose and duration should be minimized.

CONGENITAL HEART DISEASE

Knowledge of the underlying physiology associated with the infant's specific heart lesion will ultimately guide the infant's fluid needs and management. Fluid restriction is typically indicated in lesions with left-to-right shunting to manage pulmonary overcirculation. Diuretics are also commonly used in this population. Lesions with outflow tract obstructions will typically respond well to liberal fluid volumes.

Careful attention must be paid to meeting the nutritional needs of infants with congenital heart disease. Surgical outcomes can be improved by providing optimal nutrition, but this can be difficult to achieve in the face of increased metabolic demands, poor mesenteric perfusion, and delayed enteral feeding.[26]

PERSISTENT PULMONARY HYPERTENSION

Fluid management in the infant with persistent pulmonary hypertension is crucial, because hypovolemia can exaggerate right-to-left shunting, leading to worsening disease. Once euvolemia is achieved there is no additional benefit to repeated volume boluses. Hypoglycemia and hypocalcemia should be avoided, because these states can also exacerbate pulmonary hypertension.[51]

NECROTIZING ENTEROCOLITIS

Necrotizing enterocolitis often results in a shocklike state in the infant. Capillary integrity and lymphatic drainage is often compromised, leading to fluid accumulation in the interstitium and diffuse bowel or other tissue edema (the "third space"). As effective circulating volume is diminished, antidiuretic hormone is released and the renin-angiotensin-aldosterone system is activated, leading to sodium and free water retention. Management is aimed at maintaining adequate intravascular volume and perfusion with the use of volume expanders, vasopressors, and/or inotropes. Corticosteroids may also be useful to mitigate the effects of capillary leak. Discontinue all potassium-containing fluids because the combination of oliguria and bowel necrosis can quickly result in hyperkalemia.

If an oral-gastric tube is placed to facilitate intestinal decompression, monitor output closely and consider partially replacing this volume every 8 to 12 hours. Gastric fluid is typically sodium rich, so the sodium loss should be replaced as well. Strictly monitor fluid intake and output and attempt to maintain adequate urine output.

CONGENITAL ADRENAL HYPERPLASIA

The most common form of congenital adrenal hyperplasia is caused by the absence of 21-hydroxylase, which is required to produce aldosterone. Whereas affected females typically present at birth with ambiguous genitalia, males classically present in crisis at 1 to 3 weeks of life with profound hyponatremia, hyperkalemia, and metabolic acidosis. Treatment is initially guided at correcting electrolyte abnormalities. Sodium bicarbonate administration at 1 to 2 mEq/kg may be most useful in correcting hyperkalemia, hyponatremia, and acidosis. Additional treatment strategies for hyponatremia and hyperkalemia are discussed earlier in this chapter. Long-term treatment is aimed at appropriate replacement of mineralocorticoids and glucocorticoids.

RENAL DYSFUNCTION/RENAL DISEASE

Acute renal failure is most often caused by (1) extrinsic factors such as perinatal asphyxia, shock, and heart failure; (2) intrinsic factors such as congenital or acquired lesions; and (3) obstructive uropathy, including urethral obstruction or extragenitourinary mass. Oliguria or anuria usually occurs initially.

During initial oliguria, electrolyte-free glucose infusion should be limited to IWL and urine output. Frequently, this entails providing total fluids of 50 to 80 ml/kg/day. Recovery is usually associated with natriuresis (excessive urinary sodium loss) and osmotic diuresis. This may develop rapidly with sodium losses as high as 20 mEq/kg/day. Body weight and fluid losses must be carefully and frequently measured, at least every 12 hours.

Nonrenal losses, such as gastrointestinal drainage, must also be measured. Ideally, fluid and electrolyte therapy is directed toward maintaining the current weight or a weight loss of 1% per day until recovery is nearly complete. This may be accomplished initially by ordering replacement of IWL as a basal fluid order and replacing a percentage of additional fluid losses on a per-volume basis. The choice of fluid used for replacement depends on the electrolyte content of the fluid lost. Thus it may be helpful to measure urinary sodium and potassium loss concentrations and urine volume, recognizing that any "spot check" of these electrolytes will not fully reflect the loss over a 24-hour period.

Serial determination of serum electrolytes will help refine the fluid orders. As the patient recovers and renal function normalizes, transition to more standard fluids and electrolytes should occur. The renal ability of the patient to concentrate urine must be evaluated serially. If the patient remains in high-output renal failure and fluids are restricted, dehydration may occur. Dehydration will result in weight loss, increased serum electrolyte concentration, and hypernatremia with dilute urine. Weight change during renal failure demands careful reevaluation of the fluid plan.

ASPHYXIA

Perinatal depression can result in renal insult and acute tubular necrosis leading to decreased urine output. SIADH may also occur following perinatal asphyxia, further reducing urine output. Fluids must be restricted to avoid fluid overload. The use of therapeutic hypothermia for treatment of hypoxic-ischemic encephalopathy may further worsen fluid retention and the risk of hyponatremia.[44] Fluid restriction to as low as 30 to 40 ml/kg/day may be required, because this amount should replace only insensible losses. Potassium supplementation should be avoided. As the kidney recovers from acute tubular necrosis, a polyuric phase may ensue with large sodium losses. Urine output must be monitored closely, urinary sodium quantified, and fluid replacement adjusted accordingly.

Major Surgery

Surgical trauma is superimposed on the normal metabolic responses of the neonate. The type and extent of surgery and the gestational and postnatal age of the infant determine the clinical impact. In healthy term infants, negative balance of water, electrolytes, nitrogen, and calories with associated weight loss occurs during the first 3 to 5 days followed by transition to positive balance and weight gain by 7 to 10 days. Parallel transition times for preterm infants vary enormously. Deficits may exist as a result of delayed diagnosis, with external loss or internal loss. "Third space" losses can be significant, with peritoneal losses a notorious source of deficit underestimation.

Predicting the metabolic response to surgery is difficult, reflecting wide variation among individual patients, even patients with similar lesions. Uncontrollable and immeasurable variables prevent a standardized postoperative physiologic response for neonates, especially those weighing less than 2 kg. Thermoregulation is a particular challenge for operative procedures. The patient is draped and shielded from radiant heat sources. Measuring and managing the patient's internal temperature with evaporative heat and water loss complicating the situation is difficult once the incision is made. Transport incubators, prewarmed operating rooms, radiant warmers, warming pads, and prewarmed solutions may help achieve thermoneutrality. Intraoperative fluid balance is rarely precise despite the clinicians' best efforts. Blood loss on sponges, drapes, and other objects should be measured, but IWL from open body cavities is difficult to estimate.

The principles of postoperative management are as follows:

- Monitor clinical and chemical variables frequently, at least every 4 to 6 hours; evaluate fluid balance and measure drainage.
- Recognize that insensible water losses may include "third space losses." These include water lost into the lumen of the bowel or into the peritoneum secondary to peritonitis, resulting in the loss of both water and electrolytes from the intravascular compartment. At least a proportion of the fluids used to anticipate these losses should contain high sodium content similar to plasma. Clinical judgment is used to estimate the third space losses, because they cannot be measured. Serial evaluations of

blood pressure, heart rate, urine output, and skin perfusion together may help determine if the volume prescribed is sufficient.

- Provide parenteral nutrition early if significant enteral feedings (less than 50 kcal/kg) cannot be achieved by 3 to 5 days postoperatively. Gastrointestinal motility returns rapidly in term infants compared with adults. Almost all VLBW infants require parenteral nutrition after surgery.

Diuretics and Electrolytes

Diuretics represent one of the most common classes of drugs administered to sick neonates and infants. Electrolyte disturbances are the most common adverse effects of diuretic therapy and can lead to a variety of consequences. Clinical indications for the use of diuretics in neonates and infants include BPD, congenital heart disease, and renal failure. The classes of diuretics most commonly used in this age group include loop diuretics, thiazides, and potassium-sparing diuretics. A discussion of the mechanism of action, diuretic efficacy, and common side effects follows.

LOOP DIURETICS

Loop diuretics bind to one of the chloride binding sites on the $Na^+/K^+/2Cl^-$ transporter, thus inhibiting reabsorption of sodium and chloride in the thick ascending limb of the loop of Henle. Water passively follows the movement of sodium and thus allows for diuresis.

Furosemide is the most widely studied diuretic in neonates and is consequently the prototype loop diuretic. It produces a 10-fold to 35-fold increase in sodium excretion and a 10-fold increase in urine flow. Therefore hyponatremia, hypochloremia, and hypovolemia are common with chronic use of furosemide. Hypokalemia is also of significant concern with chronic use of furosemide. The mechanism of potassium loss is due to blockage of tubular reabsorption of potassium and increased aldosterone production in the presence of sodium losses.[9]

In addition to potassium losses, furosemide also promotes urine calcium and magnesium excretion. The reabsorption of these cations is decreased because of furosemide's ability to eliminate the transepithelial potential difference. Chronic hypercalciuria leads to hypocalcemia and the possibility of renal calcifications and nephrocalcinosis. Compensatory mechanisms lead to increased parathyroid hormone secretion with associated bone resorption, bone demineralization, osteopenia, and possibly rickets.

Bumetanide is another loop diuretic commonly used in neonates and infants. It is 40 times more potent than furosemide. Side effects are the same as those seen with furosemide.

THIAZIDES

Hydrochlorothiazide and chlorothiazide are the most widely used thiazide diuretics in neonates and infants. Thiazides exert their effect by blocking the Na^+-Cl^- transporter at the distal convoluted tubule, collecting tubule, and early collecting duct. Because only a small portion of sodium reabsorption occurs in the distal tubule, thiazide diuretic efficacy is limited.

Chronic use of thiazide diuretics leads to electrolyte disturbances, although usually they are less severe than with loop diuretics. Hyponatremia and hypokalemia are the most common side effects. Hypokalemia is the result of greater sodium-potassium exchange that occurs secondary to a higher concentration of sodium found in the distal tubule.

Whereas loop diuretics promote calcium loss, thiazide diuretics can increase serum calcium concentrations by increasing renal calcium reabsorption both proximally and distally.[36] This decrease in urinary calcium can be used to reverse loop diuretic–induced renal calcifications.

POTASSIUM-SPARING DIURETICS

Whereas loop and thiazide diuretics directly alter sodium reabsorption via direct inhibition of sodium transporters, potassium-sparing diuretics such as spironolactone competitively antagonize the aldosterone receptor. The primary binding site is the principal cell of the cortical collecting tubule. Aldosterone enhances sodium reabsorption in the collecting tubule and promotes potassium secretion. Therefore antagonizing aldosterone results in diminished sodium reabsorption with a consequent increase in serum concentrations of potassium and hydrogen. However, spironolactone inhibits the reabsorption of less than 2% of filtered sodium and is thus not an effective primary diuretic. The major use is to prevent urinary potassium loss induced by other diuretics.

Hyperkalemia is the primary electrolyte disturbance to monitor with the use of spironolactone. This side effect is usually not of great concern because spironolactone is frequently used in conjunction with other potassium-wasting diuretics. Spironolactone should be avoided in renal failure.

COMPLICATIONS

Excessive fluid administration (greater than 180 ml/kg/day) has been associated with BPD and PDA. Inadequate fluid administration has been associated with dehydration, decreased urine output, hypernatremia, poor tissue perfusion, and, potentially, tissue damage.

PARENT TEACHING

The need for and presence of an IV line in a newborn may be frightening for the parents. Clear, medically and physiologically sound explanations (in nonmedical jargon) of the need for fluid and electrolyte support for their infant help allay parents' fears (Box 14-3). Scalp vein IV lines are of particular concern because a common

---

BOX 14-3 | **PARENT TEACHING**
PARENT TEACHING ABOUT FLUID AND ELECTROLYTE MANAGEMENT

- Most babies cannot be fed immediately and will require intravenous (IV) fluids.
- Umbilical venous and arterial catheters must be removed in a few days.
- IV fluids will be given through percutaneous central venous catheters, peripheral IV lines, or surgically placed lines.
- Scalp IV lines go only into subcutaneous veins, not into the brain.
- Placing the IV line will hurt only during the procedure and will be painless afterward.
- Peripheral IV lines are subject to infiltration, which may be serious if the fluid is hyperalimentation fluid or contains calcium.
- Central venous catheters (percutaneously or surgically placed) carry the risks of thrombosis, infection, or infiltration into body cavities such as the pleura or pericardium.
- IV fluids will be discontinued as soon as enteral nutrition is sufficiently advanced.

misconception is that the needle is positioned in the infant's brain. Explain to parents that scalp vein IV lines are in the large veins of the head and not the brain and that an IV line in the head may stay in longer, thus decreasing the need for multiple vein punctures, and allows the infant mobility of all four extremities. In answer to the question "Does it hurt?" a truthful answer is "Yes, when it is put in, but not after it is in the vein." Explaining the strategies used to decrease pain associated with IV line placement may also help allay their concerns.

The concept of the use of central venous catheters should be presented to the parents early in the hospital course if a delay in enteral nutrition is anticipated. The advantages are fewer painful procedures, increased mobility of the patient, and decreased risk for infiltrate. These should be clearly explained in lay language. Explaining the potential complications such as infection, thrombosis, and the specific risk for the extravasation of fluid into body cavities, pleura, and pericardium is also necessary. Potential infiltration of peripheral IV sites should be addressed *prospectively* with parents. Erythema and edema are expected.

Sloughing of the skin occasionally occurs in VLBW infants and is more common on the feet and hands than on the scalp. Well-illustrated parent education materials often are very helpful when explaining these situations to parents.

Including parents in the care of their sick neonate requires an explanation about the importance of measuring intake and output. Inadvertent disposal of diapers and giving fluids that are not recorded should be prevented, emphasizing the importance of saving diapers for the infant's nurse. "A little spitting up" after feeding may be inappropriately dismissed if parents are not instructed in the importance of telling the nurse and saving it for evaluation.

REFERENCES

For a full list of references, scan the QR code or visit http://booksite.elsevier.com/ 9780323320832.

GLUCOSE HOMEOSTASIS

PAUL J. ROZANCE, JANE E. McGOWAN, WEBRA PRICE-DOUGLAS, AND WILLIAM W. HAY, JR.

During intrauterine life, the fetus depends on the constant transfer of glucose across the placenta to meet its glucose requirements. After birth, neonates must maintain their own glucose homeostasis by producing and regulating their own glucose supply. This requires activation of a number of metabolic processes, including gluconeogenesis (synthesis of glucose from nonglucose precursor substrates) and glycogenolysis (release of glucose via breakdown of glycogen stores), as well as intact regulatory mechanisms for glucose metabolism and an adequate supply of metabolic substrates.

FETAL PHYSIOLOGY

Throughout gestation, maternal glucose provides the principal source of energy for the fetus via facilitated diffusion across the placenta. Fetal glucose uptake varies directly with maternal glucose concentration; fetal glucose concentration usually is about 70% of the maternal value. Changes in maternal metabolism, including increased caloric intake and decreased sensitivity of the maternal tissues to insulin, augment maternal glucose production and provide the additional glucose necessary to meet fetal energy demands. With normal maternal glucose concentrations and rates of glucose supply to the fetus, the fetus produces little, if any, glucose, although the enzymes for gluconeogenesis are present by the third month of gestation.[105] If fetal energy demands cannot be met, however, as is the case when maternal fasting or even starvation is severe enough to produce maternal and fetal hypoglycemia, the fetus is capable of adapting by using alternate substrates, such as ketone bodies, for energy production. In addition, data from animal models suggest that, under these conditions, there may be fetal glucose production.[81] Even in the basal state, the fetus relies on fuels such as lactate and amino acids to meet up to 25% to 30% of its energy demands, whereas lipids are used primarily for fat production.

Fetal glycogen synthesis begins as early as the ninth week of gestation, but the majority of fetal glycogen is produced in the third trimester. The major sites of glycogen deposition are skeletal muscle (greater than 90% of body glycogen), liver (the only organ whose glycogen can be released for use by other organs), lung, and heart.[112] By 40 weeks of gestation, hepatic and skeletal muscle glycogen contents are several times adult levels. By contrast, lung and cardiac muscle glycogen stores decrease as the fetus approaches term, although these stores are still sufficiently large to be of physiologic significance. Survival in animals exposed to anoxia and human infants after asphyxia, for example, is directly related to cardiac glycogen content. The decrease in lung glycogen, which begins at 34 to 36 weeks' gestation, may be related to ongoing developmental processes, such as the synthesis of surfactant.

In addition to glycogen, the human fetus also stores energy as fat in adipose tissue.[109] Most triglyceride synthesis occurs during the third trimester. By 40 weeks' gestation, the human fetus has a body fat content of about 16%, making it the fattest of all terrestrial newborn mammals. The human placenta transports some free fatty acids, although the amount transported to the fetus is not sufficient to account for the amount of adipose tissue present; therefore the fetus also must synthesize triglycerides, using glycerol derived from glucose, as well as fatty acids transported across the placenta. Conditions in which fetal glucose supply is reduced will result in

---

PURPLE type highlights content that is particularly applicable to clinical settings.

less adipose tissue accumulation, as well as reduced glycogen stores.

Insulin is a major stimulus for fetal growth.[44] Fetal pancreatic insulin content and glucose-stimulated insulin secretion increase over the second half of gestation to levels comparable to those found in neonates.[75] Fetal insulin secretion is augmented by higher glucose concentrations; increased concentrations of amino acids add to this effect.[45] Increased concentrations of insulin increase fetal glucose and amino acid utilization and glucose oxidation rates without increasing total fetal oxygen consumption.[36,58,137] This implies that other substrates, primarily amino acids, become available for nonoxidative metabolism when glucose and insulin are plentiful; such conditions promote tissue accretion and growth.

Fetuses of diabetic mothers who have very unstable plasma glucose concentrations during late gestation have an increased islet cell response to hyperglycemia compared with controls, releasing more insulin than normal fetuses at any given blood glucose concentration.[74] The higher insulin levels in turn lead to increased growth consisting primarily of adipose tissue, producing the *macrosomia* typically seen in infants of diabetic mothers (IDMs).

In contrast, fetuses with intrauterine growth restriction (IUGR)[76] have reduced numbers of pancreatic islets and beta cells and produce less-than-normal amounts of insulin in response to glucose and amino acid stimulation. In IUGR fetal sheep, hepatic insulin resistance develops,[128] augmenting hepatic glucose production. Such conditions can lead to postnatal hyperglycemia. Recent studies in IUGR fetal sheep also show increased insulin sensitivity to glucose disposal in peripheral tissues (e.g., skeletal muscle)[82,133,136] and secretion from individual islets that further increase when norepinephrine activity, which is increased in IUGR fetuses in response to hypoxia, is blocked.[21,137] These observations may account for the apparent hyperinsulinemia that occasionally occurs in such IUGR infants several days after birth[22] when oxygenation is restored and norepinephrine concentrations diminish, contributing to their common risk of hypoglycemia. Not surprisingly, therefore, glucose homeostasis in IUGR neonates is highly variable.

It also is interesting to note that although correction of acute insulin deficiency promotes growth, exogenous insulin appears to have little effect on growth in human newborns or animal models with chronic insulin deficiency, suggesting that insulin infusion to promote growth in growth-restricted infants is unlikely to be beneficial and may lead to additional complications.

The related pancreatic hormone glucagon, which, like insulin, does not cross the placenta, has been detected as early as 9 to 16 weeks of gestation.[101] In postnatal life, glucagon is a potent inducer of gluconeogenic enzymes, the opposite of insulin, which suppresses gluconeogenesis.[105] In fetal life, glucagon plays a much less important role in regulating glucose metabolism than insulin, reflecting the developmental insensitivity of fetal glucagon receptors. As a result, the insulin-to-glucagon effectiveness ratio in the fetus is high, which is important in preferentially maintaining glycogen synthesis and suppressing gluconeogenesis.

NEONATAL PHYSIOLOGY

At birth, the newborn infant is removed abruptly from its glucose supply and blood glucose concentration falls. Several hormonal and metabolic changes occur at birth that facilitate the adaptation necessary to maintain glucose homeostasis. Catecholamine levels increase markedly right after birth, possibly as a response to the decrease in environmental temperature, as well as to the loss of the placenta, which is responsible for as much as 50% of the clearance of circulating fetal epinephrine.[127] Glucagon concentrations and receptor sensitivity also increase, reversing the relatively high insulin/glucagon effectiveness ratio characteristic of fetal life.[116] The increased glucagon and norepinephrine concentrations activate hepatic glycogen phosphorylase, which induces glycogenolysis. Simultaneously, the decreasing glucose concentration and perinatal surge in fetal cortisol secretion stimulate hepatic glucose-6-phosphatase activity. Together these changes lead to an increase in hepatic glucose release.[31] Increased catecholamines also stimulate lipolysis, releasing fatty acids that can be metabolized to provide precursors for gluconeogenesis, as well as providing energy in the form of adenosine triphosphate (ATP) and cofactors such as nicotinamide adenine dinucleotide phosphate that enhance the activity of gluconeogenic enzymes. Catecholamine release also activates brown fat triglyceride turnover, producing heat necessary for postnatal thermoregulation. The normal postnatal decrease in insulin effects and increase in glucagon effects induce synthesis of phosphoenolpyruvate carboxykinase (PEPCK), which is considered the rate-limiting enzyme in hepatic gluconeogenesis. The concentrations of PEPCK and other gluconeogenic enzymes continue to increase over the first 2 weeks of life, regardless of gestational age. These changes act in concert to provide glucose to replace the supply previously received via the placenta.

Maintenance of glucose homeostasis depends on the balance between hepatic glucose output and glucose utilization by the brain and peripheral tissues. Hepatic glucose output is a function of rates of glycogenolysis and gluconeogenesis. Peripheral glucose utilization varies with the metabolic demands placed on the neonate. Studies in normal human newborn infants using several different methods have determined that the steady-state glucose production/utilization rate in a term neonate is 4 to 6 mg/min/kg, approximately twice the weight-specific rate measured in adults.[35] As in the fetus, it appears that approximately half of this glucose is oxidized to CO_2 during normal metabolic processes, whereas the remainder is used in nonoxidative pathways, such as glycogen and fat synthesis. Perinatal glucose utilization increases (1) during hypoxia, because of the inherent inefficiency of anaerobic glycolysis[86]; (2) in the presence of hyperinsulinemia, which increases glucose uptake by insulin-sensitive tissues[72]; (3) in newborns with respiratory distress, because of increased muscle activity[100]; and (4) during cold stress, which leads to increased sympathetic nervous system activity with subsequent release of norepinephrine, epinephrine, and thyroid hormone, which increase metabolic rate.[23] If rates of glycogenolysis and gluconeogenesis do not match the rate of glucose utilization because of failure of the hormonal control mechanisms or variability of substrate supply, disturbances of glucose homeostasis occur. These disturbances are recognized clinically by the presence of hypoglycemia or hyperglycemia.

HYPOGLYCEMIA

Definition

The absolute blood or plasma glucose concentration that defines hypoglycemia as a pathologic condition remains difficult to establish and has not been determined. Furthermore, there is no absolute correlation between blood or plasma glucose concentrations, clinical signs or symptoms, and either short-term or long-term sequelae. Instead, "reference" glucose concentrations generally reflect the lower limit of the normal range in a specific population of newborn infants, determined by statistical analysis of data collected in that population. Thus there is no consensus about threshold glucose concentrations below which diagnostic evaluation or treatment is mandated or that identify those infants likely to have adverse neurodevelopmental outcome.

Published definitions of hypoglycemia range from a blood glucose concentration of less than 20 mg/dl in preterm infants and less than 30 mg/dl in term infants to a plasma concentration of less than 45 mg/dl.[24-26] Some sources have even suggested raising the lower limit of normal to 50 to 70 mg/dl, although others have emphasized that such higher concentrations should be used primarily as target values during treatment for relatively severe and symptomatic hypoglycemia, rather than thresholds for instituting treatment.[24] Published reports fail to distinguish between threshold glucose concentrations below which physiologic responses may occur (and below which clinical monitoring may be indicated) and those below which pathologic consequences are likely to develop (thus requiring aggressive treatment). In 1992 the majority of pediatricians in one survey in the United Kingdom defined a safe glucose concentration to be at least 2 mmol/L (36 mg/dl) in blood or 2.5 mmol/L (45 mg/dl) in plasma.[73,74] Figure 15-1 shows that 95% of normal term infants have a blood glucose concentration of more than 30 mg/dl in the first 24 hours of life and more than 45 mg/dl after 24 hours of life.[117] A number of current references use 40 to 45 mg/dl as the lower limit of "normal" plasma glucose concentrations in the first 72 hours of life. By 72 to 96 hours of age mean plasma glucose concentrations are very similar to those seen in older children and adults.*

Using these definitions of hypoglycemia, the overall incidence has been estimated at 1.3 to 4.4 per 1000 live births. Differences in incidence figures probably reflect variable inclusion of data from symptomatic versus asymptomatic infants.

---

*References 4, 24, 65, 88, 89, 114, 116, 123.

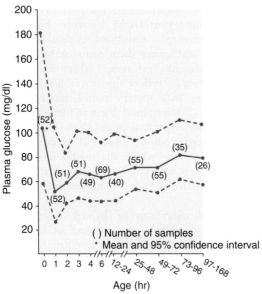

FIGURE 15-1 Plasma glucose concentrations during the first week of life in healthy appropriate-for-gestational-age term infants. (From Srinivasan G, Pildes RS, Cattamanchi G, et al: Plasma glucose values in normal neonates: a new look, *J Pediatr* 109:114, 1986.)

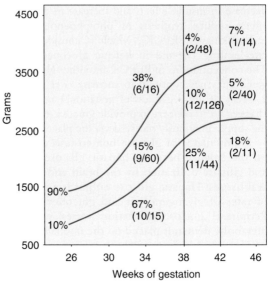

FIGURE 15-2 Incidence of neonatal hypoglycemia (blood glucose less than 30 mg/dl) by birth weight and gestational age. (From Lubchenco LO, Bard H: Incidence of hypoglycemia in newborn infants classified by birth weight and gestational age, *Pediatrics* 47:831, 1971.)

In preterm infants, the incidence of hypoglycemia is increased; estimates range from 1.5% to 5.5% (Figure 15-2). The incidence of hypoglycemia in term infants with IUGR may be as high as 25%, with an even higher rate seen in preterm small-for-gestational-age (SGA) infants.[84]

Hypoglycemia also may be defined clinically as the glucose concentration in a neonate that is associated with clinical signs (often called "symptoms") that resolve when glucose is administered. This value is difficult to determine, however, because the clinical signs of hypoglycemia are nonspecific and may not be noticed initially. From a physiologic point of view, an infant may be said to be hypoglycemic when glucose supply is inadequate to meet demand. Unfortunately, no method is available to establish this value in a given infant. Infants with increased glucose utilization demand or limited capability to alter glucose delivery (which is a function of both blood supply and glucose concentration) are at increased risk for impaired organ function at low blood glucose concentrations. Specifically, animal studies have shown that insufficient glucose supply may contribute to neuronal death, augment functional deficits, and

increase the risk for long-term neurologic injury in the presence of concurrent cerebral hypoxia and/or ischemia. Clinical studies suggest that this may be true also in newborn infants, although it is not clear whether the low glucose concentrations in cases of hypoxia and ischemia contributed directly to worse outcomes or were simply a marker for those infants with more significant metabolic compromise during hypoxia–ischemia who were, therefore, more likely to have worse outcomes. Furthermore, it remains unclear whether earlier detection of hypoglycemia, such as in the delivery room, in this population could modify subsequent neurologic outcome.[107]

Rather than defining hypoglycemia as an absolute blood glucose value, some investigators have suggested using specific glucose concentrations as an indicator that further management of low glucose concentrations is warranted. Threshold values are based on evidence available in the literature (see further discussion under Treatment later in this chapter).[24] This approach considers the overall metabolic and physiologic status of the infant when determining what constitutes an acceptable blood glucose concentration. Some infants may undergo metabolic derangements at glucose concentrations above the "hypoglycemic" threshold, whereas others may be able to tolerate lower concentrations of blood glucose without developing metabolic stress. An infant with polycythemia, for example, may have a normal blood glucose concentration but decreased cerebral delivery of glucose because of reduced plasma flow. In contrast, breastfed infants have normal substrate delivery to the brain even with "hypoglycemic" blood glucose values, because they have increased plasma concentrations of ketone bodies compared with formula-fed infants, though these concentrations are still lower than what is observed in fasting children.[55,68] Concentrations of ketones are even lower in preterm and IUGR/SGA infants than in term infants who are feeding normally, suggesting that preterm birth and IUGR are associated with less capacity to generate alternate brain energy substrates. This decreased capacity might increase the vulnerability of such infants to cerebral energy deficits when plasma glucose concentrations are decreased.[55,56]

In summary, the definition of the blood glucose concentration at which intervention is indicated must be tailored to the clinical situation and the particular characteristics of a given infant. Kalhan and Peter-Wohl[65] suggested that further investigation and treatment should be instituted in the symptomatic infant at blood glucose concentrations of less than 45 mg/dl, whereas asymptomatic term infants with known risk factors should be treated if their blood glucose concentration is less than 36 mg/dl.[66,76] Several authors suggest that these thresholds for intervention should be higher in preterm infants and lower in breastfed full-term infants.[24,54] Additionally, the American Academy of Pediatrics' Fetus and Newborn Committee has recommended different guidelines for late preterm infants and term SGA, large-for-gestational-age (LGA), and IDM infants, emphasizing initial screening, feeding if tolerated, and prompt (within 1 hour) reassessment for clinical signs and repeat measurement of glucose concentrations.[1] However, it is important to recognize that there have been no systematic studies to demonstrate the risks or benefits of using any specific blood glucose concentration as a threshold for intervention in neonatal hypoglycemia. Given the apparently wide range of glucose values associated with normal neonatal outcomes, as well as the inherent inaccuracies in measuring glucose concentrations and the absence of a specific level below which injury inevitably occurs, any individual blood glucose measurement should be considered a one-point-in-time-only representation of the balance between glucose supply and utilization rather than as an absolute indicator of glucose sufficiency or insufficiency.

Hypoglycemic Neuronal Injury and Neuropathology

A schema of how hypoglycemia can contribute to neuronal injury is presented in Figure 15-3. Hypoglycemic brain damage in the newborn infant occurs predominantly in gray matter structures, although severe hypoglycemia in newborn infants may also be associated with white matter injury, particularly when the hypoglycemia occurs simultaneously with hypoxic-ischemic injury.[106,134] Pathologic studies of such severely hypoglycemic newborn infants have shown widespread neuronal injury in cerebral cortex, hippocampus, basal ganglia, thalamus, brainstem, and spinal cord. Late neuropathologic lesions associated with severe and prolonged low glucose concentrations include microcephaly associated with cortical atrophy and diffuse neuronal loss, as well as astrogliosis. Abnormalities may also be seen in white matter, whereas the cerebellum is generally spared.

Neuroimaging of Hypoglycemic Injury

Magnetic resonance imaging (MRI) performed 2 to 3 weeks after severe hypoglycemia demonstrates abnormal signals in the cortex, often most apparent in the occipital lobes.[9] More recent neuroradiologic investigations have shown a much wider variety in the pattern of injury involving both white matter and gray matter as a consequence of severe neonatal hypoglycemia.[18,124] Radiographically defined lesions after severe hypoglycemia in the newborn period can be transient and not associated with long-term neurologic consequences, indicating that follow-up MRI scans should be considered to determine the permanency of the lesions.

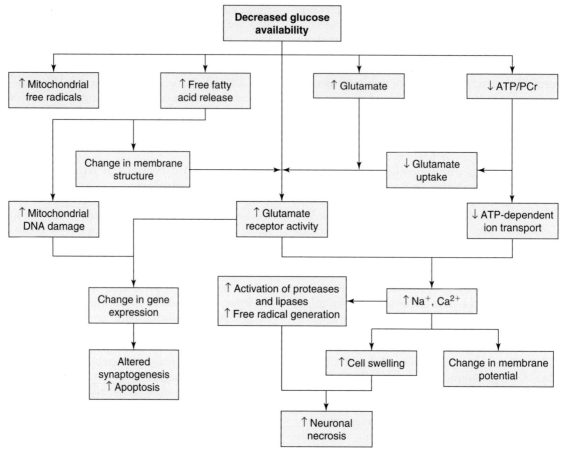

FIGURE 15-3 Proposed mechanism for the pathogenesis of hypoglycemic brain injury in the newborn. *ATP,* Adenosine 5'-triphosphate; *DNA,* deoxyribonucleic acid; *PCr,* phosphocreatine. (From McGowan JE: Role of glucose in cerebral function. In Hay WW Jr, editor: *Semin Neonat Nutr Metab* 4:2-3, Columbus, Ohio, 1997, Ross Products.)

HYPERGLYCEMIA

Definition

Hyperglycemia in newborns is usually defined, based on population data, as a blood glucose concentration of more than 125 mg/dl (greater than 150 mg/dl plasma) in a term infant or more than 150 mg/dl in blood in a preterm infant. Unlike neonatal hypoglycemia, there are no reported "clinical" definitions of hyperglycemia (i.e., the appearance of physiologic disturbances associated with a specific high blood glucose concentration). The incidence of statistically defined neonatal hyperglycemia is difficult to determine; estimates range from 5.5% of all infants receiving intravenous (IV) infusions of $D_{10}W$ to as high as 40% in infants weighing less than 1000 g who are receiving IV dextrose infusions. Dweck and Cassady[39] noted that 86% of infants with birth weights under 1100 g were hyperglycemic, and of these infants, 84% had one or more serum glucose concentrations greater than 300 mg/dl. In 2006, Blanco and colleagues[15] found that 88% of infants with birth weights less than 1000 g had at least one blood glucose concentration greater than 150 mg/dl in the first week of life.

BOX 15-1

BOX 15-1 INDICATIONS FOR ROUTINE MONITORING OF BLOOD GLUCOSE FOR PREVENTION OF NEONATAL HYPOGLYCEMIA

Maternal Conditions

- Presence of diabetes or abnormal result of glucose tolerance test
- Preeclampsia and pregnancy-induced or essential hypertension
- Previous macrosomic infants
- Substance abuse
- Treatment with beta-agonist tocolytics
- Treatment with oral hypoglycemic agents
- Late antepartum to intrapartum administration of intravenous glucose

Neonatal Conditions

- Prematurity
- Intrauterine growth restriction
- Perinatal hypoxia-ischemia
- Sepsis
- Hypothermia
- Polycythemia-hyperviscosity
- Erythroblastosis fetalis
- Iatrogenic administration of insulin
- Congenital cardiac malformations
- Persistent hyperinsulinemia
- Endocrine disorders
- Inborn errors of metabolism

ETIOLOGY OF HYPOGLYCEMIA AND HYPERGLYCEMIA

Hypoglycemia

The causes of hypoglycemia can be grouped into several broad categories based on the mechanisms producing the hypoglycemia (Box 15-1[103]; Table 15-1). These categories include inadequate substrate supply, abnormal endocrine regulation of glucose metabolism, and increased rate of glucose utilization. There also are several proposed causes for which mechanisms are not well defined.

INADEQUATE SUBSTRATE SUPPLY

If substrate availability is inadequate, hepatic glucose output will not meet metabolic demands. Most often this results from subnormal fat and glycogen stores that consequently do not provide sufficient energy to maintain glucose homeostasis until gluconeogenesis reaches adequate levels. Because most hepatic glycogen is accumulated during the third trimester, infants born preterm have diminished glycogen stores. In the past, infants with IUGR secondary to placental insufficiency also were considered to be at risk for decreased glycogen accumulation, presumably because of diminished transfer of glycogen precursors (e.g., glucose, lactate) across the placenta. In these infants, relative hypoxemia caused by placental dysfunction also could stimulate increased production of adrenaline and noradrenaline, leading to increased glycogen breakdown and further compromising substrate supply. Evidence from more recent animal studies and human observations, however, suggest that, because of increased glucose uptake mechanisms in response to glucose deficiency (e.g., increased expression of cell membrane glucose transporters), muscle and hepatic glycogen stores are normal or even increased in IUGR infants.[19,82,94,104,129]

Postnatally, catecholamine- and glucagon-stimulated glycogenolysis rapidly depletes glycogen supplies at a time when gluconeogenesis is still impaired because of low levels of PEPCK and other gluconeogenic enzymes, resulting in hypoglycemia. After the first few postnatal days, preterm infants may still be at risk for hypoglycemia even though glycogen stores are adequate, because of low levels of hepatic microsomal glucose-6-phosphatase activity. Activity of this enzyme in preterm infants is low before birth and, in some infants, can remain low for several months after birth.[105,122,123] Because this enzyme catalyzes the dephosphorylation of glucose-6-phosphate to glucose and regulates the final step in hepatic glucose production, the decreased activity could contribute to diminished glucose production from both glycogenolysis and gluconeogenesis. Infants with low hepatic glucose-6-phosphatase activity may not be symptomatic with the initial episode of hypoglycemia, but can become symptomatic if the hypoglycemia persists.

Up to 18% of preterm infants have problems in maintaining normoglycemia at the time of discharge if a feeding is omitted or delayed.[50] Inadequate cortisol secretion in very preterm infants, particularly during periods of stress, also has been cited as a cause of limited activation of gluconeogenic enzymes. The underlying mechanisms for cortisol deficiency are not clear, but may be related

TABLE 15–1	NEONATAL HYPOGLYCEMIA: ETIOLOGY AND TIME COURSE	
MECHANISM	CLINICAL SETTING	EXPECTED DURATION
Decreased substrate availability	Intrauterine growth restriction	Transient
	Prematurity	Transient
	Reduced glycogen stores	Transient
	Reduced fat stores	Transient
	Reduced ketogenesis	Transient
	Glycogen storage disease	Prolonged
	Inborn errors (e.g., fructose intolerance)	Prolonged
Endocrine disturbances		
• Hyperinsulinemia	Infant of diabetic mother	Transient
	Persistent hyperinsulinism of infancy	Transient
	Congenital hyperinsulinism (HI) • Recessive K_{ATP} HI • Focal K_{ATP} (focal adenomatosis) HI • Dominant K_{ATP} HI • Dominant glucokinase (GCK) HI • Dominant glutamate dehydrogenase (GDH) HI • Short-chain 3-hyroxyacyl-CoA dehydrogenase (SCHAD) HI	Prolonged
	Beckwith-Wiedemann syndrome	Prolonged
	Erythroblastosis fetalis	Transient
	Exchange transfusion	Transient
	Islet cell dysplasias	Prolonged
	Maternal beta-agonist tocolytics	Transient
	Improperly placed umbilical artery catheter	Transient
	Inadvertent insulin administration	Transient
• Other endocrine disorders	Immaturity of hepatic enzymes necessary for glucose production	Transient
	Reduced or failed counterregulation	Prolonged
	Hypopituitarism	Prolonged
	Hypothyroidism	Prolonged
	Adrenal insufficiency	Prolonged
Increased utilization	Increased brain weight to body weight and liver weight ratio with increased brain consumption of glucose	Prolonged
	Perinatal asphyxia	Transient
	Hypothermia	Transient
Miscellaneous/multiple mechanisms	Sepsis	Transient
	Congenital heart disease	Transient
	Central nervous system abnormalities	Prolonged

to a lack of adrenal stimulation as a result of limited hypothalamic-pituitary axis activity.

ABNORMALITIES OF ENDOCRINE REGULATION

Hyperinsulinemia is the most common endocrinologic disturbance producing neonatal hypoglycemia and may be the most common cause of the infrequent cases of persistent hypoglycemia in infants. Excessive insulin secretion in the newborn increases glucose utilization by stimulating cellular glucose uptake in insulin-dependent tissues, including muscle and liver; brain glucose uptake, however, does not appear to be significantly altered by increased insulin levels. At the same time, the high circulating insulin concentrations promote continued glycogen synthesis and inhibit both glycogenolysis and gluconeogenesis, impairing the infant's glucogenic response to the increased glucose demand and decreasing plasma glucose concentrations. Suppression of ketone body production from free fatty acids by high levels of insulin also might limit the availability of alternative fuels for cerebral metabolism, thereby contributing to the increased risk for adverse long-term outcomes in this patient population.

The most common clinical situation in which hyperinsulinemia occurs is in the infant of a diabetic mother (IDM). In utero, the fetus becomes hyperglycemic because of increased transfer of glucose across the placenta during episodes of maternal hyperglycemia. The fetal pancreatic beta cells are stimulated by the increased fetal glucose concentration to produce increased quantities of insulin. The pancreatic islet beta cells also appear to become abnormally sensitive to increases in glucose concentration after repeated hyperglycemic stimuli. Before birth, the increase in cellular glucose uptake in response to the increased insulin secretion is matched by the increased availability of glucose from the mother. After delivery, the maternal source of glucose is abruptly removed, whereas the hyperinsulinemia persists, producing hypoglycemia. The decrease in glucose concentration after birth is a result of insulin-stimulated peripheral glucose uptake, as well as inhibition of gluconeogenesis and glycogenolysis by the high insulin concentrations. Although some studies have reported other abnormalities in glucose metabolism in IDMs, Cowett and colleagues[28] found no difference in glucose kinetics in IDMs versus controls,

perhaps because maternal diabetic control was well maintained during pregnancy in the group studied. A large review of pregnancies in diabetic mothers found no association between the incidence of neonatal hypoglycemia and the number of episodes of maternal hyperglycemia (a reflection of the degree of control) late in pregnancy.[57] The incidence of neonatal hypoglycemia in IDMs correlates better with intrapartum, rather than antepartum, maternal glucose concentrations. The results of these studies emphasize that it is a sudden increase in glucose concentration that stimulates insulin secretion after a longer period in utero during which the fetal pancreatic beta cells have been sensitized to hypersecrete insulin as a result of repeated episodes of hyperglycemia.[29]

The incidence of hypoglycemia in IDMs ranges from 15% to 75%; these infants usually are asymptomatic. The large and comprehensive HAPO study has shown (1) that the complications typically associated with IDMs, including neonatal hypoglycemia, may be seen in women without overt gestational diabetes but who have glucose values on formal glucose tolerance testing at the upper end of the "normal" range; and (2) that the incidence correlates with increased glucose values. This suggests that there is a continuum of abnormal glucose tolerance during pregnancy that is associated with increased fetal insulin secretion, with gestational diabetes representing the most severe degree of disturbed glucose homeostasis.[93,132]

Other causes of islet cell hyperplasia and resultant hyperinsulinemia include (1) severe erythroblastosis fetalis,[10] possibly resulting from inactivation of insulin by glutathione released from hemolyzed red blood cells; (2) exchange transfusion,[108] in which insulin release is stimulated by the high dextrose content of commonly used blood preservative agents; and (3) in utero exposure to drugs such as beta-agonist tocolytics.[99] In utero exposure to valproate and postnatal exposure to indomethacin also may result in hypoglycemia, but the mechanisms responsible are not known.

Idiopathic hyperinsulinism (i.e., increased, persistent insulin secretion without a known predisposing factor) may occur as a result of altered regulation of insulin secretion in pancreatic beta cells.[50,61] Two general forms of persistent idiopathic hyperinsulinism are recognized: (1) prolonged neonatal hyperinsulinism and (2) congenital (genetic) hyperinsulinism. Prolonged idiopathic neonatal hyperinsulinism appears to be common, although not well recognized or understood. Affected neonates usually have some evidence of stress before or during delivery, such as low birth weight (LBW) with IUGR (this disorder may affect 10% or more of IUGR/SGA infants), birth asphyxia, or maternal preeclampsia. Prolonged neonatal hyperinsulinism usually manifests in the first days after birth and often may be severe, requiring high dextrose infusion rates providing up to 15 mg/kg/min of glucose, or occasionally more. Prolonged neonatal hyperinsulinism also may last several weeks to months, does not respond well to glucocorticoids or frequent feedings, but can be treated with diazoxide at doses of 5 to 10 mg/kg/day.[8,60]

Congenital (genetic) persistent hyperinsulinism is the most common form of persistent hypoglycemia in neonates and infants and also is the most difficult to diagnose and treat.[66] The pancreatic abnormalities observed may be diffuse or focal, depending on the mutation present. Although the overall incidence of *persistent hyperinsulinemic hypoglycemia* (PHIHG) is low (approximately 1 in 50,000 births), the incidence of the inherited forms may be as high as 1 in 2500 infants in certain genetically homogeneous populations.[51] Depending on the degree of hyperinsulinemia in utero, these infants also may be macrosomic at birth. Most often, infants with PHIHG present with repeated episodes of hypoglycemia in the immediate neonatal period, followed by severe, recurrent hypoglycemia after the first few days of life, often after discharge from the newborn nursery.[59] Recognizing such infants requires prolonged evaluation of an infant's capacity to maintain normal blood glucose concentrations between feedings after initial episodes of hypoglycemia are noted.

At least eight different genes have been associated with congenital hyperinsulinism.[102] Mutations in several regions on the short arm of chromosome 11 have been found in approximately 50% of infants with PHIHG; these mutations most often are inherited in an autosomal recessive pattern. Most affected infants have abnormalities of either the SUR1 or the Kir6.2 component of the K_{ATP} complex. Because the K_{ATP} complex, which is the site of diazoxide action, is disrupted by the mutations, these infants usually do not respond to diazoxide treatment. Octreotide (long-acting somatostatin) can be more helpful in the short term, but near-total (95% to 98%) pancreatectomy usually is necessary.

Pancreatectomy often requires continuous feedings and even insulin therapy,[102] as well as replacement of pancreatic enzymes. Infants who have this form of hyperinsulinism typically are large for gestational age (LGA), present with early neonatal hypoglycemia, and often require high rates of IV glucose infusion.

Hyperinsulinism resulting from a focal pancreatic lesion *(focal adenomatosis)* may occur in 50% of patients with congenital hyperinsulinism.[115] In this disorder, a localized clone of beta cells expresses a paternally derived mutation in the gene for either SUR1 or Kir6.2 because of loss of heterozygosity for the maternal allele. The adenomas are small—3 to 5 mm in diameter. The clinical course of these infants is similar to that of infants with hyperinsulinism due to widespread mutations of the pancreatic K_{ATP} channel. Localization of the focal adenomatous region of the pancreas via positron emission tomography (PET) with ^{18}F-fluoro-L-dopa may allow definition of the abnormal region of the pancreas, thereby guiding limited resection and avoiding more extensive, often near-total pancreatectomy.[16,77]

Several other mutations lead to genetic forms of PHIHG, including mutations in genes coding for glucokinase *(GCK HI)*, glutamate dehydrogenase *(GDH)*, hexokinase *(HK1)*, hydroxyacyl-CoA dehydrogenase *(HADH)*, and the nuclear transcription factors *HNF1A* and *HNF4A*.[102] These different genetic disorders are much less common and have variable presentations, usually later in the neonatal period or even in early infancy.

In addition to hyperinsulinemia, global endocrine disturbances also can result in hypoglycemia.[63] These disturbances include a range of abnormalities of the hypothalamic-pituitary axis, the most severe being *panhypopituitarism*. Such infants frequently have growth hormone deficiency and hypothyroidism in addition to severe hypoglycemia. If pituitary dysfunction has resulted from a structural central nervous system (CNS) lesion, other neurologic problems, including abnormal muscle tone and neonatal seizures, may be present. Adrenal failure and hypoglycemia can occur as a result of adrenal hemorrhage, often in association with neonatal sepsis. Isolated endocrine defects, including primary hypothyroidism and cortisol deficiency, also may be associated with hypoglycemia.

Infants with *Beckwith-Wiedemann syndrome* also are macrosomic and hyperinsulinemic; in addition, they have other associated anomalies, including macroglossia, which may cause airway obstruction, and omphalocele.[40] Asymptomatic hypoglycemia may occur in 30% to 50% of infants with Beckwith-Wiedemann syndrome and usually resolves in the first 3 days of life. However, up to 5% of affected infants may have persistent, frequently symptomatic hypoglycemia.[32] Infants with Beckwith-Wiedemann syndrome have been found to have mutations in the short arm of chromosome 11, the same region in which mutations associated with other hyperinsulinemic syndromes have been identified.

ENZYMATIC AND GENETIC DISORDERS[64]

Hormone Deficiencies.[64] Hypoglycemia resulting from abnormal hormone production sometimes manifests in the neonatal period. Growth hormone and cortisol are counterregulatory hormones (i.e., they oppose the actions of insulin) and increase blood glucose concentrations by reducing glucose uptake in muscle tissue and stimulating lipolysis and gluconeogenesis during hypoglycemia. Although the counterregulatory effects of cortisol and growth hormone are less important than those of glucagon and catecholamines, hypoglycemia is a common complication of growth hormone and cortisol deficiency. Appropriate hormone replacement is the treatment of choice. It is of interest that several cases of panhypopituitarism and hyperinsulinemia have been reported in children.

Enzyme Deficiency Conditions.[64] Hereditary disorders associated with deficiencies of specific enzymes that regulate substrate mobilization, interconversion, or utilization of carbohydrate, fat, or amino acids individually are rare disorders but collectively are frequently associated with hypoglycemia. These disorders are almost always inherited as autosomal recessive traits. Because of the interactions of fat, carbohydrate, and amino acid metabolism in the maintenance of normal fuel homeostasis, abnormalities in the metabolism of a single substrate can have primary and secondary effects on other metabolic pathways.

Defective Carbohydrate Metabolism[64]

Glycogen Storage Diseases. In these inherited disorders, hypoglycemia results not from inadequate glycogen stores but, rather, from one of several enzyme deficiencies that prevent or limit glycogenolysis and release of glucose into the circulation. The glycogen storage diseases (I to VII) are inherited autosomal recessive defects,

characterized by a deficient or abnormally functioning enzyme involved in the formation or degradation of glycogen in liver or muscle.

Fructose 1,6-Diphosphatase Deficiency. Hepatic fructose 1,6-diphosphatase deficiency results in a defect in gluconeogenesis. The initial signs and symptoms can be similar to those of glycogen storage disease type I (i.e., failure to thrive, hepatomegaly, lactic acidosis, and hypoglycemia).

Pyruvate Carboxylase and Phosphoenolpyruvate Carboxykinase Deficiencies. Pyruvate carboxylase and PEPCK are key gluconeogenic enzymes. Patients with pyruvate carboxylase deficiency are severely retarded and die early in infancy, and some have neuropathologic evidence of subacute necrotizing encephalopathy. Deficiency of hepatic phosphoenolpyruvate carboxykinase is a rare disorder; hypoglycemia is a common feature, although not clearly associated with defects of hepatic gluconeogenesis.

Galactose-1-Phosphate Uridylyl Transferase Deficiency (Classic Galactosemia). Infants with classic *galactosemia* are intolerant of products containing galactose. These infants have hypoglycemia, failure to thrive, sepsis, diarrhea, and vomiting after meals containing galactose. Postprandial hypoglycemia seems to be caused by inhibition of phosphoglucomutase by galactose-1-phosphate, thereby resulting in sudden inhibition of glycogenolysis. Today, most infants with galactosemia are identified based on the results of routine neonatal screening.

Defective Amino Acid Metabolism. Several other inborn errors of metabolism, including propionic and methylmalonic acidemia and glutaric aciduria, may present with hypoglycemia in the first week of life.[98] Hypoglycemia and profound hypoalaninemia are observed in patients with classic *maple syrup urine disease* (branched-chain alpha-keto acid dehydrogenase deficiency) at times when their branched-chain amino acids and alpha-keto acids are markedly elevated.

Defective Fatty Acid Metabolism. A group of rare but severe metabolic disorders resulting in hypoglycemia and hypoketonemia are associated with abnormalities in fatty acid oxidation and ketone body formation.[64] During periods of fasting or intercurrent illness, free fatty acids (FFAs) are mobilized from adipose tissue. FFAs are utilized directly by body tissue (e.g., heart, skeletal muscle, gut, skin) or undergo beta-oxidation in the liver with the resultant production and release of ketone bodies, which can partly replace glucose in many tissues such as the brain, and acetyl coenzyme A (CoA) and reducing equivalents (NAD/NADH), which provide energy fuel for the gluconeogenesis process. Oxidation of FFA includes activation of fatty acids by acyl-CoA synthetase, carnitine-dependent transport into the mitochondrial matrix, and mitochondrial beta-oxidation of the fatty acids. Infants and children with disorders of fatty acid oxidation often exhibit profound hypoglycemia and altered level of consciousness, which may not improve despite normalization of the plasma glucose concentration.

Other markers of impaired fatty acid oxidation are absolute or relative hypoketonemia, marked increase in plasma FFA concentrations, hypotonia, hepatomegaly with microvesicular fat accumulation, elevated plasma activities of both liver and muscle enzymes, congestive heart failure, rhabdomyolysis, and, frequently, cerebral edema. Although the pathophysiology of the hypoglycemia in these children is not known, two mechanisms have been suggested: (1) decreased hepatic glucose production; or (2) more commonly understood, accelerated rates of glucose utilization, because glucose might serve as the primary substrate for all tissues in the absence of ketone body availability and defective FFA oxidation. These disorders should be considered in infants and children with severe hypoglycemia, decreased plasma concentrations of free and total carnitine, and relatively low plasma ketone body concentrations in combination with very high FFA concentrations.

INCREASED GLUCOSE UTILIZATION

Some term infants may have normal energy stores at birth and intact regulating mechanisms but may be stressed by one of several conditions so that the available supplies do not meet their energy requirements. An asphyxiated newborn is one common example. During and after asphyxia, when tissue oxygen supply is limited, the neonate relies largely on anaerobic metabolism for energy production. Because this process is relatively inefficient, more glucose is metabolized to produce the amount of energy necessary than would be used under aerobic conditions. As a result, glucose produced by lipolysis and glycogenolysis is rapidly consumed. Hypoxic-ischemic damage to the liver may further impair synthesis of gluconeogenic enzymes and thus delay the normal postnatal onset of gluconeogenesis. Elevated insulin concentrations also may be present, providing an additional cause for the

hypoglycemia.[30] Other conditions in neonates that lead to a shift from aerobic to anaerobic metabolism, thus predisposing the infant to hypoglycemia, include hypotension, severe lung disease with hypoxemia and hypoventilation, and septic shock.

Hypothermia may result in hypoglycemia through rapid depletion of brown fat stores for nonshivering thermogenesis and secondary breakdown and exhaustion of glycogen stores. Hypothermia is most often seen in infants born at home, but milder degrees may occur in the delivery room. Hypoglycemia also has been observed in some infants with sepsis. A study done in several such infants found that they had an increased rate of glucose disappearance in response to an IV glucose infusion, suggesting an increased rate of glucose utilization.[78] Stimulation of glucose utilization may be a result of circulating endotoxins, which increase the rate of glycolysis.

Several other factors also contribute to the risk for hypoglycemia in infants with other identified risk factors. Preterm infants with respiratory distress syndrome (RDS), for example, have increased metabolic demands because of the increased work of breathing. Chronic hypoxia in IUGR fetuses stimulates catecholamine secretion, which can deplete glycogen stores. Infants with IUGR and hypoglycemia may have increased rates of glucose disappearance when receiving an IV glucose infusion, as well as reduced fat mobilization in response to hypoglycemia, compared with normoglycemic SGA newborns. Because of the increased brain weight/liver weight and brain weight/body weight ratios in all newborns (12% in term newborns for the latter comparison vs. 2% in adults), cerebral glucose requirements are markedly higher relative to the liver's capacity to respond than in the adult, even if glycogen stores are normal for size (Figure 15-4).[75] This is especially true in infants with asymmetric growth restriction. In addition, increased insulin sensitivity has been reported in SGA newborns within the first 48 hours of life.[11,111] These observations indicate that disturbances in glucose metabolism in addition to lower-than-normal energy stores may be present in some growth-restricted infants.

Hyperglycemia

Hyperglycemia is most common during the first week after birth (Box 15-2).[103] Typically, a neonate

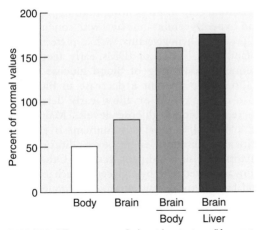

FIGURE 15-4 Differences in organ/body weight ratios in small-for-gestational-age infant compared with appropriate-for-gestational-age counterpart. (From Lafeber HN, Jones CT, Rolph TP: Some of the consequences on intrauterine growth retardation. In Visser HKA, editor: *Nutrition and metabolism of the fetus and infant,* Boston, 1979, Martinus Nijhoff.)

BOX 15-2	ETIOLOGIC FACTORS IN NEONATAL HYPERGLYCEMIA

- Iatrogenic (e.g., during intravenous glucose infusion)
- Decreased insulin production (e.g., with increased catecholamine production in very-low-birth-weight or intrauterine-growth-restricted infant; catecholamine infusion side effect)
- Decreased insulin sensitivity (e.g., with increased catecholamine production in very-low-birth-weight infant or transient diabetes mellitus; catecholamine infusion side effect)
- Sepsis
- Methylxanthine side effect
- Glucocorticoid side effect

---

with hyperglycemia is an LBW infant (less than 32 weeks' gestation and less than 1200 g birth weight), often one with IUGR, who cannot tolerate an IV glucose infusion at the usual rate of 4 to 8 mg/kg/min (i.e., D10W at 60 to 100 ml/kg/day). This relative glucose intolerance appears to be caused by general immaturity of the usual regulatory mechanisms, including absolute or decreased insulin release in response to glucose, insulin resistance (both peripheral, leading to decreased glucose utilization, and hepatic, leading to increased glucose production), and glucose intolerance caused by diminished basal glucose transport capacity.[39] These infants also have decreased insulin-sensitive tissue (e.g., skeletal muscle

and fat) as a fraction of body weight. There also is some evidence of abnormal insulin processing by the pancreatic beta cells such that more immature forms of insulin (proinsulin and proinsulin split products) are released. Because these immature forms of insulin are much less active in stimulating the insulin receptor, they may contribute to a relative insulin resistance in these infants.[95] Some investigators also have reported that, unlike adults, most preterm and term infants fail to suppress endogenous glucose production despite the administration of an adequate exogenous supply (e.g., IV infusion)[20,27]; however, other investigators did not measure any glucose production in premature infants receiving IV glucose at a rate of more than 2 mg/kg/min.[139]

Hyperglycemia also may be iatrogenic in an extremely low-birth-weight (ELBW) infant (less than 750 g) who requires excess water to replace fluid lost through insensible water losses and who receives excess glucose along with the infused water because it is necessary to provide an isotonic IV solution. The risk for developing hyperglycemia is significantly increased with decreasing birth weight (up to 18 times greater in infants with birth weights less than 1000 g than among those weighing 1000 to 2000 g), as well as with an increasing rate of glucose infusion, even if the absolute infusion rate remains within the accepted range.

Delay in initiating enteral feedings may be an additional risk factor. The incidence of hyperglycemia is higher in LBW infants receiving all of their nutrition parenterally than in those who receive at least a part of their nutrition enterally, and prolonged intravenous nutrition may contribute to insulin resistance.[95,120]

The rate at which the glucose concentration is increased in IV solutions, including intravenous nutrition, also may contribute; hyperglycemia is increasingly common at glucose infusion rates greater than 6 to 8 mg/kg/min (normal basal glucose utilization rates are 4 to 6 mg/kg/min). The presence of illness (e.g., sepsis), treatment with corticosteroids, and RDS that requires mechanical ventilation are associated with increased risk for developing hyperglycemia, most likely because of increased circulating catecholamine concentrations that lead to increased lipolysis and glycogenolysis and inhibit pancreatic insulin secretion and insulin action.

Several other etiologic factors must be considered in infants with hyperglycemia. Increased blood glucose concentrations have been reported in association with sepsis.[13] Intravenous lipid infusions also may produce hyperglycemia if given rapidly at rates of more than 0.25 g/kg/hr; however, current practice is to administer lipids at a slower rate.[135] Methylxanthines are frequently used to treat apnea in preterm infants and may be a cause of hyperglycemia. This problem has been well documented after theophylline overdose but may occur also with appropriate administration. One study, for example, found that blood glucose concentrations in infants with therapeutic theophylline levels were higher than in untreated control subjects, with glucose concentrations in the hyperglycemic range in two treated infants.[118] Neonates undergoing surgical procedures also are at increased risk for hyperglycemia, probably because of a combination of the large quantities of glucose-containing fluids and blood products that may be administered during the procedure and the effects of stress-related hormones.

NEONATAL DIABETES

Neonatal diabetes is rare, and 40% to 50% of cases are due to *transient neonatal diabetes mellitus* (TNDM). TNDM is associated with IUGR, and may be difficult to distinguish from hyperglycemia due to increased levels of catecholamines and other stress hormones and related decreased insulin secretion and sensitivity. Genetic mutations or epigenetic anomalies in the chromosome region 6q24 have been identified in 70% of patients with TNDM.[113,126] In TNDM, unlike true diabetes mellitus, ketosis does not develop. Most cases self-resolve, but insulin therapy may be necessary. *Permanent neonatal diabetes mellitus* (PNDM) also occurs, although this is a rare disorder, with incidence estimated at 2 to 3 per 100,000 live births. Only about 25% of infants with PNDM have IUGR. Causes include mitochondrial diseases, pancreatic hypoplasia or aplasia, abnormal pancreatic glucokinase activity, and mutations of pancreatic K_{ATP} channel. Neonatal diabetes may be associated with other abnormalities including developmental delay, skeletal dysplasias, and intestinal atresia.

PREVENTION OF HYPOGLYCEMIA AND HYPERGLYCEMIA

Recognition of those infants at risk for disturbances in glucose homeostasis is the most important step in preventing both hypoglycemia and hyperglycemia. In infants with conditions predisposing to hypoglycemia, such as preterm infants, infants with IUGR, or IDMs, early feeding and frequent monitoring of blood glucose concentrations may prevent a decrease in blood glucose concentration or allow early detection of decreased blood glucose levels. Maintenance of a neutral thermal environment is especially critical to minimize energy expenditure in those infants at risk for hypoglycemia. Other conditions associated with hypoglycemia, such as asphyxia and hypothermia, may be avoided through appropriate obstetric and neonatal intervention. As many as 70% of infants who were requiring transport may not have had appropriate glucose evaluations documented in the referral centers.[33] A prompted intervention (STABLE Pretransport Stabilization Self-Assessment Tool [PSSAT])[33] may result in significant improvement in glucose monitoring.

Hyperglycemia occurs most often in preterm infants receiving high rates of IV glucose. In a very-low-birth-weight (VLBW) infant, hyperglycemia may be avoided by starting IV glucose infusions at rates of 2 to 3 mg/kg/min and checking blood glucose concentrations frequently (as often as every 3 to 4 hours) while the infant continues to receive IV glucose. However, hyperglycemia may be unavoidable in a very immature infant. There is some evidence that starting amino acid infusions shortly after birth in very preterm infants may limit the development of hyperglycemia, perhaps by increasing insulin production and secretion and also by promoting protein turnover and its attendant glucose (energy) requirements.[17,131] Introduction of small-volume enteral feedings as soon as possible may also reduce the incidence or duration of hyperglycemia in VLBW infants by stimulating incretin secretion and increasing glucose metabolism.[7,71]

DATA COLLECTION

History

The history of any neonate must include a detailed prenatal and family history. Important maternal risk factors associated with neonatal hypoglycemia are listed in Box 15-1. Other important data include a history of family members with atypical diabetes or other abnormalities of glucose homeostasis, family history of metabolic disease, and previous unexplained stillbirths.

The most important information to be obtained from the infant's history is gestational age, Apgar scores, and details of events in the delivery room, especially any findings that suggest the presence of significant perinatal compromise. An infant with a history of any of the conditions listed in Box 15-1 or Table 15-1 should be considered at high risk for developing a problem with glucose homeostasis.

Physical Examination

Careful measurement of birth weight and head circumference in combination with accurate gestational age assessment will establish whether the infant is preterm, LBW, SGA, or LGA and thus at increased risk for hypoglycemia. IDMs frequently have small heads relative to their general macrosomia and have been described as having "tomato facies" because of plethora and increased buccal fat. The physical findings associated with Beckwith-Wiedemann syndrome have already been described. The presence of midline facial defects, such as cleft lip or hypertelorism, may indicate the presence of a CNS malformation with associated pituitary dysfunction. Glycogen storage diseases should be considered in infants with hepatomegaly.

Clinical Signs

Signs of neonatal hypoglycemia are nonspecific and extremely variable (Box 15-3).[103] They include general findings, such as abnormal cry, poor feeding, hypothermia, and diaphoresis; neurologic signs, including tremors and jitteriness, hypotonia, irritability, lethargy, and seizures; and cardiorespiratory disturbances, including cyanosis, pallor, tachypnea, periodic breathing, apnea, and cardiac arrest. These features also occur in preterm infants and in neonates with sepsis, intraventricular hemorrhage, asphyxia, hypocalcemia, congenital heart disease, and structural CNS lesions, among other causes. In the presence of any of the preceding signs, however, hypoglycemia always should be considered, because the diagnosis of insufficient brain energy supply can be made relatively easily and prompt treatment is essential.

Hyperglycemia usually is asymptomatic and most often is diagnosed on routine screening of the infant at risk.

BOX 15-3   CLINICAL SIGNS OF HYPOGLYCEMIA

- Mild to moderate changes in level of consciousness*
- Stupor or lethargy*
- Tremulousness*
- Irritability*
- Coma
- Seizures (depend on duration, repetitive occurrence, and severity of hypoglycemia)
- Respiratory depression or apnea, leading to cyanosis
- Hypotonia, limpness, inactivity
- High-pitched cry
- Poor feeding (after previously feeding well)
- Hypothermia

*Most frequent, and should be alleviated with correction of low glucose concentrations.

If a problem with glucose homeostasis is suspected, documentation of the aforementioned data, history (see Box 15-1), physical examination, and clinical signs (see Box 15-3) must reflect ongoing monitoring and measures taken. The use of risk assessments, guidelines, or protocols that consider the data just mentioned is encouraged (Figure 15-5).

Laboratory Data

When hypoglycemia is suspected, the plasma or blood glucose concentration must be determined promptly. Ideally, this determination should be made with one of the laboratory enzymatic methods, such as the glucose oxidase or hexokinase method, but even bedside reagent test strip glucose analyzers (i.e., glucometers) can be used if the test is performed carefully with awareness of the more limited accuracy of these devices. Although more expensive, some blood gas analyzers have the capability of measuring glucose concentrations as accurately as laboratory enzymatic methods, and if present in the nursery or as a portable device may offer the optimal combination of short turnaround time and accuracy.[62] In the clinical setting, early and rapid determination of glucose concentrations in the high-risk or symptomatic neonate is essential.[46] Prompt detection of hypoglycemia permits early treatment and potentially helps prevent long-term neurologic sequelae.[25] Although laboratory measurements of glucose

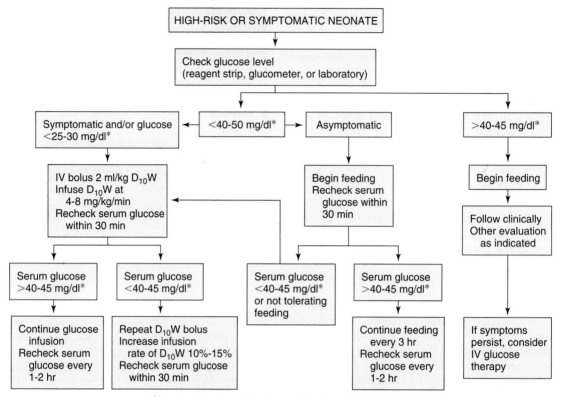

Levels arbitrary and not "normal" or "hypoglycemic."

FIGURE 15-5 Decision tree for management of neonate with acute hypoglycemia. *IV*, Intravenous.

concentrations are the most effective methods for detecting hypoglycemia, results may not be available for up to 1 hour—far longer than appropriate for diagnosing hypoglycemia and thereby delaying the initiation of treatment. Rapid measurement methods available to the clinician are described earlier in this chapter. The sample of blood can be obtained from a warmed heelstick or venipuncture specimen.

These methods can be useful in screening infants in whom abnormal glucose concentrations are suspected if the user is aware of their limitations. The accuracy of test strip results depends in part on the technique used. An adequate sample must be placed on the test strip pad, and the timing of reading the result is critical. Recently developed devices automatically read the result at the appropriate time, reducing one source of error. Hospital personnel should be trained and certified in the use of test strip methods and the bedside instruments

used to quantify glucose concentration. With proper technique, test strip results demonstrate a reasonable correlation with actual blood glucose concentrations, but the variation from the actual blood glucose value may be as much as 10 to 20 mg/dl. A number of studies have compared the results obtained with specific commercial products with results obtained with laboratory methods.[6,49,87] Regardless of the test strip or instrument used, correlations with actual blood glucose concentrations are lowest at the lower glucose concentrations at which neonatal hypoglycemia must be accurately determined. Several studies have shown that use of test strips alone may fail to detect from 11% to as many as 67% of infants with statistically defined hypoglycemia.[48,49,79] There also is a significant incidence of false-positive results.

Because of the limitations of these methods, whenever a diagnosis of hypoglycemia is suspected by test strip or glucometer results, the blood glucose concentration should be confirmed by a specimen sent to the chemistry laboratory for prompt (STAT) determination and reporting. Although laboratory results are more accurate and reliable than screening methods, a long delay in processing the specimen can result in a falsely low level as the erythrocytes in the sample metabolize the glucose in the plasma. This problem can be avoided by transporting blood in a tube containing a glycolytic inhibitor. *Treatment of suspected hypoglycemia, however, should not be postponed until confirmation is obtained from the laboratory. Also, if hypoglycemia is suspected on the basis of clinical symptoms, initial treatment should be instituted even if the test strip result is "normal."* If the actual value is abnormal, a delay in therapy could be harmful; if the actual value is within the normal range, therapy can be stopped without serious side effects.

Most cases of neonatal hypoglycemia have an identifiable cause (e.g., maternal diabetes or IUGR). In a term infant with no known risk factors for hypoglycemia, sepsis must be considered as the most likely cause of hypoglycemia and an appropriate evaluation should be performed. Of those infants without an identifiable cause, most have idiopathic hypoglycemia, which resolves spontaneously within 2 to 5 days, and no further evaluation is needed. However, in rare cases, hypoglycemia persists beyond the first week of life with no obvious cause detected, requiring a logical and rapid approach to diagnosis of the particular form of persistent hypoglycemia. The diagnostic evaluation of these infants should include (1) simultaneous determination of glucose and insulin concentrations, as well as alternate substrates, such as ketones and FFAs; (2) evaluation of pituitary function, including measurement of thyroid-stimulating hormone (TSH), thyroxine (T_4), adrenocorticotropic hormone (ACTH), cortisol, and growth hormone levels; and (3) appropriate studies to diagnose inborn errors of metabolism, such as lactate and pyruvate concentrations. Ideally, these studies should be obtained during an episode of hypoglycemia. Once hypoglycemia is identified in a neonate as persistent, a fasting study should be performed to measure plasma insulin concentration when plasma glucose concentration drops below 45 to 50 mg/dl. If this fasting study demonstrates hyperinsulinism, treatment should be immediately instituted.[66]

TREATMENT

Hypoglycemia

Early identification of an infant at risk for developing hypoglycemia and institution of prophylactic measures to prevent its occurrence constitutes the best treatment for this disorder. The goals are to recognize at-risk infants, evaluate early and frequently for decreasing glucose concentrations, treat when indicated, and provide glucose and enteral feeding as needed to achieve and maintain glucose concentrations in the range that most normal infants develop via their own homeostatic mechanisms within 6 to 12 hours after birth.

A decision tree suggesting guidelines for management of infants with hypoglycemia is shown in Figure 15-5. Although most asymptomatic infants can be managed with early and frequent feedings (by breastfeeding or with expressed milk, with donor milk when appropriate as for very preterm infants, or with formulas), all symptomatic neonates should receive treatment with IV dextrose infusion to provide glucose at an initial rate of 4 to 6 mg/kg/min. In some circumstances (symptomatic neonates with glucose concentrations of 20 mg/dl or less glucose and or with very severe clinical signs, such as seizures and/or coma), it may be useful to use a "minibolus" of 200 mg/kg dextrose (2 ml/kg of $D_{10}W$) plus the dextrose infusion regimen originally described by Lilien and colleagues.[80] Advantages of the minibolus regimen include the following: (1) There is a lower incidence of hyperglycemia immediately after the minibolus bolus than is observed with use of boluses of solutions with higher dextrose concentrations; (2) the slower rate of administration decreases the insulin response to glucose infusion, thus lowering the risk for rebound hypoglycemia after the bolus; and (3) glucose concentration reaches the normal range more quickly than if continuous infusion is started without a preceding bolus (Figure 15-6). Rapid normalization of blood glucose may be particularly beneficial in severely symptomatic infants, although no data confirm this assumption. The suggested infusion rates cover the range of hepatic glucose production in normal term newborns. In IDMs with asymptomatic hypoglycemia, the initial minibolus can be eliminated and the infusion rate kept at the minimum necessary to produce and

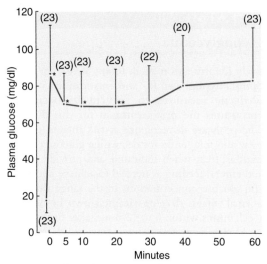

FIGURE 15-6 Plasma glucose response to glucose "minibolus" followed by continuous glucose infusion (8 mg/min/kg) as therapy for neonatal hypoglycemia. (From Lilien LD, Pildes RS, Srinivasan G, et al: Treatment of neonatal hypoglycemia with minibolus and intravenous glucose infusion, *J Pediatr* 97:295, 1980.)

maintain normal blood glucose concentrations; this practice helps prevent an excessive insulin response to the sudden increase in glucose concentration produced by the minibolus. When glucose infusion rates are being calculated, it is important to remember that commercially prepared glucose solutions actually contain glucose in its hydrated form (molecular weight [MW] 198, versus MW 180 for anhydrous glucose), which lowers the actual glucose content of the solution by approximately 8%. Thus $D_{10}W$ contains approximately 9.2 g of glucose per deciliter.

Once the infant's glucose requirement has been determined, the glucose infusion should be maintained at that level until blood glucose concentrations are stable and in the desired range. The target blood glucose concentration during IV therapy should be above the "hypoglycemic threshold" defined for that particular infant; for example, if hypoglycemia is defined as 40 mg/dl, glucose concentrations should be maintained at or above 50 mg/dl.[24]

Adjusting therapy to maintain a blood glucose concentration higher than the "diagnostic" threshold allows a margin of safety in the absence of any data establishing a correlation between specific glucose concentrations in this range and long-term outcome. There is no evidence that diagnosis or treatment thresholds for preterm infants should differ from those for term infants.

If the infant was being fed before IV therapy was instituted, feedings may be continued. However, the calculated minimum glucose requirement should be provided by the IV infusion alone rather than by the combination of glucose infusion and feedings. In infants who were not previously fed, feedings can be instituted when clinically indicated. There are several advantages to feeding a hypoglycemic infant during treatment with IV glucose. In the hyperinsulinemic infant, galactose (one of the components of lactose) stimulates less insulin release than glucose and therefore helps stabilize blood glucose concentrations. Continuation of oral feedings also aids in the process of weaning the infant off IV glucose. When feedings are well tolerated, the IV infusion generally can be slowly tapered if the glucose concentration and clinical status remain stable. Although enteral feeding has the theoretical risk for augmenting insulin secretion and subsequent hypoglycemia as a result of the food-stimulated release of gut peptides that may potentiate insulin release from the pancreas, there is no evidence that withholding feedings actually prevents this potential problem. It probably is better to continue breast milk or formula feedings using smaller, more frequent amounts or continuous gastric infusion than to stop enteral feedings and trying to maintain normoglycemia exclusively with IV glucose.

A recent study from Auckland, New Zealand, showed that a 40% oral dextrose gel, 200 mg/kg placed on the buccal mucosa, could restore normal glucose concentrations, reduce the recurrence rate of low glucose concentrations, and allow enteral feeding, particularly breastfeeding, to continue or even advance.[53] Such therapy seems appropriate for the term or late preterm infant with transient hypoglycemia, and probably for SGA, LGA, and IDM infants who are otherwise clinically stable.

Rare cases, such as infants with severe, refractory hyperinsulinemic hypoglycemia, or associated severe pathophysiologic conditions, such as adrenaline secretion and emesis, might preclude enteral feedings until glucose concentrations are stabilized and the associated adverse clinical conditions have resolved.

T A B L E 15-2	ADJUNCT THERAPIES FOR HYPOGLYCEMIA	

THERAPY	EFFECT	DOSAGE
Corticosteroids	Decrease peripheral glucose utilization Enhance gluconeogenesis	Hydrocortisone 5-15 mg/kg/day or Prednisone 2 mg/kg/day
Glucagon	Stimulates glycogenolysis Releases glycogen from hepatic stores when insulin concentrations are normal	30 mcg/kg IV or IM 300 mcg/kg if hyperinsulinism is present
Diazoxide	Inhibits insulin secretion	15 mg/kg/day
Somatostatin (long-acting: octreotide acetate)	Inhibits insulin and growth hormone release	5-10 mcg/kg every 6-8 hr
Pancreatectomy	Decreases insulin production/secretion	

From McGowan JE: Neonatal hypoglycemia, *Pediatr Rev* 20:6-15, 1999.
IM, Intramuscular; *IV*, intravenous.

ADJUNCTIVE THERAPY

See Table 15-2 for a summary of adjunct therapies for hypoglycemia.

Glucagon. Glucagon, 30 mcg/kg IV or intramuscular (IM), releases glycogen from hepatic stores when insulin concentrations are normal. However, IDMs and other infants with hyperinsulinemia may require much larger doses, up to 300 mcg/kg IV, to produce a response. Administration of glucagon may be useful diagnostically, because failure to respond to glucagon administration with an increase in serum glucose concentration suggests depletion of hepatic glycogen stores or a glycogen storage disorder. Glucose infusion should be maintained after glucagon is administered, because there is a risk for rebound increased insulin secretion in response to the glucagon-produced surge in glucose production. In addition, the rapid but transient increase in glucose concentration immediately after glucagon injection may produce a false sense that the hypoglycemia has resolved, even though the underlying cause still exists. Continuous infusions of glucagon have been used to treat refractory hypoglycemia.[19]

Other Agents. Glucocorticoids (hydrocortisone), somatostatin, and diazoxide have been used to treat hypoglycemia in refractory cases. Glucocorticoids can be used to reduce peripheral glucose utilization and increase gluconeogenesis, particularly when glucose infusion rates of 12 to 15 mg/kg/min or more are needed to maintain normal glucose concentrations. Somatostatin and diazoxide, which suppress insulin release, are most often used in infants with islet cell dysplasias.[66]

Miscellaneous. In infants with hypoglycemia caused by a specific medical problem, therapy should be directed toward alleviating the underlying illness. This includes administration of antibiotics to treat sepsis, partial exchange transfusion to reduce hyperviscosity, hormone replacement in cases of hypopituitarism, and dietary intervention for metabolic disorders. A trial of diazoxide should be initiated in infants who have been identified as having hyperinsulinism. If diazoxide is not effective at a maximum dose of 15 mg/kg per day divided into two doses per day for 2 to 3 days, it may be stopped and octreotide could be tried. However, medical therapy alone fails to control hypoglycemia in 40% to 90% of infants with severe PHIHG.[34] If octreotide is not successful, surgical management is generally necessary. Before surgery, imaging procedures should be performed to determine whether the pancreatic abnormalities are focal or diffuse. Focal disease generally is cured with partial pancreatectomy, whereas diffuse disease requires near-total pancreatectomy and then treatment of the exocrine and endocrine deficiencies that invariably result.[43]

Hyperglycemia

GLUCOSE

Most cases of hyperglycemia can be treated by reducing the neonate's IV glucose infusion rate. This approach, when combined with other measures such as early use of IV amino acids, commonly reduces glucose concentrations into more acceptable ranges within 24 hours. Many LBW infants will tolerate glucose infusions at rates as low 4 mg/kg/min with normal glucose concentrations, although Zarif and colleagues[138] reported that more than 40% of infants weighing less than 1000 g had a blood glucose concentration higher than 125 mg/dl while receiving glucose at an average rate of 4.4 mg/kg/min. VLBW infants with high fluid requirements resulting from large insensible water losses through the skin may require a combination of water and glucose intake that could be administered only by using a hypotonic solution such as $D_{2.5}W$ to avoid hyperglycemia. The use of a low glucose concentration in the IV infusate necessitates the addition of sodium (e.g., $D_{2.5}W$ has approximately 130 mOsm/L, requiring the addition of sodium chloride to produce an isotonic solution with 280 mOsm/L), which may further complicate management of fluids and electrolytes. A VLBW infant needs adequate caloric intake (50 to 60 kcal/kg/day) to avoid a negative nitrogen balance and tissue catabolism. These needs often cannot be met without resultant hyperglycemia. If the glucose is only mildly elevated (e.g., concentrations of 150 to 200 mg/dl) and the infant has no evidence of adverse effects, reducing the rate of IV glucose administration may not be necessary, because increasing amino acid infusions and enteral feeding generally promote insulin and incretin production and promote glucose utilization. There is little evidence, however, to determine whether this practice will lead to better or worse outcomes; such infants should have repeated glucose measurements made to ensure that the hyperglycemia resolves.

LIPID AND AMINO ACIDS

Intravenous lipid infusion rates can be decreased to help reduce hyperglycemia. This limits the contribution of FFAs produced by lipid metabolism that, on oxidation, generate energy to drive gluconeogenesis (acetyl CoA and reducing equivalents, NAD/NADH). Decreasing lipid supply also limits the competition of fatty acids with glucose for oxidation, as well as the direct enhancement of gluconeogenic enzymes in the liver and thus the production of glucose. Limiting lipid supply also reduces the supply of glycerol, which is the primary support for gluconeogenesis in newborn infants. As with reducing the glucose infusion rate, reducing lipid infusion rates also reduces energy supply; the risks of reducing energy intake to lower glucose concentrations, versus those of the hyperglycemia itself, are uncertain.

Amino acid infusions should be started early to promote insulin secretion and enhance protein turnover with its obligatory energy (hence, glucose) requirements.[17,131] Amino acids do not contribute measurably to enhancing gluconeogenesis, even though they provide more substrate.[121]

INSULIN INFUSION

Because of the foregoing considerations, some authors have suggested the use of a continuous insulin infusion in the infant who cannot tolerate infusion of glucose solutions with concentrations greater than 5 g/dl (e.g., D_5W).[14,37] Infusion of insulin at rates of 0.2 to 0.8 mU/kg/min (0.01 to 0.05 U/kg/hr) for 12 to 24 hours may improve glucose tolerance. However, insulin avidly binds to plastic IV tubing; thus the actual rate of insulin administration may be difficult to determine and may vary over time. Although various methods, such as priming the tubing with insulin-containing solution or albumin, have been proposed, these have not been shown to be consistently effective.[125]

Hypoglycemia during administration of exogenous insulin can be avoided by starting with a low infusion rate (0.05 to 0.1 mU/kg/min) and increasing the rate by 10% to 20% every 60 to 90 minutes until the glucose concentration is less than 200 mg/dl. Blood glucose concentrations should be monitored every 15 to 20 minutes during initiation of the insulin infusion, and an IV glucose infusion should be maintained to avoid any abrupt changes in blood glucose concentration and to allow rapid correction of glucose concentration if it starts to fall below "normal" values. Use of insulin infusion has been reported to improve tolerance to glucose infusions, resulting in increased carbohydrate intake and weight gain.[5,12] Most of the weight gain is fat, however, and there is risk for fatty infiltration and secondary inflammation in the liver and heart when insulin and glucose infusions are maintained for long periods. Such insulin treatment inhibits glucose production, though not as readily as in adults.[20] The effect of insulin to promote glucose utilization is modest in very preterm infants, given the small amount of insulin-sensitive tissue (primarily skeletal muscle) per body weight. Acutely, insulin infusion has been noted to increase lactate production, with lactate concentrations up to threefold greater than baseline, and may be associated with metabolic acidosis. Administration of glucose and insulin at high rates also enhances CO_2 production, which might lead to hypercarbia in infants with respiratory disease. Also, episodes of hypoglycemia can occur even with careful monitoring during insulin infusion. The use of insulin to prevent hyperglycemia in neonates has been evaluated in a randomized prospective study, which showed no obvious benefit and considerable morbidity, particularly a significant increase in the incidence of hypoglycemic episodes. The authors of this study and an editorial commentary concluded that chronic insulin infusion cannot be recommended and must be used cautiously even in cases of acute hyperglycemia.[12,67] This is especially true because there are no clinical studies that have demonstrated a cause-and-effect relationship between brief periods of neonatal hyperglycemia and adverse long-term outcomes.

MISCELLANEOUS

In addition to specific measures to lower the blood glucose concentration, close attention must be paid to fluid balance in the hyperglycemic infant, because, theoretically, hyperglycemia can induce an osmotic diuresis. However, this is rarely seen at blood glucose concentrations less than 400 mg/dl or when hyperglycemia occurs intermittently and for brief periods. Finally, as in hypoglycemia, efforts should be made to treat any underlying etiology, such as sepsis.

COMPLICATIONS

Hypoglycemia

The outcome for infants with neonatal hypoglycemia appears to be related to the duration, repetitive occurrence, and severity of the hypoglycemia, as well as the underlying etiology. Those with *asymptomatic hypoglycemia* usually have a normal neurodevelopmental

outcome. Furthermore, although learning disabilities and abnormal electroencephalograms without seizure disorders occasionally have been reported in infants who had asymptomatic hypoglycemia, there is no evidence that treatment prevents such abnormal outcomes.[52] *Symptomatic hypoglycemic* infants (primarily those with severe, protracted, and recurrent neurologic abnormalities such as seizures and coma associated with plasma glucose concentrations below 20 to 25 mg/dl for several hours or more) have a poorer prognosis, with abnormalities ranging from learning disabilities to cerebral palsy and persistent or recurrent seizure disorders, as well as mental retardation of varying degrees.[42] Prompt initiation of treatment is thought to be associated with a more positive outcome, although this has not been well documented.

In preterm infants, data indicate that hypoglycemia may adversely affect long-term outcome.[38,70,85] A follow-up study of more than 600 former preterm infants found significantly lower mental and motor indices in those with five or more documented episodes of moderate hypoglycemia (defined as a blood glucose concentration less than 45 mg/dl) during the neonatal period. This difference remained significant even when confounding factors such as intraventricular hemorrhage (IVH), need for ventilator support, and asphyxia were considered. However, differences in cognitive function were less apparent at school-age follow-up in the same cohort of patients, and a newer study designed to replicate the former did not confirm any adverse outcomes associated with hypoglycemia in preterm infants.[130] Hypoglycemic preterm infants who were also SGA were found to have lower scores on psychometric tests at both 3 years and 5 years of age, with a greater effect seen in those infants with recurrent hypoglycemia. These results indicate that further long-term studies in preterm infants are needed.

The incidence of neurodevelopmental abnormalities in IDMs ranges from 0% to 35%; the lower figures are from more recent studies and may represent improvement in obstetric and neonatal care. Most of the long-term follow-up studies have not shown an association between the presence of neonatal hypoglycemia and later neurodevelopmental impairment.[57,110] Instead, outcome has been related to such factors as prematurity, presence of congenital anomalies, congenital iron deficiency, and degree of control of maternal disease.

However, Stenninger and colleagues[119] found that IDMs who were hypoglycemic as newborns (glucose less than 27 mg/dl) had an increased frequency of deficits in attention, motor control, and perception at 8 years of age compared with both IDMs without hypoglycemia and normal newborn controls. A number of other neonatal complications are associated with maternal diabetes, including polycythemia, which may add to disturbances of glucose homeostasis; hypocalcemia secondary to maternal hypoparathyroidism; dystocia secondary to macrosomia; and congenital anomalies. Infants of mothers with severe diabetic vasculopathy, in contrast to most IDMs, may have IUGR caused in part by decreased placental blood flow, with hypoglycemia resulting from inadequate glycogen and fat stores as occurs in all cases of IUGR rather than hyperinsulinemia alone.

Adverse neurologic outcomes have been reported in as many as 40% to 50% of infants with PHIHG, possibly because these infants cannot effectively generate ketone bodies, which could serve as an alternative source of energy for cerebral metabolism during periods of hypoglycemia.[90-92] In addition, infants with PHIHG who require a greater than 95% pancreatectomy often develop glucose intolerance or even frank diabetes mellitus later in life.[83] Hypoglycemia secondary to hypopituitarism also is associated with a poor outcome; often this results from other CNS or endocrine dysfunction, rather than from the hypoglycemia itself.

Hyperglycemia

Although there is no direct evidence, it has been postulated that hyperglycemia in the preterm infant can increase the risk for IVH by causing rapid changes in osmolarity with resultant rapid fluid shifts within the brain and germinal matrix. Increased mortality rate in hyperglycemic premature infants compared with their normoglycemic counterparts has been reported, although hyperglycemia may have been a marker for those infants with more severe illness rather than a direct cause of the increased mortality rate.[3] Increased morbidity may be seen in the form of greater difficulty with fluid and electrolyte management because use of dextrose-containing fluids must be limited, as well as problems establishing adequate nutrition. Several studies also suggest an association between hyperglycemia in ELBW infants and increased incidence of retinopathy of prematurity,[47] perhaps due to increased production of reactive oxygen species and reduced angiogenesis and secondary neuronal necrosis, but no definitive cause-and-effect relationship has, as of yet, been demonstrated.★

Infants with TNDM usually recover spontaneously within the first week; persistent insulin resistance is extremely rare. However, those infants with chromosomal mutations have an increased incidence of adult-onset diabetes later in life.[113] No neurologic sequelae have been directly attributed to the presence of transient hyperglycemia in these neonates.

PARENT TEACHING

Parent teaching should begin before delivery, with emphasis placed on good nutrition and early and regular prenatal care. Teaching also should include information about those conditions that increase the risk for hypoglycemia (e.g., IUGR associated with maternal cigarette smoking and poor maternal nutrition). Regular prenatal care ensures the early detection of potentially serious problems, including preeclampsia, gestational diabetes, and abnormal fetal growth.

Prenatal teaching is especially important in the woman with known diabetes mellitus, because overall outcome (although not necessarily the incidence of hypoglycemia) is directly related to the degree of control before and during pregnancy. Breastfeeding information and encouragement to breastfeed must be included in the prenatal education. In addition, the possibility of neonatal hypoglycemia and requirement for IV therapy can be discussed with the parents before delivery so that they will be aware that the infant may require a longer hospital stay even if delivered at term.

If IV therapy is selected to treat neonatal hypoglycemia, regardless of cause, a thorough explanation of the treatment plan must be given to the parents at the time therapy is instituted. Frequent progress reports should be provided to resolve unanswered (and often unasked) questions and relieve parental anxiety. Parents of children with islet cell dysplasias need to be aware of the clinical signs of hypoglycemia and emergency treatment measures that can be instituted, because

---

★References 2, 41, 46, 63, 69, 96, 97.

recurrent hypoglycemia may occur in these cases. Parents of infants with inborn errors of metabolism also need counseling with regard to prognosis, as well as genetic counseling about risks for recurrence in future pregnancies.

Acknowledgments

Supported by NIH grants R01 DK088139 (PJR, PI; WWH, Co-I) and K08 HD060688 (PJR, PI); Bill and Melinda Gates Foundation Grand Challenges Exploration Grant OPP1061082 (WWH, PI); NIH Training Grant T32 HD007186-32 (WWH, PI and PD); NIH K12 HD068372 (WWH, PD); NIH UL1TR001082 (WWH, Co-PD).

REFERENCES

For a full list of references, scan the QR code or visit http://booksite.elsevier.com/ 9780323320832.

16 TOTAL PARENTERAL NUTRITION

STEVEN L. OLSEN, MARY KAY LEICK-RUDE, JARROD DUSIN, AND JAMIE ROSTERMAN

otal parenteral nutrition (TPN) support for critically ill newborns was first reported four decades ago.[37] However, in the modern era of neonatal care, TPN continues to be a critical aspect of intensive newborn care. Availability of TPN has been one of the developments responsible for improved outcome of neonatal surgical patients.[93,97,100] Increased survival of extremely preterm infants has provided new challenges for neonatal parenteral nutrition.[27] Current evidence would suggest that early nutritional support is important to prevent postnatal growth restriction, which has been commonly recognized in these infants.[38]

A neonatal service that uses TPN has the best results if it includes an experienced "nutrition team," comprising a neonatologist, surgeon, nutrition support nurse, pharmacist, dietitian, and social worker, with each member playing a vital role to make TPN a safe and effective therapy.

This chapter discusses the nutritional needs of the high-risk newborn, specific indications for TPN, and guidelines for formulation and administration of intravenous (IV) nutritional solutions. It also provides an overview of mechanical, infectious, and metabolic complications, with emphasis on prevention and early identification.

PHYSIOLOGY

Fuel Stores

During periods of fasting, tissue stores of energy provide the major source of fuel for the body. Carbohydrate is stored in the liver and muscle as glycogen. Stable blood sugar levels are maintained by hormonal regulation of glycogen production (glycogenesis) and breakdown to glucose (glycogenolysis). Newborns, particularly those who are growth restricted or preterm, have low glycogen stores and often have insufficient regulatory mechanisms.[118]

The body's greatest energy stores are in the form of fat, which provides a calorie yield of 9 kcal/g when metabolized. In addition to normal deposits of adipose tissue, newborns (and hibernating adult animals) have unique stores called brown fat. These stores, which are anatomically located between the scapulae, in the axillae and mediastinum, and around the adrenal glands, protect the body from hypothermia through nonshivering thermogenesis[83] (see Chapter 6).

Protein makes up lean body mass. Although protein generally is not used as an energy source postnatally, in fetal life, amino acids are oxidized apparently for energy.[123] This may be true for brief periods postnatally, but extended periods of protein catabolism (breakdown of endogenous substrates), such as during times of starvation, may lead to body dysfunction, as noted later.

The Effects of Insufficient Nutrition

The last trimester of gestation is a time of rapid fetal growth, with active transplacental transport of most nutritional substrates. Preterm delivery interrupts the nutritional supply and abruptly results in a catabolic state, which, if prolonged, may alter growth potential. It is unclear whether it is possible to achieve in utero growth rates for the postnatal preterm infant, but reestablishment of an anabolic state and maintenance of micronutrient sufficiency are necessary.[50,123] During this period of neonatal life, the rapidly growing brain is responsible for

PURPLE type highlights content that is particularly applicable to clinical settings.

much of the nutritional requirements. Inadequate early nutrition may have irreversible effects on later neurodevelopmental outcomes.[73]

Postnatal growth restriction also is associated with neonatal medical complications, including apnea, ventilator dependence, and chronic lung disease.[27] Immune responses may be depressed with increased susceptibility to infection (see Chapter 22). Protein malnutrition is most frequently seen in extreme preterms and may contribute to poor growth potential and long-term morbidity in these infants.[27,123,124] Poor postnatal growth for most extremely low-birth-weight (ELBW) infants has emphasized the need for additional strategies to improve nutrition for this population.[34,35]

One strategy is to initiate parenteral nutrition within the first hours after birth. Even though the exact benefits and harms are unknown, providing early, increased energy and protein support have been associated with improved short-term growth outcomes. Longer-term outcomes, such as reductions in the incidence of common neonatal morbidities, increased brain growth, and improved neurodevelopmental outcomes, are more difficult to directly link to early parenteral nutrition. There is no evidence that early parenteral nutrition increases morbidity or mortality risks, but also unclear is the influence of early nutritional support on the incidence of childhood obesity and the risk for cardiovascular disease and metabolic syndrome in adults.[79]

Nutritional Requirements of the Neonate

CALORIC

Caloric requirements for preterm infants, including very-low-birth-weight (VLBW) and small-for-gestational-age (SGA) infants, are approximately 110 to 130 kcal/kg/day.[139] Caloric requirements for near-term and term infants are 90 to 120 kcal/kg/day. These estimates are based on enteral intake (see Chapter 17). Parenteral requirements are about 20% less, or approximately 80 to 100 kcal/kg/day. Factors affecting caloric requirements include the infant's gestational age, chronologic age, weight, activity level, body temperature, ambient temperature, underlying disease, and degree of stress. Infections, including nosocomial, may also contribute to additional caloric needs.[126] Resting energy expenditure is an estimate of the approximate range of basic energy needs and is approximately 45 kcal/kg/day in infants less than 900 g and 50 kcal/kg/day for infants larger than 1000 g.[139] Physical activity, which usually is infrequent in preterm infants, contributes less than 10% to the energy needs.[71] However, in pathologic states, such as with repetitious seizures or neonatal abstinence syndrome, increased activity may increase caloric needs. An elevation of body temperature increases caloric expenditure by approximately 12% for each degree Celsius above 37.8° C (100° F). Metabolic demands of surgery and postoperative healing, or severe cardiac or pulmonary distress, may increase caloric requirements by as much as 30% and chronic failure to thrive by 50% to 100%. In addition, postnatal dexamethasone therapy may slow weight and linear growth rates and potentially may negatively affect brain growth.[27,81,116]

WATER

Water requirements vary with gestational and postnatal age (postconceptual age) and environmental conditions (e.g., care in an incubator versus radiant heat warmer, use of phototherapy) (see Chapter 14).

ELECTROLYTE AND MINERAL

Sodium requirements are minimal for the first days of life. After 1 week, the average requirement is 3 to 4 mEq/kg/day. Large renal losses (greater than 5 mEq/kg/day) may occur in very immature infants (less than 28 weeks of gestation) in the first weeks of life. Potassium and chloride requirements are approximately 2 mEq/kg/day and 3 to 4 mEq/kg/day, respectively. Glucosuria with resulting osmotic diuresis may increase sodium and potassium urinary losses.[41]

Calcium is an important cofactor in hemostasis, enzyme function, muscle contraction, and cell membrane stability. In the newborn, 98% of calcium is stored in the bone. The initial calcium requirement is 1 mEq/kg/day to maintain calcium homeostasis and to avoid irritability and tetany associated with low serum ionized calcium levels. In utero, the accretion rate is 4 to 5 mEq/kg/day, which the growing preterm infant should receive in addition to adequate phosphorus and vitamin D to avoid osteopenia, rickets, and bone fractures.[137] Excess calcium intake may cause central nervous system (CNS) depression or signs of renal toxicity.

The phosphorus requirement for the growing preterm infant is 40 to 60 mg/kg/day (31 mg = 1 mmol). Bone contains 80% of the body's phosphorus. Low phosphorus intake causes increased renal calcium excretion and a depletion of bone calcium phosphate. Low phosphorus intake or chronic furosemide diuretic therapy also may lead to hypercalciuria and nephrolithiasis.[36] Because phosphorus is a major constituent of cellular energy function (adenosine triphosphate, 2,3-diphosphoglycerate, creatinine phosphate), severe depletion may result in muscle paralysis, respiratory failure, and interruption of important cellular functions, such as the hemoglobin-oxygen dissociation curve and leukocyte activity.

Magnesium is essential for intracellular enzyme systems. The requirement is 0.25 to 0.5 mEq/kg/day.[5] Magnesium deficiency states mimic hypocalcemia, manifesting as irritability, tremulousness, tetany, and cardiac dysrhythmias. Magnesium excess may manifest as lethargy, hypotonia, and delayed stooling.

CARBOHYDRATE

During fetal life, glucose is the primary source of energy.[123] At birth, the preterm infant has only a small supply of glycogen, the storage form of glucose (equivalent to about 200 kcal of energy). Glucose is particularly important for the CNS, because other substrates are not available. Initially, a glucose infusion rate (GIR) of 6 mg/kg/min is sufficient to meet metabolic needs of the newborn infant. Requirements are greater for infants who are stressed (e.g., from sepsis or hypothermia) or hyperinsulinemic (e.g., infants of diabetic mothers or infants with Beckwith-Wiedemann syndrome).

With long-term parenteral nutrition, at least 50% of total caloric requirement should be provided as carbohydrate (GIR 8 to 10 mg/kg/min), generally as dextrose (calculated as 3.4 kcal/kg of hydrated carbohydrate). Preterm infants, especially ELBW patients, who receive early and higher amino acids in their parenteral nutrition, have been shown to decrease glucose concentrations.[2] To avoid metabolic consequences of excessive glucose loads, a GIR of more than 13 mg/kg/min (19 g/kg/day of glucose) should be avoided.

PROTEIN

The quantity of daily nitrogen required by a term newborn infant, based on estimates from breast milk intake, is approximately 325 mg/kg/day (approximately 2 g/kg/day of protein).[6,43] Requirements for preterm infants are much higher, as indicated by in utero accretion rates during the latter half of pregnancy. At 28 weeks' gestation, the fetus requires 350 mg/kg/day of nitrogen. This figure declines to 150 mg/kg/day by term gestation. When the estimated accretion rate is added to the obligatory postnatal nitrogen excretion, the requirement for a 28-weeks'-gestation preterm infant may be calculated to be approximately 495 mg/kg/day (3.1 g/kg/day of protein). If one assumes parenterally administered amino acids are converted to body proteins at 75% efficiency, the estimated parenteral amino acid requirement would be as high as 3.7 g/kg/day.[40,51,124]

In fetal life, protein is actively transported from the mother's circulation across the placenta in quantities greater than needed for accretion, with the excess being oxidized by the fetus or placenta for energy.[122] Clinicians have found that increasing protein intake postnatally at all energy intake levels above 40 kcal/kg/day results in increased protein accretion. Current evidence indicates that protein intake up to 4 g/kg/day is safe with no clinically significant increase in azotemia, acidemia, or hyperaminoacidemia.[95] Although more studies are looking at higher amino acid administration, further investigations are needed to determine safe upper limits for maximum protein administration beyond that level.[20]

Studies have shown that administration of amino acids shortly after birth decreases protein catabolism, which is extremely important, particularly for VLBW infants.[40,122] Early amino acid administration is also associated with reductions in hyperkalemia and hyperglycemia.[15,20,84] Based on the current evidence, providing VLBW infants with 3 g/kg/day of protein on the first day of life is safe.[34,132] Many units have created a "stock" or "starter TPN (protein-containing) solution" to achieve the goal of providing 2 to 3 g/kg/day of protein immediately after admission to the neonatal intensive care unit (NICU) to promote anabolism. Although current studies support the early use of parenteral protein nutrition, further investigation is needed to document the effect of this supplementation on post-NICU long-term growth and development.[79]

The quality of the amino acid mixture infused is important for efficacy and safety.[1] Although there is no formulation specifically for preterm infants, pediatric solutions provide greater quantities of essential amino acids and result in plasma amino acid levels similar to those of postprandial breastfed infants. An essential amino acid is one that cannot be synthesized in adequate quantity to meet the requirements for normal growth and development. The differentiation between essential and nonessential amino acids is not clear in newborn infants, because the ability to synthesize some amino acids may vary with the clinical situation or stage of maturity. Lysine and threonine are essential in their entirety. There is a high requirement for branched-chain amino acids (e.g., leucine, isoleucine, valine) in the growing newborn. These are metabolized primarily in skeletal muscle.[52,78]

Methionine is an essential sulfur-containing amino acid that is metabolized to cysteine and taurine. For preterm infants of less than 32 weeks' gestation, cystathionase activity is insufficient for cysteine synthesis.[135] Some investigators have found that cysteine supplementation results in greater nitrogen retention, and for this reason it is recommended for short-term supplementation for high-risk preterms, although the effects of prolonged use have not been fully investigated.[113] Cysteine is not stable in amino acid solutions, so cysteine hydrochloride supplements must be added separately to the parenteral nutrition. Taurine is a nonprotein amino sulfonic acid that is converted from cysteine by cysteine sulfonic acid decarboxylase. Taurine concentrations are low in infants who have received nonsupplemented TPN infusions. Taurine deficiency may have a detrimental effect on the developing nervous system. It is a general practice to add taurine to TPN for VLBW infants because this may prevent cholestasis in some newborns by more effectively conjugating bile salts and creating soluble end-products.[53,115,134]

Tyrosine is another amino acid that appears to be essential in the newborn period. It is present in small amounts in most amino acid solutions, although one manufacturer uses a soluble form, *N*-acetyl-L-tyrosine, which infants slowly metabolize to tyrosine.[98] Tyrosine is a byproduct of phenylalanine metabolism, so supplementation has an effect on the phenylalanine requirement. Histidine is considered to be an essential amino acid for newborns, with the lowest levels evident in preterm infants. Arginine may be essential only for the newborn with reduced arginine synthetase activity. This amino acid is thought to facilitate clearance of nitrogenous waste products by "priming the urea cycle." Use of amino acid infusate with insufficient arginine has been associated with hyperammonemia.[48] Glutamine also has been considered a conditionally essential amino acid; however, in a randomized trial, no benefit was shown for parenteral glutamine in relation to days to enteral feedings, incidence of necrotizing enterocolitis (NEC), or growth rates.[94]

Nonessential amino acids make up the largest percentage of the amino acid pool in the fetal body. The desired quantities of these amino acids for parenteral solutions are not known. It is thought that they should be provided in a balanced formulation. Pediatric solutions differ from adult solutions by providing glutamic acid and aspartic acid with lower glycine concentrations.[1,129]

FAT

Long-chain fatty acids are essential in the newborn for brain development and appear to be important for gene expression and other molecular mechanisms.[131] Essential fatty acids (EFAs) include linoleic and linolenic and, in the newborn, arachidonic acid.[5] Biochemical evidence of EFA deficiency may be seen in less than 1 week in VLBW infants receiving a deficient diet, and the administration of parenteral glucose and amino acids may accelerate these abnormalities.[123] EFA deficiency results in an imbalance in fatty acid production with an overproduction of nonessential fatty acids. Clinical manifestations appearing at variable times after biochemical changes of EFA deficiency include scaly dermatitis, poor hair growth, thrombocytopenia, failure to thrive, poor wound healing, and increased susceptibility to bacterial infection. Clinical manifestations of EFA deficiency can be avoided if 3% to 4% of caloric intake is supplied as linoleic acid (approximately 0.5 g/kg/day of IV lipid).[42]

In addition to preventing EFA deficiency, lipid emulsion is a concentrated source of nonprotein calories, which promotes nitrogen retention. Preterm infants appear to have limited capability to oxidize fatty acids. This limitation may be related to deficiency of carnitine, which, in the form of acylcarnitine, promotes transfer of fatty acids into mitochondria, where oxidative metabolism occurs. However, a systematic review of randomized studies found no benefit for carnitine supplementation on weight gain, lipid utilization, or ketogenesis, so routine supplementation is not recommended.[22]

VITAMINS

The biologic role of vitamins, signs and symptoms of deficiency states, and recommended oral requirements are available in Chapter 17. Although there is not a multivitamin formulation specifically for preterm infants, the American Society for Clinical Nutrition (ASCN) has suggested that preterm infants receive 40% to 65% of the daily recommended vitamin doses for term infants and children.[110] These guidelines may result in excessive intakes of some water-soluble vitamins, particularly pyridoxine and riboflavin. Although preterm infants have limited stores of lipid-soluble vitamins because of low body fat, potential toxicity from excess administration is a concern. Vitamin A is a lipid-soluble vitamin important for tissue growth, protein synthesis, and epithelial differentiation. Vitamin A may be administered more effectively in lipid emulsion rather than dextrose amino acid solutions.[5,31] However, vitamin A supplementation has been proven to be effective in lowering chronic lung disease rates only when given by intramuscular injections three times per week.[33,130]

Vitamin E is a lipid-soluble biologic antioxidant that is deficient in preterm infants. However, daily parenteral intake of 2 to 3 mg/kg has been associated with serum levels generally in the recommended range of 1 to 2 mg/dl. Pharmacologic doses have been tried unsuccessfully for prevention of bronchopulmonary dysplasia and retinopathy of prematurity, and IV high-dose vitamin E may increase risk for sepsis.[18] Therefore, aiming for tocopherol levels greater than 3.5 mg/dl is not recommended. Vitamin K production by intestinal flora is impaired by insufficient enteral feedings and use of broad-spectrum antibiotics in infants on long-term TPN. Vitamin K is provided at the recommended dosage through parenteral pediatric multivitamin solutions.[5]

TRACE MINERALS

Although trace minerals are relatively scarce (less than 0.01% of the weight of the human body by definition), they play an important role in normal growth and development.[140] Early supplementation of selenium has shown a reduction in sepsis events.[21] Deficiencies of both zinc and copper have been identified in infants on long-term TPN not supplemented with trace minerals. Postsurgical infants with ongoing gastrointestinal losses may have negative zinc balance even if given usual zinc replacement in TPN.[109]

Manifestations of deficiency and recommendations for intake are provided in Chapter 17. Parenteral recommendations are lower than enteral, which are based on physiologic requirements. For infants not receiving frequent blood transfusions, iron therapy may be necessary by 2 months of age. Infants receiving erythropoietin therapy need additional iron supplementation, given either enterally or parenterally.[77]

INDICATIONS

Parenteral nutrition, including protein supplementation and carbohydrate at basal levels, should begin on the first day of life for preterm infants not being fed, as well as for other newborns who are not likely to tolerate enteral feedings within a few days. A preterm infant has limited nutritional stores and quickly develops negative protein balance without early supplementation. TPN continues to be a critical aspect of long-term management for neonatal surgical patients.[100] When parenteral nutrition solutions are administered through a peripheral vein, caloric intake is limited because the fluid osmolarity should not exceed 900 mOsm/L, which results in relatively limited concentrations of carbohydrate (less than 12.5% dextrose) and amino acids (less than 3%). Some recommend even more conservative limits on osmolarity for peripheral lines (500 mOsm/L).[55] When used with lipid emulsions, peripheral parenteral nutrition (PPN) allows caloric intake of about 70 to 80 kcal/kg/day and protein intake of 2.5 to 3.0 g/kg/day. This level of nutritional intake prevents catabolism and, in some cases, results in moderate growth. PPN usually is adequate for term newborns with transient bowel disease (such as may be seen after the repair of a small omphalocele) or for larger preterm infants whose enteral feedings are delayed for a few days. PPN is used commonly to supplement nutrition in newborns who are receiving partial enteral feedings. When caloric needs can be met by PPN, this route is preferred to the central route, because the catheter insertion risks of central catheters are avoided and generally the risk for infection is less.

If parenteral nutritional duration is longer than 1 week, administration of TPN solution through a central line is recommended. The placement of a central line for parenteral nutrition allows a higher carbohydrate load to be used, giving more calories with less fluid. In preterm infants at risk for a patent ductus arteriosus and pulmonary edema, diminishing fluid intake and improving nutritional status may be important aspects of management. Specific indications for TPN by a central catheter include the following:

- ELBW infants (less than 1000 g birth weight) and others who do not tolerate a significant volume of enteral feeding within the first week of age or who cannot receive adequate caloric intake by PPN
- Infants who have had gastrointestinal surgery and will have a significant delay in enteral nutrition, such as those with a gastroschisis, bowel resection after NEC, or meconium peritonitis
- Infants with chronic gastrointestinal dysfunction, such as intractable diarrhea

DATA COLLECTION

Monitoring Growth

Weight loss or insufficient weight gain is the initial effect of inadequate caloric intake. Linear growth, although less affected, is diminished after long periods of poor nutrition. Because of "brain sparing," head circumference growth is the least affected. Measurements should be obtained in a standardized fashion and recorded weekly.

Fetal weight gain in utero at each week of gestation is currently used as the standard to assess adequacy of postnatal growth. In the midtrimester (24 to 27 weeks' gestation), expected weight gain is 1.5% of body weight.[123] Charts are available to monitor postnatal growth rates based on data from a large preterm population, although

for long-term monitoring, use of growth curves from normal populations may be more appropriate, as available from the World Health Organization (WHO).[136]

Minimum monitoring of growth should consist of the following:

- Weigh daily, or more frequently in ELBW infants with rapidly changing extracellular fluid status. Maintenance of a thermostable environment with minimal handling of ELBW infants can be achieved through the use of in-bed scales. Strict attention to consistency of technique during the weighing process is essential to obtain accurate, reliable measurements.[128] Monitoring weight gain on a weekly basis in grams per kilogram of weight gained daily (g/kg/day) may help in reducing postnatal growth restriction and positively affect long-term neurodevelopmental outcome. An ideal rate of weight gain for ELBW infants appears to be 18 to 21 g/kg/day.[39]
- Measure length weekly.
- Measure head circumference weekly.

Biochemical Monitoring

In addition to anthropometric measurements, biochemical parameters may be monitored to assess nutritional adequacy. Periodic assessment of calcium, phosphorus, and alkaline phosphatase levels is important to detect metabolic disturbances associated with osteopenia.[137] Tests for protein malnutrition include serum total protein, albumin, transferrin, retinol-binding protein, and transthyretin (prealbumin); the latter two are suggested primarily for preterm infants.[6,43] Routine clinical use of these measurements awaits greater definition of normal variation and independent effects of systemic illness and medications.

Biochemical monitoring of the infant's physiologic status is necessary to avoid complications of TPN. Usefulness of the laboratory data should be balanced with the economic costs and risks from iatrogenic blood losses for the infant (Table 16-1).

When serum electrolyte levels are abnormal, urinary electrolyte levels may be useful to clarify sodium and potassium requirements (e.g., if body sodium is depleted, low urine concentration would be expected).

T A B L E 16-1	METABOLIC MONITORING FOR INFANTS RECEIVING PARENTERAL NUTRITION	

	FREQUENCY	
VARIABLE	ACUTE	STABLE
Electrolytes, BUN	Daily	2×/wk
Calcium, phosphorus	Weekly	Biweekly
Alkaline phosphatase	—	Biweekly
Serum glucose screen	q8hr	Daily
Urine glucose	q8hr	Daily
Hemoglobin/hematocrit	Daily	Weekly
Liver function:		
Bilirubin	2×/wk	PRN
Transaminase	Weekly	Biweekly
Triglyceride*	—	Weekly

BUN, Blood urea nitrogen; *PRN*, as needed.
*When on lipid emulsion.

TREATMENT

Vascular Access

UMBILICAL ARTERY CATHETERS AND UMBILICAL VEIN CATHETERS

Umbilical artery catheters (UACs) and umbilical vein catheters (UVCs) are commonly placed in sick newborns to provide vascular access for IV fluids, blood samplings, and blood pressure monitoring. Because of the risks for thromboembolic and infection complications, these lines generally are removed as soon as possible when no longer needed. Optimally UACs should not be left in place greater than 5 days, although UVCs can be used up to 14 days if managed aseptically.[29,44,85]

PERIPHERAL AND MIDLINE CATHETERS

If continued venous access is necessary after this time, a peripheral, midline, or peripherally inserted central catheter (PICC) can be placed. The type of line used is determined by the anticipated length of time needed and the osmolarity of the substances to be infused.[55]

Peripheral IV lines are indicated for short-term IV access. A midline catheter, which is threaded to the proximal portion of an extremity or neck, can provide longer IV access than a peripheral IV line when prolonged peripheral strength TPN is indicated. Midline catheters appear to be associated with lower rates of phlebitis than short peripheral catheters and with lower rates of infection and cost than central lines.[70]

PERIPHERALLY INSERTED CENTRAL CATHETERS

A PICC line can provide maximal nutritional intake when long-term parenteral access is necessary.[3] Percutaneous placement of a 1.9-Fr to 3.0-Fr Silastic (silicone) or polyurethane catheter can be performed routinely in even the smallest of neonatal patients by trained nurses and physicians.[87,91,106] The catheter usually is placed in the antecubital or axillary veins in the arms; however, leg, scalp, or external jugular veins may be used to achieve central access. Veins that may be needed for percutaneous central line placement should not be sites for routine venipuncture (see Chapter 7).

Percutaneous line placement involves stabilization of the vein, maximum barrier precautions (sterile gloves, gown, large drape, masks), and antiseptic preparation of the skin with 2% chlorhexidine or povidone-iodine and alcohol product.[65,85,107] Infrared vein detectors or ultrasound may be used as adjuncts to identify appropriate veins for PICC cannulation.[19,92] Fully equipped prepackaged kits are available for this procedure from a number of manufacturers. Most kits include an insertion needle that is used to puncture and tunnel through the subcutaneous tissue before entering the vein. Once the needle is within the vein, the catheter, which has been flushed with heparinized saline solution, is passed through the needle into the vein and advanced to a premeasured distance, which is the estimated location of the superior vena cava.[55] The catheter tip position should be documented radiographically. The addition of heparin to IV fluids is commonly used by practitioners to prevent occlusion of vascular catheters. However, there is no indisputable evidence for this practice.[104,105]

BROVIAC CATHETER

Large-bore Silastic catheters (Broviac) are placed surgically in infants in whom the percutaneous method is not successful and long-term access is anticipated. Generally, the catheters are placed in the internal or external jugular veins or common facial vein by cutdown and threaded to a central venous site, but can also be placed via the femoral vein. The distal end is tunneled subcutaneously and exited through the anterior chest wall or thigh if placed in the leg.[80] The catheter must be secured and dressed under sterile conditions.

OTHER VASCULAR ACCESS OPTIONS

Other sites that may be used for TPN infusion on a short-term basis include subclavian, jugular, and femoral veins. Some centers use a UVC for short-term parenteral nutrition when another site is not feasible.

Composition of Infusate

CARBOHYDRATE

The prime source of calories for the neonate usually is dextrose. Peripherally, 10% to 12% solution is used. When central access is obtained, a 15% to 30% dextrose concentration may be used. The glucose load is increased if either the infusion rate or glucose concentration of the infusate is increased. Too rapid an increase in glucose load may exceed an infant's carbohydrate tolerance and result in hyperglycemia. A rapid decrease in the infusion rate or the glucose concentration of the infusate may result in hypoglycemia.

When calculating caloric intake, use the following:

$$1 \text{ g dextrose} = 3.4 \text{ kcal}$$

or

$$100 \text{ ml/kg of } D_{10}W = 34 \text{ kcal/kg}$$

or

$$100 \text{ ml/kg of } D_{30}W = 102 \text{ kcal/kg}$$

The glucose infusion rate (GIR) can be calculated as follows:

$$\text{GIR (mg/kg/min)}$$
$$= \frac{[\text{g glucose/day} \times 1000}{1440 \text{ (min/day)}]} / \text{weight (kg)}$$

Endogenous glucose production is approximately 4 mg/kg/min. Parenteral nutrition infusions should start with a GIR between 5 and 6 mg/kg/min for VLBW and ELBW infants.[127]

Daily increases in dextrose concentration or fluid volume to increase carbohydrate administration by 2.0 mg/kg/min usually are tolerated. ELBW infants may be carbohydrate intolerant, and initial GIR should be lower (4 or 5 mg/kg/min) for these infants. An insulin infusion may be considered for ELBW infants experiencing persistent hyperglycemia with physiologic glucose infusion rates.[41] Glucose infusion rates should not exceed 13 mg/kg/min unless severe hypoglycemia is ensuing. Blood glucose determinations and screening for glucosuria should be performed several times each day when glucose delivery is initiated or altered.

LIPIDS

Lipid emulsion at a rate of 0.5 to 1 g/day/100 kcal is sufficient to prevent EFA deficiency; however, additional lipids should be provided to supplement nonprotein caloric intake and support growth.[123] Lipids should never make up more than 50% of total caloric intake. Fat emulsions should be given cautiously, beginning with 0.5 to 1 g/kg/day and advanced 0.5 g/kg every 1 to 2 days as tolerated to 3 g/kg/day maximum. Fat emulsions are available as either 10% or 20%, but the 20% concentration is universally used for VLBW infants, because its lower phospholipid concentration results in lower plasma levels of triglyceride and cholesterol and less fluid administration (Table 16-2).[96]

Emulsified fat particles are similar in size and metabolic rate to naturally occurring chylomicrons. Most are cleared through passage in the adipose and muscle tissue. The capillary endothelial lipoprotein lipase hydrolyzes triglycerides and phospholipids, generating free fatty acids (FFAs), glycerol, and other glycerides. Most of the FFAs diffuse into the adipose tissue for reesterification and storage. A small portion circulates to be used by other tissues for fuel or for conversion by the liver into very-low-density lipoprotein. Extremely preterm and SGA infants with decreased adipose tissue have prolonged clearance of fat emulsion. In general, because complications of lipids are related to delay in clearance, lipids should be infused over a 24-hour period to provide the lowest hourly rate.[96] Faster rates than 0.2 g/kg/hr for lipid infusions have been associated with hyperlipidemia.[127] The rate-limiting step for lipid clearance is the metabolism by lipoprotein lipase. The use of heparin stimulates the release of this enzyme and may enhance clearance of IV lipids. Carbohydrate

TABLE 16-2	COMPOSITION OF FAT EMULSIONS	
COMPOSITION	INTRALIPID (CLINITEC) 20%	LIPOSYN II (ABBOTT) 20%
Fatty Acid Distribution (%)		
Linoleic acid	50	54.5
Oleic acid	26	22.4
Palmitic acid	10	10.5
Linolenic acid	9	8.3
Stearic acid	3.5	4.2
Components (%)		
Soybean oil	20	20
Safflower oil	—	—
Egg phospholipids	1.2	1.2
Glycerin	2.25	2.5
Caloric contents (kcal/dl)	200	200
Osmolarity (mOsm/L)	260	292

also must be administered with fat to facilitate fatty acid oxidation and to promote FFA clearance.

AMINO ACID SOLUTION

There are multiple amino acid solutions available for neonatal and infant parenteral use. Each solution is sterile, is hypertonic, and contains crystalline amino acids. Each solution provides a mixture of essential and nonessential amino acids and may or may not contain taurine and a soluble form of tyrosine. The amino acid formulation provides a well-tolerated nitrogen source for nutritional support. The essential amino acids typically found in formulations are leucine, isoleucine, lysine, valine, histidine, phenylalanine, threonine, methionine, tryptophan, and cystine. The nonessential amino acids that are typically included are alanine, arginine, proline, glutamic acid, serine, glycine, and aspartic acid. The composition of amino acid varies by manufacturer.

A minimum quantity of energy substrates must be provided for effective utilization of parenteral protein. For ELBW infants, approximately 40 kcal/kg/day of carbohydrates or fat and 1.5 g/kg/day of protein are necessary for resting metabolic needs to prevent catabolism. However, urinary protein losses are greatest for preterm infants, so additional supplementation is needed to prevent protein deficits. For each gram of protein provided above the basal amount, approximately 10 kcal of nonprotein energy is needed.[34,40,123]

Contraindications to amino acid administration include untreated anuria, hypersensitivity to the solution, or inborn errors of metabolism, including those involving branched-chain amino acid metabolism, such as maple syrup urine disease and isovaleric acidemia.

ELECTROLYTES

Sodium and potassium may be supplied with chloride, acetate, or phosphate anions. The daily chloride requirement is approximately 3 mEq/kg/day and should be balanced with acetate to avoid alkalosis or acidosis (acetate is converted to bicarbonate). Amino acid preparations also supply anions that must be recognized to calculate a balanced anion solution. For example, TrophAmine supplies 1 mEq of acetate per gram of protein. On the other hand, cysteine addition to the TPN solution reduces the pH, necessitating buffering with acetate.

MINERALS

Phosphorus may be provided as sodium or potassium phosphate. Calcium may be provided as 10% calcium gluconate (9.7 mg of elemental calcium/100 mg of salt). Both calcium gluconate and potassium phosphate have relatively high levels of aluminum and should be used judiciously for chronic TPN in infants with renal dysfunction (see discussion of aluminum toxicity under Trace Elements later in this chapter).[54] When preparing a solution with both calcium and phosphate, care must be taken to avoid calcium phosphate precipitation, which may limit the intake of these important minerals. Magnesium is supplied as magnesium sulfate.

If one is using a potassium phosphate solution at pH 7.4, 4.4 mEq of potassium supplies 93 mg of elemental phosphorus (3 mM). When a solution of sodium phosphate is used at pH 7.4, 4.0 mEq of sodium is given with each 93 mg of elemental phosphorus.

CALCIUM

- Because of increased risk for precipitation, calcium chloride generally should not be used (but may be considered for an infant at risk for aluminum toxicity).
- An elevation in ambient temperature, increased storage time, rise in pH, and

decrease in protein or glucose concentration may increase the likelihood of precipitation. The addition of cysteine, which lowers solution pH, may enhance calcium and phosphate solubility.[129]

- When one is preparing the solution, calcium and phosphate salts should be added separately, but not in sequence, during the last stages of solution mixing. The solubility of the added calcium should be calculated from the volume at the time the calcium is added, not the final volume.
- The use of a physiologic ratio of calcium to phosphorus (1.8:1) in the TPN solution allows increased concentration of these minerals.[88,112]

VITAMINS

A preparation approximating the American Medical Association's recommended formulation of IV vitamins is available (MVI-Ped). The daily recommended dose is one vial for infants weighing more than 3 kg, 65% vial for infants 1 to 3 kg, and 30% vial for infants less than 1 kg.[5]

TRACE ELEMENTS

Zinc is supplied as zinc sulfate. Serum zinc levels usually approximate the maternal levels at birth and decline over the first week of life. Zinc supplementation should be considered from the time parenteral nutrition is initiated.[21] It may be important to initiate zinc intake earlier in neonates with intestinal loss, such as after gastrointestinal surgery.

Copper is supplied as cupric sulfate. Approximately two thirds of stored copper is accumulated during the last trimester. Therefore, a preterm infant may need early supplementation but a term infant has adequate hepatic stores for at least several weeks.

Because copper is excreted through the biliary system, this mineral should be removed from parenteral fluids for infants with cholestasis.[140]

Selenium, manganese, and *chromium* salts are commonly provided in long-term parenteral nutrition. Supplementing very preterm infants with selenium is associated with reduction in sepsis.[32] Manganese supplementation should not be provided to infants with cholestasis. The chromium dose may be reduced or discontinued in an infant with impaired renal function. Some studies have suggested that manganese and chromium should not be provided in parenteral nutrition.[21,49]

Traces of aluminum are incorporated into parenteral solutions during processing.[64] Although aluminum is not known to have a physiologic role in the body, high aluminum levels have been associated with bone disease, encephalopathy, anemia, and hepatic cholestasis and may contribute to neurodevelopmental damage in preterm infants on chronic parenteral nutrition.[14] Infants with disturbance of renal clearance are at greatest risk for aluminum loading. The U.S. Food and Drug Administration requires manufacturers to report the aluminum content of parenteral products.[54]

Definitions of safe and potentially toxic levels of contamination are available.[7] Clinicians should attempt to reduce aluminum intake and should monitor levels for infants at highest risk.[4]

Table 16-3 outlines a suggested composition for a TPN solution (guideline only). Even in the most knowledgeable hands, accurate calculation and ordering of parenteral nutrition for preterm or ill infants is a complex task. Online TPN ordering programs are available in many units to assist the clinician with this task. Use of such programs has been shown to decrease order entry errors.[69] The Case Study illustrates considerations in writing orders for TPN solutions.

CASE STUDY

The following case example illustrates considerations in writing orders for total parenteral nutrition (TPN).

History

A male infant born at 26 weeks of gestation at 900 g is now 10 days old and unable to be fed because he has developed necrotizing enterocolitis (NEC). Because there will be a prolonged delay in enteral alimentation, a central vein catheter is placed for TPN. He is currently receiving $D_{10}W$ at 140 ml/kg with maintenance electrolytes. His current weight is 850 g. Serum electrolytes and blood glucose are normal. The approach to calculating TPN requirements is as follows.

Caloric Requirement

Because the patient has already had a significant postpartum period without adequate nutrition, achieving caloric intake necessary for growth is a very important part of his care. The infant will probably

Continued

CASE STUDY—cont'd

require 100 kcal/kg or more for tissue repair and growth. We will begin with approximately 60 to 70 kcal/kg (the birth weight is used until weight gain is established) and advance the intake daily to reach this level.

Carbohydrate

Initially, a dextrose load just above what has been previously tolerated should be used. Thus the patient may receive $D_{12.5}W$ at approximately 140 ml/kg/day; the volume could vary depending on the infant's fluid requirements.

This represents:

$$12.5 \text{ g /dl} \times 140 \text{ ml/kg} = 17.5 \text{ g glucose/kg}$$

$$17.5 \text{ g glucose/kg} \times 3.4 \text{ kcal/g glucose} = 60 \text{ kcal/kg}$$

Fat

Lipid emulsion should be added to increase the caloric intake, starting with 1.0 g/kg/day.

$$5 \text{ ml/kg } 20\% \text{ lipid emulsion } (1.0 \text{ g} \times 2 \text{ kcal/ml} = 10 \text{ kcal/kg/day}$$

Thus the total nonnitrogen calories on the first day of TPN is 70 (60 + 10).

Protein

Provision of protein nutrition is critical to this preterm infant for growth and to repair damaged tissues. The initial amino acid replacement is 2.5 to 3 g/kg/day.

Electrolytes

The patient should receive maintenance sodium ion (approximately 3 mEq/kg) and potassium ion (2 to 3 mEq/kg) unless there are excessive renal or gastrointestinal losses.

Anions

Balancing anions is the next consideration. The 3 g/kg of amino acids, if given as TrophAmine, adds approximately 3 mEq/kg of acetate to the solution (1 mEq acetate/1 g amino acids). If 3 mEq/kg of potassium is provided as potassium chloride, the solution has balanced anions.

Giving 3 mEq/kg of sodium as sodium phosphate provides approximately 2.2 mM/kg of elemental phosphorus:

$$(3 \text{ mM PO}_4/4 \text{ mEq Na}^+) = (3 \text{ mEq Na}^+/\text{kg}) = 2.25 \text{ mM PO}_4$$

Minerals, Vitamins, and Trace Elements

Calcium, magnesium, phosphorus, vitamins, and trace elements should be ordered at this point. Calcium initially should be started at 2 to 3 mEq/kg/day but may be increased as tolerated with growth to 4 to 5 mEq/kg/day.

Use of an online TPN ordering program may assist the clinician by automating many of these calculations.[69]

TPN Orders

Thus the TPN orders would be written for this patient as follows:

125 g Dextrose ($D_{12.5}W$) with the Following per Liter to Run 5.3 ml/hr	Quantity Provided per kg/Day (in 140 ml):
20 g amino acids	2.8 g amino acids
20 mEq potassium as potassium chloride	2.8 mEq K$^+$
	2.8 mEq Cl$^-$
20 mEq sodium as sodium phosphate	2.8 mEq Na$^+$
15 mM phosphate*	2.1 mM Phos
20 mEq calcium	2.8 mEq Ca^{2+}
2 mEq magnesium	0.3 mEq
21.7 ml MVI-Ped	3 ml/day
1.3 ml trace element solution†	0.18 ml

Run 20% lipid emulsion at 0.14 ml/hr for 24 hr (approximately 0.5 g/kg of lipids/day).
*3 mM of sodium phosphate = 4 mEq sodium; if potassium phosphate is used, 3 mM of potassium phosphate = 4.4 mEq potassium.
†Commercially available trace element solution (Multitrace4—Neonatal, includes zinc, copper, manganese, and chromium).

Progression

On subsequent days, the dextrose concentration and lipids would be advanced slowly to increase the caloric intake to requirement as tolerated. The quantity of protein would also be increased to about 4 g/kg/day.

Preparing the Solution

Solutions should be prepared in the hospital pharmacy under a laminar flow hood in a work area isolated from traffic and contaminated supplies. There should be quality control checks to monitor for sterility breaks in equipment, personnel, environment, and solutions.

Because many additives potentially can be insoluble in combination, a mixing sequence should be established that separates the most incompatible ingredients. Storage increases the risk for microbial contamination; therefore TPN solutions should be prepared on the day they are needed.[75] However, to be able to provide an amino acid infusion to preterm infants immediately after

TABLE 16-3	**SUGGESTED COMPOSITION FOR DAILY INTRAVENOUS NUTRITION REGIMEN**

COMPONENT	DAILY AMOUNT
Calories	
Dextrose 3.4 kcal/g	10-15 g/kg
Lipids 2.0 kcal/ml (20%) solution	1-3 g/kg
Protein (6.25 g protein = 1 g N_2)	3.5-4 g/kg
Electrolytes	
Sodium	3 mEq/kg
Potassium	2-3 mEq/kg
Chloride	3-4 mEq/kg
Acetate	3 mEq/kg
Phosphate	2 mM/kg
Calcium	3 mEq/kg
Magnesium	0.3 mEq (range 0.25-0.5 mEq/kg) or 20 mg/kg (range 10-40 mg/kg) of elemental magnesium
Vitamins	
MVI-Ped	1 vial*
Vitamin A	0.7 mg
Thiamine (B_1)	1.2 mg
Riboflavin (B_2)	1.4 mg
Niacin	17 mg
Pyridoxine (B_6)	1 mg
Ascorbic acid (C)	80 mg
Ergocalciferol (D)	10 mcg
Vitamin E	7 mg
Pantothenic acid	5 mg
Cyanocobalamin	1 mcg
Folate	140 mcg
Vitamin K	200 mcg
Trace Elements	
Zinc (zinc sulfate)[†]	300 mcg/kg
Copper (cupric sulfate)[†]	20 mcg/kg
Manganese sulfate[†]	5 mcg/kg
Chromium chloride[†]	0.2 mcg/kg
Selenium	2 mcg/kg

*MVI Pediatric (Astra Pharmaceuticals), reduced amount provided for very-low-birth-weight infants (see text).

[†]As Multitrace-4 Neonatal (American Regent Laboratories, Inc.).

admission, some units maintain a "stock" amino acid solution (10% dextrose with 2 to 3 g of amino acids per 100 ml).[120]

Administering the Total Parenteral Nutrition Solution

Proper administration of the TPN solution is as important as its preparation in preventing complications. The label on the solution always should be checked to correctly identify the patient, using at least two identifiers, and to verify current formulation order.

Standardized procedures must be established to avoid infectious complications from solution contamination. Solutions on the nursing units may be returned to the pharmacy for additives before hanging, but no additives should be placed in the solution once it is hanging. The bag or bottle of TPN solution should be changed every 24 hours, and the tubing administration sets should be changed no more frequently than every 72 to 96 hours. Lipid emulsions and tubing should be changed every 24 hours.[9,55,65,74,85] Polyvinyl chloride tubing and IV bags containing phthalates should be avoided to reduce potential toxicity from plasticizers.[56,86]

Exposure of TPN to light generates peroxides, which induce vasoconstriction and oxidant stress associated with bronchopulmonary dysplasia. Photoprotection of bags, syringes, and tubing used to deliver TPN and lipids may reduce the oxidant effect on the lungs and mesenteric blood flow. Light shielding also appears to diminish oxidative stress and alterations of lipid metabolism, resulting in lower levels of triglyceride and better substrate delivery. Amber-colored tubing may be used for this purpose.[24,45,60,61]

Changes in TPN infusion rates result in changes in glucose delivery to the newborn and may lead to hypoglycemia or hyperglycemia if the glucose homeostatic mechanisms do not adjust fast enough. Reactive hypoglycemia may occur if the glucose load is abruptly reduced or discontinued such as from loss of vascular access or rapid decrease in dextrose concentration or infusion rate.[11] Parenteral nutrition solutions must infuse at a constant rate via an infusion pump. Infusion rates should not be rapidly increased or decreased. If the parenteral nutrition infusion is suddenly discontinued because of a clotted catheter or accidental removal, an appropriate solution with dextrose should be infused via a peripheral vein and blood glucose should be monitored closely.

Use of parenteral nutrition may increase an infant's risk for hyperglycemia during surgery. Because rapid fluid infusions may be necessary during operative procedures, the TPN solution should be discontinued and replaced with a physiologic infusate during the perioperative period. After surgery, TPN should be as when the patient is euglycemic, with recent evidence of early postoperative protein tolerance and improved protein balance.[97]

Tapering of the TPN solution occurs as the infant begins to tolerate enteral feedings. When the patient is taking approximately two thirds of the necessary calories enterally, the central line may be removed.

Administering Fat Solution

Rapid infusion of the fat emulsion may exceed its clearance rate from the body and accentuate complications; therefore fat emulsions should not be infused faster than 0.15 g/kg/hr.[5,96] Lipids generally are given through a Y-site connection to bypass the filter in the TPN line or may be given through a separate venous site. However, some hospitals use a combined dextrose, amino acid, and lipid solution known as three-in-one or total nutrient admixture (TNA).[99,110] A 1.2-micron filter is used with this solution to remove certain drug precipitates (Ca/PO_4), air, and *Candida,* but is not effective in removing bacteria. The decision to use TNA should be approached with caution in infants. Lipid emulsions increase the pH of the TPN solution, limiting the amount of calcium and phosphorus that can be delivered because of the risk for precipitation. Precipitates are particularly difficult to detect in TNA, which is a milky solution. High concentration of calcium and low pH of the solution also can disrupt TNA, causing it to "crack" and leading to separation of oil from the rest of the solution. One must store the admixture emulsion at an ambient temperature below 28° C to prevent coalescence.[67]

When administering lipids to ill infants receiving other infusions, care must be taken to ensure that medications are compatible with lipids or medications must be provided by a separate IV route to prevent precipitation.

COMPLICATIONS

Mechanical Complications

Pneumothorax, hemothorax, hydrothorax, air embolism, thromboembolism, catheter misplacement, cardiac perforation, and tamponade are all recognized complications of Broviac, subclavian, or jugular catheter insertions. Potential mechanical complications of percutaneous central lines include catheter occlusion, accidental dislodgement, erythematous tracking, phlebitis, thrombosis, superior vena cava syndrome, catheter migration, and catheter entrapment or breakage.[82,87,89,90] A pleural or pericardial effusion may be blood or chyle or may be a signal that the catheter has eroded into the pleural or pericardial space. The effusion may be the infusate. Therefore chest x-ray examination is necessary to document correct catheter placement before a hypertonic solution is instilled, with the superior vena cava the preferred catheter tip location.

The preceding complications may occur at any time while the catheter is present. Documentation of catheter position should be repeated if there is any history of pulling or tension on the catheter or any apparent change in its external position or change in the clinical condition associated with the preceding complications.

Any signs of catheter malfunction require troubleshooting and assessment for potential interventions to salvage the line. Some clinicians will flush a partially occluded line with a thrombolytic agent, such as recombinant tissue plasminogen activator (rt-PA).[59,114] The risk of this practice must be weighed against the benefits of maintaining the central line. In most cases, if the catheter is a temporary line, it may be better to remove it and place a new line in another site.

Infectious Complications

Infections associated with the central line may occur from contamination of the solution, tubing connections, or hubs. Although organisms may contaminate the solution during preparation, usually colonization occurs with entry into the line or bag. Intermittent administration of medications, removal of blood samples through the line, or multiple tubing changes provide opportunity for organisms to contaminate the solution.

Rigid criteria for sterile preparation of the solutions are mandatory (see Preparing the Solution earlier in this chapter).

An in-line 0.22-mcm membrane filter, which is incorporated into the IV tubing, is capable of trapping bacteria and fungi (although not endotoxin) and should help minimize the risk for septicemia from a contaminated IV bag. In addition, filters lessen the risk for an air embolism. An in-line filter setup is available that decreases the number of connections.

Nothing should be added to the TPN solution after it leaves the pharmacy.

AVOIDING LINE COLONIZATION

Use of a dedicated central line team for placement, monitoring, maintenance, and troubleshooting has been found to improve line outcomes and reduce the incidence of neonatal catheter-related bloodstream infections. Line insertion and maintenance bundles, which include hand hygiene, skin antisepsis, maximal barrier precautions, strict adherence to proper hub care, and daily review of line necessity, are also important for avoiding line complications. In addition, pay attention to the following to avoid line colonization.[55,85,102,106,119]

- When changing IV fluids, one should avoid bleed-back into the catheter.
- Line setups should be designed to minimize the number of ports and connections.[63]
- Generally, medications should not be given into injection ports in the IV tubing but, rather, should be given into a dedicated heparin-locked Y-site entry port. Stopcocks are not recommended.
- The source of an infection is usually contamination with an organism that has colonized the hub or surrounding skin. Scrupulous attention to hand hygiene and disinfection of catheter tubing, hubs, ports, and connections by vigorous rubbing with 70% alcohol before tubing changes or entry are critical infection prevention strategies.[62,63,87,102]

Dressings are not routinely changed on PICC lines. If the dressing becomes nonocclusive or moistened, the site should be cleaned according to hospital protocol and redressed with a sterile transparent dressing.[55,106,107] This should be performed using sterile gloves. The exposed catheter should be remeasured to ensure that it was not inadvertently moved during this process. Dressings are changed routinely on Broviac, subclavian, jugular, and femoral catheters. Dressing changes are recommended at least weekly or more frequently if drainage is noted or the dressing is no longer occlusive.

EVALUATING INFANTS FOR INFECTIOUS DISEASE COMPLICATIONS

Central line–associated bacteremia represents an important source of nosocomial infections in the intensive care nursery. The prevalence of this complication varies by unit based on patient demographics, including birth weight, gestational age, diagnoses (proportion of surgery and medicine), and care practices.

Bacteremia must be considered in a newborn with a central line in place who exhibits signs of sepsis (e.g., temperature instability, lethargy, poor skin perfusion, increased cardiopulmonary distress, apnea). Some neonatal infections may be treated successfully with the line in place. However, if the infant remains systemically ill, even if the blood culture result is negative, the central line should be removed.[16]

Altered immune function by lipid deposition in macrophages and the reticuloendothelial system must be considered in infants with sepsis. *Malassezia furfur* is a lipophilic, opportunistic fungal organism that may cause sepsis in infants receiving long-term lipid infusions.[111] Although this organism is infrequently seen, it may contaminate the line and appear as a white film. This organism often will not grow in routine blood culture media. Specific culture techniques are necessary when *Malassezia* is suspected.[26]

Guidelines for management of an infant with a central line in place with suspected sepsis are as follows:

- The infant should be evaluated for potential sources of infection, including a general physical examination looking for non–TPN-related sources and inspection of peripheral and central venous sites for erythema.
- Laboratory assessment should include (1) complete blood cell count with platelet count and (2) aerobic blood cultures. Other cultures, including urine, tracheal aspirate,

and cerebrospinal fluid, may be indicated, based on clinical findings. A blood fungal culture should be considered if the infant has had preceding antibiotic treatment or signs of fungal infection.[12,13,57]

- A chest x-ray evaluation should be performed if the infant demonstrates signs of respiratory distress or there is a need to reassess catheter position.
- Consider decreasing or discontinuing lipid infusion until the infection has been treated for 24 to 48 hours.[8,108]
- If the infant is critically ill, the central line should be removed immediately. If the infant is stable, treatment may be considered through the line.
- A positive blood culture generally is considered to indicate bacteremia or sepsis in a newborn with a central line in place. However, the coagulase-negative *Staphylococcus*, an opportunistic organism that is a common cause of catheter-related sepsis, also is normal skin flora and frequently contaminates blood cultures. Use of ancillary diagnostic tools, such as the C-reactive protein levels and complete blood counts, are helpful to distinguish false-positive results from true infections. Some clinicians also recommend obtaining two cultures (two peripheral, or one peripheral and one from the line) before starting antibiotics. If both yield positive results, catheter-related sepsis is confirmed.[76]
- If bacteremia is documented but the sepsis signs are improved, the catheter may remain in place while being used for antibiotic treatment. One should be sure that the antibiotics are compatible with the TPN solution (to avoid stopping the TPN during the antibiotic infusion). A follow-up blood culture and close clinical monitoring are necessary to document that the infection has been treated adequately.

If a central line is pulled because of sepsis, a new central line should not be placed for 48 to 72 hours.

Metabolic Complications

GLUCOSE METABOLISM

Hyperglycemia may occur with increased carbohydrate load, especially in ELBW infants who may have inadequate endogenous insulin production or decreased sensitivity to insulin. *Hyperglycemia* is arbitrarily defined as a blood glucose concentration greater than 125 mg/dl (6.9 mmol/L) or a plasma or serum blood glucose concentration greater than 150 mg/dl (8.3 mmol/L).[101] Elevated blood sugar may lead to hyperosmolality and osmotic diuresis, resulting in dehydration. Manifestations include polyuria, glucosuria, and excessive weight loss. Serum sodium is not a reliable measure of serum osmolality if there is hyperglycemia. Direct measurement or estimate by use of the following formula is necessary:

$$\text{Serum osmolality} = (1.86)\,\text{Na}^+ + (\text{BUN}/2.8) + (\text{Glucose}/18)$$

Transient glucose intolerance may be seen with stress. If hyperglycemia occurs without apparent change in glucose infusion, the possibility of sepsis, pain, hypoxemia, intraventricular hemorrhage (especially if the infant is less than 34 weeks of gestation), glucocorticoid administration, or inadvertent increase in carbohydrate administration (mistake in preparation or rate of infusion) should be considered. Glucose intolerance also may be accentuated during infusions of lipid emulsion, especially in an ELBW infant. Discontinuation of the lipid infusion without alteration of the carbohydrate load will often eliminate hyperglycemia in this situation. Some ELBW infants remain hyperglycemic even on reduced carbohydrate intakes. Controversy still remains over the use of a continuous insulin infusion to attain adequate caloric intake. A recent Cochrane review of neonatal hyperglycemia and insulin treatment showed no improvement in outcomes with continuous insulin infusion compared with reduced glucose infusion rates.[17] Treatment with insulin varies, but the usual infant dose is 1 U/kg/min and should be reserved for severe hyperglycemia, with clinical symptoms and resistance to other medical management changes.[41] Routine use of insulin to promote growth in the preterm infant is not advised because of side effects.[10]

Hypoglycemia may result from an abrupt interruption of glucose infusion or excessive exogenous insulin administration. Manifestations of hypoglycemia include apnea, lethargy, jitteriness, and seizures. If these signs occur immediately after an interruption of the TPN infusion, an IV glucose infusion must be initiated at once, followed by close monitoring of the blood glucose to allow appropriate glucose administration. The glucose concentration of the infusate may usually be safely decreased by 5 g/dl every 12 hours. Blood glucose values should be monitored hourly until stable after each change.

AMINO ACID METABOLISM

Hyperammonemia may be seen in preterm infants given excessive protein loads. Hyperammonemia will occur also in an infant with a congenital metabolic disturbance, such as a urea cycle defect, when challenged with an amino acid load. Hyperammonemia may manifest as somnolence, lethargy, seizures, and coma. Biochemical screening is necessary to identify this complication before symptoms appear.

Azotemia may occur before hyperammonemia, but blood urea nitrogen (BUN) elevation in the first week of life of a preterm infant is usually associated with dehydration and has not been a reliable marker of protein excess.[34,132] Therefore, although daily monitoring is common in the first week, rising BUN is not an indication by itself to decrease the protein load.

CHOLESTASIS

Infants receiving TPN for more than 2 weeks frequently develop cholestatic jaundice (direct bilirubin greater than 2 mg/dl).[25,117,121] The risk appears to be greatest for the least mature infants and those receiving the longest period of TPN without enteral feeding. The cause appears to be multifactorial, including lack of bile flow stimulation, delayed enteral feedings, malnutrition, or inflammation after localized or generalized infection.[138] More recently, IV fat emulsions, particularly polyunsaturated fatty acid, are thought to contribute to cholestasis.[125] Serum amino transferases often are normal early in the clinical course. Serum albumin and prealbumin levels usually remain normal. An abnormality in hepatic synthetic function or early rise in isoenzyme levels should lead the clinician to investigate other forms of liver disease. The differential diagnosis of cholestatic jaundice includes the following:

- Bacterial sepsis
- Congenital viral infection
- Postpartum acquisition of cytomegalovirus
- Neonatal hepatitis
- Bile duct obstruction, such as biliary atresia or choledochal cyst
- Galactosemia
- Cystic fibrosis
- Alpha$_1$-antitrypsin deficiency

Management of cholestatic jaundice should include (when possible) the following:

- Increase enteral feedings as tolerated and decrease proportionately the parenteral nutrition
- Dose reduction of soybean-based IV fat emulsion[28,133]
- Eliminate copper and manganese from trace minerals in TPN
- Protect solutions from light by covering the bag and IV tubing to reduce levels of light-induced toxic peroxides[60,66]
- Trial of an agent that induces bile flow[23,72]
- For infants with short bowel syndrome, control intestinal bacterial overgrowth[58]
- Consider an alternative type of fat emulsion[47,68]

LIPID METABOLISM

High-risk infants, including preterm and SGA low-birth-weight infants, may demonstrate intolerance to fat emulsion infusions. Hyperlipidemia may result, causing elevation of triglyceride, FFA, and lipoprotein levels. In extreme cases, lactescence may be visible in serum on a spun blood specimen (increased plasma turbidity). For screening, a triglyceride level should be checked after initiation of therapy and then weekly and doses adjusted based on results. Steroid therapy may elevate the triglyceride level.[103] Transient hyperglycemia may result from lipid infusion. This complication is usually dose related and rarely requires treatment.[30]

Competitive displacement of bilirubin by FFA theoretically may increase the risk for kernicterus in preterm infants with hyperbilirubinemia. However, studies of preterm infants have indicated that lipid infusions may be used in jaundiced infants but attention to the infusion rate and monitoring of FFAs are necessary.[96]

PARENT TEACHING

In-Hospital Total Parenteral Nutrition

Clinicians caring for an ill newborn must be attentive to the involvement and emotional state of the parents. There remain a number of concerns for child abuse, foster placement, and relinquishment among infants who have been cared for in the NICU compared with healthy term newborns, especially when care has been prolonged and complex.

Clinical conditions or policies that promote separation of parents from their infant increase the risk for bonding problems. When a newborn infant cannot be fed orally, an important, normal part of the infant's care is no longer available for the parents. The placement of a central line may be frightening to parents and result in less handling and caregiving. Infants requiring continuous care, including TPN, should have primary nursing (one regularly scheduled nurse), and the parents should have regular and consistent communication with a primary physician. Care providers should attempt to keep the parents involved in other parts of the infant's care, because the parents are unable to feed the infant. Parents should be fully informed about the purpose and appropriate care of the infant's central line so they will feel comfortable handling their infant with the line in place.[55]

Home Total Parenteral Nutrition

Home parenteral nutrition has been used in infants with congenital intestinal anomalies or after massive bowel resection for NEC. TPN is initiated in the hospital. If growing and otherwise well, the infant may be a candidate for TPN at home. Issues to be addressed include ability and willingness of parents to care for the infant at home, available financial support, adequate home setting, pharmacy support services, and additional skilled nursing care needed. The infant should have a more permanent central line placed as early in the discharge process as possible. Parent teaching should begin early, including verbal and written instruction and hands-on practice and return demonstrations (Box 16-1).

Administration of TPN at home is different from hospital administration of TPN and is typically

BOX 16-1	PARENT TEACHING
	HOME ADMINISTRATION OF PARENTERAL NUTRITION

- Strict handwashing and aseptic handling of tubing connections and hubs
- Use of infusion pump
- Monitoring of site for signs of infection, phlebitis, or leaking
- Troubleshooting for occlusion, leaking, extravasation
- Evaluation for signs of systemic infection
- Emergency response to broken or dislodged catheter, loss of electrical power
- Developmental care: oral stimulation, holding, appropriate play activities
- Dressing care and changes
- Monitoring for signs and symptoms of hypoglycemia
- Securing or taping of line to avoid dislodgement with positioning and handling

managed by a pediatric gastroenterology service in conjunction with a home infusion therapy or pharmacy service. Infants often go home on a cyclic TPN regimen (12 hr/day). An ambulatory pump improves the mobility and flexibility of the parent and infant and allows a more normal life.

Compliance and success with home TPN are greatly increased when the parents understand the need for and the appropriate way to administer TPN and how to troubleshoot and care for the catheter.[46]

REFERENCES

For a full list of references, scan the QR code or visit http://booksite.elsevier.com/ 9780323320832.

17

ENTERAL NUTRITION

LAURA D. BROWN, KENDRA HENDRICKSON, RUTH EVANS, JANE DAVIS, MARIANNE SOLLOSY
ANDERSON, AND WILLIAM W. HAY, JR.

The provision of adequate and optimal nutrition to support term and preterm infants in the neonatal intensive care unit continues to be a difficult, though important, challenge. Recent research in neonatal nutrition has provided some evidence-based guidance for clinicians, resulting in the adoption of earlier, more substantial parenteral and enteral strategies for nutrition of newborn infants, particularly those born very preterm. Other research has emphasized the importance of early enteral feeding for the best support of gastrointestinal (GI) development, somatic growth, metabolic homeostasis, prevention of infection, neurodevelopment, and future health. Together, such research has demonstrated that immediate parenteral support and early enteral feedings are fundamental and not optional in neonatal management.

This chapter provides an overview of the physiology of fetal and neonatal nutrition and growth, anatomic and functional development of the GI tract, and the fundamentals of neonatal enteral nutritional requirements. More specific details about the assessment and monitoring of growth, feeding strategies and techniques, and the possible complications of enteral feeding of at-risk infants are included. The ongoing nutritional needs of infants recovering from complications of preterm birth and other disorders also are presented, as well as the elements of providing for those needs after hospital discharge.

PHYSIOLOGY

Fetal Growth

Fetal growth is regulated by complex genetic, nutritional, endocrine, environmental, and epigenetic factors.[37,76,197] Maternal factors such as prepregnancy weight, body composition, and weight gain during pregnancy directly correlate with placental[200] and fetal size.[1,34,102,192] Maternal nutrition and the quality of the maternal diet (protein, energy, vitamins, and minerals) are critically important in the regulation of placental-fetal development and therefore directly affect fetal growth. For example, a growing body of evidence shows that maternal obesity, and even modestly increased maternal body mass index (BMI), increases the risk of perinatal complications, including fetal and neonatal death,[16] increased birth weight,[152,193] and lifelong risk of obesity in the offspring.[154] Conversely, suboptimal nutrition during pregnancy can result in low birth weight and also increases the risk of metabolic complications for offspring later in life.[21,175] The growth and function of the placenta strongly determine fetal growth by providing oxygen and essential nutrients.[47,97] Critical fetal anabolic hormones, such as the insulin-like growth factors (IGF-I and IGF-II) and insulin, are regulated by circulating concentrations of nutrients and are themselves regulators of fetal nutrient uptake and metabolism. IUGR infants, who have very little glucose supply from the placenta and have very little circulating insulin, are among the smallest of infants; infants of gestational diabetic mothers, who respond to increased maternal glucose concentrations and maternal-fetal glucose delivery with increased insulin secretion, are among the largest (Figure 17-1). Thyroid hormone also contributes to fetal growth by regulation of oxidative metabolism. Infants with other endocrine deficiencies, such as those resulting from anencephaly, panhypopituitarism, or hypothyroidism, are near normal in age-specific size at birth, indicating a complex interplay between the

PURPLE type highlights content that is particularly applicable to clinical settings.

fundamentally required supply of nutrients to the fetus and the supporting roles of the fetal endocrine milieu that regulates intrauterine growth.

Gastrointestinal Development

Enteral feeding supports GI development in the preterm infant that normally would occur during fetal life. The fetal GI tract is anatomically complete by 20 to 22 weeks after conception; functional development of the GI tract begins in utero and continues into infancy (Table 17-1). In utero, the fetal intestine is exposed to nutrients and growth factors from the mother, placenta, amniotic fluid, and the fetal tissues. The fetal GI tract is in communication with the external amniotic fluid environment by 7 weeks postconception, and early development and functional priming are supplied by growth factors, enzymes, immunoglobulins, and hormones present in that fluid.[132] Fetal swallowing can be observed as early as 11 weeks' gestation.[60] The components of the amniotic fluid, including carbohydrates and amino acids, change during development, as does the volume of amniotic fluid ingested, varying from a few milliliters per day to more than 450 ml per day, or 20% of fetal weight, late in gestation.[77,83] Amniotic fluid contains growth factors that promote intestinal mucosal cell differentiation. Such growth factors and nutrients in the amniotic fluid

stimulate production of enteric hormones that act locally to promote further gut development. The timing of the appearance of GI hormones, polypeptides, neurotransmitters, and digestive enzymes in the fetus is variable, but most are present in the GI tract by the end of the first trimester of

TABLE 17-1	DEVELOPMENT OF THE HUMAN GASTROINTESTINAL TRACT: FIRST APPEARANCE OF DEVELOPMENTAL MARKERS

DEVELOPMENTAL MARKER	WEEKS OF GESTATION
Gastrulation	3
Gut tube formed, early differentiation of foregut, midgut, and hindgut	4
Gut lumen in continuity with amniotic cavity	7
Growth of intestines into umbilical cord	7
Intestinal villus formation	9
Intestines into abdominal cavity	10
Δ glucosidase, dipeptidase, lactase enzymes	10
Glucose transporters	10
Liver lobules, bile metabolism	11
Swallowing	11
Parietal cells, pancreatic islets, bile secretion	12
Stomach fundus, body, pylorus, greater and lesser curvature	14
Gastric glands	14
Intestinal crypts, elongation of intestinal villi	14
Intestinal lymph nodes	14
Differentiation of pancreatic endocrine and exocrine tissue	14
Active transport of amino acids	14
Sucking movements	19
Superficial esophageal glands	20
Gastric motility and secretion	20
Fatty acid absorption	24
Coordination of suck and swallow	33–36

Data from Lebenthal E: The impact of development of the gut on infant nutrition, *Pediatric Ann* 16:215-216, 1987; Montgomery RK, Mulberg AE, Grand RJ: Development of the human gastrointestinal tract: twenty years of progress, *Gastroenterology* 116:702-731, 1999.

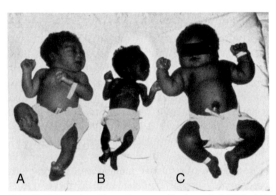

FIGURE 17-1 **Fetal nutrition and patterns of fetal growth. A,** 3200 g birth weight term appropriate-for-gestational age (AGA) infant. **B,** 1500 g term small-for-gestational age (SGA) infant who had intrauterine growth restriction (IUGR). **C,** 5200 g large-for-gestational age (LGA) macrosomic infant of a gestational diabetic mother (IDM). (Courtesy Newborn Service, University of Colorado Hospital, Denver, Colorado [W. W. Hay, Jr.].)

pregnancy. Nutrient transport systems are in place by 14 weeks for amino acids, 18 weeks for glucose, and 24 weeks for fatty acids.

After birth, the GI tract must further adapt for mucosal growth and differentiation, peristalsis, digestion of food, and absorption of nutrients. Some GI functions are "switched on" at birth (e.g., decrease in intestinal permeability, increase in mucosal lactase activity), regardless of the length of gestation. Others, however, are intrinsically "programmed" to occur at a certain postconceptual age (e.g., the onset of peristalsis at 28 to 30 weeks and the coordination of suck, swallow, and breathing at 33 to 36 weeks). Environmental influences, including colonization of the GI tract by bacteria and the introduction of nutrients into the GI tract, also affect postnatal GI and immunologic development.[9,41,119] The microbial population within the GI tract, termed the *gut microbiome,* is acquired at birth and may even begin to develop in utero with influences from the maternal microbiome.[186] Many factors influence the development of the gut microbiome, including mode of delivery (vaginal versus cesarean section), early exposure to antibiotics, maternal health conditions (such as diabetes or obesity), and the composition of the diet: breastmilk versus formula, high versus low protein formulas, cow versus human milk supplements, degree of protein hydrolysis, and inclusion of long chain–polyunsaturated fatty acids (LC-PUFAs), particularly docosahexaenoic acid (DHA).[40,124] Importantly, evidence shows that establishment of the gut microbiome during infancy may influence the development of obesity later in life.[167]

Infants born before term have both anatomic and functional limits to the digestion and tolerance of enteral feedings. Neurologic maturation is important not only for coordination of sucking, swallowing, and breathing during feeding but also for GI motility. Peristalsis in the esophagus is immature and bidirectional in the preterm infant, with forward movement of food to the stomach developing only near term.[95] Abnormal esophageal peristalsis and transient relaxations of the lower esophageal sphincter muscle likely contribute to the common problem of *gastroesophageal reflux* seen in preterm infants. Enteral feeding promotes the ongoing maturation and development of the GI tract in both term and preterm infants.[39] Once enteral feedings are established, gastric emptying rate is similar in term and preterm infants.[143,191]

Intestinal motor activity in the preterm infant is immature and disorganized compared with that in term infants, with term infants having distinct fasting phases of GI quiescence, nonmigrating motor activity, and migrating motor complexes. After feeding, term infants show a dramatic increase in the intensity of motor activity that is not observed in preterm infants. A measure of GI motility is provided by the passage of stool within 24 hours of birth in more than 95% of full-term infants; however, the more preterm the infant, the greater the delay in passing the first stool. Coordinated, mature GI motility and peristalsis with feeding develop in the preterm infant between 33 weeks and term.

Digestion occurs in the lumen of the intestine. Nutrient absorption occurs at the enterocyte interface (microvillus membrane). Protein digestion and absorption are remarkably efficient in the preterm infant despite the fact that *enterokinase,* a rate-limiting enzyme in the activation of pancreatic proteases via activation of *trypsinogen,* at 26 to 30 weeks' gestation has only 6% of the activity found in the term newborn and 10% of adult activity. In the newborn, protein digestion is aided by the activity of brush border enterocyte cytosolic peptidases. Carbohydrate absorption is limited initially by a relative deficiency of lactase, which splits lactose into glucose and galactose. Lactase in the infant of less than 34 weeks' gestation is present at only about 30% of the activity found in the normal term infant, although lactose intolerance is rare in these infants, particularly when they are fed human milk.[178] Lactase functional activity increases with feeding and approaches term levels by 10 days after birth in most preterm infants.[179] Human milk feedings increase lactase activity more than formulas. Twenty percent of dietary lactose may reach the colon in neonates. Lactose lowers fecal pH, a beneficial effect in that it promotes *Bifidobacterium* and *Lactobacillus* proliferation. Preterm infants malabsorb 10% to 30% of dietary fat because of a small bile acid pool size and relative lack of pancreatic lipase.[122] Some compensation is provided by lingual and gastric lipases, as well as the lipase present in human milk. Despite relative deficiencies in many enzymes important in nutrient processing, the preterm infant usually can digest and absorb complex nutrient mixtures such as human milk quite effectively.

Postnatal Growth of Preterm Infants

After birth, usual nutritional regimens, even when provided more aggressively, fail to produce growth rates in preterm infants that mimic normal rates of intrauterine growth, the accepted goal of nutrition for the preterm infant.[59,161] A variety of complications contribute to this growth failure, but the primary problem is that most preterm infants are fed less protein and calories immediately after birth than are needed to support normal fetal rates of protein accretion and body growth. In addition, the preterm infant is exposed to environmental factors that increase energy expenditure, including low relative humidity and radiant and convective heat losses, as well as energy-consuming demands of breathing, resistance to gravity, and the processes of digestion, absorption, and synthesis of nutrients into body structure. Stress-induced hormones that are catabolic in sick infants, particularly corticosteroids and catecholamines, limit the production and action of anabolic growth factors, particularly insulin and IGFs, further preventing normal rates of growth and weight gain at rates comparable to those of healthier infants of the same gestational age. Overall, however, even in sick or physiologically unstable infants, the principal factor causing postnatal growth failure, as well as worse neurodevelopmental outcome, is delayed and inadequate intake of protein and energy.[59,64,67]

After birth, all infants lose excess extracellular salt and water. Term infants usually lose 5% to 8% of birth weight by the third day of life. In extremely low-birth-weight (ELBW; less than 1000 g birth weight) preterm infants, normal diuresis and common fluid management strategies to limit fluid overload over the first 10 to 14 days of life usually produce a net loss of body weight. Such infants may lose 8% to 15% of birth weight, though fluid management among institutions varies considerably. Currently, mild fluid restriction that does not lead to dehydration appears safe and might decrease the incidence and/or severity of a patent ductus arteriosus, necrotizing enterocolitis (NEC), and bronchopulmonary dysplasia (BPD), and even reduce the risk of death.[22,148] Further weight loss and failure to gain weight are exacerbated by inadequate nutritional support, particularly of protein and energy. Relative fluid restriction during later stages of enteral feeding can be accomplished in milk-fed infants by concentrating nutrients in milk with human milk fortifiers or preterm or postdischarge formula powder. Deficits accumulated daily during early neonatal life may take weeks to months to replenish. Serial measurements of body length and head circumference are particularly useful in the newborn period, because linear growth and head circumference represent lean mass growth and have the potential to help predict neurodevelopmental outcome.[157] Employing validated methods, such as recumbent length boards, and training staff on correct technique will improve the validity of these measurements (Box 17-1).[53] More recent methods to assess body composition in the neonate include dual x-ray absorptiometry and air displacement plethysmography, which partition new tissue accrual into water, fat, and lean body mass components, thus helping to define needs for additional specific nutrients (protein, lipids, carbohydrates) for body growth (even during the early postnatal period of fluctuating water weight).[66] These methods are not usually available for routine clinical use and are used primarily as research tools.[164] Thus, assessment of postnatal growth is limited to following the trajectories of height, weight, and head circumference and calculating BMI or Ponderal Index (weight in grams $\times$ 100/length in centimeters^3) (Figure 17-2). Improving the capacity to accurately assess body composition, however, is fundamental for determining optimal nutrition. With current feeding practices and nutritional regimens, preterm infants develop less lean tissue than the normally growing fetus in utero. Body fat content varies among studies, from similar fat mass compared with infants born at term to excess body fat, with the excess distributed more to the intraabdominal region.[98] Early provision of both adequate calories and protein to sustain optimal nutrition is difficult without the addition of parenteral nutrition for preterm infants and sick infants of all gestational ages (see Chapter 16).

BOX 17-1 GROWTH MONITORING

1. *Weight* is subject to large variations based on fluctuations in fluid balance (e.g., presence or absence of edema, congestive heart failure, renal failure) and attached equipment (e.g., intravenous lines and boards, endotracheal tubes). Infant weight should be measured daily as follows:
   a. Use the same scale and weigh infant naked or using supportive weighing method as possible. Supportive weighing, or swaddled weights, help ensure an infant's physiologic and behavioral stability during the weighing procedure. Remove "attached" equipment if possible, or weigh similar items separately and subtract from total weight. Swaddled weights are equal to the naked weight after the weight of the diaper and blanket are subtracted. Unswaddled weights still can be used to improve accuracy for very small infants or if swaddling puts the infant at risk or interferes with the infant's care needs. In-bed scales are useful for ELBW infants or infants who become unstable with handling. An electronic scale that averages several measurements reduces movement artifact and may be useful for active infants.
   b. Reference standards for the weights of nursery equipment (e.g., diapers, intravenous boards, tubing, endotracheal tubes) should be available for nursery use.
   c. Weigh the infant at the same time daily, preferably before a feeding.
   d. Record the infant's weight, the time of weight measurement, and the scale used on the chart. Energy (calories) and fluid intake should be recorded on the same chart. This information combined with biochemical parameters (e.g., serum electrolytes, hemoglobin, albumin) and the physical examination provides the best overview of the infant's nutritional status. Once weekly a daily weight should be plotted on the appropriate preterm or term growth chart. Weekly review of the infant's weight change provides useful information on trends in overall growth or weight loss that may be overlooked in the daily charting.
2. *Crown-heel length and head circumference* are measured and recorded on admission and at least weekly thereafter. Accurate length measurements are difficult to obtain without special equipment such as a length board, but accuracy can be improved by repeated measurements and

use of the tonic-neck reflex to straighten the hip and knee. Length and head circumference monitoring are just as important as, if not more important than, weight measurements. Increase in length reflects lean mass growth and head circumference is used as an indicator of brain growth. Both measurements are predictors of neurodevelopmental outcome.[157,163]
   a. To measure the crown-heel length, two people are required for measuring patients using the statiometer: one registered nurse (RN) and one assistant. The assistant may be another RN, other NICU care team member, or parent. Position infant supine on board with head at stationary head piece and feet facing movable foot piece. The assistant positions infant's head against head piece by securing head and shoulders between hands. The top of the patient's head should touch the stationary head piece. Eyes should be facing straight up. Avoid hyperextension of the patient's neck. The RN straightens the infant's body along the center of the board. Apply gentle pressure to patient's knees and hold legs in place. Using free hand, slide foot piece until it is positioned firmly against infant's heels. Toes should point directly up. Measurements with one lower limb extended may result in less patient discomfort than when both lower limbs are extended.[156] Repeat three times.
   b. Head circumference is obtained using a paper or soft tape measure. Record the largest measurement obtained with the tape placed over the frontal, parietal, and occipital prominences.
3. *The Ponderal index* (or weight-length index; see Figure 17-2) is used to assess "quality" of growth. The Ponderal index is calculated as the weight in grams multiplied by 100, divided by the cube of the length in centimeters. True organ growth and tissue accretion are accompanied by increases in both weight and length and can be evaluated partly using the Ponderal index.
4. *Biochemical monitoring* of the growing infant may include periodic measurement of serum electrolytes, calcium, phosphorus, alkaline phosphatase, total protein, albumin, and hemoglobin. These data can be used to help prevent specific deficiencies in the diet, such as hyponatremia in preterm infants with excessive renal solute losses or hypophosphatemia with increased alkaline phosphatase as seen in rickets and osteopenia.

Assessment of Growth and Nutritional Status

The generally accepted goal of postnatal nutrition for preterm infants is to achieve and maintain the normal rate of intrauterine growth (Figure 17-3). Unfortunately, there is no clear standard for normal fetal growth. Many growth curves have been developed from anthropometric measurements taken at birth in populations of infants born at different gestational ages.[70,149] Because preterm birth is not a normal outcome, cross–sectional anthropometric

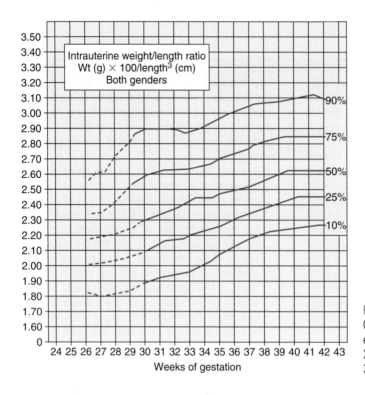

FIGURE 17-2 Ponderal index. (From Lubchenco L, Hansman C, Boyd E: Intrauterine growth in length and head circumference as estimated from live birth at gestational ages from 26 to 42 weeks. Reproduced with permission from *Pediatrics* 37:403-408, 1966. © American Academy of Pediatrics.)

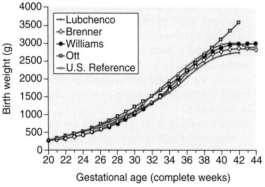

FIGURE 17-3 Fetal growth by selected references.

measurements obtained at birth do not accurately describe normal growth parameters for any given gestational age. Growth curves based on serial ultrasound measurements of fetuses who were born at term in healthy condition provide continuous, rather than cross-sectional, data that correlate better with the expected fetal growth rate of a particular fetus or newborn[38,194] (Figure 17-4). Such intrauterine growth data are not yet available, however. Most rely, therefore, on growth charts derived from birth weights and ultrasound-validated gestational ages to monitor growth trajectories in preterm infants. The most recent of these are based on data from nearly 4 million births.[69] For the average, appropriately grown, preterm infant, expected weight gain is approximately 15 to 20 g/kg/day.

We lack good methods to assess nutritional adequacy over time in very small infants. Rates of change in anthropometric measurements provide some retrospective information, but they do not tell us what an infant needs to maintain a normal growth rate (see Box 17-1). Too often, growth charts simply document continuing and all too often worsening growth, highlighting the failure to provide adequate nutrition during the previous days to weeks. Indirect calorimetry offers some advantage for determining at least the energy requirements for growth, but instruments that are clinically practical and sufficiently accurate to quantify nutrient metabolism in tiny infants are not yet available. Similarly, application of stable isotope methodology to measure utilization and oxidation rates of individual nutrients remains confined to large medical centers with expensive and sophisticated mass spectrometry facilities. Evaluation of an

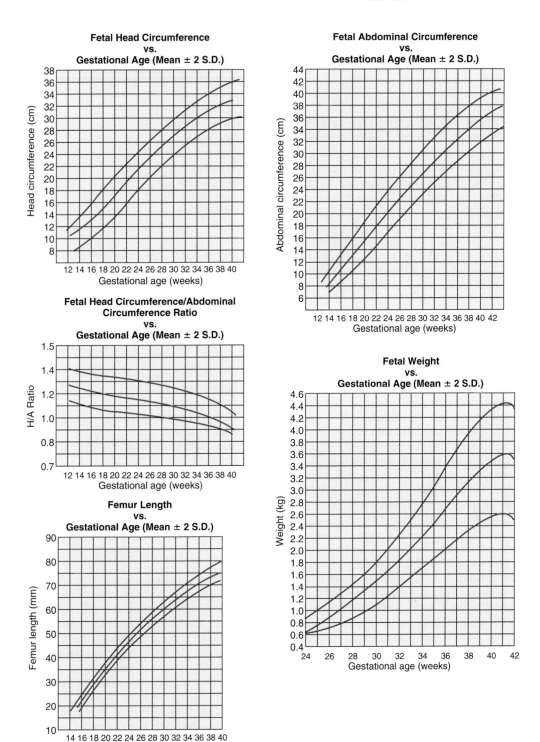

FIGURE 17-4 Composite of serial fetal body measurements by ultrasound examination. *H/A,* Head/abdominal circumference; *S.D.,* standard deviation.

individual infant's immediate nutrient requirements and responses to the administration of different mixtures and amounts of nutrients remains an elusive but still necessary goal.

NUTRITIONAL REQUIREMENTS

Nutritional requirements should be considered in general categories: energy (or calories), protein, carbohydrate, fats, minerals and solutes, and vitamins. Water requirements and limits also must be considered when designing nutrition support strategies. The source, complexity, and constituents of these nutrients are important, as well as the route of administration. Box 17-2 lists commonly used nutritional conversion factors and formulas. See Chapter 16 for parenteral nutrition and Chapter 18 for breastfeeding.

Energy

Negative energy balance is frequent in preterm infants because they have limited energy stores, high energy expenditures, and low intake. Energy requirements are determined by an infant's total energy expenditure, energy excretion, and energy stored in new tissue as growth. Total energy expenditure can be subdivided into contributions of basal metabolic rate, activity, thermoregulation, and the energy costs of digestion and metabolism. Energy excretion is composed of fecal and urinary losses, as well as heat lost by radiation and evaporation. Feeding infants under thermoneutral temperature conditions in humidified incubators, starting at admission to the neonatal intensive care unit (NICU), substantially decreases energy expenditure in preterm infants. Estimates of energy requirements for growing preterm infants are shown in Table 17-2. The large range of these estimates reflects the variability of infant activity and environmental conditions. Therefore it is essential to adjust nutrient delivery to individual requirements. In general, muscle activity does not contribute much to total energy expenditure,[187] though older studies of infants with BPD did seem to support this. Today, however, respiratory distress in such infants is less common and less severe, partly due to improved respiratory care. Most such infants also are tightly swaddled and do not move much.[89]

Caloric requirements for the healthy term breastfed infant average 90 to 100 kcal/kg/day.[86]

BOX 17-2	COMMONLY USED CONVERSION FACTORS AND FORMULAS

Energy
   1 kcal = 4.184 kJ
Gross energy (kcal/g)
   Protein = 5.65
   Carbohydrate = 3.95
   Fat = 9.25
Metabolizable energy (kcal/g)
   Protein = 4
   Carbohydrate = 4
   Fat = 9
Protein
   Total protein (g/dl) = total nitrogen (g/dl) × 6.25
Vitamins
   1 International unit vitamin A = 0.3 retinol equivalent
      = 0.3 mcg retinol
      = 1.8 mcg beta-carotene
   400 International units vitamin D = 10 mcg vitamin D
   1 International unit vitamin E = 1 mg DL-α-tocopherol
Minerals
   1 mEq Na = 1 mmol Na = 23 mg Na
   1 mEq K = 1 mmol K = 39 mg K
   1 mEq Cl = 1 mmol Cl = 35 mg Cl
   2 mEq Ca = 1 mmol Ca = 40 mg Ca
   1 mmol P = 31 mg P
Osmolarity (mOsm/L) = Osmolality (mOsm/kg H_2O) × kg H_2O/L solution
Renal solute load (mOsm/dl) = [Protein (g/dl)] × 4 + [Na + K + Cl (mEq/dl)]
Potential renal solute load (mOsm/dl) = [Protein (g/dl)] × 5.7 + [Na + K + Cl (mEq/dl)] + [P (mg/dl)/31]

Formula-fed term infants need slightly more, up 100 to 110 kcal/kg/day, due to less efficient nutrient absorption from the GI tract, although still lower than the energy requirements of preterm infants. Caloric requirements for very-low-birth-weight (VLBW) preterm infants (less than 1500 g) are 110 to 130 kcal/kg/day for enterally fed preterm infants, but slightly lower due to better efficiency, 85 to 95 kcal/kg/day, for parenterally fed infants.[84] Increased energy requirements can be anticipated during sepsis, acute and chronic respiratory illness when increased work of breathing and other motor activity is documented and is excessive, and recovery

TABLE 17-2	ESTIMATED DAILY ENERGY REQUIREMENT (kcal/kg) FOR ENTERALLY FED PRETERM INFANTS		
FACTOR	AMERICAN ACADEMY OF PEDIATRICS	EUROPEAN SOCIETY OF GASTROENTEROLOGY AND NUTRITION	RANGE
Energy Expenditure			
Resting metabolic rate	40-50		45-50
Activity	0-5		15-20
Thermoregulation	0-5		
Synthesis	15		
Energy stored	20-30		
Energy excreted	15		29-41
Total requirements	105-120	110–135	105-131

Data from American Academy of Pediatrics Committee on Nutrition: Nutritional needs of the preterm infant. In Kleinman RE, editor: *Pediatric nutrition handbook*, ed 6, Elk Grove Village, Ill, 2009, AAP, pp 79-112; European Society of Paediatric Gastroenterology, Hepatology and Nutrition, Committee on Nutrition of the Preterm Infant (Agostoni C, Buonocore G, Carnielli VP, et al): Enteral nutrient supply for preterm infants: commentary from the European Society for Pediatric Gastroenterology, Hepatology, and Nutrition Committee on Nutrition, *J Pediatr Gastroenterol Nutr* 50:85, 2010; Zeigler EE: Meeting the nutritional needs of the low-birth-weight infant, *Ann Nutr Metab* 58:8, 2011.

from surgery (Figure 17-5). Daily caloric intake should be calculated for each infant during periods of growth or when recovering from illness in the NICU. A useful approach for calculating caloric intake is shown in Box 17-3.

Protein

Protein accretion is critical for normal growth. The amounts and types of protein necessary for optimal growth in preterm infants have been difficult to establish. Metabolic balance studies support a need for higher protein intakes in the growing preterm infant than in the term infant. Throughout the normal period of breastfeeding, the concentration of protein in human milk decreases; however, the preterm infant's need for protein continues to be much higher than the term infant. Mature human milk provides adequate protein for the slower growth rates during this period of development; such slower growth rates of term infants

determine the recommended goals of 2 to 2.5 g/kg/day of protein. Such protein intakes, however, are not adequate to meet the recommended goals of 3.5 to 4 g/kg/day for preterm infants that are determined by their much higher fractional protein accretion rates.[7,13,42] In one study, preterm infants receiving protein and energy supplementation during enteral feedings (to as much as 3.6 g/kg/day protein and 149 kcal/kg/day energy) had increased gains only in length and head circumference in relation to increased protein intake. In the same study, extra energy increased primarily weight and triceps skinfold thickness, demonstrating the need for protein to grow bone, brain, and lean body mass, whereas excess energy leads primarily to increased fat deposition (Figure 17-6).[100,101] These benefits unique to protein and energy have since been supported by Cochrane Reviews of the literature.[71,108,109]

Preterm infants, especially those born very preterm and of extremely low birth weight and who develop growth failure in the NICU, are at higher neurodevelopmental risk.[75] Previous studies that did not provide adequate protein and energy did not clearly establish long-term benefits to developmental outcome with particular feeding strategies. More recent studies of preterm infants maintained on diets fortified with protein and energy, however, have shown improved neurodevelopmental test scores in early life. Neurodevelopmental outcome, which is improved in most preterm infants who receive breastmilk, appears to be even better when human milk is supplemented with protein and energy.[117,118] More recent studies have shown that such benefits extended into adolescence, when previously preterm infants have increased brain size, caudate nucleus volume, and intelligence quotient (IQ) in direct relation to their protein and energy intake during their postnatal period.[90,93,94]

Human milk from an infant's own mother is unique and the preferred source of protein for that newborn. There are times when mother's own milk is not available. In such situations, donor human milk (DHM) is a valid alternative. DHM is a viable substitute when obtained from established milk banks that follow protocols established by the Human Milk Banking Association of North America (www.hmbana.org).[26,85] Human milk contains whey-predominant protein (whey:casein ratio of 70-80:30-20), whereas cow's milk has a whey:casein

	Normal Requirements		Likely Changes in Requirements with Illness						
	Well Term	Well Preterm	RDS	CLD	CHD Cyanotic	CHD CHF	Sepsis	NEC/SBS	IUGR
Free water (mL/kg)	100 to 120	120 to 140	↓	↓	∅	↓	↑	↑	↑
Energy (kcal/kg)	100	120	↑	↑↑	↑	↑↑	↑↑	↑↑	↑
Carbohydrate (g/kg)	10	12 to 14	↑	↓	↑	↑	↑	↑	↑
Protein (g/kg)	1.5 to 2.2	3.0 to 4.0	∅	↑	↑	↑	↑↑	↑	↑
Fat (g/kg)	3.3 to 6	4 to 7	∅	↑	↑	↑	∅	↑↑*	↑
Calcium (mg/kg)	45 to 60	120 to 230	∅	↑↑•♦	↑◊	↑•◊	∅	↑*	↑
Iron (mg/kg)	1	2 to 4	∅	↑♦	↑	∅	∅	↑	↑
Vitamin A (IU/kg)	333	700 to 1500	↑◊	↑◊	∅	∅	∅	∅	∅

∅ No change.

* Particularly with loss of the terminal ileum.

• Particularly with calciuric diuretics such as furosemide.

◊ Particularly if postoperative.

♦ In <1500-g preterm infants.

FIGURE 17-5 Daily nutritional requirements and changes with illness. *CHD,* Congenital heart disease; *CHF,* congestive heart failure; *CLD,* chronic lung disease; *IUGR,* intrauterine growth restriction; *NEC,* necrotizing enterocolitis; *RDS,* respiratory distress syndrome; *SBS,* short bowel syndrome. (Modified from Thureen PJ, Hay WW Jr: Conditions in preterm infants requiring special nutritional management. In Tsang R, Lucas A, Uauy R, Zlotkin S, editors: *Nutritional needs of the preterm infant: scientific basis and practical guidelines,* Baltimore, 1993, Williams & Wilkins.)

BOX 17-3 CALCULATING DAILY CALORIC INTAKE (kcal/kg/day)

Conversion Factors
20 kcal/oz = 0.67 kcal/ml
24 kcal/oz = 0.80 kcal/ml
1 kcal = 1 calorie
1 oz = 30 ml

Calculation
1. Add total daily feeding intake (in ml)
2. Divide total intake (ml) by the infant's weight (kg). This equals enteral intake in ml/kg/day.
3. Multiply ml/kg/day intake by kcal per ounce of feeding.
4. Divide by 30 ml

This equals enteral intake in kcal/kg/day.

---

ratio of 18:82. Whey protein is particularly rich in essential and conditionally essential amino acids. Milk and colostrum expressed from mothers of preterm infants is somewhat higher in protein than milk from mothers of term infants, but both have higher protein concentrations at the onset of lactation than later during full or mature lactation. Nonetheless, fortification of preterm maternal milk with protein (as well as calcium, phosphorus, sodium, potassium, and lipid) usually is necessary to promote growth rates approximating those of normal human fetuses, particularly in ELBW and VLBW preterm infants.[168]

Given the multiple benefits of mother's milk feeding for preterm infants, including provision of antimicrobial factors and improved feeding tolerance, mother's milk feeding with protein and energy supplementation (e.g., with Enfamil Human Milk Fortifier produced by Mead Johnson Nutritionals or Similac Human Milk Fortifier produced by Abbott Nutrition) is highly recommended (Table 17-3).[4] A human milk–based fortifier, Prolact+ H2MF (Prolacta Bioscience, Monrovia, Calif.), also is available.

An average protein intake of 3.5 g/kg/day is recommended for most preterm infants born before 30 weeks' gestation. Protein requirements are higher (4.0 g/kg/day) in ELBW infants (i.e., less than 27 weeks' gestation and less than 1000 g) to meet the higher protein synthesis

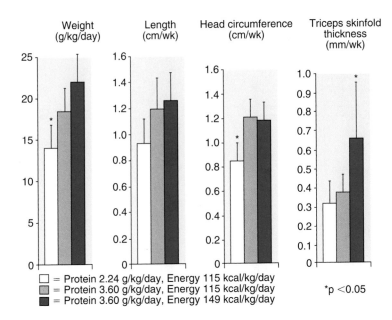

FIGURE 17-6 Growth rates with varying protein and energy intakes. (From Kashyap S, Schulze KF, Forsyth M, et al: Growth nutrient retention and metabolic response in low-birth-weight infants fed varying intakes of protein and energy, *J Pediatr* 113:713-721, 1988; Kennaugh JM, Hay WW Jr: Nutrition of the fetus and newborn, *West J Med* 147:435-448, 1987.)

and growth requirements at this stage of gestation; 4.0 to 4.5 g/kg/day may be necessary to compensate for accumulated protein deficits. A mainstay of nutrition for preterm infants has been the use of preterm formulas when human milk is not available. Newer generation "high protein" formulas are now available that contain higher protein contents than standard preterm formulas (3.3 to 3.6 g/100 kcal) and are recommended to increase protein delivery for very small and very preterm infants at greatest risk for undernutrition[36] (see Table 17-3) (Box 17-4). Term infants do not require protein or energy supplementation unless their dietary fluid is restricted because of illness (e.g., congestive heart failure).

The amino acid profile in the newborn diet is as important as the amount of protein provided. Growth rate of lean body mass is determined directly by the intake of the essential amino acids. Conditionally, or developmentally, essential amino acids (those that are uniquely required in larger amounts at certain developmental stages and cannot be synthesized at sufficient rates for requirements [e.g., cysteine, taurine, histidine, arginine, lysine]) also are important to the infant, especially if preterm. Normal growth, energy metabolism, and immune function depend on appropriate availability of these amino acids. Particularly in the rapidly growing infant, growth requirements may not be met by the relatively limited intake of essential amino acids common with most current nutritional regimens or by the limited biosynthesis of conditionally essential amino acids.

Fat

Human neonates are unique among neonatal mammals in having a relatively high white fat content of 12% to 18% of body weight at term. The term infant also has stores of brown fat, which are necessary for neonatal thermogenesis. In utero fat deposition occurs predominantly during the last 12 to 14 weeks' gestation. Thus infants born preterm before fat deposition has occurred have insufficient fat stores for use as energy and for thermogenesis. Dietary fats also are important to sustain growth, provide essential fatty acids, and promote the absorption of fat-soluble vitamins. Newborn infants absorb fat less efficiently than older children. Preterm infants demonstrate even greater deficiencies in fat digestion and metabolism. Pancreatic lipase and bile acids are less available for fat digestion and absorption. Lingual and gastric lipases, present in greater amounts in term newborn oral-pharyngeal secretions than in the preterm infant, compensate for deficient pancreatic lipase, as

TABLE 17-3   COMPOSITION OF PRETERM HUMAN MILK AND HUMAN MILK FORTIFIERS

| | MATURE PRETERM HUMAN MILK (28 DAYS, APPROXIMATE per 100 ml*) | COW'S MILK–DERIVED HUMAN MILK FORTIFIERS (PER 4 PACKETS OR VIALS) | | | | | HUMAN MILK–DERIVED HUMAN MILK FORTIFIER (PER 20 ml) |
		ENFAMIL HUMAN MILK FORTIFIER POWDER†	ENFAMIL HUMAN MILK FORTIFIER ACIDIFIED LIQUID†	SIMILAC HUMAN MILK FORTIFIER POWDER‡	SIMILAC HUMAN MILK FORTIFIER CONCENTRATED LIQUID‡	SIMILAC HUMAN MILK FORTIFIER EXTENSIVELY HYDROLYZED PROTEIN CONCENTRATED LIQUID‡	PROLACT+4 H²MF
Energy (kcal)	67-75	14	30	14	27	28	28
Protein							
Amount (g)	1.3-1.8	1.1	2.2	1	1.4	2	1.2
Source	Human milk	Milk protein isolate and whey protein isolate hydrolysate	Whey protein isolate hydrolysate	Nonfat milk and whey protein concentrate	Nonfat milk and whey protein concentrate	Casein hydrolysate	Human milk
Fat							
Amount (g)	3-3.9	1	2.3	0.36	1.06	0.84	1.8
Source	Triglycerides	MCT oil (70%) Soy oil (30%)	MCT oil Soy oil High oleic sunflower oil	MCT oil	MCT oil, *M. alpina* oil, *C. cohnii* oil	MCT oil, soy oil, coconut oil, *M. alpina* oil, *C. cohnii* oil	Triglycerides
Carbohydrate							
Amount (g)	6-11	<0.4	<1.2	1.8	3.23	3	1.8
Source	Lactose and glucose	Mineral salts and corn syrup solids	Mineral salts	Corn syrup solids	Corn syrup solids	Maltodextrin, modified corn starch	Lactose and glucose
Minerals							
Calcium (mg)	25	90	116	117	140	120	103
Phosphorus (mg)	13	50	63	67	80	68	53.8
Sodium (mEq)	0.9±0.2	0.7	1.2	0.65	0.9	0.8	37
Potassium (mEq)	1.2±0.3	0.7	1.15	1.61	2.12	2	50
Chloride (mEq)	1.5±0.2	0.4	0.8	1.07	1.51	1.6	29
Iron (mg)	0.2	1.44	1.76	0.35	0.43	0.44	0.1
Zinc (mg)	0.3	0.72	0.96	1	1.21	1.24	0.7
Magnesium (mg)	3	1	1.84	7	8.6	8.4	4.7

Other Characteristics

Potential renal solute load (mOsm/100 mL)	12.6	24	25.8	23.1	23.1	25.6	N/A
Osmolality (mOsm/kg water)	290	+35 (above human milk when mixed)	+36 (above human milk when mixed)	+95 (above human milk when mixed)	+95 (above human milk when mixed)	+160 (above human milk when mixed)	+<70 (above human milk when mixed)§
pH			~4.3 product alone ~4.7 at normal dilution				
Emulsifier						Gellan Gum	

This table lists the major constituents; refer to product inserts for a complete listing of vitamins, minerals, and trace elements.

MCT, Medium-chain triglyceride.

*Data from Klein CJ: Nutrient requirements for preterm infant formulas, *J Nutr* 132:1395S, 2002.

†Mead Johnson Nutritionals, Evansville, Indiana.

‡Ross Products Division, Abbott Nutrition, Columbus, Ohio.

§Sullivan S, Schanler RJ, Kim JH, et al: An exclusive human milk based diet is associated with a lower rate of necrotizing enterocolitis than a diet of human milk and bovine milk-based products, *J Pediatr* 156:562, 2010.

BOX 17-4	INDICATIONS FOR USING HIGH-PROTEIN PRETERM FORMULAS

- Weight <1500 g
- Fluid-/volume-restricted infants
- Promotion of wound healing
- Cumulative deficit of protein intake
- Inadequate growth in length and/or head circumference
- Unfortified human milk feeds (e.g., direct breastfeeding or use of donor milk)

does mammary gland lipase if the infant is receiving breastmilk, but even these are reduced in the preterm infant. Current recommended intakes for dietary fat consist of 40% to 52% of total calories (4.4 to 5.7 g/100 kcal).

Long-chain polyunsaturated fatty acids (LC-PUFAs) are essential for normal growth and development, particularly of the retina and brain (especially affecting cognition). LC-PUFA supplementation, therefore, has been a topic of much discussion and research in recent years. Of particular interest are the n-3 and n-6 essential fatty acids, alpha-linolenic acid (ALA) and linoleic acid (LA), and their metabolites, docosahexaenoic acid (DHA) and arachidonic acid (ARA), respectively.[123] Both term and preterm human milk contain considerable quantities of ALA. The term infant can synthesize DHA from its precursor ALA, but whether the synthesized amount is sufficient for growth and development in preterm infants remains uncertain. Human milk also contains preformed LC-PUFAs. In an effort to make formula more like the gold-standard human milk, manufacturers in the United States have added DHA and ARA to both term and preterm infant formulas. This also has made clinical cases of essential fatty acid (EFA) deficiency relatively rare. When severe and prolonged enough, EFA deficiency can lead to a clinical syndrome consisting of dermatitis (especially in the perianal region), thrombocytopenia, infection, and failure to thrive, and characterized by an increased triene/tetraene ratio (increased nonessential trienoic:ETA $20:3\omega9$ to decreased essential tetraenoic:AA $20:4\omega6$).[82]

LC-PUFA supplementation is thought to be safe for both term and preterm infants.[68,72,91,106] The evidence for long-term benefit, however,

particularly for term infants, has been mixed.[87] A recent Cochrane review concluded that the majority of randomized controlled trials have not shown a beneficial effect of LC-PUFA supplementation on the neurodevelopmental outcomes of term infants.[180] For preterm infants, in whom PUFAs are particularly important for growth, brain, and visual development and who have not had the opportunity for late gestation accumulation of fats, there may be benefit and little risk with supplementation.[72,73,105,169] A recent systematic analysis of the literature found only a trend for LC-PUFAs to reduce the risk of BPD and NEC.[205] Areas of ongoing research include maternal supplementation of LC-PUFAs to promote fetal growth and improve the length of gestation, exploration of the effects of LC-PUFAs on preventing NEC, and the relationship of neonatal fat composition to the development of atherosclerosis in later life.

Some fats (e.g., essential fatty acids) are essential for normal infant growth.[105] The amount of medium-chain triglycerides (MCTs) also is important for fat nutrition due to their greater absorptive capacity, especially in the underdeveloped GI tract of preterm infants (MCTs do not require bile salts for absorption and can be directly absorbed into the portal venous circulation). This offers theoretical advantages for the preterm infant, although there is little evidence that inclusion of MCTs improves energy or protein/nitrogen absorption or retention, or growth of the healthy preterm infant.[199] The content of MCTs varies considerably among current feedings for preterm and term infants: expressed human milk, 2%; fortified human milk, 2% to 18%; preterm formula, 40%; and term formula, 8%. The considerable variability in milk MCT content parallels that of fat content of human milk and occurs because of interindividual variations and changes in milk fat content during the day, throughout lactation, and within one feeding (foremilk to hind milk). MCTs do improve fat absorption and energy intake in infants with hepatic dysfunction or short bowel syndromes. Excess MCTs can lead to diarrhea and dicarboxylic acid excretion.

Carbohydrates

Carbohydrate reserves begin to accumulate as glycogen in the developing fetus as early as the start of the second trimester. Most of this glycogen (as much as 90% of total body glycogen in term infants) serves local cellular needs in different organs, whereas hepatic glycogen specifically provides glucose for other glucose-dependent tissues, primarily the brain. Immediately after birth, with cessation of glucose supply from the placenta, the neonate must use stored glycogen for energy. The newborn can exhaust the supply of stored glucose from the liver within 12 hours of birth under severely stressful conditions (e.g., hypoxia, hypotension, increased catecholamine and glucagon release) if milk/formula or IV glucose is not provided. The normal glucose utilization rate in the term newborn is 4 to 6 mg/kg/min. The brain accounts for most of the glucose used in the whole body, especially in preterm and asymmetrically growth-restricted infants, who have a larger-than-normal brain:body-weight ratio.

The predominant carbohydrate in human milk is lactose, a disaccharide composed of glucose and galactose. Glucose has a central role in energy metabolism. Galactose provides 50% of the calories derived from lactose; its major metabolic role is in energy storage, because the newborn liver readily incorporates galactose from the portal circulation into hepatic glycogen.

Provision of 40% to 50% of total caloric intake as carbohydrate (10 to 12 g/kg/day) prevents accumulation of ketone bodies and other adverse metabolic effects (e.g., hypoglycemia) in the newborn. This amount of carbohydrate generally is supplied as lactose in human milk or commercial formulas. Preterm formulas have reduced lactose content, 40% to 50% of the total carbohydrate, and human milk fortifiers provide little to no lactose. If there are signs of lactose intolerance, such as frequent loose stools, abdominal distention or apparent cramping, or positive stool reducing substances (Clinitest), a lactose-free infant formula may be considered (Table 17-4). Use of such nonlactose products should be reserved for those rare infants with clinically proven lactose intolerance.

Vitamins

Vitamins are organic substances that are present in trace amounts in natural food sources and are essential to normal metabolism. Lack of vitamins in the diet produces well-recognized deficiency states in adults. The biologic roles of many vitamins are not completely understood in preterm infants, and recognition of clinical deficiency states often is difficult. Certain vitamins have received close attention in neonatology, in particular vitamin C for its role in enhancing iron absorption from the GI tract, vitamin K for prevention of hemorrhagic disease of the newborn,[12] vitamin D for the prevention of rickets,[2] and vitamins A and E as antioxidants.[88] Vitamin A supplementation has been shown in some studies to decrease chronic lung disease in ELBW infants.[55]

Because vitamins have a central role in many metabolic processes, signs of vitamin deficiency can be nonspecific, such as lethargy, irritability, and poor growth. Table 17-5 is a summary of the recommended vitamin intake for enterally fed infants. For comparison, the average vitamin content of term human milk and commercial infant formulas is included in Table 17-4. Routine supplementation of vitamins above the recommended doses is not advised because of possible toxicity and lack of clearly demonstrated benefits. For example, the recommended dose of vitamin D for preterm infants, once they have reached full enteral feeds and weigh more than 1500 g, is 400 IU/day, up to a maximum of 1000 IU/day.[2]

Minerals and Trace Elements

The content of minerals in human milk is the gold standard for mineral requirements in term infants. Mineral requirements for the preterm infant have been estimated from in utero accretion rates. Preterm infants are relatively lacking in some important minerals (e.g., iron, calcium, zinc), because their accumulation occurs mostly in the third trimester. Published recommendations for selected daily intakes in healthy, enterally fed preterm infants are shown in Tables 17-5 and 17-6.[104] Supplementation with calcium and phosphorus to achieve the recommended intakes (a Ca:P ratio of 1.7:1, by weight) has been shown to decrease the incidence of metabolic bone disease in preterm infants.[2] Mineral supplementation of human milk or use of an enriched preterm formula (as shown in Table 17-7) usually is necessary to achieve the recommended mineral requirements.

TABLE 17-4 COMPARATIVE NUTRITIONAL COMPOSITION OF TERM INFANT FEEDINGS PER 100 kcal

	MATURE HUMAN MILK (28 days)	ENFAMIL NEWBORN	ENFAMIL INFANT†	COW'S MILK–BASED WITH INTACT PROTEIN			LACTOSE FREE / SOY PROTEIN–BASED	
				SIMILAC ADVANCE STAGE 1‡	SIMILAC ADVANCE STAGE 2‡	SIMILAC SENSITIVE (LACTOSE FREE)	ENFAMIL PROSOBEE LIPIL†	SIMILAC ISOMIL ADVANCE‡
Nutrient density (kcal/oz)	20	20	20	20	19	19	20	19
Energy (kcal)	98-110	100	100	100	100	100	100	100
Protein								
Amount (g)	1.8	2.1	2	2.07	2.07	2.14	2.5	2.45
% Total calories	7	8	8	8	8	8.5	10	10
Source	Human milk	Nonfat milk, whey protein concentrate	Nonfat milk protein concentrate	Nonfat milk and whey protein concentrate	Nonfat milk and whey protein concentrate	Milk protein isolate	Soy protein isolate and L-methionine	Soy protein isolate and L-methionine
Fat								
Amount (g)	4.3-4.9	5.3	5.3	5.4	5.6	5.4	5.3	5.46
% Total calories	50	48	48	49	50	49	48	49
Source	Triglycerides	Palm olein, Soy oil, Coconut oil, High oleic sunflower oil, Single cell oil products (DHA and ARA)	Palm olein, Soy oil, Coconut oil, High oleic sunflower oil, Single cell oil products (DHA and ARA)	High oleic safflower oil, Soy oil, Coconut oil, Single cell oil products (DHA and ARA)	High oleic safflower oil, Soy oil, Coconut oil, Single cell oil products (DHA and ARA)	High oleic safflower oil, Soy oil, Coconut oil, Single cell oil products (DHA and ARA)	Palm olein, Soy oil, Coconut oil, High oleic safflower oil, Single cell oil products (DHA and ARA)	High oleic safflower oil, Soy oil, Coconut oil, Single cell oil products (DHA and ARA)
Linoleic acid (mg)	440-1500	860	800	1000	1000	1000	860	1000
Carbohydrate								
Amount (g)	10-11	11.2	11.3	10.8	10.7	10.7	10.6	10.4
% Total calories	40-44	45	45	43	43	43	42	42
Source	Lactose and glucose	Lactose	Lactose	Lactose	Lactose	Maltodextrin and sugar	Corn syrup solids	Corn syrup and sucrose

Minerals

Calcium (mg)	39-45	73	78	78	82	88	105 (5.2)	110 (5.5)
Phosphorus (mg)	18-24	43	43	42	44	59	69	79
Ca:P ratio	1.9-2.1	1.8	1.8	1.8	1.8	1.5	1.5	1.4
Sodium (mg [mEq])	18-26 [0.8-1.1]	27 [1.2]	27 [1.2]	24 [1]	25 [1.1]	32 [1.4]	36 [1.6]	44 [1.9]
Potassium (mg [mEq])	60-80 [1.5-2]	108 [2.8]	108 [2.8]	105 [2.7]	110 [2.8]	110 [2.8]	120 [3.1]	110 [2.8]
Chloride (mg [mEq])	55-63 [1.6-1.8]	63 [1.8]	63 [1.8]	65 [1.8]	68 [1.9]	68 [1.9]	80 [2.3]	65 [1.8]
Iron (mg)	0.05-0.75	1.8	1.8	1.8	1.9	1.9	1.8	1.9
Zinc (mg)	0.2-0.3	1	1	0.75	0.79	0.79	1.2	0.79
Magnesium (mg)	4.5-5	8	8	6	6	6	8-11	7.9

Vitamins

Vitamin A (international units)	110-320	300	300	300	300	300	300	300
Vitamin D (international units)	3-3.2	75	60	60	75	60	60	60
Vitamin E (international units)	0.3-0.6	2	2	1.5	1.5	1.5	2	1.5
Vitamin K (mcg)	0.3	9	9	8	8	8	8-9	11
Vitamin C—ascorbic acid (mg)	5.6-6	12	12	9	9	9	12	9
Vitamin B$_1$—thiamine (mcg)	29-31	80	80	100	100	100	80	63
Vitamin B$_2$—riboflavin (mcg)	49-51	140	140	150	160	160	90	95
Vitamin B$_6$ (mcg)	10-46	60	60	60	63	63	60	63
Folic acid (mcg)	2.5-18	16	16	15	16	16	16	16

Other Characteristics

Potential renal solute load (mOsm)	14	19.1	18.6	18.7	20.5	20.3	23	23.2
Osmolality (mOsm/kg water)	290-305	300	300	310	310	200	200	200

Data from Klein CJ, editor: Nutrient requirements for preterm infant formulas, *J Nutr* 132:1395S, 2002; Koletzko B, Uauy R, Poindexter B, editors: *Nutritional care of premature infants,* 2014, S. Karger AG, pp 64-81 (*World Rev Nutr Diet* 110:64-81, 2014).

This table lists the major constituents; refer to product inserts for a complete listing of vitamins, minerals, and trace elements.

ARA, Arachidonic acid; *DHA,* docosahexaenoic acid.

†Mead Johnson Nutritionals, Evansville, Indiana.

‡Abbott Nutrition, Columbus, Ohio.

TABLE 17-5   COMPARATIVE NUTRITIONAL COMPOSITION OF HYDROLYZED INFANT FEEDINGS PER 100 kcal

	PARTIALLY HYDROLYZED		EXTENSIVELY HYDROLYZED			COMPLETELY HYDROLYZED		
	ENFAML GENTLEASE	SIMILAC TOTAL COMFORT	ENFAMIL NUTRAMIGEN	SIMILAC EXPERT CAREALIMENTUM	ENFAMIL PREGESTIMIL	ENFAMIL PURAMINO	ELECARE (FOR INFANTS)	NUTRICIA NEOCATE INFANT DHA/ARA
Nutrient density (kcal/oz)	20	19	20	20	20	20	20	20
Energy (kcal)	100	100	100	100	100	100	100	100
Protein								
Amount (g)	2.3	2.32	2.8	2.75	2.8	2.8	3.1	2.8
% Total calories	9	9	11	11	11	11	15	11
Source	Partially hydrolyzed nonfat milk and whey protein concentrate solids (soy)	Whey protein hydrolysate	Casein hydrolysate, L-cystine, L-tyrosine, L-tryptophan	Casein hydrolysate, L-cystine, L-tyrosine, L-tryptophan	Casein hydrolysate, L-cystine, L-tyrosine, L-tryptophan	Free L-amino acids	Free L-amino acids	Free L-amino acids
Fat								
Amount (g)	5.3	5.4	5.3	5.54	5.6	5.3	4.8	5.1
% Total calories	48	49	48	48	48	48	43	46
Source	Palm olein, soy, coconut, and high oleic sunflower oils; Single cell oil products (DHA and ARA)	High oleic safflower oil, soy and coconut oil; Single cell oil products (DHA and ARA)	Palm olein, soy, coconut and high oleic sunflower oils; Single cell oil products (DHA and ARA)	Safflower oil, MCT oil, soy oil; Single cell oil products (DHA and ARA)	MCT oil, soy oil, corn oil, and high oleic safflower oil or sunflower oil; Single cell oil products (DHA and ARA)	Palm olein, coconut, soy and high oleic sunflower oils; Single cell oil products (DHA and ARA)	Safflower oil, MCT, soy oil; Single cell oil products (DHA and ARA)	MCT, high oleic sunflower oil, sunflower oil, canola oil; Single cell oil products (DHA and ARA)
Oil ratio (approximate)	44:19.5:19.5:14.5	40:30:29	44:19.5:19.5:14.5	38:33:28	55:25:10:7.5	44:19.5:14.5	39:33:28	N/A
Linoleic acid (mg)	800-860	1000	860	1900	940	860	840	738
Carbohydrate								
Amount (g)	10.8	11	10.3	10.2	10.2	10.3	10.7	10.8
% Total calories	43.5	42	41	41	41	41	42	43
Source	Corn syrup solids	Corn syrup solids, sugar, galacto-oligosaccharides	Corn syrup solids	Sugar, modified tapioca starch	Corn syrup solids	Corn syrup solids, modified tapioca starch	Corn syrup solids	Corn syrup solids

Minerals

Calcium (mg)	82	105	94	105	94	94	116	116
Phosphorus (mg)	46	70	52	75	52	52	84.2	82.2
Ca:P ratio	1.8:1	1.5:1	1.8:1	1.4:1	1.8:1	1.8:1	1.4:1	1.4:1
Sodium mg (mEq)	36 (1.6)	46 (2)	47 (2)	44 (1.9)	47 (2)	47 (2)	45 (2)	39.1 (1.7)
Potassium mg (mEq)	108 (3.1)	121 (3.1)	110 (2.8)	118 (3)	110 (2.8)	110 (2.8)	150 (3.9)	109 (2.8)
Chloride mg (mEq)	63 (1.8)	68 (1.9)	86 (2.4)	80 (2.3)	86 (2.4)	88 (2.5)	60 (1.7)	79.9 (2.2)
Iron (mg)	1.8	1.9	1.8	1.8	1.8	1.8	1.8	1.5
Zinc (mg)	1	0.79	1	0.75	1	1	1.15	1.1
Magnesium (mg)	8	6	8–11	7.5	8	11	84	10.3

Vitamins

Vitamin A (international units)	300	300	300	300	350	300	273	280
Vitamin D (international units)	60	60	50	45	50	50	60	72.9
Vitamin E (international units)	2	1.5	2	3	4	2	2.1	1.4
Vitamin K (mcg)	9	8	8-9	15	12	8	13	8.8
Vitamin C—ascorbic acid (mg)	12	9	12	9	12	12	9	10.7
Vitamin B_1—thiamine (mcg)	80	100	80	60	80	80	210	140
Vitamin B_2—riboflavin (mcg)	140	160	90	90	90	90	105	110
Vitamin B_6 (mcg)	60	63	60	60	60	60	84.2	112
Folic acid (mcg)	16	16	16	15	16	16	29.5	13.3

Other Characteristics

Potential renal solute load (mOsm)	21	22.5	25	25.3	25	25	18.7	16.8
Osmolality (mOsm/kg water)	220-230	200	260–320	370	260-280	350	350	340

This table lists the major constituents; refer to product inserts for a complete listing of vitamins, minerals, and trace elements.
ARA, Arachidonic acid; *DHA*, docosahexaenoic acid; *MCT*, medium-chain triglycerides.
†Mead Johnson Nutritionals, Evansville, Indiana
‡ Abbott Nutrition, Columbus, Ohio.

TABLE 17-6	**RECOMMENDED ENTERAL MINERAL AND VITAMIN INTAKE FOR INFANTS**	
	TERM (per 100 kcal)	PRETERM (per 100 kcal)
Minerals		
Calcium (mg)	50-140	123-185
Phosphorus (mg)	20-70	82-109
Ca:P ratio by weight	1.1-2:1	1.7-2:1
Sodium		
mg	25-50	39-63
mEq	1.1-2.2	1.7-2.7
Potassium		
mg	60-160	60-160
mEq	1.5-4.1	1.5-4.1
Chloride		
mg	50-160	60-160
mEq	1.4-4.6	1.7-4.6
Magnesium (mg)	4-17	6.8-17
Iron (mg)	0.2-1.65	1.7-3
Zinc (mg)	0.4-1	1.1-1.5
Manganese (mcg)	1-100	6.3-25
Copper (mcg)	60-160	100-250
Iodine (mcg)	8-35	6-35
Selenium (mcg)	1.5-5	1.8-5
Fluoride (mcg)	0-60	Maximum 25
Chromium (mcg)	—	—
Molybdenum (mcg)	—	—
Vitamins		
Vitamin A (mcg RE)	60-150	204-380
(international units)	203-506	679-1265
Vitamin D (international units)	40-100	75-270
Vitamin E (mg α-TE/100 kcal)	0.5-(5 mg α-TE/g PUFA)	2-8
Vitamin K (mcg RE)	1-25	4-25
Vitamin C — ascorbic acid (mg)	6-15	8.3-37
Pantothenic acid (mcg)	300-1200	300-1900
Biotin (mcg)	1-15	1-37
Vitamin B_1 — thiamine (mcg)	30-200	30-250
Vitamin B_2 — riboflavin (mcg)	80-300	80-620
Vitamin B_3 — niacin (mcg)	550-2000	550-5000
Vitamin B_6 — pyridoxine (mcg)	30-130	30-250
Vitamin B_{12} — cobalamin (mcg)	0.08-0.7	0.08-0.7
Folate (mcg)	11-40	30-45

RE, Retinol equivalents.
Data from Klein CJ, editor: Nutrient requirements for preterm infant formulas, *J Nutr* 132:1395S, 2002; Greer FR: Vitamins. In Thureen PJ, Hay WW Jr, editors: *Neonatal nutrition and metabolism,* ed 2, Cambridge, 2006, Cambridge University Press.

COMPOSITION OF ENTERAL FEEDINGS

Human Milk

The ideal enteral diet for almost all term newborn infants is human milk,[8] which provides sufficient energy, protein, fat, carbohydrate, micronutrients, and water for normal growth. Contraindications to the use of human milk, which are rare, are found in Box 17-5. The development of a beneficial GI flora, characterized by a large prevalence of bifidobacteria and lactobacilli, is strongly supported by human milk feedings.[40,116,125,126] In addition, human milk, unlike formulas, provides a variety of antimicrobial factors that protect against infections and NEC,[117,173,181] such as secretory immunoglobulins (IgA), leukocytes, complement, lactoferrin, and lysozyme.[142] Human milk also contains hormones and growth factors such as epidermal and nerve growth factors, IGF-I and IGF-II, erythropoietin, prolactin, calcitonin, steroids, thyrotropin-releasing hormone, and thyroxine.[174] These milk hormones and trophic factors play active roles in organ maturation, growth, and health. Several essential and conditionally essential amino acids are present in high concentrations in human milk. The protein and fat components of human milk are readily digestible, and human milk contains large numbers of enzymes that aid in nutrient digestion and processing (e.g., lipase). Exclusive human milk feeding of infants at high risk may reduce the risk for developing atopic disease or milk protein allergy in infancy.[80,114] There also are obvious psychological benefits to a mother who provides her own milk for her sick infant (see Chapter 18). Human milk also is advantageous for enhancing neurodevelopment, including vision, mental scales (particularly cognition), motor scales, behavior, and hearing. Preterm infants breastfed at discharge have less subnormal neurodevelopment at 2 to 5 years of age.[172] These effects last into infancy,[196] childhood,[118] and even into adolescence.[92] Thus, as clearly stated by the American Academy of Pediatrics, human milk is the recommended basis of nutrition for the preterm infant[14]: All preterm infants *should* receive human milk; human milk should be fortified with protein, minerals, and vitamins to ensure optimal nutrient intake for infants weighing less than 1500 g at birth; and pasteurized donor human milk, appropriately fortified, *should* be used if mother's own milk is unavailable or its use is contraindicated.

TABLE 17-7 MINERALS AND TRACE ELEMENTS IN NEONATAL NUTRITION

MINERAL OR ELEMENT	BIOLOGIC ROLE	DEFICIENCY STATE	RECOMMENDED INTAKE FOR GROWING PRETERM INFANTS
Sodium	Growth and tissue accretion, body fluid equilibrium, cellular energy, electrical charge balance	Poor growth, fluid imbalance, hypotension, neurologic dysfunction, lethargy, seizures	3-5 mEq/kg/day
Potassium	Growth and tissue accretion, acid-base balance, cellular energy, electrical charge balance	Myocardial damage, dysrhythmia, hypotonia, muscle weakness	2-3 mEq/kg/day
Chloride	Growth and tissue accretion, cellular energy, electrical charge balance	Failure to thrive, muscle weakness, alkalosis, vomiting	3-5 mEq/kg/day
Calcium	Bone and tooth formation, fat absorption, nerve conduction, muscle contraction	Osteomalacia, tetany, dysrhythmias, seizures	200 mg/kg/day
Phosphorus	Bone and tooth formation, energy transfer compounds	Rickets, neuropathy, weakness	100-140 mg/kg/day
Magnesium	Metalloenzymes, cellular electrical charge balance	Hypocalcemia, hypokalemia, diarrhea, tremor, arrhythmia	5-10 mg/kg/day
Iron	Hemoglobin formation, metalloenzymes	Anemia, apathy	2 mg/kg/day after 1 month of age
Zinc	Metalloenzymes, DNA-RNA synthesis, wound healing, host defenses	Growth restriction, dermatitis, alopecia, diarrhea, delayed wound healing, hypogonadism	1.2-1.5 mg/kg/day
Copper	Metalloenzymes, protein metabolism	Neuropathy, anemia, neutropenia, osteoporosis, depigmentation of hair and skin	100-200 mcg/kg/day
Manganese	Metalloenzymes, carbohydrate metabolism, antioxidants, hemostasis	Neurologic dysfunction, defects in lipid metabolism, reduced coagulants, growth restriction in animals	10-20 mcg/kg/day
Chromium	Carbohydrate metabolism, component of nucleic acids	Impaired glucose tolerance, impaired growth	2-4 mcg/kg/day
Selenium	Metalloenzymes, antioxidants	Cardiomyopathy, anemia, myositis	1.5-3 mcg/kg/day
Iodine	Thyroid hormone synthesis	Hypothyroidism, goiter, cretinism	1 mcg/kg/day
Molybdenum	Metalloenzymes	Neurologic and visual dysfunction, growth restriction in animals	2-3 mcg/kg/day

DNA, Deoxyribonucleic acid; *RNA,* ribonucleic acid.
From Kleinman RE, editor: *Pediatric nutrition handbook,* ed 6, Elk Grove Village, Ill, 2009, American Academy of Pediatrics.

The preterm infant will not grow at the normal rate of fetal growth on human milk alone, however, because of the special nutritional requirements addressed previously. In fact, the larger the fraction of total feeding provided by just human milk without supplementation, the greater the reduction in final weight at term gestational age.[49] Recommended daily requirements for energy, protein, calcium, sodium, phosphorus, magnesium, iron, zinc, and several vitamins necessary to meet the normal rate of in utero growth usually will not be achieved in the growing "healthy" preterm infant who is fed with unsupplemented human milk. The preterm infant with respiratory distress,

BOX 17-5	CONTRAINDICATIONS TO BREASTFEEDING

- Untreated maternal miliary tuberculosis or brucellosis, active herpes virus lesions on the breast, or acute H1N1 pneumonia, or acute varicella (*Note:* Expressed milk can be used because there is no concern about these infectious organisms passing through the milk and breastfeeding can be resumed when a mother with tuberculosis is treated for a minimum of 2 weeks and is documented that she is no longer infectious.)
- Maternal human immunodeficiency virus (HIV) infection
- Galactosemia
- Maternal drug abuse (e.g., narcotics, phencyclidine, cocaine, cannabis) (*Note:* This contraindication is relative; mothers who test positive for such drugs should be enrolled in drug reduction programs rather than stopping breastfeeding, particularly among mothers with preterm infants, in whom the advantages of mother's milk generally outweigh the risks of addiction and neurodevelopmental defects in the infant.)

From American Academy of Pediatrics, Section on Breastfeeding: Breastfeeding and the use of human milk, *Pediatrics* 129:e827, 2012.

infection, excessive heat losses, GI disorders, or surgery has even greater nutritional needs. Nonetheless, milk from mothers of preterm infants has more protein and sodium than milk obtained at term and occasionally provides for adequate growth in larger and healthier preterm infants who have the capacity to take in larger volumes, at times over 200 ml/kg/day. This is particularly important when feeding preterm infants with donor human milk.

Donor human milk is a pasteurized product from accredited milk banks and used when maternal milk is insufficient or unavailable, because of the multitude of benefits associated with the use of human milk in preterm infants. Donor milk is pasteurized to prevent infections, but this removes most of the antiinfective properties of milk. Nevertheless, infection rates and NEC rates are much lower with donor milk than formulas and even pasteurized human milk does not lead to a significant increase in infections.[139] There may be differences in milk composition as well, especially in protein content, but also energy, lactose, and fat content, and particularly between human milk donated by women later in lactation after having delivered term infants compared with milk expressed by mothers delivering preterm infants[201] (see Chapter 18). Donor milk in the United States also is low in DHA content, as much as 50% to 75% of

milks from women in other parts of the world whose natural diets include more fish and vegetable oils that contain ALA and DHA.[17] Donor milk is an appropriate choice for VLBW preterm infants whose maternal milk is unavailable[48] and has a greater than 75% improvement in feeding tolerance compared with formulas.[31] The lowest rates of NEC and possibly related sepsis have been found in preliminary studies with an exclusive breastmilk diet, consisting of mother's milk and/or donor milk supplemented with "human" Human Milk Fortifier (Prolacta),[109,184] particularly compared with formula-fed infants.[54]

There also is a growing interest in the use of *probiotics*, principally *Lactobacillus* species and *Bifidobacterium*, to assist in colonization of the preterm infant's gut with bacteria that might promote a more normal gut flora, replenish such flora after antibiotic use, and reduce the risk of GI disorders associated with abnormal gut flora, principally NEC. Several international trials support the use of probiotics to reduce the risk of NEC. Use of probiotics in individual institutions might be considered if the NEC rate, particularly of surgical NEC and/or death from NEC, is relatively high (greater than 2%) despite efforts to reduce the risk of NEC. Such efforts to reduce NEC include the use of exclusive breastmilk feeding (mother's own or donor), restricted use of antibiotics (in both mother and infant), and promotion of early trophic or gut priming feedings with colostrum or mother's milk or donor milk. A recent multicenter collaborative U.K. trial and an updated Cochrane meta-analysis[20] that included 24 trials from around the world showed that there is a significant decrease in NEC and all-cause mortality rate with the use of probiotics.[10] Probiotic preparations containing either lactobacilli alone or in combination with bifidobacteria were found to be effective. Length of stay was 3 to 4 days shorter. Although there remains risk for probiotic-related sepsis, especially in the most vulnerable ELBW infants, this has only rarely been reported and only in case reports outside of the trials noted, particularly the U.K. trials and those reported in the Cochrane review noted above. Recommendations for developing local institutional protocols to use probiotics have been published.[185]

The nutritional composition of term human milk is compared with commercial term infant formulas in Table 17-4. The nutrient content of "mature" preterm human milk is compared with fortified preterm human milk and preterm formulas in Table 17-8. Use of commercially available supplements to human milk that provide additional

TABLE 17–8	COMPARATIVE NUTRITIONAL COMPOSITION OF PRETERM FEEDINGS PER 100 kcal

| | MATURE PRETERM HUMAN MILK (UNFORTIFIED)* | PREMATURE INFANT FORMULAS | | | | POSTDISCHARGE FORMULAS | |
		ENFAMIL PREMATURE †	ENFAMIL PREMATURE 24 CAL HIGH PROTEIN†	SIMILAC SPECIAL CARE WITH IRON‡	SIMILAC SPECIAL CARE 24 HIGH PROTEIN‡	ENFAMIL ENFACARE †	SIMILAC EXPERT CARE NEOSURE‡
Nutrient density (kcal/oz)	19-21	20 or 24	24	20 or 24	24	22	22
Energy (kcal)	100	100	100	100	100	100	100
Protein							
Amount (g)	2.2 ± 0.2	3	3.5	3	3.3	2.8	2.8
% Total calories	8	12	14	12	13	11	11
Source	Human milk	Whey protein concentrate and nonfat milk	Whey protein concentrate, nonfat milk	Nonfat milk, whey protein concentrate	Nonfat milk, whey protein concentrate	Nonfat milk, whey protein concentrate	Nonfat milk, whey protein concentrate
Fat							
Amount (g)	5.4 ± 0.9	5.1	5.1	5.43	5.43	5.3	5.5
% Total calories	44-52	44	44	47	47	47	49
Source	Triglycerides	MCT oil Soy oil High oleic vegetable oil Single cell oil products (DHA and ARA)	MCT oil Soy oil High oleic vegetable oil Single cell oil products (DHA and ARA)	MCT oil Soy oil Coconut oil Single cell oil products (DHA and ARA)	MCT oil Soy oil Coconut oil Single cell oil products (DHA and ARA)	High oleic oil Soy oil MCT oil Coconut oil Single cell oil products (DHA and ARA)	Soy oil Coconut oil MCT oil Single cell oil products (DHA and ARA)
Oil ratio (approximate)	99	40:30:27:2:1	40:30:27:2:1	50:30:18.3: 0.25:0.4	50:30:18.3: 0.25:0.4	34:29:20:14: 2.2:0.8	44.7:29:24.9: 0.25:0.4
Linoleic acid (mg)	440-1500	810	810	700	700	950	750
Carbohydrate							
Amount (g)	10 ± 0.6	11	10.5	10.3	10	10.4	10.1
% Total calories	40-44	44	42	41	40	42	40
Source	Lactose, glucose	Corn syrup solids, lactose	Corn syrup solids, lactose	Corn syrup solids, lactose	Corn syrup solids, lactose	Corn syrup solids, lactose	Corn syrup solids, lactose

Continued

TABLE 17-8	COMPARATIVE NUTRITIONAL COMPOSITION OF PRETERM FEEDINGS PER 100 kcal—cont'd

	MATURE PRETERM HUMAN MILK (UNFORTIFIED)*	PREMATURE INFANT FORMULAS				POSTDISCHARGE FORMULAS	
		ENFAMIL PREMATURE †	ENFAMIL PREMATURE 24 CAL HIGH PROTEIN†	SIMILAC SPECIAL CARE WITH IRON‡	SIMILAC SPECIAL CARE 24 HIGH PROTEIN‡	ENFAMIL ENFACARE †	SIMILAC EXPERT CARE NEOSURE‡
Minerals							
Calcium (mg)	37-44	165	165	180	180	120	105
Phosphorus (mg)	19-21	83	83	100	100	66	62
Ca:P ratio	1.9-2.2:1	2:1	2:1	1.8:1	1.8:1	1.8:1	1.7:1
Sodium mg (mEq)	30-37 (1.3-1.6)	58 (2.5)	58 (2.5)	43 (1.9)	43 (1.9)	35 (1.5)	33 (1.4)
Potassium mg (mEq)	78-85 (2-2.2)	98 (2.5)	98 (2.5)	129 (3.3)	129 (3.3)	105 (2.7)	142 (3.6)
Chloride mg (mEq)	63-82 (1.8-2.3)	90 (2.5)	90 (2.5)	81 (2.3)	81 (2.3)	78 (2.2)	75 (2.1)
Iron (mg)	0.2	1.8	1.8	1.8	1.8	1.8	1.8
Zinc (mg)	0.5	1.5	1.5	1.5	1.5	1.25	1.2
Magnesium (mg)	4.4-4.9	9	9	12	12	8	9
Vitamins							
Vitamin A (mcg RE) (international units)	104-125 (345-416)	375 (1250)	375 (1250)	375 (1250)	375 (1250)	135 (450)	105 (350)
Vitamin D (international units)	3-3.2	240	240	150	150	80	70
Vitamin E (international units)	1.9	6.3	6.3	4	4	4	3.6
Vitamin K (mcg)	0.3	8	9	12	12	8	11
Vitamin C— ascorbic acid (mg)	5-6.25	20	20	37	37	16	15
Vitamin B_1—thiamine (mcg)	200	200	200	250	250	200	175

TABLE 17-8	COMPARATIVE NUTRITIONAL COMPOSITION OF PRETERM FEEDINGS PER 100 kcal — cont'd						

| | MATURE PRETERM HUMAN MILK (UNFORTIFIED)* | PREMATURE INFANT FORMULAS | | | | POSTDISCHARGE FORMULAS | |
		ENFAMIL PREMATURE †	ENFAMIL PREMATURE 24 CAL HIGH PROTEIN†	SIMILAC SPECIAL CARE WITH IRON‡	SIMILAC SPECIAL CARE 24 HIGH PROTEIN‡	ENFAMIL ENFACARE †	SIMILAC EXPERT CARE NEOSURE‡
Vitamins — cont'd							
Vitamin B₂ — riboflavin (mcg)	270-310	300	300	620	620	200	150
Vitamin B₆ (mcg)	18-20	150	150	250	250	100	100
Folic acid (mcg)	12	40	40	37	37	26	25
Other Characteristics							
Potential renal solute load (mOsm)	18.7	27	30	27.8	27.8	24.5	25.2
Osmolality (mOsm/kg water)	290	275-300	300	258–280	280	250	250

This table lists the major constituents; refer to product inserts for a complete listing of vitamins, minerals, and trace elements.

ARA, Arachidonic acid; *DHA*, docosahexaenoic acid; *MCT*, medium-chain triglycerides.

*Klein CJ, editor: Nutrient requirements for preterm infant formulas, *J Nutr* 132:1395S, 2002; Koletzko B, Uauy R, Poindexter B, editors: *Nutritional care of premature infants,* 2014, S. Karger AG, pp 64-81 (*World Rev Nutr Diet* 110:64-81, 2014).

†Mead Johnson Nutritionals, Evansville, Indiana.

‡Abbott Nutrition, Columbus, Ohio.

energy, protein, vitamins, and minerals is recommended.[100] Nutrient composition of these fortifiers is shown in Table 17-3. Most of the new formulations of the commercially available fortifiers now use hydrolyzed cow's milk protein, which might lead to less GI intolerance and possibly NEC.

Formulas

Cow's milk–derived formulas have been modeled after the composition of human milk to provide biologically available protein mixtures with appropriate protein:energy ratios for normal growth. In general, formulas designed for term infants contain 20 kcal/oz and are adequate to meet the needs

of term infants with an intact GI tract and "normal" fluid requirements. A whey and casein mixture approximating that of human milk is preferred. Preterm formulas contain whey:casein ratios of 60:40 and have higher protein contents than those of term formulas (2.4 g/100 ml in preterm formula versus 2 g/100 ml in term formula or human milk). Preterm formulas also contain less lactose as a carbohydrate source and substitute corn syrup solids for lactose to provide approximately 42% to 44% of the calories derived from this carbohydrate (largely sucrose). Preterm formulas provide some of the fat in the form of MCTs because of the ease with which they are absorbed. Calcium (Ca) and phosphorus (P) content is increased, with a Ca:P ratio of 1.8 to 2:1, which provides for improved bone mineralization. Other minerals and vitamins also are present in higher concentrations in preterm formulas to reflect the special nutritional needs of the VLBW infant. Preterm formulas are available in 20 and 24 kcal/oz preparations, with similar osmolalities and renal solute loads. Newer generations of high-protein preterm formulas containing approximately 2.8 g/100 ml may be indicated for VLBW preterm infants who are not growing well, have experienced a cumulative deficit of protein intake, have inadequate growth in length and/or head circumference, or are fluid/volume restricted.[36]

Soy protein formulas should be reserved for term infants with galactosemia, severe lactose intolerance, hereditary lactase deficiency, vegan families, or those who have IgE-mediated cow's milk protein allergy. Soy-derived formulas should not be used for preterm infants because of the poorer quality of protein, lower digestibility and bioavailability, and lower calcium and zinc accretion rates seen with these formulas.[27] In addition, there are concerns for all infants about the concentrations of phytates, aluminum, and phytoestrogens that these formulas contain.[6,190] If necessary, a protein hydrolysate formula should be used for preterm infants with protein intolerance. For term infants, formulas derived from protein hydrolysates should be reserved for infants who are allergic to cow's milk proteins and are not breastfed or do not tolerate soy-derived formulas. Soy formulas have no role in the prevention of atopic disease. In contrast, extensively hydrolyzed formulas may delay or prevent atopic dermatitis in infants at high risk and who are not breastfed.[80] In general, families with a strong history of cow's milk protein allergy should be encouraged to breastfeed. The compositions of hydrolyzed formulas (partially, extensively, and completely) are shown in Table 17-5.

Elemental formulas are used in infants with malabsorption, abnormal GI tracts, or severe protein allergy. The protein source in these formulas is derived from free amino acids, 52% of the fat is from MCT oil, and many are lactose free. Use of elemental formulas generally is indicated in the infant with severe liver disease and fat malabsorption, with short bowel syndrome (e.g., after NEC with surgical resection), or with dysmotility syndromes (e.g., in gastroschisis). Occasionally, elemental formulas are useful after a severe episode of infectious gastroenteritis with mucosal injury and resulting protein or lactose intolerance. It is not necessary to use an elemental formula in the routine care of VLBW infants. Most recent evidence also suggests that there is no benefit in feeding tolerance, enteral intake, or growth when preterm infants are fed a partially hydrolyzed whey preterm infant formula,[74] although there is some evidence for benefit in certain circumstances.[131,161] A variety of other modified formulas are available for infants with special nutritional needs due to inherited enzyme deficiencies.

In some circumstances, infants require fluid restriction (e.g., because of pulmonary edema, congestive heart failure, or renal failure) while on full enteral feedings. Caloric delivery and nutritional support can be maintained by increasing the caloric density of feedings when feeding volumes cannot be tolerated or fluid intake must be limited. This can be done by adding human milk fortifiers to the milk or formula to achieve acceptable concentrations and intakes of these nutrients. Liquid formula concentrates, including liquid protein modular and oils, also are used to increase the caloric density of infant feedings. Powdered infant formulas should *not* be used for feeding or fortification in hospitalized newborns in an intensive care unit, unless no alternative is available, because of information linking *Cronobacter sakazakii* infections in neonates to the use of powdered infant formulas (Food and Drug Administration [FDA] recommendation, 4-11-02). Caloric densities of greater than 24 kcal/oz can be achieved with fortification, although infants tolerate these supplements in a highly individual fashion and should be monitored for signs of feeding intolerance (e.g., abdominal distention, increased stooling, presence of fat or carbohydrates [e.g., lactose] in the stool). The distribution of calories should maintain a balance of protein, fat, and carbohydrate at about 10%, 45%, and 45%, respectively. Increasing caloric density of feedings also necessitates less water delivery to the infant and generally leads to an increase in formula osmolality as well. Therefore careful monitoring of feeding tolerance, electrolytes, and fluid balance (renal function) is necessary on a high–caloric density feeding regimen.

FEEDING TECHNIQUES

Gavage Feeding

Gavage feedings are indicated in infants requiring endotracheal intubation, continuous positive airway pressure (CPAP), or those with an immature, weak, or absent suck, swallow, or gag reflex (Box 17-6). Most infants tolerate intermittent feedings delivered slowly over 30 to 60 minutes, commonly termed *slow bolus feedings.* Feedings should run in slowly, either by gravity or infusion pump. Studies indicate that such an intermittent "slow" infusion (e.g., 3 hours of volume given over 1 hour out of three) improves gastric emptying and duodenal motility.[18,57] Some institutions use continuous feedings for infants recovering from NEC or infants with short bowel syndrome, congenital heart

disease, or intolerance of bolus feedings. However, a summary of randomized controlled trials did not find consistent differences regarding the effectiveness of continuous versus intermittent bolus nasogastric feedings, with the exception of a small subset of patients less than 1000 g who gained weight faster and tended toward earlier discharge when fed by the continuous tube feeding method.[160] Regardless of feeding method, gavage tube position must be checked carefully using auscultation over the stomach and aspiration techniques. Bedside testing of gastric aspirate pH[146] and/or abdominal

---

BOX 17-6 GAVAGE FEEDING GUIDELINES

Equipment

1. Breastmilk/formula in syringe (4-hour amount, or unit protocol, maximum).
2. Tape, optional transparent dressing.
3. Lubricant, optional.
4. Stethoscope.
5. For intermittent feeding: infant feeding set with syringe, medicine cup, 4-Fr to 8-Fr gavage tube.
6. For indwelling feeding tubes: infant less than 1 kg, 4-Fr tube; greater than 1 kg, 5-Fr to 6-Fr tube (tube size may also depend on placement [i.e., oral versus nasal], amount of feeding, and rate of delivery of feeding). Short-term feeding tube (generally made of polyvinyl chloride [PVC]) should be changed every 24 to 72 hours. Long-term feeding tube (made of polyurethane) should be changed at least once every week. *Note:* Always follow manufacturer's recommendations.
7. Syringe pump and extension tubing as needed.

Feeding Tube Insertion

1. Wash hands and assemble equipment in a clean area.
2. Measure for tube placement by placing tip of feeding tube at the tip of nose, draw to base of ear, then to halfway between the xiphoid process and the umbilicus.
3. Mark tube with indelible ink pen to indicate the distance from the tip of the tube to the corner of the mouth or edge of the naris.
4. Insert tube (swaddling the infant may help with tolerance of this procedure).
   NEVER FORCE THE TUBE.
   Oral placement (usually for infants less than 1 kg, those on nasal CPAP or ventilator, those with high oxygen need, or those with excoriated nares): insert tip into the oropharynx, gently pushing tube in a downward arc into the esophagus until reaching the premeasured mark.

Nasal placement (generally preferred for infants greater than 1 kg with mature or strong gag reflex and infants who are breastfeeding or nippling): moisten tip with water or lubricant. Insert tip gently into one nostril and advance slowly as above.

5. Gastric tube tip placement is verified by auscultation or abdominal radiograph or pH measurement of gastric aspirates. The tube landmark should be checked with every caregiving procedure to determine that it is still visible and at the correct location.
6. Soft Silastic tubes are generally used for transpyloric feedings and require the use of a stylet for insertion. The tube must be inspected visually and by flushing with water before insertion to ensure that it has not been perforated by the stylet. The stylet is removed after insertion and is stored in package by the bedside. Tip placement usually is verified by radiographic imaging.

Securing Feeding Tube

1. Intermittent feeding tubes can be taped to the cheek.
2. Indwelling tubes must be taped securely to the face, leaving the landmark visible. For tubes placed nasally, a narrow piece of tape may be placed along the tubing on the upper lip, with a transparent dressing applied over the tube on the cheek.

Feeding

1. Aspirate entire stomach contents to assess quantity, as well as color and appearance.
2. To prevent loss of electrolytes, slowly return aspirate to the stomach. Exceptions to this include aspirates that are bloody or "coffee ground," green or bright yellow, or fecal appearing or contain large amounts of mucus. Do not refeed, and discuss feeding plan with physician or practitioner. Also report aspirates of undigested formula if amount is more than one half of the feeding or occurs more than once or if there is a change in abdominal assessment. Reducing the feeding by the amount of the refed aspirate is recommended for one or two feedings.

Continued

BOX
17-6   GAVAGE FEEDING GUIDELINES — cont'd

3. Instill human milk or formula via intermittent gavage feeding:

Detach syringe from feeding tube and remove plunger; reattach syringe to feeding tube. Pour the predetermined amount of milk into the syringe. Flow may begin spontaneously or require a gentle nudge from the plunger. Allow feeding to run in slowly by gravity. Never push a feeding. The higher the syringe is held, the faster the feeding will flow (about 8 inches is ideal). For most infants, a feeding should run in over 30 minutes. Gavage sets may be rinsed carefully and used for up to 24 hours unless labeled "single use only" or manufacturer's directions indicate otherwise.

4. Intermittent gavage feeding via indwelling feeding tube:

Check aspirate and feed as above. When feeding is complete, instill 1 to 2 ml sterile water to clear tubing of residual food and cap or close off the tube by attaching syringe with plunger.

5. Continuous drip feedings via indwelling feeding tube:

Check feeding tube placement and feeding residuals every 2 to 4 hours using stopcock, which is placed between the feeding tube and the extension tubing. Check ink landmark on feeding tube hourly to ensure proper placement of the tube. Prepare up to 4 hours of breastmilk or formula (or amount according to institutional studies of bacterial growth). Fill syringe with predetermined feeding amount plus enough to prime the extension tubing. Place syringe into syringe pump and program to deliver feeding at desired rate. To help prevent loss of milk fat by settling, place syringe in an upward vertical position and use minibore tubing.

Care, Assessment, and Documentation

1. Assess infant's tolerance of feeding tube placement. If gagging occurs, attempt to insert tube down one side of the oropharynx rather than down the middle. If the infant becomes apneic, bradycardic, or cyanotic during feeding tube placement, pause to allow recovery or remove the tube and allow infant to rest before trying again. If these symptoms occur during the feeding, stop the feeding by lowering the syringe or stopping the pump. If recovery occurs quickly, resume feeding slowly and observe. If distress continues or recurs, stop feeding and inform the physician or practitioner.

2. Change short-term (PVC) feeding tube every 24 to 72 hours (or manufacturer's recommendations).

3. Change long-term nasal feeding tube (polyurethane) to opposite nostril weekly. Discard and replace tube after 4 weeks (or manufacturer's recommendations).

4. Document all details of the feeding and the infant's tolerance, proper placement of the indwelling feeding tube, and when feeding tube or equipment is to be changed.

---

radiographs are generally reserved for transpyloric tube placement. Prolonged oral or nasal gastric tube feedings cause adverse oral stimulation and promote GER and problems of oral aversion. Some neonates require gastrostomy tube placement after certain surgical procedures or if oral feeding failure is expected to be prolonged (see Chapter 28).

For most infants, intragastric feedings are preferred to transpyloric feedings. Current data available do not provide any evidence of benefit of transpyloric feeding for preterm infants, and some evidence for harm exists, including a higher risk of GI disturbances and mortality.[198] Even when indicated because of severe GER with aspiration, transpyloric feedings have additional complications, including malabsorption and diarrhea, altered gut microbiome, and intestinal perforations requiring surgery. Use of transpyloric feeding should be restricted to short-term use in those infants who cannot tolerate gastric feedings because of excessive GER with aspiration, pneumonia, and apnea.

Extended infusion times and pump position may lead to significant (up to 50%) fat and calcium losses when gavage feeding human milk.[28,33,170,192] Increased exposure of milk to plastic in the form of extension tubing and milk transfer systems, as well as the syringe design, also can contribute to these losses. Positioning eccentric syringes horizontally or with the tip angled upward, minimizing the length of extension tubing, streamlining feed preparation, and shortening infusion time as medically appropriate can mitigate these losses.[33,140,170,192] Some data indicate that the type of human milk fortification also has an effect.[28,170] More research is needed in this area as use of breastmilk in the NICU setting increases.

Oral Feeding

Development of appropriate neuromuscular coordination is necessary to successfully initiate oral feedings. Criteria for initiating oral feeding must

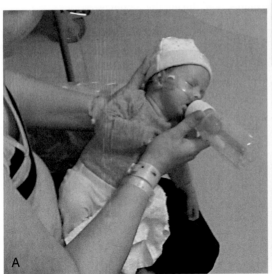
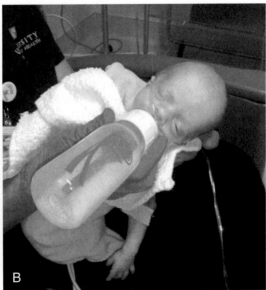

FIGURE 17-7 Both panels (**A** and **B**) show the semielevated side-lying (ESL) position when introducing bottle feedings to the preterm infant.[45,153]

be individualized, because components of sucking, swallowing, and respiration and their coordinated activity mature at different rates and times in preterm infants.[11] In general, coordination of suck, swallow, and breathing emerges at about 34 weeks of corrected gestational age (range 32 to 36 weeks).[35] Aspiration is a serious risk in an infant of any gestational age who does not have a neurologically mature swallow, gag, or cough reflex. Tachypneic infants with labored respirations also are at increased risk for aspiration; thus, oral feeding usually is not possible unless the respiratory rate is less than 60 breaths/min (although oral/nasal gastric tube feeding, at least of small, gut priming feedings, can be started in such infants, especially if mother's colostrum or milk is available, rather than waiting until the respiratory distress resolves). Neonates with craniofacial malformation (e.g., cleft lip or palate, choanal stenosis or atresia, mandibular hypoplasia) are at increased risk for aspiration.

Use of different nipple shapes and sizes and bottles that allow for infant-driven flow may facilitate safe oral feeding. Recent evidence has advocated the use of the semielevated side-lying (ESL) position when introducing bottle feedings to the preterm infant rather than the semielevated

recumbent position (ESU). ESL positioning better mimics the breastfeeding position and allows for better coordination of breathing with swallowing[45,153] (Figure 17-7, A). As infants mature, they can be transitioned to ESU positioning. Pacing of the feeding also can assist infants as they transition through the process of learning how to orally feed (also see Chapters 13 and 18). *Semidemand, cue-based,* or *infant-driven* feedings result in an earlier attainment of full oral feedings in premature infants.[103,115,128,176] Swallowing exercises, including placement of a milk bolus (0.05 to 0.2 ml) on the tongue where the bolus rests before entering the pharynx, also facilitate the attainment of independent oral feeding.[113] Gastrostomy tube placement may be necessary if oral feedings are not adequately established (see Chapter 28).

The ability to suck on a pacifier, fingers, or a gavage tube does not ensure the infant's ability to perform nutritive sucking. An infant who is successful at oral feeding should exhibit an active suck, coordinated swallow with breathing, minimal fluid loss around the nipple, and completion of feeding within 15 to 30 minutes.[177]

Coordination of sucking with breathing is the first lesson for the preterm infant. Stress behaviors (e.g., increase or decrease in respiratory or heart rate, decreased oxygen saturation, color change, gagging, choking, emesis, fatigue, irritability, or a "panicked look") should be treated with a rest period or cessation of the feeding. Provider *pacing* is important until the infant learns to self-pace feedings. Strategies to facilitate oral feedings also include a relaxed caregiver, a quiet environment with subdued light, and a snugly wrapped infant (see Chapter 13). A too rapid change to oral feeding can result in insufficient nutrition and potential failure to gain weight appropriately, primarily because the infant tires with feeding and is unable to take in a sufficient amount of food. Diligent attention is warranted, and nipple feedings often have to be limited and gavage feedings continued to prevent dehydration and undernutrition. Box 17-7 provides infant-driven feeding scales, an approach to determine infant readiness to nipple feed, quality of the feeding, and caregiver techniques used during the nipple feeding.

FEEDING INTOLERANCE AND COMPLICATIONS

Assessment for signs of feeding intolerance is imperative; although some feeding complications are mild and respond to nursing interventions, others are more serious and require more intervention. Feeding intolerance frequently is the first sign of illness (e.g., hypoxia, dyspnea, congestive heart failure, sepsis, NEC). At first, such signs often are subtle; thus, the caregiver should be constantly aware of any change in the infant's overall condition and feeding tolerance.

BOX 17-7 **INFANT-DRIVEN FEEDING SCALES**

Infant-Driven Feeding Scales (IDFS) help to determine infant readiness to nipple feed, quality of the feeding, and caregiver techniques used during the nipple feeding. These scales help caregivers determine if infants are ready to nipple feed, a way to assess the quality of the feeding, and what techniques are used to deliver that nipple feeding. The scales may help make nipple feeding more consistent among caregivers and promote feeding success.

Infant-Driven Feeding Scales (IDFS) — Readiness Score Description

1. Alert or fussy before care. Rooting and/or hands to mouth behavior. Good tone.
2. Alert once handled. Some rooting or takes pacifier. Adequate tone.
3. Briefly alert with care. No hunger behaviors. No change in tone.
4. Sleeping throughout care. No hunger cues. No change in tone.
5. Significant change in heart rate, respiratory rate, O_2 saturations/requirements, or work of breathing outside safe parameters.

   If the infant receives a score of 1 or 2, the infant is ready to nipple feed. For any score higher than 2, the infant is gavage fed. The nurse would then reassess infant behavior at the next feeding. If nipple feeding readiness is determined, the next two scales are used to document quality of feeding and techniques used during feeding.

Infant-Driven Feeding Scales (IDFS) — Quality Score Description

1. Nipples with a strong coordinated suck, swallow, and breathing (SSB) throughout feed.
2. Nipples with a strong coordinated SSB but fatigues with progression.
3. Difficulty coordinating SSB despite consistent suck.
4. Nipples with a weak/inconsistent SSB. Little to no rhythm.
5. Unable to coordinate SSB pattern. Significant change in heart rate, respiratory rate, O_2 saturations/requirements, work of breathing outside safe parameters or clinically unsafe swallow during feeding.

Infant-Driven Feeding Scales (IDFS) — Caregiver Techniques Score Description

A. *Modified Side-lying:* Position infant in inclined side-lying position with head in midline to assist with bolus management.
B. *External Pacing:* Tip bottle downward/break seal at breast to remove or decrease the flow of liquid to facilitate SSB pattern.
C. *Specialty Nipple:* Use nipple other than standard for specific purpose (i.e., nipple shield, slow-flow, Haberman).
D. *Cheek Support:* Provide gentle unilateral support to improve intraoral pressure.
E. *Frequent Burping:* Burp infant based on behavioral cues, not on time or volume completed.
F. *Chin Support:* Provide gentle forward pressure on mandible to ensure effective latch/tongue stripping if small chin or wide jaw excursion.

From Waitzman KA, Ludwig SM, Nelson CLA: Contributing to content validity of the Infant-Driven Feeding Scales (IDFS). *Newborn Infant Nurs Rev* 14(3):88-91, 2014. Used with permission.

Residuals

The feeding tube is aspirated every 2 to 4 hours before a feeding to determine whether gastric emptying is adequate. Incompletely digested aspirates of less than 50% of the previous feeding, 2 to 4 ml/kg, or a 1-hour volume if on continuous feedings may be normal and generally should be refed to the infant (Figure 17-8). Increasing residuals, abdominal distention, or both, and the disruption of the infant's feeding plan can indicate *feeding intolerance*.[133] The infant should be evaluated for excessive air in the intestines, for example, from CPAP-assisted breathing, and for cow's milk protein intolerance. In more serious cases with progressively larger residuals, intestinal obstruction or NEC should be considered. If such serious disorders are not discovered, feedings can be started again with decreased feeding volumes and/or slower rates of feeding and feeding advancement. Medications such as metoclopramide or erythromycin have been used to accelerate bowel motility and improve feeding tolerance and weight gain.[121,144] An association has been observed between erythromycin exposure in young infants and hypertrophic pyloric stenosis and thus should only be considered when therapeutic benefits

outweigh the risks.[120] Changing the infant's position from supine to prone has been shown to decrease residuals.[44] Placing the infant in the right lateral recumbent position also aids in gastric emptying. Due to gastric outlet sphincter incompetence, bile staining of gastric residuals is common. Frank blood, increasing bile in progressively increasing residual volumes, bilious emesis, and other signs of intestinal obstruction and/or NEC should be evaluated promptly.

Emesis

Infants with emesis always should be evaluated for intestinal obstruction or diseases that produce ileus, such as NEC and sepsis. With persistent emesis or increasing amounts of bilious emesis, feedings should be held and the infant should be evaluated for sepsis, NEC, obstruction (including Hirschsprung's disease, malrotation, and midgut volvulus, with or without congenital bands, and microcolon in infants of diabetic mothers), metabolic disorders, or increased intracranial pressure. Postoperative emesis and abdominal distention may indicate a stricture, partial obstruction from subclinical continued NEC, or inflammatory abscess. Emesis also results from an overdistended

Assessment of Gastric Residuals

>50% of amount of feeding given in 3 hr or >2-4 ml/kg

<u>Evaluate Infant</u>
Activity
Abdominal examination and girth measurement
Increased apnea or bradycardia
Increased oxygen requirement

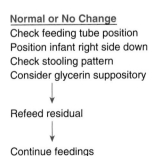

<u>Normal or No Change</u>	<u>Abnormal or Second Residual in 24 hr</u>
Check feeding tube position	Evaluate with abdominal radiograph
Position infant right side down	Consider infection screen
Check stooling pattern	Discard residual
Consider glycerin suppository	Hold feedings
↓	Reevaluate frequently
Refeed residual	↓
↓	Normal findings
Continue feedings	↓
	Restart feedings after 24 hr
	Consider reducing feeding volumes by 20%

FIGURE 17-8 Assessment of gastric residuals.

stomach, severe GER, a poorly positioned feeding tube, gastric irritation from enterally administered medications, drug withdrawal, or overstimulation in a very small infant. Interventions include allowing the feeding to flow more slowly by use of a smaller gavage tube, instilling the feeding over a longer period, decreasing feeding volumes, prone positioning, giving medications at the end of the feeding, or modifying a stressful environment (see Chapter 13). Auscultation, pH testing of gastric aspirates, or abdominal radiographs should be used to assess feeding tube position.

GASTROESOPHAGEAL REFLUX

GER should be suspected in an infant with irritability, emesis, apnea and bradycardia, respiratory deterioration, refusal to eat, or otherwise unexplained blood in the stools.[3] The use of histamine-2 (H-2) receptor blocker therapy and/or suppression of the (H^+, K^+)-ATPase enzyme system at the secretory surface of the gastric parietal cell for GER or feeding intolerance in infants is not supported by good evidence. H-2 blockers have been implicated in neonatal sepsis for being permissive to pathologic organisms by eliminating the barrier function of gastric acid.[79] Studies have reported decreased NEC with the acidification of feedings,[150] and there is an association between use of H-2 blocker therapy and NEC.[81]

Abdominal Distention

Abdominal distention with or without palpable or visible loops of bowel is a sign of poor gastric motility, ileus, constipation, or "gas." Variations in abdominal circumference of up to 1.5 cm can occur and, without other clinical signs of illness, may be normal. If the abdomen remains soft and nontender, prone positioning may be comforting, allowing gas and stool to pass. Persistent abdominal distention, pain with palpation, and discoloration of the overlying skin are signs of pathology (e.g., anatomic obstruction or infection) and require investigation. An abdominal x-ray examination is indicated in these patients. Abdominal girth is measured every 4 to 8 hours to document increased distention. Place paper or cloth tape around the abdomen at a consistent point marked on the abdomen.

Abdominal distention is a common complication in infants treated with CPAP. These infants are prone to excess accumulation of air in their stomach and ultimately their intestines, which can present as visible bowel loops. This is a benign condition that can be alleviated by the placement of an 8-French or larger orogastric (OG) tube to allow for continuous venting of gastric air.[30]

Diarrhea

Diarrhea, or frequent water-loss stools, indicates intolerance of the caloric density of feedings, transient lactase deficiency, use of highly osmotic medications, or other pathology, including, rarely, allergy. Stool culture for bacterial or viral pathogens and stool Clinitest should be performed if the infant also appears ill or if there is blood in the stool. In lactose malabsorption, short-term use of a non–lactose-containing formula or protein hydrolysate formula should result in return to normal stools.

Intermittent Rectal Bleeding/Food Protein–Induced Proctocolitis/ Eosinophillic Allergic Colitis

Asymptomatic and otherwise well newborns can pass stool noted to contain bright red blood. Pathologic factors including NEC, malrotation, Hirschsprung's disease, anal fissures, and blood clotting disorders should be investigated, as indicated. A short period of withholding feeds with supplemental intravenous (IV) fluids can be undertaken. Commonly the cause is cow's milk protein. If pathology is ruled out, oral feedings can be resumed with a hypoallergenic formula or with mother's own milk after she has been on an elimination diet. The elimination diet in the mother should continue for 2 weeks but in severe cases up to 4 months before the suspected allergen is reintroduced.[15,96]

Apnea and/or Bradycardia

Apnea and/or bradycardia frequently occur during or after feeding. These signs are the result of vagus nerve stimulation by the passage or presence of a feeding tube, gastric distention, or GER, or occur with abdominal distention and compromise of lung volumes or airway obstruction. In most cases, it is the apnea that triggers GER by decreasing lower esophageal sphincter tone.[3] Interventions to decrease vagal stimulation include changing to an OG gavage tube, decreasing feeding volume, and feeding more slowly. Achieving improved treatment of apnea often alleviates the GER.

Poor Growth

Growth is an essential requirement for the preterm infant. When normal growth does not occur, all possible factors should be considered, but most commonly, the infant has not been fed sufficient amounts of nutrition. If this is the case and the infant is not sick in some obvious way, he or she should be fed more, primarily by increasing protein and energy delivery.[84] Factors that increase caloric expenditure, such as thermal instability or over-stimulation, should be considered as causes of growth failure. Preterm infants always should be cared for in a thermoneutral environment, wearing a hat or other form of head covering (because large amounts of heat are lost from the surface of the head). Additional clothing, bundling or wrapping in soft blankets, supportive positioning, and grouping of care and stimulation to conserve energy often help improve growth.

Danger Signs

Gross amounts of bile in the gastric aspirate, bilious emesis, and progressively increasing abdominal distention can be a sign of significant ileus, obstruction, or NEC. The presence of blood in the stools or gastric aspirate, a tense or tender abdomen, and abdominal wall erythema are more ominous signs of feeding intolerance and may indicate frank NEC (Box 17-8). The presence of these signs and symptoms warrants a careful physical examination and usually further investigation including x-ray examinations. Feedings should be postponed while these signs and symptoms are being investigated. Other useful studies include a complete blood count with differential to evaluate extent of blood loss, presence of thrombocytopenia (a marker of necrotic bowel), and change in white blood cell count as evidence of infection. Although feeding of human milk may help protect against developing NEC and 5% to 10% of cases of NEC occur in infants who

---

BOX 17-8 | **CRITICAL FINDINGS**
DANGER SIGNS REQUIRING IMMEDIATE ATTENTION

1. Gross bile in the gastric aspirate with evidence of intestinal obstruction
2. Presence of blood in the stools or gastric aspirate
3. Tense or tender abdomen
4. Abdominal wall erythema
5. Unexplained anemia, thrombocytopenia, and neutropenia

---

have never been fed enterally, NEC can occur in *any* infant. Abnormal abdominal distention or grossly bilious or bloody gastric aspirates should be investigated carefully regardless of feeding status.

THE PRETERM INFANT

Much progress has made in providing nutritional support for ELBW (less than 1000 g) and VLBW (less than 1500 g) preterm infants. The nutritional requirements of these very small infants are marked, unique, incompletely understood, and frequently inadequately provided for, despite improvements in both the quality and quantity of nutrients in currently used IV and enteral nutrient regimens (Box 17-9). Also, many of these infants are growth restricted at birth. Thus their nutritional needs for normal rates of metabolism and growth are very likely to differ from those of normal-growth infants. Table 17-9 shows enteral intake recommendations for stable, growing preterm infants.

In spite of increasingly aggressive in-hospital nutritional management, the majority of infants born preterm experience postnatal growth restriction during their NICU stay, in large part due to inadequate nutrient intakes.[46,51,63,67,182] In fact, the fraction of these infants who are small for gestational age at discharge is several-fold greater than the fraction at birth (Figure 17-9).[65] There is increasingly strong evidence that early nutritional support of preterm and growth-restricted infants can have lasting consequences for improved neurodevelopmental outcome.[32,62,64] Such observations have important implications. First, we cannot now think of "early" nutrition of these small infants simply in terms of providing immediate

BOX 17-9	SPECIAL NUTRITIONAL CONDITIONS IN EXTREMELY LOW-BIRTH-WEIGHT INFANTS

1. Minimal energy reserves (both carbohydrates and fat)
2. Intrinsically higher metabolic rate (greater relative mass of more metabolically active organs: brain, heart, liver)
3. Higher protein turnover rate (especially when growing)
4. Higher glucose needs for energy and brain metabolism
5. Higher lipid needs to match the in utero rate of fat deposition
6. Excessive evaporative rates (immature skin)
7. Occasionally very high urinary water and solute losses (depending on intake and renal maturation)
8. Low rates of gastrointestinal peristalsis
9. Limited production of gut digestive enzymes and growth factors
10. Higher incidence of stressful events (hypoxemia, respiratory distress, sepsis)
11. Metabolic effects of medications used frequently (steroids, antibiotics, sedatives, catecholamines)
12. Abnormal neurologic outcome if not fed adequately

Modified from Thureen PJ, Hay WW Jr: Conditions in preterm infants requiring special nutritional management. In Tsang R, Lucas A, Uauy R, Zlotkin S, editors: *Nutritional needs of the preterm infant: scientific basis and practical guidelines*, Baltimore, 1993, Williams & Wilkins.

nutrient needs just for metabolic maintenance (e.g., glucose to prevent hypoglycemia); we also must consider that early nutrition, both prenatally and postnatally, has biologic effects that have lasting or lifelong significance. Second, we can no longer regard nutritional practices in preterm infants as simply a matter of personal choice. The major impact of sufficient early nutritional support on long-term outcome should be a stimulus to new research that defines consistent approaches to the nutrition of preterm infants to optimize their future health and development.

Concerns about the safety of enteral feeding of preterm infants have frequently delayed the initiation of feedings, despite the fact that there is little or no evidence that withholding enteral feedings decreases NEC.[135] Furthermore, the absence of enteral feeding leads to GI mucosal atrophy.[141] Evidence is accumulating that strongly supports early initiation (within the first 2 days of life) of low-volume enteral feedings ("minimal enteral nutrition" or "trophic feeds" or "gut priming"), especially with human colostrum and

milk. Minimal enteral feedings represent the administration of small feeds, less than 24 ml/kg/day, over a short but defined period of time (various feeding advancement protocols among different institutions define how many days to remain on minimal enteral nutrition before advancing to full enteral feeds) to promote GI development, motility, and function in the preterm infant. Enteral feedings are associated with surges in gut hormone production that mediate trophic effects on GI growth and mucosal maturation, including gastrin, enteroglucagon, motilin,[129] and lactase activity.[178] Animal studies have shown that minimal enteral feeding strategies trigger maturation of motor function in the intestine.[24,151] Absorption of nutrients is improved with increased amount and length of villous absorptive surface. Trophic feeding has been shown to improve energy intake, weight gain, head circumference gain, feeding tolerance, and time to reach full enteral feedings.[61,127,129] The potential advantages of minimal enteral feeding are listed in Box 17-10. Nearly all studies support the use of minimal enteral feedings, although a recent Cochrane review could not define specific benefits or exclude harmful effects of minimal or trophic enteral feedings for VLBW infants.[134] Early trophic or gut priming feedings have not, however, increased the risk of NEC, particularly when mother's milk is used, and should be considered the standard of practice. Minimal enteral feedings should begin within the first 2 days of life, range from 6 to 24 ml/kg/day, and be given every 4 to 6 hours for 3 to 5 days in VLBW infants.

Following minimal enteral nutrition, transition to nutritive enteral feedings can proceed (see Table 17-9), with continuous assessment of feeding tolerance. Mother's colostrum/milk is the preferred initial feeding choice, but, if necessary, donor human milk or full-strength formula may be used as an alternative for minimal enteral feeding. Although most infants benefit from early enteral feeding, those who are asphyxiated with persistent hypoxemia and metabolic acidosis, hypotensive with or without need for blood pressure medications, persistently and severely hypoxemic, symptomatic with a patent ductus arteriosus, or clearly septic and with evidence of NEC should not be fed enterally. These infants should be managed with aggressive full parenteral nutrition.

TABLE 17–9		ENTERAL INTAKE RECOMMENDATIONS FOR STABLE, GROWING PRETERM INFANTS PER 100 kcal*				

		CONSENSUS RECOMMENDATIONS BY THE AUTHORS OF THIS CHAPTER				
		INFANT WEIGHT <1000 g	INFANT WEIGHT >1000 g	AAP† <1000 g	AAP† 1000-1500 g	ESPGHAN‡
Water	ml	125-167	125-167	107-169	104-173	—
Energy	kcal	100	100	100	100	100
Protein	g	3-3.16	2.5-3	2.5-3.4	3.4-4.2	3.6-4.1 (<1 kg) 3.2-3.6 (1-1.8 kg)
Carbohydrate	g			6-15.4	5.4-15.5	10.5-12
Lactose	g	3.16-9.5	3.16-9.8	—	—	—
Oligomers	g	0-7	0-7	—		—
Fat	g			4.1-6.5	4.1-6.5	4.4-6
Linoleic acid	g	0.44-1.7	0.44-1.7	0.467-1.292	0.462-1.309	0.35-1.4
Linolenic acid	g	0.11-0.44	0.11-0.44	—	—	>0.05
18:2/C18:3		>5	>5	5-15	5-15	—
Vitamin A	International units	583-1250 1250-2333	583-1250 1250-2333	467-1154	538-1364	360-740
Vitamin D	International units	125-333§	125-333§	100-308	150-400	800-1000/day
Vitamin E	International units	5-10	5-10	4-9.2	4.6-10.9	2-10
Vitamin K	mcg	6.66-8.33	6.66-8.33	5.3-7.7	6.2-9.2	4-25
Ascorbate	mg	15-20	15-20	12-18.5	13.8-21.8	10-42
Thiamine	mcg	150-200	150-200	120-185	138-218	125-275
Riboflavin	mcg	200-300	200-300	167-277	192-327	180-365
Pyridoxine	mcg	125-175	125-175	100-162	115-191	41-273
Niacin	mg	3-4	3-4	2.4-3.7	2.8-4.4	3.45-5.0
Pantothenate	mg	1-1.5	1-1.5	0.8-1.3	0.9-1.5	>0.3-1.9
Biotin	mcg	3-5	3-5	2.4-4.6	2.8-5.5	>1.5-15
Folate	mcg	21-42	21-42	17-38	19-45	32-90
Vitamin B$_{12}$	mcg	0.25	0.25	0.2-0.23	0.23-0.27	0.08-0.7
Sodium	mg	38-58	38-58	46-88	53-105	63-105
Potassium	mg	65-100	65-100	52-90	60-106	60-120
Chloride	mg	59-89	59-89	71-192	82-226	95-161
Calcium	mg	100-192	100-192	67-169	77-200	110-130
Phosphorus	mg	50-117	50-117	40-108	46-127	55-80
Magnesium	mg	6.6-12.5	6.6-12.5	53-11.5	6.1-13.6	7.5-13.6
Iron	mg	1.67	1.67	1.33-3.08	1.54-3.64	1.8-2.7

Continued

TABLE 17-9	ENTERAL INTAKE RECOMMENDATIONS FOR STABLE, GROWING PRETERM INFANTS PER 100 kcal — cont'd					

		CONSENSUS RECOMMENDATIONS BY THE AUTHORS OF THIS CHAPTER				
		INFANT WEIGHT <1000 g	INFANT WEIGHT >1000 g	AAP[†] <1000 g	AAP[†] 1000-1500 g	ESPGHAN[‡]
Zinc	mcg	833	833	337-2308	769-2727	1000-1800
Copper	mcg	100-125	100-125	80-115	92-136	90-120
Selenium	mcg	1.08-2.5	1.08-2.5	0.9-3.5	1.4-1	4.5-9
Chromium	mcg	0.083-0.42	0.083-0.42	0.07-1.73	0.08-2.05	0.027-1.12
Manganese	mcg	6.3	6.3	0.5-5.8	0.5-6.8	6.3-25
Molybdenum	mcg	0.25	0.25	0.2-0.23	0.23-0.27	0.27-4.5
Iodine	mcg	25-50	25-50	6.7-46.2	7.7-54.5	10-50
Taurine	mg	3.75-7.5	3.75-7.5	3-6.9	3.5-8.2	—
Carnitine	mg	~2.4	~2.4	~1.9-2.2	~2.2-2.6	—
Inositol	mg	27-67.5	27-67.5	21-62	25-74	4-48
Choline	mg	12-23.4	12-23.4	9.6-12.5	11.1-25.2	7-50

Note: ESPGHAN states that "no specific recommendations are provided for infants with a weight below 1000 g, because data are lacking for this infant group for most nutrients, except for protein needs."

*120 kcal/kg/day was used where conversion was made from per kg recommendations.

[†]American Academy of Pediatrics, Committee on Nutrition. American Academy of Pediatrics Committee on Nutrition: Nutritional needs of the preterm infant. In Kleinman RE, editor: *Pediatric nutrition handbook,* ed 6, Elk Grove Village, Ill, 2009, AAP, pp 79-80.

[‡]European Society of Paediatric Gastroenterology, Hepatology and Nutrition, Committee on Nutrition of the Preterm Infant: Enteral nutrient supply for preterm infants: commentary from the European Society for Pediatric Gastroenterology, Hepatology and Nutrition Committee on Nutrition, *J Pediatr Gastroenterol Nutr* 50:85, 2010.

[§]Aim = 400 international units/day.

Few controlled trials support any given feeding strategy. Although older studies indicated that rapid advances to large feeding volumes were poorly tolerated by preterm infants,[25] more recent evidence indicates that progressive feeding advances in both volume and concentration with supplements can proceed more promptly in most preterm infants.* The following guidelines reflect a general approach to the advancement of enteral feedings (Table 17-10); clinical judgment should be used in following any feeding schedule. In general, the smaller the infant, the greater attention should be paid to feeding tolerance, although larger, more mature infants certainly can develop serious feeding intolerance and, in some cases, even NEC.

After a period of minimal enteral feedings, advancement to full nutritive enteral feedings for the infant who weighs less than 2000 g should proceed in increments of 20 to 30 ml/kg/day. Full feedings of human milk or formula (approximately 160 ml/kg/day) usually can be achieved over 7 to 10 days (see Table 17-10). In most cases, breastmilk should be fed to the infant in the order in which it is collected, with the colostrum given first. An alternative for infants who cannot tolerate large volumes of feedings is hind milk (see Chapter 18), which has increased fat content and may be given preferentially to increase energy delivery. Once the infant is tolerating increasing amounts of enteral feeding (practice is variable, ranging from 50 to 100 ml/kg/day of enteral nutrition), breastmilk can be fortified with the addition of human milk fortifiers (see Table 17-3).

*References 43, 99, 107, 136, 166, 188.

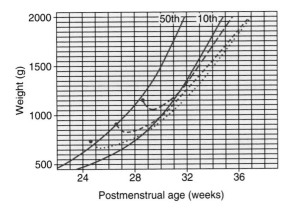

— Intrauterine growth (10th and 50th)
···· 24-25 weeks
—·— 26-27 weeks
—— 28-29 weeks

FIGURE 17-9 Average body weight versus postmenstrual age in weeks for infants with gestational ages 24 to 25 weeks *(dotted line)*, 26 to 27 weeks *(short dashes)*, and 28 to 29 weeks *(long dashes)*. The reference intrauterine growth curves were plotted using the smoothed 10th and 50th percentiles birth weight data reported by Alexander G, Himes JH, Kaufman RB, et al: A United States national reference for fetal growth, *Obstet Gynecol* 87:163-168, 1996. (From Ehrenkranz RA, Younes N, Lemons JA, et al: Longitudinal growth of hospitalized very low birth weight infants. Reproduced with permission from *Pediatrics* 104:280-289, 1999, © American Academy of Pediatrics.)

BOX 17-10 | ADVANTAGES OF MINIMAL ENTERAL FEEDING

- No increase in incidence of necrotizing enterocolitis
- Decreased sepsis
- Decreased permeability of mucosa to foreign antigens
- Increased intestinal peptides and hormones
- Increased mucosal thickness and villi
- Maturation of intestinal motor activity
- Improved feeding tolerance
- Improved bone mineralization
- Earlier achievement of full enteral feedings
- Improved weight gain
- Shorter hospital stay
- Reduced requirement for supplemental oxygen

Thus progression to full enteral feedings of fortified human milk or 24 kcal/oz preterm infant formula occurs over about 2 weeks in the smallest, most preterm infants. During this time, parenteral nutritional support is tapered to maintain from birth at least 3.5 g/kg/day protein, 30% to 54% of total calories from fat, and 40% to 60% of total calories from carbohydrate. If feedings have been interrupted, higher amounts of feeding and concentrations of nutrients, particularly protein (up to 4.5 g/kg/day), can be used to catch up. Infants weighing 500 to 1500 g fed on an every-2-hour interval have been shown to achieve full enteral feedings with subsequently less parenteral nutrition then those who were fed on a 3-hour schedule.[58] Firm experimental support for any specific feeding guidelines for preterm infants is sorely lacking; however, implementation of standardized feeding regimens has been shown to decrease the risk of NEC by up to 84% and reduce variability in nutrition outcomes.[155,183] One theory on the mechanism behind this improvement is the increased consistency in feeding management and decreased likelihood of advancing "too fast." Another possibility is that the process of development and implementation of the guideline leads to reviewing current evidence and increased awareness of feeding tolerance and early signs of NEC by staff.

Late–Preterm Infant

The late-preterm infant, born at $34^{0/7}$ to $36^{6/7}$ weeks of gestation, represents the population of preterm infants now accounting for more than 70% of all preterm births. Although generally these babies are larger and healthier than less mature newborns, NICU admission is frequent for feeding issues. These infants have intact, functional digestive and absorptive functions, but motility and intestinal colonization may be delayed. Of particular clinical importance is the immaturity of oromotor tone, function, and neural integration. Infants born between 33 and 36 weeks of gestation may initially seem to feed well but cannot maintain successful feeding during the first week of life. Poor feeding, therefore, is common in this group of babies, potentially contributing to problems of hypoglycemia, hyperbilirubinemia, and excessive postbirth weight loss (see Chapter 5). The ideal nutrition for these infants, as with those infants born more preterm, is breastmilk, preferably mother's own. A significant amount of brain growth and development occurs between 34 and 40 weeks' gestation, including a 50% increase in cortical volume,[5] which could be compromised

TABLE 17–10 EXAMPLE OF FEEDING ADVANCEMENT GUIDELINES

GESTATIONAL AGE (weeks)	DOF 1	DOF 2	DOF 3	DOF 4	DOF 5	DOF 6	DOF 7	DOF 8	DOF 9	DOF 10
≤25 6/7	≤20	≤20	≤20	≤20	≤20	≤50	≤80 Fortify	≤110	≤140	160
26-28 6/7	≤20	≤20	≤20	≤50	≤80 Fortify	≤110	≤140	160		
29-31 6/7	≤20	≤20	≤50	≤80 Fortify	≤110	≤140	160			
32-33 6/7	≤20	≤50	≤80 Fortify	≤110	≤140	≤160				
34-35 6/7	≤40	≤80 Fortify PRN	≤120	160						

DOF, Day of feeds.
- Intake amounts presented as ml/kg/day.
- Gray shaded boxes represent minimal enteral feedings (trophic feedings).
- Patients may nipple bottle feeds up to the maximum feeding volume, or breastfeed as able. Patients should not initially be placed on ad lib nippling or advanced at higher volumes, due to increased risk for feeding intolerance.
- Breastmilk is preferred. Donor milk or formula is also acceptable if breastmilk is not available or parental choice of formula.

Infants deemed at higher risk (two or more risk factors) may have feeding amounts reduced or initiated at GI priming volumes with advancement as medically appropriate. *Perinatal risk factors* include 5-minute Apgar score <5, umbilical venous gas or infant's first blood gas with metabolic acidosis (pH <7.2, base deficit >10 mEq/L), nonreassuring fetal heart rate tracing as indication for delivery, asymmetric IUGR or IUGR with reversed or absent end-diastolic flow, monochorionic twin gestation with twin-twin transfusion syndrome, severe polycythemia with hyperviscosity.

Neonatal risk factors include significant cardiovascular instability (chest compressions, vasoactive agent requirement, or multiple boluses of crystalloid or colloid), significant apnea (>1 per hour requiring intervention defined as vigorous stimulation with supplemental oxygen and bag-mask ventilation, any >4 per hour, or >6 total in 24 hours requiring intervention), symptomatic patent ductus arteriosus, antibiotic treatment greater than 7 days, prolonged NPO status greater than 7 days.

Source: K. Hendrickson, MS, RD, CNSC, CSP, in conjunction with NICU Quality Leadership, University of Colorado Health, Aurora, Colorado.

if suboptimal amounts of nutrition are delivered. Thus it is reasonable even in such late-preterm infants to fortify mother's milk or donor human breastmilk, or use preterm formulas, particularly if growth is compromised by illness and/or until the infant is taking full enteral feedings appropriate for a term infant.[158]

THE INTRAUTERINE GROWTH-RESTRICTED INFANT

Many preterm infants have experienced intrauterine growth restriction (IUGR) and thus are often born small for gestational age as well as preterm. Their nutritional needs for normal rates of metabolism and growth are very likely to differ from those of normally grown infants.[56] Nutritional support for the small-for-gestational-age infant requires separate consideration, because decreased size-for-dates occurs with various pathologic conditions or no pathology at all. Small size at birth is related to any number of diseases or abnormalities, both intrinsic and extrinsic to the fetus and newborn. Early events in gestation, including chromosomal and genetic abnormalities or early infection, lead to symmetric growth restriction. In contrast, asymmetric growth restriction occurs in response to late placental insufficiency or other insults that restrict nutrient supply to the fetus. Many completely healthy and normal infants are constitutionally small. Complicating these issues is the fact that preterm infants often are growth restricted at birth (i.e., whatever led to IUGR also contributed to processes that caused or promoted preterm birth). Such infants require more individualized management, because they may not tolerate advancing enteral feedings as well as normally grown infants and do not necessarily respond to increased nutrient intake with appropriate rates of growth.[32,162] Overfeeding an IUGR infant has been considered a cause of adult diseases such as obesity, insulin resistance, diabetes, and cardiovascular disease.[78]

In general, IUGR infants are likely to have increased energy needs due to low stores of energy, nutrients, and minerals.[29,56,138,165,189] Hypoglycemia, hyperglycemia, increased need for heat production, and increased risk for GI ischemia and NEC are more likely in the early postnatal period in these infants than in their normally grown peers.[23,204] These problems require anticipatory nutritional monitoring and management. Early parenteral glucose, protein, and energy supplementation is necessary while cautious enteral feedings are started.[195] Refeeding syndrome has been shown to occur in VLBW infants with IUGR born to mothers with preeclampsia. *Refeeding syndrome* occurs on initiation of enteral or parenteral nutrition, following a period of malnutrition or starvation. Laboratory markers of refeeding syndrome are hypophosphatemia, hypokalemia, hyperglycemia, and hypomagnesemia.[130,171]

CHANGES IN NUTRITIONAL REQUIREMENTS WITH ILLNESS

Studies in adult patients have shown dramatic changes in nutritional requirements depending on type of illness, degree of illness, surgery, and premorbid nutritional status. Although these changes are not well studied in neonates, preliminary data and clinical experience indicate that similar changes should be expected in ill infants. In fact, these patients have even greater nutritional needs because of requirements for growth and development. The overriding observation from all studies, however, is that ELBW and VLBW preterm infants are underfed during the early postnatal period and that this undernutrition, combined with additional stresses from various diseases, increases the risk for long-term adverse neurologic sequelae.[163] The value of achieving a specific body composition and growth rate is less certain. There remains a critical need for determining the right quality, as

well as quantity, of nutrients for these infants. The effects of common disease states on the nutrient requirements in preterm and term infants are shown in Figure 17-5.

Acute and chronic respiratory diseases are the most common illnesses in neonates. Acute respiratory problems, such as respiratory distress syndrome, pneumonia, and aspiration, all increase the infant's metabolic needs for energy and protein. Energy requirements are met by increasing carbohydrate and fat delivery. However, the metabolism of excessive carbohydrate feeding (greater than 12.5 mg/kg/min) may be detrimental to pulmonary status by increasing oxygen consumption and carbon dioxide production, increasing respiratory work, and adding to respiratory failure. Lipid is a good alternative source of concentrated energy because its metabolism has a lower respiratory quotient and produces less carbon dioxide. Lipids provide dense calories for volume and prevent essential fatty acid deficiency. Protein wasting and catabolism with illness increase the infant's requirement for exogenous support. Adequate provision of amino acids, especially branched-chain amino acids, prevents catabolism of body protein stores, including respiratory and diaphragmatic muscle protein, and may improve minute ventilation by decreasing carbon dioxide production.

Infants with *chronic lung disease and bronchopulmonary dysplasia* present difficult nutritional problems.[137] Poor nutrition is associated with abnormal lung development, increased toxic effects of oxygen, decreased surfactant production, and increased risk for infection. Although energy and metabolic demands are increased in these patients, many routine management strategies make the disease process worse. Excessive fluid volumes increase pulmonary edema and contribute to lung injury. Increased work of breathing limits intake. Steroid therapy and chronic disease have negative effects on protein balance. Diuretic use can waste calcium and potassium. Decreasing the proportion of energy provided by carbohydrates has been shown in older infants with chronic respiratory disease to decrease lipogenesis and therefore carbon dioxide production. Vitamin supplementation should be provided at the estimated advisable intake.

Congenital heart disease, especially when accompanied by cyanosis or congestive heart failure, significantly impairs nutritional status and growth. These infants have increased *basal metabolic needs* and experience the additional catabolic stress of early surgery. Nutritional management also is complicated by underlying hypoxemia, diuretic therapy, respiratory distress, malabsorption, and delicate fluid balance. Mineral derangement is common postoperatively with diuretic therapy and suboptimal intake. Iron supplementation is necessary to provide for increased erythropoiesis with chronic hypoxemia.

Good nutritional status can decrease the risk for infection and sepsis, as well as improve recovery in neonates. Normal immune response depends on adequate protein energy, micronutrients, and trace elements. Although not well studied in this population, it appears that the metabolic requirements of septic infants, especially for energy and amino acids, are much greater than the requirements of otherwise similar, but uninfected, infants.

The infant with NEC or short bowel syndrome is at additional risk for malnutrition because of malabsorption and increased nutrient losses. During the acute illness, these patients must receive adequate parenteral nutrition. Recovery needs to be supported by gradual increases in enteral nutrition and slowly decreasing parenteral supplementation. Of particular concern are excessive water losses with electrolyte imbalance and malabsorption of fats and fat-soluble vitamins.

Any infant recovering from perinatal hypoxic-ischemic injury or "asphyxia" with significant evidence of shock (low blood pressure, poor circulation, and metabolic acidosis) should probably not receive enteral feedings for 24 to 72 hours to allow recovery of the bowel from the ischemic injury. In preterm infants, such delays might decrease the risk for NEC. Infants with milder forms of such pathology probably can be given minimal enteral feedings with own mother's colostrum or breastmilk, which potentially could improve gut development after injury and colonize the gut with a more favorable microbiome.

Neonates who have undergone surgery are at increased risk for nutritional deficiencies resulting from the stresses of illness and surgery and possible abnormal nutrient and water losses. In these infants, enteral feedings are preferred because they are safe and more economical, preserve the integrity of the intestinal mucosa, and promote continued development of the GI tract. After a surgical procedure, the infant is often nil per os (NPO) status for 3 to 14 days until the return of intestinal motility

and function (e.g., stooling, lack of abdominal distention, decreased gastric aspirates, absence of bilious aspirates). The method of feeding chosen, rapidity of feeding advancement, formula composition, and type of feeding depend on the infant's general medical condition, GI function, and type of surgery. The choice of formula for the postsurgical neonate depends on bowel integrity. An infant recovering from mild NEC may be started on human milk or regular formula. With serious or surgically treated NEC, human milk is preferred but an elemental or hydrolysate formula may be used.

DEVELOPMENTAL SUPPORT

The importance of developmentally supportive feeding cannot be overlooked when discussing infant nutrition. Preterm birth resulting in delayed introduction of feeding skills, surgical interventions for congenital or genetic abnormalities sometimes necessitating alternative feeding methods such as gastrostomy tube feedings, and prolonged interruption of normal feeding patterns are all examples of the impact that hospitalization can have on patients and their families.[50]

Being aware of the impact that prolonged hospitalization can have on feeding is the first step in being able to provide support and guidance to families of fragile infants. By using a team approach, the family can help support their infant in attaining and strengthening feeding skills in preparation for discharge and hopefully prevent or minimize long-term feeding difficulties that often are associated with an extended hospital stay, such as loss of feeding skills and feeding aversion issues.

A *supportive feeding team* should include the parents, physicians, nurse practitioners, lactation specialists, dietitians, occupational and physical therapists, developmental specialists, and nursing staff educated in the developmental support of infants with specialized feeding needs. This support should start as soon as an infant is admitted and continue beyond discharge to promote the best possible outcome with regard to feeding ability.

FAMILY SUPPORT

Parents of the NICU patient may feel overwhelmed by their infant's illness, appearance, and uncertain future. Loss of control of the infant's care and unclear parental roles make bonding difficult and add to feelings of helplessness, frustration, and isolation. It is imperative that the health care team be supportive of the parents as caregivers. This support can begin with education about early feeding practices in the nursery and anticipated infant growth and development. Feeding is an excellent way to involve parents in their infant's care. Parents should be involved in discussions of feeding practices and food choices. Scheduling oral feedings for parent visits enables them to actively participate in their infant's care. During gavage feedings, parents should be encouraged to hold their infant and support the pacifier to encourage nonnutritive sucking. Frequent communication about the ups and downs of feeding the sick newborn, as well as weekly progress updates on growth charts, is helpful.

A mother's ability to provide breastmilk remains the one aspect of care that she alone can do for her infant. Preterm birth and prolonged illness, as well as the inability to breastfeed the infant directly, are major barriers to successful breastfeeding. Lactation support in the NICU increases mothers' success at maintaining lactation through discharge from the NICU. Guidelines for expression and collection of human breastmilk, gavage feeding of human milk, and identification of oral feeding readiness all are essential elements of lactation support and success (see Chapter 18).

FEEDING THE PRETERM INFANT AFTER HOSPITAL DISCHARGE

Many preterm infants are still preterm when they are discharged from the NICU, and most are small for their corrected gestational age (i.e., they are growth restricted) and at significant risk for growth failure in the postdischarge period, especially if they are discharged before the expected delivery date.[65,110] These infants require continued attention to nutritional support after hospital discharge.[111,147] It is recommended that mother's own milk be used exclusively for the first 6 months of life, with continuation of breastfeeding for 1 year or longer as mutually desired by mother and infant.[104] However, postdischarge feeding practices, including the question of whether to fortify human milk, vary widely because evidence is conflicting.

For VLBW, formula-fed preterm infants who are of subnormal weight at the time of discharge, expert consensus guidelines support the use of postdischarge transitional formula and close nutritional follow-up.[111,145] These products are intermediate between preterm and term formulas in their energy, protein, calcium, phosphorus, vitamin, and mineral contents (see Table 17-7 for nutritional composition). These recommendations are supported by some evidence that has shown that providing preterm infants with a formula containing higher protein and energy contents after discharge results in improved growth.[202] Furthermore, use of a transitional formula for 6 months after discharge increases lean mass without increasing percent body fat at 1 year and decreases body fat, truncal fat, and fasting insulin concentrations at 2 years.[52,159] However, few trials have assessed neurodevelopmental outcomes, and those that have do not detect any significant differences in developmental indices at 18 months' corrected age.[203] Thus preterm infants discharged home with a normal weight for postmenstrual age could be fed similarly to term infants of similar gestational age.[145]

Guidance on how to feed the breastfed, preterm infant is scarce. Limited available data do not provide convincing evidence that multinutrient fortified breastmilk compared with unfortified breastmilk following hospital discharge affects important outcomes, with the exception of a small but significant effect on length at 12 months of age.[202] However, human-milk–fed preterm infants often accrue the greatest nutritional deficits by discharge and are at continued risk of growth deficiencies postdischarge.[147] Thus, preterm infants who are discharged on breastmilk feedings can be supplemented with powder formula fortification of mother's milk (22 to 24 kcal/oz) if growth is suboptimal at the time of discharge or in the immediate postdischarge period.

Preterm infants with significant chronic lung disease or other chronic conditions that might increase energy expenditure are likely to need increased protein and energy delivery after discharge to maintain adequate growth. For all preterm infants, attention should be paid to other possible nutrient deficiencies including calcium, phosphorus, iron, vitamins, and LC-PUFAs. Feeding postdischarge preterm formulas or breastmilk with higher concentrations of calcium and phosphorus results in improved bone mineralization.[112] All preterm infants also should receive iron supplementation and close surveillance of iron status.[19] Regardless of milk type, demand feeding should be initiated before discharge to document adequate growth on the chosen feeding regimen. Close monitoring of growth (weight, length, and head circumference for age, indices of body proportionality) and feed intake should be performed at discharge and regularly after discharge using appropriate growth curves.

REFERENCES

For a full list of references, scan the QR code or visit http://booksite.elsevier.com/9780323320832.

18 BREASTFEEDING THE NEONATE WITH SPECIAL NEEDS

SANDRA L. GARDNER AND RUTH A. LAWRENCE

Human milk has been recognized as the gold standard for infant nutrition for centuries. Published studies from 1918 on have confirmed that problems develop when human milk is replaced with artificial formulas made from the milk of other species. Milk of other species that is fed to human infants has been known to contribute to increased infant mortality risk. Over the years, increasing research has confirmed the presence of the antiinfective properties of human milk, which protect against infections of the gastrointestinal tract, the upper and lower respiratory tracts, and the urinary tract, as well as against otitis media, bacteremia, bacterial meningitis, botulism, and necrotizing enterocolitis (NEC), leading to lower infant mortality rates.[11,15,165] In numerous studies, human milk also has been shown to have a protective effect against sudden infant death syndrome, type 1 and type 2 diabetes, obesity, Crohn's disease, ulcerative colitis, lymphoma, childhood leukemia, allergic diseases, asthma, chronic digestive disorders, heart disease, and hypertension.[11,178] Breastfeeding also enhances cognitive and visual development and neurodevelopment.[188,236] Studies show less of a pain response in full-term infants undergoing heel lance when they were breastfed before, during, and after the procedure. Breastfeeding as a nonpharmacologic intervention for procedure-related neonatal pain is highly recommended[9] (see Chapter 12). In preterm infants, human milk provides both short-term and long-term advantages (Table 18-1) in a dose-dependent relationship—the more breastmilk the preterm receives, the more benefits received.[130,225,227,255,267,294]

Because of a lack of experience and knowledge about breastfeeding, a new mother who is discharged early (24 to 48 hours) from the hospital may find it challenging to initiate breastfeeding for her healthy newborn infant. The mother of a newborn with special needs, such as a preterm infant, a sick term newborn, or an infant with a congenital anomaly, may have even more difficulty in establishing breastfeeding because of the stress of separation and concerns about the infant's well-being (see Chapter 29). The tremendous benefits of providing human milk for all infants, but especially the premature, outweigh any apparent difficulties. In 2011, 30.8% of NICUs reported that 90% or more of their infants received human milk feedings, an increase from 2007 (21.2%) and 2009 (26.7%).[257] Human milk feedings (i.e., mother's own milk; donor human milk) need to be a priority for all preterm infants in NICUs.*

Healthy People 2020,[331] the health policy statement for the United States, states the following goal about breastfeeding: 81.9% of women breastfeeding in the early postpartum period, at least 60.6% still breastfeeding their infant at 6 months, and 34.1% breastfeeding their infant at 1 year of age. A report published by the Institute of Medicine,[145] the American Academy of Pediatrics (AAP) Section on Breast Feeding,[15] the Academy of Breastfeeding Medicine,[3] and the U.S. Surgeon General's *Call to Action to Support Breastfeeding*[329] states that (1) all infants in the United States should be breastfed, (2) "human milk is uniquely superior for infant feeding,"[145] (3) "infants should be exclusively breastfed for 5 to 6 months,"[15] and (4) "breastfeeding is the ideal method of feeding and nurturing infants."[329] The policy statement by the AAP provides additional recommendations for

---

*References 15, 24, 96, 171, 172, 225, 227, 253.

PURPLE type highlights content that is particularly applicable to clinical settings.

TABLE 18-1 ADVANTAGES OF BREASTFEEDING AND HUMAN MILK INTAKE FOR PRETERM INFANTS[223,225,294,326]

BENEFIT	COMMENT
Protection from NEC*	Formula-fed infants developed NEC 6-10 times more often than infants receiving only human milk. Infants ≥30 weeks' gestation: incidence of NEC 20 times more in formula-fed than in human milk–fed infants.
	Lower incidence of intestinal perforations and less severity of NEC with human milk intake before NEC.
	Dose-dependent relationship between human milk intake and reduced risk for NEC/death after 2 weeks of life in ELBW preterms.[226]
	Exclusive human milk diet fortified with human milk fortifier significantly lowers rates of NEC and severity of NEC compared with human milk or formula diet fortified with bovine-based fortifier.[317]
Protection from infection or sepsis†	Lowered infection and severity of infections in hospitalized ELBW, VLBW, or LBW infants fed human milk,[105,144,255,295] resulting in shortened LOS. Skin-to-skin care customizes human milk by production of antibodies against NICU-specific pathogens.[277]
	Lower intestinal permeability with human milk versus formula feedings; >75% human milk intake resulted in 3.8-fold lower intestinal permeability compared with <25% or no human milk intake.[321]
	A dose-response relationship between consumption of human milk and sepsis: every 10-ml/kg/day increase in human milk consumption decreased the risk of sepsis by 19%.[255]
	Use of mother's milk for oral care of ventilated premature infants was not associated with decrease in ventilator days, LOS; reduced positive tracheal aspirates/positive blood cultures not statistically significant.[322]
Increased feeding tolerance[213]	Decreased protection if formula feeding added to human milk feedings. Increased rehospitalization: sevenfold for formula-fed compared with 0-1 for infants who are breastfed (both partially and completely).
	Whey protein in human milk is more digested, which results in more rapid gastric emptying and less gastric residual.[40] Fat globules in human milk provide optimal absorption.[21] It is possible to achieve complete enteral feedings by 6 weeks of age in VLBW infants fed own mother's milk (compared with VLBW infants fed donor milk or formula).[187] Formula-fed infants: increased vomiting, gastric residuals, and longer time to achieve complete enteral feedings.[187] Early enteral feeding with human milk is as well tolerated in preterms treated with indomethacin for PDA as in matched controls.[34]
Earlier attainment of full enteral feedings,[307] which is associated with a significant reduction in late-onset sepsis among extremely premature infants[282]	Preterms ≤1250 g receiving at least 50% human milk attained earlier full enteral feeding.
Decreased risk for later allergy	Lower incidence of allergic symptoms (especially eczema) at 18 months in human milk–fed preterm infants.[186]
Improved retinal function[69,249,295]	Better retinal function, depending on omega-3 fatty acid concentration (found in human milk, but not previously in formula) in enteral feedings. Less ROP and less severe ROP in human milk–fed compared with formula-fed infants.[200,251]
Improved neurocognitive development‡ and brain growth[146]	Long-term advantages: higher intelligence quotients at 30 months,[338] 5 years,[267] and 7-8 years of age[139]; better development at 18-22 months of age[188,236,337]; and better behavioral scores (orientation/engagement, motor regulation, and total scores).[337]
	Faster brainstem maturation—resulting in better control of breathing.[17]
	Early supplementation of human milk with DHA/ARA for VLBW associated with better recognition, memory, and problem-solving skills at 6 months.[132]
Suppression of oxidative stress	Oxidative DNA damage in VLBW infants is suppressed at 14 and 28 days of age by measuring urinary 8-O HdG excretion.[301] Reduced incidence of BPD/CLD.[296,337]
	Antiinflammatory and antioxidant properties of human milk may protect premature infants from white matter injury.[163,350]

TABLE 18–1	ADVANTAGES OF BREASTFEEDING AND HUMAN MILK INTAKE FOR PRETERM INFANTS — cont'd

BENEFIT	COMMENT
Reduced health care costs[255]	A dose-response relationship between consumption of human milk and cost savings: NICU costs lowest in VLBW infants with the highest intake of human milk in the first 28 days of life.[255] Lower risk of NEC and sepsis (see above). Earlier attainment of full enteral feedings (see above). Shorter LOS.[296] Fewer hospital admissions up to 30 months of age.[337]
Reduced heart disease in later life and features predictive of metabolic syndrome[304]	Lower cardiorespiratory levels and LDL to HDL ratios in adolescents born premature who were fed human milk.

Modified from Meier P, Brown L: Breast feeding for mothers and low birth weight infants, *Nurs Clin North Am* 31:351, 1996.
ARA, Arachidonic acid; *BPD,* bronchopulmonary dysplasia; *CLD,* chronic lung disease; *DHA,* docosahexaenoic acid; *DNA,* deoxyribonucleic acid; *ELBW,* extremely low-birth-weight; *HDL,* high-density lipoprotein; *LBW,* low-birth-weight; *LDL,* low-density lipoprotein; *LOS,* length of stay; *HdG,* hydroxy-deoxy-guanosine; *NEC,* necrotizing enterocolitis; *NICU,* neonatal intensive care unit; *PDA,* patent ductus arteriosus; *ROP,* retinopathy of prematurity; *VLBW,* very-low-birth-weight.
*References 180, 187, 200, 268, 295, 297, 306.
†References 223, 226, 255, 295, 296, 321.
‡References 39, 69, 99, 132, 267, 309, 337, 338.

high-risk infants, including preterm infants. It states that the "hospitals and physicians should recommend human milk for premature and other high-risk infants either by direct breastfeeding or using the mother's own expressed milk." The statement continues by recognizing that maternal support and education, mother-infant skin-to-skin contact, and direct breastfeeding as early as possible are keys to success. State-by-state breastfeeding data on the percentage and length of breastfeeding are available from the Centers for Disease Control and Prevention (CDC) in its Breastfeeding Report Card.[54] In 2013, the CDC reported that 77% of mothers in the United States were discharged from the hospital breastfeeding their newborns—the highest rate in more than a decade.

The goal of this chapter is to give the health care provider the skill and knowledge to support the breastfeeding dyad, especially when it involves the neonate with special needs.

PHYSIOLOGY OF BREASTFEEDING

Nutritional Value of Breastmilk

The components of breastmilk vary with the (1) stage of lactation, (2) time of day, (3) sampling time during a feeding, and (4) extremes of maternal nutrition. In addition, there is variation among individuals.[157,178]

Colostrum is produced immediately at delivery and within 5 days gradually changes to transitional milk with increased lactose and finally mature milk by 2 weeks with an increasing concentration of fat. Colostrum contains higher ash content and higher concentrations of sodium, potassium, chloride, protein, fat-soluble vitamins, and minerals than does mature milk. Colostrum has a lower fat content, especially of lauric and myristic acids, than does mature milk. This milk is yellowish, thick, and rich in antibodies, has specific gravity between 1.040 and 1.060, and contains 67 kcal/dl. During the first day of life, full-term healthy breastfeeding neonates ingest a total of 15 ml (±11 ml) divided among 10 feeding sessions.[293] Multiparas and women who have previously breastfed have more colostrum during the first few days than do women who have not.

Transitional milk is produced between 7 and 10 days postpartum, remains high in protein and lower in fat, and has a dramatic increase in water content compared with colostrum. Among mothers, the high variability of transitional milk accounts for 67 to 75 kcal/dl.

Mature milk is produced after 10 days postpartum and contains 75 kcal/dl. By the second week of life, maternal milk production averages about 30 ml/hr (i.e., 750 to 800 ml/day). During a feeding, the relative content of protein and the absolute content of fat increases. Morning feedings have a higher fat content than do afternoon and evening feedings. Foremilk is lower in fat and energy content than hindmilk. Severely malnourished mothers have been shown to produce less milk, and water-soluble vitamins may be affected by deficient diets, as may occur in strict vegetarians.

Human Milk versus Cow's Milk

Cow's milk differs significantly from human milk. Cow's milk has 18 parts whey to 82 parts casein, whereas human milk has 60 parts whey to 40 parts casein. Casein is composed of proteins with ester-bound phosphate, high proline content, and low solubility at a pH of 4 to 5. Casein forms curd by combining with calcium caseinate and calcium phosphate. The cysteine and taurine content is low in cow's milk but high in human milk, whereas the methionine content is high in cow's milk and low in human milk (the human infant lacks the enzyme to digest methionine). Human milk also has lower levels of aromatic amino acids, phenylalanine, and tyrosine. Human milk contains 6.8 g/dl of lactose, and cow's milk contains 4.9 g/dl of lactose. Sodium, phosphorus, calcium, magnesium, citrate, and total ash content are higher in cow's milk, but potassium and the calcium:phosphorus ratio is higher in human milk. Formula attempts to mimic human milk but still lacks cholesterol, omega-3 fatty acids, enzymes, antibodies, lactoferrin, and other protective antiinfective properties.

Human milk contains more iron than unsupplemented cow's milk but less iron than supplemented cow's milk. Only 10% of iron is absorbed from formula, whereas about 80% is absorbed from human milk. Iron in formula encourages the growth of *Escherichia coli* and inactivates lactoferrin. Cow's milk has a mean pH of 6.8, osmolality of 350 mOsm, and 221 mOsm renal osmolar load. Human milk has a mean pH of 7.1, osmolality of 286 mOsm, and 79 mOsm renal osmolar load.

Cow's milk forms indigestible curds much more easily and thus delays gastric emptying. The newborn cannot handle certain proteins well because cow's milk lacks specific enzymes necessary for metabolism. These enzymes are readily available in human milk. However, 95% of human milk protein is nutritionally available to term infants, whereas the gastrointestinal immaturity of the preterm infant enables four to six times higher daily losses of human milk protein if human milk is pasteurized or has cow's milk–based fortifier added. Some human milk proteins are immunoglobulins, which have a protective effect on the gut and are preserved by antiproteases from being digested (i.e., are found in stool). In very-low-birth-weight (VLBW) infants, the antiproteases persist so that there are more immunoglobulins and lactoferrin in the stool early on (i.e., six and four times more immunoglobulin A (IgA) and lactoferrin, respectively). This is a function of the milk of mothers who deliver prematurely, not a deficiency of VLBW gut. Iron is more bioavailable in human milk, and iron absorption from human milk is more efficient, but cow's milk has a higher concentration of zinc and contains more fluorine than does human milk. Human milk, however, contains a ligand specific to zinc absorption, and thus more zinc actually is absorbed and used. Human milk has been used as a therapy for zinc deficiency (see Chapter 17 for other human milk components).

Preterm versus Term Breastmilk

Significant evidence exists that there are many differences in the breastmilk that a mother produces when she has a preterm infant compared with breastmilk produced for a term infant[162]: (1) Preterm breastmilk has increased protein content; (2) the types of protein, predominantly whey, have a more physiologic balance of amino acids and contain many antiinfective properties; (3) the lipid content in preterm breastmilk is more specific for the preterm neonate (i.e., an increased supply of medium-chain to intermediate-chain fatty acids); (4) lactose, the major carbohydrate in breastmilk, has increased absorption in preterm infants; and (5) IgA concentrations are higher (see Chapter 17 for a comparison of preterm and term breastmilk).

In the neonatal intensive care unit (NICU), four critical exposure periods for premature infants to human milk have been identified: (1) colostrum in the transition from intrauterine to extrauterine life, (2) transition from colostrum to mature milk in the first month of life, (3) the amount of human milk feeding throughout the NICU stay, and (4) human milk feeding after discharge.[223] Colostrum is rich in bioactive factors that promote growth and maturation, as well as protection of the immature intestinal tract of infants.[223,225] Mothers of the least mature preterm infants produce the most protective colostrum and produce colostrum for a longer period of time in order to protect their vulnerable offspring.[223,278]

The Immunologic Value of Breastmilk

Because human milk protects neonates through its many antiinfective properties, breastfed infants have decreased morbidity compared with bottle-fed infants.[116,235] The immunologic benefits of human milk depend on dose, duration, and exclusivity.[121,130] The main defense factors in human milk are (1) antimicrobial agents, (2) antiinflammatory factors, and (3) immunomodulators and leukocytes. In addition to providing protective agents, the components in human milk also modulate the development of the newborn's own immune functions.[116] Bioactive factors in human milk and their functions are listed in Table 18-2.

The highest concentration of immunoprotective factors is found in colostrum, which should be pumped, preserved, and fed to a neonate with special needs.[125,280] Pumped milk should be labeled chronologically so that it is fed to preterm infants in the same sequence in which it was collected. In this fashion, the preterm infant receives the high concentration of protective qualities that have been shown to protect the gastrointestinal and respiratory systems. Clinical guidelines for colostrum feeding in the NICU are presented in Box 18-1.[223]

Providing colostrum to the oral cavity of the preterm infant stimulates the development and response of the neonate's own immune system.[278,279] Colostrum as oral immune therapy has been studied in seven small studies, of fair quality, and recently reviewed.[109] In this review findings of colostrum as oral therapy include the following: (1) safe, feasible with very low to no risk; (2) less use of total parenteral nutrition; (3) promotes early enteral feeding; and (4) preterms less likely to be growth restricted at 36 weeks' postmenstrual age.[109] Although no difference in infectious outcomes were found, this was attributed to small sample sizes and low statistical power. Well-designed randomized controlled trials of sufficient size are needed to provide definitive evidence of colostrum as oral immune therapy, appropriate dose, duration of therapy, and

impact on neonatal morbidities such as sepsis, NEC, pneumonia, chronic lung disease, and retinopathy of prematurity.[109] Box 18-2 is an adapted protocol for oral care with colostrum.

Enteral intake in the first month of life constitutes the second critical period when benefits listed in Table 18-1 are seen in VLBW and extremely low-birth-weight (ELBW) preterms in a dose-dependent relationship to human milk intake.[223,267] The normal microflora found in the neonatal gastrointestinal tract is the first line of defense against many pathogenic bacteria. After birth, the first exposure of the neonatal gut is to the maternal vaginal flora, and colonization continues with development of an environment of flora by 1 week of age. However, colonization of the gastrointestinal tract of preterm and sick neonates is altered by cesarean birth, antibiotics, delayed enteral feeding, separation from mother, and presence in an NICU. With breastfeeding or provision of breastmilk, containing both prebiotics and probiotics, the dominant flora are *Bifidobacterium* and *Lactobacillus,* which suppress pathogens. Breastmilk has been shown to be effective in reducing the colonization with *Klebsiella, Enterobacter,* and *Citrobacter.*[98] In addition, paracellular pathways between enterocytes in the preterm infant's intestine are closed, thus inhibiting the passage of bacteria and toxins from gut lumen to the bowel wall. When infants are provided formula, the growth of bifidobacteria is very slow and at the end of the first week, there is only one tenth the concentration compared with that in infants fed breastmilk. During this critical period, even small amounts of formula interrupt both of these processes.[223]

There are conflicting results from research as to whether reduction of antiinfective activity occurs with the use of breastmilk fortifier. Older studies showed that fortifier does not decrease antiinfective properties of human milk,[126,179,296] whereas a more recent study showed that human milk fortifier with iron reduced the bacteriostatic action of the fortified breastmilk against *E. coli,* in vitro.[52] Continued surveillance in the use of fortifiers is recommended.[296]

The fourth critical period of human milk intake for preterm infants is the total amount and/or exclusive human milk feeding during their NICU stay.[223] Research shows that extremely premature infants (i.e., ELBW, VLBW) exhibit benefits of human milk intake listed in Table 18-1 based

T A B L E **18-2**	**BIOACTIVE FACTORS IN HUMAN MILK**

COMPONENT	FUNCTION
Antibodies	
Secretory IgA (slgA)	Attaches to mucosal epithelium of digestive tract, thus preventing attachment of pathogens,[167,281] slgA against enteric, respiratory, and viral pathogens, as well as specific pathogens to which the mother has been exposed; highest concentration in colostrum peaks during first 3-4 days postpartum; present in mature milk through first year of life.[47,294] Antiallergic properties: inhibits absorption of macromolecular antigens from neonatal small intestine.
Major Nutrients **Protein**	
slgA, IgM, IgG	Immune protection.
Lactoferrin	Binds iron, thwarts growth of pathogens (e.g., bactericidal, antiviral), modulates cytokine function, and is antiinflammatory; highest levels in colostrum; present in mature milk through first year of life.[167] May attenuate iron-induced oxidation products in preterms.[270]
Lysozyme	Destroys pathogens (e.g., gram-positive and few gram-negative bacteria) by cell wall lysis; human milk contains 300 times the concentration in cow's milk; concentration increases with prolonged lactation.[281]
Casein	Inhibits microbial adhesion to mucous membranes of respiratory and gastrointestinal tracts. Promotes growth of *Lactobacillus bifidus*, the normal intestinal flora for breastfed infants, and inhibits pathogens[183]; by 1 month of age, *Bifidobacterium* level in infants fed human milk is 10 times that of formula-fed infants.
Adiponectin	Regulates metabolism; possible protection against obesity.
Fibronectin	Enhances antimicrobial activity of macrophages[281]; assists in repair of intestinal tissue damage by immune reactions.
Carbohydrate	
Oligosaccharides	Bind to microorganisms (microbial ligands), thus preventing pathogens from attaching to respiratory mucosal surfaces.[294]
Glycoconjugates mucin and lactadherin	Microbial and viral ligands.[70] Provide receptor site binding for organisms so that the organism is made less harmful or passes from the body in the stool.[281]
Fat	
Free fatty acids (FFAs)	Disrupt and destroy lipid-enveloped virus, bacteria, and protozoa.[125]
Minor Nutrients	
Nucleotides	Enhance T-cell maturation, antibody response to vaccines, intestinal maturation, repair after diarrhea and natural killer cell activity; promote growth of *Lactobacillus bifidus*.
Vitamins	
A, C, E, D	Antiinflammatory: scavenges oxygen radicals. Vitamin D content of breastmilk is 25 IU/L or less. For prevention of rickets and vitamin D deficiency, all breastfed infants should be given supplemental vitamin D (e.g., 400 IU/day) beginning within the first few days of life.[16]
Enzymes	
Amylase	Digestion of polysaccharides.
Bile salt–dependent lipase	Production of FFAs with antibacterial/protozoan activity. Assists with fat digestion.
Catalase	Antiinflammatory: degrades H_2O_2.
Glutathione peroxidase	Antiinflammatory: prevents lipid peroxidation.
Lipase	Breaks down triacylglycerols.
Platelet-activating factor (PAF) acetyl hydrolase	Degrades PAF, a potent cause of ulceration; protects against necrotizing enterocolitis.

	TABLE 18-2	BIOACTIVE FACTORS IN HUMAN MILK — cont'd

COMPONENT	FUNCTION
Growth Factors	
Epithelial growth factors	Enhances maturation of gut epithelial barrier; limiting penetration by foreign antigens, thus decreasing immune stimulation.[281]
Transforming growth factors	Alpha: promotes epithelial cell growth.
	Beta: suppresses lymphocyte function: antiinflammatory; prevents allergic reaction.
Hormones	
Prolactin	Enhances B- and T-lymphocyte development; affects differentiation of intestinal lymphoid tissue.
Cortisol, thyroxine, insulin	Promotes maturation of neonatal intestine and development of intestinal host-defense mechanisms.
Erythropoietin	Influences erythropoiesis, gut maturation, apoptosis, neurodevelopment, and immunity.[298]
Cells	
B lymphocytes	Synthesize IgA and other antibodies targeted against specific pathogens.
Macrophages	90% of cells in breastmilk; phagocytize microorganisms and kill bacteria in neonatal intestine; produce lysozyme, lactoferrin, and complement.
Neutrophils	Phagocytize bacteria in neonatal gastrointestinal tract.
T lymphocytes	Phagocytosis against organisms in gastrointestinal tract; mobilize other host defenses; antigens introduced into maternal respiratory and/or gastrointestinal systems stimulate development of antibodies in breastmilk; incorporation into neonatal tissue bestows short-term adoptive immunity.[179]
Cytokines	Modulate functions and maturation of immune system.
Proinflammatory: interleukins 1-beta, 6, 8, 12; interferon-gamma; tumor necrosis factor—alpha	Enhances inflammation.
Antiinflammatory: interleukin 10; tumor growth factor—beta	Suppresses function of macrophages, natural killer cells, and T cells.

Modified from Hamosh B: Bioactive factors in human milk, *Pediatr Clin North Am* 48:69, 2001.
IU, International units.

on their total intake of human milk. Those infants with the highest doses benefited most in both short- and long-term outcomes.[295,296,337,338]

Banked human milk (donor milk) can be used if the mother is unable or unwilling to provide sufficient quantities of breastmilk.[15,96] Human milk banks in the United States have rigorous guidelines for donations and adhere to strict quality controls.[15]

Normal Lactation

Breast development during pregnancy is stimulated by luteal and placental hormones—lactogen, prolactin, and chorionic gonadotropin.[244] Production of breastmilk depends on both mammogenesis and lactogenesis. Mammogenesis is the growth and development of the glandular tissue of the breast and the differentiation of secretory epithelial cells or lactocytes during pregnancy.[127] Estrogen stimulates growth of the milk collection (ductal) system, whereas progesterone stimulates growth of the milk production system. These hormones, however, inhibit the initiation of breastmilk production in significant quantity. With the birth of the infant, the hormones of pregnancy decline abruptly when the placenta is delivered, permitting the initiation of milk secretion. There is some speculation that mammogenesis and lactogenesis I may be truncated with the birth of preterm infants, especially

---

BOX 18-1

CLINICAL GUIDELINES FOR COLOSTRUM FEEDING IN THE NICU

- Colostrum should be the first feeding received by the newborn infant.
- Colostrum may be used for minimal enteral nutrition (trophic feeds).
- Colostrum can be safely administered to the oropharynx either before or with minimal enteral nutrition.
- Give exclusive colostrum feedings for the first 3-4 days; then alternate colostrum with fresh mature human milk (to protect the infant from NICU organisms through the enteromammary pathway).
- Store colostrum in small, sterile, food-grade containers that are easy to recognize in the refrigerator/ freezer.
- Number the colostrum containers in the order of pumping; feed to baby in the order of pumping.
- Dilute small, expressed drops of colostrum with 1-2 ml of sterile water so that drops of colostrum are removed from container and/or to achieve desired feeding volume. Dilution of colostrum is not necessary for any other reason.
- Do not mix colostrum with formula or fortifier.
- Pumping colostrum may be facilitated by a combination of hand expression and breast pumping.
- Avoid formula feeding during the introduction and advancement of colostrum. Formula may exert a separate detrimental effect on gastrointestinal integrity during this critical time.

Adapted from Meier PP, Engstrom JL, Patel AL, et al: Improving the use of human milk during and after the NICU stay, *Clin Perinatol* 37:217, 2010.

BOX 18-2

ORAL CARE WITH COLOSTRUM[109,223,313]

Teach mother hand expression and place colostrum in small breastmilk containers.

Use fresh colostrum if possible; otherwise, refrigerated/frozen can be used.

Use colostrum in the order that it was pumped.

Using universal precautions, saturate a sterile cotton swab with colostrum (about 0.2 ml).

Before feeds or with scheduled cares if on nothing-by-mouth status: Parents/nurse paints the tongue, gums, and cheeks with colostrum.

Document.

---

the VLBW premature infant. In addition, cesarean section delivery may affect lactogenesis II as it affects the hormone balance stimulated by labor. Breast growth varies greatly during pregnancy, and it is unclear how much breast tissue is necessary to support full lactation. Many factors other than breast size affect milk production, such as stress and fatigue, both of which are increased when a preterm infant is born.

If a woman aborts as early as 16 weeks, her breasts secrete colostrum; therefore mothers are prepared to breastfeed any viable infant.[178]

Estrogen and progesterone function as inhibitors to actual milk production because they inhibit the breast receptors for prolactin. Therefore stimulation of the breast before delivery does not create milk but may induce uterine contractions because oxytocin is released. Once the infant and placenta are delivered, stimulation of the nipple becomes effective in producing milk.

Stimulating the nipple by the infant's sucking action causes an increase in the prolactin released in the bloodstream and induces the synthesis and release of oxytocin, which is initiated by nipple stimulation and other sensory pathways (Figure 18-1). The amount of prolactin is directly related to the quantity and quality of nipple stimulation; because prolactin stimulates the synthesis and secretion of milk, the surges in prolactin levels are related to the quantity of milk. A decrease in the quality of stimulation causes a decrease in prolactin surges and thus a decrease in milk production. Studies show that overweight/obese mothers have a diminished prolactin response to infant suckling (e.g., less milk production) in the first postpartum week.[272] These mothers may benefit from earlier lactation counseling and support that will enable them to continue breastfeeding.[272,305]

Adequate prolactin secretion controls the maintenance of milk supply. The sooner the infant nurses, the sooner the milk comes in and becomes established. Initially, production of milk is on a more consistent basis because the basal level of prolactin is very high immediately after birth. Maintenance of milk depends on adequate stimulation of the breast and removal of milk on a regular and frequent basis. Initially, a newborn needs to nurse for a longer time to stimulate milk production and letdown. As the infant grows, sucking becomes more efficient, with the infant stimulating sequential letdowns early in the nursing period, thereby shortening the length of nursing. Establishing a generous milk supply is critical in long-term maintenance. Research has demonstrated that for mothers who are separated from their infants, pumping both breasts

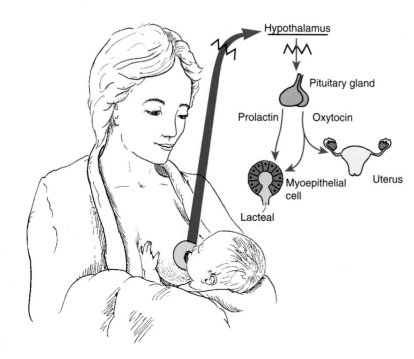

FIGURE 18-1 Ejection reflex arc, or letdown reflex. Infant suckling stimulates mechanoreceptors in the mother's nipple and areola that send the stimuli along the nerve pathways to the hypothalamus. Stimulation of the posterior pituitary releases oxytocin that (1) stimulates myoepithelial cells of the breast to contract and eject milk and (2) stimulates the uterus to contract. Stimulation of the anterior pituitary releases prolactin, which is responsible for milk production in mammary alveoli. (Modified from Lawrence RA, Lawrence RM: *Breast feeding: a guide for the medical profession*, ed 5, St Louis, 1999, Mosby.)

simultaneously stimulates a higher prolactin surge with increased milk supply than pumping one breast at a time.[133,150,242]

PSYCHOLOGIC VALUES OF BREASTFEEDING

The short-term advantage of breastfeeding is early mother-infant contact. The *en face* position of breastfeeding enhances this contact. During the first 1 to 2 hours after birth, the infant's suckling and touching of the mother's areola increases maternal attentiveness to the baby's needs for at least the first week of life. Because several studies show that maternal analgesia alters the infant's initial breastfeeding behavior, the mother's behavior may also be altered. Early contact—whether by breastfeeding or another physical means—sometimes must be delayed or modified in a sick neonate. Prolactin and oxytocin affect the initiation of maternal behavior and are involved in stress management in humans. Oxytocin has been shown to reduce depression and anxiety in lactating mothers compared with nonlactating mothers.[210] Feldman and Eidelman[99] found that providing breastmilk functions to initiate

a more optimal bonding process between mothers and their premature infants by operating on physiologic, behavioral, and representational (mood) systems. Maternal depression as measured by the Beck Depression Inventory was reduced significantly when mothers provided more than 75% of breastmilk nutrition for their preterm infant.[99] Two more recent studies also show that breastfeeding is associated with a reduced risk of postpartum depression that is maintained over the first 4 months of the postpartum period.[123,319]

The long-term psychologic effect for the mother of unrestricted nursing appears to be a more even mood cycle as a result of elevated prolactin, oxytocin, and endorphin levels,[332] which enhance coping mechanisms associated with caring for a new family member by diminishing maternal stress responses to physical, intrapersonal, or interpersonal stress.[118] Providing her own milk, including pumping and gavaging breastmilk and eventual feeding at the breast, enhances maternal attachment and maternal behaviors[118,154,323] and enables the mother to contribute to her infant's care (see Chapter 29). Proximity of mother and infant, as well as the infant's initial experience at the breast, contributes to maternal and infant regulation and the establishment of innate behaviors and emotional and social ties between mother and infant.[323] Kavanaugh and colleagues[154] described rewards to the mother from breastfeeding as follows:

- Knowing that she is providing the healthiest nutrition
- Enhancing closeness between her and her preterm infant
- Perceiving her preterm infant's contentment and tranquility during breastfeeding
- Convenience for the mother
- Giving her a tangible claim to her preterm infant

All physicians and nurses who admit infants to the NICU should educate, encourage, support, and assist mothers who wish to breastfeed their infants.[223,230,231] Use of kangaroo care (see Chapter 13) in the NICU facilitates early initiation of breastfeeding and increases maternal confidence, competence, and breastfeeding duration. If the infant is able to take oral nourishment, he or she can be breastfed at 1000 to 1200 g and about 28 weeks' gestational age (see Chapter 13, Box 13-14).

Neurobehavioral Development in Premature Infants

The positive impact of breastfeeding on neurobehavioral and cognitive development in infants has been posited for several decades. Two theories have been proposed to explain improved neurobehavioral development: nutritional content of breastmilk that improves neurologic growth, and the effect of breastfeeding on mother-infant relationship that indirectly supports cognitive development. Evidence continues to mount demonstrating positive effects of human milk in the preterm infant. Breastfeeding increases maternal responsiveness and higher levels of synchrony observed between mothers and preterm infants, hence leading to higher cognitive outcomes. A study of 86 preterm infants with mean gestational age at birth of 30 weeks and average birth weight of 1300 g found that amount of breastmilk provided made a significant impact on the neurodevelopment of the infant when assessed at 37 weeks and 6 months of corrected age. The preterm infants who received more than 75% of their nutrition from breastmilk demonstrated a more mature neurodevelopmental profile at

37 weeks corrected for gestational age and higher mental and psychomotor skills at 6 months of corrected age.[99] An observational cohort study of the relationship between breastfeeding, early weight gain, and neurodevelopment resulted in an "apparent breastfeeding paradox."[287] In the studied cohorts only 16% and 19% of very preterm infants breastfed at discharge from the NICU. On follow-up the breastfed infants' initial weight gain was characterized as "suboptimal" but their neurodevelopmental outcomes were better than the very preterm infants who were not breastfed.[287]

FACILITATING SUCCESSFUL BREASTFEEDING

Although breastfeeding is a normal, natural function, it is not a reflex but, rather, a highly complex interaction and interdependence between mother and infant. To be successful, the breastfeeding dyad must synchronize their behavior and physiology and receive support from their environment. Delayed breastfeeding may be as successful as immediate feeding when (1) problems are prevented, (2) the mother receives support and encouragement in maintaining her milk supply, and (3) everyone is patient and knowledgeable about teaching the infant to suckle. Initiating breastfeeding as early as possible is important to prevent problems. Thorough evaluation of the effectiveness of the nursing couple is important in achieving adequate nutrition and breastfeeding success. Knowledgeable health care providers and licensed, certified lactation consultants, where available, can perform these evaluations.[75,263] Development of an evidence-based and mother-friendly breastfeeding service has been shown to dramatically improve the volume of mother's milk that is available and to prolong the duration of milk provision for preterm infants.[225]

Sucking

Sucking is a primitive reflex appearing as early as 15 to 16 weeks' gestation. Although isolated components of feeding behaviors (e.g., root, suck, swallow, gag) are all present early in gestation, they are not effectively coordinated for bottle feedings before 32 to 34 weeks' gestational age (see Chapter 13, Table 13-2). The infant can coordinate suck and swallow while breastfeeding as early as 28 weeks' gestation. Two distinct types of sucking, nonnutritive and nutritive, develop in the human infant.

Nonnutritive Sucking

Nonnutritive sucking (NNS) is sucking activity in which no fluid or nutrition is delivered to the infant. Characterized by short bursts of rapid motion, pauses, and few swallows, nonnutritive sucking has a stabilizing effect on physiologic responses (i.e., better oxygenation; quieter, more restful behavior; decreased tension; increased insulin and gastrin secretion that may stimulate digestion and storage of nutrients; and improved readiness for oral feedings) (see Chapter 13). Because there is no bolus of fluid to swallow, nonnutritive sucking results in an alternation of inspiration and expiration without the regular apneic periods of nutritive sucking. However, even in NNS when the occasional swallow of saliva is necessary, there is a maturational progression of swallow-breath interaction from central apnea to obstructive apnea to attenuated breathing.[274]

Nutritive Sucking

Nutritive sucking, used by an infant when fluid or nutrition is available, is characterized by an organized, rhythmic pattern that is about half the rate of nonnutritive sucking (i.e., one per second). During nutritive sucking, each milk expression is followed by a reflexive swallow and an occasional brief pause. In a term neonate, rates of sucking range from 40 to 100/min. Nutritive sucking provides the neonate with positive reinforcement, which encourages a steady level of behavior. A variety of factors affect nutritive sucking, including maternal anesthesia and/or analgesia, length of labor, type of delivery, gestational age, birth weight, age (in hours), severity of illness, infant state, type of fluid, disorders of the central nervous system, and individual variations.*

Although nutritive sucking is associated with faster heart rate (when bottle feeding), little information is available describing energy requirements of nutritive sucking. The findings of one study

suggest that, during bottle feeding, preterm infants expend significantly less energy to suck the same volume than do full-term infants.[148] Bottle feeding requires *more* energy than breastfeeding in all infants.[148]

Two patterns of nutritive sucking have been identified: continuous sucking and intermittent sucking.[199] *Continuous sucking* occurs at the beginning of bottle feeding, when the suck is strong and continuous for at least 30 seconds.[196,199] *Intermittent sucking,* an alternation of sucking bursts with periods of pause/no sucking,[196,199] occurs first during breastfeeding, followed by continuous sucking (with breastmilk letdown).[198,218] Breathing and oxygenation are affected more during continuous than during intermittent sucking,[324] even in full-term infants who can exhibit apnea and bradycardia with feeding.[195]

An increasing level of organization of nutritive sucking occurs with increasing gestational age, maturity, and experience.*

Preterm sucking patterns exhibit more sucking-to-breathing ratio (2:1 to 4:1) than well-coordinated sucking breathing ratios (e.g., 1:1) of full-term newborns.[259] By 32 to 34 weeks' postconceptual age (PCA), there is a change in sucking bursts (i.e., increase in number of sucks, number of suck bursts and pressure; decrease in time between sucking bursts). This developmental maturation[50] enables nutritive sucking to take less time and is less tiring. For infants having feeding difficulties or a preterm who is not progressing as expected in feeding ability, there is a quantitative instrument, the Medoff-Cooper Nutritive Sucking Apparatus (M-CNSA), that provides a continuous record of the negative pressure generated during a 5-minute feeding assessment. The M-CNSA augments clinical evaluation as it objectively measures nutritive sucking parameters and enhances clinical decision making.[340]

Nutritive sucking requires coordination between suck, swallow, and breathing. During coordinated sucking bursts, suck/swallow/breathing occur in a 1 second:1 second:1 second sequential pattern. The lack of a suck, swallow, and breathing ratio of 1:1:1 contributes to a preterm infant's apnea with feeding, a reflexive protection of the airway.[198,263,274,324] Although suck/swallow is achieved

---

*References 104, 112, 174, 198, 206, 210, 211, 248, 259, 269, 303.

*References 104, 112, 174, 198, 206, 210, 211, 248, 259, 269, 303.

by 32 weeks' gestation,[212] respiration may still not be well coordinated so the preterm infant may develop apneic episodes with bottle feeding.[263,274,324] With increasing PCA and neuromuscular maturity, *consistent* coordination of suck-swallow-breathe (with bottle feeding) occurs by 35 to 37 weeks' PCA.[104]

Sucking patterns of full-term, preterm, and preterm infants with bronchopulmonary dysplasia (BPD) have recently been studied. All full-term infants had a normal sucking pattern soon after birth, but bottle feeding was found to contribute to arrhythmic sucking over a 10-week period of time after birth.[72] Small-for-gestational-age (SGA) preterm infants were found to develop normal sucking patterns later than appropriate-for-gestational-age (AGA) preterms; by term-equivalent no SGA infants and 38% of AGA preterms had normal sucking behaviors.[73] Abnormal sucking in the SGA infants included incoordination and dysfunctional sucking patterns. Compared with preterms without BPD, preterms with BPD had more incoordination of sucking, swallowing, and breathing (36% vs. 15%).[74]

A randomized study of early introduction of oral (bottle) feeding (e.g., within 48 hours of full tube feedings) found the following[303]:

- Transition time to all oral feedings was significantly shorter.
- Oral feeding was introduced 2.6 weeks earlier.
- Total oral feeding was achieved at earlier postmenstrual age (PMA) (e.g., 54% of 33-week-PMA infants versus 12.5% of control group infants).
- Weight gain and discharge weights were similar in both groups.
- Episodes of feeding-related bradycardia and desaturations were similar for both groups.
- The early feeding group was discharged 10 days earlier than the control group.

In this study and others, researchers postulate that feeding opportunities in young infants provide them with practice and *experiential* opportunities to develop their oral motor skills and coordination of suck-swallow-breathe.[103,201,303]

Human nutritive suckling is composed of five separate yet interrelated processes: rooting, orienting, suction, expression, and swallowing (Figure 18-2).[45] *Rooting,* the tactile stimulating of the infant's face and lips, elicits the head to turn toward the stimulus. Stimulation of the center of the lower lip enables the infant to root by coming

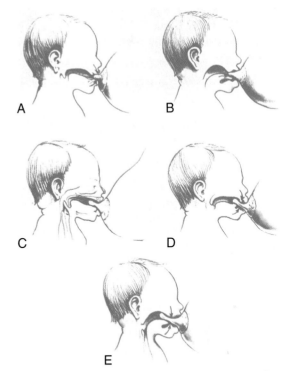

FIGURE 18-2 Normal suckling. **A,** Infant grasps breast (note *arrows* showing jaw action). **B,** Tongue moves forward to draw nipple in. **C,** Nipple and areola move toward palate as glottis still permits breathing. **D,** Tongue moves along nipple, pressing it against hard palate, creating pressure. **E,** Ductules under areola are milked, and flow begins because of peristaltic movement of tongue. Glottis closes and swallow follows. (From Lawrence RA, Lawrence RM: *Breast feeding: a guide for the medical profession,* ed 6, St Louis, 2005, Mosby.)

forward extending the tongue, drawing in the nipple and areola, and latching on, rather than turning the head to one side. *Orienting,* or *latching on,* occurs when the tongue draws the nipple and areola into an elongated teat and compresses it against the hard palate.[128]

Suction, the application of negative pressure in the infant's mouth, holds the nipple and areola in place.[128] At the beginning of breastfeeding, a strong suction stretches and shapes the nipple, but only moderate suction is necessary to maintain adequate grasp of the nipple. During the feeding, occasional bursts of suckling enable milk to be expressed. *Expression* of milk occurs when the peristaltic motion of the tongue[128] stimulates the release of oxytocin, which stimulates myoepithelial

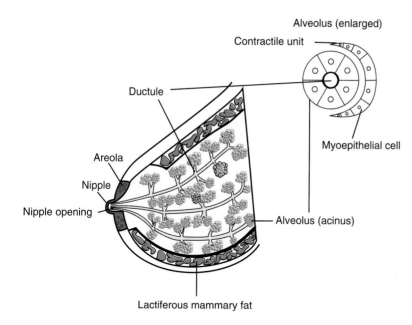

Alveolus (enlarged)

Contractile unit

Ductule

Areola

Nipple

Nipple opening

Myoepithelial cell

Alveolus (acinus)

Lactiferous mammary fat

FIGURE 18-3 Structure of human breast during lactation based on ultrasound findings. (Redrawn figure from Ramsey DT, Kent JC, Hartmann RA, et al: Anatomy of the lactating breast redefined with ultrasound imaging, *J Anat* 206:525, 2005. With permission of Wiley-Blackwell Publishing.)

cells surrounding the milk ducts (Figure 18-3) to contract, and milk is ejected from the ducts. The lips should be flanged out to create a seal as peristaltic motion of the tongue stimulates milk ejection. After maximal compression of the nipple with peristaltic motion, milk is expressed from the lactiferous sinuses.

Swallowing milk occurs as the peristaltic motion of the tongue triggers peristaltic motion of the posterior pharynx (reflexive swallowing)[128] and propulsion down the esophagus (which also shows peristalsis). These peristaltic motions coordinate suck and swallow so breastfeeding infants do not choke, unless letdown reflex is excessive. Swallowing milk also inhibits respiration (thus protecting the airway) and reflexively initiates the expression cycle of jaw and tongue movements. Therefore nutritive suckling is primarily expression and swallowing of milk. During nursing, just enough suction to keep the nipple in proper position is used, even during the expressive phase of suckling. Breastfeeding is an infant-regulated system; milk flow depends on the active suckling by the infant. When an infant pauses to regain physiologic stability, the flow of milk from the breast ceases.

Ultrasonographic studies of full-term infants' breastfeeding note (1) an elongation to twice the resting size of the maternal nipple; (2) formation of a passive seal by the neonate's oral cavity; (3) milk ejection coinciding with the downstroke of the tongue and jaw, creating negative pressure by oral cavity enlargement; and (4) multiple milk ejections occur during breastfeeding that may not be sensed by the mother.[271] Ultrasonographic studies of full-term infants bottle feeding note (1) less elasticity and less elongation of artificial nipples (compared with human nipple); (2) similar mechanism used to suckle artificial nipples as used to breastfeed, which is quickly replaced by the thrusting motion to close the holes and control the flow; and (3) milk expression dependent on a vacuum phenomenon by oral cavity enlargement rather than by nipple compression.[128]

Artificial nipples have also been shown to vary in their rate of milk flow.[192,194,196] Nipple hole size, rather than the type of nipple,[192,197] has been found to be the major determinant in the variability in milk flow.[194] With an artificial nipple, fluid flows into the posterior oropharynx by gravity (Figure 18-4). Artificial nipples and bottles are gravity-regulated systems requiring the infant to actively inhibit milk flow to permit swallowing and breathing. In an attempt to regulate milk flow and prevent choking or gagging, infants may clench their jaws or obstruct the nipples' holes with their tongues in a thrusting motion. Orthodontic nipples result in physiologic

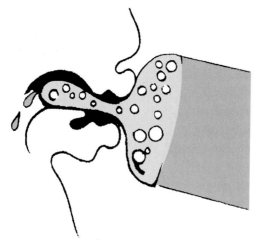

FIGURE 18-4 Artificial nipple. (From Lawrence RA, Lawrence RM: *Breastfeeding: a guide for the medical professional,* ed 6, St Louis, 2005, Mosby.)

stability and more effective feeding behavior in some infants.[88] A study comparing breastfeeding and bottle feeding with two delivery systems (soft-walled and rigid-walled bottles/nipples) found better coordination of suck/swallow/breathing, better oxygen saturations, and a feeding pattern more like breastfeeding when the soft-walled system was used.[115]

PREVENTION OF BREASTFEEDING PROBLEMS

Problems with breastfeeding may be with the mother or with the neonate or may arise from a combination of problems in the dyad. Lack of information about common problems in the early weeks of breastfeeding is a common reason for breastfeeding failure.[311] In descriptive studies addressing breastfeeding problems, mothers have frequently identified concerns related to sore nipples, breast discomfort, and inadequate milk supply.[51,80] Breastfeeding problems should be prevented. To solve a breastfeeding problem, the mother must be observed feeding the infant.

Maternal Problems

INADEQUATE MILK SUPPLY
Inadequate milk supply, a major problem for both mother and infant, is the most commonly

cited reason for discontinuation of breastfeeding in the NICU and after discharge.[51,136,153,216] Predictors of maternal perception of inadequate milk supply at 8 to 12 weeks postpartum (after preterm birth) include inadequate milk supply at 6 weeks postpartum, unemployment, and infant hospital discharge after postpartum day 42.[136] Initially, some neonates with special needs are unable to breastfeed. In this common situation, the most compelling breastfeeding issue is establishing an adequate milk supply without the neonate's assistance[135,223] (Table 18-3). Preterm mothers are three times more likely to produce an inadequate milk supply at 6 weeks than are full-term mothers.[135] Because low milk volume in the first week of life is related to continued low production,[135] developing a very early program of education and support for the mother will help her establish an early milk supply and prevent low milk volume.

Initiating, establishing, and maintaining a milk supply must be accomplished mechanically when the infant is unable to breastfeed. Because milk production depends on adequate and frequent expression, maternal education is the key to establishing an adequate supply (see Table 18-3). Mothers should be encouraged to provide their milk for their compromised infants and should be educated about the benefits of human milk feedings for their fragile infant so that they are able to make an informed choice and decision.* A parent-focused video about the importance of human milk and the science that supports human milk as the best source of nutrition is available.[288]

The mother who wants to or is willing to breastfeed should be instructed about initiating and maintaining a milk supply until the infant can breastfeed. In general, instruction includes information about pumping, which is individualized to the mother's situation. Milk production through pumping should be encouraged early and regularly to (1) collect colostrum, which is rich in antiinfective properties; (2) ease initial engorgement associated with lack of regular stimulation and maintain continued stimulus to produce milk; (3) provide quality nutrition for the neonate; and (4) alleviate concerns about available volume once the infant begins breastfeeding. The early postpartum

---

*References 185, 217, 225, 230, 231, 280, 311.

T A B L E 18-3	CRITICAL FINDINGS
	FACTORS THAT INFLUENCE THE MOTHER'S MILK SUPPLY AND SUCCESSFUL BREASTFEEDING OF THE PRETERM INFANT

ENHANCES	REDUCES	COMMENTS
Early initiation of pumping, preferably with a double-pumping setup and breast massage[150,241]	Immediate separation at birth, delayed initiation of pumping or feeding at the breast[48,239]	Initiate within 2-3 hours of birth, if possible; pumping both breasts simultaneously is associated with higher prolactin levels, milk yield, fat concentration, and maternal preference.[133,150,223] Provide volume-based containers for storing milk from each pumping episode.[223]
Frequent milk expression with complete breast emptying at each session	Failure to express frequently or incomplete emptying of the breasts	5-8 expressions/day (every 3-4 hr) [241]: duration of pumping >100 min/day (about 15-20 minutes with double-pump setup); longest nonpumping interval <6 hours.[58] Maintain a pumping log.[241]
Rest, relaxation, and stress management (see Chapters 29 and 30)	Fatigue, anxiety, stress (i.e., maternal illness; stress, noise and lack of privacy in NICU; return to work, more commitments in and outside the home, maternal dislike of breastfeeding) [48,239]	Inverse relationship between maternal anxiety scores and milk volume for mothers of preterm infants; uninterrupted sleep of at least 6 hours.[179,332] Privacy for breast pumping: 55% of mothers preferred to pump at home for more privacy; more mothers pumped in their preterm's single-family room.[89]
Adequate nutrition	Inadequate nutrition	At least 60% of recommended daily allowances produces milk of adequate quantity and quality to promote infant growth.[55]
Medications Use of galactogogues[5] (metoclopramide, oxytocin, reserpine, phenothiazines, domperidone)	Bromocriptine, antihistamine, oral contraceptives (especially estrogen and progesterone combination)	Knowledge of maternal medication use enables effective counseling.
Herb Fenugreek		Two or three capsules two or three times per day; maternal diarrhea; lowers blood glucose; may increase asthma symptoms; maple syrup smell to sweat, urine, milk; colic.[121] Less weight loss and greater milk volume at 3 days of age in infants whose mothers took fenugreek.[327]
Positive feedback to mother regarding infant growth; infant's condition improving	Worsening infant's condition	Mothers report feeling rewarded by infant's growth while receiving expressed mother's milk by gavage.[216]
Skin-to-skin contact (kangaroo care)[66,180,241]	Parental separation	Maternal reinforcement of lactation, maternal behaviors, confidence, and attachment; ensures maternal exposure to pathogens in NICU so that her immune system is stimulated to produce environmentally specific antibodies that are passed in maternal milk and protect the preterm.
Educational information (e.g., video, brochure) readily available for both mothers and fathers[3,12,241,308,318] of preterm infants within the first 24 hours after birth[241]	No verbal or written information for parents; conflicting opinions and advice about breastfeeding[217,223]	Decision about type of pump, frequency; written instructions on collection and storage per NICU protocol; information about maternal rest, fluid intake, and nutrition. Positive effects of breastfeeding, advantages of human milk to preterm infant; how to interpret infant cues and behaviors.[202,247,318]

Continued

TABLE 18-3	CRITICAL FINDINGS — cont'd	
	FACTORS THAT INFLUENCE THE MOTHER'S MILK SUPPLY AND SUCCESSFUL BREASTFEEDING OF THE PRETERM INFANT	

ENHANCES	REDUCES	COMMENTS
Herb — cont'd		
Knowledgeable professional care providers (e.g., primary nurses, lactation specialists, physicians, peer support) who educate, support, and assist[3,12,42] through consistent, practical advice[180,217,223]	Nonsupportive care providers and/or inconsistent advice and information; no alignment between NICU routines and parents' needs[12]	Prevention of maternal problems (e.g., inadequate supply,[48] sore nipples, engorgement) through self-education and professional interaction and education enhances success and prevents discontinuation of breastfeeding.
Initiation of breastfeeding before bottle feeding	Initiation of bottle feeding before breastfeeding[48] Small size, fragility, medical complications of premature infant[239]	Early breastfeeding is less stressful than early bottle feeding[43,104,214–216,218,345] because of difference in the patterns of sucking and breathing; during bottle feedings, preterm infants alternate short bursts of sucking with breathing and do not breathe within sucking bursts; during breastfeeding, breathing is integrated within sucking bursts.[215] Test weighing (i.e., weighing before and after breastfeeding, with differences in weight representing milk intake [1 g = 1 ml]) using electronic scales is a reliable method of documenting milk intake in preterm infants.[220,223] For specific problems, maximizing milk intake may be assisted by lactational support devices (i.e., nipple shields; lactation supplementer) and/or breast pump stimulation of the opposite breast during infant feeding.[179,216,223]
Simultaneous feeding and caregiving schedules for multiples (see Chapter 13)		For multiples: Introduce simultaneous feeding as soon as possible, encourage maternal independence with position suggestions, comfort measures, experimenting, and verbalizing what mother needs or wants.[247] Need for privacy, taking babies out of NICU, rooming-in with father to assist with care and feeding.[247] Lactation support devices and/or breast pump stimulation of the opposite breast during infant feeding.[295]

Modified from Schanler R, Hurst N: Human milk for the hospitalized preterm infant, *Semin Perinatol* 18:476, 1994.
NICU, Neonatal intensive care unit.

period in the hospital is the optimal time to teach pumping methods, while support and encouragement are readily available.

BREAST DISCOMFORT

Maternal problems include engorgement, painful nipples, and cracked nipples.[275] A primipara is at high risk for developing engorgement. Frequent emptying of the breast is the best prevention.

Engorgement occurring in the early postpartum period is characterized by general breast swelling, usually in both breasts in a well, afebrile woman.[7] A little engorgement is normal. Areolar engorgement blocks the nipple and makes grasping the areola difficult for the infant. Gentle breast massage and manual expression of a small amount of milk soften the areola so the infant is able to "latch on." When the body of the breasts and the areolae become excessively engorged and painful, the goal of management is to make the mother comfortable so that nursing may continue. Supporting the breasts is crucial, and the mother should wear a well-fitting but adjustable brassiere 24 hours a day.[179] Applying cold packs between nursing decreases pain and swelling. Pain relievers also may be prescribed. Applying heat (packs or a warm shower) and expressing some milk before feeding help initiate milk flow.

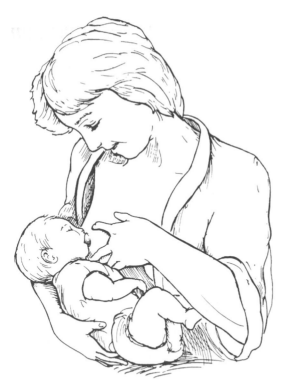

FIGURE 18-5 Proper positioning for breastfeeding infant tummy-to-tummy facing the mother.

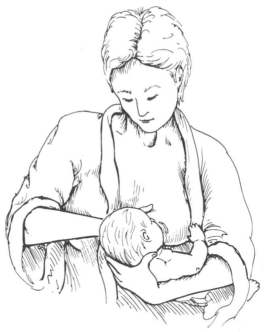

FIGURE 18-6 Football hold in breastfeeding. Pillows may be used for support.

A nursing infant, manual expression, or an effective pump helps initiate and maintain milk flow. Breast massage before and during breast pumping/feeding also facilitates milk flow.

Prenatal stimulation of the nipple by pulling or rolling (to toughen it for breastfeeding) is not recommended because of the possibility of initiating uterine contractions and premature labor.[179]

Breastfeeding should *not* be painful. When it is, the problem is most often an incorrect latch. Sore nipples are another major discomfort and concern for the new mother. The initial grasp of the nipple by the infant or with pumping can be uncomfortable. Poor positioning of the infant, however, can cause painful and eventually cracked nipples. Prevention and treatment involve educating the mother about careful positioning of the infant facing the mother, looking directly at the breast, and tummy-to-tummy with her (Figure 18-5). Changing the infant's position on the nipple at different feedings is helpful.

Positioning the infant correctly at the breast assists in the prevention of sore nipples.[44] There are three common positions that can be used with breastfeeding: the cradle hold (see Figure 18-5), the football hold (Figure 18-6), and lying down. Initially, the cradle or football hold allows the most control for the mother and infant to learn breastfeeding. Breastfeeding in the lying-down position becomes easier once latch-on techniques are developed.

Nipple care involves keeping nipples clean and dry. Clear water (no soap or alcohol) is all that is necessary to keep the nipples clean. Drying nipples well, not using plastic nursing pads, and exposing nipples to air and dry heat (sunlight, light bulb sauna, or a low setting on a hair dryer) are comforting. Using ointments may be helpful, especially in dry climates. If used, a small amount (i.e., one drop) should be gently massaged into the nipple after the feeding. Purified lanolin (if there is no allergy to wool), A&D ointment, or vitamin E may be used to treat, but will not prevent, sore nipples. A randomized clinical trial (RCT) found that use of breast shells and lanolin cream to treat sore nipples promoted healing and prevented infections.[28] Another RCT comparing the use of hydrogel dressings with lanolin ointment in the prevention and treatment of sore nipples found a greater reduction in pain, no infections, and earlier discontinuation of therapy in the hydrogel dressing group.[83]

Severe and/or persistent nipple pain may be caused by bacterial or yeast infection, which should be promptly treated. Yeast infection of the breast (Table 18-4) manifests as a burning sensation in the nipples, stabbing pain throughout the breast, and edema/shiny skin or flaking skin on the nipple/areola.[237] A significant risk factor for yeast infections of the breast and oral thrush in the baby is the use of bottles in the early postpartum period.[237] In one study, yeast infection was associated with cessation of breastfeeding (in 65% of infected mothers) by 9 weeks postpartum because of pain with feeding.[237]

Another recognized cause of nipple pain is Raynaud's phenomenon of the nipple, which is often misdiagnosed and mistreated as a yeast infection.[19] Twenty percent of childbearing-age women may have Raynaud's, and symptoms are exacerbated by cold temperatures.[19] Raynaud's phenomenon of the breast, associated with a history of breast surgery, is characterized by extreme or severe nipple pain with breastfeeding; nipple blanching, cyanosis, or erythema; and accompanying throbbing pain, burning, and paresthesia. Treatment includes (1) preventing and/or decreasing exposure to cold and emotional stress, (2) avoiding vasoconstrictive drugs (e.g., nicotine), (3) using nifedipine for its vasodilator effects[11] (see Table 18-7), and (4) including fish oil and evening primrose oil in the mother's diet.[178] If the mother does not have Raynaud's of fingers or toes, it is unlikely she has it of the breast.

In the past, nipple shields were not recommended because they are awkward for the mother, are confusing for the infant, and decrease milk production by 50%. Modern ultrathin nipple shields concentrate the immature (preterm or late preterm) infant's suction pressure in the tunnel of the shield, stimulate milk flow, and stimulate milk removal.[220,223] Use of silicone nipple shields has been found to be a useful tool in treatment of sore nipples and latch-on problems and as a bridging technique to direct breastfeeding.[311] One study showed that for preterm infants, use of a nipple shield increased breastmilk intake and promoted longer duration of breastfeeding.[219] Breast pumping after use of nipple shields is necessary to express residual milk, maintain adequate milk supply, and obtain milk for supplemental feeding.[225,311] Nipple shields are also helpful if the mother's nipple is too large for her infant's mouth. Use of nipple shields to facilitate and support breastfeeding is certainly preferable to cessation of breastfeeding.[60]

Flat or inverted nipples may be difficult for the infant to grasp and result in maternal engorgement, decreased milk supply, infant frustration, and suboptimal infant breastfeeding behavior[80] (Figure 18-7). Inverted nipples may be treated by using a breast pump to draw out the nipple before attempting to latch the baby onto the nipple.

Neonatal Problems

Ideally, no term or preterm infant who will be breastfed should ever be fed with an artificial nipple, but this is not always possible, especially for a sick premature infant who requires prolonged hospitalization. However, teaching a premature infant to suck often starts long before nutrition is obtained from a nipple. When a premature infant is gavage fed, swabbing the cheeks, tongue, and gums with colostrum familiarizes the infant with the smell and taste of mother's milk and provides oral immune therapy.[109] In addition, stable preterms who are gavage fed should be held for feedings and offered a pacifier, which may teach the infant to equate satiety with sucking. Using a pacifier provides nonnutritive sucking that calms and soothes the preterm infant and also provides the opportunity to develop sucking skill. A recent RCT in preterm infants showed no influence of pacifier use on any breastfeeding outcome (e.g., breastfeeding at discharge or several months later).[84] These findings agree with an RCT of reducing pacifier use in term infants that showed no effect on early weaning.[164]

When the mother is present for gavage feeding, she can administer oral colostrum,[109] hold the infant, and offer the breast instead of an artificial nipple. If it is necessary to avoid swallowing any fluid, the breast can be prepumped. Placing the infant in direct skin-to-skin contact with the mother's breast enables nuzzling and licking behaviors and teaches that relief from hunger and the breastfeeding position are associated. Because increased stimulation creates an

TABLE 18-4 PERINATAL COMPLICATIONS AND BREASTFEEDING

COMPLICATIONS	BREASTFEED		COMMENTS
	YES	NO	
Maternal Complications			
Cesarean section	X		Regional anesthesia enables contact and feeding in recovery room. Pain medication is best given after feeding so levels peak before next feeding.
Pregnancy-induced hypertension	X		Preterm or small-for-gestational-age infants may be delivered, making delayed breastfeeding and pumping necessary. Maternal drugs may affect infant (see Table 18-7).
Venous thrombosis and pulmonary embolism	X		Depending on mother's ability; radioactive materials may be used for diagnosis, and pulmonary embolism anticoagulants may be used for therapy (see Table 18-7).
Bacterial Infections			
Urinary tract	X		Choice of antibiotics is important (see Table 18-7).
Mastitis[18]	X		Continued emptying of breast (i.e., nursing baby or breast pump), bed rest, antibiotic therapy that is safe for infant, application of heat and cold, and use of analgesics are therapeutic.
Sexually transmitted diseases	X		No contraindication once mother is treated appropriately.
Tuberculosis	X	X	Culture-positive mothers must be separated from their infants regardless of mode of feeding; may pump and provide breastmilk because tubercle bacillus is not passed through milk but through respiratory contact.[179]
	X		After therapy, when it is safe for mother to contact infant, it is safe to breastfeed directly.
Diarrhea	X		Proper handwashing should be done and breastfeeding continued.
Viral Infections			
Cytomegalovirus (CMV)	X		Both virus and protective antibodies occur in breastmilk; the relative incidence and severity of CMV infection acquired from breastmilk in low-birth-weight (LBW) infants is low.[232] For preterm infants with lower concentration of transplacental antibodies: freeze milk (which decreases viral titer) for 3-7 days before feeding (for the first few weeks) until antibodies received via milk increase.[104,109]
Enterovirus	X		Maternal antibodies in breastmilk protect infants from enteroviral infections, especially if the infant was breastfed for >2 weeks.[292]
Rubella	X		Isolate infected infant from other infants and susceptible personnel. Mother is not contagious postpartum and need not be isolated from infant.
			Rooming-in may be considered.
Rubella immunization	X		There is no known adverse effect on infant.
Herpes simplex virus (HSV)	X	X	May breastfeed if there is no active lesion on breast. Strict handwashing, as well as covering of genital lesions, is necessary. Rooming-in supports breastfeeding while isolating infant from others in nursery.
Varicella (chickenpox)	X	X	If mother has chickenpox within 6 days of delivery, isolate mother and do not allow her to breastfeed until she is no longer contagious. Infant should be separated regardless of mode of feeding.
Measles (rubeola)	X	X	If infant has measles, may isolate mother and infant together and allow breastfeeding. Mothers with postpartum measles have breastfed, and neonates have acquired mild disease. Secretory antibodies are probably present in milk in 45 hours. Mother exposed before delivery without active disease should be isolated from infant, because 50% of infants contract disease.
Hepatitis	X		Hepatitis A: may breastfeed as soon as mother receives gamma globulin.
	X		Hepatitis B antigen has been found in breastmilk, but transmission by this route is not well documented. Both infants of chronic HBsAg carriers and those with acute hepatitis should receive high-titer hepatitis B immunoglobulin and hepatitis vaccine, and breastfeeding is permitted.
	X		Hepatitis C virus (HCV) infection rate is 4% in both breastfed and bottle-fed infants; breastfeeding permitted: HCV-positive women do not increase the infection risk to their infants.

Continued

| TABLE 18-4 | PERINATAL COMPLICATIONS AND BREASTFEEDING — cont'd | | |

| | BREASTFEED | | |
COMPLICATIONS	YES	NO	COMMENTS
Viral Infections — cont'd			
Human immunode-ficiency virus (HIV), acquired immunode-ficiency syndrome (AIDS)	X		Breastfeeding is absolutely contraindicated in mothers who are HIV positive and living in developed countries where safe alternatives are available.[14,178,179] The risk for HIV transmission with exclusive breastfeeding has recently been studied in the developing world. Exclusive breastfeeding decreases the risks of HIV transmission (14.1% at 6 weeks and 19.5% at 6 months of age) and mortality (6.1% at 3 months of age) compared with infants who received solids in addition to breastfeeding.[68] World Health Organization recommends that mothers receive antiretroviral therapy while breastfeeding, not breastfeed, or if breastfeeding without antiretroviral therapy to breastfeed for 12 months.[346]
Human T-cell leukemia virus type I (HTLV-I)		X	Infected lymphocytes found in breastmilk; unknown if able to cause disease. Current U.S. position: breastfeed-ing is contraindicated.[179]
West Nile virus	X		Transmission through human milk occurs but is rare.[137]
Parasitic Infections			
Toxoplasmosis	X		No transmission of toxoplasmosis has been demonstrated in humans. Antibodies are present in breastmilk.
Fungal Infections			
Candida albicans infection of the nipple/ breast	X		Antifungal topical medication (nystatin) for the mother and simultaneous oral nystatin for the infant. Persistent yeast infections are treated with oral fluconazole (see Table 18-7).
Other Infections			
Trichomoniasis		X	Metronidazole is contraindicated for infant; milk may be pumped and discarded until therapy is completed. Mother's dose can be modified so she can pump and discard milk for 24-48 hours.
Other Maternal Complications			
Anemia	X		Severe maternal anemia, but not mild to moderate anemia, adversely affects the iron status of breastmilk. Maternal nutritional status significantly influences fetal iron status but not breastmilk iron content.[166]
Diabetes	X		Lactation is antidiabetogenic. Lactosuria must be differentiated from glycosuria.
Thyroid disease	X	X	Radioisotopes and thiouracil are found in breastmilk and may adversely affect infant. Mother who is taking propylthiouracil can breastfeed. Neither hypothyroidism nor hyperthyroidism is contraindication alone.
Cystic fibrosis	X	X	May cause nutritional drain on mother. Milk composition is normal. The Cystic Fibrosis Association has guidelines for lactation.
Smoking	X	X	Nicotine interferes with letdown and is excreted in milk. Of mothers who smoke, breastfed infants are healthier than bottle-fed infants.
Opiate withdrawal	X		One small study. See "Methadone" in the "Other Substances" section in Table 18-7.
Neonatal Complications **Medical**			
Diarrhea	X	X	Maintain breastfeeding in infectious diarrhea unless milk is source of infection. Congenital lactase deficiency is rare but requires lactose-free formula.
Respiratory disease	X	X	Breastmilk by gavage may be used if infant's condition permits.
Galactosemia		X	Galactose (lactose)–free diet is required.

TABLE 18-4	**PERINATAL COMPLICATIONS AND BREASTFEEDING — cont'd**		

	BREASTFEED		
COMPLICATIONS	**YES**	**NO**	**COMMENTS**
Neonatal Complications — cont'd			
Inborn errors of metabolism (e.g., phenylketonuria)	X	X	Combination of breastmilk and special formula may sometimes be used. Careful monitoring of blood and urine levels of the amino acid is required.
Acrodermatitis entero-pathica	X		Low plasma zinc levels are corrected by human milk and zinc sulfate supplementation.
Down syndrome	X		Hypotonia and poor suck reflex contribute to poor letdown and inadequate supply. Proper positioning, manual expression to begin feeding, and supporting the breast so infant does not lose nipple are helpful. Support from another mother with an infant with Down syndrome is helpful.
Hypothyroidism	X		Enough T_3 may be ingested to avoid serious symptoms.
Hyperbilirubinemia	X		May have slightly higher bilirubin than bottle-fed infant. There is no evidence that supplements are beneficial (see Chapter 21).
Breastmilk jaundice	X	X	Uncommon occurrence; diagnosis of exclusion; if all other causes are excluded, a temporary cessation of breastmilk may be indicated (see Chapter 21).
Cystic fibrosis	X		Increased losses of and lower electrolyte content of breastmilk may cause electrolyte imbalance, which is less likely than with formulas.
Surgical			
Cleft lip and/or palate	X		Associated lesions, size, and position of defect influence successful feeding. Positioning and stabilizing breast in infant's mouth may help seal defect. Consult plastic surgeon.
Gastrostomy	X		If gastrostomy feedings are used, expressed breastmilk is appropriate.
Partial obstruction (meconium plug, ileus, Hirschsprung's disease)	X		If oral feedings are indicated, breastmilk is feeding of choice because of digestibility and mild cathartic effect.
Necrotizing enterocolitis	X		Breastfeeding may be partially protective and may be used when feeding resumes.
Gastrointestinal bleeding	X		Most common cause is maternal bleeding from nipple. Perform Apt test to differentiate fetal from adult hemoglobin.
Central nervous system	X		Weak suck and uncoordinated suck and swallow may be problems; however, infants with malformations may breastfeed more effectively than bottle feed.
Omphalocele repair	x		If oral feedings are indicated, breastmilk is feeding of choice because of digestibility.[312]
Congenital diaphrag-matic hernia	x	x	Breastfeeding is deferred until surgery and ECMO are completed. Mother initiates pumping and storing until baby is able to have enteral nutrition.[314]

Data from American Academy of Pediatrics: *Report of the committee on infectious disease,* ed 29, Elk Grove Village, Ill, 2012, The Academy; Lawrence RA, Lawrence RM: *Breast feeding: a guide for the medical profession,* ed 7, St Louis, 2010, Mosby.
ECMO, Extracorporeal membrane oxygenation.

increased milk supply, it is possible to breast-feed multiple infants. In the early weeks, it will be difficult and time consuming, but eventually it can become faster and more convenient than bottle feeding. Two infants can be fed at the same time, in the cradle position or in the football hold position (Figure 18-8). A study of breastfeeding twins found that mothers preferred simultaneous feeding using the football hold (possibly because of the bias of the observers because not all mothers of twins agreed).[157] Infants should change breasts with each feeding, because one may

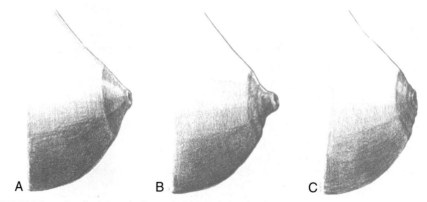

FIGURE 18-7 Inverted nipples. **A,** Normal and inverted nipples may look similar when nipple is not stimulated. **B,** Normal nipple protrudes when stimulated. **C,** Inverted nipple retracts when stimulated. (Courtesy Jimmy Lynne Scholl Avery.)

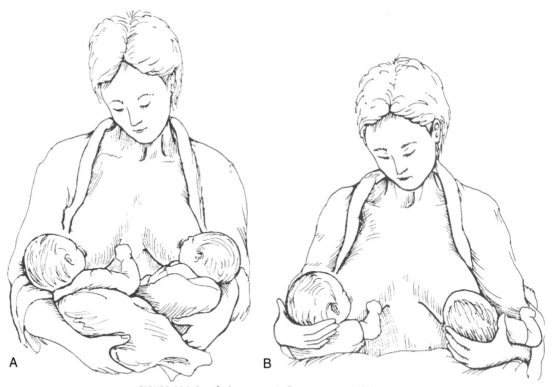

FIGURE 18-8 Breastfeeding twins. **A,** Cradle position. **B,** Football hold position.

have a stronger suck than the other and each breast should receive an equal amount of stimulation.

Understanding the mechanisms of suckling is essential to preventing, assessing, and intervening in neonatal suckling problems. Infants are born ready to suckle the breast.[72] Arrhythmic sucking has been found in full-term infants who bottle feed.[72] Nipple confusion describes the difficulty of infants who have been fed with artificial nipples before learning to breastfeed.

The infant who has learned to feed from a bottle nipple often sucks incorrectly at the breast, preventing milk flow.

The infant's confusion creates frustration and crying, which may inhibit milk letdown. The best means for preventing nipple confusion is to enable the infant to learn breastfeeding *before* bottle feeding is established[243] (see Table 18-3).

Assessment of the problem includes evaluating the method of feeding and possibly using alternative nutritional methods (gavage feedings) until the cause is determined. If the infant is bottle fed, choking may be a result of a soft nipple, a fast flow that the infant cannot control, or a nipple that is too long for the infant's (particularly the preterm infant's) mouth. If the mother is breastfeeding and the ejection is strong, the first rush of milk could cause choking, which may be prevented by manual expression of a small amount (several spurts) of milk before offering the nipple to the infant. Collins and colleagues[64] studied the effect of bottles, cups, and dummies (pacifiers) on breastfeeding in preterm infants using an RCT. Included in the study were 319 preterm neonates born at 23 to 34 weeks' gestation, with 303 included in the final analysis. The primary outcome measure was continuation of any breastfeeding on discharge home from the NICU. The results demonstrated that there were no significant differences with the use of a dummy (pacifier). However, infants randomized to cup feeds were more likely to be fully breastfed on discharge home but had a longer length of stay in the hospital (cup = 59 days; bottle = 48 days). Cup feeding did not show a difference in the incidence of any breastfeeding at discharge. On the other hand, Howard and colleagues[140] found in a cohort of 750 healthy newborns that early use of a pacifier did decrease success and duration of breastfeeding through 1 year. A more recent study of pacifier restriction in term newborns, without restriction of formula use, resulted in a drop of exclusive breastfeeding rates to 68% from 80% when pacifiers were routinely used.[152] Two systematic analyses of nine studies found that cup feeding cannot be recommended over bottle feeding as a supplemental method for breastfeeding because (1) there is no significant benefit in maintaining breastfeeding beyond hospital discharge, (2) dissatisfaction of parents and staff with the method, and (3) there is an unacceptable consequence: longer length of stay with cup feeding.[65,102] Longer length of stay in

the NICU is associated with low rates of exclusive breastfeeding in VLBW infants.[190] A recent RCT comparing cup and bottle feeding in late preterm infants who were breastfeeding found no increase in hospital stay and increased breastfeeding at discharge, 3 months, and 6 months in the cup-fed group.[348]

Some suckling problems result from the sequelae of perinatal events (e.g., low Apgar score, preterm low-birth-weight [LBW], small-for-gestational-age [SGA], large-for-gestational-age [LGA], late-preterm infants, infant of a diabetic mother [IDM], and multiple births)[72,73,147] or of physical disorders (e.g., hyperbilirubinemia, hypoglycemia, cardiorespiratory conditions, sepsis, neuromotor/developmental problems, and structural abnormalities of the oral cavity)[33,74,178,243] and represent developmental delays. These suckling difficulties require diagnostic evaluation of the underlying cause and appropriate intervention.[33,178,243]

Late-preterm infants (e.g., $34^{0/7}$ to $36^{6/7}$ weeks' gestation) (see Chapter 5) are often poor feeders because of their developmental immaturity in coordination of suck-swallow-breathe and because they are awake less frequently, give fewer if any cues of readiness to feed, and are easily fatigued and fall asleep before a feeding is completed.[108,224] Being a late-preterm infant is an independent risk factor for breastfeeding difficulties and lack of exclusive breastfeeding at 4 months of age.[184,224,240] All of these problems contribute to poor stimulation of the breast, incomplete breast emptying, and inadequate milk production. While in the hospital, lactation assistance should focus on strategies to initiate and maintain maternal milk supply and provide adequate fluids and calories for the late-preterm infant.[108] Hallmarks of breastfeeding the late-preterm infant include proper positioning; use of breast pump, nursing supplementer (Figure 18-9), or nipple shield; waking every 2 to 3 hours to feed (for 8 to 12 breastfeedings a day); use of skin-to-skin care; weights before and after breastfeeding; and use of alternative methods of enteral nutrition.[6,108,184,224] Collaboratively creating a feeding plan with parents that they understand and are able to carry out at home is essential before discharge.[6,27,93,224] A Canadian study of late-preterm and term infants found a longer hospital stay for late preterms, initial breastfeeding difficulties, and higher readmission rates by 4 months.[205] Although this study found earlier cessation of breastfeeding at 4 months,[205] another Canadian study, in the same region, found that being a late preterm and readmission were not factors influencing the predominance of breastfeeding at 2 months, especially if parents had a positive encounter with a health care provider about breastfeeding.[209] In a U.S. study, low breastfeeding initiation rates among mothers of late-preterm infants was due more to sociodemographic variables (i.e., age, marital status, smoking, ethnicity, education, participation in WIC) than to the fact of late-preterm birth.[79]

Some mothers may not establish or may have difficulty maintaining an adequate milk supply, yet infants with problems require an easily obtainable milk supply. The Lact-Aid Nursing Trainer system (see Figure 18-9) addresses a variety of breastfeeding problems, including suckling defects.[29] Expressed breastmilk (EBM) or formula is contained in a presterilized, disposable bag suspended between the mother's breasts by a cord, and the liquid is delivered by a thin, flexible tube attached to the bag. The end of the tube is placed against the mother's nipple to enable the infant to suckle the tube and nipple at the same time. This device provides the correct rate of flow and volume of liquid that

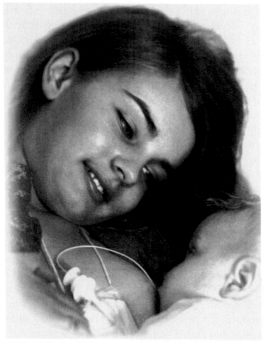

FIGURE 18-9 Lact-Aid Nursing Trainer. (Courtesy Lact-Aid International, Inc.)

elicits the reflexes of swallowing and expression. The Lact-Aid trainer provides oral therapy and nutritional supplementation for the infant and the mammary stimulus necessary to enhance the mother's lactation.[178] It is effective in managing low milk production in the mother that has resulted from separation, delayed breastfeeding, poor technique, or other correctable problems, and the device gives nutritional and oral therapy to an infant who is slow in gaining weight or has a suckling dysfunction.

CAUTION: To prevent the spread of serious infections, the Lact-Aid trainer should never be borrowed, rented, or loaned from another mother.

Problems with the letdown reflex may originate with the mother, the neonate, or both. The mother's emotional state may interfere with letdown—a tense mother will not have a letdown reflex. Often, especially in breastfeeding a premature infant, this is because of fear of failure or a lack of privacy. Knowledge of the mechanisms of lactation can help the mother avoid a fear of failing. Give the mother as much privacy and the least stressful environment possible when she is pumping her breasts and breastfeeding. If a mother experiences a weak or delayed letdown, she should massage the colostrum or milk down to the nipple before putting the infant to the breast. Infants with a poor suck, such as preterm infants or infants with Down syndrome or a neurologic deficit, understimulate the breast and do not trigger the letdown reflex. Use of the Lact-Aid trainer provides oral therapy, improves these infants' suckling ability, and facilitates a successful nursing relationship. The breast also can be stimulated with a good pump between feedings to increase the milk supply.

DATA COLLECTION AND INTERVENTION

Establishment of Breastfeeding

AVAILABLE FEEDING AND SUCKLING NEONATE

Infants who have been admitted to a NICU often present a dilemma to care providers as to the most favorable time to begin putting the infant to the breast. Research shows that direct breastfeeding, especially for the first oral feeding in the NICU, is associated with an increase in (1) frequency of later breastfeeding, (2) duration of breastmilk feedings, (3) success with breastfeeding in the hospital, and (4) breastmilk feedings at discharge.[260] Because combination human milk and formula feedings have been shown to result in earlier breastfeeding cessation, prompt initiation of breastfeeding in the NICU benefits the mother-infant breastfeeding dyad.[138] A recent randomized study of oral stimulation (15 minutes for at least 10 days before oral feeding) provided to preterm infants resulted in significantly higher breastfeeding rates (70% vs. 45.6%) at discharge.[31]

In the NICU, the infant's current physical status, plus considerations of nutrition and energy expenditure, helps determine the decision to initiate enteral feedings.[160] In a national survey, criteria used to determine readiness for oral feedings included the following: (1) 75% used gestational age (e.g., 34 weeks by 60%) or weight (e.g., 1500 g by 50%); and (2) infant behavioral cues (e.g., sucking behaviors)[302] (Table 18-5). A more recent survey of enteral feeding practices found that gestational age was the leading criteria used to initiate feedings.[116] Few empiric data support the contention that either weight or gestational age affects the ability of a preterm infant to suckle effectively because the suck and swallow will automatically be coordinated by the peristaltic motion at the breast. In the earlier survey, a majority (85% to 93%) responded that bottle feeding is started first, before breastfeeding.[302] Professional caregivers believe and teach parents that breastfeeding is too stressful and requires more energy and exertion than bottle feeding.[341] Contrary to physiologic evidence, progression of nutritional support for the preterm has proceeded from intravenous fluids → total parenteral nutrition → gavage (continuous → intermittent) → bottle feeding (at 1500 to 1800 g or 34 to 35 weeks' PCA) → breastfeeding (after bottle feeding without distress). Problems arising from this approach include the following*:

- Delay in initial oral feedings, slower attainment of full oral feedings
- Establishment of a sucking method that may not easily transfer to breastfeeding (i.e., bottle feeding alone has been found to contribute to arrhythmic sucking in full-term infants)[72]

- Initiation of breastfeeding when discharge is imminent so the mother receives little, if any, breastfeeding assistance and support
- Each additional week of hospitalization reduces the likelihood of the infant transitioning to direct breastfeeding by 14%

An *Early Feeding Skills (EFS) Assessment* checklist has been developed to assess both oral feeding readiness and oral feeding skills in preterm infants.[325] To individualize interventions, an infant's developmental stage regarding specific feeding skills (e.g., the ability to remain engaged in feeding; to organize oral-motor functioning; to coordinate swallowing and breathing; and to maintain physiologic stability) is profiled. Content validity and intrarater and interrater reliability have been established. The EFS is being tested for predictive, concurrent, and construct validity.[325]

Use of a breastfeeding protocol[316] without use of bottle feeding (either before breastfeeding or to supplement breastfeeding) is associated with the longest duration of breastfeeding.[28] An RCT of this protocol in which nasogastric (NG) supplementation was compared with bottle feeding for a transition to feeding at the breast found that NG supplementation was associated with feeding from the breast at discharge, 3 days, 3 months, and 6 months compared with preterm infants supplemented with bottle feeding.[161] In this same study, earlier age at initiation of breastfeeding also was associated with successful and longer duration of breastfeeding.[161] Other protocols for transitioning from gavage to breast have been proposed but not tested in an NICU population.[246] After discharge from the NICU, mothers wean their preterm infants from the breast because of (1) infant resistance to latching on, (2) weak suck, (3) refusing the breast, and (4) difficulty with latch-on.[134] If the sucking pattern learned with bottle feeding impedes breastfeeding, health care providers should promote early, exclusive breastfeeding to prolong the duration of preterm breastfeeding after discharge.[28,43,161,263]

Maturation of feeding skills depends on developmental changes in the infant's central nervous system coupled with experiential learning.* Experiential learning through a prefeeding oral stimulation program has been shown to improve preterm infants'

---

*References 104, 122, 202, 216, 265, 303, 310, 311, 341.

*References 43, 50, 103, 206, 248, 259, 263, 303, 311, 316.

TABLE 18–5	CRITICAL FINDINGS
	READINESS FOR INITIATION OF ORAL FEEDINGS: RESEARCH BASIS

BREASTFEEDING	CRITERIA	BOTTLE FEEDING
Preterm	←Gestational/ Postconceptual Age→ ←Weight→	*Preterm*
28-32 weeks: Better able to coordinate suck, swallow, and breathing.[214,215,218]		34-35 weeks: PCA is a developmental guideline—based on belief that sucking pattern is similar to that of full-terms*; infants may be ready at an earlier age (i.e., 28-34 weeks).[159,212] Coordination of respirations with sucking and swallowing is consistently achieved by infants >37 weeks PCA.[147,206,259,335]
<1500 g: Better able to coordinate suck, swallow, and breathing.[214–216,218]		1500-1800 g: Traditional criteria without research basis.
Full-Term	←Mechanics of Sucking→	*Full-Term*
Ultrasound study shows human nipple elongates to twice its resting length; neonatal cheeks act as a passive seal for the oral cavity. Sucking pressures of −50 to −155 mm Hg.[264]		Higher maximum pressure and number of sucks or bursts; greater suck widths and greater intake/suck. Able to alter sucking to accommodate nutrient composition, nipple, and hole size to minimize energy expenditure[198] and autoregulate milk flow by controlling pressure generated during sucking.[198] Regulates sucking pressure by coordination of various oral motor structures so that intraoral pressure is controlled to enable milk flow in a manageable fashion.
Preterm		*Preterm*
Sucking pressures of −2.5 to −15 mm Hg.[264]		Burst width (interburst and intersuck width) similar to that of full-term infant.[148,210,211] At the beginning of a feeding, preterms generate weaker sucking pressure within the oral cavity that changes over time to pressures and duration in the same range as for term infants, because of neural maturation[50] and sucking experience.
Full-Term	←Energy Expenditure→	*Full-Term*
50% of feeding obtained in first 2 min; 80%-90% by 4 min; last 5 min, minimal obtained from each breast.[264]		86% of feeding obtained in first 4 min of sucking.[174] Generate larger negative pressure with sucks with higher energy expenditure.[148] Able to alter sucking to accommodate nutrient composition, nipple and hole size to minimize energy expenditure[198] and autoregulate milk flow by controlling pressure generated during sucking.[198]
Preterm		*Preterm*
After 34 weeks: 70%-80% of feeding ingested in first 6 min, then intake sluggish, rest periods increase; and sucking and nourishment decrease. At 36-37 weeks: Sucking standards are similar to those in mature neonate.[248] The younger the gestational age, the higher the variability.[248] Longer duration of breastfeeding than bottle feeding.[214,218] No differences in duration of breastfeeding versus bottle feeding.		40% of total volume ingested in first min, less energy to suck same volume as full-term infant.[148] Infants born 26-29 weeks' gestational age benefit from restricted milk flow (i.e., milk is obtained only with active sucking; no milk flows to infant by gravity or high-low nipples during rest periods). At initiation of oral feeding (with restricted milk flow), an intake of 1.5 ml/min and a proficiency of 30% (e.g., intake of 9 ml in first 5 min; intake of 30 ml in 20 min) are indicative of earlier attainment of full oral feeding.[174] Consumes an average of 2.6 ml/min of feeding.[259]

TABLE 18-5	CRITICAL FINDINGS—cont'd
	READINESS FOR INITIATION OF ORAL FEEDINGS: RESEARCH BASIS

BREASTFEEDING	CRITERIA	BOTTLE FEEDING
Preterm		*Preterm*
At 35 weeks' CA: Small volume of milk intake in same duration of feeding; fed less efficiently and with fewer suck bursts.[104]		At 35 weeks' CA: Greater volume of milk intake in same duration of feeding with more sucking bursts; fewer single sucks, better nipple seal.[104]
Preterm	←Temperature→	
Skin temperature higher (than when bottle feeding) because of bodily contact with mother.[59,214,218] No temperature change before feeding (ac) or after feeding (pc).		
Preterm	←Weight Gain→	*Preterm*
Less weight gain after breastfeeding compared with bottle feeding.[122]		No difference in weight gain between experimental self-demand feeding protocol and control group (standard care).[201]
	← Heart Rate→	*Preterm*
		Bradycardia occurred with bottle feeding but not breastfeeding; bradycardia possibly related to faster milk flow and interference with breathing[214,218]; apnea and bradycardia with bottle feeding in otherwise healthy preterms.[206]
Full-Term	← Coordination of Suck, Swallow, and Breathing→	*Full-Term*
Swallowing occurs nonrandomly between breaths and does not interfere with breathing.[115]		Suck, swallow, breathe in a 1:1:1 pattern.[206] Alteration of breathing pattern—prolongation of expiration and shortening of inspiration.[199,218] No difference in sucking frequency or pressure when bottle feeding expressed milk or formula. Differences in sucking and/or breathing patterns attributed to nutrient delivery rather than nutrient composition.[197] Soft-walled delivery system results in significantly higher oxygen saturation, better coordination of suck/swallow/breathe and feeding behaviors more like breastfeeding than use of hard-walled delivery system.[115]
Preterm	← Coordination of Suck, Swallow, and Breathing→	*Preterm*
Different patterns of sucking bursts and better coordination, breathing is integrated within sucking bursts.[215]		Initial feedings at 32-34 weeks are characterized by periods of apneic suckle alternating with respirations; as PMA increases, the percentage of apneic swallows decreases and suck-swallow-breathing is more synchronized.[112,335] High-flow nipples result in apnea[198,300] or bradycardia.[192-194,196] Do not breathe within sucking bursts but in alternate short bursts of sucking with breathing.[218] Consistently achieved by infants 36-37 weeks' PCA.[335] Use of orthodontic nipples results in physiologic stability and effective feeding behavior in some preterms.[88] At 34 weeks' PCA, sucking pattern primarily expression component; with maturation, experience, endurance, and strength gains, there is a shift to more frequent use of term sucking pattern.[303] Not necessary to wait for full-term sucking pattern for successful oral feeding.[103,303]

Continued

TABLE 18-5	CRITICAL FINDINGS — cont'd
	READINESS FOR INITIATION OF ORAL FEEDINGS: RESEARCH BASIS

BREASTFEEDING	CRITERIA	BOTTLE FEEDING
Full-Term	*← Oxygen Saturation→*	*Full-Term*
No desaturation with feeding.[124] 18% of pc saturations <90%.		No desaturation with feeding.[199] 29% of pc saturations <90%. More oxygen desaturations (<90%) than breastfeeding.[197]
Preterm		*Preterm*
No difference in oxygenation with breastfeeding versus bottle feeding[214,218]; no pc decline of oxygenation; oxygenation more stable than with bottle feeding — fewer desaturations.[88] Desaturations (<90%) in 21% of breastfeedings.[59] With BPD, saturation higher than with bottle feeding.[59]		Decreased oxygenation during initial sustained sucking, but oxygenation increased as sucking pattern modulated.[283] 32-36 weeks: Range of 94%-97% with feeding, with sucking decreased saturation from 2.5%-16% (range 80%-100%).[212] Fluctuations and sharper decrease in saturation with bottle feedings versus breastfeeding[59,214,218,283]; 10 min pc saturation 50% below baseline.[59] Desaturations (>90%) in 38% of bottle feeding.[59] Desaturation in VLBW infants at discharge: average of 10.8 events during feeding; 20% of feeding time with saturations less than 90% Behavioral cues of desaturation are unreliable; changes in breathing and sucking pauses to regulate breathing pattern and increase oxygenation may occur.
	←Hypercapnia→ (elevated Pco_2)	*Preterm*
		34-35 weeks: Increased Pco_2 depresses sucking and swallowing so that respirations may supersede feeding in preterms with increased respiratory drive (e.g., BPD).
Preterm	*←Behavioral Cues→*	*Full-Term and Preterm*
32 weeks: Increased feeding in active/alert and quiet/alert.	←Quiet, alert→state before and during feedings associated with more successful feeding behaviors.[37,201,206,207] Offer pacifier for NNS (or pacifier with music[347] or mother's voice[61]) ac to promote awake behavior at beginning of feeding.[259,263] NNS ac associated with better oral feeding ability.[45] ←NNS pattern of sucking develops before nutritive pattern; mature NNS pattern not reliable cue for readiness to orally feed.[174,259] ←Cues include[15,206,303]→ Oral behaviors — sucking on pacifier, fingers, feeding tube. Rooting reflex, hand-to-mouth behaviors, mouthing movements. Presence of gag reflex. *←Behavioral State→* Changes — arousal from sleep, quiet alert state ac.[207] Exhibits stability in autonomic, motoric, and behavioral states. Able to self-regulate, interact, and tolerate outside stimuli.[206] ←Crying→fussing and demanding to feed — a late sign.	Motor behavior: Change in arm posture (flexion) with feeding.

ac, Before feeding; *BPD*, bronchopulmonary dysplasia; *CA*, corrected age; *NNS*, nonnutritive sucking; *pc*, after feeding; *PCA*, postconceptual age; *PMA*, postmenstrual age; *VLBW*, very-low-birth-weight.
*References 103, 174, 201, 206, 212, 259.

sucking behaviors before actual oral feeding.[31] A recent randomized study of oral stimulation (15 minutes for at least 10 days before oral feeding) resulted in significantly higher breastfeeding rates (70% vs. 45.6%) at discharge.[31] Studies show that preterm infants are able to breastfeed far earlier (less than 1500 g or 28 to 36 weeks' gestation) than they can bottle feed.[214-216,218,311] A comparison of studies of breastfeeding and bottle feeding shows less oxygen desaturation, warmer skin temperature, no bradycardia, and better coordination of sucking and breathing with breastfeeding compared with bottle feeding (see Table 18-5). According to these research data, the ability of the preterm infant to breastfeed without alterations in homeostasis occurs *before* the ability to safely bottle feed. Oxygenation is more stable with breastfeeding, because the type of sucking pattern (e.g., intermittent) and the flow of milk at the beginning of breastfeeding may be easier for the VLBW infant to control and regulate.[193,300] In VLBW infants, breathing is compromised (e.g., desaturations, increase in heart and respiratory rates) more during continuous sucking than during intermittent sucking.[300]

When an NG tube is in place, a VLBW infant has even poorer oxygenation, shallower breathing, and inability to increase tidal volume.[300] The postfeeding period enables recovery of oxygen saturation and end-tidal CO_2 to the prefeeding levels.[300]

Health care providers and parents should closely observe VLBW infants during the continuous sucking period (e.g., the first minute of bottle feeding,[324] with letdown during breastfeeding) for apnea, oxygen desaturation, and heart rate changes. Recommendations for continuous sucking periods include (1) not allowing breathing pauses of more than 10 seconds, (2) monitoring oxygen saturation and heart rate for continuous sucking of more than 30 seconds, and (3) interrupting sucking by withdrawing the nipple for breathing pauses and desaturations.[177,300] Desaturations, especially in the first minute of bottle feeding, during the continuous sucking period, still occur in VLBW infants nearing discharge.[324]

Skin-to-skin (kangaroo) care provides a safe, effective alternative method of caring for premature infants (see Chapter 13). Use of kangaroo care has been shown to improve lactation for mothers of preterm infants.[104,311] During skin-to-skin contact, the infant may initiate nonnutritive suckling at the breast.[225,241] Nonnutritive time at the breast is used to accustom both mother and baby to each other and the pleasant sensory stimuli at the breast. Nonnutritive suckling at the breast improves maternal letdown, enhances attachment and bonding, and shortens transition time to and lengthens the duration of breastfeeding.[263,311] As the preterm matures, nonnutritive suckling is replaced by hunger cues, latching on, and effective nutritive suckling. Both AGA and SGA infants (700 to 2450 g) benefit from early (sometimes starting at birth) and sustained breastfeeding as follows (see Chapter 13):

- More mothers breastfeed and are more confident.
- More frequent feedings are given.
- More milk is produced.
- Infants breastfeed longer (e.g., at 1 month after discharge, breastfeeding rates increased from 11% to 50%).
- There is less bradycardia than with gavage or bottle feeding.
- There is better weight gain and earlier discharge.

Both maternal and neonatal responses to breastfeeding should be monitored.[263,311] Adequate milk volume is available when the milk ejection (letdown) reflex occurs. Breast massage may assist in bringing down the milk, thus making it easier for the infant to obtain. Letdown may be felt by the mother or observed as a change in the rhythm of infant suckling and audible swallowing. After letdown is established, the infant expends little energy in suckling. He or she only needs to coordinate swallowing and breathing with an occasional burst of sucking. The nurse should be available during the initial breastfeeding to provide support to the mother, to ensure that the infant exhibits no signs of distress (e.g., color changes, bradycardia, oxygen desaturation, drop in temperature), and to provide guidance for the mother if the infant chokes with letdown. The nurse also needs to reinforce to the mother that the infant's sucking pattern will be a pattern of bursts and pauses. The pauses are present in all infants and provide rest periods for the infant.

The infant's respiratory status should be reviewed. Infants requiring supplemental oxygen can breastfeed. If the infant requires 35% oxygen or less, oxygen may be delivered through a nasal cannula to ensure adequate, consistent oxygenation. This will eliminate another source of concern for the mother: having to worry about juggling the blow-by oxygen line. If the infant has not been placed on a nasal cannula previously, the nurse should initiate the cannula and then assess oxygenation using a pulse oximeter before the feeding begins. The infant's temperature status requires review. Attention should be directed toward preventing hypothermia with infants who require significant thermal support. The infant should be swaddled, and a hat should be placed on his or her head to prevent heat loss.

Duration of breastfeeding should be based on cues of satiety, such as sucking cessation or falling asleep, or cues of physiologic instability or fatigue. Frequency of breastfeeding can be progressed, as can frequency of bottle feeding: from one breastfeeding per day to one per shift to every other breastfeeding. If the mother is available with this progression, bottle feeding may be deferred until breastfeeding is well established, or bottle feeding may be avoided altogether. When the infant is taking all nutrition orally, the mother can be encouraged to breastfeed as often as possible and institute an ad lib schedule.[217,311] If the mother is available, the infant should breastfeed as often as necessary and supplementation should not be provided. However, if the breastmilk supply is insufficient, using a Lact-Aid Nursing Trainer provides nutritional supplementation and mammary stimulation to increase maternal milk supply. Total intake should be estimated to ensure adequate calories. If the infant weighs less than 1500 g, it may be necessary to augment calories, protein, and calcium with human milk fortifiers (fortifiers made from human milk are preferred to cow's milk fortifiers) (see Chapter 17).[2,81,168] Exclusive use of human milk, fortified with human milk fortifier, results in lower rates and severity of NEC in extremely premature infants compared with the use of human milk or preterm infant formulas with bovine milk fortifier.[317] There are limited data to support multinutrient fortification of human milk after hospital discharge and little data to show that important outcomes are affected, including growth rate during infancy.[349] Fortification also interferes with feeding at the breast.[349]

Families and staff often fear that the infant will not get enough during a breastfeeding. This concern is especially predominant when infants have been hospitalized for prematurity and fluids and calories have been scrutinized closely. Health professionals should be sensitive to such concerns and refrain from employing methods such as weighing infants before and after feedings or using gavage tubes to attempt to determine the exact amount of breastmilk ingested during the feeding. With today's electronic NICU scales, however, test weighing (before and after feeding) (see Table 18-3) is accurate, if necessary.[122,220,225] Test weighing reassures mothers (and professionals) that preterm infants are receiving adequate intake while nursing and is associated with a higher exclusive breastfeeding than merely estimating breastfeeding intake.[95,143,223]

Health professionals should also focus on cues that can be used during and after hospitalization by both caregivers and the family.[122] These cues include the infant's satisfaction after the feeding (asleep or fussy), the frequency of feedings, voiding pattern (minimum of six to eight wet diapers per day, weighing diapers, and checking specific gravity), and palpation of the mother's breasts before and after feeding. Trends in weight gain also can demonstrate the success of the mother-infant dyad in breastfeeding.

A small infant may have difficulty taking a large nipple into the mouth. The mother should shape her nipple by compressing behind the areola to allow more of the nipple to be placed in the infant's mouth. The thumb and index finger or the first two fingers should be parallel to the infant's nose and chin. The breast must be soft enough to be compressed in this manner. The mother should hold the infant close for the comfort of both, with the infant's entire body, not just the head, turned toward the mother's body (see Figure 18-5).

A nipple shield allows the infant to get a nipple in the mouth but increases the amount of sucking necessary to obtain milk and decreases the amount of stimulation received at the nipple. Supervised temporary use of silicone nipple shields has been found to be a successful bridging technique for the infant to transfer to direct breastfeeding (after only a few sessions of shield use).[275] Use of a nipple shield should be followed by breast pumping to express residual milk, maintain adequate milk supply, and obtain milk to freeze for supplemental feeding.

Because nonnutritive suckling does not stimulate prolactin secretion and milk production, infants should not be placed on an empty breast to feed. Without positive reinforcement (i.e., milk) for their efforts, infants soon learn that the breast does not give milk, become frustrated, and refuse to feed. The Lact-Aid trainer may be used to initiate proper suckle and supplement intake in a small premature infant who is able to nurse (see Prevention of Breastfeeding Problems earlier in this chapter).

Supplementing breastfeedings with bottle-fed formula is inefficient in terms of energy and calories, because the infant expends energy, and thus calories, to feed twice. More energy-efficient and calorically efficient methods of initiating breastfeeding include offering smaller, more frequent feedings; supplementing by gavage feeding[77]; and using a lactation supplementing device. Breastmilk fortifiers (see Chapter 17) should be used when the mother's milk is not nutritionally adequate for the infant's requirements.[81] Breastmilk substitutes, such as donor milk, should be used when the mother does not provide sufficient volume; donor milk also needs fortification to meet the nutritional needs of VLBW premature infants[344] (see Chapter 17).

UNAVAILABILITY OF A FEEDING OR SUCKLING NEONATE

If premature birth or neonatal or maternal illness delays the onset of breastfeeding, the mother experiences a decrease in her milk production. Depending on how long breastfeeding has been delayed, mammary involution and the return of menstrual hormonal cycles may inhibit breastfeeding. A preterm infant or one who is ill may be weak and tire easily, and thus adequate lactation is not established.

If a neonate is unable to feed at the breast, breastmilk must be produced through artificial stimulation of the breast. The mother should establish a regular routine of breast massage[150,311] and pumping soon after the infant's birth. A comfortable chair with armrests or a pillow often helps, and the mother should be assured of privacy during breastfeeding and breast pumping. It is often necessary for the care provider to help the mother start and to encourage her routine. Each breast should be pumped every 2 to 4 hours, preferably with a double pumping system to enhance milk supply.[133,150] Mothers should increase pumping

time up to 15 to 20 minutes as the milk comes in, with the suction pressure increased as tolerated. At the beginning of pumping, mothers should awaken to pump at night to establish a good milk supply. Sleep and rest are necessary for good milk supply; however, the mother should not sleep when breasts are engorged because this will decrease the supply. Mothers should be advised that if their infant were with them, they would be feeding every 2 to 4 hours around the clock and therefore should develop that pattern to establish an adequate supply.

CAUTION: Mothers should be counseled about the potential risks of using breast shells or breast pump kits that have been used by other women. Breast shells, breast pump kits, and lactation aids are intimate-care items and are meant for use with one mother and one baby. Breast pump attachments and collection devices must be appropriately cleaned.[71]

Induction Aids. Various induction aids using tactile and mechanical principles are available to assist the mother in lactating and relactating. Knowledge of the different systems and their advantages and disadvantages enables the health care provider to help the mother choose the most helpful aid.

Breast massage (gentle, tactile stimulus usually in a circular motion using increasing pressure) before breastfeeding or pumping may help unplug breast ducts and enable milk to flow more easily.

Breast massage during pumping provides the important tactile stimulation that is missing without the infant's nursing and facilitates prolactin release and milk yield.[178]

Hand Expression. Once the breastmilk supply has been established, hand expression (Figure 18-10) is the simplest and most cost-effective way to collect milk; however, prolactin secretion and milk yields are less than with a pulsatile breast pump.[351] Combining hand expression of colostrum and hands-on pumping results in greater milk production for pump-dependent mothers of preterm infants.[238] Some mothers find hand expression esthetically unsatisfactory, and they should use other methods.

Mechanical Devices. Breast pumps work by application of negative pressure (e.g., −50 to −155 mm Hg) and compression in a suck-release pattern

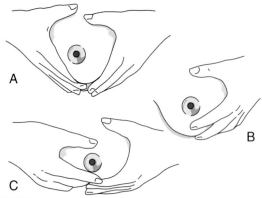

FIGURE 18-10 Breast massage. **A,** Place hands with palms toward chest at breast. Encircle breast with fingers and thumbs. **B** and **C,** Applying pressure, move hands forward, overlapping as they near nipple. Stop posterior to areola. Continue for 1 to 2 minutes or until milk is on nipple. Repeat on opposite breast. (From Lawrence RA, Lawrence RM: *Breastfeeding: a guide for the medical professional,* ed 6, St Louis, 2005, Mosby.)

(e.g., rate of 40 to 50 suck-release cycles/min) by fitting the nipple cup (or flange) over the maternal nipple and areola.[38] Nonautomated pumps are regulated by the number of times the mother manually exerts and releases pressure. Three types of nonautomated pumps are available: (1) bicycle horn pumps, which should never be used; (2) cylinder pumps; and (3) trigger or handle pumps.[38] Nonautomated pumps are best for occasional use. Automated pumps (either fully or partially) exert more negative pressure, permit the greatest number of cycles per minute, and are the pumps of choice for establishing and maintaining lactation for a preterm or sick infant.[38,311] A randomized trial comparing a novel manual breast pump (with compressive action on the areola) with a standard electric pump, used by mothers of preterm infants, found that the manual pump produced greater milk flow, resulted in greater total milk volume, was preferred by most mothers, and was more cost effective.[100] Breast pumps that mimic the sucking pattern of the human infant result in greater amounts of pumped milk and are more efficient, comfortable, and convenient.[221] Automated pumps are available in the NICU and for home rental use. Health insurance (both public and private) may reimburse for pump rental.

Serum prolactin levels and increased milk yield more closely parallel those with natural infant suckling when an intermittent, pulsative pump is used.[351] Just as nursing twins simultaneously results in a greater prolactin response, pumping both breasts simultaneously is more convenient and provides higher prolactin release (and higher milk yield) and saves time.[133,351]

To increase milk supply when the infant is not nursing, the pump should be used frequently (see Table 18-3). Because the breast pump is not as efficient as the suckling infant,[38] before initiating pumping, the mother may find that tactile stimulation and breast massage help increase the milk supply. Looking at the infant's picture or listening to a tape recording of the infant's cry stimulates her milk production with a pump.

Beginning on the low or normal pump setting and carefully breaking the suction at the breast with a finger help prevent sore nipples. Painful engorgement is relieved by pumping each breast just enough to obtain relief. Nipple or areolar engorgement must be relieved so that the infant is able to grasp and suckle the nipple.

Lactoengineering. To increase caloric density of EBM to improve growth/weight gain in VLBW infants, the pumping process can be altered to increase lipid content. Because the lipid content of hindmilk (e.g., milk expressed after letdown or later in the pumping session) is two to three times higher than the lipid content of foremilk, selectively feeding hindmilk to VLBW infants has been shown to increase growth and weight gain.[294] For VLBW infants with a consistent weight gain of less than 15 g/kg/day, hindmilk feedings may be initiated until a consistent weight gain of more than 30 g/kg/day is achieved.[333]

To express hindmilk, breast pumping is interrupted an average of 2 to 5 minutes after milk ejection has begun. This milk is collected and labeled "foremilk." Pumping is resumed until about 2 minutes after milk flow has ceased. This milk is placed in a separate container labeled "hindmilk." Another method of lactoengineering is to individualize the milk fractionation procedure by use of a "creamatocrit" that accurately estimates lipid and caloric content of EBM.[117,222] A small sample (less than 1.0 ml) of pumped breastmilk is aliquoted into two capillary tubes that are sealed and centrifuged for 5 minutes. The lipid and cream layer rises to the top of the tubes and can be quantitated as a percentage of breastmilk volume using a hematocrit reader and converted to estimates of lipid concentration and caloric density using published regression equations.[222] One study showed that mothers are able to cost-effectively and accurately perform creamatocrit assays; the mothers enjoyed the responsibility and increased involvement in their infant's care.[117] It is interesting to note that low-income mothers with fewer years of formal education and skilled rather than professional occupations were the most accurate in their performance of creamatocrits.

DONOR HUMAN MILK

Human milk banks that collect, store, and distribute milk to infants other than those of the donating mother exist around the world. This support is not available to some NICUs; others intentionally choose not to store or use donor milk.[254,334] The reservations about storing/using donor milk generally involve lack of knowledge (i.e., advantages, concerns about adequate nutrition, safety, parental receptiveness, cost).[96,254] Recognition of human milk as the best nutrition for preterm infants has increased research into donor milk and the growing use of pasteurized donor human milk in NICUs worldwide.[15,53,96,254] A recent survey of U.S. Level III NICUs found increasing use (42% of directors reporting donor milk use), especially in larger NICUs and among those in the West and Midwest.[254] Another recent study showed a marked increase in the use of donor milk for preterm infants, especially in the first 2 weeks of life, from 8% to 77% in two urban U.S. hospitals from 2006 to 2011.[78] For preterm infants, use of donor milk dramatically increases human milk intake, decreases formula intake, does not alter mother's milk intake,[78] and is associated with higher rates of exclusive breastfeeding of VLBW preterms at discharge.[24,96]

The World Health Organization (WHO), United Nations International Children's Emergency Fund (UNICEF), AAP,[15] Academy of Breastfeeding Medicine,[3] European Society for Pediatric Gastroenterology, Hepatology, and Nutrition (ESPGHAN),[96] and World Association of Perinatal Medicine all endorse the use of donor human milk.[227] The increased use of donor milk has increased the importance and existence of human milk banks.[96,156,250] Adequate screening of human milk donors (for cytomegalovirus [CMV], human immunodeficiency virus [HIV], and other viruses) is essential because of the possibility of milk-borne pathogens (e.g., CMV,

HIV, herpes simplex virus, human papillomavirus, hepatitis B and C virus).[84,173,250] All donor milk must be pasteurized, which eradicates bacteria with 93% of pooled samples sterile after pasteurization in one study.[173] Milk banks ship human milk when necessary. Human milk banks are listed in Box 18-3.

Donor human milk should *only* be provided by a human milk bank.[15,96,250] Two recent studies of purchases of human milk from the Internet found microbial contamination[155] and milk arriving above the recommended frozen and refrigerated temperatures.[110,111] Seventy-four percent (74%) of the Internet milk was colonized with gram-negative bacteria

---

BOX 18-3 **HUMAN MILK BANKS IN NORTH AMERICA**

Not-for-Profit Milk Banks
- California: Mothers' Milk Bank, www.mothersmilk.org
- Canada:
  British Columbia: Women's Milk Bank, www.bcawomens.ca
  Ontario: Human Milk Bank, www.milkbankontario.ca
  Calgary: Mothers' Milk Bank, www.calgarymothersmilkbank.ca
  Quebec: www.hem-quebec.qc.ca/lait-maternal
- Colorado: Mothers' Milk Bank, www.rmchildren.org/milkbankcolorado
- Florida: Mothers' Milk Bank of Florida, www.milkbankofflorida.org
- Indiana: Mothers' Milk Bank, Inc., www.immb.org
- Iowa: Mothers' Milk Bank of Iowa, www.uichildrens.org
- Kansas: Kansas City Regional Human Milk Bank, www.saintlukeshealthsystem.org
- Massachusetts: Mothers' Milk Bank of New England, www.milkbankne.org
- Michigan: Bronson Mothers' Milk Bank, www.bronsonhealth.com/mothers-milk-bank
- Mississippi: Mothers' Milk Bank of Mississippi, www.msmilkbank.org
- North Carolina: Wake Med Mothers' Milk Bank and Lactation Center, www.wakemed.org
- Ohio: Mothers' Milk Bank of Ohio, www.ohiohealth.com
- Oregon: Northwest Mothers' Milk Bank, www.nwmmb.org
- Texas:
  Mothers' Milk Bank of Austin, www.milkbank.org
  Mothers' Milk Bank of North Texas, www.texasmilkbank.org

For-Profit Milk Bank
- California: Prolacta Bioscience, www.prolacat.com

or had too high an overall bacterial count.[155] No samples were HIV positive, but 21% of the Internet samples were positive for CMV DNA.[155] Parents should be cautioned that human milk obtained without adequate screening, use of proper collection and storage techniques, and pasteurization poses an increased risk as a source of acquired infection for their preterm and/or medically compromised neonate.[110,111,155]

Nutritional analysis of donor human milk may optimize its use in feeding of preterm infants[67,96] (Box 18-4). In addition, the method of administration of donor human milk alters its nutritional content. When three feeding methods (bolus/gravity gavage; syringe pump gavage over 1 hour and 2 hours) were compared, lipid loss was significant in the timed feedings compared with the bolus method.[49]

Outcomes of premature infants fed donor human milk are compared with outcomes from mother's own milk and formula in Table 18-6. Use of donor breastmilk to feed preterm infants and the resulting decrease in the incidence of NEC has been shown to be a cost-effective and clinically effective strategy.[106] Currently three RCTs are being conducted comparing fortified donor human milk feedings for VLBW/ELBW preterm infants (either as a supplement to maternal milk or in place of maternal milk that is minimal or nonexistent) compared with preterm formula. All of these trials are assessing neurodevelopmental outcomes at 18 to 22 and 22 to 26 months.[85-87]

COMPLICATIONS OF BREASTFEEDING

Many complications other than prematurity may pose difficulties with breastfeeding. Information on perinatal complications and breastfeeding is shown in Table 18-4.[15,178] Because of the significant benefits of breastmilk, infants with special needs should be encouraged and mothers should be assisted in breastfeeding. Many principles used with the preterm and other variations of feeding styles and techniques may help facilitate these infants and their mothers in enjoying a successful breastfeeding experience.

Consultation with or referral to a certified licensed lactation consultant or specialist also may be helpful.[263] Many NICUs have such an expert on their staff.

BOX 18-4 **NUTRITIONAL ANALYSIS OF DONOR HUMAN MILK COMPARED TO MOTHER'S OWN MILK[96,172]**

Differs from Mother's Own Milk
- Oligosaccharide amount and content[191]
- Lower protein levels[67]
- Pasteurization:
  - Decrease in cytokines, lactoferrin, lysozyme, leukocytes, lymphocytes, phosphatases, and growth factors[62,273]
  - Inactivation of maternal T and B cells, macrophages, neutrophils[62]
  - Reduction of secretory immunoglobulin A (sIgA) by 28% to 60%[62]
  - Reduction of immunoglobulin A and G by 33% to 40%[250]
  - Modest decrease in protein (6%) and fat (8%);[62] reduction of fat absorption by infant recipient[10]
  - Higher concentration of free fatty acids than in fresh milk[62]
  - Kills bacterial pathogens such as *Staphylococcus aureus*, *E. coli*, etc.
  - Inactivates cytomegalovirus
  - Slightly affects content of vitamins (A, D, E, B_2, and B_6); choline, niacin, and pantothenic acid[10]
  - Significantly decreases thiamine (25%), biotin (10%), and vitamin C (35%)[10]
  - Reduces nitrogen retention[10]
- After first year of lactation[256]:
  - Increased concentration of lysozyme
  - Decreased concentration of zinc and calcium

Similar to Mother's Own Milk
- Does not meet nutritional requirements of preterm infants; fortification required
- Pasteurization:
  - No decrease in cytokines, chemokines, and growth factors[119]
  - No change in long-chain polyunsaturated fatty acids (DHA/ARA),[30] monoglycerides/free fatty acids, linoleic/alpha-linoleic acid[250]
  - Oligosaccharide amount and content[36]
  - No effect on protein, fat, and carbohydrate levels[62]
- After first year of lactation[256]:
  - Stable concentrations of protein, lactose, iron, copper, lactoferrin, and secretory immunoglobulin A (sIgA)

Misappropriation of Breastmilk

Misappropriation of breastmilk (giving the wrong expressed breastmilk to the wrong infant) does occur. As a distillate of human blood, human milk may contain infectious bacteria (e.g., *Klebsiella*, *Staphylococcus*, methicillin-resistant *Staphylococcus aureus*) and viruses (e.g., HIV, hepatitis virus,

TABLE 18-6	OUTCOMES OF PREMATURE INFANTS FED DONOR HUMAN MILK*

COMPARED WITH MOTHER'S OWN MILK	COMPARED WITH PRETERM FORMULA
Higher risk of slower growth both with and without fortification[†] in VLBW premature infants	Lower short-term rates of weight gain and growth[268,295]
Better weight and length gain; similar head circumference growth with early aggressive fortification of human milk with HHMF[120]	Feeding of choice (if mother's own milk unavailable) for GI problems (i.e., anomalies, NEC, short gut syndrome) for protective qualities and increased feeding tolerance[342]
Additional protein supplementation of donor human milk may be needed in VLBW infants[62]	Less feeding intolerance, including GE reflux[23,268]
	Less nosocomial infection, including UTI and diarrhea[129,185,208,268,297]
	Less NEC[‡] (4-6.5 times less likely[129,208]; decreased by 79%[46]; 3% in HM versus 21% in preterm formula[70]
Shorter LOS of premature infants fed entirely with maternal milk[295]	Shorter length of stay (LOS)[15,70,297] No difference in LOS between maternal milk–fed infants supplemented with either donor milk or preterm formula[295]
	Fewer days on TPN (28 days vs. 36 days)[70]
	Less morbidity[342]
	Neurodevelopmental outcomes: Similar outcomes when unfortified donor milk group compared with preterm formula group[188] Better outcomes (i.e., higher scores on mental and psychomotor development) when donor milk group compared with *term* formula group[188] VLBWs fed unfortified donor milk performed poorly on task of orientation to inanimate stimuli compared with group fed *term* formula[328]

GE, Gastroesophageal; *GI*, gastrointestinal; *HM*, expressed human milk; *HHMF*, human milk–derived human milk fortifier; *NEC*, necrotizing enterocolitis; *TPN*, total parenteral nutrition; *UTI*, urinary tract infection; *VLBW*, very low birth weight.
*References 15, 24, 25, 62, 92, 96, 172.
[†]References 18, 63, 114, 189, 295, 317.
[‡]References 23, 70, 200, 268, 295, 297, 317.

CMV, herpes virus) to which the infant given the wrong milk may be exposed. Both staff and parents involved in such an event experience psychologic stress and anxiety.[90] Human milk has also been mistakenly administered by the intravenous instead of the enteral route, resulting in a range of consequences from no sequelae to death.[290] Unit practices to prevent these occurrences include the following[10,90,181,290,326]:

- Use tubing for enteral feedings that is incompatible with intravenous tubing/connections.
- Check milk containers for two identifiers.
- Two nurses verify milk for administration; both nurses sign that verification has occurred.

- Two nurses verify and sign (that milk has been verified) at transfer and at discharge.
- Use commercial bar-coded devices.

Drugs in Breastmilk

Table 18-7 provides information about specific drugs excreted in breastmilk.[178,291] The most current and comprehensive information about the transfer of drugs and therapeutics into human milk is available at LactMed at www.toxnet.nlm.nih.gov. Protein binding, degree of ionization, molecular weight, and solubility of drugs influence the passage of drugs into milk. Protein-bound drugs and drugs of large molecular weight (greater than 200) are less likely to pass into milk. Conversely,

TABLE 18-7 DRUGS EXCRETED IN BREASTMILK

DRUGS	BREASTMILK	CONSIDERATIONS IN INFANT
Analgesics		
Heroin, codeine, meperidine, fentanyl, morphine, pentazocine, oxycodone, dextropropoxyphene	Appears in variable amounts. FDA warning[330] about mothers who rapidly metabolize codeine (because of a genetic predisposition), resulting in increased morphine levels in their breastmilk and morphine overdose to breastfeeding infants. Mothers who rapidly metabolize codeine will become so sleepy that they are unable to care for themselves or their infant. Rapid metabolizers of codeine include (1) 1%-10% in whites, (2) 3% in blacks, (3) 1% in Asians and Hispanics, (4) 16%-28% in North Africans, Ethiopians, and Saudi Arabians, and (5) those positive for *CYP2D6* genotype with genetic testing.	Symptoms of depression and floppiness have been associated with these drugs.[151,170] Sleepiness, difficulty breastfeeding, limpness, hypotonia, and respiratory distress. Severe, life-threatening events (respiratory arrest) caused by morphine overdose have occurred.
Aspirin	Safe on a single-dose schedule, although it passes into milk in low concentration.	In a deliberate overdose, metabolic acidosis resulted from an accumulation in the infant; use cautiously because of the risk for Reye's syndrome.
Acetaminophen	Appears in small amounts.	Well tolerated.
Ibuprofen	Appears in small amounts.	Well tolerated.
Sumatriptan succinate	Appears in small amounts.	Well tolerated.
Antibiotics and Sulfa Drugs		
Sulfa drugs	Appear in breastmilk and may interfere with bilirubin binding in neonate; infants with G6PD deficiency may develop hemolysis.	Should not be used for breastfeeding mother in the first month if infant is jaundiced or if infant has G6PD deficiency.
Chloramphenicol	Appears in breastmilk.	Contraindicated in nursing mother because infant may accumulate drug and develop "gray baby syndrome."
Penicillins (ampicillin, amoxicillin)	Small amounts in breastmilk.	Disruption of gastrointestinal (GI) flora, allergic sensitization/reactions. Observe for thrush, diarrhea, and rash. Breastmilk assists recolonization of normal gut flora.
Tetracycline	Appears in breastmilk at 50% of serum level.	Infants may develop stained and mottled teeth when therapy exceeds 10 days; should be given only for life-threatening maternal infections. Discontinue breastfeeding during treatment.
Antifungals		
Metronidazole/tinidazole	Appears in breastmilk in levels equal to serum levels.	Side effects include decreased appetite, vomiting, blood dyscrasia, and animal evidence of tumorigenesis. Mother's dose can be modified (e.g., 2 g single-dose therapy) so she can pump and discard milk for 24 hours.
Antimalarial (chloroquine)	Very small amounts appear in breastmilk.	Observe for GI symptoms (vomiting, diarrhea); hypotension.
Cephalosporins (cephalexin, cephalothin)	Very small amounts appear in breastmilk.	Rash and sensitization are possible. Also may affect bacterial flora — diarrhea, thrush.
Fluconazole (Diflucan)	Excreted into breastmilk in small amounts (1% of the maternal dose; <5% of the therapeutic pediatric dose).	Considered safe for nursing infants.
Fluoroquinolones (levofloxacin, norfloxacin, ofloxacin, ciprofloxacin)	Varying levels in breastmilk — use with caution.	Pseudomembranous colitis — observe for GI symptoms (vomiting, diarrhea). Tooth discoloration; phototoxicity. Arthropathy in animals.

TABLE 18-7 DRUGS EXCRETED IN BREASTMILK—cont'd

DRUGS	BREASTMILK	CONSIDERATIONS IN INFANT
Anticholinergics		
Atropine, scopolamine, synthetic quaternary ammonium derivatives	Atropine appears, but quaternary ammonium derivatives do not appear in breastmilk.	The neonate of nursing mother receiving atropine should be observed for tachycardia, constipation, and urinary retention.
Cimetidine	Appears in higher concentration than in serum.	No reported effects, although may suppress gastric activity, inhibit drug metabolism, and produce central nervous system stimulation. Use with caution until more information about antiandrogenic effects.
Anticoagulants		
Heparin and warfarin (Coumadin)	Do not appear in breastmilk.	
Antithyroidal Agents		
Iodide	Passes into milk. May affect thyroid activity and cause goiters.	Not contraindicated during breastfeeding.
Thiouracil	Higher concentration in maternal milk than in blood.	Neonatal problems include suppression of thyroid activity and agranulocytosis. If breastfed, infant should be given thyroid supplement, and thyroid function should be followed.
Propylthiouracil	Appears in small amounts (<0.3% of maternal dose).	No reported effects on infant. Follow with T_3, T_4, and TSH.
Anticonvulsants		
Phenobarbital, phenytoin, carbamazepine (Tegretol), and valproic acid (Depakene)	All appear in small amounts.	Sedation is possible, but rarely are clinical symptoms significant enough to cause adverse effects. Accumulation may occur because of long half-life of valproic acid.
Lamotrigine	Mean milk-to-plasma ratio 41.3% with a nonsignificant trend toward higher levels in breastmilk 4 hours after maternal dose.[245]	Infant plasma concentrations were 18.3% of maternal plasma concentrations, with a theoretical infant dose of 0.51 mg/kg/day and a relative infant dose of 9.2%.[245] Mild thrombocytosis was the only adverse event noted.
Cardiovascular Drugs		
Digoxin	Appears in small amounts.	Appears to be safe.
Reserpine	Appears in breastmilk.	Symptoms include diarrhea, lethargy, nasal stuffiness, bradycardia, and respiratory difficulties; contraindicated in breastfeeding.
Propranolol, metoprolol, labetalol	Appear in breastmilk in varying degrees; safest beta blockers with breastfeeding.	Observe for beta blockade—respiratory depression, bradycardia, or hypoglycemia.
Verapamil, diltiazem	Appear in varying amounts in breastmilk.	Appear to be safe.
Nifedipine	90% of the dose unavailable for transfer to breastmilk because of binding to plasma proteins.[19] One to 3 hours after maternal dosing, low levels (<1-10.3 mcg/L) appear in breastmilk.[121]	Appears to be safe.

Continued

TABLE 18-7	DRUGS EXCRETED IN BREASTMILK — cont'd	

DRUGS	BREASTMILK	CONSIDERATIONS IN INFANT
Cathartics		
Aloin, cascara sagrada, and anthraquinone preparations	Appear in breastmilk.	Colic and diarrhea are possible side effects.
Contraceptives		
Birth control pills (combined; progestin only; minipill)	Appear in breastmilk with peak levels 2 hours after intake.	Combined: may alter the quality and quantity of milk — suppress lactation, shorter breastfeeding, and slower weight gain. Progestin only or minipill: no alteration of milk volume or infant weight gain. Avoid progestins in pump-dependent mothers of premature infants to avoid affecting milk supply.[223] Unknown long-term risk for cancer — no evidence in past 30 years.[178]
Medroxyprogesterone (Depo-Provera)	Increased prolactin levels before/after sucking.	No adverse effects — 3-month injection (increased protein and quantity of milk); 6-month injection (increased quantity but decrease in protein, fat, calcium).[178]
Birth control implant (IMPLANON)	Small amount of hormone passes into breastmilk. Best to delay implant until 4 weeks postpartum.	Small number of children studied for 3 years after breastfeeding — no effects on growth and development.
Barrier methods (diaphragm, condoms, foams, cervical cap)	No chemicals to be excreted into breastmilk.	No effects on infant.
Diagnostic Radioactive Compounds		
^{67}Ga, ^{125}I, and ^{64}Cu	Appear for 24-48 hours.	Check half-life of specific compound. Pump and discard; then resume breastfeeding.
Diuretics		
Hydrochlorothiazide	May suppress lactation.	Inadequate milk; no significant risks are present; compatible with breastfeeding.
Immunosuppressant		
Azathioprine	One small study ($n = 10$ mothers; 31 breastmilk samples) found small levels (1.2 and 7.6 ng/ml) of 6-mercaptopurine (6-MP) in breastmilk samples at 3 and 6 hours after azathioprine ingestion.	Potential risks of bone marrow suppression, increased risk for infections and pancreatitis. No signs of clinical immunosuppression in the small study.
Psychotherapeutic Agents		
Lithium	Appears in breastmilk; infant serum level is 10%-50% of mother's level.	Contraindicated in pregnancy; controversial during lactation. Cyanosis, hypotonia, electrocardiogram changes. Evaluate lithium levels. Inhibits cyclic $3',5'$-AMP, a substance significant to brain growth.
	A small study ($n = 10$ mother/baby pairs) found the average breastmilk concentration of lithium to be 0.35 mEq/L with an infant trough concentration of 0.16 mEq/L.[336]	Carefully selected mothers may breastfeed a healthy infant while taking lithium: (1) maternal mood stable, (2) simple medication regimen and/or monotherapy with lithium, and (3) a pediatrician collaborating to monitor the infant.[336]

TABLE 18-7	DRUGS EXCRETED IN BREASTMILK — cont'd	

DRUGS	BREASTMILK	CONSIDERATIONS IN INFANT
Psychotherapeutic Agents — cont'd		
Olanzapine	Small amount (1.02%). Avoid breastfeeding during peak levels within 5 hours after dose.[107]	No adverse effects. Monitor for drowsiness and sedation; developmental milestones, especially if combination antipsychotics used.
Haloperidol	Low levels in breastmilk.	Monitor for drowsiness and sedation; developmental milestones, especially if combination antipsychotics used.
Risperidone	Low levels in breastmilk.	Little data; another antipsychotic agent preferred during breastfeeding.
Phenothiazines	Appear in small amounts.	Evaluate each drug separately; observe for sedation.
Diazepam (Valium)	Appears in breastmilk and may accumulate in infant because it is detoxified in liver.	Poor feeding, weight loss, hypoventilation, and drowsiness may be seen. Low incidence of toxicity and adverse events.
Tricyclic antidepressants (amitriptyline, nortriptyline, desipramine)	Appear in minimal amounts (<1%)	Careful considerations to select the safest for the infant. Nortriptyline may be the preferred choice.
Selective serotonin reuptake inhibitors (SSRIs) (fluoxetine, sertraline, paroxetine, citalopram, escitalopram)[127]	Appear in varying amounts. Fluoxetine — high levels, highly lipid bound. Produces the highest proportion (22%) of infant levels that are elevated above 10% of the average maternal level.[41] Citalopram produces elevated levels in 17% of infants.[41]	Sertraline is the drug of choice after birth because plasma levels are low (<2 ng/ml).[82,233,339] May alter short-term and/or long-term central nervous system development and function. Slower growth curve or weight gain with fluoxetine.[56] Most infants may continue breastfeeding when mother is treated with 20–40 mg daily.[94] Citalopram — minimize maternal dose to decrease elevated infant levels.[339] Paroxetine levels are also low.[339] Escitalopram — somnolence and sedation in young infants.
Serotonin-norepinephrine reuptake inhibitors (SNRI) (duloxetine, venlafaxine, desvenlafaxine)	Appears in breastmilk in low levels	Monitor for drowsiness, sedation, adequate weight gain, and developmental milestones, especially if combination antipsychotics used.
Stimulants		
Amphetamines (methamphetamine*)	Amphetamine concentration 3-7 times higher in breastmilk than in maternal plasma on the 10th and 42nd days of life.[315]	Stimulation of the infant — poor sleeping patterns and irritability. Infant death and SIDS-like syndrome reported with methamphetamine intake of mother.[20] Small amounts of amphetamine in infant's urine.[315]
Caffeine	Appears in small amounts (<1%) but may accumulate in infant.	Symptoms include jitteriness, wakefulness, and irritability. May alter iron concentration in milk and iron deficiency anemia at 1 month of age.
Theophylline	Appears in moderate amounts.	Irritability, jitteriness, and wakefulness may be seen in infant.
Cocaine*	Appears in breastmilk.	Cocaine intoxication: neurotoxicity (e.g., irritability, hyperactive reflexes, tremulousness, and mood lability) and seizures have been reported (see Chapter 11).[57,58]
Other Substances		
Buprenorphine†	Appears in low concentrations; poor oral bioavailability of drug in infants.	Monitor for drowsiness, adequate weight gain, and developmental milestones. Observe for sedation and withdrawal symptoms.

Continued

TABLE 18-7	DRUGS EXCRETED IN BREASTMILK — cont'd	

DRUGS	BREASTMILK	CONSIDERATIONS IN INFANT
Other Substances — cont'd		
Methadone[†]	Appears in breastmilk, concentration low (range 21.0 to 46.2 ng/ml).[149] Peak methadone levels occur in 4 hours after oral administration; the maximum amount secreted into breastmilk is approximately 2.2% of the mother's dose.[179] Milk-to-plasma ratios range from 0.05-1.89.[126]	Management depends on maternal dosing for methadone maintenance.[13,203] Observe for sedation, withdrawal. Studies have found that breastmilk intake is associated with less neonatal abstinence syndrome (NAS) and less use of pharmacologic treatment, regardless of type of drugs and gestation.[1,8,149]
Naltrexone[†]	Minimally excreted into breastmilk	Monitor for drowsiness, adequate weight gain, and developmental milestones. Observe for sedation and withdrawal symptoms.
Ethanol (alcohol)	Quick equilibration between serum and breastmilk levels.	Large quantities associated with lethargy, drowsiness, and affected motor development. The deficit in motor development was not replicated in a study of 18-month-olds exposed to moderate alcohol use during breastfeeding.[182] May inhibit milk letdown reflex and suppress lactation. Avoid nursing within 2-3 hours of alcohol intake.
Marijuana*	May reach high concentrations. THC, the active ingredient in marijuana, is absorbed and metabolized by the infant.	THC, the active ingredient in marijuana, is absorbed and metabolized by the infant.[8] May decrease prolactin levels, milk supply, and motor development. Exposure to secondary smoke. Avoid breastfeeding for several hours after use.[178] Long-term effects on development are unknown.[8]
Nicotine	Appears in breastmilk in proportion to number of cigarettes smoked and/or time from last cigarette. Smoking reduces the transport of iodine into breastmilk. Mothers should receive iodine supplement.[175]	Irritability; failure to thrive may result because of suppression of lactation. Effects of secondary smoke: increased incidence of upper respiratory infections, otitis media, bronchitis, pneumonia, and SIDS. Avoid smoking in the same room with the infant. Infants whose mothers smoke are at increased risk for iodine deficiency–induced brain damage if the mother does not receive iodine supplementation.[175]
Herbal tea mixtures (containing anise, fennel, licorice, galega) used to stimulate lactation (i.e., mother's milk tea)	Essential oils found in anise and fennel appear in breastmilk.	Difficulty feeding; growth failure, hypotonia; lethargy; vomiting; weak cry; poor suck; decreased reaction to painful stimuli.[286]
Fenugreek Ginseng Comfrey	Appears in breastmilk; milk has a maple syrup smell. No data on amount in breastmilk. No data on amount in breastmilk; caution use in any form.	Urine may have a maple syrup smell. May cause neonatal androgen effect and hirsutism. Associated with veno-occlusive disease and hepatotoxicity and is carcinogenic. Contraindicated in breastfeeding.
Silicone breast implants	Silicon in cow's milk has been shown to be 10 times higher and even higher in commercial infant formulas than in mothers with silicone implants.[299] Breastfeeding mothers with silicone implants are similar to mothers without implants with respect to levels of silicon in their blood and breastmilk.[299]	No adverse effects.

TABLE 18-7	DRUGS EXCRETED IN BREASTMILK—cont'd	
DRUGS	BREASTMILK	CONSIDERATIONS IN INFANT
Respiratory Drugs		
Inhalants (steroids—budesonide)	Lower levels of budesonide (mean ratio of 0.46) in milk than in maternal plasma.[97]	Negligible systemic exposure to inhaled corticosteroids[97]: Mean infant dose 0.3% of daily maternal dose; average infant plasma concentration 1/600th of maternal plasma concentration.

Modified from Sachs HC and the Committee on Drugs: Transfer of drugs and therapeutics into human milk: an update on selected topics, *Pediatrics* 132:e796, 2013; Lawrence RA, Lawrence RM: *Breast feeding: a guide for the medical profession*, ed 7, St Louis, 2010, Mosby; LactMed: www.toxnet.nlm.nih.gov.
*3′,5′-AMP, 3′,5′-*Adenosine monophosphate; *FDA,* Food and Drug Administration; *G6PD,* glucose-6-phosphate dehydrogenase; *SIDS,* sudden infant death syndrome; T_3, triiodothyronine; T_4, thyroxine; *TSH,* thyroid-stimulating hormone.
*Drug of abuse; contraindicated during breastfeeding—hazardous to both mother and infant.
†Food and Drug Administration–approved drug for opiate withdrawal

lipid-soluble drugs pass more easily into the milk. Because breastmilk is slightly acidic compared with plasma, weakly alkaline compounds are present in equal or greater amounts in breastmilk compared with plasma. Weakly acidic compounds have a higher concentration in plasma than in breastmilk.

Several factors influence the drug effect on the infant. Most drugs appear in milk, but drug levels usually do not exceed 1% to 2% of the ingested dose and do not depend on the milk volume.[178] The clinical dose of a drug to the infant can be calculated by the following formula[121]:

$$D - \text{infant} = \text{Drug concentration in milk} \\ (\text{at } C - \max, \text{ or } C - av) \times \text{Volume of milk ingested}$$

Drug transfers through breastmilk may be minimized by feeding the infant before taking oral medications. Many variables, such as gastric emptying, pH, and effects of intestinal enzymes, affect absorption. Finally, the chronologic and gestational ages of the infant affect the maturity of the systems involved in excretion and detoxification (see Chapter 10).

PARENT TEACHING

Parent teaching has been discussed throughout this chapter because it is essential to a successful breastfeeding experience for both mother and infant (Box 18-5).

> **BOX 18-5**
> **PARENT TEACHING**
> **KEY POINTS FOR SUCCESSFUL BREASTFEEDING**
>
> - Breastmilk is the best milk for preterm or sick neonates. Teach parents the benefits and advantages of breastmilk for their infant(s).
> - Teach parents how to interpret their infant's cues/behaviors of self-regulation and stress (see Chapter 13), hunger, and satiety.
> - Teach parents proper collection/storage/transport of pumped breastmilk; proper care and cleaning of breast pump supplies to prevent infection.
> - Teach mothers self-care: need for rest, diet, and fluid intake for lactation.
> - Provide anticipatory guidance about pumping and a dwindling milk supply (see Figure 18-11).
> - Teach parents realistic expectations for the first feeding at the breast and that breastfeeding is a learned behavior for both mother and preterm or sick infant.
> - Provide positive feedback, support, and encouragement to mother for pumping and with feeding at the breast.
> - Teach parents the importance of their involvement in their infant's care, especially in skin-to-skin (kangaroo) care and its benefits for both mother and preterm infant.

Before a premature or sick infant is actually nursed at the breast, the colostrum and breastmilk may have to be pumped and fed to the infant. If the mother's production is adequate, no supplementation is necessary. Before collecting the mother's milk, perform the following:

- Screen the mother (by history) for disease.
- Screen the mother (by history) for drugs that she has taken.
- Instruct the mother in sterile technique.

Proper collection and storage must be discussed with each family so that stored milk does not cause infections. Breast pumps can be a potential source of contamination, and therefore instructions on proper cleaning are paramount. D'Amico and colleagues[71] describe a process used for review and updating procedures to decrease this risk in an NICU. A written handout of pumping, storing, and thawing practices is helpful. Often the mother pumps and collects the milk, and the father transports it to the NICU (see Chapter 29). In addition, fathers assist with pumping, assume more daily domestic duties, and provide moral support to pumping mothers.[308] Methods of treatment and storage are listed in Box 18-6. A recent study of

---

BOX 18-6 TREATMENT AND STORAGE OF BREASTMILK

Treatment

1. Heat: Significant loss of lysozyme, lactoferrin, immunoglobulins, lactoperoxidase, lymphocyte function, complement, phagocytosis, and macromolecules may occur. Fat content altered (approximately 13%) by milk sterilization.[15,101] Pasteurization (Holder method: 62.5° C for 30 minutes)[141] does not alter fatty acid composition, but fat absorption by small preterm infants may be reduced from inactivation of bile salt lipase.[167]
2. Lyophilization: Effects are similar to those of heat treatment.
3. Freezing: Limited information; cells are not viable, but there is no effect on IgA content. Fat content is altered by freezing and thawing.

Storage

1. Use sterile glass or hard food-grade plastic containers (to ensure minimal loss of immunologic properties and fat-soluble vitamins)[22,181] with an airtight lid (to maintain closed system).[10] Milk stored in plastic bags may lose immune components and/or become contaminated.[326] Use a new container for each expression. Place amount for one feeding/container
2. Label with name, date, and time of collection, so that oldest milk is used first and colostrum is fed in the order in which it was pumped.[10,181]
3. Store in refrigerator for 24 hours (at 0° to 4° C [32° to 39.2° F]) or for longer periods (−18° C [0° F]).

---

how U.S. mothers of healthy babies store and handle expressed breastmilk found practices (e.g., microwaving milk and rinsing bottle nipples with water instead of cleaning with soap and water) that may pose a health risk to infants.[169]

Rewarming techniques include (1) placing frozen milk in a room-temperature water bath, in a hot-water bath, in a microwave oven, or under cold running water and then tepid water or (2) using commercially available devices.[10,181] Slow room-temperature rewarming is a concern because of bacterial overgrowth, especially if thawing is prolonged. Most nurseries use room-temperature water bath rewarming to avoid exposure to the high temperatures of the hot-water bath and the microwave. Microwaving is contraindicated—*never* use microwave heating of breastmilk because of the destruction of antiinfective properties (e.g., lysozyme and secretory IgA), resulting in an overgrowth of bacteria, and possible "hot spots" in the liquid.[10,15,181,266] The Human Milk Banking Association of North America recommends warming feedings to body temperature for preterm infants.[141,181] However, research shows a range of temperatures at which feedings are actually delivered, from a low of 21.8° C[91] to a high of 46.4° C.[176] Commercial warming devices are either waterless or heat milk with water (below the level of the container lid).

Fresh breastmilk is preferable for feedings because it has the greatest amount of immunologic properties. If the mother visits the infant at feeding time, she may pump her breasts and the breastmilk can be immediately fed to the infant, if the infant cannot be put to breast.

Maternal Care

A mother may be so concerned about the welfare of her infant that she spends most of her time at the hospital and receives inadequate rest, which is a common cause of milk production problems. The care plan includes encouraging, educating, and suggesting to the mother that she go home and rest, which may require someone to assist with the care of the newborn's siblings. The stress of having a sick infant and the time spent at the hospital may mean that the mother does not receive adequate nutrition.

It is necessary to add about 600 kcal to the nonpregnant diet and to replace elements, such as calcium, minerals, and fat-soluble vitamins, used in producing milk. The recommended dietary increases are even greater than those during pregnancy.[343] Adequate fluid intake (six to eight glasses of water, skim milk, or other noncaffeine liquids) should be consumed every day. Certain components of breastmilk (e.g., quantity, protein and calcium content) do not vary with the mother's diet, whereas others (e.g., fatty and amino acids, lysine, methionine, water-soluble vitamins) vary with maternal intake.

A mother's diet does not have much effect on the quality of the breastmilk (unless malnutrition intervenes) but affects the mother's overall health. She should be reminded to eat a balanced diet. Vegetarian diets should be supplemented with about 4 mg of cyanocobalamin (vitamin B_{12}) per day to prevent neurologic impairment in the breastfed infant.[55]

Anticipatory Guidance and Realistic Expectations

Anticipatory guidance is essential for mothers who are breastfeeding preterm infants. Mothers must be informed in the beginning that their milk supply may dwindle, even though they closely adhere to the pumping schedule. This is normal, because most pumps do not stimulate the breast as efficiently and physiologically as the suckling infant. Use of breast pumps that mimic the sucking pattern of the human infant result in greater amounts of pumped milk and are more efficient, comfortable, and convenient.[221,271] When the pumping regimen begins, explaining and drawing the mother a picture (Figure 18-11) of what is commonly experienced helps alleviate guilt caused by a dwindling milk supply. A rather sparse supply of milk does not mean she cannot nurse the infant, because the milk supply builds in response to the infant's nutritive suckle. The parent should be taught that there is no correlation between the amount of breastmilk expressed and the amount of milk a mother actually lets down when the infant is at the breast.

Breastfeeding problems may be particularly detrimental to the mother's perception of breastfeeding success. Disappointment with the breastfeeding experience may result from unrealistic expectations about breastfeeding the preterm infant. Establishing realistic parental expectations for the first time the infant breastfeeds decreases disappointment from unattainable goals. Breastfeeding, like parenting, is not instinctual but, rather, is a learned behavior for both the mother and the infant. No one, including the health care provider, should expect immediate latch-on and vigorous sucking. The first several attempts at breastfeeding may consist only of direct skin contact, nuzzling, and licking behaviors by the infant and cuddling and positioning by the mother.[241] Any actual sucking is an "extra" reward but should not be anticipated.

Facilitating Breastfeeding Success

Emotional support during breastfeeding of a normal or sick infant facilitates a successful experience for both the mother and the infant.[252] Mothers are more successful with breastfeeding when they have a positive attitude toward breastfeeding, are confident in their ability, and have support from significant others (both professional and lay).[252,311] Breastfeeding support programs in the NICU result in improved breastfeeding rates at discharge. Use of peer counselors and lactation consultants has been shown to positively influence the provision of breastmilk to infants in the NICU.[225,252]

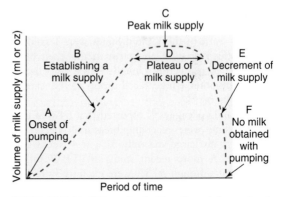

FIGURE 18-11 Establishing and maintaining milk supply by pumping. **A,** Pumping begins. **B,** Milk supply is established and increases. **C,** Peak or maximum volume of milk is established and plateaus. **D,** Gradually, supply begins to dwindle and may totally cease. **E** and **F,** The volume of milk and time period for decline in supply to begin and end in no milk production is an individual process. Some women begin and end this cycle in days or weeks; others are able to pump for months. Even if the supply dwindles to no milk, nutritive *suckling* of the infant with a Lact-Aid Nursing Trainer in place (see Figure 18-9) will reestablish the supply.

In one NICU, 73% of mothers of VLBW infants initiated breastfeeding, and breastfeeding outcomes of low-income black mothers were 63% with an evidence-based support program.[225] Support groups with mothers who have had similar experiences are helpful in supplementing support obtained from significant others and professionals.

The incidence and duration of breastfeeding preterm or sick newborns vary among NICUs[228,262,311] and among countries. In the United States in 1995, only 32% to 38% of mothers of LBW infants initiated breastfeeding compared with 62% of all mothers. During the same period, 75% of mothers of hospitalized newborns in Switzerland succeeded in breastfeeding their infants: 50% exclusively and 25% partially breastfed.[142] There is an inverse relationship between gestational age and duration of breastfeeding, with most mothers (more than 50%) abandoning breastfeeding before their infants are discharged from the hospital.[158,216,228] In a German cohort study, the average duration of breastmilk feedings in VLBW infants was one third of that of a matched group of term infants.[158] Early cessation of breastmilk feeding (e.g., during initial hospitalization) in VLBW infants was associated with the mother's smoking and low level of parental education. In the same study, prolonged breastmilk feeding was associated with multiple pregnancies, infants of less than 29 weeks' gestation, maternal age greater than 35 years, and spontaneous pregnancy.[158] Another study found that white mothers born in the United States were less likely to breastfeed preterm and term infants than black mothers born in the United States and mothers of any other ethnic/racial group in the state of Massachusetts.[228]

Hill and colleagues[134] reported that 54% of preterm infants were receiving breastmilk or breastfeeding at discharge and only 51% at 4 weeks after discharge. A more recent study of VLBW infants found that although 30.5% were exclusively receiving human milk at discharge, only 10% were exclusively feeding at the breast.[76] A descriptive study of nutritional intake in the first 6 months of life in 31 mothers of LBW preterms found that whereas 70% of the infants were receiving breastmilk at 40 weeks' PCA, only 26% were still fed some breastmilk at 6 months of PCA.[352] The "Breast milk Early Saves Trouble (BEST) Program" (initiated to improve use of breastmilk in the first week of life in preterms less than 2000 g) resulted in 50% (vs. 33%) of preterms receiving EBM, 82% (vs. 74%) of babies receiving some breastmilk, and 33% (vs. 2%) of preterms receiving banked breastmilk; trends of more mothers breastfeeding and more discharged home breastfeeding also occurred.[235] Another study of the transition from bottle feeding/breastfeeding to exclusive breastfeeding for preterms of 30 to 35 weeks' gestational age (GA) in the first 4 weeks after hospital discharge found the following[345]:

- Sixty percent received exclusive breastmilk in the first week.
- In weeks 2 to 4, 56% to 59% received breastmilk exclusively.
- The number of feedings directly at the breast was initially low and increased over the first 4 weeks (e.g., 60% were fed directly at the breast less than 50% of the time in the first week; by the fourth week, 23% were exclusively breastfed and another 27% were primarily breastfed).
- Fifty percent of these infants were primarily breastfed by 1 month after discharge.

Establishing an adequate milk supply was a key factor in successful transition from primarily bottle feeding at discharge (e.g., 60% of the infants were discharged when direct breastfeeding was less than 50% of the time) to primarily breastfeeding at home.[345] The most common reason cited by mothers for discontinuation of breastfeeding (both in the hospital and after discharge) is inadequate milk supply (or "not getting enough").[51,80,153,216,345] Early initiation and establishment of adequate feeding at the breast before discharge encourages both mothers and professionals that exclusive breastfeeding is successful. However, the early postdischarge period may be significantly stressful for mothers, because the breastfeeding pattern of a preterm infant may predispose to underconsumption (i.e., inability to compensate for inadequate intake in one feeding by increasing the number or intake of subsequent feedings), result in behaviors indicative of inadequate intake, and require nutritional supplementation.[153]

Education and training about the many facets of breastfeeding are essential for medical and nursing staff.* Education about human milk use in the NICU has been shown to change NICU nursing staff's knowledge and attitudes.[35,113,180] Staff attitudes and behaviors are important to breastfeeding families and

---

*References 3, 15, 113, 131, 180, 223, 234, 258, 261, 276, 320.

affect the breastfeeding experience,[4,234,258,276,320] as well as increasing human milk feeding rates.[113,180,229] A multidimensional approach to such education includes providing the staff with manuals, guides, and other educational materials, as well as scheduling routine classes, in-service training, and workshops. Moreover, professionals with clinical expertise should be identified; these resource personnel can increase the staff's competency in counseling and assisting breastfeeding families.

Evidence-based protocols addressing breastfeeding can outline a consistent approach for staff, as well as provide resource material that addresses successful strategies for handling common problems. Protocols can also reduce the amount of incorrect information that is disseminated.[223] A number of protocols, including a model hospital policy[4] for managing breastfeeding issues, have been developed by the Academy of Breastfeeding Medicine and are available from their website (see **www.bfmed.org**).

Providing a breastfeeding program for preterm infants that is grounded in evidence-based practices demonstrates strong success. The Rush Mother's Milk Club is an evidence-based NICU lactation program in which 98% of mothers provide milk for their infants, even though 50% of these mothers initially intended to breastfeed.[225] This program provides assistance to low-income mothers who are a group known to have low breastfeeding rates. Among these mothers the average amount of human milk provided to VLBW infants exceeded 60 ml/kg/day and total human milk intake was 71% of total enteral feeding volume.[225] Success of the Rush Mother's Milk Club is attributed to (1) consistent information about the science of human milk, lactation, and breastfeeding; (2) use of breastfeeding peer counselors[223,284,285]; (3) use of more physiologic breast pumps[221,271]; (4) use of evidence-based milk expression protocols[223]; (5) protection, storage,

and safe handling of expressed milk; and (6) use of developmentally based transitioning to feeding at the breast.[225]

One study showed that longer length of stay in the NICU (with kangaroo care and the Baby Friendly initiative) is associated with lower rates of exclusive breastfeeding in VLBW infants after discharge.[190]

A study of lactation counseling for mothers (some who intended to breastfeed and others who intended to formula feed) of VLBW preterms showed that more mothers decided to pump breastmilk, mainly because of the health benefits for their infant.[305] In mothers who intended to formula feed, there was an 85% milk expression rate; in mothers intending to breastfeed, the rate was 100%. Black and Hispanic mothers pumped at 95% and 93% rates, respectively. All mothers believed that pumping was worth the effort and appreciated the help they received; none felt more stress or anxiety. Reasons given by the mothers for ceasing to pump included (1) low milk supply, (2) returning to school or work, and (3) inability to pump as often as needed. Success in breastfeeding infants who were in the NICU depends on family support, timely breastfeeding information, and a supportive NICU environment.[32]

Breastmilk is the best milk, especially for a sick or premature infant. By understanding normal lactation, the health care provider can support the breastfeeding dyad when breastfeeding is delayed or disrupted.

REFERENCES

For a full list of references, scan the QR code or visit http://booksite.elsevier.com/ 9780323320832.

19 SKIN AND SKIN CARE

CAROLYN LUND AND DAVID J. DURAND

The skin is a large organ in premature and term infants, comprising at least 13% of body weight in contrast to 3% of the body weight in adults.[67] Skin functions include thermoregulation, barrier against toxins and infections, water and electrolyte excretion, fat storage and insulation, and tactile sensation.

Like many other organs, the skin of a premature infant is immature. The combination of immaturity with the need for intensive care monitoring and procedures places premature infants at risk for skin trauma and loss of skin integrity. Skin trauma and skin immaturity have serious consequences for infants in the neonatal intensive care unit (NICU), including problems in thermoregulation, fluid and electrolyte balance, diversion of calories for tissue repair, discomfort, potential toxicity from absorbed substances, and increased risk for infection.

This chapter reviews the physiology of term and premature infants' skin, the differences in structure and function related to skin immaturity, and prevention and treatment strategies to promote optimal skin integrity for infants in the NICU.

PHYSIOLOGY

There are three layers to the skin: the epidermis, the dermis, and the subcutaneous layer (Figure 19-1). The *epidermis* is comprised of the stratum corneum, a nonliving layer, and the basal layer. The *stratum corneum* is formed of lipids and protein in "brick and mortar" configuration. The basal layer of the epidermis replaces the stratum corneum with cells called *keratinocytes*. Approximately every 26 days, keratinocytes migrate from the basal layer to the exfoliated layers of the stratum corneum. In addition to keratinocytes, *melanocytes* are also found in the basal layer.

The *dermis,* a woven layer of collagen and elastin fibers, is 2 to 4 mm thick at birth. It contains nerves, blood vessels, and hair follicles. Sensations of heat, touch, pressure, and pain originate in the dermal layer. Sebaceous glands and sweat glands are located in the dermis, as well as in the subcutaneous layer of the skin. Sweat glands become mature in term infants during the first week of life, whereas maturation in premature infants occurs between 21 and 33 days and perhaps even longer in extremely premature infants.

The *subcutaneous layer* is composed of fatty connective tissue, with fat deposition occurring primarily during the last trimester of pregnancy. This layer provides heat insulation and functions as a calorie reservoir.

The skin of a normal term infant is covered with *vernix caseosa,* a "cheesy" substance composed of water (80%), lipids and proteins,[105,119,124] sebum from sebaceous glands, broken-off lanugo, and desquamated cells from the amnion. Vernix production begins at the end of the second trimester, accumulates on fetal skin in a cephalocaudal manner,[53,57] and protects the fetus against maceration from the amniotic fluid and chafing caused by crowding in utero. Vernix detaches from fetal skin as the levels of pulmonary surfactant rise, resulting in a progressive increase in the turbidity of the amniotic fluid.[57,99] Leaving residual vernix intact may be beneficial after delivery, because the presence of vernix produces earlier acidification of the skin, facilitates colonization by normal bacterial flora, and serves as a natural moisturizer for the skin.[109,124,131]

The skin of premature infants is thinner than that of term infants and may appear transparent or even gelatinous in extremely immature

PURPLE type highlights content that is particularly applicable to clinical settings.

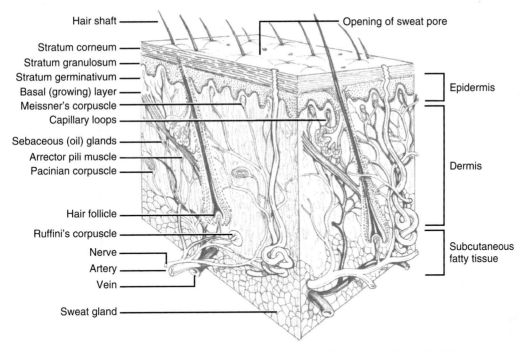

Hair shaft

Stratum corneum
Stratum granulosum
Stratum germinativum
Basal (growing) layer
Meissner's corpuscle
Capillary loops

Sebaceous (oil) glands
Arrector pili muscle
Pacinian corpuscle

Hair follicle

Ruffini's corpuscle
Nerve
Artery
Vein

Sweat gland

Opening of sweat pore

Epidermis

Dermis

Subcutaneous
fatty tissue

FIGURE 19-1 Cross section of skin layers and anatomic structures. (From *Principles of infant skin care*, Skillman, NJ, 1994, Johnson & Johnson.)

infants. There is usually a ruddy, red appearance caused by the underdeveloped stratum corneum, making skin color a poor tool for assessing the oxygenation status of very immature infants. There are fewer wrinkles on skin surfaces than in term infants, and the skin is covered by lanugo to varying degrees, depending on maturity; these fine hairs cover the upper back, arms, and forehead. The amount of *vernix caseosa* depends on the gestational age at birth. The subcutaneous layer in premature infants is often edematous because of an excess of cutaneous water and sodium (see Chapter 14).

ETIOLOGY

Term Newborn Skin Variations

Although the basic skin structures are the same in all term newborns without dermatologic disease, there may be cutaneous variations seen on physical examination. These variations (Table 19-1) are not considered pathologic, but it is useful for clinicians

to know them, because many parents ask the significance of physical variations as they examine their newborn.

Physiologic and Anatomic Differences in Premature Skin

There are developmental differences in skin physiology and anatomy between skin of full-term and premature infants compared with skin of older children and adults. This section discusses these differences and identifies the implications for care.

UNDERDEVELOPMENT OF THE STRATUM CORNEUM

The *stratum corneum*, the nonliving layer of the epidermis that is responsible for controlling evaporative heat loss and transepidermal water loss (TEWL), contains 10 to 20 layers in adults and term infants. Term infants have been shown to have lower transepidermal water loss than adults, with the lowest levels seen on the first day of life.[134] Despite reports of normal barrier function at birth, other

TABLE 19-1	NORMAL VARIATIONS OF TERM NEWBORN SKIN

VARIATION	DESCRIPTION
Linea nigra	Line of increased pigmentation from umbilicus to genitalia
Mongolian spots	Irregular, blue-gray, bruise-like spots Usually seen over sacrum and buttocks, may extend over back and shoulders Caused by pigmented cells in dermis Most common in infants with darker pigmentation
Lanugo	Fine, downy hair over back, shoulders, and face Shed at 32-36 weeks' gestation
Milia	White, pinhead-size bumps over chin, cheeks, nose, and forehead Tiny epidermal cysts If on palate, called *Epstein's pearls*
Miliaria	Caused by retention of sweat from edema in stratum corneum that blocks sweat glands Most common is rubra (prickly pear), but there are also clear versions
Harlequin sign	Color of half of body turns deep red whereas the other half is pale Caused by immature autoregulation of blood flow
Vernix caseosa	Gray-white, cheesy substance that protects fetal skin in utero Gradually diminishes near term
Cutis marmorata	Mottling caused by vasomotor immaturity
Erythema toxicum neonatorum	Small, firm white or yellow pustules with erythematous margin Most often seen on trunk, arms, and perineal area Benign condition seen in 30%-70% of newborns
Acne neonatorum	Acne-like rash seen in newborns at several weeks of age Caused by stimulation of sebaceous glands by maternal hormones More common in males Instruct caregivers not to use creams, lotions, or ointments because they can worsen the rash
Transient neonatal pustular melanosis	Resembles miliaria but present at birth Most frequently found on face, palms of hands, soles of feet Not infectious or contagious
Café-au-lait spots	Irregularly shaped oval lesions If large size (>4 × >6 cm), or if >6 in number, associated with neurofibromatosis

studies indicate that infant skin is prone to higher percutaneous absorption and prone to irritant and contact dermatitis, which has prompted others to maintain that barrier function is not fully developed in the term neonate and young infant.[51,58,101] The infant stratum corneum is 30% thinner than adult, with the overall epidermis 20% to 30% smaller. *Keratinocyte* cells are small, with a higher cell turnover rate that may explain some observations of faster wound healing in infant skin.[119]

Premature infants have fewer layers of *stratum corneum* depending on their gestational age; at less than 30 weeks' gestation, it may contain only two or three layers (Figure 19-2), and extremely premature infants of less than 24 weeks' gestation are just beginning to develop the stratum corneum.[54,58,60] Another function of the stratum corneum—protection against toxins and infectious agents such as bacteria and viruses—is minimal in premature infants,

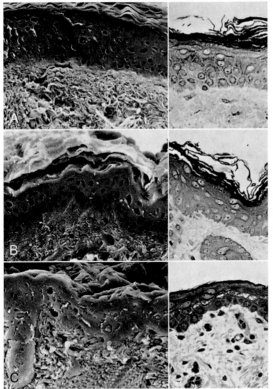

FIGURE 19-2 Photomicrograph of the stratum corneum in an adult **(A)**, a term newborn **(B)**, and a premature infant of 28 weeks' gestation **(C)**. Note fewer layers of stratum corneum in the premature infant. (From Holbrook KA: A histological comparison of infant and adult skin. In Maibach HI, Boisits EK, editors: *Neonatal skin: structure and function,* New York, 1982, Marcel Dekker.)

leaving them vulnerable to percutaneously transmitted infections and toxicity from topically applied substances.

The transition from the aquatic, intrauterine environment to the atmospheric, external environment has been thought to result in accelerated maturation of the stratum corneum and more mature function after the first 10 to 14 days of life.[41,52] However, other authors cite a slower process in premature infants less than 27 weeks' gestation, with rates of TEWL nearly double adult levels even at 28 days of life.[116] Premature infants of 23 to 25 weeks' gestation have losses 10 times higher than term infants initially, and they continue to have elevated heat and water loss resulting from immature barrier function for a longer period.[2] The maturation process can take as long as 8 weeks in an infant of 23 weeks' gestation.[65]

DERMAL INSTABILITY

The dermis is made of collagen and elastin fibers in a gel matrix, providing mechanical strength, protection, and elasticity to the skin. The dermis of the term newborn is thinner than the adult dermis and has a higher water content.[59,78] Collagen deposition in the dermis increases with advancing gestational age, preventing fluid from accumulating in this layer. Premature infants have a tendency to become edematous, because they have less collagen and fewer elastin fibers in the dermis.

Both term and premature infants may be prone to necrotic injury from excessive edema because of alteration in blood flow and perfusion to the epidermis. Edematous infants need protection from pressure and ischemic injury, including routine turning and the use of surfaces to minimize pressure points such as water beds and gelled mattresses or pads.[9]

DIMINISHED COHESION BETWEEN EPIDERMIS AND DERMIS

Numerous fibrils connect the epidermis to the dermis at the *dermo-epidermal junction*. These fibrils are more widely spaced and fewer in number in the premature infant[59] (Figure 19-3) but become stronger with advancing gestational and postnatal age. Genetically abnormal fibrils at this junction are found in certain types of the genetic disorder *epidermolysis bullosa,* a blistering skin condition that occurs with even minimal trauma. Premature infants also are prone to blistering from injury, although this decreases as they mature. Diminished cohesion also places premature infants at risk for injury from adhesive removal. Particularly if extremely aggressive adhesives are used, there may be a stronger bond of the adhesive to the epidermis than of the epidermis to the dermis, and epidermal stripping may result during adhesive removal.[86]

SKIN pH

The ability of the skin surface to form and maintain an acid surface is a function of various chemical and biologic processes. An acid skin surface with a pH less than 5 has been documented extensively in adults and children.[17] This *acid mantle* contributes to the stratum corneum's innate immune function by inhibiting the growth of pathogenic microorganisms.[72,133]

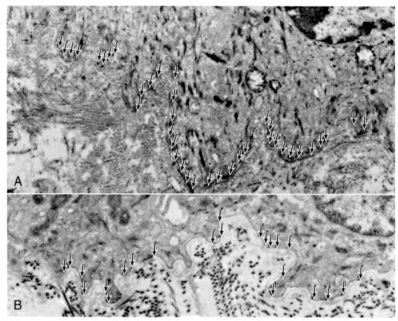

FIGURE 19-3 **A** and **B,** *Arrows* indicate fibrils called *hemidesmosomes,* which anchor the epidermis to the dermis. **B,** They are fewer in number and more widely spaced in the premature infant. (From Holbrook KA: A histological comparison of infant and adult skin. In Maibach HI, Boisits EK, editors: *Neonatal skin: structure and function,* New York, 1982, Marcel Dekker.)

Term newborns are born with a relatively alkaline skin surface, measuring a mean pH of 6.34. Within 4 days the pH declines to a mean of 4.95.[17] Skin pH measurements have been reported in premature infants of varying gestational ages, and the pH was above 6 on the first day, decreasing to 5.5 during the first week, and gradually declining to 5 during the first month.[43] Bathing and other skin care practices alter skin pH; it may take an hour or longer to regenerate the acid mantle after bathing with an alkaline soap. Of note, skin that is occluded by wearing diapers has been shown to have a pH of 6, which is known to be a risk factor in the development of diaper dermatitis.[132] This may occur because an alkaline skin surface may reduce stratum corneum integrity and enhance susceptibility to mechanical damage.[132]

PREVENTION

During daily skin care practices such as bathing, emollient use, antimicrobial skin disinfection, and adhesive removal, the skin of newborns is at risk for trauma or disruption of normal barrier function. This is particularly true of newborns in the NICU, who may have been born prematurely or may be critically ill or require surgery.

This section reviews basic skin care practices in terms of impact on skin integrity, preventing potential toxicity, and reducing exposure to potentially sensitizing chemicals. Recommendations for preventing trauma, protecting immature barrier function, and promoting skin integrity supported by scientific evidence are presented. These recommendations also are integrated into an evidence-based skin care guideline for health professionals.[9]

Bathing

Among the purposes of bathing the newborn are overall hygiene, esthetics, and protection of health care workers by removing blood and body fluids. Bathing, however, is not an innocuous procedure. Bathing full-term infants immediately following birth can compromise thermal and cardiorespiratory stability. When environmental controls are in place (i.e., stable ambient temperatures of 80° F) and free of drafts, bathing need not compromise thermal stability.[20,25,93]

For stable full-term infants, the first bath can safely be given when the axillary temperature is 36.9° C (98.2° F) or higher.[18,128] For the late-preterm infant (34 to 36⁶/⁷ weeks' gestation), maintaining a stable axillary temperature is necessary, and this frequently takes longer than for the full-term infant.[10,40,79] Younger premature infants can be gently cleansed at soiled areas with warm water and cotton balls or cloths. Do not rub the skin; use a rinsing technique instead.[9] Delay the bath if the infant is not physiologically stable, because bathing has been shown to destabilize vital signs and temperature in premature infants.[104]

Bathing with antiseptic soaps and cleansers is still practiced in some nurseries. Bathing full-term neonates with chlorhexidine gluconate reduced skin colonization with microorganisms in some areas, such as the axilla, but not in the groin.[31] In premature infants, bathing with chlorhexidine gluconate reduced skin colonization only transiently.[112] Although daily chlorhexidine gluconate baths have been shown to decrease infections in pediatric intensive care unit patients older than 2 months of age,[96] this practice has not been studied in NICU patients due to potential for toxicity with repeated full-body exposure. Antimicrobial cleansers are not endorsed by the American Academy of Pediatrics and American College of Obstetricians and Gynecologists[4,5] because of concern for skin irritation and toxicity, as well as the potentially negative effect it may have on normal skin colonization.

Soaps made with lye and animal fats are alkaline, with a pH above 7.0. Cleansing bars and liquids made with synthetic detergents are formulated to a neutral or mildly acidic pH (5.5 to 7.0). All soaps and cleansers are at least mildly irritating and drying to skin surfaces[125,126] and disrupt the skin surface pH. In addition, the degree to which the skin is irritated also depends on the length of contact and the frequency of bathing.

The recommendation is to select cleansers that have neutral or mildly acidic pH (5.5 to 7.0) and to bathe the infant no more than every other day.[9] Although the use of water alone for bathing the newborn has been advocated by some, several randomized controlled studies show no difference between water and mild baby wash products, in terms of skin colonization,[32,94] hydration of the stratum corneum, pH of the skin surface, and barrier function measured by TEWL.[74] In addition, there may be some advantage in using mild cleansers to remove soils, such as feces.[20]

The effects on skin parameters of bathing in small premature infants has not been studied to date. In an effort to reduce alterations in skin pH, dryness, and irritation in premature infants less than 32 weeks, cleanse with warm water baths during the first week, using soft cotton cloths, cotton balls, or the caregiver's hands.[9] Skin colonization with bacteria does not increase with bathing as infrequently as every 4 days.[105] Less frequent bathing may offer other advantages for premature infants, who have demonstrated physiologic and behavioral disruptions during sponge baths.[105] Immersion bathing, even of stable infants on ventilators or nasal continuous positive airway pressure, may be soothing and less stressful.[3]

Immersion bathing places the infant's entire body, except the head and neck, into warm water (38° C [100.4° F]), deep enough to cover the shoulders. A study of immersion versus sponge bathing in 102 newborns for their first and subsequent baths showed that the immersion-bathed infants had significantly less temperature drop and appeared more content, and their mothers reported more pleasure with the bath; there was no difference in cord healing scores with either immersion or sponge bathing.[25] In another study of late-preterm infants, immersion bathing resulted in improved temperatures.[79] Immersion bathing is also beneficial from a developmental perspective.[3,7] Stable premature infants, after umbilical catheters are removed, and term infants with umbilical clamps in place can be bathed safely in this way.[79] Bathing is an excellent time to educate parents about how to physically care for their baby and also may integrate information about their baby's neurobehavioral status and social characteristics.[66]

Emollients

The skin surface of term newborns is drier than that of adults but becomes gradually better hydrated as the eccrine sweat glands mature during the first year of life.[98,111] Maintaining the hydration of the *stratum corneum* is necessary for an intact skin surface and normal barrier function. Skin that is dry, scaly, or cracking not only is uncomfortable but can also be a portal of entry for microorganisms. Products used to counteract dryness are called moisturizers, emollients, or lubricants. Common emollients include mineral oil, petrolatum, and lanolin and its derivatives. Emollients are sometimes divided into oil-in-water or water-in-oil emulsions. Emollient use to prevent dermatitis and improve skin integrity has been studied in several randomized, controlled trials in premature infants. In one report,[70] premature infants of 29 to 36 weeks' gestation were treated with Eucerin cream daily and had less dermatitis as measured by a visual grading scale but no differences in direct measurements of TEWL with an evaporimeter. In a later study, premature infants of both shorter gestation and younger postnatal age were treated with Aquaphor ointment, a water-miscible oil-in-water preparation that contains neither dyes nor perfumes. In this study there was improvement in both TEWL and visual scale dermatitis. No increases in skin surface temperatures or thermal burns were seen, even when the emollient was applied to infants under radiant heaters or phototherapy lights. In addition, cutaneous cultures revealed no increase in bacterial or fungal colonization on skin treated with emollients. It was noted that a smaller number of treated infants had positive blood or cerebrospinal fluid culture results compared with control subjects, although the study was not large enough to prove this effect.[102]

A large, randomized controlled trial of 1191 infants with birth weights of 501 to 1000 g was conducted to determine whether twice-daily application of Aquaphor ointment would reduce combined outcome measures of mortality and sepsis. Although skin integrity appeared improved with routine emollient use, no effect was seen in the outcomes of sepsis plus mortality. Of note, an increase in coagulase-negative *Staphylococcus epidermidis* bloodstream infections was seen in infants with birth weights below 750 g, although the mechanism and relationship to emollient use are not clearly understood.[39] Several other studies have not reported higher infection rates when comparing emollient therapy with no treatment,[16,68] and report benefits in fluid and electrolyte balance, as well as less dermatitis.

The benefits of emollient use must be carefully weighed against the risk of infection. In general, emollients can be safely used to treat skin with excessive dryness, cracking, or fissures on an as-needed basis. They also may be effective in reducing TEWL and evaporative heat loss, although other methods, such as using a high-humidity environment or transparent adhesive dressings, also are available for this purpose. Avoiding products with perfumes or dyes is prudent, because these can be absorbed and are potential contact irritants.[28] Small tubes or jars for single-patient use are recommended to prevent contamination with microorganisms.[9]

Skin Disinfectants

Decontamination of skin before invasive procedures such as venipuncture and placement of umbilical catheters and chest tubes is common practice in NICU nurseries. However, there are anecdotal reports of skin injury, including blistering, burns, and sloughing, from disinfectants including isopropyl alcohol, povidone-iodine, and alcohol-containing chlorhexidine use in premature infants.* Several prospective studies of routine povidone-iodine use in intensive care nurseries[76,103,118] and one study of presurgical skin preparation of infants under 3 months of age[97] found alterations in iodine levels and thyroid effects from povidone-iodine exposure as a result of absorption through the skin. Although one study did not find alterations in thyroid function from iodine absorption in neonates,[49] the study period (10 days) may be too short a period of time to see this effect.

Another important aspect of skin disinfection is how effectively disinfectant solutions reduce colonization and infection rates. Blood culture contaminants in a pediatric emergency department were lower when a chlorhexidine-containing disinfectant was used, compared with povidone-iodine.[90] Garland and colleagues[45] reported that chlorhexidine reduced catheter colonization in neonates while inserting peripheral intravenous (IV) lines (4.3% with chlorhexidine vs. 9.3% with povidone-iodine).

A number of studies support the efficacy of chlorhexidine-containing solutions in preventing colonization and infections in adults with central venous catheters.[29] Large studies determining the best disinfectant for neonates with central venous catheters are not available. Chlorhexidine

---

*References 22, 51, 69, 87, 108, 113, 115.

gluconate (CHG) disinfection has been shown to reduce colonization with microorganisms in peripheral IV catheters in a large number of neonates.[45] A pilot study of 47 infants comparing 2% CHG/isopropyl alcohol with povidone-iodine for percutaneously inserted central catheters in infants greater than 1500 g and over 7 days old found no difference in bloodstream infection, sepsis evaluations, and skin irritancy but was terminated by the sponsor and was not powered to look at colonization rates.[46] In a sequential study in a single NICU, the rate of positive blood cultures and number of true infections was unchanged when the unit switched from povidone-iodine to chlorhexidine gluconate for skin disinfection.[75] Of note, the typical dwell time for central catheters in many of the studies is 7 to 10 days, whereas peripherally inserted central catheters in neonates are often in for 3 weeks or longer; it is possible that techniques for aseptic care of catheter hubs, caps, connectors, and IV tubing may prevent infection from the intraluminal route, which may be the primary source of catheter-associated bloodstream infection in this population.[95]

CHG is currently available in the United States as a 2% aqueous skin preparation in 4-oz bottles, as a tincture (2% or 3.15% CHG in 70% isopropyl alcohol) in single-use packaging, and as a wipe containing 0.5% CHG in 70% isopropyl alcohol. According to Food and Drug Administration (FDA) regulations, chlorhexidine-isopropyl products are now labeled "use with care in premature infants or infants less than 2 months of age. These products may cause skin irritation or chemical burns."[42] However, the combination of two disinfectants (CHG and isopropyl alcohol) has a significant potential for skin injury in very-low-birth-weight (VLBW) infants and cannot be recommended in these patients. All CHG products should not be allowed to come in contact with the eyes or ears, per manufacturer's recommendations, because of reports of damage to these structures. However, careful use before scalp IV or central line insertion is acceptable, if splashing or using excessive amounts of CHG is avoided. CHG is applied in two consecutive wipings, or for a 30-second scrubbing period, and then is removed with sterile water or saline solution when the procedure is completed. Aqueous CHG may not dry, but can be wiped with sterile gauze after the application.[9,71]

Many nurseries have chosen to continue the use of povidone-iodine disinfectants because of the lack of single-use CHG products that do not contain isopropyl alcohol. Povidone-iodine is available in a 10% aqueous solution in a variety of single-use applications. It is also applied in two consecutive wipings, or for a 30-second scrubbing period, and then is allowed to dry for at least 30 seconds before the procedure. Any solution should be completely removed after the procedure using sterile water or saline solution to prevent any further absorption. Disinfection with isopropyl alcohol is questionable in the NICU, because it is less effective than either povidone-iodine or chlorhexidine and can be irritating and drying to skin surfaces.

The risks and benefits of routine skin antisepsis in infants is a subject that clearly deserves further investigation. Although there are insufficient comparative data on the costs, risks, and benefits of skin antisepsis regimens to mandate standard practice, the use of alcohol pledgets alone provides the least-effective antimicrobial activity. Both povidone-iodine and isopropyl alcohol carry significant risks of percutaneous toxicity.[51] The potential for subclinical toxicities must be considered with all products used on small newborns, so, when several topical therapeutic options are available, the one with the least potential for toxicity should be chosen. In addition, disinfectants should be removed completely from the skin with water or saline to prevent further absorption and contact.

The routine use of antimicrobial sprays, creams, or powders for umbilical cord care has not been shown to be more effective in preventing infection, compared with dry cord care.[136] The use of antibiotic ointments and antiseptics can prolong the time to cord separation, and it seems to have no beneficial effect on the frequency of infection.[8,64,136] A study of 1811 newborns randomized to receive either routine isopropyl alcohol with each diaper change or natural drying found no umbilical infections in either group, and time to cord separation was reduced from 9.8 days in the alcohol-treated group to 8.16 days in the natural-drying group.[37] Another study randomized 766 newborns to receive either triple dye applied to the umbilical cord immediately after delivery, followed by twice-daily applications of isopropyl alcohol, or "dry care" without any treatment. Infants in the dry care group were more likely to be colonized with bacteria than those in the treatment group, and one infant in the dry care group developed omphalitis on the third day of life. The days to cord separation were not reported.[63]

Recommendations for umbilical cord care include washing hands before handling the cord, and, if the cord becomes soiled with urine or stool, cleansing with water, drying with absorbent gauze, and keeping the diaper folded down and away from the umbilical stump to prevent contamination.[9] The development of omphalitis is not necessarily related to cord disinfection, because it also occurs in infants who have received topical disinfectants. However, vigilant attention to the signs and symptoms is necessary by health professionals, and parents need guidance about how to manage the umbilical cord and when to consult their health care provider.[36]

Adhesive Application and Removal

One of the most common practices in the NICU is the application and removal of adhesives that secure endotracheal tubes, IV devices, and monitoring probes and electrodes. A research utilization project involving 2820 premature and term newborns found that adhesives were the primary cause of skin breakdown among NICU patients.[84] Changes in TEWL and skin barrier function are seen in adults after 10 consecutive removals of adhesive tape[77] and after one removal of adhesive tape in premature infants.[52] Types of damage from adhesive removal include epidermal stripping, tearing, maceration, tension blisters, chemical irritation, sensitization, and folliculitis.[56,92]

Adhesive removers are sometimes used to prevent discomfort and skin disruption from adhesive removal. There are three categories of adhesive removers: alcohol/organic-based solvents, oil-based solvents, and silicone-based removers.[19] The alcohol/organic-based removers contain hydrocarbon derivatives or petroleum distillates that have potential or proven toxicities. Toxicity is a major concern, especially in premature infants with their underdeveloped stratum corneum, increased skin permeability, larger surface area/body weight ratio, and immature hepatic and renal function. A case report of toxic epidermal necrosis in a premature infant resulted from the use of a solvent in this category.[62] Mineral oil, petrolatum, and citrus-based products may be helpful in removing adhesives

but cannot be used if the site must be used again for reapplication of adhesives, such as with the retaping of an endotracheal tube. Silicone-based removers form an interposing layer between adhesive and skin, evaporate readily after application, and do not leave a residue.[19] The use of silicone-based removers has been advocated for patients with extremely fragile skin, such as infants with epidermolysis bullosa.[120] Future studies with this type of remover with neonates is encouraged. Removing adhesives with water-soaked cotton balls sometimes helps, and gently pulling the adhesive parallel to the skin surface rather than straight up at a 90-degree angle may facilitate removal with less skin trauma.[86]

Skin bonding agents, or "tackifiers," promote adherence; examples of these products include tincture of benzoin and Mastisol. Unfortunately, they may create a stronger bond between adhesive and epidermis than the fragile cohesion of the epidermis to the dermis; when the adhesive is removed, epidermal stripping may result. Alcohol-free skin barrier films, composed of silicone, are reported to reduce skin trauma from repeated adhesive removal.[19] In addition to reports of the positive effects when using this skin protectant to tape IV lines in newborns, one study of premature infants showed both skin protection and the additional benefit of reducing TEWL.[21,61]

Hydrocolloid skin barriers such as Hollihesive and DuoDERM are used as a "platform" between skin and adhesive. Studies initially described less visible trauma to skin with hydrocolloid barriers.[35,82,91] However, a controlled trial of a hydrocolloid barrier (Hollihesive), plastic tape (Transpore), and hydrophilic gelled adhesive found that significant skin disruption, as measured by TEWL and visual inspection, occurred after removal of both the pectin barrier and plastic tape.[83] Because the adhesives were left in place 24 hours before removal in this study, there may be a time effect of peak adhesive aggressiveness that was reached. Significant changes were measured after a single adhesive application and removal in all three weight groups studied (less than 1000 g, 1001 to 1500 g, and greater than 1501 g), indicating that even larger premature infants are at risk for skin injury from tape removal. Despite this finding, hydrocolloid adhesive products continue to be used in the NICU because they mold well to curved surfaces and adhere even with moisture.

Prevention of skin trauma from adhesive removal includes minimizing tape use when possible by using smaller pieces, backing the adhesive with cotton, and delaying tape removal until adherence is reduced. Hydrocolloid adhesives may prove helpful, because they mold and adhere well to body contours and often attach better in moist conditions. As with tape, removal of hydrocolloids should be delayed, if possible, until the adherence lessens. The use of soft gauze wraps to secure probes and hydrogel electrocardiogram electrodes and hydrogel tapes is helpful. *Silicone-based adhesive* products have been shown to improve adherence to wounds and reduce discomfort when removal is necessary.[38,50] Silicone tapes, the newest class of adhesives, are very gentle to skin, but do not adhere well to plastic materials and cannot be used to secure critical tubes and appliances[92]; however, they may prove beneficial if developed for other adhesive products in neonates, such as electrodes or sensors.

DATA COLLECTION

History

The gestational age and postnatal age of neonates in the NICU are both important considerations for determining appropriate skin care practices. Premature infants of lower gestational ages have underdeveloped skin layers and function. With advancing postnatal age and maturation there is improved skin integrity and skin barrier function.

Reviewing the maternal history for any dermatologic diseases is also important. Many of the most severe skin diseases, such as forms of *congenital ichthyosis* or *epidermolysis bullosa,* are inherited disorders. A positive family history will alert the clinician to the potential for developing these rare disorders.

Signs and Symptoms

A thorough daily examination of all skin surfaces reveals the state of skin integrity for neonates in the NICU. Early signs such as skin abrasions or small excoriations may call for either diagnostic or treatment procedures. A scoring tool, such as the *Neonatal Skin Condition Score* (NSCS) (Box 19-1), used in the Association of Women's Health, Obstetric,

---

BOX 19-1 THE NEONATAL SKIN CONDITION SCORE

Dryness
1 = Normal, no sign of dry skin
2 = Dry skin, visible scaling
3 = Very dry skin, cracking/fissures

Erythema
1 = No evidence of erythema
2 = Visible erythema <50% body surface
3 = Visible erythema >50% body surface

Breakdown
1 = None evident
2 = Small localized areas
3 = Extensive

Note: Perfect score = 3; worst score = 9.

From Lund C, Osborne J, Kuller J, et al: Neonatal skin care: clinical outcomes of the AWHONN/NANN evidence-based clinical practice guideline, *J Obstet Gynecol Neonatal Nurs* 30:41, 2001.

---

and Neonatal Nurses (AWHONN)/National Association of Neonatal Nurses (NANN) research-based practice project,[81,82,84] has been extensively used in both premature and full-term infants, with validity and reliability established.[84] This scoring system can be integrated into skin care protocols to identify neonates with excessive dryness, erythema, or skin breakdown.[9] Risk factors for skin injury in individual patients are listed in Box 19-2. In the first week of life in extremely low-birth-weight infants (less than 30 weeks, under 1000 g), there may be problems with thermoregulation (see Chapter 6) and dehydration (see Chapter 14) because of the large evaporative heat losses and transepidermal water losses through the immature stratum corneum.

Laboratory Data

With the many skin excoriations in both small and large neonates that result from traumatic events such as adhesive removal or pressure necrosis, there is the potential for infection through this portal of entry in the skin. In VLBW infants it may be useful to obtain a skin culture, Gram stain, or potassium hydroxide

BOX 19-2 RISK FACTORS FOR SKIN INJURY

- Gestational age <32 weeks
- Edema
- Use of paralytic agents and vasopressors
- Multiple tubes and lines
- Numerous monitors
- Surgical wounds
- Ostomies
- Technologies that limit movement: high ventilation, extracorporeal membrane oxygenator

preparation[13,14] for early detection of microorganisms that can lead to systemic illness in these immunocompromised patients. A skin surface culture is helpful if the skin breakdown cannot be traced to a traumatic injury, because the origin of the breakdown often is linked to infection, especially with fungal infections[110] or *staphylococcal scalded skin syndrome.* A more comprehensive workup for infection may be indicated if there is evidence of clinical deterioration in infants with extensive skin breakdown (see Chapter 22).

TREATMENT

Skin Excoriations

Skin excoriations are cleansed with warmed sterile water or half–normal saline solution; a 20- or 30-ml syringe with a Teflon IV catheter attached can be used to gently débride the excoriation. This technique is effective in flushing out debris and dead tissue from an infected or "dirty" wound, allowing a better surface for healing. Moistening the tissue every 4 to 6 hours aids the healing process, because drying of tissue actually impedes the migration of cells. Once the wound surface is clear, other dressings or ointments can be used.

Ointments are sometimes used because of their antibacterial or antifungal properties and also because covering the wound with a semiocclusive layer promotes healing by facilitating the migration of epithelial cells across the surface. *Only if*

extensive bacterial colonization is suspected, Polysporin, Bacitracin, or Bactroban ointment is used sparingly every 8 to 12 hours. Many dermatologists do not recommend the use of Neosporin because of the potential for developing later sensitization to this ointment, although sensitization to Bacitracin is being reported with increasing frequency.[89] Overuse of antimicrobial ointments can be a problem in promoting more resistant strains of bacteria. Petrolatum ointment can be used to cover surface excoriations if not infected. If fungal infection is suspected, Nystatin ointment is used, and it also can be applied to surrounding intact skin to prevent extension of the infection. In general, ointments are preferable to creams for this use because of better adherence and healing properties.

Transparent adhesive dressings are made from a polyurethane film backed with adhesive that is impermeable to water and bacteria but allows air flow. Uses include wound care and dressings for IV devices, including central venous lines and percutaneous silicone catheters. Other types of dressings used in wound management include *hydrogels* (dressings and gel) and *hydrocolloid dressings* (DuoDERM) and *silicone* (Mepitel), which promote moist healing.[12,44] It is best to avoid placing hydrogel dressings on intact skin surfaces, because they can macerate the skin and actually reduce barrier function. *Hydrocolloid dressings* are used over uninfected wounds and can be left in place for 5 to 7 days while healing takes place. Another wound treatment is amorphous hydrogel applied directly onto the wound from a tube. *Amorphous hydrogel,* such as DuoDERM Gel and IntraSite, consists of 80% to 90% water making it soothing to skin while keeping the wound moist, a cellulose polymer that extracts and traps fluid; and propylene glycol, which rehydrates tissue.44 *Silicone dressings* are very effective in covering skin breakdown and can be used together with antimicrobial or petrolatum ointment.

Surgical wounds that open or dehisce are infrequent but require expert wound management. Nutrition is often a part of the process in getting these wounds to heal, as is the prevention of infection.[48] Often the surgeon or a wound and ostomy specialist will design the appropriate wound management program for these situations.

Intravenous Extravasations

Prevention of tissue injury from IV extravasations includes taping IV devices with transparent dressings or plastic tape so that the insertion site is clearly visible, and observing the site with appropriate documentation every hour. If the IV device is placed in a limb, the tape that secures it to the rigid board should be placed loosely over a bony prominence, such as the elbow or knee, and not on skin in close proximity to the insertion site. This allows extravasated fluid and medications to expand over a larger surface and not remain in a small, constricted area, which can result in greater tissue injury. Alternatively, leaving the extremity free of the rigid board is the practice for some NICUs, with success. Using central venous lines, such as percutaneously inserted central venous catheters, to infuse highly irritating solutions and medications is also recommended. Many nurseries limit the glucose concentrations in peripheral lines to 12.5% and the amino acid concentrations to 2%. Use of continuous infusion of calcium in IV fluids is debatable, because it is extremely irritating to the intima of the vein; when used, the concentration of calcium gluconate should be limited to 200 mg/100 ml. In some NICUs, calcium solutions are never infused continuously through peripheral veins.

If IV fluid has extravasated into surrounding tissue, the IV device should be removed and the extremity elevated. Use of moisture, heat, or cold is not recommended, because the tissue is vulnerable at this point to further injury.[23] Hyaluronidase (Amphadase, Vitrase, Hylenex) can be extremely helpful if administered within an hour of extravasation (see Chapter 10). This medication is an enzyme that causes a breakdown of interstitial barrier and allows the diffusion of the extravasated fluid over a larger area to prevent tissue necrosis.[15,73,107,114] The dose of hyaluronidase is 15 to 20 units diluted to 1 ml, although in one study using an animal model, 150 units was used without harmful effects.[73] It is administered in five injections, inserted subcutaneously around the periphery of the extravasation site (Figures 19-4 and 19-5), and ideally is administered within 1 to 2 hours of the extravasation. Extravasations that may benefit from administration of hyaluronidase include any with evidence

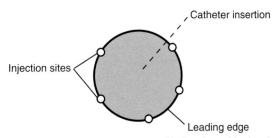

FIGURE 19-4 Technique for administration of hyaluronidase and/or phentolamine. A total volume of 1 ml is administered at five sites subcutaneously (0.2 ml each) around the periphery of the intravenous extravasation.

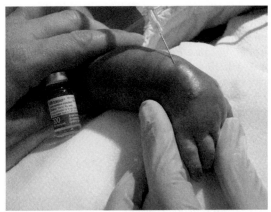

FIGURE 19-5 Hyaluronidase (Vitrase) being administered to extravasation in hand using 27-gauge needle.

of blanching, discoloration, or blistering, or extravasations involving hypertonic or calcium-containing solutions, even if the site appears relatively undisturbed. The use of an extravasation scale for treatment of IV extravasations may improve communication and consistency of providing appropriate immediate care.[6,117]

Calcium-containing solutions may cause deep tissue injury even when epidermal tissues are not involved. In addition to hyaluronidase administration, creating multiple puncture holes over the area of swelling and gently squeezing or letting the extravasated fluid leak out can facilitate the removal of the infiltrate and prevent skin sloughs.[30] Saline washout is another technique described to facilitate the removal of extravasated irritants from tissues surrounding an IV site.[27,33,47]

Hyaluronidase is not recommended in the extravasation of vasoconstrictive medications such as dopamine, because the vasoconstriction could extend with its use. Phentolamine (Regitine) is used in this case, because it directly counteracts the action of dopamine. The method of delivery is the same as for hyaluronidase, with the total dose (0.5 mg) diluted to 1 ml, injected in five sites subcutaneously around the periphery of the extravasation.[135]

When tissue injury occurs after extravasation, treating the wound with techniques using *moist healing* principles facilitates healing without scarring. There has been success using a generous application of amorphous hydrogel and placing the extremity in a plastic bag, the so-called *bag/boot method*.[122] This method is also beneficial immediately after hyaluronidase injections and multiple puncture technique for 12 to 24 hours, because it facilitates the ongoing flow of the irritating vesicant. In most cases, skin grafts can be avoided by the use of appropriate wound healing techniques. In all cases of tissue injury, open wounds should be considered a portal of entry for infection, and topical or systemic treatment should be considered.

Diaper Dermatitis

A common skin disruption that occurs in neonates and infants is *diaper dermatitis* (diaper rash). This term encompasses a range of processes that affect the perineum, groin, thighs, buttocks, and anal area of infants who are incontinent and wear some covering to collect urine and feces. Diaper dermatitis can be caused by many different mechanisms, but the condition of the skin has a direct role in the progression of skin injury. Review articles provide an excellent background for current evidence-based care in the prevention of and treatment for diaper dermatitis.[1,55]

The pathogenesis of diaper dermatitis is partly related to the degree of wetness of the skin. Skin that is moist and macerated becomes more permeable and susceptible to injury because wetness increases friction. In addition, moisture-laden skin is more likely to contain microorganisms than dry skin.

Another component in the process of skin injury from diaper dermatitis is the effect of an alkaline pH. Normal skin pH is acidic—ranging between 4.0 and 5.5—but can become alkaline when it is diapered.[125,127] The increased pH of the skin increases its vulnerability to injury and penetration by microorganisms, as well as stimulating fecal enzyme activity. Specifically, both protease and lipase in stool can injure the skin, which is made up of protein and fat components. These enzymes can quickly cause significant injury to the epidermis and are responsible for the contact irritant diaper dermatitis that is commonly seen.

Strategies for preventing diaper dermatitis include maintaining a skin surface that is dry and has a normal (acidic) skin pH. Frequent diaper changes are recommended, especially in the newborn period. Insufficient evidence exists to support any specific type of diaper for preventing diaper dermatitis.[11] However, superabsorbent gelled diapers with breathable covers have been shown to keep skin surfaces dryer by "wicking" the moisture away from the skin and separating urine from feces.[26,34] Use of powders is discouraged because of the risk of inhalation of particles into the respiratory tract.

After skin injury from diaper dermatitis has occurred, protecting injured skin to prevent reinjury is the primary goal of treatment. Topical treatment for diaper dermatitis involves ointments and creams containing a variety of ingredients. Most contain zinc oxide and petrolatum, and are generally similar in composition.[55,130] Generous application of protective skin barriers that contain zinc oxide can prevent further injury while allowing skin to heal. Once skin excoriations occur, keeping skin open to air may not be effective, because the already impaired tissue may be reinjured with fecal contact, and dryness is counterproductive to healing. It is not necessary or desirable to completely remove skin barrier products with diaper changes, because this may disrupt healing tissue. Instead, remove as much waste material as possible and reapply the barrier generously to the affected areas with each diaper change. Another class of barrier products are *semipermeable barrier films,* designed to repel moisture and protect the skin from irritants.[55,129] Although these products are FDA approved for use in infants greater than 30 days of age, they can be used "off label" and have been beneficial for neonatal ostomy care.[123]

If *Candida albicans* is involved in the diaper dermatitis, it is necessary to use an antifungal ointment or cream. Antifungal preparations include Mycostatin, miconazole, clotrimazole, and ketoconazole in ointment or cream forms; ointments are preferable to coat the skin and repel moisture. If the dermatitis is both fungal and a contact irritant dermatitis, it may be necessary to layer the ointment with the antifungal preparation: (1) Mycostatin powder is used, (2) followed by an application of alcohol-free skin protectant to seal the powder onto the skin surface, and (3) a generous application of a skin barrier cream is then done, such as zinc oxide or pectin paste.

Occasionally infants may experience extremely severe diaper dermatitis from intestinal malabsorption syndromes or if there is constant dribbling of stool (i.e., decreased or lack of rectal innervation [myelomeningocele, bladder exstrophy, or following a "pull-through" procedure for Hirschsprung's disease]). With malabsorption, stool not only is more frequent, but also may have a high pH because of rapid transit through the small intestine resulting in significant amounts of undigested carbohydrates and stool enzymes. Severe diaper dermatitis in this case can be a symptom of a more severe nutritional deficiency, or even dehydration, and needs thorough medical evaluation.

While optimal nutritional therapy is being addressed with special diets or parenteral nutrition, skin protection from injury should be initiated. Products that contain pectin without alcohol (such as Ilex, a nonalcohol pectin paste) may provide a sturdier barrier for these infants than zinc oxide preparations. The skin should be thoroughly cleansed before a very thick application of the pectin paste. Then it is necessary to apply a greasy ointment because the pectin-based paste may adhere to the diaper. When the infant has a stool, it is not necessary to completely remove the barrier paste; the stool can be wiped away as much as possible before reapplying the thick paste barrier. The skin will heal under this protective covering as long as it is protected from reinjury.[80] If fungal infection is a component of the dermatitis, antifungal therapy must be instituted in addition to the protective barriers. In this case, Mycostatin powder attached with alcohol-free skin protectant is the first layer; then the barrier cream is applied as described previously.

COMPLICATIONS

Improper handling of newborn skin (and injudicious use of products) can cause damage, prevent healing, and interfere with normal maturation processes. Other compromised skin integrity can lead to infection, pain and discomfort, and diversion of calories for tissue repair. Other dangers include toxicity from topically applied substances that are readily absorbed by small infants with a large surface area to body weight ratio, as well as immature renal and hepatic function that cannot detoxify chemicals readily.

Injury from infiltrated IV solutions can cause skin injury and occasionally deep tissue necrosis with both muscle and nerve damage. Factors that increase the risk of injury from IV extravasations include length of time between extravasation and treatment; hypertonic solutions, such as those with high calcium, potassium, amino acid, or glucose solutions; medications such as nafcillin that are irritating to veins; and the use of mechanical pumps for infusions. There may be an added risk for injury in patients with poor perfusion to extremities and in limbs that have been secured with restricting adhesives that obstruct venous return.

If the epidermis has been injured, it can easily become a portal of entry for infection. Thus a contact irritant diaper dermatitis can progress to a fungal or staphylococcal infection. *Staphylococcus aureus* can cause pustule formation at hair follicles and is a rare complication of diaper dermatitis. The mechanism for fungal diaper dermatitis is still debated. Some researchers believe that *Candida albicans* infection is a secondary invasion to skin that has been previously injured, whereas others see this organism as a primary cause of skin disruption.[106]

Candida albicans diaper dermatitis causes an intense inflammation that is bright red and sharply demarginated in the inguinal folds, buttocks, thighs, abdomen, and genitalia, often with satellite lesions that extend the rash over the trunk (Figure 19-6).

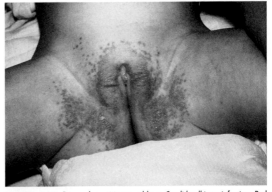

FIGURE 19-6 Diaper dermatitis caused by a *Candida albicans* infection. Red pustular satellite lesions extend into the periphery.

Candida albicans can be harbored in the gastrointestinal tract, necessitating oral therapy if lesions are found in the mouth.

PARENT TEACHING

It is the responsibility of professionals to teach parents informally during caregiving procedures such as bathing, cord care, and diaper changes and to prepare written materials about appropriate skin care practices for their infant after discharge from the NICU (Box 19-3). Parents will need education about the normal mechanisms of cord healing, including the range of appearance in umbilical cords, because some cords can appear very moist and soggy. The cord can be cleansed with water if it becomes soiled with urine or stool.[9] Inform parents that minimal use of skin care products is optimal, and may reduce the incidence of contact sensitization to chemicals.[24,28,88] It is also extremely useful to educate parents about the mechanisms that are involved in diaper dermatitis so that prevention is stressed and appropriate interventions are selected depending on the underlying cause. A parent education handout in PDF form, based on the AWHONN *Evidence-Based Neonatal Skin Care Guideline*,[100] is now available online (www.health4mom.org).

Developmental differences in the anatomy and physiology of neonatal skin affect skin integrity for term and premature infants in the NICU. Prevention is the primary focus of care, and decisions about the best way to provide basic skin care and hygiene based on current research are essential for care providers, both professionals and parents.

BOX 19-3 **PARENT TEACHING**

APPROPRIATE SKIN CARE PRACTICES

- Baby needs to be bathed only two or three times per week. Sponge bath with water between tub bathings.
- Use on the skin only products that have as few additives and as little fragrance as possible; minimal skin care products reduce the incidence of contact sensitization of the skin by added chemicals.
- Do not use powder because of inhalation into baby's lungs.
- Prevent diaper rash by frequently changing wet and soiled diapers, cleansing diaper area, and using diapers that "wick" moisture away from the skin. If baby's skin becomes red and irritated with one brand of disposable diaper, try another brand.
- Treat diaper rash by using protective skin barriers (e.g., zinc oxide) with each diaper change to prevent further injury and allow skin to heal. Clean waste from skin barrier but do not clean off the skin barrier because this may disrupt skin healing.
- Diaper rash caused by a yeast infection requires antifungal medication.
- Umbilical cord dries and falls off within 7 to 10 days. Turn diaper back away from the cord until it falls off; as the cord separates, a small amount of blood stain may be on the diaper. Keep cord area clean, and rinse with water if it becomes soiled with urine or stool. Call the health care provider immediately if the cord develops an area of red, warm-to-touch skin at the base, a foul odor, or drainage from the base of the cord.

REFERENCES

For a full list of references, scan the QR code or visit http://booksite.elsevier.com/9780323320832.

20 | NEWBORN HEMATOLOGY

MARILYN MANCO-JOHNSON, CHRISTOPHER McKINNEY, RHONDA KNAPP-CLEVENGER, AND JACINTO A. HERNÁNDEZ

RED BLOOD CELLS

Physiology

Red blood cells (RBCs) transport and deliver oxygen to vital organs and body tissues. Red blood corpuscles are simple cells composed of a membrane encasing hemoglobin with an energy system to fuel the cells. Hemoglobin is the protein in RBCs that carries oxygen, binding and releasing it based on concentration differences. Ex utero, RBCs absorb oxygen by diffusion in the lungs, where the oxygen tension of the alveolar air is higher than that of the capillary blood, and release it from the systemic capillaries, where the oxygen tension is now higher than that of surrounding tissues. In utero, oxygen diffuses to the fetus from the placental venous circulation.

Fetal red cells contain a unique hemoglobin (fetal hemoglobin, *hemoglobin F*) in which the two beta chains of adult hemoglobin *(hemoglobin A₁)* are replaced by two gamma chains. *Fetal hemoglobin* has a higher affinity for oxygen than does adult hemoglobin, allowing fetal red cells to compete successfully for available oxygen. Normal fetal red cells are characterized by an increased mean corpuscular hemoglobin (MCH), mean corpuscular volume (MCV), hemoglobin, and hematocrit. After birth with the transition to air breathing and a higher blood oxygen tension, the hypoxic stimulus driving fetal red cell production in the bone marrow

is removed. The plasma concentration of *erythropoietin,* the hormone that stimulates bone marrow production of RBCs, falls. The number of circulating *reticulocytes,* which are young RBCs in the circulation, decreases. Subsequently, the hemoglobin and hematocrit diminish until a new equilibrium is reached. Postnatal changes in red cell production include an increase in the ratio of hemoglobin A to hemoglobin F and an increase in levels of the red cell enzyme *2,3-diphosphoglycerate* (2,3-DPG). 2,3-DPG promotes the release of oxygen to tissues by decreasing hemoglobin affinity to oxygen within tissues. Oxygen delivery in the neonate is enhanced by increases in the concentrations of hemoglobin A and red cell concentration of 2,3-DPG.

The production of hematopoietic cells is first seen within the yolk sac in the 14-day embryo and disappears by the eleventh week of gestation.[25] *Hematopoiesis* in other tissues results from colonization by stem cells derived from the yolk sac.[9] By the fifth to sixth week, embryonic erythropoietic activity is present in the liver. The liver becomes the primary source of RBC production by 8 to 9 weeks.[14]

Between the eighth and twelfth weeks the spleen and lymph nodes are involved in erythropoiesis.[19] Other tissues and organs involved in erythropoiesis include the kidney, thymus, and connective tissue. Erythropoiesis is found in the bone marrow at 10 to 11 weeks. This activity increases rapidly until the twenty-fourth week, when bone marrow

---

PURPLE type highlights content that is particularly applicable to clinical settings.

erythropoiesis replaces liver erythropoiesis. There is no evidence of erythropoietin production before the tenth week.[81] After the tenth week of gestation, erythropoietin production rises and appears to stimulate red cell production in the bone marrow during the third trimester.[23] Initially, erythropoietin is produced in the fetal liver, and by the last trimester, production relocates to the kidneys. The level of erythropoietin gradually rises to significant levels after the thirty-fourth week of gestation.[19] Elevated erythropoietin levels can be found when the fetus is hypoxic.[9]

In more than 90% of healthy term infants the hematocrit range is 48% to 60% and the hemoglobin range is 16 to 20 g/dl.[12] Changes in the blood count at the time of birth are shown in Table 20-1.[15,19] Normally after a term birth, hemoglobin concentrations fall from a mean of 17 g/dl to approximately 11 g/dl by 2 to 3 months of age. This nadir in RBC values is called *physiologic anemia of the newborn* and is a normal process in the adaptation to extrauterine life.

Several factors should be considered in the interpretation of hematocrit values in the newborn, including age of the infant (both in hours and in days), site of blood collection, and method of analysis. Hematocrit changes significantly during the first 24 hours of life; it peaks at 2 hours of age and then progressively drops, with decreases determined at 6 and 24 hours of age.[64] The method used to determine hematocrit can significantly affect the value. *Capillary hematocrit* measurements are highly subject to variations in blood flow; hematocrit results generally are highest in capillary blood and lowest in arterial samples, with venous intermediate.[36,50,74] Prewarming the site minimizes the artifactual increase in the hematocrit. When obtaining blood counts, note that in both term and preterm infants there can be as much as a 20% difference between the hematocrit obtained from a capillary puncture (commonly termed *heelstick*) and the hematocrit of blood drawn from a central vein.

Interpretation of blood count parameters requires understanding of the source of the comparison values. Normal ranges are generally derived from large populations of healthy subjects where major confounding medical conditions, including personal and family history, can be excluded. The newborn infant, particularly the preterm baby, is at risk for many complicating conditions, such as infection, hypoxia, and inflammation, and it is difficult to determine that a preterm infant is healthy at birth. In settings such as this, reference ranges are often used. Reference ranges determine values of a parameter of interest in a population that has no known confounding illness. Reference ranges for most blood tests in term and preterm infants are derived from relatively small sample sizes. Robert Christensen and his colleagues from the Intermountain Healthcare System, a large primary care–based health network, have derived reference ranges of various blood indices from a very large population of infants (greater than 20,000 infants). This group reported for otherwise healthy extremely preterm infants that the lower 5% of hemoglobin was slightly less than 10 g/dl and the hematocrit slightly under 30% for otherwise healthy infants less than 28 weeks of gestation. In comparison, the lower limits for infants 32 weeks of gestation and greater was 13 g/dl and 40% (Figure 20-1).[31]

Pathophysiology of Anemia

Anemia is a deficiency in the concentration of red cells and hemoglobin in the blood and results in tissue hypoxia and acidosis. Anemia is defined by a hemoglobin or hematocrit value that is greater than 2 standard deviations below the mean for postconceptional and postnatal age. For a normal full-term infant in the first week of life,

TABLE 20-1	CHANGES IN ERYTHROPOIESIS AROUND THE TIME OF TERM BIRTH	
	IN UTERO	POSTDELIVERY
Oxygen saturation (%)	45*	95
Erythropoietin levels	High	Undetectable
Red cell production	Rapid	<10% (by day 7)
Reticulocyte count (%)	3-7	0-1 (by day 7)
Hemoglobin (g/dl)	16.8	18.4
Hematocrit (%)	53	58
MCV (fL)	107	98 (by day 7)
MCHC (g/dl) [4,7]	31.7	33 (by day 7)

MCHC, Mean corpuscular hemoglobin concentration; *MCV,* mean corpuscular volume.
*Mean values represented.

hemoglobin values less than 13 g/dl would be considered anemia.

Determination of the cause of anemia is important to direct treatment. Anemia in the newborn results from one or more of the following basic mechanisms:

- Blood loss (acute or chronic)
- Decreased red cell production
- Shortened red cell survival

BLOOD LOSS

Acute and chronic blood losses are the most common causes of anemia in the neonate. Blood loss can occur in utero, perinatally, or postnatally. Some degree of fetomaternal blood mixing occurs in 50% of all pregnancies.[15] Blood loss usually is insignificant; however, in about 8% of pregnancies, the transfer of blood is estimated to be between 0.5 and 40 ml, and in 1% of pregnancies the volume of blood transfused to the mother is greater than 40 ml.[23] The total blood volume of the fetus is approximately 90 ml/kg. Large blood loss can cause profound asphyxia and death; determination of a profound drop in hemoglobin and hematocrit may lag by hours when blood volume is equilibrated. Anemia caused by chronic blood loss is better tolerated, because the neonate is able to compensate for the gradual loss in red cell mass. There is a large differential for blood loss in the neonate (Box 20-1).

Fetomaternal transfusion is a common cause of occult blood loss in the fetus. The **Kleihauer-Betke** acid elution test is the method used to confirm the presence of fetal blood cells in the maternal circulation.[80] Fetal cells retain red staining of hemoglobin after fixing, whereas adult cells (also called *ghost cells*) are very pale because hemoglobin has been eluted. The volume of fetal blood in the maternal circulation is estimated by counting fetal red cells on the maternal blood smear under light microscopy. Ten fetal cells per 30 fields viewed under high power are equal to 1 ml of fetal blood.

Twin-to-twin transfusion is another cause of occult blood loss and is seen in 15% to 30% of all monochorionic twins with abnormalities of placental blood vessels.[70] The anemic twin is on the arterial side of the placental vascular malformation. The clinical significance of twin-to-twin transfusion depends on the duration of blood transfer. With chronic transfusion, a 20% weight discordance similar to that observed with placental insufficiency can be found; the recipient twin (i.e. the plethoric or polycythemic one) usually suffers greater morbidity.[32]

Intracranial bleeding associated with prematurity, later birth order of a multiple-gestation delivery, rapid delivery, breech delivery, and massive cephalohematoma can cause anemia. Other forms of neonatal hemorrhage predisposing to anemia include

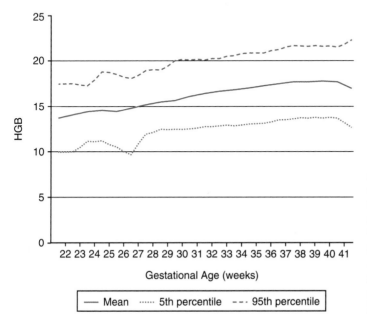

FIGURE 20-1 Reference ranges (5th percentile, mean, and 95th percentile) are shown for blood hemoglobin concentrations obtained during the first 6 hours after birth among patients 22 to 42 weeks' gestation. Values were excluded if the diagnosis included abruption, placenta previa, or known fetal anemia, or if a blood transfusion was given before the first hemoglobin was measured. (From Joplin J, Henry E, Wiedmeier SE, Christensen RD: Reference ranges for hematocrit and blood hemoglobin concentration during the neonatal period, *Pediatrics* 123:e333-337, 2009).

BOX 20-1	CAUSES OF BLOOD LOSS IN THE NEONATE

1. Hemorrhage before birth
   a. Fetomaternal
      Traumatic amniocentesis or periumbilical blood sampling
      Spontaneous
      Chronic gastrointestinal bleeding
      Blunt trauma to the maternal abdomen
      Postexternal positioning
   b. Twin-to-twin
   c. External
      Abruptio placentae
      Placenta previa
2. Hemorrhage during birth
   a. Placental malformation
      Chorangioma
      Chorangiocarcinoma
   b. Hematoma of the cord or placenta
   c. Rupture of a normal umbilical cord
      Precipitous delivery
      Entanglement
   d. Rupture of an abnormal umbilical cord
      Varices
      Aneurysm
   e. Rupture of anomalous vessels
      Aberrant vessel
      Velamentous insertion of the cord
      Communicating vessels in the multilobular placenta
   f. Incision of placenta during cesarean section
3. Internal fetal or neonatal hemorrhage
   a. Intracranial
   b. Giant cephalohematoma, caput succedaneum
   c. Pulmonary
   d. Retroperitoneum
   e. Subcapsular liver or spleen
   f. Renal or adrenal
4. External neonatal hemorrhage
   a. Delayed clamping of the umbilical cord
   b. Gastrointestinal
   c. Iatrogenic from blood sampling

Modified from Luchtman-Jones L, Schwartz A, Wilson D: Hematologic problems in the fetus and neonate. In Fanaroff A, editor: *Neonatal-perinatal medicine: diseases of the fetus and infant,* vol 2, St Louis, 1997, Mosby.

umbilical, retroperitoneal, adrenal, renal, and gastrointestinal bleeding, as well as ruptured liver or spleen.

Swallowed maternal blood may be confused with gastrointestinal (GI) bleeding. The Apt test is used to distinguish swallowed maternal blood from neonatal blood and is based on alkali resistance of fetal hemoglobin.[4] A 1% solution of sodium hydroxide is added to 5 ml of diluted blood. Fetal hemoglobin remains pink, but adult hemoglobin becomes yellow.

Iatrogenic blood loss results from blood sampling with inadequate replacement. A survey performed in the intensive care nursery of the University of California at San Francisco found that an average of 38.9 ml of blood was removed for laboratory tests during the first week of life.[61] For premature infants, whose blood volume can be as little as 50 ml, anemia is commonly caused by blood draws. The majority of red cell transfusions given in nurseries are directly related to frequent blood sampling.[50]

DECREASED RED CELL PRODUCTION
Anemia caused by decreased production of red cells tends to develop slowly, allowing time for physiologic compensation. Affected infants may have few signs of anemia other than pallor. The reticulocyte count will be low and inappropriate for the degree of anemia.

Worldwide, iron deficiency is the leading cause of anemia in infancy and childhood. Iron-deficiency anemia can occur at any time when growth exceeds the ability of the stores and dietary intake to supply sufficient iron for erythropoiesis. Iron storage at birth is directly related to body weight. Typically infants are born with iron stores sufficient to support new RBC production until they double their birth weight.[52] Infants who are fed exclusively breastmilk or iron-enriched formula and cereal are less likely to develop iron-deficiency anemia.

Premature infants have iron stores adequate for less than 3 months postnatally because of low birth weight, faster rate of growth, and iatrogenic blood losses. Iron supplementation is necessary early in preterm infants to prevent anemia (Table 20-2).

Iron deficiency causes a hypochromic, microcytic anemia. The peripheral smear shows small, pale red cells with a large variety of shapes and sizes resulting in an increased relative distribution of width.

TABLE 20-2	RECOMMENDED IRON SUPPLEMENTATION FOR THE NEONATE	
GROUP	DOSE (mg/kg/day)	INITIATION, DURATION
Full term	1	4 mo to 3 yr
Preterm, low birth weight	2	2 mo to 1 yr, then
	1	1 yr to 3 yr
Very low birth weight	4	2 mo to 1 yr, then
	1	1 yr to 3 yr

The platelet count is increased and may be greater than $1,000,000/\mu l$. Mild forms of iron deficiency may be confused with other causes of anemia, including infection and thalassemia. A therapeutic trial of iron can be used to diagnose iron deficiency.

Anemia of prematurity is common in infants born at less than 35 weeks' gestation. This is a normocytic, normochromic anemia appearing between 2 and 6 weeks characterized by a low reticulocyte count and an inadequate response to erythropoietin.[62] If hemoglobin levels drop below 10 g/dl, the infant may display decreased activity, poor growth, tachypnea, and tachycardia. Randomized placebo-controlled trials demonstrate that preterm infants can respond to erythropoietin with decreased amount of blood transfused if they are also supplemented with iron.[47] Because preterm infants currently receive fewer red cell transfusions compared with the past two decades, they are at increased risk for iron deficiency. Although the Academy of Pediatrics recommends 2 to 4 mg/kg/day elemental iron for preterm infants and 4 to 6 mg/kg/day for preterm infants receiving concomitant erythropoietin, higher doses for prevention of iron deficiency may be associated with improved outcomes.[33]

Iron deficiency with or without accompanying anemia has been associated with cognitive and behavioral deficits.[43] One longitudinal study followed patients diagnosed with iron deficiency in early infancy for 10 years and found higher rates of psychomotor impairment and specific cognitive deficits, including spatial memory, selective recall, and attention.[38] Possible biologic mechanisms for this effect of iron deficiency include impairment of iron-dependent cytochromes, decreased myelination, and alterations in neurotransmitter systems, which have been demonstrated in iron-restricted animal models.

Hypothyroidism, deficiency of transcobalamin II, and inborn errors of cobalamin utilization cause macrocytic anemia because of decreased and ineffective bone marrow production. Metabolic causes of anemia are important to diagnose and treat because deficiencies can cause permanent neurologic and cognitive deficits.

Constitutional pure red cell aplasia is also known as *Diamond-Blackfan anemia.*[37] Diamond-Blackfan anemia is caused by more than 200 unique mutations in ribosomal protein genes.[8] This normocytic or macrocytic anemia manifests at birth in 10% and by 1 month in 25% of affected infants. Signs and symptoms include pallor, anemia, and reticulocytopenia. In red cell aplasia the platelet count may be moderately elevated and the leukocyte count may be slightly decreased. Bone marrow examination is normocellular with few erythroid precursors. Thirty percent of affected infants demonstrate congenital anomalies, primarily of the head, face, eyes, and thumb. The syndrome can have autosomal dominant or recessive inheritance. As infants grow older, characteristics of fetal erythropoiesis persist, including elevations in fetal hemoglobin, *i* antigen, and red cell adenosine deaminase, as well as fetal patterns of red cell enzymes. Seventy percent of affected infants respond to corticosteroid therapy, particularly if treatment is initiated early in infancy. Infants who do not respond to steroids require long-term RBC transfusion therapy and are at risk for subsequent iron overload. In Diamond-Blackfan anemia the erythrocyte progenitors do not respond to erythropoietin, but often respond to stem cell factor and, to a lesser degree, interleukin-3. *Fanconi's anemia* is a congenital syndrome of progressive bone marrow failure with autosomal recessive inheritance.[2] At birth, infants may be recognized by one or more of the associated congenital defects, which include microcephaly; short stature; absent or abnormal thumb; and other cutaneous, musculoskeletal, and urogenital abnormalities. Thrombocytopenia and an elevated MCV usually are the first hematologic abnormalities, but they are seldom recognized in the neonatal period. The underlying defect in Fanconi's anemia is an inability to repair damaged deoxyribonucleic acid. Chromosomal breakage analyses and specific molecular diagnosis have been used for prenatal diagnosis. Diamond-Blackfan and Fanconi's anemias have been successfully treated with bone marrow transplantation. Infants with genetic hemoglobin mutations of alpha or gamma chains that result in production of hemoglobins with decreased oxygen affinity will have lower hemoglobins without signs of tissue hypoxia.

B19 parvovirus exerts an inhibitory effect on bone marrow production of red cells.[77] Infection with B19 parvovirus during pregnancy can cause hydrops fetalis, the clinical syndrome caused by severe intrauterine anemia of any cause and consisting of congestive heart failure, massive skin edema, and intrauterine demise, especially during the first two trimesters. Early detection of parvovirus infection in pregnant women and serial examinations with ultrasonography are important to diagnose and monitor the condition. Affected fetuses have been supported successfully with intrauterine transfusions of RBCs. Postnatal infection with parvovirus does not cause anemia in most infants unless they have preexisting shortened RBC survival. Infants with congenital or acquired immunodeficiency may become anemic because of an inability to clear parvovirus.

SHORTENED RED BLOOD CELL SURVIVAL

Adult RBCs circulate for an average of 120 days. Normal neonatal RBCs have a circulating half-life reduction of 20% to 25% compared with the RBCs of older children or adults. Survival of RBCs of premature infants is reduced by approximately 50%. Senescent RBCs are removed from the circulation by the reticuloendothelial system. Bilirubin is produced by degradation of the heme moiety of hemoglobin, and RBC iron is recycled. Many conditions accelerate removal of RBCs from the circulation.

Hemolysis is a term for RBC destruction that is premature in terms of expected life span of the red cells relative to postconceptual age. *Hyperbilirubinemia* is evident in most cases of hemolysis. Reticulocytosis is usually found. However, in the presence of chronic illness, nutritional deficiency, or congenital infection, the reticulocyte count may be lower than expected for the degree of anemia. In the most severe cases of intrauterine hemolysis the outcome is *hydrops fetalis* (Box 20-2).

BOX 20-2   CAUSES OF SHORTENED RED CELL SURVIVAL IN THE NEONATE

1. Isoimmune-mediated hemolysis
   a. Rh incompatibility
   b. ABO incompatibility
   c. Minor blood cell antigen incompatibility
2. Infection
   a. Bacterial sepsis
   b. *Campylobacter jejuni*
   c. *Clostridium welchii*
   d. Rubella
   e. Cytomegalovirus
   f. Epstein-Barr virus
   g. Disseminated herpes
   h. Malaria
   i. Toxoplasmosis
   j. Syphilis
3. Microangiopathic and macroangiopathic
   a. Cavernous hemangioma (Kasabach-Merritt)
   b. Renal vein thrombosis
   c. Disseminated intravascular coagulation
   d. Severe coarctation of the aorta
   e. Renal artery stenosis

4. Vitamin E deficiency
5. Congenital red cell membrane disorders
   a. Hereditary spherocytosis
   b. Hereditary elliptocytosis
      i. Hereditary poikilocytosis
      ii. Hereditary pyropoikilocytosis
      iii. Hereditary stomatocytosis
   c. Infantile pyknocytosis
6. Congenital red cell enzyme disorders
   a. Glucose-6-phosphate dehydrogenase deficiency
   b. Pyruvate kinase deficiency
7. Congenital hemoglobinopathies
   a. Alpha and gamma chain defects including thalassemias; structural abnormalities; unstable hemoglobin
8. Metabolic disorders
   a. Galactosemia
   b. Organic aciduria; orotic aciduria
   c. Prolonged or recurrent acidosis
9. Liver disease

Isoimmune hemolytic anemia occurs when fetal cells, bearing antigens of paternal origin that the mother does not possess, enter the maternal circulation and stimulate production of immunoglobulin G (IgG) antibodies. The IgG antibodies are transferred across the placenta, coat fetal RBCs, and mediate their removal from the circulation through the reticuloendothelial system.

The major fetal RBC antigens responsible for isoimmune hemolytic anemia include the Rh (also called D) antigen in an Rh-negative mother and the blood group A and B antigens in a group O mother. *Kell, Duffy,* and *Kidd antigens* can also cause isoimmune hemolytic anemia. Sources of maternal sensitization to fetal RBC antigens include chorionic villus sampling, amniocentesis, abortion, rupture of an ectopic pregnancy, maternal blood transfusion, and fetomaternal transfusion. Anti-Rh antibodies derived from plasma of previously sensitized donors are given to Rh-negative mothers at 28 weeks of gestation, at delivery, and at the time of any of the previously mentioned events. These antibodies coat any fetal red cells present in the maternal circulation and prevent them from initiating the maternal immune response. Thus they provide a form of passive immunization. With widespread use of Rh immunoglobulin (Ig) in Rh-negative mothers, the rate of anti-Rh Ig formation dropped from 17% to 9% to 13%.[5,77] The rate of Rh hemolytic disease in the United States is 1 case per 1000 live births.[11] The persistence of Rh isoimmunization may be attributed to failures in administering Rh Ig to all women at risk and incorrect dosing. Women who receive no prenatal care and women who develop silent antenatal sensitization compose two populations that are difficult to reach with prevention strategies.

ABO hemolytic anemia is more common than Rh hemolytic disease but less severe. Unlike Rh disease, hemolysis secondary to ABO incompatibility can occur during the first pregnancy because A and B antigens are ubiquitous in foods and bacteria, causing sensitization. Most isoimmune hemolytic diseases that are not related to ABO or Rh incompatibility are caused by sensitization to minor blood group antigens Kell, Duffy, Lewis, Kidd, M, or S. Mothers should be screened at 34 weeks for antibodies to these minor blood group antigens.

Congenital bacterial and *viral infections* may cause hemolytic anemia and bone marrow suppression with reticulocytopenia. Microspherocytes may be very prominent.

Microangiopathies and *macroangiopathies* are characterized by red cell fragmentation, shortened red cell survival, and thrombocytopenia. Coagulation proteins are also consumed in cavernous hemangiomas and disseminated intravascular coagulation (DIC).

Vitamin E is a fat-soluble vitamin that functions as an antioxidant. Deficiency of vitamin E manifests with hemolytic anemia, reticulocytosis, thrombocytosis, and edema of the lower extremities.[62] Diets high in polyunsaturated fatty acids and iron increase requirements for vitamin E. With current supplementation of infant formulas and parenteral nutrition with vitamin E, prevention of vitamin E deficiency using a water-soluble form of tocopherol is not currently necessary.

Shortened red cell survival secondary to an intrinsic red cell defect is a rare but important cause of shortened red cell survival in the neonate. Because even normal neonates have shortened red cell survival and hyperbilirubinemia, the presentation of these syndromes in the neonate often is more severe than in older affected family members. Affected infants usually present with anemia and hyperbilirubinemia. Splenomegaly develops later in infancy or early childhood. A preliminary diagnosis of constitutional red cell defect is made by family history and careful inspection of the peripheral smear. Abnormalities of red cell shape, including spherocytes, elliptocytes, pyknocytes, "bite cells," target cells, and other bizarre morphologic structures, are often characteristic of the specific red cell defect.

Constitutional defects in red cell membranes cause lifelong hemolytic anemia. *Hereditary spherocytosis* is the most common red cell membrane defect, usually is inherited as an autosomal dominant trait, and primarily affects infants of Northern European descent. *Pyropoikilocytosis,* an infantile form of the mild membrane defect *hereditary elliptocytosis,* is characterized by striking red cell pyknocytes and fragments on peripheral smear with evidence of mild hemolysis. Typical elliptocytes may not become apparent until a few months of life.

Glucose-6-phosphate dehydrogenase (G6PD) is the first rate-limiting enzyme in the pentose phosphate pathway of red cell energy metabolism. This enzyme is important in the production of nicotinamide adenine dinucleotide phosphate (NADPH), which maintains cellular systems in a reduced state. G6PD deficiency is the most common inherited disorder of red blood cells and is transmitted as an X-linked recessive trait; therefore affected infants are overwhelmingly male. There are many isoforms of abnormal G6PD enzymes. The Mediterranean type produces severe hemolysis, whereas the form found in African Americans usually is mild. Infants are asymptomatic until challenged with oxidant stresses from infections or drugs. Agents associated with hemolysis in G6PD-deficient infants are shown in Box 20-3. *Pyruvate kinase deficiency* is the second most common RBC enzyme defect and can have a clinical presentation similar to G6PD. It may be inherited in either an autosomal dominant or recessive fashion and thus may be seen in female or male infants.

Hemoglobinopathies are inherited disorders resulting from gene mutations that affect quantity or quality of hemoglobin chains. The clinical expression of a hemoglobinopathy is dependent on the affected globin chain, the developmental stage of globin synthesis, and the amount and function of alternate hemoglobins. Hemoglobinopathies presenting at birth affect either the alpha or gamma chain of hemoglobin. Hemoglobin beta chains are not produced until 3 months of postnatal age; therefore defects of beta chains, such as *sickle cell anemia* and *beta-thalassemia,* do not present in the nursery. The *thalassemias* are disorders manifested by absence or decrease of specific globin proteins.[32] Because there are four genes controlling alpha globin synthesis (two on each allele of chromosome 16), clinical presentations may range from asymptomatic (one alpha hemoglobin gene deletion) to abnormalities incompatible with life (absence of production from all four alpha hemoglobin genes).[71] Most infants with moderate to severe anemia related to alpha-thalassemia have a three-gene deletion. Alpha globin is an essential component of both hemoglobin F and hemoglobin A. Alpha thalassemia may be detected on universal newborn screening by the presence of hemoglobin Barts in the neonatal period, which is composed of four gamma chains. Hemoglobin Barts is replaced later by the compensatory hemoglobin, hemoglobin H, which is a beta-chain tetramer. In Western societies there has been a dramatic decline in the incidence of new births with severe

---

BOX 20-3 SOME AGENTS REPORTED TO PRODUCE HEMOLYSIS IN PATIENTS WITH G6PD DEFICIENCY

Drugs and Chemicals Clearly Shown to Cause Clinically Significant Hemolytic Anemia in G6PD Deficiency

Acetanilid
Methylene blue
Nalidixic acid (NegGram)
Naphthalene
Niridazole (Ambilhar)
Phenylhydrazine
Primaquine
Pamaquine
Pentaquine
Sulfanilamide
Sulfacetamide
Sulfapyridine
Sulfamethoxazole (Gantanol)
Thiazolsulfone
Toluidine blue
Trinitrotoluene

Drugs Probably Safe in Normal Therapeutic Doses for G6PD-Deficient Individuals (Without Nonspherocytic Hemolytic Anemia)

Acetaminophen (Paracetamol, Tylenol, Tralgon, Hydroxyacetanillid)
Acetophenetidine (Phenacetin)
Acetylsalicylic acid (aspirin)
Aminopyrine (Pyramidon, Amidopyrine)
Antazoline (Antistine)
Antipyrine
Ascorbic acid (vitamin C)
Benzhexol (Artane)
Chloramphenicol
Chlorguanidine (Proguanil, Paludrine)
Chloroquine
Colchicine
Diphenhydramine (Benadryl)
L-dopa

Menadione sodium bisulfite (Hykinone)
Menaphthone
p-Aminobenzoic acid
Phenylbutazone
Phenytoin
Probenecid (Benemid)
Procaine amide hydrochloride (Pronestyl)
Pyrimethamine (Daraprim)
Quinidine
Quinine
Streptomycin
Sulfacytine
Sulfadiazine
Sulfaguanidine
Sulfamerazine
Sulfamethoxypyridazine (Kynex)
Sulfisoxazole (Gantrisin)
Trimethoprim
Tripelennamine (Pyribenzamine)
Vitamin K

From Beutler E: *Hemolytic anemia in disorders of red cell metabolism,* New York, 1978, Plenum.
G6PD, Glucose-6-phosphate dehydrogenase.

thalassemia syndromes because of the widespread use of molecular diagnostic techniques by couples at risk.

Methemoglobin contains an oxidized form of heme iron, Fe^{3+}, which renders it incapable of reversible binding to oxygen. Constitutional methemoglobinemia presenting in the neonatal period is caused either by deficiency of the red cell enzyme *methemoglobin reductase* or by an *M hemoglobinopathy* of the gamma chain of hemoglobin. Infants with either of these disorders present with cyanosis of the skin and mucous membranes but are otherwise usually asymptomatic. *Acquired methemoglobinemia* can be life-threatening due to severe hypoxemia. Normal newborn infants are at risk for developing toxic/acquired methemoglobinemia from environmental toxins and pharmacologic agents because neonatal RBCs contain lower levels of the enzyme *NADH-methemoglobin reductase.* In addition to the ingestion of nitrates, Xylocaine and its derivatives, aniline dyes, and dapsone are the most common drugs precipitating methemoglobinemia.

Data Collection

HISTORY

Information obtained should include maternal history of illness and dietary intake during pregnancy, delivery type, hemorrhage, transfusion or iron therapy, and any abnormal occurrences during birth. A careful family history includes specific questioning about anemia, iron or transfusion therapy, pallor, jaundice, splenomegaly, splenectomy, gallstones, cholecystectomy, or congenital malformations in the parents, grandparents, siblings, aunts, uncles, and cousins of the infant.

SIGNS AND SYMPTOMS

In performing a physical examination of a newborn with anemia, attention should be paid to the infant's cardiovascular function, general vigor, and signs of pallor, jaundice, skin lesions, hepatosplenomegaly, lymphadenopathy, and congenital malformation (Box 20-4).

LABORATORY DATA

The diagnosis of anemia is based on the hemoglobin and hematocrit in comparison with normal values established for postconceptional and postnatal age. Initial laboratory evaluation of anemia should include a complete blood count with careful attention to the RBC indices, reticulocyte count,

and review of the peripheral blood smear. Additional laboratory testing depends on the characterization of the anemia (Table 20-3). If the peripheral smear suggests a constitutional RBC abnormality by severe anisocytosis, poikilocytosis, spherocytes, blister cells, bite cells, or elevated relative distribution of width, obtain an ACD tube (yellow) for assay of G6PD, pyruvate kinase, and other red cell enzymes and an EDTA tube (lavender) for assay of red cell membrane proteins and hemoglobin electrophoresis before transfusing the baby. A clinical decision tree in the evaluation of anemia is shown in Figure 20-2.

Treatment of Anemia

If acute blood loss is suspected and the infant is pale and limp at birth, blood pressure should be obtained and monitored, perfusion should be assessed, intravenous (IV) fluids started at 20 ml/kg, and oxygen administered. A catheter should be inserted into the umbilical artery to measure blood gases. Blood should be obtained for complete blood count (CBC), reticulocyte count, Coombs' test, blood type, fractionated bilirubin, and serum screen for blood group antibodies. Because infants less than 4 months of age rarely produce antibodies against blood group antigens, maternal serum can be used in the antibody screen.

Once the infant's condition stabilizes, a decision can be made about transfusion based on clinical status. If the infant is anemic with signs of hypoxemia or has underlying pulmonary or cardiac disease, transfusion of 10 ml/kg of RBCs over 2 to 3 hours may be given to increase

---

BOX 20-4	CRITICAL FINDINGS
	SIGNS AND SYMPTOMS OF ANEMIA IN THE NEONATE

1. Acute anemia (with hemorrhage, anemia may not be present initially; hemodilution develops over 3 to 4 hours)
   a. Hypovolemia, hypotension
   b. Hypoxemia, tachypnea
   c. Tachycardia
2. Chronic anemia (may be well compensated)
   a. Pallor, metabolic acidosis, poor growth
   b. High-output congestive heart failure
   c. Persistent or increased oxygen requirement
   d. Iron deficiency with hypochromia, microcytosis

TABLE 20-3	CHARACTERIZATION OF ANEMIA
CHARACTERIZATION	**TEST**
Blood loss	Kleihauer-Betke on maternal sample
	Apt test on gastric blood from infant as indicated
Bone marrow production	Reticulocyte count
	Platelet and white blood cell count
	Erythropoietin level
	T_3, T_4, TSH
	Bone marrow aspirate and biopsy
	Fetal hemoglobin iAg, MCV
Iron deficiency	Ferritin, iron, and iron-binding capacity
Antibody mediated	Maternal and infant blood type
	Direct and indirect Coombs' tests
Hemolysis	Bilirubin
	Coagulation tests (if sepsis or liver disease is suspected)
	Osmotic fragility, specific determinations of red cell membrane proteins, enzymes, hemoglobin, and ceruloplasmin as indicated
Infection	Culture and serologies as appropriate
Microangiopathy, macroangiopathy	DIC screen
Vitamin E deficiency	Vitamin E level
Metabolic disorder	pH, lactate, pyruvate
	Galactosemia screen

DIC, Disseminated intravascular coagulation; *MCV*, mean corpuscular volume; *TSH*, thyroid-stimulating hormone.

oxygen-carrying capacity (see diagnosis of congenital red cell defects in Laboratory Data section earlier). Normally, larger quantities of blood should not be given in one transfusion. Most blood banks at institutions with neonatal intensive care units have protocols for neonatal blood transfusion and will give leukodepleted, either type-specific or O-negative uncrossmatched red cells if the antibody screen is negative.[54] Blood used for transfusion should be less than 7 days old and negative or reduced for cytomegalovirus (CMV). Irradiation of RBCs and other blood cell products to prevent graft-versus-host disease is recommended for intrauterine transfusions or neonatal exchange transfusion and for infants with congenital or acquired immune deficiency. For infants with continuing hemorrhage requiring massive transfusion exceeding one blood volume, transfusions of fresh frozen plasma (FFP)

are necessary to replace clotting factors and prevent the consumptive coagulopathy that results from massive transfusion of stored blood. Platelet transfusions may also be needed.

An order from a physician or nurse practitioner is necessary for any blood transfusion. Parental consent should be obtained by the physician before transfusion. In the neonatal intensive care nursery a policy of "double-checking" blood is essential to ensure that the proper blood is being administered to the infant. Blood should be warmed and administered through a blood filter of 40 μm or finer. Fresh blood can be administered through a 25-gauge needle without significant hemolysis.

Directed donor programs are used in hospitals for nonemergent blood transfusions, especially in small preterm infants. In most cases biologic parents are able to serve as directed donors for

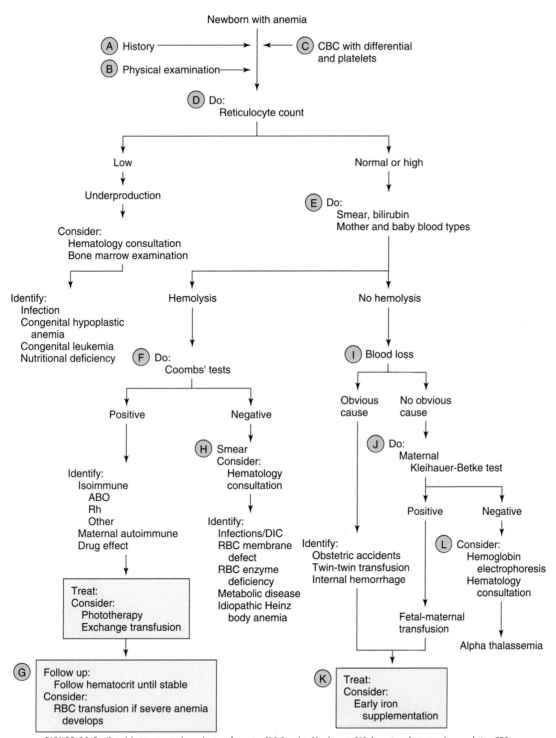

FIGURE 20-2 Clinical decision tree in the evaluation of anemia. *CBC,* Complete blood count; *DIC,* disseminated intravascular coagulation; *RBC,* red blood cell. (From Lane PA, Nuss R: Anemia in the newborn. In Berman S, editor: *Pediatric decision making,* ed 3, St Louis, 1996, Mosby.)

Continued

A. In the history, document any prenatal infections or drug use. Also note any history of maternal vaginal bleeding, placenta previa, abruptio placentae, or umbilical cord rupture, constriction or velamentous insertion, as well as cesarean, breech, or traumatic delivery. Obtain a family history of neonatal jaundice, anemia, splenomegaly, and unexplained gallstones.

B. In the physical examination, note tachypnea, tachycardia, peripheral vasoconstriction (acute blood loss), and hepatosplenomegaly (chronic anemia, intrauterine infection, congenital malignancy). Jaundice appearing before 24 hours of age suggests significant hemolysis.

C. A hematocrit less than 45% during the first 3 days of life is abnormal and requires explanation. The mean corpuscular volume (MCV) at birth is normally above 95. An MCV below 95 suggests alpha-thalassemia or chronic intrauterine blood loss (as with fetal maternal transfusion). Rarely, a low MCV may be seen with hemolytic disease caused by hereditary elliptocytosis or pyropoikilocytosis. The presence of neutropenia or thrombocytopenia suggests the possibility of infection. Except in an emergency, no anemic newborn should receive a blood transfusion before adequate diagnostic studies.

D. Normal reticulocyte values are 3% to 7% during the first day of life and 1% to 3% during the second and third days. A low reticulocyte count in the presence of significant anemia suggests bone marrow failure.

E. An indirect hyperbilirubinemia, abnormal peripheral blood smear, or ABO or Rh incompatibility between the mother and infant suggests hemolysis.

F. Perform direct and indirect Coombs' tests. ABO isoimmunization is usually associated with a negative direct and a positive indirect Coombs' test.

G. Infants with immune hemolysis have varying degrees of hemolysis, which may continue for 3 months. Severe, life-threatening anemia may develop in infants with Rh sensitization; such infants require close follow-up with serial hematocrit measurements until the hemolysis resolves.

H. Examine the peripheral blood smear. Spherocytes suggest ABO isoimmunization, hereditary spherocytosis, or infection (e.g., cytomegalovirus). Red cell fragmentation suggests intravascular hemolysis (infection, disseminated intravascular coagulation [DIC]). Consider infection or DIC in any ill newborn with hemolysis, particularly if thrombocytopenia is also present.

I. Review the obstetric history and examine the placenta for clues to the cause of fetal blood loss.

J. Perform a Kleihauer-Betke test to detect fetal red cells in the maternal circulation. False-negative results occur when an ABO incompatibility results in the rapid clearance of the infant's red cells from the maternal circulation.

K. Newborns with significant prenatal or perinatal blood loss are at risk for iron deficiency during the first 6 months of life.

L. Anemic infants without evidence of hemolysis or blood loss whose mothers have a negative Kleihauer-Betke test may have alpha-thalassemia, especially if the MCV is below 95. Ethnic groups affected most often include South and Southeast Asians, Mediterraneans, and Africans. The diagnosis of alpha-thalassemia may be confirmed with a hemoglobin electrophoresis that shows hemoglobin Barts.

REFERENCES

Ballin A, Brown EJ, Zipursky A: Idiopathic Heinz body hemolytic anemia in newborn infants, *Am J Pediatr Hematol Oncol* 11:3, 1989.

Blanchette VS, Zipursky A: Assessment of anemia in newborn infants, *Clin Perinatol* 11:489, 1984.

Oski FA: Anemia in the neonatal period. In Oski FA, Naiman JL, editors: *Hematologic problems in the newborn,* ed 3, Philadelphia, 1982, Saunders.

Oski FA: The erythrocyte and its disorders. In Nathan DG, Oski FA, editors: *Hematology of infancy and childhood,* ed 4, Philadelphia, 1993, Saunders.

FIGURE 20-2, cont'd.

their neonates. Preparation of directed donations is more costly than standard blood units and requires the same time for testing. At this time there are no scientific data that suggest directed donor programs increase blood safety. Some immunologic incompatibilities may exist between maternal and paternal donors; therefore the following guidelines should be considered for parental donors[19]:

- Mothers should not provide blood components containing plasma. If maternal red cells are transfused, they should be washed.
- Fathers are not recommended as blood cell (red, white, or platelet) donors for their newborns unless maternal serum is shown to lack cytotoxic antibodies.
- All parental blood components should be irradiated before transfusion to the infant.

Equipment necessary for blood transfusion includes a filter, extension tubing, and a pump. Except in extreme emergencies, blood should be administered through a peripheral catheter rather than through an umbilical artery catheter (UAC). It is essential to confirm that the unit of blood infused matches the typed blood bank form and assigned number, patient name, and patient hospital number. The expiration date and time must be respected. IV tubing used for blood transfusion should be flushed with 0.45% normal saline solution before it is used for infusing blood products.

Blood bags should not be used for more than 4 to 6 hours after opening. Vital signs should be obtained and recorded every 15 minutes during blood transfusion. Careful observations should be made for reactions, including increased temperature, diaphoresis, irregular respiration, bradycardia, restlessness, and pallor. Transfusions should be stopped promptly if any of these signs are present. All materials used for blood transfusion should be disposed of properly.

Infants who are anemic as a result of acute or chronic external blood loss who do not require transfusion therapy should be treated with iron replacement 6 mg/kg/day until the blood count is normal and two additional months to replace stores.

Infants who are born with *isoimmune hemolytic anemia* are often treated with exchange transfusion. In this procedure, catheters placed in central and peripheral veins are used to remove the infant's blood in small aliquots and replace it with packed red cells usually reconstituted with FFP. General guidelines for aliquot volumes are as follows:

- 3 kg : 20 ml per aliquot
- 2 kg : 15 ml per aliquot
- 1 kg : 5 ml per aliquot

Infants who are treated for isoimmune hemolytic anemia with intrauterine transfusions may be born with normal or near-normal hematocrit and bilirubin levels. Exchange transfusion is often used early after delivery to remove antibody and decrease postnatal hemolysis. Hyperbilirubinemia can be managed using phototherapy (see Chapter 21).

Data regarding the use of IV immunoglobulin (IVIG) for treatment of hemolytic disease of the newborn are conflicting. Multiple prospective, randomized clinical trials have shown no decrease in the need for exchange transfusion or rate of associated complications.[65,59] Additionally, there is some evidence that high dose IVIG administration is associated with increased rates of necrotizing enterocolitis.[22] Therefore there is no consensus for the routine use of IVIG in severe hemolytic disease of the newborn at this time.

Prevention of Anemia

Many forms of neonatal anemia are preventable. Improved fetal monitoring and obstetric care may prevent anemia caused by blood loss during delivery.

Administering Rh Ig to unsensitized Rh-negative mothers within 72 hours of delivery of an Rh-positive infant prevents most cases of hydrops fetalis in subsequent pregnancies. For previously sensitized Rh-negative mothers carrying Rh-positive fetuses, amniocentesis performed between 20 and 22 weeks' gestation may allow for intrauterine transfusion of Rh-negative RBCs and possible early delivery of a nonhydropic infant. For severe thalassemia syndromes and sickle cell anemia, prenatal diagnosis is possible. Intrauterine transfusions are also appropriate for infants with alpha-thalassemia major.

Hemolysis may be prevented in infants with significant G6PD deficiency by avoiding administration of drugs known to present an oxidative stress to the red cells.

Low-birth-weight (LBW) premature infants are at high risk for late-onset anemia because of low endogenous production of erythropoietin, exacerbated by phlebotomy losses for laboratory surveillance. Inadequate nutrition and other factors also may play a significant role. Strategies for minimizing blood donor exposure related to anemia of prematurity include decreasing the number of blood draws, using the absolute minimum quantity of blood possible for testing, and using satellite packs (aliquots of a larger unit from a single donor) for transfusion.

LBW premature infants often undergo transfusion because they are critically ill and have the highest blood sampling loss in relation to their weight. In an attempt to reduce the number of transfusions and donor exposure, most centers have implemented more restrictive transfusion guidelines, with very encouraging results. Recombinant human erythropoietin (r-HuEPO) has been successfully used to decrease the severity of anemia and lessen the use of blood transfusion in small premature infants. Erythropoietin has not been universally adopted for prevention of anemia of prematurity. Recent Cochrane Database meta-analyses suggest that the potential clinical benefit of erythropoietin administration is more limited.[1,51] The meta-analysis[51] found that despite the decrease in total number of transfusions, total transfused volume and donor exposures were not significantly decreased. In addition, this analysis also suggests an association between r-HuEPO and retinopathy of prematurity. Benefits of therapy other than decreased exposure to blood transfusion are also unknown at present.

Potential improvements in organ maturation or infant growth because of higher sustained levels of hemoglobin, and improved neural development are speculative at present. The cost of a 6-week course of therapy with r-HuEPO is comparable in most institutions with that of conventional therapies with blood replacement.

Treatment with EPO may be considered in infants of birth weight 800 to 1300 g. Infants with a birth weight of less than 800 g may receive so many transfusions early in their hospital course that treating with r-HuEPO may confer no substantial additional benefit. Infants with a birth weight of more than 1300 g rarely require blood transfusion.

If the decision is made to treat with r-HuEPO, therapy can begin when infants are stable and able to tolerate iron supplementation, usually when tolerating approximately 60% of caloric requirements by enteral feedings. The recommended dose is 200 to 250 U/kg r-HuEPO given IV or subcutaneously, three times weekly. The reticulocyte count should be monitored to document an adequate response. Oral iron supplementation should be initiated at the time of therapy, beginning with 2 mg/kg/day of elemental iron and increasing to 6 mg/kg/day as tolerated. A baseline hematocrit measurement and reticulocyte count should be obtained and followed weekly. Dosing should be adjusted to maintain a reticulocyte count above 6%. Supplemental vitamin E, 15 to 25 IU/day, and folic acid, 100 mcg/kg/day, may be given at the start of therapy. Treatment is continued for 6 weeks or until 36 weeks' postconceptual age. Once treatment is discontinued, hematocrit levels should be monitored every other week until stable.[46,47]

The *treatment of methemoglobinemia* is methylene blue, 1 to 2 mg/kg given IV over 5 to 10 minutes or orally; this therapy is ineffective in infants with deficient NADPH or G6PD, as well as M-hemoglobinopathies. Treatment of methemoglobinemia in G6PD-deficient infants consists of ascorbic acid, 200 to 500 mg/kg/day.[30,57]

POLYCYTHEMIA AND HYPERVISCOSITY

Physiology

Neonatal polycythemia in a term infant is defined by a peripheral venous hemoglobin and hematocrit more than 2 standard deviations (SDs) above the mean; this translates to a hemoglobin greater than 22 g/dl and a hematocrit greater than 65%.[27] Viscosity is related to but not identical to hematocrit. The viscosity of blood increases linearly with hematocrit up to a hematocrit of 60% and then increases exponentially, but inconsistently, thereafter.[39] Although viscosity may be measured directly, required instrumentation is not widely available in clinical laboratories and hematocrit is often used as a surrogate for viscosity. Blood sampling at 12 hours' postnatal age seems ideal to determine hematocrit and viscosity for diagnosis of polycythemic hyperviscosity.[76] Capillary hematocrit can be used as a screening test, but a central venous sample should be analyzed to confirm an abnormally high capillary hematocrit because these values may differ by as much as 20%.[36]

Pathophysiology

The pathophysiology of polycythemia can be attributed to either hyperviscosity or increased RBC mass. *Hyperviscosity* is a syndrome of circulatory impairment resulting from increased resistance to blood flow. Complications of polycythemia and hyperviscosity include respiratory distress, congestive heart failure, neurologic signs, and sequelae such as significant motor and mental retardation and cerebral palsy. Thromboemboli, arterial ischemic stroke, necrotizing enterocolitis, and acute tubular necrosis are additional complications. Complications related to increased RBC mass include hypoglycemia and hyperbilirubinemia.

Polycythemia can result from a large number of perinatal complications, as shown in Box 20-5. Polycythemia and hyperviscosity result from chronic hypoxia, such as that associated with intrauterine growth restriction. However, the cause of polycythemia and hyperviscosity in otherwise normally developed term infants is unknown. Although delayed cord clamping and umbilical cord milking have been cited as the most frequent cause of polycythemia in term infants, two recent randomized clinical trials in term and near-term infants refute this assertion.[3,72] Infants in these two trials demonstrated higher hemoglobin and increased ferritin levels with less anemia than infants undergoing early cord clamping, without cord milking. There was also no difference in the incidence of polycythemia or jaundice.[3,72]

BOX 20-5	CAUSES OF NEONATAL POLYCYTHEMIA

1. Placental transfusion
   a. Delayed cord clamping (may increase the blood volume and red cell mass of the infant by as much as 55%)
   b. Twin-to-twin transfusion
2. Intrauterine hypoxia/placental vascular insufficiency
   a. Intrauterine growth restriction syndrome
   b. Maternal diabetes
   c. Maternal smoking
   d. Maternal hypertension syndromes
   e. Maternal cyanotic heart disease
3. Fetal factors
   a. Trisomy 13, 18, 21
   b. Hyperthyroidism
   c. Neonatal thyrotoxicosis
   d. Congenital adrenal hyperplasia
   e. Beckwith-Wiedemann syndrome
4. High altitude
5. Idiopathic

In up to one third of *monochorionic twins* there is a significant transfusion of blood from one twin into the other defined as a discrepancy in the infants' blood counts of greater than 5 g/dl of hemoglobin. Usually, the recipient twin is larger and prone to cardiorespiratory symptoms, hyperviscosity, and hyperbilirubinemia, whereas the donor twin is smaller, anemic, and at risk for congestive heart failure.[77] Blood viscosity correlates better with symptoms than does hematocrit.[55] In addition, clinical signs and symptoms may be related to an underlying condition instead of polycythemia per se.

Data Collection

HISTORY

In addition to a complete history of the pregnancy and delivery, questions should be directed to pertinent maternal medical conditions, including insulin-dependent diabetes mellitus, hypertension, and heart disease. Additional maternal risk factors include cigarette smoking and living at high altitude. Fetal risk factors include documented intrauterine growth restriction and delayed cord clamping.

SIGNS AND SYMPTOMS

Newborn infants with hematocrit values of greater than 65% to 70% may manifest symptoms because of increased viscosity.[76] Physical examination may be normal except for plethora and, occasionally, cyanosis. Neurologic findings may include lethargy, irritability, hypotonia, tremor, seizures, and poor suck. Tachypnea, tachycardia, and respiratory distress may be present. Poor GI function is common with abdominal distention, decreased bowel sounds, and poor feeding.

LABORATORY DATA

The diagnosis of polycythemia is based on hemoglobin and hematocrit in comparison with two standard deviation normal values for postconceptual and postnatal age. The diagnosis of hyperviscosity may be based on direct viscosity measurement but usually is assigned based on polycythemia in the presence of consistent clinical signs and symptoms. Affected infants often have thrombocytopenia, hyperbilirubinemia, and hypoglycemia. Tests of thyroid and adrenal function to rule out hyperthyroidism and adrenal hyperplasia should be performed with appropriate clinical indication. Chromosome analysis should be considered for babies with dysmorphic features.

Treatment

Therapy for polycythemia should be based on the presence of clinical signs and symptoms consistent with hyperviscosity and not laboratory values alone. Traditionally, treatment of polycythemia aims to decrease blood viscosity through phlebotomy or partial exchange transfusion with replacement of removed RBC volume with volume expanders. Supportive care measures should also include IV fluids to treat hypoglycemia and phototherapy to treat hyperbilirubinemia. Although partial exchange transfusion may increase short-term cerebral blood flow,[21] the long-term benefits (follow-up at greater than 2 years) appear to be negligible with no difference in neurodevelopmental outcomes in patients who were managed conservatively with observation and fluids.[48,49]

Neurologic sequelae in babies with hyperviscosity appear to be related to prenatal risk factors for fetal asphyxia as much as or more than hematocrit at birth.[58] Additionally, there may be a relationship between partial exchange transfusion and increased

GI morbidity, that is, necrotizing enterocolitis.[53] In general, all peripheral hematocrits greater than 65% need to be checked and confirmed in a central venous sample. Asymptomatic infants with a hematocrit 60% to 70% may be monitored closely with adequate hydration and glucose levels. Some centers recommend that partial exchange transfusion in asymptomatic patients be limited to patients with repeated venous hematocrit measurements greater than 70%.[6,60] For symptomatic patients, conservative treatment aimed at plasma expansion using early feeding or IV fluids may be attempted. However, partial exchange transfusion should be strongly considered in patients with significant cardiopulmonary or neurologic symptoms and those with a central venous hematocrit greater than 70%.

FFP has not shown greater efficacy than saline in initial correction in hematocrit or viscosity, or in improvement in outcome. In a randomized controlled trial, Roithmaier and colleagues[56] showed that partial exchange transfusion using crystalloid solution (Ringer's solution) was as effective as partial exchange transfusion using a colloid (plasma) in decreasing the hematocrit of polycythemic neonates. Crystalloid solutions are preferable to colloids because they are less expensive and are free of the risk for transmitted infection. Exchange transfusion often requires placement of an umbilical venous catheter (UVC). Risks of umbilical catheterization in polycythemic infants include portal vein thrombosis, phlebitis of the portal vein, and decreased plasma volume (if phlebotomy is used alone). In addition, infants with polycythemia and hyperviscosity are at increased risk of spontaneous large vessel thrombosis, especially renal vein thrombosis and stroke. Symptomatic infants and asymptomatic infants with confirmed venous hematocrit greater than or equal to 70% may be treated with partial exchange transfusion using crystalloid.

COAGULATION

Physiology

When a blood vessel is torn, blood clots form at the site of vessel injury through a series of carefully controlled cellular and enzymatic reactions. First, *platelets,* which are small, platelike blood cells without

nuclei, adhere to the damaged endothelium both directly through membrane integrin *glycoprotein (GP)1α* and by linkage through the von Willebrand protein *(von Willebrand factor [vWF])* via *GP 1β IX* to *collagen,* which is exposed beneath the blood vessel lining. The platelets release adenosine diphosphate (ADP), which, in addition to collagen, recruits more platelets to the activation process. Activated platelets express a receptor for the blood protein fibrinogen, *GPIIb/IIIa,* which binds to adjoining platelets and links them.

Fibrinogen is a contractile protein that pulls platelets together, forming a tightly woven net over the vessel tear. *vWF, fibronectin, and thrombospondin* similarly link activated platelets through the *GPIIb/IIIa receptor.* This is known as a *platelet plug* and is responsible for the initial cessation of bleeding, especially in mucous membranes of the nose, mouth, throat, and GI and genitourinary tracts. At the same time, *thromboxanes* produced by the platelet prostaglandin pathway stimulate platelet aggregation, vasoconstriction, and decreased local blood flow.

Figure 20-3 shows the sequential reactions in activation of coagulation known as the *clotting cascade.*[42] The coagulation proteins in blood are inert proenzymes called *zymogens* until they are activated. The primary activation process involves exposure of a potent membrane glycoprotein receptor for clotting activation called *tissue factor,* for which the tissue factor pathway of coagulation activation is named. Tissue factor is normally hidden in the subendothelium and becomes exposed by vascular injury or is presented on the intact surface of monocytes and endothelial cells through the inflammatory process. Small amounts of circulating *activated factor VII (FVIIa)* in the plasma bind to exposed tissue factor and form a complex that results in the sequential activation first of factor X and then of factor II (also called *prothrombin*). These biochemical reactions are similar in that they take place preferentially on procoagulant phospholipid surfaces of activated endothelial cells and platelets at the site of injury, involve calcium-dependent binding to the surface, and can be accelerated by cofactors (*activated factors VIII [FVIIIa] and V [FVa]*).

The contact activation pathway is an alternative route to factor X activation. In this pathway, factor XII is activated by contact with negatively charged subendothelial collagen or by acidosis, cold, or heat injury. Activated factor XII subsequently activates factors XI and IX. *Prekallikrein* and

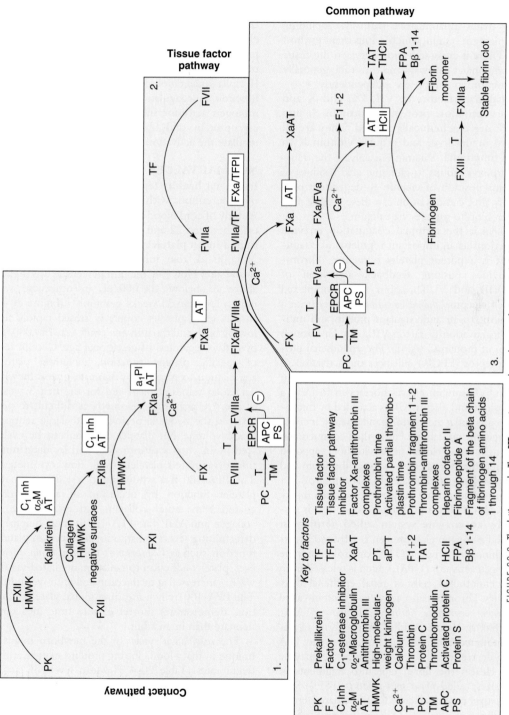

FIGURE 20-3 The clotting cascade. The aPTT screening test and coagulation test factors are included in panels 1 and 3. The PT test factors are shown in panels 2 and 3. Proteins encased in boxes inhibit the procoagulant reactions. *EPCR*, Endothelial protein C receptor.

high-molecular-weight *kininogen* serve as cofactors for activation. Contact activation initiates clot lysis and also many inflammatory pathways, including the complement system, which is important for host defense. There is cross-activation between the tissue factor and contact pathways and thus each generally is not functioning completely independently.

Procoagulant factors II, VII, IX, and X and regulatory proteins, protein C, protein S, and protein Z are biochemically related. They are all produced in the liver and require vitamin K to become functional. Vitamin K catalyzes the transfer of carboxyl groups to glutamic acid residues in the gamma position of vitamin K–dependent proteins; only after carboxylation can these unique proteins then bind to surfaces via calcium.

Thrombin is the terminal coagulation enzyme and functions as an important regulator of coagulation. It is a potent platelet activator. Thrombin provides positive feedback activation of factors VIII and V. Thrombin, when complexed to the cell receptor, *thrombomodulin,* changes from a procoagulant to an anticoagulant protein and initiates the inactivation of factors VIIIa and Va through activation of protein C (APC). The endothelial protein C receptor (EPCR) enhances the activation of protein C and complements the important protein C system.[18] Thrombin cleaves fibrinogen to form a sticky fibrin strand. Factor XIII is activated by thrombin and cross-links the fibrin strand, greatly increasing its strength and stability. Fibrin then contracts and forms a tight dense clot. A fibrin clot holds apposed surfaces together for about a week as thrombin and other growth factors stimulate fibroblasts to grow.

Ultimately, scar tissue bridges the original injury. When a blood clot is no longer needed, it is dissolved by an enzyme system called *fibrinolysis.* The blood zymogen plasminogen is activated by tissue plasminogen activator (TPA) or urokinase-type plasminogen activator (UPA), which is released from vascular endothelial cells or renal epithelial cells, respectively. Thrombin also activates a protein called the *thrombin activatable fibrinolytic inhibitor* (TAFI), which removes lysine residues from fibrin resulting in inhibited binding of plasminogen and TPA to fibrin decreasing fibrinolysis. The active enzyme plasmin cleaves the fibrin clot into fragments of various sizes, called *fibrin split products* (FSPs). Split products that contain factor XIII–mediated cross-linked fibrin are called *D-dimer fragments.* Several proteins are responsible for regulating the coagulation process and ensuring that these powerful enzymes are not activated in the systemic circulation, causing uncontrolled blood clotting. The most important of these regulatory proteins are antithrombin, protein C, and the protein C cofactor protein S. Heparin cofactor II, alpha$_2$-macroglobulin, and alpha$_1$-antitrypsin also function as coagulation regulatory proteins. Plasminogen activator inhibitor (PAI), histamine-rich glycoprotein, and fibrin binding of plasminogen regulate the activation of fibrinolysis.

NORMAL VALUES

In general, healthy term and preterm infants have platelet counts within the normal adult range. A study of cord blood from more than 34,000 deliveries between 22 and 42 weeks of gestation determined mean platelet counts ranging from 200 to 250,000/μL that increased slightly with gestational age. However, the fifth percentile was slightly above or below 100,000/μL in otherwise well infants less than 33 weeks' gestation[12] (Figure 20-4). In this study, platelet counts increased rapidly following birth and the fifth percentile was 150,000/μL by 7 days regardless of gestational age. Certain tests of specific platelet function, including platelet aggregation to physiologic agonists, give somewhat decreased values at birth and for the first 3 weeks of age.[66] Classical aggregometry is difficult to perform in the neonatal period due to large required blood volume, but platelet function can be evaluated by in vitro activation followed by determination of activated platelets using flow cytometry.[67] The PFA-100 is a whole blood test that estimates platelet function by occlusion of a membrane coated with either collagen and epinephrine or collagen and ADP. The PFA-100 is most helpful in determining severe constitutional defects in platelet function, such as *Glanzmann's thrombasthenia.* However, platelet adhesion to collagen, mediated via the vWF, is increased at birth compared with well adults. The PFA-100, which measures global platelet function, demonstrates shorter closure time in a term neonate than in an adult.

The *coagulation system* of the newborn infant is unique in that blood clotting proteins mature at different rates (Table 20-4).[29] Mean levels of factors V and VIII and fibrinogen are within the normal adult range by 20 weeks of fetal development. Very low levels of these clotting proteins are never normal. The level of the vWF is elevated above adult

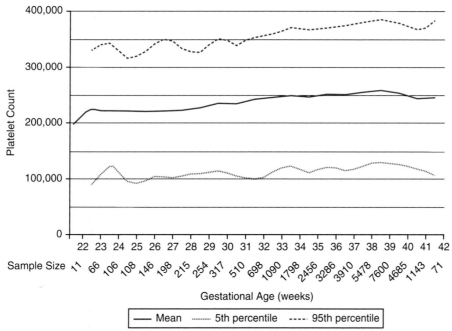

FIGURE 20-4 Reference ranges for platelet counts on the day of birth according to gestational age 22 to 43 weeks. Values were excluded from infants diagnosed with bacterial or fungal sepsis, necrotizing enterocolitis (NEC), or extracorporeal membrane oxigenation (ECMO). (From Christensen RD, Henry E, Del Vecchio A: Thrombocytosis and thrombocytopenia in the NICU, *J Matern Fetal Neonatal Med* 25:15-17, 2012.)

normal values at birth and the neonatal vWF protein subunits, called *multimers,* include ultralarge forms, which makes the protein more adherent to platelets and vessel walls. Fetal fibrinogen differs from the adult molecule in its increased content of sialic acid. This prolongs the thrombin time (TT) of the neonate, although the role of fetal fibrinogen as a risk factor for neonatal bleeding is unlikely. Vitamin K–dependent factors II, VII, IX, and X and protein C and protein S develop very slowly. Factor IX does not reach its full adult potential until 9 months of age; protein C may not reach adult levels until puberty. It is very difficult to determine if these proteins are genetically deficient during the neonatal period.

The clotting system is evaluated using a hemostasis screen, which includes testing for the activated partial thromboplastin time (aPTT), prothrombin time (PT), TT, fibrinogen concentration, and platelet count. A test of platelet function, such as the platelet function analyzer (PFA-100), can be included but is not standard. The aPTT may be within the adult range at term birth or may be slightly prolonged and achieve the adult range by 2 months. The aPTT of a stable preterm infant with a birth weight of less than 1000 g is often extremely prolonged, without signs of excessive bleeding.

The PT is usually near normal at birth, may prolong slightly by day 3, and reaches adult normal values by day 5. The TT is slightly prolonged because of fetal fibrinogen until 3 weeks of age. Fibrinogen mean is within the normal adult range at birth in stable term and preterm infants. However, a recent report of 175 preterm infants (excluding infants with early-onset infection, confirmed alloimmune thrombocytopenia or confirmed congenital coagulopathy such as hemophilia) showed a wide range of values with the 5th percentile of fibrinogen activity at 71 mg/dl and the 95th percentile at 535.[13] Global coagulation assays demonstrate that neonatal plasma generates less thrombin than adult plasma, but thrombin activity is generated following a shorter lag time than that determined in adult plasma.[68] Early thrombin generation in neonatal plasma, which is exaggerated in preterm plasma, has been related primarily to deficiencies in tissue

| TABLE 20-4 | COAGULATION FACTOR VALUES* FOR FETUS AND NEWBORN INFANT | | | | | | | | |

AGE-GROUP	I (mg/dl)	II	V	VII	VIII:C	vWF:Ag	IX	X	XI
Fetus (~20 wk)	96	0.16	0.70	0.21	0.50	0.65	0.10	0.19	—
	(40)	(0.10)	(0.40)	(0.12)	(0.23)	(0.40)	(0.05)	(0.15)	—
Preterm newborn (25-32 wk)	250	0.32	0.80	0.37	0.75	1.50	0.22	0.38	0.20
	(100)	(0.18)	(0.43)	(0.24)	(0.40)	(0.90)	(0.17)	(0.20)	(0.12)
Preterm newborn (33-36 wk)	300	0.45	0.82	0.59	0.93	1.66	0.41	0.44	—
	(120)	(0.26)	(0.48)	(0.34)	(0.54)	(1.35)	(0.20)	(0.21)	—
Term newborn (37-41 wk)	240	0.52	1	0.57	1.50	1.60	0.35	0.45	0.42
	(150)	(0.25)	(0.54)	(0.35)	(0.55)	(0.84)	(0.15)	(0.30)	(0.20)
Older infant (age and level when adult value is approximated)	340	0.97	1	0.90	0.93	1.13	0.7	0.55	0.52
	(21 days)	(45-60 days)	(1 day)	(21 days)	(1-2 days)	(1 wk)	(6 mo)	(6 wk)	(6 wk)

From Hathaway WE, Bonnar J: *Hemostatic disorders of the pregnant woman and newborn infant,* New York, 1987, Elsevier Science.

AT-III, Antithrombin III; *HMWK,* high-molecular-weight kininogen; *PK,* prekallikrein; *vWF,* von Willebrand factor.

Values (data taken from references discussed in text) are expressed in units per milliliter compared with normal adult subject reference plasma (100% = 1 U/ml); the mean and lower limit of range (or −2 SD) are shown.

*Clotting activity or chromogenic substrate methods (except protein C:Ag, protein S:Ag) in subjects in the first 24 hours of life.

†Cord blood. All other values are venous. All subjects received vitamin K at birth.

factor pathway inhibitor (TFPI) and secondarily to decreased antithrombin and impaired activity of protein C.[16,17]

Pathophysiology

THROMBOCYTOPENIA

Thrombocytopenia is a general term that denotes a decreased number of platelets in the infant's blood. Thrombocytopenia is the most common coagulation disorder in the neonate. Determine whether the infant appears well or ill. The causes of thrombocytopenia in an otherwise well infant differ from those in an acutely ill neonate (Box 20-6).

A well-appearing infant is likely to suffer from *neonatal alloimmune thrombocytopenia (NAIT),* in which the platelets are coated by circulating antibody and rapidly cleared from the circulation

by the spleen and liver. Alloimmune thrombocytopenia develops when the mother is negative for a platelet antigen, usually PLA-1, for which the father is positive. Fifty percent of recognized cases of NAIT occur in a mother's first infant. Subsequent infants can be more severely involved. Presentations of NAIT range from asymptomatic infants in whom a low platelet count is detected coincidentally on a blood count to fatal cases of intracranial hemorrhage with onset in utero. Infants of mothers with *idiopathic thrombocytopenic purpura* (ITP) may have a low platelet count because the maternal antibody crosses the placenta to the infant but usually do not develop life-threatening hemorrhage.

Constitutional thrombocytopenia is rare. Affected infants often manifest congenital skeletal malformations of the hands and arms. *Thrombocytopenia–absent radius (TAR) syndrome* is a

XII	PK	HMWK	XIII	PLASMINOGEN	ALPHA$_2$-ANTIPLASMIN	AT-III	PROTEIN C: Ag	PROTEIN S:Ag
—	—	—	≈0.30	—	—	0.23	0.10	—
—	—	—	—	—	—	(0.12)	(0.06)	—
0.22	0.26	0.28	0.11–0.40	0.35	74	0.35	0.29	—
(0.09)	(0.14)	(0.20)	—	(0.20)	(≈50)	(0.20)	(0.21)	—
0.25	0.33	—	—	0.38	73	0.40	0.38	—
(0.09)	(0.23)	—	—	(0.26)	(≈50)	(0.25)	(0.23)	—
0.44	0.35	0.64	0.61	0.49	83	0.56	0.50[†]	0.24[†]
(0.16)	(0.16)	(0.50)	(0.36)	(0.25)	(≈65)	(0.32)	(0.30)	(0.10)
1	0.86	0.82	1	1	1	0.82	0.82	—
(14 days)	(6 mo)	(6 mo)	(1 mo)	(6 mo)	(1 wk)	(3-6 mo)	(24 mo)	—

rare but well-characterized platelet syndrome. A bone marrow examination is important to evaluate the megakaryocyte pool. In *Bernard-Soulier syndrome* the platelet number is moderately decreased and giant platelets are seen on the peripheral smear. Infants with *trisomy 21 (Down syndrome)*, trisomy 18, or trisomy 13 can manifest abnormal platelet counts without apparent illness. The bone marrow of infants with Down syndrome is highly reactive. Other features of trisomy 21 should be present.

Infants with *large-cavernous hemangiomas* and *arteriovenous malformations* can also trap platelets and consume fibrinogen. Clues to these syndromes include skin hemangiomas; bruits over the liver, spleen, or brain; and high-output congestive heart failure with a structurally normal heart. *Kaposiform hemangioendothelioma (KHE)* is a specific vascular tumor associated with a severe, often life-threatening coagulopathy with platelet and fibrinogen trapping resulting in severe thrombocytopenia and hypofibrinogenemia that is known as the *Kasabach-Merritt phenomenon (KMP)*. KHE, the subject of a recent National Institute of Health Consensus Conference,[20] presents with affected infants showing a very low platelet number and fibrinogen with elevated D-dimer. Bleeding, including intracranial hemorrhage, can be life-threatening.

Sick infants usually manifest moderate thrombocytopenia. Bacterial and viral infections are the most common cause of thrombocytopenia in the newborn infant and must be excluded in any thrombocytopenic neonate. The infant of a mother with chorioamnionitis often demonstrates thrombocytopenia in the cord blood. Thrombocytopenia develops in most infants with

BOX 20-6	CAUSES OF THROMBOCYTOPENIA IN THE NEWBORN INFANT

1. Well infant
   a. Immune
      Alloimmune thrombocytopenia (NAIT)
      Maternal idiopathic thrombocytopenia purpura
   b. Constitutional
      Thrombocytopenia–absent radius syndrome
      Amegakaryocytic thrombocytopenia
      Wiskott-Aldrich syndrome
      Fanconi's anemia
      Bernard-Soulier syndrome
      Autosomal dominant thrombocytopenia
2. Sick infant
   a. Respiratory distress syndrome
   b. Bacterial sepsis
   c. Viral infection
   d. Necrotizing enterocolitis
   e. Hyperviscosity
   f. Disseminated intravascular coagulation
3. Infant appearing either well or sick
   a. Kasabach-Merritt (giant hemangioma) syndrome
   b. Trisomy 21, 18, 13
   c. Leukemia
   d. Thrombosis

NAIT, Neonatal alloimmune thrombocytopenia.

respiratory distress severe enough to require mechanical ventilation. The lowest platelet counts are usually found about day 3 of life, and normal counts recover by day 10 if the infant's course is not complicated by infection or thrombosis. Infants of less than 32 weeks' gestation with respiratory distress syndrome and severe thrombocytopenia are at increased risk for intracranial hemorrhage.

Thrombosis in a neonate often presents with an idiopathic falling platelet count. Thromboses are most commonly found at the tips of UACs and UVCs and can be diagnosed with ultrasound. An infected clot should be suspected in an infant with diagnosed catheter-related thrombosis and alterations in temperature, respiratory stability, or cardiovascular stability. Spontaneous thrombosis in the newborn most commonly manifests as renal vein or cerebral sinovenous thrombosis and arterial ischemic stroke.

Heparin-induced thrombocytopenia (HIT) has been described in neonates, especially babies with significant heparin exposure associated with cardiac surgery, cardiopulmonary bypass, or extracorporeal membrane oxygenation (ECMO). HIT is caused by antibodies that develop against a complex of heparin with platelet factor 4 on the platelet surface. When HIT is suspected all heparin must be promptly removed, including solutions used to flush catheters. *Direct thrombin inhibitors* can be used to anticoagulate infants during cardiac procedures or surgery. *Argatroban* and *bivalirudin* have been studied in the neonate with spontaneous hemorrhage, including intracranial hemorrhage, a major risk.[78,79]

DISSEMINATED INTRAVASCULAR COAGULATION

Thrombocytopenia in an ill infant is often part of the larger syndrome of DIC.[26] In DIC, activation of blood clotting proteins is initiated by tissue factor from bacterial products (endotoxin) or inflammation (cellular expression through protease activatable receptors) or through the contact system. The activation of clotting proteins leads to a hypercoagulable state and thromboses form, especially in the small vessels of the liver, spleen, brain, lungs, kidneys, and adrenal glands. The bone marrow and liver partially compensate by releasing platelets and clotting factors into the circulation. However, the regulatory system of coagulation is immature in term and preterm neonates. The capacity to neutralize activated clotting proteins is quickly exhausted, and the resulting deficiencies of platelets and clotting factors is called *consumptive coagulopathy.* Protein C deficiency is a major contributor to DIC in the newborn infant. Depletion of procoagulant proteins leads to bleeding and paradoxic bleeding, and thrombosis can occur simultaneously. DIC predisposes a preterm infant to intracranial hemorrhage. Venous thrombosis of the germinal matrix occurs as the initial lesion, followed by postthrombotic hemorrhage. Bleeding is also seen in the skin, around indwelling catheters, endotracheal tubes, and chest tubes; into the lungs and other parenchyma; and in the urine and stool.

LIVER FAILURE

The coagulopathy of liver failure is complex and includes thrombocytopenia, platelet dysfunction, decrease in synthesis of coagulation proteins in the liver, and enhanced fibrinolysis. Severe liver disease is characterized by a markedly abnormal PT in excess of aPTT prolongation. Liver failure in the neonatal period can result from viral hepatitis or rare metabolic disorders such as infantile hemochromatosis. Other signs of liver dysfunction, such as hepatomegaly, jaundice, and elevated liver enzymes, are present. Infants with liver dysfunction manifest bleeding into the skin, GI tract, retroperitoneum, and cranium. Invasive procedures, such as liver biopsy, can provoke severe bleeding.

CONGENITAL PLATELET DYSFUNCTION

Genetic platelet function defects causing severe bleeding in the neonatal period are rare. *Glanzmann's thrombasthenia* is an autosomal recessive disorder resulting from a severe deficiency or dysfunction in the platelet fibrinogen receptor GPIIb/IIIa. Severe neonatal bleeding, including intracranial hemorrhage, can occur. Platelet number is normal in this syndrome. Absent receptors can be determined by flow cytometry and genetic mutations have been determined, but all cases can be diagnosed by severe abnormalities on platelet aggregation studies or PFA-100.

Platelet storage pool disorders can be suspected from abnormal granule staining on the peripheral smear. *Hermansky-Pudlak syndrome* is a recessively inherited syndrome characterized by absence of platelet-dense granules and oculocutaneous albinism. *Chédiak-Higashi disease* is characterized by large, dysfunctional platelet granules. In *gray platelet syndrome,* the alpha granules are absent and the platelets have a pale appearance on the peripheral smear. Acquired platelet dysfunction can cause bleeding in the first several days of life in an infant after maternal use of aspirin or other drugs affecting platelet function shortly before delivery.

VITAMIN K DEFICIENCY

The most important bleeding syndrome in the otherwise stable neonate is hemorrhagic disease of the newborn, caused by vitamin K deficiency.[35] There is a tenfold gradient in vitamin K concentration between the maternal and fetal plasma. It is not known why fetal levels of vitamin K are maintained at low levels physiologically, but it has been speculated that because high levels of vitamin K are mutagenic in vitro, low levels of vitamin K may

be protective during the rapid cellular proliferation and differentiation in utero. Marginal fetal vitamin K levels are further compromised by maternal use of anticonvulsants or warfarin. Approximately 3% of cord blood samples from normal term pregnancies show biochemical evidence of noncarboxylated clotting proteins related to vitamin K deficiency.[63] *Early hemorrhagic disease of the newborn* presents within the first 24 hours of life with skin bruising, massive cephalohematoma, GI tract bleeding, or intracranial hemorrhage. Classic hemorrhagic disease of the newborn presents between 1 and 7 days of life; *late vitamin K deficiency* occurs between 1 week and 2 months of life. Intracranial hemorrhage caused by vitamin K deficiency is the leading cause of cerebral palsy in Southeast Asia. The recommendation of the American Academy of Pediatrics is to give every neonate 1 mg of vitamin K by intramuscular injection;[7] this is adequate to prevent bleeding in most infants (see Chapter 5). Vitamin K prophylaxis can be achieved with use of an oral vitamin K preparation. However, because oral therapy requires multiple doses over the first 6 weeks of life, it is difficult to ensure compliance and protect all infants using this formulation. Recommendations for oral vitamin K can be found in the European and Japanese literature (and in Chapter 5) where oral vitamin K repletion is more commonly practiced.[73] Vitamin K concentrations are physiologically very low in human breastmilk; cow's milk contains 10 times the amount of vitamin K (1.5 and 15 mg/L, respectively), but the bioavailability of vitamin K is greatly enhanced in infants receiving only breastmilk and greatly reduced in cow's milk. Infants fed breastmilk are at increased risk of vitamin K deficiency during the first week of life when milk production and fluid volume ingested may be low. In addition, infants with fat malabsorption caused by cystic fibrosis, alpha$_1$-antitrypsin deficiency, or biliary atresia and infants treated with prolonged courses of antibiotics are at increased risk of late vitamin K deficiency. All infants with late-onset vitamin K deficiency should be evaluated for a fat malabsorption syndrome.

HEMOPHILIA AND OTHER CONGENITAL BLEEDING DISORDERS

The *hemophilias* are a group of lifelong bleeding disorders caused by genetic deficiencies of one or more coagulation proteins. Factor VIII deficiency causes 80% of the hemophilias, and factor IX deficiency causes most of the remainder. Both factors VIII and IX are encoded on the X chromosome; thus deficiency states are manifested with carrier mothers (who manifest no or a mild bleeding disorder) and affected sons. Deficiencies of other coagulation factors are inherited as autosomal traits with severe bleeding manifested with homozygous or compound heterozygous deficiency. Most infants with hemophilia appear to tolerate labor and a routine vaginal delivery with no undue problems. However, intracranial hemorrhage has been documented in approximately 1% to 4% of infants with hemophilia as a result of birth trauma.[10,34] Current recommendations call for vaginal delivery in the absence of complications; however, cesarean section should be elected if needed to avoid prolonged or difficult labor. Use of vacuum extraction or forceps to assist delivery should be avoided. Approximately 50% of male infants with severe hemophilia will hemorrhage from a circumcision. The absence of procedure-related bleeding in the neonatal period does not exclude hemophilia, because hemostasis can be supported by physiologically increased platelet function around birth. Prolonged bleeding from the umbilical cord stump is suggestive of factor XIII deficiency. Spontaneous intracranial hemorrhage also occurs in infants with homozygous deficiency of factors V, VII, X, or XIII or fibrinogen.

Data Collection

HISTORY

A history of maternal bleeding, medical and obstetric diagnoses, and medications should be elicited for every infant at birth. A careful family history for bleeding disorders in the parents, grandparents, siblings, aunts, uncles, and cousins should be taken as part of every admission evaluation. Specific questions must be asked about excessive bleeding with surgeries (including dental procedures), menses, childbirth, traumas, and spontaneous bleeding events. Efforts should be made to obtain confirmatory medical records for any positive response. Procedures, including circumcision, should not be performed until the possibility of a bleeding disorder in the infant is excluded. The administration of vitamin K to the infant should be confirmed by review of the nursing notes.

SIGNS AND SYMPTOMS

Thrombocytopenia usually manifests with small, flat hemorrhages into the skin called *petechiae* that do not blanch with pressure. Petechiae may be concentrated in skin creases of the neck and axilla and around the site of a tourniquet or may be scattered over the entire body. More severe thrombocytopenia results in large *ecchymoses,* which are flat bruises. Infants with severe thrombocytopenia may hemorrhage into the central nervous system or GI tract.

Bleeding with coagulation disorders causes palpable *hematomas* of the skin and scalp. Large cephalohematomas are common and can result in a decreased hematocrit. Intracranial, retroperitoneal, intraperitoneal, GI, and genitourinary bleeding may occur. Bleeding with surgeries or procedures may be immediate or delayed. Three quarters of infants affected with severe hemophilia are diagnosed in the first month of life.

Hemangiomas are dark red raised lesions that blanch with pressure. KHE tumors are usually solitary indurated tumors with a pebbly rough surface and indistinct margins. The lesions may be associated with hypertrichosis or increased sweating. *Arteriovenous malformations* may not have skin manifestations but may have overlying swelling and warmth; an overlying bruit may be heard.

LABORATORY DATA

Any infant with bleeding signs should be evaluated with a hemostasis screen and a platelet count. The CBC should be obtained with attention to all cell lines. The peripheral smear should be carefully inspected for evidence of giant platelets or platelet clumping in the feathered edge of the smear. The results of the hemostasis screen in the healthy infant and during many states of illness are shown in Table 20-5. The possibility of hemophilia should be excluded by specific assay of factor VIII and factor IX. Severe *von Willebrand disease* can present with severe bleeding in the neonatal period and is diagnosed by a vWF activity that is 10 IU/dl. In addition, fibrinogen and factors XIII, alpha$_2$-antiplasmin, and plasminogen activator inhibitor-1 (PAI-1) should be assayed in a term infant with unexplained significant hemorrhage, such as intracranial hemorrhage. Platelet function should be assessed with a screening test, such as the PFA-100, bleeding time, or aggregation studies, if Glanzmann's or a similar congenital

TABLE 20-5	**COAGULATION RESULTS IN NORMAL NEONATES AND NEONATES WITH BLEEDING SYNDROMES**					

DESCRIPTION	PTT	PT	TT	F$_{IB}$	D-DIMER	P$_{LT}$ C$_T$
Healthy term	N-↑	N-↑	↑	NL	Neg	NL
Healthy preterm	↑↑	N-↑	↑	NL	Neg	NL
Vitamin K deficiency	↑↑	↑↑↑	↑	NL	Neg	NL
Liver disease	↑↑	↑↑↑	↑↑-↑↑↑	↓	Pos	↓
Hemophilia	↑↑↑	N-↑	↑	NL	Neg	NL
DIC	↑↑↑	↑↑	↑↑	↓	Pos	↓↓

Fib, Fibrogen; *N,* normal; *P$_{LT}$ C$_T$,* platelet count; *PT,* prothrombin time; *PTT,* partial thromboplastin time; *TT,* thrombin time; ↑, mildly prolonged; ↑↑, moderately prolonged; ↑↑↑, severely prolonged; ↓, decreased.

platelet dysfunction is suspected. Tests should be sent for HIT for infants who develop thrombocytopenia or a decrease in platelet count by 50% on heparin therapy in the absence of other obvious cause.

Treatment

THROMBOCYTOPENIA

Therapy for thrombocytopenia depends on the overall health and stability of the neonate, as well as the cause of the thrombocytopenia. In immune thrombocytopenia, antibodies that are affecting neonatal platelets also may cause rapid destruction of transfused platelets. Management of fetal and neonatal alloimmune thrombocytopenia has been recently reviewed.[69] Platelet antibodies in infants with NAIT do not react against maternal platelets, and washed maternal platelets are an effective therapy for affected infants with severe bleeding. Thrombocytopenia in this disorder, as well as maternal autoimmune thrombocytopenia, responds well to IVIG. Infants with alloimmune thrombocytopenia are likely to receive incompatible platelets from a random donor, and platelet transfusions, when needed, must be from a donor who shares maternal antigen profile if time and availability permit. If HIT is suspected, heparin should be stopped promptly, a blood sample sent for HIT testing, and alternative anticoagulation (e.g., with *argatroban* or *bivalirudin*) should be substituted, until test results are obtained. Although there have been no prospective randomized clinical trials, infants with KHE and KMP have been treated with steroids and vincristine, either agent along with antifibrinolytic agents (epsilon-aminocaproic acid or tranexamic acid), platelet inhibitors (aspirin, ticlopidine, clopidogrel), or interferon-α.[20] There is currently an ongoing clinical trial using sirolimus for vascular malformations that include KHE.

The primary support of most other thrombocytopenic infants is replacement transfusions of platelets, which are derived from CMV-reduced donor units. A stable, otherwise healthy infant can tolerate a platelet count as low as 20,000/µL without undue risk of serious bleeding. However, any infant who is less than 30 weeks of gestation, mechanically ventilated, on ECMO therapy, with indwelling UACs or UVCs, with chest tubes, or septic or otherwise unstable will require a platelet count of 50,000/µL to prevent or treat bleeding.

DISSEMINATED INTRAVASCULAR COAGULATION

Transfusion of platelets into infants with thrombosis or DIC may aggravate the platelet consumption unless specific therapy of the underlying condition also is administered. The primary treatment of DIC is reversal of the trigger (Box 20-7). Adequate ventilation, support of circulation and perfusion, treatment of sepsis, and general supportive care usually interrupt the DIC process within 48 hours. Routine infusion of FFP into infants with DIC without clinical bleeding does not improve infant outcomes, although infants with active bleeding require replacement of coagulation proteins and platelets to maintain minimal hemostatic levels.[26] Replacement of coagulation regulatory proteins in FFP or anti-thrombin (AT) concentrate or inhibition of coagulation activation with low-dose heparin is helpful in some cases.

BLEEDING DISORDERS

Infants with vitamin K deficiency are treated with vitamin K 1 mg by slow IV push or subcutaneous injection. FFP, 10 to 15 ml/kg, may be given to control active bleeding.

Neonates with severe liver disease can be treated for active bleeding or prepared for liver biopsy using transfusions of FFP and platelet concentrates. Parenteral administration of vitamin K should be confirmed; ongoing replacement may be necessary if there is fat malabsorption. There is no benefit to treating babies with liver disease and abnormal clotting tests but without clinical bleeding signs.[26] A recombinant preparation of activated factor VII (rFVIIa, NovoSeven, Novo Nordisk, Copenhagen, Denmark) has been used to control bleeding in the neonate in the setting of liver failure with encouraging results. Concentrates of vitamin K–dependent clotting factors purified from human plasma (prothrombin complex concentrates) and subjected to viral inactivation techniques are also available. These concentrates may be dosed at much smaller volumes than FFP and may be clinically useful for situations in which close attention must be paid to volume status. Consultation with a regional hemophilia treatment center about use

and availability of these specialized products is strongly recommended.

Treatment of congenital coagulation factor deficiencies is based on the deficient factor. The most specific and viral-safe product available should be used. Factor VIII or IX should be replaced in a bleeding neonate (or for surgery) using recombinant proteins. Factor VII may be replaced using rFVIIa in low doses of 15 to 25 mcg/kg every 6 to 12 hours. Viral-inactivated, human plasma–derived concentrates are available for vWF, fibrinogen, factor XIII, AT, and protein C. Factors II (prothrombin) and X may be replaced using prothrombin complex concentrates; a hemophilia center pharmacist should be consulted for factor concentrations in specific brands and lots. Factor XIII and fibrinogen may be replaced in cryoprecipitate. Replacement of factor V and other clotting proteins usually requires FFP. Desmopressin (DDAVP), a synthetic vasopressin that stimulates release of endothelial stores of factor VIII and the von Willebrand protein, is generally not used in the neonate because of the possibility of seizures related to hyponatremia in this age-group. Antifibrinolytic agents are effective for babies with severe deficiency of PAI-1. The hemophilia center should be involved in the diagnosis and management of all infants with congenital bleeding disorders.

Prevention and Parent Teaching

Mothers should be instructed during pregnancy that vitamin K deficiency is routinely prevented with an intramuscular (IM) injection of vitamin K to the neonate. Primary care providers should be careful to document administration of vitamin K, especially for infants born at home. For babies whose parents refuse IM vitamin K, even after education, oral supplementation should be offered.[73]

Bleeding in an infant with a bleeding disorder can be minimized by exerting care to prevent undue trauma. IM injections and other invasive procedures should be avoided if at all possible, although vitamin K may be safely administered to infants with severe hemophilia if a small-bore needle is used and care is taken not to Z-track the needle under the skin. The infant should be handled in as gentle a manner as possible. Pressure for holding and placement of a tourniquet should be minimized. Extreme care should be taken with arterial puncture.

Replacement platelet or clotting factor infusions should be considered before any necessary invasive procedure. Parents should be educated about the nature of the bleeding disorder and its cause in their infant. They should know whether this is a time-limited complication of the neonatal course or a long-term concern. Infants with constitutional thrombocytopenia or coagulopathy are at lifelong risk of bleeding. The risk of platelet sensitization and the consequent aim to minimize platelet exposure must be conveyed to the parents. Any other family member at risk of having a genetic thrombocytopenia or bleeding disorder should be identified, screened, and counseled.

Education of families about hemophilia or constitutional thrombocytopenia begins as soon as the diagnosis is established. Nurses should instruct parents about routine infant care and recognition of possible bleeding events in coordination with the hemophilia nurse coordinator.

THROMBOSIS

Pathophysiology

Thrombosis is an uncommon problem in pediatric patients, with increased incidence noted both in the neonatal period and after puberty. Physiologic correlates of the neonate's increased predisposition to thrombosis are shown in Boxes 20-8 and 20-9.

The most common sites of spontaneous thrombosis in the neonate are the renal veins, the central nervous system (CNS), the superior and inferior vena cava, and the aorta. Catheters placed for critical care support are associated with an increased risk of thrombosis.

Thrombosis in the stable term infant most often presents in the first few days of life and may be of fetal onset. In contrast, stroke and other thromboses in preterm infant are more often related to indwelling catheters and other underlying medical conditions; as such, presentation is often delayed.

PURPURA FULMINANS

Purpura fulminans is a syndrome of skin necrosis from thrombosis in the postcapillary venules caused by severe deficiencies of protein C or protein S.[28,40] Most cases are caused by homozygous or compound heterozygous genetic defects. Protein C or protein S is usually below the laboratory limit of detection. Screening coagulation tests are often

---

BOX 20-8 PROTHROMBOTIC CHARACTERISTICS OF NEONATAL BLOOD

- Increased hematocrit values
- Increased concentration and size of von Willebrand factor multimers
- Increased concentration of circulating tissue factor in preterm infants
- Low concentrations of physiologic anticoagulants, antithrombin, protein C, protein S, and tissue factor pathway inhibitor
- Low concentration of the fibrinolytic protein plasminogen
- Small-caliber, reactive blood vessels

BOX 20-9 PATHOLOGIC CONDITIONS PREDISPOSING TO THROMBOSIS IN THE NEONATE

- Hypotension
- Hyperviscosity
- Severe genetic and acquired deficiencies of antithrombin, protein C, protein S, and plasminogen[49,50]
- Genetic mutations in factor V and prothrombin; elevations in homocysteine and lipoprotein(a)
- Mechanical obstruction by catheters
- Maternal diabetes mellitus

---

normal initially but DIC quickly develops and can be controlled only by replacement of the missing protein. Purpura fulminans is uniformly fatal if untreated. Rarely, acquired deficiencies from maternal lupus anticoagulants can mimic these genetic syndromes.

Purpura fulminans complicating bacterial sepsis or meningitis has a similar pathophysiology to genetic deficiency and is caused by acquired consumption of protein C and protein S at the endothelial cell surface. Purpura fulminans associated with infection usually manifests at a later age and is less fulminant than the genetic syndromes.

THROMBOCYTOSIS

Inflammation following infection is the most common cause of *thrombocytosis* in the neonatal period. Thrombocytosis occurs with iron-deficiency anemia. An iron-deficient neonate may have suffered from chronic blood loss in utero, either by hemorrhage into the placenta, to a twin, or with GI bleeding. Following interruption of platelet consumption by thrombus, which occurs with successful implementation of anticoagulation, infants may often manifest thrombocytosis from increased bone marrow synthesis and release. *Neuroblastoma,* a malignancy of neural crest cells, and Down syndrome may also be associated with thrombocytosis. *Primary thrombocytosis* is a very rare syndrome that is seldom diagnosed in the neonatal period.

Data Collection

HISTORY

A history of thrombosis, including deep vein thrombosis, pulmonary embolism, heart attack, or stroke in persons under age 50 years in the parents, grandparents, siblings, aunts, uncles, and cousins of the infant, raises suspicion of genetic thrombophilia. Many family members affected with heterozygous deficiencies of antithrombin, protein C, or protein S are asymptomatic. A history of fetal or neonatal death with thrombosis is helpful. Maternal obstetric complications have been linked to thrombophilia. A maternal history of severe or recurrent preeclampsia, severe intrauterine growth restriction, three first-trimester losses, or any fetal death beyond 10 weeks' gestation indicates potential genetic thrombophilia. Maternal abnormalities of fibrinogen are associated with early pregnancy loss, as well as placental abruption. Maternal diabetes mellitus and placental transfer of antiphospholipid antibodies are causes of acquired neonatal thrombophilia.

SIGNS AND SYMPTOMS AND LABORATORY DATA

Thrombosis. Signs of decreased organ perfusion and subsequent dysfunction indicate the possibility of a thrombosis. The classic presentation of renal vein thrombosis includes hematuria, thrombocytopenia, and hypertension. Palpably enlarged kidneys may be noted on physical examination. The presence of unilateral or bilateral flank masses on the initial physical assessment indicates prenatal occurrence of renal vein thrombosis. *Stroke* usually presents with seizures during the first 24 hours of life. *Aortic thromboses* present with cool, pale extremities, decreased pulses and capillary refill, and upper extremity hypertension.

Confirmation of thrombosis is made with ultrasound examination of the renal veins and other abdominal vasculature, inferior vena cava and aorta, renal scan, and computed tomography or magnetic resonance imaging and angiography of the brain. Classic signs of arterial emboli include purple toes or fingers.

Purpura Fulminans. Purpura fulminans is a dramatic syndrome that usually manifests within hours of birth. Infants develop patchy areas of skin thrombosis over the trunk and buttocks, usually in dependent areas. The lesions are palpable and initially dark red, and quickly become dusky purple and then black; an eschar forms. The lesions are exquisitely painful. Most infants with severe protein C deficiency manifest a white light reflex of the eyes from in utero thrombosis of the primary vitreal veins with subsequent retinal detachment, hemorrhage, and blindness.

Imaging studies of the brain show evidence of CNS infarction in many infants. Renal vein thrombosis is not uncommon.

Thrombocytosis. Infants rarely manifest signs of thrombocytosis. Occasionally, platelet counts of greater than $2,000,000/\mu L$ are associated with cerebral ischemia and may manifest as poor feeding, irritability, lethargy, or a focal neurologic deficit.

LABORATORY EVALUATION

Before initiation of anticoagulation, a CBC including platelets and coagulation studies should be obtained. Because infants have physiologically prolonged baseline aPTT values, low and variable levels of antithrombin, and accelerated drug clearance, anticoagulation with heparin products should be monitored using an anti-Xa activity level, if at all possible. If anti-Xa levels are subtherapeutic on high doses of unfractionated heparin, consider checking an antithrombin level. In addition, infants who are refractory to the anticoagulant effects of unfractionated heparin often manifest an enhanced response to low-molecular-weight heparin. Screening for inherited thrombophilia should be guided by clinical presentation and family history.

Treatment

THROMBOSIS

The optimal therapy for neonatal thrombosis has not been determined. Two approaches include anticoagulation with unfractionated or low-molecular-weight heparin to prevent propagation of the clot or fibrinolytic therapy to dissolve

Anticoagulant Therapy

Unfractionated Heparin

Term infants: 100 U/kg bolus

25-50 U/kg/hr maintenance; adjusted to maintain anti-Xa activity level of 0.3-0.7 U/ml

Preterm infants: 50 U/kg bolus

15-35 U/kg/hr maintenance; adjusted to maintain anti-Xa activity level of 0.3-0.7 U/ml

Low-Molecular-Weight Heparin (Enoxaparin)

1.5 mg/kg subcutaneously every 12 hours; adjusted to maintain anti-Xa activity level of 0.5-1 U/ml 4 hours after injection

Consider FFP 10 ml/kg or AT concentrate 50-150 units/kg q 24-48 hr to enhance heparin effect, if heparin resistant

Fibrinolytic Therapy

Tissue Plasminogen Activator (TPA)

0.1-0.5 mg/kg/hr for 4-12 hr (bleeding risk is greater at the higher doses) or 0.06 to 0.12 mg/kg/hr for 12-48 hr

Fibrinolytic therapy has been given to neonates both as higher-dose, shorter infusions and lower-dose, longer-term infusions. The higher-dose infusions may be more effective in thromboses that are acute, arterial, and smaller in volume (e.g., aortic or cardiac). Lower, longer infusions may be more efficacious in larger, older, or venous thromboses (e.g., subclavian or extensive vena cava).

Contraindications to TPA: Intracranial hemorrhage, surgery or ischemia (poor Apgar scores) in previous 10 days; surgery within 7 days; invasive procedures within 72 hours; seizures within 48 hours; active bleeding.

Concomitant with TPA, may give heparin 10 U/kg/hr (no bolus) or enoxaparin 0.5 mg/kg every 12 hours subcutaneously

Consider FFP 10 ml/kg every 24 hours to replace plasminogen

Term infants show the highest dose requirements for unfractionated and low-molecular-weight heparin with increased volume of distribution and more rapid plasma elimination. Extremely preterm infants show the lowest dose requirements.

AT, Antithrombin; *FFP*, fresh frozen plasma; *TPA*, tissue plasminogen activator.

the clot, as shown in Box 20-10. In the absence of any significant contraindications, anticoagulation remains the standard of care for most neonatal thromboses. Neonates are relatively heparin resistant compared with older children and adults and have baseline antithrombin levels about 50% of the predicted value for adults.[44] Additionally, heparin has accelerated clearance and increased volume of distribution in the neonate, which can make it more difficult to achieve therapeutic anti–Xa levels.[47,63]

Off-label use of antithrombin concentrate has been increasing in this population to help achieve therapeutic anticoagulation in heparin-resistant neonates.[75] Newer anticoagulants have been developed that do not require antithrombin for therapeutic action, such as DTI. Several prospective studies, which included infants less than 6 months of age, have been conducted using either *bivalirudin* or *argatroban*.[78,79] These studies found low rates of clinically significant bleeding complications with early clot resolution, although severe bleeding, including intracranial hemorrhage, is an important risk of DTI, especially in sick preterm infants.[78,79] Large, prospective trials into the use of bivalirudin and argatroban in the neonatal population are needed. DTI should only be used in consultation with hematology.

Fibrinolytic therapy is intended to restore blood flow rapidly. However, the risk of hemorrhage is greater with fibrinolytic therapy, especially in preterm infants. Oozing around catheters is the most common bleeding complication of thrombolytic therapy, but the most important complication is CNS bleeding, which occurs most often in infants with brain ischemia from a previous episode of asphyxia or hypotension. Fibrinolytic therapy, if deemed acceptably safe, may be indicated for life- or limb-threatening aortic thrombosis and thromboses affecting shunts in infants with complex congenital heart disease.[24]

Thrombolytic therapy can be considered for bilateral renal vein thrombosis, although it should be recognized that many episodes of renal vein thrombosis have onset in utero and clots may be too organized for effective thrombolysis. Kidney enlargement and certain imaging features can be used to estimate age of clot. Long-term anticoagulation with warfarin or low-molecular-weight heparin is necessary only in the small proportion of infants who have an ongoing trigger for thrombosis or who have experienced a thrombus recurrence.

PURPURA FULMINANS

The treatment of neonatal purpura fulminans due to genetic thrombophilia is replacement of the deficient regulatory protein. A recombinant antithrombin protein produced in transgenic goats is Food and Drug Administration (FDA) approved for use (ATryn, GTC Biotherapeutics, Inc.). Viral-inactivated, human plasma–derived concentrates of protein C and antithrombin are FDA approved for severe deficiencies. Protein S and plasminogen for replacement are currently available only in FFP. The hemophilia center staff members are the best resources for information on the availability and safety of existing replacement proteins. FFP may be administered while confirmatory laboratory assays are being performed, using 10 ml/kg every 8 to 12 hours. Prophylactic replacement with protein C concentrate is currently available for infants with severe genetic protein C deficiency, although some infants may be medically managed with anticoagulation alone after the neonatal period and up until puberty.

Infants with acquired deficiencies of protein C or S due to autoantibodies may respond to IVIG or steroids in addition to plasma replacement. Infants with sepsis and purpura fulminans may require FFP or protein concentrate until antibiotics have successfully controlled their infection.

Parent Teaching

Parents of infants with severe genetic deficiencies of protein C or S require intensive teaching about administration and monitoring of anticoagulation therapy, observation for early lesions of purpura fulminans or bleeding, and care and rehabilitation of early lesions, which may lead to blindness, skin necrosis, and other lesions. Parents of children without severe thrombophilia, but who will be discharged to home on anticoagulation, require similar teaching about administration and monitoring of anticoagulation therapy and observation for bleeding complications.

WHITE BLOOD CELLS

Physiology

White cell production in the fetus begins relatively late in human gestation (14 to 16 weeks) and appears to be limited to the bone marrow, in contrast to erythropoiesis, which is found earlier in liver, spleen, and lymph nodes. The neutrophil reserve pool size is extremely small during the second trimester and increases slowly during gestation. At 18 to 20 weeks, the fetal total white count is approximately 4000 with 5% neutrophils.[41] This increases to 8.5%, or

350 absolute neutrophil count, by 26 to 30 weeks. Developmental levels of total granulocytes and neutrophils are shown in Figure 20-5. Thus the baby born at extreme prematurity has severely limited neutrophil capacity and is at increased risk for overwhelming bacterial infection.

White cell counts rise after normal delivery with a peak at 12 hours, and gradual decline over the subsequent 48 hours, as shown in Figure 20-6. Neutrophil counts must be evaluated with respect to postconceptual and postnatal age.

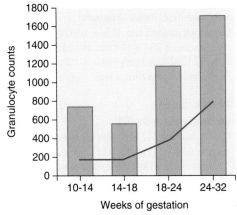

FIGURE 20-5 Mean and range of neutrophil counts at 10 to 14, 14 to 18, 18 to 24, and 24 to 32 weeks' gestational age. (From Thomas DB, Yoffe JM: The cellular composition of foetal blood, *Br J Haematol* 8:290, 1962.)

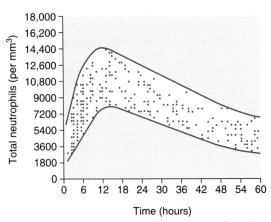

FIGURE 20-6 The total neutrophil count reference range in the first 60 hours of life. (From Monroe BL, Weinberg AG, Rosenfeld CR, et al: The neonatal blood count in health and disease. I. Reference values for neutrophilic cells, *J Pediatr* 95:89, 1979.)

Pathophysiology of Neutropenia

As with anemia, the etiology of neutropenia in the neonate can be divided into decreased production and shortened survival. Decreased production of neutrophils can result from maternal hypertension. Constitutional disorders causing neutropenia are rare, but most result in a predisposition to infections. *Reticular dysgenesis* is a severe defect leading to absent production of all myeloid cells, including neutrophils, monocytes, macrophages, and lymphocytes. *Kostmann's syndrome* is an autosomal recessive disorder resulting in severe neutropenia with monocytosis and eosinophilia. *Shwachman-Diamond* is another autosomal recessive syndrome of neutropenia associated with short stature, metaphyseal dysostoses, and pancreatic exocrine insufficiency. *Myelokathexis* is a disorder of intramedullary destruction and release of small numbers of neutrophils with abnormal morphology into the peripheral circulation. In *dyskeratosis congenita,* an X-linked disorder consisting of nail dystrophy, hyperpigmented dystrophic skin, and leukoplakia, one third of children develop neutropenia. In *cartilage-hair hypoplasia,* an autosomal recessive syndrome of short-limbed dysostosis, one fourth of children develop neutropenia or lymphopenia. There are genetic forms of *familial neutropenia* that are more mild and less symptomatic. Most benign congenital neutropenia is not associated with infection and is not often detected in the neonatal period.

Increased destruction of neutrophils is mediated by antibodies, infection, or inflammation. *Congenital acquired neutropenia* can result from maternal lupus or drugs, and is found in severe isoimmune hemolytic anemia. *Neonatal isoimmune neutropenia,* similar to NAIT, occurs in about 1 in 1000 live births, and often is an incidental finding on the CBC. Most neutropenia developing in the neonatal nursery results from infection or other stresses, including respiratory distress syndrome and intracranial hemorrhage.

The most common severe congenital disorder of neutrophil function is *chronic granulomatous disease* (CGD). CGD has an autosomal recessive inheritance and is characterized by normal neutrophil number but a failure of the granulocytic respiratory burst, and results in recurrent infections with organisms that produce catalase, such as *Staphylococcus aureus, Pseudomonas aeruginosa,* and *Burkholderia cepacia* (also known as *Pseudomonas cepacia*). Fungal infections, including *Aspergillus* species and *Candida albicans,* also occur in patients with CGD.

Data Collection

HISTORY

History should include questioning about maternal gestational complications, hypertension, collagen vascular disorders, and medications. Family history of previously affected infants and information about predisposition to or death during childhood from infections are important.

SIGN AND SYMPTOMS

Signs and symptoms of neutropenia follow primarily from related secondary infections. Although older infants may manifest fevers and aphthous ulcers with neutropenia, these are rarely apparent in newborn infants.

LABORATORY DATA

The CBC should be obtained with attention to all cell lines. The peripheral smear should be carefully inspected for evidence of abnormal neutrophil morphology.

Treatment

Infants with neutropenia must be evaluated for sepsis and other infections, and treated with appropriate antimicrobial agents while cultures are pending. Immune neutropenia responds to IVIG and steroids. CGD can be treated with granulocyte colony-stimulating factor and γ-interferon. Replacement IVIG has a role in defects that also affect lymphocyte production of antibodies. The role of transfused granulocytes is controversial and its use is most indicated for overwhelming infections with gram-negative organisms in severely neutropenic babies.

Prevention and Parent Teaching

The sequelae of some severe genetic neutropenias can be prevented with bone marrow transplantation. Important adjuvant approaches for all neutropenic babies include careful attention to hygiene when touching babies, infant skin care to prevent infections and avoid skin trauma, and recognition of early signs. Most acquired neutropenias in neonates are of short duration. Parents of babies with congenital neutropenia must be instructed about the diagnosis, underlying defect, available treatments, and long-term prognosis.

REFERENCES

For a full list of references, scan the QR code or visit http://booksite.elsevier.com/ 9780323320832.

21 NEONATAL HYPERBILIRUBINEMIA

BEENA D. KAMATH-RAYNE, ELIZABETH H. THILO, JANE DEACON, AND JACINTO A. HERNÁNDEZ

Unconjugated hyperbilirubinemia is the most common condition requiring evaluation and treatment in neonates, but for most newborns it is a benign postnatal transitional phenomenon of no overt clinical significance. Neonatal hyperbilirubinemia is manifested by jaundice, the yellow-orange tint usually detected visually in the sclera and skin of infants with total serum bilirubin concentration between 6 and 7 mg/dl. Despite the cause-and-effect relationship, the terms *neonatal hyperbilirubinemia* and *neonatal jaundice* are used fairly interchangeably. All infants experience a rise in their serum bilirubin concentration after birth because of brisk bilirubin formation and an immature liver that cannot clear the bilirubin from the blood. It is estimated that about 60% to 80% of normal newborns will appear clinically jaundiced during the first week of life.[22,35,48] Despite this, the incidence of extreme hyperbilirubinemia and kernicterus is low[11,65] (Box 21-1).

Severe hyperbilirubinemia, defined as total serum bilirubin above the 95th percentile for age in hours, occurs in 8% to 9% of infants during the first week of life.[8,9] Experience has shown the dangers of excessive concentrations of unconjugated bilirubin, such as the development of bilirubin encephalopathy and the devastating and irreversible effects of kernicterus. An understanding of the pathophysiology and clinical significance of hyperbilirubinemia is critical in the care of newborn infants. This chapter provides the reader with a basic overview of the multiple causes and contributing factors in the development of hyperbilirubinemia; describes the diagnosis, clinical significance, and complications of

hyperbilirubinemia; and discusses current treatment modalities and their complications.

PATHOPHYSIOLOGY

To understand the pathophysiology and clinical significance of hyperbilirubinemia, normal bilirubin metabolism in the newborn must be reviewed (Figure 21-1). A newborn has a rate of bilirubin production of 8 to 10 mg/kg/24 hr, which is 2 to 2.5 times the rate in adults. Red blood cells in newborns have a shortened life span of 70 to 90 days, compared with 120 days in adults, and the newborn has a higher red cell mass per kilogram weight compared with the adult. Because the catabolism of *1 g of hemoglobin yields 35 mg of bilirubin*, this accelerated red blood cell breakdown produces most of the bilirubin (75% to 85%) in newborns. The remaining 15% to 25% of bilirubin is derived from nonerythroid heme proteins found principally in the liver, and heme precursors in the marrow and extramedullary hematopoietic areas that do not go on to form red blood cells (referred to as "early peak" or "shunt" bilirubin).

Bilirubin metabolism is initiated in the reticuloendothelial system, principally in the liver and spleen, as senescent or abnormal red blood cells are removed from the circulation. The enzyme *heme oxygenase* will act on heme to produce biliverdin, and *biliverdin reductase* will then convert biliverdin into bilirubin. This bilirubin, in its unconjugated or indirect-reacting form, is released into the plasma, where it is bound to albumin for

PURPLE type highlights content that is particularly applicable to clinical settings.

transport. Exhaled carbon monoxide is an end product of these pathways.

At a normal plasma pH, bilirubin is very poorly soluble and binds tightly to circulating albumin, which serves as a carrier protein. Albumin contains one high-affinity site for bilirubin and one or more sites of lower affinity. Bilirubin binds to albumin in a molar ratio of between 0.5 and 1 mole of bilirubin per mole of albumin. A bilirubin/albumin molar ratio of 1 corresponds to approximately 8.5 mg bilirubin/g of albumin. This ratio is likely to be lower in a sick very-low-birth-weight (VLBW) infant, who is also likely to have a lower serum albumin concentration.[16] It is important to note that the total serum bilirubin (TSB) is the concentration of albumin-bound bilirubin; the concentration of unconjugated, unbound bilirubin ("free bilirubin") is potentially more important in prediction of neuronal injury, but measurement is not yet commercially available.[3]

Bilirubin bound to albumin is carried to the liver and dissociates from circulating albumin before entering the liver cell. The process of entering the liver cell occurs partly by a passive process of carrier-mediated diffusion involving the sinusoidal transporter SLCO1B, and partly by mediation by organic anion transporter proteins (OATPs). In the liver cell cytoplasm, the unconjugated bilirubin is bound to glutathione-S-transferase A, also known as *ligandin,* or with B-ligandin (Y protein). These

are major intracellular transport proteins, and their bilirubin binding ability helps keep the potentially toxic unbound portion low. Z protein, another hepatic cytoplasmatic carrier, also binds bilirubin but with lower affinity.[29,64] Conjugation occurs within the smooth endoplasmic reticulum of the cell. This reaction, catalyzed by the enzyme *uridine diphosphate glucuronosyl transferase (UGT-1A1),* leads to the formation of water-soluble compounds called *bilirubin glucuronides.* UGT-1A1 is the predominant isoenzyme, and arises from the *UGT1* gene complex on chromosome 2(2q37).[63] In addition to UGT-1A1, conjugation requires glucuronic acid synthesized from glucose. Conjugated bilirubin is then actively secreted into bile and passes into the small intestine.

Conjugated bilirubin is not reabsorbed from the intestine, but the mucosal brush border of the newborn contains the enzyme *beta-glucuronidase,* which can convert conjugated bilirubin back into glucuronic acid and unconjugated bilirubin, which may be absorbed. This pathway constitutes the enterohepatic circulation of bilirubin and contributes significantly to an infant's bilirubin load.[22]

Factors That Affect Bilirubin Levels

The ability of albumin to bind bilirubin is affected by a number of different factors, including plasma pH, free fatty acid concentrations, and certain drugs, particularly sulfonamides and ceftriaxone. Albumin binding of unconjugated bilirubin may be important in the prevention of bilirubin toxicity, by limiting the amount of unbound, unconjugated bilirubin available for causing neuronal damage.[3,40,47] Consequently, serum albumin concentration may be measured as an estimate of available binding capacity, perhaps allowing a better estimation of the concentration at which aggressive phototherapy and exchange transfusion should be considered in a particular infant.[5]

Newborn monkeys have been shown to be deficient in the intracellular Y and Z proteins for the first few days of life, and this also may occur in the human newborn. The hormonal (estrogen) environment of the infant may inhibit liver function and bilirubin secretion. A rise in bilirubin levels shortly after birth is also partially attributable to a relative deficiency of UDPGT activity (0.1% of adult levels at 30 weeks of gestation, 1% of

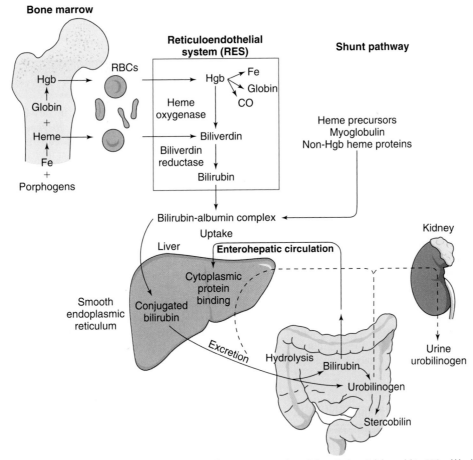

FIGURE 21-1 Bilirubin physiology: pathways of bilirubin production, transport, and metabolism. *Fe,* Iron; *Hgb,* hemoglobin; *RBC,* red blood cells; *CO,* carbon monoxide. (Adapted from Gartner LM, Hollander M: Disorders of bilirubin metabolism. In Assali NS, editor: *Pathophysiology of gestation,* vol 3, New York, 1972, Academic Press.)

adult levels by 40 weeks of gestation). Enzyme activity increases rapidly after birth independent of the infant's gestational age, achieving adult concentrations by 14 weeks of age.[63]

Certain ethnic groups, including Eskimo, Asian, and Native American, have an increased incidence and severity of hyperbilirubinemia for reasons that are not completely understood, but are likely related to genetic polymorphisms involving UGT-1A1 activity.[24,64] The presence of *beta-glucuronidase* in the bowel lumen during fetal life enables bilirubin to be reabsorbed and transported across the placenta for excretion by the maternal liver; its presence in the neonate, however, contributes to an excessive enterohepatic circulation of bilirubin.

Physiologic Jaundice

Debate and controversy remain over efforts to define normal or physiologic ranges of TSB concentrations in normal full-term newborn infants, because the data are affected by multiple variables. Traditionally, a distinction has been made between physiologic jaundice and hyperbilirubinemia that is either pathologic in origin or severe enough to be considered for further evaluation and intervention. This entity has been called *nonphysiologic,* although frequently, no disease is identified as being causative.[33] Data from multiple studies consider that the 97th percentile of maximal TSB concentration in healthy mature newborns is 12.4 mg/dl for formula-fed infants and 14.8 mg/dl for breastfed infants.[4,9,45] Any TSB elevation exceeding 17 mg/dl should be presumed pathologic and warrants investigation for a cause and possible therapeutic intervention, such as phototherapy.

In the normal full-term newborn, the clinical course of physiologic jaundice is characterized by a rapid and progressive increase in TSB concentration from about 2 mg/dl in cord blood to a mean peak of 5 to 6 mg/dl between 3 and 4 days of life *(phase I physiologic jaundice)*. This is followed by a rapid decline to about 3 mg/dl toward the end of the first week of life and then continues with a period of minimal, slowly declining TSB concentration until reaching the normal adult level of less than 2 mg/dl at the end of the second week of life *(phase II physiologic jaundice)*. Several criteria have been proposed that can be used to exclude the diagnosis of physiologic jaundice in a full-term infant: (1) clinical jaundice in the first 24 hours of life, (2) TSB concentration that increases more than 0.2 mg/dl per hour, (3) TSB concentration exceeding the 95th percentile for age in hours, (4) direct serum bilirubin levels exceeding 1.5 to 2 mg/dl, or (5) clinical jaundice persisting for more than 2 weeks. However, absence of these criteria does not guarantee that the jaundice is physiologic.

ETIOLOGY OF HYPERBILIRUBINEMIA

Bilirubin concentrations rise in newborn infants by three main mechanisms: increased production (accelerated red blood cell breakdown), decreased excretion (transient UGT-1A1 insufficiency),[50] and increased reabsorption (enterohepatic circulation) (Box 21-2). The normal pathways of bilirubin metabolism described earlier account for much of the increase in bilirubin concentrations in newborn infants; however, the following circumstances deserve special attention for infants who have a more prolonged hyperbilirubinemia.

From a management perspective, it is helpful to describe severe hyperbilirubinemia according to its time of onset, early (first 24 to 48 hours) or late (after 48 to 96 hours), to determine its specific etiology. In general, early-onset severe hyperbilirubinemia is associated with increased bilirubin production, whereas later-onset hyperbilirubinemia is often associated

---

BOX 21-2   CAUSES OF HYPERBILIRUBINEMIA

Overproduction
- Hemolytic disease of the newborn (antibody-mediated hemolysis: Rh, ABO, Kell, Duffy)
- Hereditary hemolytic anemia
  - Membrane defects (spherocytosis, elliptocytosis, pyknocytosis)
  - Hemoglobinopathies
  - Enzyme defects (G6PD deficiency)
- Polycythemia
- Extravascular blood
  - Swallowed
  - Bruising or enclosed hemorrhage (e.g., cephalhematoma)
- Increased enterohepatic circulation (prematurity, delayed feedings, bowel obstruction)

Slow Excretion
- Decreased hepatic uptake
  - Decreased sinusoidal perfusion
  - Ligandin deficiency and SLCO1B1 deficiency

- Decreased conjugation
  - UGT-1A1 deficiency (Crigler-Najjar syndrome, Gilbert syndrome)
  - Enzyme inhibition, such as the Lucey-Driscoll syndrome
- Inadequate transport out of hepatocyte
- Biliary obstruction (Dubin-Johnson syndrome, Rotor syndrome, biliary atresia)

Combined (Overproduction and Slow Excretion)
- Bacterial infection
- Congenital intrauterine infection

Breastfeeding
- Breastfeeding jaundice ("lack of breastmilk" jaundice)
- Breastmilk jaundice

Physiologic

Miscellaneous
- Galactosemia
- Hypothyroidism
- Infant of diabetic mother

with delayed bilirubin elimination with or without increased bilirubin production (Figure 21-2).[31]

Overproduction of Bilirubin

HEMOLYTIC DISEASE OF THE NEWBORN

Hemolytic disease of the newborn may occur when blood group incompatibilities such as Rh, ABO, or minor blood groups exist between a mother and her fetus (see also Chapter 20). The classic example of hemolytic disease of the newborn has been erythroblastosis fetalis occurring as a result of Rh incompatibility. Fifteen percent of the white population is Rh negative. When an Rh-negative mother is sensitized to the Rh antigen following a blood transfusion or a fetal-maternal contamination during pregnancy, delivery, abortion, or amniocentesis, the presence of the Rh antigen induces maternal antibody production. Because prior sensitization with the Rh antigen is necessary for antibody production, the first Rh-positive infant usually is not affected. Once a mother is sensitized, an anamnestic response to further exposure causes maternal immunoglobulin G (IgG) to cross the placenta into the fetal circulation where it reacts with the Rh antigen on fetal erythrocytes. These antibody-coated cells are recognized as abnormal and destroyed by the fetal spleen. This results in increased amounts of heme requiring metabolic degradation. As the destruction of erythrocytes and production of bilirubin progress, severe anemia and congestive heart failure can ensue, progressing to hydrops fetalis. Fortunately, the use of anti-D gamma globulin (RhoGAM), particularly antenatal administration at 26 to 28 weeks' gestation to prevent sensitization of nonsensitized pregnant Rh-negative women, has markedly decreased the incidence of Rh isoimmunization and the resulting hyperbilirubinemia in newborn infants.

Early-onset hyperbilirubinemia (age < 72 hours)		Late-onset hyperbilirubinemia (age >72 hours and <2 weeks)
First 24 hours of life	**First week of life**	**>1 week of life**
Direct Coombs' positive: • Isoimmune erythroblastosis fetalis • Rhesus disease • Minor blood group incompatibilities • ABO (often the direct Coombs' is negative)	Benign idiopathic jaundice (physiologic; <40th percentile)	Prolonged idiopathic jaundice (breast milk jaundice; TSB <13 mg/dL)
	Sepsis (viral or bacterial)	Sepsis (viral or bacterial)
	Increased enterohepatic circulation	Functional gastrointestinal tract abnormality
Direct Coombs' negative: • G6PD deficiency • Intrinsic red blood cell defect • Spherocytosis • Elliptocytosis • Hemoglobinopathies	Disorders of bilirubin metabolism: • UGT1A1 gene polymorphisms (delayed conjugation) • Co-inheritance of UGT1A1 polymorphism with G6PD deficiency, ABO incompatibility, spherocytosis • Crigler-Najjar syndrome: I and II • Gilbert syndrome • Others Metabolic disorders: • Galactosemia • Alpha$_1$-antitrypsin deficiency • Storage diseases • Others	
	Enclosed hemorrhages: • Cephalohematoma • Subaponeurotic hemorrhage • Bruising	Cystic fibrosis Hypothyroidism

FIGURE 21-2 Differential diagnosis of severe neonatal hyperbilirubinemia based on pathophysiology and timing at presentation. *G6PD*, Glucose-6-phosphate dehydrogenase; *TSB*, total serum bilirubin. (Modified from Smitherman H, Stark AR, Bhutani VK: Early recognition of neonatal hyperbilirubinemia and its emergent management, *Semin Fetal Neonatal Med* 11:214, 2006.)

With the widespread use of RhoGAM, the most frequent cause of hemolytic disease of the newborn is now ABO blood group incompatibility. ABO incompatibility is limited to mothers of blood group O and affects infants of blood group A or B. All group O individuals have naturally occurring anti-A and anti-B (IgG) antibodies, so specific sensitization is not necessary. The resulting hyperbilirubinemia in the newborn is highly variable and generally milder than that seen with Rh incompatibility. Although some 15% of pregnancies are a "set-up" for ABO incompatibility (mother O, baby A or B), only 33% of these infants show a positive direct antiglobulin test (DAT), and only 15% of these, or 5% of the "set-ups," have clinically significant hemolysis and hyperbilirubinemia. If the DAT is negative, these infants, as a group, do not have an increased incidence of significant hyperbilirubinemia compared with non-ABO incompatible infants.[63]

HEREDITARY HEMOLYTIC ANEMIAS

Erythrocytes with abnormal membranes or containing abnormal hemoglobin variants have increased rates of red blood cell destruction. Individuals with *membrane defects*, such as spherocytosis, elliptocytosis, stomatocytosis, and pyknocytosis, cannot maintain the integrity of red blood cells because of abnormal osmotic fragility (generally increased) and an increased rate of splenic destruction (see Chapter 20). A mean corpuscular hemoglobin concentration greater than 36 g/dl may be a clue to the diagnosis of hereditary spherocytosis.[63]

Glucose-6-phosphate dehydrogenase (G6PD) deficiency is the most common enzyme defect and is more commonly found in certain racial and ethnic groups, including East Asian, Mediterranean, and African peoples. Pyruvate kinase deficiency is much less common. G6PD deficiency affects some 400 million individuals worldwide.[12] G6PD deficiency is also common in the United States, with an estimated overall incidence of 3.4%. Up to 12.5% of African American males and 4% of African American females are G6PD deficient.[13] Although G6PD deficiency is an X-linked recessive disease, affecting males and homozygous females, heterozygous females may also be phenotypically deficient due to X chromosome inactivation. Affected infants may occasionally present with acute hemolysis and severe hyperbilirubinemia in response to exposure to an oxidative trigger (infection, starvation, or drug exposure, notably sulfonamides), but more commonly present with later-onset (end of first week of age) hyperbilirubinemia without significant anemia.[66] The combination of G6PD deficiency with Gilbert's disease (another common genetic variation involving partial UGT-1A1 deficiency) makes infants especially prone to the development of later-onset severe hyperbilirubinemia without significant hemolysis or anemia.[28,62]

Individuals with *hemoglobinopathies*, which can be diagnosed by hemoglobin electrophoresis, may also have increased splenic destruction of red blood cells, although most do not manifest clinically in the newborn period. The exceptions are the alpha-thalassemia syndromes wherein three or four of the four globin genes are affected, resulting in hemoglobin H disease (three genes affected) or homozygous alpha-thalassemia (absence of all four genes for alpha globin synthesis). Hemoglobin H disease can manifest as hemolysis and anemia in the neonate, and homozygous alpha-thalassemia regularly causes severe hemolysis, anemia, hydrops fetalis, and death.[63] A family history is important, because it may be positive in as many as 80% of cases.

POLYCYTHEMIA

Polycythemia (with a central venous hematocrit value greater than 65) is the condition in which an increased red blood cell mass, coupled with the shortened life span of these cells found in all newborns, results in an increased bilirubin load. Polycythemia may be idiopathic, or it may occur as a result of a maternal-fetal transfusion, twin-to-twin transfusion, chronic in utero hypoxia, or delayed clamping of the umbilical cord at the time of delivery.

EXTRAVASCULAR BLOOD

Enclosed hemorrhage includes cephalohematoma, subgaleal hemorrhage, cerebral hemorrhage, adrenal hemorrhage, intraabdominal or retroperitoneal bleeding, or extensive bruising. As these enclosed hemorrhages resolve, red blood cells trapped within are broken down and add to bilirubin production. Swallowed maternal blood is another possible source of increased bilirubin load.

INCREASED ENTEROHEPATIC CIRCULATION

As mentioned, the intestinal brush border contains the enzyme *beta-glucuronidase*, which can convert conjugated bilirubin back into its unconjugated (absorbable) form plus glucuronic acid. Meconium contains a substantial amount of bilirubin, estimated at 1 mg of bilirubin per 1 g of meconium, or a total load of 100 to 200 mg. Any delay in the passage of meconium, as can occur with prematurity, delayed feedings, or bowel obstruction, increases the bilirubin load that must be metabolized. Hyperbilirubinemia requiring treatment due to these causes is rarely evident in the first 24 to 48 hours of life.

Slow Excretion of Bilirubin

Infants with normal bilirubin production rates may be unable to remove this load for a variety of reasons, as described in the following conditions.

DECREASED HEPATIC UPTAKE OF BILIRUBIN

Diminished hepatic uptake of bilirubin may be a result of inadequate perfusion of hepatic sinusoids or of deficient carrier proteins (Y and Z). *Inadequate perfusion* of hepatic sinusoids occurs when there is a shunt through a persistent ductus venosus or due to an extrahepatic portal vein thrombosis, or with hyperviscosity or hypovolemia, as seen in infants with severe congestive heart failure. *Functional deficiency* of the transporter proteins may be caused by certain drugs and compounds (e.g., steroid hormones, free fatty acids, chloramphenicol) that competitively bind to them. Although Y and Z proteins are decreased in some newborn primates, no actual deficiency has yet been demonstrated in the human newborn.

DECREASED BILIRUBIN CONJUGATION

Decreased bilirubin conjugation may be a result of *UGT-1A1 deficiency*, as in the Crigler-Najjar syndrome or Gilbert syndrome.[53] These disorders are caused by defects in the *UGT-1A1* gene complex recently identified on chromosome 2. Newer thinking is that these diseases represent a continuous spectrum of severity. *Crigler-Najjar syndrome* is rare and exists in two forms with either complete (type I) or partial (type II) absence of enzymatic activity. Type I is an autosomal recessive disorder, resulting in an inactive UGT-1A1 enzyme, putting the infant at significant risk of bilirubin encephalopathy. Phototherapy becomes ineffective in preventing toxicity, and liver transplantation is the only possible cure. Type II Crigler-Najjar syndrome is characterized by

low but detectable concentrations of the enzyme and more moderate degrees of hyperbilirubinemia.[63] It is inherited as an autosomal dominant disorder and responds to enzyme induction with phenobarbital.

Gilbert syndrome is a milder and very common autosomal dominant disorder with partial UGT-1A1 enzyme activity caused by a number of polymorphisms in the *UGT-1A1 promoter sequence*, usually involving the number of TA base pair repeats. As the number of TA repeats increases above the normal 6, UGT-1A1 activity declines.[62] Approximately 9% of the U.S. population is homozygous for the promoter sequence polymorphism responsible for Gilbert's syndrome and shows a 50% reduction in UGT-1A1 activity, whereas 42% of the population is heterozygous and shows a 37% reduction in enzyme activity. Although Gilbert syndrome generally manifests after the newborn period with mild bilirubin elevation during times of stress, fasting, or intercurrent illness, it is also an important contributing factor in cases of late-onset severe hyperbilirubinemia, even in the absence of significant hemolysis.[53] In the neonate, where total serum bilirubin is a delicate balance between production and elimination, even a small decrease in bilirubin elimination can have a major impact on degree of hyperbilirubinemia. Although neither G6PD deficiency nor Gilbert syndrome alone is associated with an increased incidence of hyperbilirubinemia, both together are associated with severe hyperbilirubinemia.[13,65]

Gilbert syndrome does not lead to chronic liver inflammation or fibrosis and is therefore not life-limiting. Liver biopsy is unnecessary and histology is normal. Confirmation of the diagnosis is possible by genotyping. A variety of additional studies suggest that variations of the *UGT-1A1* genotype affects more than just bilirubin metabolism and may play a role in other diseases and in drug disposition. The clearance of lorazepam, for instance, is reduced by 20% to 40% in individuals with Gilbert syndrome.

INADEQUATE TRANSPORT OUT OF THE HEPATOCYTE

Dubin-Johnson syndrome (DJS) and *Rotor syndrome*[51] are genetically inherited conditions that are both autosomal recessive and have a similar phenotype in which individuals can conjugate bilirubin normally but cannot excrete it. In DJS, a mixed elevation in both conjugated and unconjugated bilirubin is seen, due to impairment in the biliary excretion of organic anions (except bile acids). Rotor syndrome has a different underlying mechanism, with impaired hepatocellular storage of conjugated bilirubin. Both conditions are considered benign and do not require treatment. Liver biopsy is not recommended for making the diagnosis, because it will be unlikely to show abnormalities. Urine coproporphyrin excretion is helpful to differentiate the two disorders: in DJS, coproporphyrin concentrations will be normal, but comprised predominantly of coproporphyrin I, as opposed to coproporphyrin III as seen in normal individuals. In Rotor syndrome, the total urine coproporphyrin concentration is 2 to 5 times the normal amount, with the majority being coproporphyrin I.

BILIARY OBSTRUCTION

Biliary obstruction often is seen as a diagnostic dilemma requiring differentiation between generalized hepatocellular damage and mechanical obstruction.

A variety of disorders can cause hepatocellular damage, including infections, such as hepatitis, and metabolic disorders, such as galactosemia. In the neonatal intensive care unit (NICU), the most common cause of hepatocellular damage is the use of parenteral nutrition. The mechanism is not well established, but the injury takes at least 2 weeks to develop and is especially prominent in VLBW infants. Biliary atresia or, much less frequently, a choledochal cyst can cause mechanical obstruction to bile flow, resulting in a conjugated hyperbilirubinemia with light-colored stools.

Combined Overproduction and Slow Excretion

INFECTIONS

Bacterial infections (sepsis neonatorum, especially necrotizing enterocolitis and urinary tract infection caused by toxin-producing organisms such as certain strains of *Escherichia coli*) or intrauterine viral infections can result in increased bilirubin production and decreased hepatic clearance.

Intrauterine infections, including syphilis, toxoplasmosis, rubella, cytomegalovirus, herpes simplex, coxsackie B virus, and hepatitis virus, cause clinical jaundice with evidence for hepatocellular damage (elevated liver enzymes, poor synthetic function, coagulopathy). Infants with these infections often have additional clinical signs of their infection such as thrombocytopenia and rash.

INFANT OF A DIABETIC MOTHER

The cause of hyperbilirubinemia in an infant of a diabetic mother (IDM) appears to be multifactorial. In addition to prematurity and a tendency to feed poorly, leading to delayed intestinal motility and enhanced enterohepatic circulation, an IDM may have an increased bilirubin load as a result of an expanded red blood cell mass. Erythrocyte membrane composition may be altered, and macrosomic infants often are bruised during labor and delivery. Evaluation of exhaled CO in IDM infants has consistently shown evidence for increased production of bilirubin.[34,51]

Jaundice Associated With Breastfeeding

Numerous studies have reported an association between exclusive breastfeeding and an increased incidence and severity of hyperbilirubinemia, both during the first few days of life and in the genesis of prolonged neonatal jaundice.[5,23,34,62] Breastfed infants are several times more likely to have TSB concentrations greater than 12 mg/dl than infants who are formula fed (13% vs. 4%). As such, exclusive breastfeeding, particularly if nursing is not going well and weight loss is excessive, is listed as a major hyperbilirubinemia risk factor. Promotion and support of successful breastfeeding constitutes a key element of the American Academy of Pediatrics (AAP) clinical practice guideline on the management of hyperbilirubinemia.[5] Ideally, a trained observer should evaluate all breastfed infants within 48 to 72 hours of discharge in either a home or office setting. Early discharge of breastfed infants with inadequate follow-up may result in extreme hyperbilirubinemia and kernicterus, even in the absence of hemolysis.[11]

Two separate patterns of jaundice in breastfeeding infants have been described. The first one has been termed *breastfeeding-associated jaundice* and the second *breastmilk jaundice*.

BREASTFEEDING-ASSOCIATED JAUNDICE

It is important to recognize that not all breastfed infants will receive optimal milk intake during the first few days of life; as many as 10% to 18% of exclusively breastfed newborns lose more than 10%

of birth weight.[18] It has been postulated that this early jaundice is related to decreased caloric and fluid intake from colostrum (sometimes called "lack of breastmilk" jaundice)[41] and increased enterohepatic circulation resulting from low stool output and breastmilk containing beta-glucuronidase.[5,46] Many studies show a relationship between the degree of hyperbilirubinemia and the amount of weight lost by the infant after birth.[1,62] Breastfeeding-associated jaundice, however, is not due to increased bilirubin production.

Optimal management of a breastfeeding mother and infant includes early and frequent nursing: 8 to 12 times each day. If the infant is unable to feed this frequently, the mother should be instructed in the regular use of a mechanical breast pump to improve her milk supply, and the infant supplemented with expressed breastmilk or formula to improve the infant's nutritional status and intestinal motility.

BREASTMILK JAUNDICE

Breastmilk jaundice is a benign condition that resolves without treatment. Such infants have an unconjugated hyperbilirubinemia (less than 12 mg/dl) that becomes exaggerated and persistent toward the end of the first week of life.[46] Infants with breastmilk jaundice are otherwise healthy, with normal weight gain, normal stool and urine output, a normal physical examination, and no other underlying etiology for the hyperbilirubinemia. If concentrations are higher than 12 mg/dl and persist for several weeks, other causes of hyperbilirubinemia need to be investigated. For the vast majority of infants, it is not necessary to interrupt breastfeeding, even if the bilirubin increases to concentrations that may require phototherapy.

Lactation failure is not uniformly present in affected infants, suggesting that other possible mechanisms may be operative in breastmilk jaundice. No specific inhibitor or inhibitory substance has been identified in mother's breastmilk, but animal models suggest that mature breastmilk may increase unconjugated bilirubin concentration by enhancing bilirubin uptake in the digestive tract, thereby increasing enterohepatic circulation. Breastmilk may act as an environmental modifier for selected genotypes and thereby potentially predispose to the development of marked neonatal jaundice.[58,59] It is possible that the risk of developing a TSB concentration of 20 mg/dl or higher associated with breastmilk

feeding is enhanced when combined with expression of a coding sequence gene polymorphism of the UGT-1A1 and SLCO1B1 variants.[62]

Hyperbilirubinemia in the Late-Preterm Infant

Late-preterm gestation ($34^{0/7}$ to $36^{6/7}$ weeks) is one of the most prevalent identified risk factors for the development of severe hyperbilirubinemia and kernicterus,[9,11] because these infants have an approximately eightfold increased risk of developing a TSB greater than 20 mg/dl (5.2%) compared with those born at 41 or more weeks' gestation (0.7%). Many late-preterm infants will be breastfeeding, and frequently are cared for in normal newborn nurseries, despite the fact that they remain relatively immature compared with term newborns in their capacity to handle unconjugated hyperbilirubinemia.[10]

Neonatal hyperbilirubinemia in late-preterm newborns is more prevalent, more pronounced, and more protracted in nature than it is in their term counterparts. Although late-preterm and full-term infants become jaundiced by similar mechanisms, they differ in how effectively the late-preterm infant can handle the resultant bilirubin load, demonstrating a lower hepatic bilirubin conjugation. In addition, compared with their term counterparts, late-preterm infants are considered to be at a greater risk for developing kernicterus. Indeed, late-preterm infants are over-represented in the U.S. Pilot Kernicterus Registry.[25]

Miscellaneous Causes

The following causes of hyperbilirubinemia are uncommon but important to consider in infants who have no other clear etiology to explain their elevated bilirubin levels. These conditions include hypothyroidism and galactosemia. States now require routine screening for these conditions, because early detection allows intervention before permanent adverse neurologic injury occurs. Hyperbilirubinemia, unconjugated or mixed, may be the initial sign of these conditions.

HYPOTHYROIDISM

A prolonged period of unconjugated hyperbilirubinemia can be seen in infants with hypothyroidism. The mechanism of hyperbilirubinemia in hypothyroidism is not well understood, but in some animal studies, thyroxine was needed for the hepatic clearance of bilirubin.

GALACTOSEMIA

Galactosemia is an autosomal recessive disorder characterized by increased jaundice in infants fed breastmilk or lactose-containing formulas. The mechanism of hyperbilirubinemia in galactosemia may be related to a lack of substrate for glucuronidation and the accumulation of abnormal hepatotoxic byproducts. The presence of non–glucose-reducing substances in the urine suggests galactosemia.

MECHANISMS OF BILIRUBIN NEUROTOXICITY

Identification of those infants at risk for severe hyperbilirubinemia enables clinicians to provide timely treatment to prevent neuronal injury. The AAP[5] has described risk factors for hyperbilirubinemia, which can be seen in Box 21-3. The mechanism of bilirubin neurotoxicity has been the subject of increased investigation in recent years. The most important determinants of brain injury caused by hyperbilirubinemia are the concentrations of unconjugated bilirubin and free bilirubin, the concentration of serum albumin and its ability to bind unconjugated bilirubin, the concentration of hydrogen ion (pH), and neuronal susceptibility.[49] Although the TSB concentration alone is of limited value in predicting neurologic impairment and kernicterus, the use of the bilirubin:albumin ratio does not appear to offer better result than the use of TSB alone in predicting neurodevelopmental outcomes in preterm infants.[63] Similarly, although levels of unbound, or free, bilirubin seem to be more associated with abnormal hearing tests, and may prove to be a better predictor of bilirubin toxicity, this measurement is not available clinically.[2] There is also no agreement on a "threshold" above which injury would always occur.[3] Finally, photoisomers, which account for up to 25% of circulating TSB during phototherapy, may affect albumin binding and the amount of unbound bilirubin available to enter the central nervous system; the presence and effects of these compounds are largely unknown.

BOX 21-3 | **RISK FACTORS FOR HYPERBILIRUBINEMIA IN NEWBORNS**

Major Risk Factors
- Predischarge TSB or TcB level in the high-risk zone
- Jaundice observed in the first 24 hours of life
- Blood group incompatibility with positive direct antiglobulin test, other known hemolytic disease (e.g., G6PD deficiency), elevated ETcoc
- Gestational age 35 to 36 weeks
- Previous sibling received phototherapy
- Cephalohematoma or significant bruising
- Exclusive breastfeeding, especially if nursing is not going well and weight loss is excessive
- East Asian race*

Minor Risk Factors
- Predischarge TSB or TcB level in the high intermediate-risk zone
- Gestational age 37 to 38 weeks
- Jaundice observed before discharge
- Previous sibling with jaundice
- Macrosomic infant of a diabetic mother
- Maternal age ≥25 years
- Male gender

Decreased Risk
These factors are associated with decreased risk for significant jaundice, listed in order of decreasing importance.
- TSB or TcB level in the low-risk zone
- Gestational age ≥41 weeks
- Exclusive bottle feeding
- Black race*
- Discharge from the hospital after 72 hours

From American Academy of Pediatrics, Subcommittee on Hyperbilirubinemia: Clinical Practice Guideline. Management of hyperbilirubinemia in the newborn infant 35 or more weeks of gestation, *Pediatrics* 114:297, 2004.
ETcoc, End-tidal carbon monoxide corrected; *G6PD,* glucose-6-phosphate dehydrogenase; *TcB,* transcutaneous bilirubin; *TSB,* total serum bilirubin.
*Race as defined by mother's description.

Nevertheless, unbound bilirubin induces a variety of cellular events that result in neurotoxicity. Unbound bilirubin affects neurons, astrocytes, microglia, and oligodendrocytes, resulting in increased apoptosis in all cell lines, decreased arborization by neurons, release of proinflammatory cytokines by astrocytes and microglia, and decreased myelin synthesis by oligodendrocytes.[14,64]

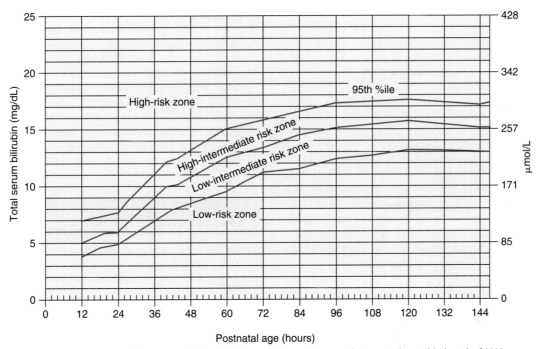

FIGURE 21-3 Nomogram for designation of risk in 2840 well newborns at 36 or more weeks' gestational age with birth weight of 2000 g or more or 35 or more weeks' gestational age with birth weight of 2500 g or more based on the hour-specific serum bilirubin levels. The serum bilirubin level was obtained before discharge, and the zone in which the value fell predicted the likelihood of a subsequent bilirubin level exceeding the 95th percentile (high-risk zone). (From Bhutani VK, Johnson L, Sivieri EM: Predictive ability of a predischarge hour-specific serum bilirubin for subsequent significant hyperbilirubinemia in healthy term and near-term newborns, *Pediatrics* 103:6, 1999.)

Interpretation of High Bilirubin Concentrations

All bilirubin concentrations should be interpreted according to the infant's age in hours. The AAP recommends a nomogram that designates risk for newborn infants at 35 weeks or greater, according to TSB obtained at varying postnatal ages in hours. The nomogram (Figure 21-3), based on work by Bhutani and colleagues,[8] designates whether an infant is at high, intermediate, or low risk for requiring further intervention for hyperbilirubinemia, based on the total serum bilirubin concentration.[5,8] Universal screening combined with use of the hour-specific bilirubin nomogram has been shown to be more accurate than a clinical risk factor scoring system alone, although the addition of gestational age to the risk assessment strategy can increase accuracy further.[31] However, the nomogram includes only infants at 35 weeks' gestation and above, was generated from a single institution, and the primary outcome measure was a TSB greater than 20 mg/dl, not the presence of bilirubin encephalopathy.[21] In addition, premature infants have a slightly later peak and are at risk for adverse neurologic outcomes at lower levels of bilirubin than older infants.

PREVENTION OF HYPERBILIRUBINEMIA

Early Feeding

Compared with infants not fed during the first 24 to 48 hours of life, infants fed earlier have lower peak bilirubin levels, likely related to a decrease in intestinal transit time and decreased enterohepatic circulation.

RhoGAM

As previously described, widespread use of Rho-GAM has proven effective in preventing the sensitization of Rh-negative mothers after delivery or abortion of Rh-positive infants. RhoGAM, or anti-D gamma globulin, provides passive protection by preventing maternal production of anti-Rh antibodies that might affect subsequent Rh-positive pregnancies, causing destruction of fetal red blood cells. Failures may occur if the amount of RhoGAM administered is insufficient compared with the load of fetal red blood cells received or if a significant fetal-maternal hemorrhage occurred before prophylaxis. Routine management of the Rh-negative mother now includes the administration of antenatal Rho-GAM in the second trimester (26 to 28 weeks), at the time of amniocentesis, and after delivery.

Phenobarbital

Phenobarbital acts to induce microsomal enzymes, increasing the levels of UGT-1A1. It also stimulates bile secretion in infants with nonobstructive cholestasis and increases the concentration of ligandin. When used in conjunction with phototherapy, however, phenobarbital does not increase the rate of decline in bilirubin levels.[17] Phenobarbital is effective when given to the mother before delivery. In infants with significant hemolytic disease of the newborn, it appears to slow the rate of rise of bilirubin and decrease the incidence of exchange transfusion. Phenobarbital treatment is indicated in infants with Crigler-Najjar syndrome type II, but is otherwise not used on a routine basis.

Heme Oxidase Inhibitors

Metalloporphyrins, compounds that are potent competitive inhibitors of the enzyme *heme oxygenase,* the initial and rate-limiting step in bilirubin production, have been investigated as possible interventions for hyperbilirubinemia in modulating bilirubin production.[52] Only tin protoporphyrin (SnPP) and tin mesoporphyrin (SnMP) have been studied in humans, to prevent neonatal unconjugated hyperbilirubinemia. Although highly efficacious, SnPP had photosensitizing properties that made it less appealing. Although SnMP is also photosensitizing, its use at lower doses reduces photoreactivity. Human trials with SnMP in preterm neonates have shown a dose-dependent reduction in peak bilirubin levels irrespective of gestational age and a reduction in the need for phototherapy.[30,42,56] The efficacy of SnMP has been well described in patients with Crigler-Najjar. Other alternative metalloporphyrins and nonmetalloporphyrins are currently being investigated; however, further trials in humans to determine long-term safety and effectiveness are necessary before widespread use can be recommended.

EVALUATION OF THE INFANT WITH HYPERBILIRUBINEMIA

The history, physical examination, and laboratory data play an important role in the evaluation of the infant with hyperbilirubinemia (Box 21-4).

History

The evaluation of a jaundiced infant begins with a complete family, perinatal, and neonatal history. The family history should include the occurrence of disorders associated with hyperbilirubinemia in other family members, particularly siblings. Need for phototherapy in a sibling is a risk factor for hyperbilirubinemia requiring intervention in the current child. A family history of early gallstones or chronic anemia is also important. The infant's course during labor and delivery should be assessed for possible infection during the pregnancy, the use of oxytocin induction for delivery, or the occurrence of an asphyxial episode during labor or delivery. A history of medications used and the infant's feeding and elimination patterns should also be obtained. The time of onset of jaundice is important, because clinical jaundice in the first 24 hours of life is considered abnormal, and likely indicates a hemolytic process.

Signs and Symptoms and Clinical Approach

A wide spectrum of signs and symptoms may occur in a jaundiced infant, often depending on the cause of the jaundice. Jaundice in a newborn usually can be detected visually at a level between 6 and 7 mg/dl. Visible icterus appears first on the head and face and progresses in a cephalocaudal

<table>
<tr><td>

BOX 21-4

EVALUATION OF UNCONJUGATED HYPERBILIRUBINEMIA IN THE NEONATE

History
- Family
- Perinatal and obstetric
- Neonatal

Physical Examination
- Pallor
- Hepatosplenomegaly
- Enclosed hemorrhage
- Petechiae
- Congenital anomalies

Laboratory Data
All Jaundiced Infants
- Maternal and infant blood type
- Coombs' test on cord blood
- Total/direct bilirubin (serial measurements)
- Complete blood count, including hematocrit, reticulocyte and platelet counts, white blood cell differential, and peripheral smear for red blood cell morphology
- Urinalysis, test for reducing substances

Selected Cases
- Protein, total/albumin

Sepsis Evaluation
- IgM
- Urine cytology for cytomegalovirus
- Viral cultures

New Techniques
- Transcutaneous bilirubinometry
- Bilirubin-binding tests

</td></tr>
</table>

An infant with hemolytic disease of the newborn may show jaundice and pallor, or may appear entirely normal at birth. *Hepatosplenomegaly* resulting from congestion and extramedullary hematopoiesis may be present. Infants affected by severe hemolytic disease of the newborn may also have pancreatic islet cell hyperplasia and may be at increased risk for hypoglycemia. Physical examination may reveal the presence of a cephalhematoma or other lesion resulting from enclosed hemorrhage. The occurrence of petechiae or purpura raises the possibility of intrauterine infection or sepsis. Congenital anomalies or syndromic appearance should be noted, because an increased incidence of jaundice is noted in aneuploidy syndromes. Jaundice and umbilical hernia may be associated with congenital hypothyroidism.

SIGNS OF BILIRUBIN TOXICITY

Hyperbilirubinemia is of clinical concern because of the potential for brain injury. Neurons are the principal target of bilirubin toxicity. The spectrum of bilirubin-induced neurologic dysfunction ranges from acute bilirubin encephalopathy to the devastating and irreversible syndrome of kernicterus.[31]

Acute bilirubin encephalopathy (ABE) describes the effects of hyperbilirubinemia seen during the hyperbilirubinemia and immediately thereafter. Clinical signs of ABE include progressive changes to an infant's mental and behavioral status, including lethargy, poor feeding, hypotonia and alternating tone followed by hypertonia, a poor Moro reflex with incomplete flexion of the extremities, and a high-pitched cry. Opisthotonos and retrocollis occur in the later stages.[12,49] As the symptoms of ABE worsen, apnea, seizures, and coma occur, which can result in death.

Kernicterus, or chronic bilirubin encephalopathy, is an irreversible and devastating brain injury[27] evidenced pathologically by yellowish staining in the deep nuclei of the central nervous system, particularly in the globus pallidus of the basal ganglia, central and peripheral auditory pathways, pontine and brainstem nuclei, subthalamic nuclei, cerebellum, and hippocampus. Compared with other forms of perinatal brain injury, in the instance of kernicterus, a clear correlation exists between etiology, pathogenesis, and symptomatology. Based on multiple studies, kernicterus has a mortality rate of 10% and at least 70% long-term morbidity.[24]

manner. The skin of the extremities, particularly the palmar and plantar surfaces, are the last skin surfaces to be affected; once the TSB approaches 15 mg/dl, all body surfaces are affected, and further elevation causes no difference in appearance. However, multiple studies show the inaccuracy of visual estimation of the degree of jaundice, even by experienced health care workers; thus all newborns should be assessed for hyperbilirubinemia with a serum or transcutaneous measurement if concern exists.

The clinical signs of kernicterus include extrapyramidal movement disorder, including dystonia and choreoathetoid movements (rapid, highly complex, involuntary, spasmodic movements); gaze abnormalities (especially paralysis of upward gaze); auditory disturbances (deafness); dysplasia of the enamel of deciduous teeth; and mild cognitive defects. The neuromotor abnormalities may be subtle, with the auditory abnormalities most apparent because the auditory pathways are the neural system most sensitive to bilirubin injury.[12]

In later life, severely affected survivors with kernicterus may exhibit choreoathetosis, spastic cerebral palsy, mental retardation, sensory and perceptual deafness, and visual-motor incoordination. It is not likely that significant mental retardation alone, without the other features, is caused by bilirubin encephalopathy. Although not yet proven, more subtle neurologic signs may include learning and behavioral problems, awkwardness, gait abnormalities, or minimal fine and gross motor incoordination.[25]

Bilirubin Toxicity in VLBW Infants. Infants with hemolytic disease and premature (especially VLBW) infants should receive phototherapy and exchange transfusion at lower bilirubin concentrations than full-term and otherwise healthy infants. Unfortunately, the "critical level" at which bilirubin toxicity occurs in either preterm or term infants has not been established. Preterm infants are more susceptible to elevated bilirubin concentrations due to less efficient hepatic conjugation, lower albumin binding capacity, and increased central nervous system sensitivity to unbound bilirubin. Although some studies have shown no neurotoxicity despite hyperbilirubinemia in preterm infants, other studies have shown significant neurodevelopmental impairment, despite only modest elevations in bilirubin concentration. Such studies are difficult to interpret due to the many confounders (gestational age, concurrent illness, etc.) in this population of infants.

Laboratory Data

The TSB level remains the recommended method on which to make clinical decisions.

Transcutaneous bilimeters are commonly used in newborn nurseries and outpatient settings to screen for hyperbilirubinemia and work by emitting a beam of light onto the skin and measuring the light reflected, which is not absorbed by bilirubin in the skin. Transcutaneous bilirubin measurements (TcB) have been shown to be valid[9]; however, regular monitoring for quality assurance by comparison with TSB measurements is necessary. In addition, different instruments can vary in their measurements, and quality checks should be performed periodically. TcB measurements are not reliable during phototherapy because of the bleaching effect of the light on skin.[12] Newer devices (such as the BiliCheck device by Phillips-Respironics or the JM-103 device by Konica Minolta/Air-Shields) are able to correct for skin melanin content and give results within 2 to 3 mg/100 ml of the TSB. Although transcutaneous devices are currently approved and recommended for the evaluation of jaundice in infants greater than or equal to 35 weeks' gestation, a systematic review of these two devices in premature infants (including less than 32 weeks' gestation) found that they were reliable in this population, with the JM-103 device demonstrating better precision.[33]

Still, most studies in term and late-preterm infants show that TcB may significantly underestimate the severity of hyperbilirubinemia. Because of the uncertain accuracy of the transcutaneous bilirubin measurement, it is not recommended to consider this device reliable at levels greater than 15 mg/dl.[12] A TSB level should be obtained whenever therapeutic intervention is considered, particularly in the following situations: (1) the TcB level is at 70% of the TSB level at which phototherapy would be instituted, (2) the TcB value is above the 75th percentile on the AAP nomogram or the 95th percentile on the TcB nomogram, and (3) at follow-up after discharge, the TcB value is greater than 13 mg/dl.[38]

ADDITIONAL LABORATORY EVALUATION

In addition to a bilirubin level, the minimum laboratory evaluation of the newborn with significant jaundice requiring treatment should include the mother's and infant's blood types, Rh status, and antiglobulin testing on cord blood. A complete blood count (CBC), including hematocrit, reticulocyte and platelet counts, white blood cell count and differential, and peripheral smear for red blood cell morphology, should be performed, seeking evidence of hemolysis. Microspherocytosis is characteristic of ABO incompatibility and hereditary spherocytosis.

Bilirubin concentration (TSB) should be measured serially and interpreted based on the infant's age in hours at the time of measurement (see Figure 21-3). A fractionated bilirubin should be obtained if the jaundice is severe, prolonged, or associated with light-colored stools. Serum albumin levels may be helpful at higher bilirubin concentrations and the bilirubin:albumin ratio considered as an additional factor in deciding when to start phototherapy or perform an exchange transfusion.

Evaluation for other potential causes of hyperbilirubinemia is essential when the etiology is not immediately clear. An elevated direct fraction of bilirubin, abnormal white blood cell count, left-shifted differential, or thrombocytopenia may suggest infection. Urinalysis, including evaluation for reducing substances, may be helpful. Infants suspected of having bacterial sepsis should receive antibiotic treatment and a complete sepsis evaluation performed. Infants suspected of having intrauterine infection should have additional tests, including immunoglobulin M (IgM), as well as blood, cerebrospinal fluid, and/or exudate from skin vesicles for viral cultures and urine for cytomegalovirus as indicated.

Infants with hemolytic disease are at risk for late anemia after discharge from the nursery, which may require treatment with erythropoietin or transfusion. These infants require close follow-up for anemia from their primary care provider.

TREATMENT

Treatment is aimed at lowering the concentration of circulating bilirubin or keeping it from increasing, thereby preventing the complications of acute bilirubin encephalopathy and kernicterus. In 2004 the AAP Subcommittee on Hyperbilirubinemia published clinical practice guidelines on the management of hyperbilirubinemia in the newborn infant 35 or more weeks of gestation that lend direction regarding the use of phototherapy and exchange transfusion (Table 21-1).[5] These guidelines and recommendations are outlined in Figure 21-4 *(phototherapy)* and Figure 21-5 *(exchange transfusion)*. Since the publication of these guidelines, several other studies suggested that combining clinical risk factors analysis with the predischarge measurements of TSB or TcB improves prediction of subsequent hyperbilirubinemia risk[10,15,31,32,45];

TABLE 21-1	PHOTOTHERAPY AND EXCHANGE TRANSFUSION CRITERIA FOR VERY-LOW-BIRTH-WEIGHT AND EXTREMELY LOW-BIRTH-WEIGHT INFANTS		
WEIGHT (g)	INITIATE PHOTOTHERAPY (mg/dl)	CONSIDER EXCHANGE TRANSFUSION (mg/dl)	
500-750	5-8	12-15	
751-1000	6-10	>15	
1001-1250	8-10	15-18	
1251-1500	10-12	17-20	

Modified from Cashore WJ: Bilirubin and jaundice in the micropremie, *Clin Perinatol* 27:178, 2000.

consequently, these recommendations were updated in a consensus-based guideline in 2009.[38] The outlined *algorithm* in Figure 21-6 represents the proposed consensus-based guidelines for the management and follow-up of hyperbilirubinemia in the newborn infant 35 or more weeks' gestation, according to predischarge bilirubin measurements, gestation, and risk factors. Similarly, a consensus-based guideline has been developed for the suggested use of phototherapy in infants less than 35 weeks' gestation.[39] Subsequently, in 2013 Wallenstein and Bhutani[57] published an expanded form of these recommendations for the management of hyperbilirubinemia in the moderately preterm infant of 32 to 34 weeks' gestation (Figure 21-7).

Phototherapy

Phototherapy is the most commonly used treatment for hyperbilirubinemia. With the widespread use of phototherapy, the use of exchange transfusion in infants with nonhemolytic hyperbilirubinemia is almost obsolete. Hospital-based studies in the United States have shown that 5 to 40 infants per 1000 term and late-preterm infants receive phototherapy before discharge from the nursery and an equal number are readmitted for phototherapy after discharge.[35] The decision to initiate phototherapy must be individualized for each newborn and should be based on the recent AAP guidelines (see discussion in legend for Figure 21-4).

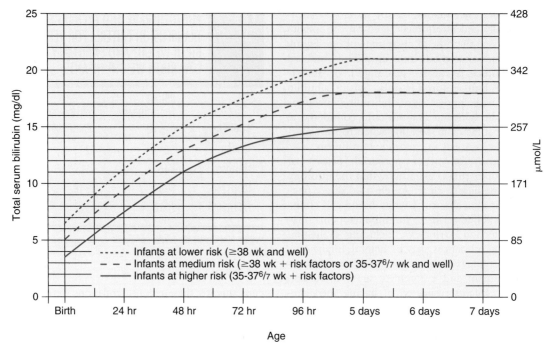

- Use total bilirubin. Do not subtract direct-reacting or conjugated bilirubin.
- Risk factors = isoimmune hemolytic disease, G6PD deficiency, asphyxia, significant lethargy, temperature instability, sepsis, acidosis, or albumin <3.0 g/dl (if measured).
- For well infants 35-37⁶/₇ weeks, can adjust TSB levels for intervention around the medium risk line. It is an option to intervene at lower TSB levels for infants closer to 35 weeks and at higher TSB levels for those closer to 37⁶/₇ weeks.
- It is an option to provide conventional phototherapy in the hospital or at home at TSB levels 2-3 mg/dl (35-50 mmol/L) below those shown, but home phototherapy should not be used in any infant with risk factors.

FIGURE 21-4 American Academy of Pediatrics (AAP) guidelines for phototherapy in hospitalized infants of 35 or more weeks' gestation. (NOTE: These guidelines are based on limited evidence, and the levels shown are approximations. The guidelines refer to the use of intensive phototherapy that should be used when the total serum bilirubin [TSB] exceeds the line indicated for each category. Infants are designated as "higher risk" because of the potential negative effects of the conditions listed on albumin binding of bilirubin, the blood-brain barrier, and the susceptibility of the brain cells to damage by bilirubin.) G6PD, Glucose-6-phosphate dehydrogenase. (From American Academy of Pediatrics, Subcommittee on Hyperbilirubinemia: Clinical Practice Guideline. Management of hyperbilirubinemia in the newborn infant 35 or more weeks of gestation, *Pediatrics* 114:297, 2004.)

RATE OF BILIRUBIN DECLINE UNDER PHOTOTHERAPY

With effective phototherapy, the infant's bilirubin level should drop at a rate of 0.5 to 1 mg percent per hour, and by 30% to 40% after 24 hours of treatment, when applied at several days of age. The rate of decline of bilirubin in the first days (early hyperbilirubinemia, likely the result of increased bilirubin production) will not be as brisk, but the rate of rise will be significantly slowed.

Bilirubin best absorbs light in the blue-green spectrum, particularly in the blue region of the spectrum near 460 nm[35]; the spectrum of light at 425 to 475 nm is therefore most effective. Phototherapy uses this light energy to change the shape and structure of bilirubin, converting it to photoisomers that can be excreted in the bile and urine without conjugation.[35] Configurational isomers are formed most rapidly (Z, E and E, Z isomers), but the reaction is reversible.[23] The most important

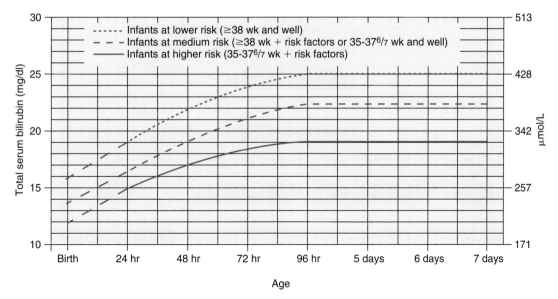

- The dashed lines for the first 24 hours indicate uncertainty due to a wide range of clinical circumstances and a range of responses to phototherapy.
- Immediate exchange transfusion is recommended if infant shows signs of acute bilirubin encephalopathy (hypertonia, arching, retrocollis, opisthotonos, fever, high-pitched cry) or if TSB is ≥5 mg/dl (85 μmol/L) above these lines.
- Risk factors: isoimmune hemolytic disease, G6PD deficiency, asphyxia, significant lethargy, temperature instability, sepsis, acidosis.
- Use total bilirubin. Do not subtract direct-reacting or conjugated bilirubin.
- If infant is well and 35-37⁶/7 weeks (median risk), can individualize TSB levels for exchange based on actual gestational age.

FIGURE 21-5 American Academy of Pediatrics (AAP) guidelines for exchange transfusion in infants of 35 or more weeks' gestation. (NOTE: These suggested guidelines represent a consensus of most of the American Academy of Pediatrics Subcommittee on Hyperbilirubinemia but are based on limited evidence, and the levels shown are approximations. During birth hospitalization, exchange transfusion is recommended if the total serum bilirubin [TSB] rises to these levels despite intensive phototherapy. For readmitted infants, if the TSB level is above the exchange level, repeat TSB measurement every 2 to 3 hours and consider exchange if the TSB remains above the levels indicated after intensive phototherapy for 6 hours.) G6PD, Glucose-6-phosphate dehydrogenase; TSB, total serum bilirubin. (From American Academy of Pediatrics, Subcommittee on Hyperbilirubinemia: Clinical Practice Guideline. Management of hyperbilirubinemia in the newborn infant 35 or more weeks of gestation, *Pediatrics* 114:297, 2004.)

of these isomers is *lumirubin,* a stable structural photoisomer. Lumirubin does not require conjugation and is rapidly excreted in both bile and urine. The production of lumirubin is an irreversible reaction that appears to be dose related, but occurs more slowly than formation of the configurational isomers. Photooxidation of bilirubin occurs much more slowly and is not as important as photoisomerization.

The efficacy of phototherapy depends on the energy output *(irradiance)* of the light source (measured with a radiometer in units of watts per square centimeter or microwatts per square centimeter per nanometer over a given wavelength band), the distance of the light source from the infant, and the surface area of the infant exposed to the light. Intensive phototherapy consists of 30 μW/cm²/nm or more.[5] Fiberoptic blankets delivering phototherapy from a high-intensity light source are available for use by themselves or in conjunction with other sources of phototherapy but are unlikely to expose an adequate surface area on a term infant to provide intensive phototherapy.[35]

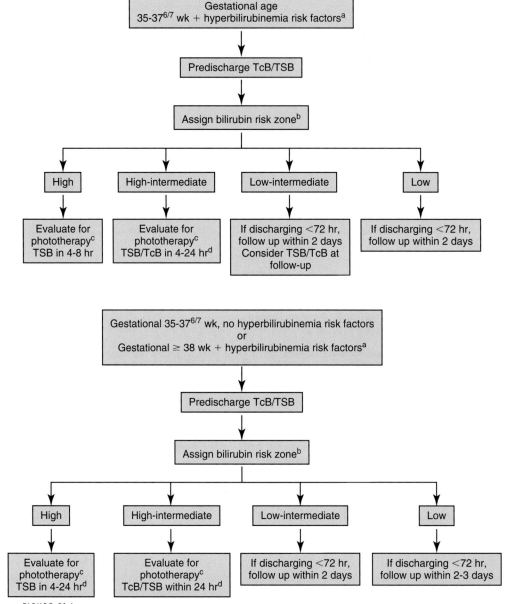

FIGURE 21-6

- Recommendation for timing of repeat TSB measurement depends on age at measurement and how far the TSB level is above the 95th percentile (Figure 21-3). Higher and earlier initial TSB levels require an earlier repeat TSB measurement.
- (a) Risk factors, (b) Figure 21-3, (c) Figure 21-4, (d) in hospital or as outpatient, (e) follow-up recommendations can be modified according to level of risk for hyperbilirubinemia.

Algorithm providing recommendations for management and follow-up according to predischarge bilirubin measurements, gestation, and risk factors for subsequent hyperbilirubinemia. Provide lactation evaluation and support for all breastfeeding mothers. (From Maisels MJ: Neonatal hyperbilirubinemia and kernicterus—not gone but sometimes forgotten, *Early Hum Dev* 85:727-732, 2009. Reproduced with permission from Maisels MJ, Bhutani VK, Bogen D, Newman TB, et al: Hyperbilirubinemia in the newborn infant 35 or more weeks' gestation, *Pediatrics* 124:1193, 2009.)

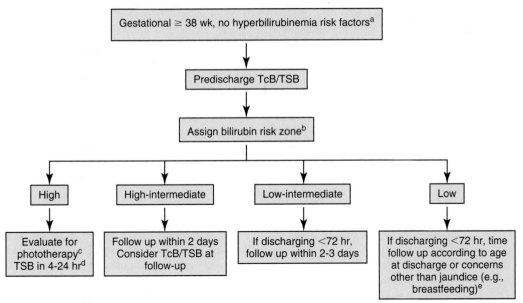

FIGURE 21-6, cont'd.

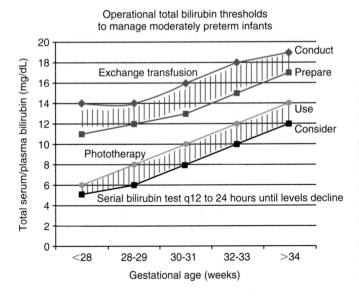

FIGURE 21-7 Suggested use of phototherapy and exchange transfusion in preterm infants less than 35 weeks' gestational age. The operational thresholds have been demarcated by recommendations of an expert panel. *The shaded bands* represent the degree of uncertainty. Recommended threshold to prepare for exchange transfusion assumes that these infants are already being managed by effective phototherapy. Increase in exposure of body surface area to phototherapy may inform the decision to conduct an exchange transfusion based on patient response to phototherapy. (From Wallenstein MB, Bhutani VK: Jaundice and kernicterus in the moderately preterm infant, *Clin Perinatol* 40:679, 2013. Adapted with permission from Maisels MJ, Watchko JF, Bhutani VK, et al: An approach to the management of hyperbilirubinemia in the preterm infant less than 35 weeks of gestation, *J Perinatol* 32(9):660-664, 2012.)

LIGHT SOURCES

The AAP describes the most commonly used phototherapy units in its 2004 guidelines. These include daylight, cool white, blue, or "special blue" fluorescent tubes or tungsten-halogen lamps in different configurations, either freestanding or as part of a radiant warming device. Most of these devices deliver enough output in the blue-green region of the visible spectrum to be effective for standard phototherapy use. The most effective light sources commercially available for phototherapy are those that use special blue fluorescent tubes or a specially designed light-emitting diode light (Natus Inc., San Carlos, Calif.). The special blue fluorescent tubes are labeled *F20T12/BB* (General Electric, Westinghouse, Sylvania) or *TL52/20W*

(Phillips, Eindhoven, The Netherlands). It is important to note that special blue tubes provide much greater irradiance than regular blue tubes (labeled *F20T12/B*). Special blue tubes are most effective because they provide light predominantly in the blue-green spectrum. At these wavelengths, light penetrates skin well and is absorbed maximally by bilirubin.[5] Fiber-optic phototherapy blankets (Wallaby Phototherapy System, Fiberoptic Medical Products, Inc., Allentown, Pa.; Biliblanket, Ohmeda, Columbia, Md.) use a high-intensity halogen light source for transmission of light by fiber-optic bundles. Irradiance and efficacy appear comparable with those for standard phototherapy. Purported advantages of these systems are elimination of the need for eye patches, exposure of greater surface area, and provision of phototherapy outside of the nursery with less interference in mother-infant bonding. These blankets are more convenient to use when phototherapy is necessary in an outpatient setting.

Physical and laboratory evaluation should be performed before initiating phototherapy in any infant. Once phototherapy has been initiated, TSB must be monitored because TcB measurement is no longer valid. Hematocrit also must be monitored in infants with hemolytic disease.

There are conflicting data in the literature on whether continuous or intermittent administration of phototherapy is most effective. Phototherapy may be interrupted during brief periods for feeding, laboratory draws, assessment of the eyes, visual stimulation, and parental contact. Table 21-2 outlines some of the nursing assessments and management to be performed in infants undergoing phototherapy.

REBOUND

After phototherapy ceases, TSB should be followed for at least 24 hours to assess for significant rebound. A rebound in the TSB of 1 to 2 mg/dl or more can occur after phototherapy is discontinued. Infants most likely to experience significant rebound are those less than 37 weeks' gestation, those with hemolytic disease, and those treated with phototherapy during the birth hospitalization, because the bilirubin is still expected to rise at the time phototherapy is discontinued.[35]

SAFETY

Despite its widespread use since 1958, questions about the safety and side effects of phototherapy

remain. However, reports of clinically significant toxicity are rare.[37] Animal studies have demonstrated a potential retinal toxicity of light. Although it is not established that this occurs in the human newborn, the possibility remains a concern and the infant's eyes should be covered while phototherapy is in use. Patches should completely cover the eyes without placing excessive pressure on the eyes and should be carefully positioned to avoid occluding the nares. Eye patches should be removed every 4 hours to permit evaluation of the infant's eyes. The patches should be left off during feedings and parental visits.

HEAT BALANCE

Infants exposed to phototherapy, particularly low-birth-weight infants and infants under a radiant warmer, may have significant increases in their insensible water losses. Infants in incubators or servocontrolled care centers may become overheated. The servocontrol probe should be shielded by an opaque covering.

Infants treated in open cribs may become cold stressed. Fluid balance must be monitored carefully in an infant receiving phototherapy. Infants under phototherapy also have increased stool water losses and may develop temporary lactose intolerance. The infant's temperature, weight, and intake and output should be monitored frequently. The presence of reducing substances in the stool can be treated with a non–lactose-containing formula.

AGGRESSIVE VERSUS CONSERVATIVE PHOTOTHERAPY

Because the concentrations of bilirubin that are detrimental to preterm infants have not been well defined, a randomized controlled trial attempted to determine whether aggressive versus conservative phototherapy led to improvement in neurodevelopmental outcome at 18 to 22 months for infants between 501 and 1000 grams.[43] Although there was no difference in survival between groups, of the surviving infants, the aggressive phototherapy group had significant decreases in rates of neurodevelopmental impairment. Of concern was that in a subgroup analysis of the smallest infants, 501 to 750 grams, the mortality rate was increased by 5% in the aggressive versus conservative phototherapy group. Although not statistically significant, this increased mortality rate was worrisome to

TABLE 21-2	NURSING MANAGEMENT OF INFANTS UNDERGOING PHOTOTHERAPY

NURSING ASSESSMENT	
AREA	PARAMETER
Physical status	Intake and output
	Color
	Location of jaundice
	Skin integrity
	Stools (character, consistency)
	Vital signs
	Infant/environmental temperature
	Hydration status
	Signs of phototherapy side effects
	Eye discharge and tearing
	Position
	Activity
Neurobehavioral status	Sleep-wake states
	Sensory threshold
	Behavioral responsiveness
	Feeding behaviors
	Consoling abilities
	Stress responses
	Interactive capabilities

NURSING MANAGEMENT	
NURSING DIAGNOSIS	INTERVENTION
Deficient Fluid Volume (Actual or Potential)	Monitor intake and output.
	Monitor hydration status (weight, specific gravity, urine output).
	Monitor stooling pattern, character.
	Maintain adequate fluid intake (oral or parenteral).
Imbalanced Nutrition: Less Than Body Requirements	Assess feeding behavior and activity.
	Monitor fluid and caloric intake, weight, abdominal girth.
	Remove eye shields during feeding.
	Hold during oral feedings as health and thermal status permit.
	Bring to alert state before feeding.
	Feed on demand if possible.
Impaired Skin Integrity	Observe color, rashes, excoriation.
	Clean skin with warm water.
	Clean perineal area after stooling.
	Turn frequently (also increases skin exposure to phototherapy).
	Ensure Plexiglas shield is in place between light source and infant to reduce exposure to ultraviolet light.

Continued

	TABLE	21-2	NURSING MANAGEMENT OF INFANTS UNDERGOING PHOTOTHERAPY — cont'd

NURSING ASSESSMENT	
NURSING DIAGNOSIS	**INTERVENTION**
Risk for Injury	Observe for side effects associated with phototherapy.
	Observe for signs of sepsis.
	Provide care to minimize side effects of phototherapy.
	Shield eyes from lights with opaque patches.
	Ensure eyelids are closed when shield is applied to prevent corneal injury.
	Remove eye shield and observe eyes regularly.
	Monitor position of eye shield to prevent occlusion of nose.
	Avoid tight headband on eye shield to reduce risk of increased intracranial pressure, especially in preterm infants.
	Observe for eye discharge, tearing.
	Shield testes and possibly ovaries (data unclear about need to do this) with diaper.
Ineffective Thermoregulation	Place in warm, thermoneutral environment.
	Monitor environmental and infant temperature.
	Observe for hypothermia and hyperthermia.
	Reduce heat losses from environmental sources.
	Use servocontrol for infants in incubator or under radiant warmer.
	Shield servocontrol thermistor from direct exposure to phototherapy lights.

From Blackburn S: Hyperbilirubinemia and neonatal jaundice, *Neonatal Netw* 14:15, 1995.

the authors and may offset any potential benefit of aggressive phototherapy in this weight category.

CHOLESTATIC JAUNDICE AND PHOTOTHERAPY

Infants who have cholestatic jaundice and are exposed to phototherapy may develop the "bronze baby syndrome," presumably caused by retention of a bilirubin breakdown product produced by phototherapy, although the mechanism is unclear. An infant with bronze baby syndrome develops a dark gray-brown discoloration of the skin, urine, and serum. There are generally no other clinical symptoms, but at least one death has been reported. After phototherapy ceases, the bronzing gradually resolves.

TRANSIENT SIDE EFFECTS

Transient skin rashes and tanning resulting from increased melanin production have been reported, as have bullous skin eruptions in infants treated with tin mesoporphyrin who are subsequently exposed to sunlight or daylight fluorescent

bulbs.[35] A study published in 2008 suggested that intensive phototherapy might increase the number of melanocytic nevi identified at school age.[35] Other potential problems include interference with biologic (circadian) rhythms and maternal-infant bonding. Although there may be some transient, short-term growth effects, long-term growth effects and development appear unaffected by phototherapy.

Intravenous Immunoglobulin

When immune-mediated hemolysis is present and the TSB is rising despite intensive phototherapy or is approaching the exchange level, intravenous immunoglobulin should be administered to the infant to decrease the severity of hemolysis. The dose is 500 mg/kg to 1 g/kg IV over 2 to 4 hours and may be repeated one time after 12 hours. This intervention has been shown in multiple trials to decrease the need for exchange transfusion by approximately 70% and is recommended for Rh isoimmunization as soon as the diagnosis is established, and for

ABO isoimmunization if the TSB continues to rise despite intensive phototherapy.[5,6] Immunoglobulin is of no benefit in non–antibody-mediated hyperbilirubinemia such as occurs in G6PD deficiency, Gilbert syndrome, or spherocytosis.

Exchange Transfusion

An exchange transfusion is indicated for correction of anemia and removal of antibody-coated red blood cells in severe hemolytic disease, or for treatment of signs of acute bilirubin encephalopathy regardless of its cause or TSB level. Phototherapy cannot be used in place of an exchange transfusion in those infants with severe hemolytic disease. A packed red blood cell exchange transfusion using type O Rh-negative blood will correct anemia, as well as remove sensitized cells and bilirubin, leading to a more complete therapy for the problem.

It must be stressed that the decision to perform an exchange transfusion must be individualized for each patient. Particularly in VLBW infants, the indications to perform an exchange transfusion vary from nursery to nursery. The recent AAP guidelines for performing exchange transfusion in infants of 35 or more weeks of gestation are shown in Figure 21-5 (see discussion in legend). Similar guidelines have recently been proposed for the preterm infant, as shown in Figure 21-7, by Wallenstein and Bhutani.[57]

Usually a double-volume exchange transfusion is performed using 160 ml/kg of appropriate whole blood product. If fresh whole blood is not available, reconstituted whole blood can be requested that can be mixed to a desired hematocrit. ABO type-specific Rh-negative blood should be used in cases with Rh incompatibility. Type O Rh-specific cells are indicated when ABO incompatibility exists. Whereas a single-volume exchange is likely to exchange 63% of the infant's blood, a double-volume exchange will exchange 86%. Further increase in the amount exchanged gives little additional benefit.

The blood bank can prepare this blood for the infant with a predetermined hematocrit, usually 50% to 55%. An exchange transfusion will reduce bilirubin levels by approximately 45% to 85%, according to various sources. Administration of 1 g/kg of 25% albumin 1 hour before the exchange transfusion has been shown in some studies to increase the efficiency of exchange by about 40%. As plasma and tissue levels equilibrate

posttransfusion, the bilirubin rises to about 60% of the preexchange level.

Exchange transfusion trays are commercially available and include a four-way stopcock, necessary tubing and syringes, 10% calcium gluconate, and a plastic bag for discarded blood.

PROCEDURE

The infant should be in the NICU for close observation during and immediately after the procedure. Feedings should be held for 2 to 3 hours before the procedure and for some time afterward. The procedure is performed by removing small aliquots of the infant's blood and replacing similar small aliquots of transfused blood product while blood pressure, heart rate, and general condition are monitored. Generally, 5- to 20-ml aliquots of blood are used, depending on the size and condition of the infant. Each aliquot should be 5% to 8% of the estimated blood volume or 5 ml/kg, withdrawn or infused at approximately 5 ml/kg/min. The entire procedure should take 60 to 90 minutes and encompass 30 to 35 cycles of withdrawal and infusion.[20] In general, a slower exchange will result in less rebound of TSB than a rapid exchange because the extravascular bilirubin may equilibrate with the plasma bilirubin more extensively.[20] The initial aliquot should be withdrawn and sent to the laboratory for bilirubin, hematocrit, calcium, and culture. Blood used in the exchange must be warmed to prevent "cold heart syndrome," which may include arrhythmia and cardiac arrest.[20]

The final aliquot from an exchange should be sent for CBC, fractionated bilirubin, calcium ion, electrolytes, culture, and repeat type and crossmatch studies for potential additional exchange transfusion. In addition to the individuals performing the exchange, one person must keep an accurate record of time, volumes withdrawn and infused, vital signs, and medications administered.

POTENTIAL COMPLICATIONS

Exchange transfusion is a procedure with many potential complications and carries a mortality risk of about 0.5%. For this reason and because so few exchange transfusions are performed today (estimated at 3/100,000 live births in the United States),[44] this procedure should be done only by personnel familiar with it and its complications, preferably in a tertiary care unit. Vascular complications are related to the use of umbilical catheters (discussed in Chapter 7). Necrotizing enterocolitis has been reported as a postexchange complication, probably as a result of bowel ischemia during the procedure, and may be related to a more rapid exchange and use of larger aliquots of blood.[20,44]

Electrolyte and glucose disturbances are related to the blood preparation used for the exchange. Citrate used as part of the anticoagulant solution binds divalent ions such as calcium and magnesium; thus laboratory evaluation of calcium and magnesium during the procedure is essential. The infant should be evaluated for hypocalcemia after each 100 ml of the exchange has been completed. Although symptomatic hypocalcemia is rare, clinical signs and symptoms include irritability, tachycardia, or prolongation of the Q-Tc interval. If hypocalcemia is detected, 1 ml of a 10% calcium gluconate solution is infused slowly under continuous electronic cardiac monitoring.

Acid-citrate-dextrose and citrate-phosphate-dextrose blood have high levels of sodium and glucose and sometimes potassium. Initial hyperglycemia may be followed by reactive hypoglycemia as a result of an insulin response. Although acidic at the time of infusion, a postexchange alkalosis may occur as citrate is metabolized to bicarbonate in the liver.

Many of the electrolyte and acid-base disturbances may be avoided by the use of fresh, heparinized blood. Bleeding may occur in an overheparinized infant but is reversible with protamine sulfate. Thrombocytopenia may occur, especially in the infant needing repeated exchange transfusions. Bacterial infection is rare, and routine antibiotic prophylaxis is not indicated. Most complications are avoidable if careful attention to technique is observed.

PARENT TEACHING

Providing parents with written information about jaundice and its therapy may be a beneficial adjunct to verbal explanations and is a key element of recent AAP guidelines on management of hyperbilirubinemia (Box 21-5). Because early discharge policies (less than 48 hours) have increased the need for outpatient evaluation or management of neonatal hyperbilirubinemia, it is important that parents feel empowered to ask questions about hyperbilirubinemia and its symptoms so

---

BOX 21-5 KEY ELEMENTS OF AAP CLINICAL PRACTICE GUIDELINE (2004): MANAGEMENT OF HYPERBILIRUBINEMIA IN THE NEWBORN INFANT 35 OR MORE WEEKS OF GESTATION

Important Points for the Management of Jaundice

- Promote and support successful breastfeeding.
- Establish nursery protocols for the identification and evaluation of hyperbilirubinemia.
- Measure the total serum bilirubin (TSB) or transcutaneous bilirubin (TcB) level on infants jaundiced in the first 24 hours.
- Recognize that visual estimation of the degree of jaundice can lead to errors, particularly in darkly pigmented infants.
- Interpret all bilirubin levels according to the infant's age in hours.
- Recognize that infants at less than 38 weeks' gestation, particularly those who are breastfed, are at higher risk of developing hyperbilirubinemia.
- Screen all infants before discharge with a TSB or TcB measurement, combined with clinical risk factors, to guide the need for additional testing to identify a cause for hyperbilirubinemia and for additional TSB measurements.
- Provide parents with written and verbal information about newborn jaundice.
- Provide appropriate follow-up based on the time of discharge and risk assessment.
- Treat newborns, when indicated, with phototherapy or exchange transfusion.

From American Academy of Pediatrics, Subcommittee on Hyperbilirubinemia: Clinical Practice Guideline. Management of hyperbilirubinemia in the newborn infant 35 or more weeks of gestation, *Pediatrics* 114:297, 2004.

---

that they can bring any concerns to the attention of health care providers.[60] This is especially true for the nursing mother, who may be questioning her ability to provide adequate nourishment for her infant. Indeed, early discharge of infants has now led to hyperbilirubinemia being the most common cause for hospital readmission in term infants.

Providing parents and families with consistent information, reassurance, and support is essential. The use of phototherapy can be distressing for parents and should be explained to them before they see the infant under phototherapy lights for the first time.

In addition, incubators, bili-masks, and phototherapy lights can all contribute to a sense of separation between parents and their infant by creating a physical and emotional barrier. Parents may avoid coming to the nursery to be with their infant. If they do come to their infant's bedside, they may be reluctant to touch or participate in care for fear of interfering with phototherapy and potentially hindering their infant's progress.

As with many disorders in newborn infants, time and energy spent providing parents with information and support can alleviate much fear, guilt, and anger. It also can help facilitate the development of a healthy family relationship in a time of crisis. Signs and symptoms of jaundice should be explained in a manner that is understandable and meaningful for parents, emphasizing that neonatal hyperbilirubinemia is usually a transient condition and one to which all infants must adapt after birth.

HEALTH SYSTEMS APPROACH TO BILIRUBIN

In the 1970s and 1980s, few health care providers had the opportunity to see a patient with kernicterus.[24] In recent times, however, rates of kernicterus have been rising; this is seen as a systems failure in neonatal services, because most infants developing kernicterus in recent times are not those with hemolytic disease, but term and late-preterm babies who have been discharged postnatally and return to a pediatrician or emergency department with symptoms of kernicterus.[7,10,27] For that reason, the Joint Commission on Accreditation of Healthcare Organizations issued Sentinel Event Alerts on kernicterus in 2001 and again in 2004.[11,19,25,26,61] However, neither hyperbilirubinemia nor kernicterus has been a reportable disease, and no reliable information source exists to produce national annual estimates,[11] but most estimates are 0.4 to 2.7 cases per 100,000 live births among infants born at or after 35 weeks of gestation[39,40] (see Box 21-1).

The root cause analysis for the reappearance of kernicterus revealed several factors. First, health services are provided by multiple providers at multiple sites, some of whom may not have a sufficient understanding of bilirubin and its potential for toxicity. Early discharge of newborn infants younger than 72 hours ensures that infants will be discharged before the natural peak of bilirubin rise in term infants and before the establishment of adequate breastfeeding; this will be accentuated in the late-preterm infant. A lack of or limited knowledge by parents and health care providers regarding hyperbilirubinemia and the early symptoms of acute bilirubin encephalopathy, and limitations within health care systems to provide appropriate predischarge screening of at-risk infants, only serves to complicate issues.[10,54,55] Inadequate screening, the inability to measure TSB easily, and a high prevalence of medical conditions that increase the risk of severe hyperbilirubinemia (UGT-1A1 polymorphisms and G6PD deficiency) may cause infants at risk for hyperbilirubinemia that will require treatment to be overlooked.[50] In addition, issues related to patient referrals, challenges with implementation of phototherapy, limited availability of whole blood, or lack of experienced personnel to perform exchange transfusions may cause delays in the treatment of infants with acute bilirubin encephalopathy.[65]

The overall aim of the published guidelines[5,38] was to promote an approach that would (1) reduce the frequency of severe hyperbilirubinemia and bilirubin encephalopathy, (2) minimize the risk for unintended harm (e.g., increased anxiety, decreased breastfeeding, unnecessary treatment for the general population), and (3) avoid excessive cost and waste. These guidelines emphasize the importance of universal predischarge screening combined with clinical risk assessment, close follow-up, and prompt intervention when indicated. By obtaining a TcB or TSB on all infants before discharge, a systems-based approach to reducing the occurrence of acute bilirubin encephalopathy is achievable. Infants with bilirubin levels above the 75th percentile for age in hours can be identified, and ongoing tracking of those with rapid rates of rise (greater than 0.2 mg/dl/hr)[12] can be arranged. Although evidence that universal predischarge screening will reduce the incidence of kernicterus is lacking, published data suggest that predischarge screening can reduce the incidence of TSB levels of 25 mg/dl or greater by facilitating the early recognition of those infants at greatest risk but may introduce the risk of overuse of phototherapy. When possible overuse of phototherapy is balanced against the permanent and devastating, though rare, occurrence of kernicterus, such a widespread approach may be seen as conferring a small, but still worthwhile, benefit.[36,38]

The 10 key elements of the 2004 AAP practice guidelines are listed in Box 21-5. Bhutani and Johnson[10] went further to recommend a five-step nationwide strategy to prevent severe neonatal hyperbilirubinemia:

- An institutional curriculum for the systems approach, including universal prenatal, predischarge, and postdischarge risk assessment of severe neonatal hyperbilirubinemia
- Advocacy for on-site services that promote breastfeeding in the context of supervised and seamless health care delivery during the first month of life
- Effective parent-provider partnerships for safer management of neonatal jaundice
- Statewide (or regional) reporting of birthing institution outcome assessment for severe neonatal hyperbilirubinemia along with outcomes for neonatal screening for other inherited disorders
- Nationwide surveillance in which all cases of severe neonatal hyperbilirubinemia are reported

REFERENCES

For a full list of references, scan the QR code or visit http://booksite.elsevier.com/9780323320832.

22 INFECTION IN THE NEONATE

MOHAN PAMMI, M. COLLEEN BRAND, AND LEONARD E. WEISMAN

A newborn infant is uniquely susceptible to infectious diseases. This chapter presents causes of infectious diseases with particular emphasis on prevention, history, presenting signs and symptoms, laboratory data, treatment, and parent teaching methods of prevention applicable to the care of the neonate. Abbreviations for this chapter are listed in Box 22-1.

PATHOPHYSIOLOGY AND PATHOGENESIS

An infection occurs when a susceptible host comes in contact with a potentially pathogenic organism. When the encountered organism proliferates and overcomes the host defenses, infection results. Sources of infection in a newborn can be divided into three categories: (1) transplacental acquisition (intrauterine infection), (2) perinatal acquisition during labor and delivery (intrapartum infection), and (3) hospital acquisition in the neonatal period (postnatal infection) from the mother, hospital environment, or hospital personnel.

In general, most infecting organisms can, under the proper circumstances, cross the placenta or ascend from the birth canal and invade the at-risk neonate. These infections may result in abortion, stillbirth, and disease present at birth or in the neonatal period.

The main goal is to prevent infections in the fetus and newborn. Unfortunately, few proven measures exist for the prevention of infections acquired via the placenta or in the perinatal period. Preventive measures are important, because most nonbacterial infections (except syphilis and possibly toxoplasmosis, cytomegalovirus [CMV] infection, and herpes simplex) do not respond to current therapy.

ETIOLOGY

Thorough data collection for diagnosis of infectious diseases includes a review of the perinatal history, signs and symptoms, and laboratory data. Intrauterine, intrapartum, or neonatal disease may be caused by a wide variety of organisms, many of which are discussed in this chapter.

SPECIFIC INFECTIOUS DISEASES

The following specific infectious diseases are grouped according to their source of infection.[113]

Transplacental (Intrauterine) Acquisition

HUMAN IMMUNODEFICIENCY VIRUS INFECTION AND ACQUIRED IMMUNODEFICIENCY SYNDROME

Prevention. The primary risk to infants for infection with human immunodeficiency virus (HIV), the causative agent of acquired immunodeficiency syndrome (AIDS), is intrauterine, intrapartum, and postpartum exposure to a mother with HIV infection. HIV has been isolated from blood and many

PURPLE type highlights content that is particularly applicable to clinical settings.

Acknowledgment: This is the second edition in which Gerry Merenstein has not contributed to this chapter. We miss him and dedicate this chapter to him for all his work on this chapter in the first six editions of this book.

AIDS	Acquired immunodeficiency syndrome
CF	Complement fixation (test)
CIE	Counterimmunoelectrophoresis
CRP	C-reactive protein
CRS	Congenital rubella syndrome
CSF	Cerebrospinal fluid
DFA	Direct fluorescent antibody
DNA	Deoxyribonucleic acid
ELISA	Enzyme-linked immunosorbent assay
FA	Fluorescent antibody (test)
FAMA	Fluorescent antibody to membrane antigen
FTA-ABS	Fluorescent treponemal antibody absorption (test)
GBS	Group B *Streptococcus*
HBsAg	Hepatitis B surface antigen
HIV	Human immunodeficiency virus
IAHA	Immune adherence hemagglutination
IFA	Indirect fluorescent antibody (test)
IHA	Indirect hemagglutination inhibition (test)
IPV	Inactivated poliovirus vaccine
IUGR	Intrauterine growth restriction
LA	Latex agglutination (test)
MHA-TP	Microhemagglutination test for *Treponema pallidum* infection
NAAT	Nucleic acid amplification test
OPV	Oral poliovirus vaccine
PCP	*Pneumocystis jiroveci* pneumonia*
PCR	Polymerase chain reaction
RNA	Ribonucleic acid
RPR	Rapid plasma reagin (test)
RT-PCR	Reverse transcriptase PCR
VDRL	Venereal Disease Research Laboratory (test)

*Formerly *Pneumocystis carinii* pneumonia.

body fluids. Epidemiologic evidence has implicated only blood, semen, vaginal secretions, and breastmilk in transmission. In countries such as the United States, where safe alternatives exist, mothers with HIV infection should be discouraged from breastfeeding.[116] HIV testing should be recommended and encouraged to all pregnant women.[5,6,139]

Because the medical history and examination cannot reliably identify all patients infected with HIV (or other bloodborne pathogens) and because during delivery and initial care of the infant, perinatal care providers are exposed to large amounts of maternal blood, standard precautions (e.g., gloves) should be consistently used for all patients when handling the placenta or infant until all maternal blood has been washed away.[5,57]

Data Collection

History. HIV infection in the mother is acquired primarily sexually or by intravenous (IV) drug abuse. Infection may be asymptomatic. Transmission from an untreated infected mother to the fetus or infant occurs in 13% to 39% of births. Approximately 40% of transmissions are before birth and the rest around the time of delivery. Two thirds of infections occurring before delivery are caused by transmission within the 14 days before delivery.[5] A high maternal plasma viral load, high cervico-vaginal viral load, low CD4$^+$ lymphocyte count, advanced maternal illness, an increase in exposure of the fetus to maternal blood, premature delivery, prolonged labor, longer duration of rupture of membranes before delivery, and mode of delivery all increase perinatal transmission of HIV infection.[6,112,138]

Signs and Symptoms. Infants with perinatally acquired HIV infection uncommonly have symptoms in the neonatal period, but the majority of these infants present with clinical illness by 24 months of life (median age at onset of symptoms is 11 to 12 months). One fifth of infants infected with HIV perinatally develop serious disease or die in the first year of life.[139] Symptoms include failure to thrive, developmental disabilities, neurologic dysfunction, hepatosplenomegaly, generalized lymphadenopathy, parotitis, persistent oral candidiasis (thrush), and chronic or recurrent diarrhea. Lymphoid interstitial pneumonia is frequently seen in these infants. HIV-infected infants commonly have osteomyelitis, septic joints, pneumonia, sepsis, meningitis, and otitis media with common organisms (e.g., *Streptococcus pneumoniae, Haemophilus influenzae* type b), and these infections may be recurrent.[112,139]

Laboratory Data. HIV nucleic acid detection by polymerase chain reaction (PCR) of DNA extracted from peripheral blood mononuclear cells is the gold standard for early diagnosis of infected infants, and results are available within 24 hours.[139] About 30% of HIV-infected infants have a positive DNA PCR assay from samples obtained within 48 hours of age; 93% have detectable HIV DNA by 2 weeks; and almost all by 1 month of age. The primary serologic laboratory test for HIV antibody is the enzyme-linked immunosorbent assay (ELISA). The Western blot test is used for confirmation of positive ELISA results. Differentiation of the child with passively acquired antibody from the infant with active infection is critical but difficult. Acquired antibody is undetectable in 75% of infants by 12 months of age and in most infants by 15 to 18 months of age. Infants have also been described with negative serology but active infection.[95] Virus isolation by culture is difficult and expensive, and p24 antigen detection is less sensitive.[86,112] The plasma HIV RNA PCR assay is currently used for quantifying the viral load but not routinely used for diagnosis. Although hypogammaglobulinemia has been reported (less than 10% of patients), hypergammaglobulinemia usually is present.

Treatment. Antiretroviral therapy with zidovudine (ZDV) alone or in combination with other antiretroviral agents reduces HIV transmission from infected mothers to their newborns.[83,94,95] ZDV should be given to infants of infected women beginning at 8 to 12 hours of life and should be continued for 6 weeks.[6,83] ZDV is administered orally at 2 mg/kg body weight/dose every 6 hours.[6] Infants born to untreated HIV-infected women should receive ZDV for 6 weeks, and 3 doses of nevirapine (NVP) in the first week of life (at birth, 48 hours later, and 96 hours after the 2nd dose), beginning as soon after birth as possible. NVP is administered orally at 8 mg/dose (for infants 1.5-2.0 kg) or 12 mg/dose (infant >2.0 kg). If the infant is confirmed to be HIV positive, ZDV is changed to a multidrug antiretroviral regimen. Infants who are perinatally infected with HIV are at high risk for developing *Pneumocystis jiroveci* pneumonia (PCP, formerly known as *Pneumocystis carinii* pneumonia) early in the first year of life. Guidelines recommend initiating prophylaxis for the prevention of PCP for all HIV-exposed infants at 4 to 6 weeks of age, regardless of their CD4+ cell count. For infants receiving ZDV, PCP prophylaxis should begin after completion of the 6-week course of ZDV. The recommended PCP prophylaxis may be provided by 150 mg/m²/day (5 mg/kg/day) of trimethoprim (TMP) and 750 mg/m²/day (25 mg/kg/day) of sulfamethoxazole (SMX) administered in two divided doses for three consecutive days in a week.[6,83,112] TMP/SMX prophylaxis should be continued through the first year of life or until HIV infection is reasonably excluded.[6,83]

Parent Teaching. Care of an infant at risk for HIV requires close and long-term follow-up. Involvement of the parents is essential to this process.

Education of the parents will maximize the success of such a care plan, and utilization of all available community resources should provide additional support. In addition to the rationale for and importance of the medical management just outlined, the parents should be counseled concerning the need for the following:

- Immunizations following the American Academy of Pediatrics schedule
- Rapid consultation with the infant's physician if he or she is exposed to varicella (may need treatment with varicella-zoster immune globulin [VZIG] within 96 hours of exposure) or measles (needs immune globulin intramuscularly regardless of immunization status)
- Rapid consultation with the physician for tetanus-prone wounds (requires tetanus immune globulin irrespective of immunization status)
- Rapid consultation with the physician for thrush, a diaper rash, or any other signs or symptoms of illness

Prevention of infections is important, and this requires good handwashing, regular bathing, appropriate food preparation skills (wash bottles, nipples, and pacifiers), and good skin care (changing diapers and moisturizing skin in other areas to prevent drying and cracking).[112]

CYTOMEGALOVIRUS INFECTION

Prevention. There are no practical methods for preventing CMV infection. Avoiding exposure is virtually impossible because of the ubiquitous and asymptomatic nature of the infections. Avoiding unnecessary blood transfusions or using CMV-seronegative blood donors, white blood cell–depleted blood products, or frozen deglycerolized blood cells has proved to be important in minimizing the occurrence of postnatally acquired CMV, particularly in premature infants.[5,112]

The question frequently arises about assignment of staff to infants with a possible diagnosis of CMV infection. Staff members who may be pregnant have heightened concern about this issue. Staff members should be aware that many infants with CMV infection are often asymptomatic and therefore not identified while in the hospital. To avoid any problems, staff members should employ good handwashing technique with all infants. Wearing gloves when handling urine and other secretions is a strategy that can also be employed by staff members who are working in the neonatal intensive care unit (NICU) and are pregnant or of childbearing age. The actual risk for an infected infant's transmitting disease to a susceptible health care worker is unknown but probably small.[112]

Data Collection

History. Congenital infections are represented by a wide spectrum of disease from asymptomatic disease to profoundly symptomatic disease. CMV infection in the mother is usually asymptomatic.[50,141]

Signs and Symptoms. An infant with CMV infection is usually asymptomatic. Congenital manifestations include intrauterine growth restriction (IUGR), neonatal jaundice (increased direct fraction), purpura, hepatosplenomegaly, microcephaly, seizures, intracerebral calcification, chorioretinitis, and progressive sensorineural hearing loss.[14]

Laboratory Data. CMV may be cultured from urine, pharyngeal secretions, and peripheral leukocytes. Isolation of the virus within 3 weeks of birth indicates transplacental acquisition. A paired sera demonstration of a fourfold titer rise or histopathology demonstration of characteristic nuclear inclusions in certain tissues can confirm infection. Examining the urine for intranuclear inclusions is not helpful. PCR detection of viral DNA in tissues and cerebrospinal fluid is also available.[112]

Treatment. Ganciclovir, foscarnet, valganciclovir, and cidofovir are the only licensed antiviral agents effective against CMV. These drugs are approved only for treatment of life- and sight-saving disease. In a randomized controlled trial that evaluated 42 neonates with congenital CMV infection involving the central nervous system (CNS), 6 weeks of IV ganciclovir therapy prevented hearing deterioration at 6 months. However, two thirds of neonates treated with ganciclovir had significant neutropenia.[35, 81] Antiretroviral therapy for congenital CMV infection with antiviral agents is recommended in infants with evidence of CNS involvement, including sensorineural hearing loss, and should be considered in infants with serious end-organ disease (hepatitis, pneumonia, thrombocytopenia).[135]

Parent Teaching. The need for good handwashing technique by parents and caregivers of infants with suspected CMV should be included in discharge instructions.

RUBELLA

Prevention. Medical personnel should ensure that all mothers have a protective hemagglutination titer

before conception. If the woman is susceptible, vaccinate her with rubella vaccine before conception and advise her that she should avoid conception for 28 days after receiving the vaccine.[89,112] If a woman is found to lack immunity to rubella during pregnancy, she should receive rubella immunization in the postpartum period even if she is breastfeeding.[48,89]

All perinatal health care workers should have rubella titers drawn to identify immunity status, and they should be reimmunized if this is not adequate. Women of childbearing age who do not have protective immune titers should be encouraged to have rubella immunization.[5,112]

Data Collection

History. Rubella in the first 4 to 5 months of pregnancy is associated with a high incidence of sequelae in the infant.[5] A mother with rubella may be relatively asymptomatic or mildly ill with respiratory symptoms with or without a rash.[112]

Signs and Symptoms. Congenital manifestations of rubella include IUGR, sensorineural deafness, cataracts, neonatal jaundice (increased direct fraction), purpura, hepatosplenomegaly, microcephaly, chronic encephalitis, chorioretinitis, and cardiac defects (especially patent ductus arteriosus and peripheral pulmonic stenosis). Less frequent manifestations include bone lesions and pneumonitis.[112]

Laboratory Data. The virus may be isolated from the throat, blood, urine, and cerebrospinal fluid (CSF). A paired sera demonstration of a fourfold titer rise, such as an indirect hemagglutination (IHA) inhibition test or an indirect fluorescent antibody (IFA) test, is diagnostic. The IHA test generally has been replaced by one of several more sensitive methods, including ELISA, or latex agglutination, and reverse transcriptase polymerase chain reaction (RT-PCR) assays.[20,112]

Parent Teaching. Infants with congenital rubella syndrome may secrete the virus for many years. This requires that discharge instructions include preventive strategies that should be employed to decrease the chance of contact of susceptible pregnant women with the infant. Parents should be informed of their responsibility to ensure that potentially seronegative women of childbearing age avoid direct contact with the infant.[112] The challenge arises to impress this on the family and at the same time avoid ostracizing the infant or negatively affecting the parent-infant attachment process. In discharge planning with these families, a collaborative approach should be employed, using community health, medical, nursing, and social work input and support. Another challenge is to impress on parents that an infant exposed to rubella during pregnancy may appear normal at birth, but the first appearance of some CNS symptoms may extend into childhood. Thus families and clinicians should keep a watchful eye on these children during the early childhood years.[89]

SYPHILIS

Prevention. Pregnant women should avoid exposure to syphilis. Monitor the serum early and late in pregnancy, and treat the mother for the appropriate stage of disease. Erythromycin, previously used in penicillin-sensitive women, is not considered adequate treatment during gestation because of 30% treatment failure rates in adults and failure to establish a cure in newborns as a result of poor transplacental passage of erythromycin. Infants born to women treated with erythromycin should be considered high risk for infection and appropriately evaluated and treated. If penicillin allergy is confirmed in the pregnant woman, acute desensitization is necessary. Desensitization can be accomplished using increasing doses of oral penicillin over 4 to 6 hours.[130]

Data Collection

History. A congenital infection may be manifested by a multisystem disease. A primary syphilitic chancre on the cervix or rectal mucosa in a mother may be unnoticed.[130]

Signs and Symptoms. An infant exposed to syphilis may be asymptomatic at birth, or virtually all organ systems may be involved. Clinical findings may include hepatitis, pneumonitis, bone marrow failure, myocarditis, meningitis, nephrotic syndrome, rhinitis (snuffles), a rash involving the palms and soles, and pseudoparalysis of an extremity.[28,112,130]

Laboratory Data. The microscopic darkfield examination identifies spirochetes from nonoral lesions. Nonspecific, nontreponemal reaginic tests, such as Venereal Disease Research Laboratory (VDRL) tests and rapid plasma reagin (RPR) tests, followed serially with a rise or absence of fall after birth, are useful for screening.[28,130] Specific treponemal antibody serologic tests, such as a fluorescent treponemal antibody absorption (FTA-ABS) test or a microhemagglutination test for *Treponema pallidum* (MHA-TP), provide diagnostic confirmation of a reactive nontreponemal test, but an FTA-ABS immunoglobulin M (IgM) test is unreliable.[28,130] False-positive results

may occur with nontreponemal tests secondary to other medical conditions or other spirochetal diseases. Therefore confirmation of diagnosis is necessary.[112] A long-bone x-ray examination showing metaphysitis or periostitis may help in diagnosing syphilis. VDRL tests on CSF are mandatory in all infants suspected of having congenital syphilis. When the diagnosis of active congenital syphilis is equivocal, often it is best to treat and ascertain the diagnosis by serial serologic determinations.[28,112,130]

Treatment. Table 22-1 outlines the treatment for syphilis.[112]

Parent Teaching. Adequate follow-up of both symptomatic and asymptomatic neonates is very important. A physical evaluation should be conducted at 1, 2, 3, 6, and 12 months. Serologic testing should be performed at 3, 6, and 12 months after completion of therapy regimen, or until titer decreases fourfold. Noninfected or adequately treated infants' titers should be decreased by 3 months and nonreactive by 6 months. If titers fail to decline or if they increase or are still present after 6 to 12 months of age, the infant should be reevaluated and retreated. Infants with neurosyphilis should have a repeat CSF examination every 6 months until it is normal and VDRL nonreactive. If CSF VDRL is still reactive at 6 months or CSF white cell count is not decreasing at each reexamination or is abnormal at 24 months, retreatment is indicated.[112]

TOXOPLASMOSIS

Prevention. Women should avoid unnecessary exposure to raw meat, cat feces, and eating fruits or vegetables not peeled or washed thoroughly. Using a pair of gloves when emptying the litter box may provide protection if the pregnant woman (or a woman attempting to become pregnant) must empty the litter box.[112] A pregnant woman (or woman attempting to become pregnant) should use hot soapy water to wash her hands immediately after exposure to any infectious source, even after wearing gloves.[19]

Data Collection

History. Congenital infections are represented by a wide range of disease, from asymptomatic disease to profound symptomatic disease, and all require treatment.[112,136] Mothers may have noted an influenza-like illness, posterior cervical adenitis, or chorioretinitis but usually lack accompanying

TABLE
22-1 **RECOMMENDED THERAPY FOR INDICATED CONDITIONS**

CONDITION	TREATMENT
Sepsis and/or Meningitis	
Initial Therapy	
Early onset	Intravenous (IV) ampicillin and gentamicin or IV amikacin (if gentamicin-resistant organisms are present in nursery, ampicillin plus cefotaxime is a suitable alternative, particularly if meningitis is present).
Late onset	IV vancomycin plus cefotaxime or IV aminoglycoside (see "Early onset").
Once Specific Organisms Are Identified	
Group B *Streptococcus*	IV ampicillin and gentamicin for 10-14 days (gentamicin may be discontinued if strain is not tolerant).
Coliform species	IV ampicillin and gentamicin for 10-14 days (cefotaxime may replace gentamicin).
Listeria monocytogenes	IV ampicillin and IV gentamicin for 14-21 days.
Enterococci	Same as for *Listeria monocytogenes*. For ampicillin resistance, use vancomycin.
Group A *Streptococcus*	IV penicillin G for 10-14 days.
Group D *Streptococcus* (nonenterococcus)	Same as for group A *Streptococcus*.
Staphylococcus aureus	IV nafcillin for 10-14 days; IV vancomycin for methicillin-resistant strains.
Staphylococcus epidermidis	IV vancomycin for 10-14 days.
Pseudomonas aeruginosa	IV ceftazidime and aminoglycoside for 10-14 days.
Anaerobes	IV metronidazole, clindamycin, or meropenem.
Pneumonia	
Group B *Streptococcus*	Same as for sepsis (respiratory distress syndrome may mimic pneumonitis and vice versa).
Staphylococcus aureus	Same as for sepsis.
Chlamydia trachomatis	Oral (PO) erythromycin for 14 days.
Pneumocystis jiroveci	PO or IV trimethoprim and sulfamethoxazole, or IV pentamidine isethionate.
Pertussis	PO or IV azithromycin for 5 days (clinical course is unchanged, but shedding of organism is diminished significantly).
Other organisms	Same as for sepsis.
Skin and Soft Tissue Infections	
Impetigo	IV or intramuscular (IM) nafcillin; PO cephalexin for 7 days (depending on clinical severity). For methicillin resistance, use vancomycin. Also consider topical mupirocin.
Group A *Streptococcus* infections	IV penicillin G for 7 days.
Breast abscess	IV nafcillin and gentamicin for 7 days pending identification of etiologic agent (change to IV penicillin if *Streptococcus* is etiologic agent; IV ampicillin or gentamicin should be used for coliform species pending sensitivities); value of surgical drainage is individualized; vancomycin for methicillin-resistant strains.
Omphalitis and/or funisitis	IV nafcillin for 7 days (penicillin may be used if infection is caused by group A or B streptococci); if gram-negative rods, consider gentamicin or cefotaxime also.
Gastrointestinal Infections	
Salmonella species	IV ampicillin for 7-10 days; or IV cefotaxime or ceftriaxone for 7-10 days depending on sensitivities (focal complications of meningitis and arthritis should be monitored closely).
Shigella species	PO trimethoprim/sulfamethoxazole or PO or IV ampicillin, depending on sensitivities.
Necrotizing enterocolitis	IV ampicillin and IV gentamicin for 2-3 weeks (if *Pseudomonas* is isolated, IV ceftazidime or piperacillin/tazobactam combination may be substituted for ampicillin); supportive measures (gastrointestinal suction) are appropriate.

T A B L E 22-1	RECOMMENDED THERAPY FOR INDICATED CONDITIONS — cont'd

CONDITION	TREATMENT
Osteomyelitis or Septic Arthritis	
Group B *Streptococcus*	IV penicillin G for 21 days minimum.
Staphylococcus aureus	IV oxacillin for 21 days minimum.
Coliform species	IV gentamicin for 21 days (IV ampicillin for 21 days minimum if organism is sensitive).
Gonococcus species	IV penicillin G for 10 days.
Unknown	IV oxacillin and gentamicin for 21 days minimum.
Urinary Tract Infections	Suspect predisposing anatomic defect if urinary tract infection; individualize workup and follow-up.
Coliform species	Gentamicin, 3 mg/kg/day divided q 8 hr for 10 days.
Enterococcus species	Ampicillin, 150 mg/kg/day divided q 8 hr for 10 days.
Miscellaneous Conditions	
Congenital syphilis	If more than 1 day of treatment is missed in either of the following regimens, the entire course should be restarted.
• Without central nervous system (CNS) involvement	IM procaine penicillin G (50,000 units/kg) daily for 10-14 days (follow-up Venereal Disease Research Laboratory [VDRL] test results should revert to negative if treatment is adequate by 1 year).
• With CNS involvement	IV aqueous crystalline penicillin G 100,000-150,000 U/kg/day, administered as 50,000 for a total U/kg/dose q 12 hr for the first 7 days of life and q 8 hr thereafter for 10 days. Repeat lumbar puncture about every 6 months until results are normal.
Toxoplasmosis	PO sulfadiazine, 100-120 mg/kg/day divided q 12 hr and PO pyrimethamine, 1 mg/kg/day divided q 12 hr (duration of treatment is debatable but should be long [i.e., months]; supplemental folic acid, 1 mg/day, should be added). Ocular, CNS, or human immunodeficiency virus (HIV) involvement may require additional therapy.
Herpes simplex infections	IV acyclovir, 20 mg/kg/dose q 8 hr, for 14 days if skin or mucous membrane involvement; 21 days if CNS involvement.
Conjunctivitis	
• *Chlamydia* species	PO erythromycin for 10 days (topical may be ineffective).
• *Gonococcus* species	IV penicillin G for 10 days; cefoxitin for penicillin-resistant strains.
Otitis media	
• In otherwise normal neonate	PO amoxicillin/clavulanic acid (Augmentin), 40 mg/kg divided q 8 hr for 10 days.
• In neonate with nosoco-mial infection	PO or IV ampicillin and IV gentamicin (if there is no response to treatment, consider diagnostic tympanocentesis; *Staphylococcus aureus* and coliform species may be present).

Data from Bradley JS, Nelson JD: *Nelson's pocket book of pediatric antimicrobial therapy: 2006-2007*, ed 16, Philadelphia, 2006, Alliance for World Wide Editing.

signs or symptoms. A history of exposure to cat feces or ingestion of raw meat occasionally may be obtained.[5,74,136]

Signs and Symptoms. Manifestations in a newborn may be prematurity, IUGR, hydrocephalus, chorioretinitis, seizures, cerebral calcifications, hepatosplenomegaly, thrombocytopenia, jaundice, generalized lymphadenopathy, and a rash.[112,136]

Laboratory Data. Isolating *Toxoplasma gondii* from blood or body fluids is difficult and tedious. Cysts may be found in the placenta or tissues of a fetus or newborn.[97] Most congenitally infected infants have a Sabin–Feldman dye test titer greater than 1:1000 at birth.

Treatment. Table 22-1 outlines the treatment of toxoplasmosis.[112]

Perinatal Acquisition During Labor and Delivery

CHLAMYDIA TRACHOMATIS INFECTION
Prevention. Eye prophylaxis with erythromycin (preferred) or tetracycline ophthalmic ointment

minimizes the development of conjunctivitis but has no effect on the subsequent development of pneumonitis.[108,112]

Data Collection

History. A mother with a *Chlamydia trachomatis* infection is usually asymptomatic during her pregnancy.[5,108]

Signs and Symptoms. Conjunctivitis may be manifested as congestion and edema of the conjunctiva, with minimal discharge developing 1 to 2 weeks after birth and lasting several weeks with recurrences, particularly after topical therapy. Infants with pneumonitis usually do not have a fever but have a prolonged staccato cough, tachypnea, mild hypoxemia, and eosinophilia. Otitis media and bronchiolitis also may occur.[108,112]

Laboratory Data. Definitive diagnosis is made by isolating the organism in tissue culture and by nucleic acid amplification tests (NAATs) (e.g., PCR). Demonstrating chlamydial antigen in clinical specimens by the direct fluorescent antibody method or enzyme immunoassay is very reliable. To enhance the likelihood of obtaining an adequate sample, scrape the lower conjunctiva (for conjunctivitis) or obtain deep tracheal secretions or a nasopharyngeal aspirate (for pneumonia). NAATs are not recommended for nasopharyngeal aspirates. Scraping conjunctival epithelial cells and demonstrating characteristic intracytoplasmic inclusion bodies by a Giemsa stain is diagnostic. Although serologic tests for conjunctivitis are unreliable, a significant titer rise in IgM-specific antibody may be reliable in cases of pneumonia. Eosinophilia (greater than 300 eosinophils/mm^3) may suggest chlamydial pneumonia.[108,112]

ENTEROVIRUS (COXSACKIEVIRUS A, COXSACKIEVIRUS B, ECHOVIRUS, AND POLIOMYELITIS) INFECTIONS

Enterovirus infections are the most commonly diagnosed viral infections in the NICU, and coxsackievirus B1 was the most common in 2007 by the National Enterovirus Surveillance System.[25,79,143]

Prevention. To prevent poliomyelitis, it is essential to maintain poliomyelitis immunity with active immunization before conception. Passive protection with pooled human serum globulin may help in selected exposures (0.2 ml/kg body weight, given intramuscularly). Routine nursery infection control procedures must be observed. It is recommended that only inactivated poliovirus vaccine (IPV) be used in the nursery. The IPV is administered intramuscularly and contains no live virus, whereas oral poliovirus vaccine (OPV) (OPV is no longer available in the United States) is administered orally and contains live but attenuated virus, which has been reported to cause infection in immunocompromised patients.[112]

Data Collection

History. Infection may occur year-round but is more prevalent from June to December in temperate climates. Most enterovirus infections are asymptomatic. Poliomyelitis is rare because of a high level of vaccine-induced immunity in most of the world.[112]

Signs and Symptoms. Mothers with enteroviral infections are usually mildly ill, with fever or diarrhea. Infants may be asymptomatic or have fever or diarrhea. Infants who acquire the infection without maternal antibody have severe disease and high mortality rates. Fever, irritability, lethargy, and rash are common. Severe disease with sepsis, meningoencephalitis, myocarditis, pneumonia, hepatitis, or coagulopathy may occur.[2] Prematurity, early onset of illness (less than 7 days), maternal history of illness, high white blood cell count (15,000/mm^3 or greater), and low hemoglobin (less than 10.7 g/dl) have been shown to be risk factors of severe infection.[88]

Laboratory Data. The virus may be isolated from the throat, rectum, or CSF. Isolating coxsackievirus A may require suckling mouse inoculation. Serologic screening is impractical because of the large number of serotypes. PCR assay for enterovirus RNA in CSF and other specimens is available and is more sensitive than viral isolation.[112]

Treatment. The antiviral agent *pleconaril* is currently being assessed in a phase 2, multicenter, randomized, placebo-controlled trial for newborns with enteroviral sepsis characterized by hepatitis, coagulopathy, or myocarditis.[1] Pleconaril has a novel mechanism of action by preventing the viral attachment and entry into the host cells and seems to be well tolerated in neonates.[3,122] Hand hygiene is paramount to control spread of enteroviral infections.[112] Intravenous immunoglobulin may be effective in severe enteroviral infection.[1,121]

GROUP B *STREPTOCOCCUS* INFECTION

Prevention. Group B *Streptococcus* (GBS) sepsis is associated with significant morbidity and mortality risks. The Centers for Disease Control and Prevention (CDC) recommends universal screening of pregnant women at 35 to 37 weeks' gestation and the use of intrapartum prophylactic antibiotics in colonized women to prevent GBS sepsis. Pregnant women who are GBS positive are treated with penicillin or ampicillin during labor or, if allergic to penicillin, treated with cefazolin. Clindamycin is generally not recommended unless culture results indicate sensitivity due to resistant GBS strains in up to 20% of cultures and a limited ability to reach bactericidal levels in amniotic fluid and in fetal circulation.[34,36,67,92]

Intrapartum prophylactic antibiotics are also indicated if the GBS status of the mother is unknown and one or more intrapartum risk factors exist (see History following).[83]

Treatment with antibiotics for less than 4 hours is inadequate to prevent the transmission of GBS.[91] It is estimated that use of these guidelines results in an 80% reduction in the number of neonates affected by early-onset GBS sepsis.[5,9,17,23,112]

Data Collection

History. Maternal history of any risk factors that include (1) gestation less than 37 weeks, (2) rupture of membranes for 18 hours or longer, (3) a maternal temperature of 38° C (100.4° F) or higher, (4) a history of GBS bacteriuria during the current pregnancy, or (5) a previous infant with GBS infection warrants intrapartum antibiotics.

Signs and Symptoms. Symptoms of early-onset GBS are seen within the first 24 hours of life.[17,23] Table 22-2 depicts clinical and laboratory findings of early-onset GBS infection.

Laboratory Data. New screening tests have been developed and validated for rapid identification of GBS, including pigmented enrichment broths, chromogenic agars, DNA probes, and NAATs, such as PCR.[9] A full sepsis evaluation including a lumbar puncture is indicated for any newborn who demonstrates signs of infection.

Treatment. An updated treatment algorithm has been developed to manage at risk infants with the intention of preventing GBS infection (Figure 22-1). Table 22-1 outlines the antibiotic treatment of GBS infection.

Complications. Use of the updated treatment algorithm has been shown to reduce the number of early-onset sepsis evaluations and antibiotic exposure without increasing the rate of onset of GBS infection.[5,9,23,99,112]

Parent Teaching. See Early Onset Bacterial Disease, Parent Teaching on p. 555 and Parent Teaching on p. 562.

TABLE 22-2	MATERNAL AND INFANT CLINICAL CHARACTERISTICS OF EARLY-ONSET GBS DISEASE								
GBS STATUS	ROM >18 hr	ANY FEVER	FEVER >100.4° C	INTRAPARTUM ANTIBIOTICS	TERM	PRETERM	ILL-APPEARING	ABNORMAL WBC COUNT	CRITICALLY ILL/DIED
Negative (n = 16)	7 (44)	8 (50)	3 (19)	2 (12)	14 (88)	2 (12)	11 (69)	12 (75)	5 (31)
Positive (n = 5)	3 (60)	2 (40)	1 (20)	2 (40)	2 (40)	3 (60)	4 (80)	2 (40)	2 (40)
Unknown (n = 4)	0 (0)	2 (50)	1 (25)	0 (0)	1 (25)	3 (75)	4 (100)	4 (100)	4 (100)
			5 (20)	4 (16)	17 (68)	8 (32)	19 (76)	18 (72)	11 (44)

Numbers in parentheses indicate percentage of total for each category (GBS negative, positive, or unknown and total cases). ROM indicates rupture of membranes; abnormal WBC count. Adapted from Puopolo KM, Madoff LC, Eichenwald EC: Early-onset group B streptococcal disease in the era of maternal screening, *Pediatrics* 115:1240, 2005.
GBS, Group B *Streptococcus*; *ROM*, rupture of membranes; *WBC*, white blood cell.

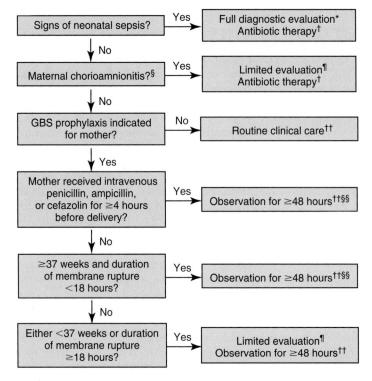

FIGURE 22-1   Algorithm for secondary prevention of early-onset group B streptococcal (GBS) disease among newborns. (From CDC: Prevention of perinatal group B streptococcal disease, revised guidelines from CDC, 2010, *MMWR* 59:1, 2010.)

* Full diagnostic evaluation includes a blood culture, a complete blood count (CBC) including white blood cell differential and platelet counts, chest radiograph (if respiratory abnormalities are present), and lumbar puncture (if patient is stable enough to tolerate procedure and sepsis is suspected).

† Antibiotic therapy should be directed toward the most common causes of neonatal sepsis, including intravenous ampicillin for GBS and coverage for other organisms (including *Escherichia coli* and other gram-negative pathogens) and should take into account local antibiotic resistance patterns.

§ Consultation with obstetric providers is important to determine the level of clinical suspicion for chorioamnionitis. Chorioamnionitis is diagnosed clinically and some of the signs are nonspecific.

¶ Limited evaluation includes blood culture (at birth) and CBC with differential and platelets (at birth and/or at 6–12 hours of life).

†† If signs of sepsis develop, a full diagnostic evaluation should be conducted and antibiotic therapy initiated.

§§ If ≥37 weeks' gestation, observation may occur at home after 24 hours if other discharge criteria have been met, access to medical care is readily available, and a person who is able to comply fully with instructions for home observation will be present. If any of these conditions is not met, the infant should be observed in the hospital for at least 48 hours and until discharge criteria are achieved.

¶¶ Some experts recommend a CBC with differential and platelets at age 6–12 hours.

TABLE 22-3 ACCEPTABLE METHODS OF PASSIVE IMMUNIZATION IN NEWBORNS

DISEASE	INDICATIONS	WHEN TO USE	PRODUCT	DOSE
Hepatitis A	Active infection in mother or close family contacts	As soon as possible	HSIG	0.02-0.04 ml/kg body weight given IM
Hepatitis B	Mothers with acute type B infection or who are antigen (+)	As soon as possible (within 12 hr)	HBIG*	0.5 ml IM
Tetanus	Inadequately immunized mothers with contaminated infant (e.g., dirty cord)	As soon as possible	TIG	250 units given IM (optimal dose not established)
Varicella	Administer as soon as possible to infant born to a mother who develops lesions <5 days before delivery, within 7 days after delivery, or when/if infant is exposed to varicella-zpster virus any time during the initial hospitalization.	Within 10 days	ZIG	2 ml given IM

Modified from Remington JS, Klein JO, editors: *Infectious diseases of the fetus and newborn infant,* ed 5, Philadelphia, 2001, Saunders; with addition from Updated recommendations for use of VariZIG–United States, 2013. *MMWR* 62(28):574-576, 2013.
HBIG, Hepatitis B immune globulin; *HSIG,* human serum immune globulin; *IM,* intramuscularly; *TIG,* tetanus immune globulin (human); *ZIG,* zoster immune globulin.
*Should be used in conjunction with active immunization with hepatitis B virus (HBV) vaccine (see Table 22-4).

TABLE 22-4 ACCEPTABLE METHODS OF ACTIVE IMMUNIZATION IN NEWBORNS

DISEASE	INDICATION	WHEN TO USE	PRODUCT	DOSE
Hepatitis B	HBsAg positive or HBsAg negative	3 separate doses: at birth*; at 1 month; and at 6 months	Recombivax HB	0.5 ml given IM
			Engerix-B	0.5 ml given IM
Pertussis	To control outbreak in nursery	As soon as possible	Pertussis vaccine†	0.25-0.5 ml administered subcutaneously
Tuberculosis	Selected infants at risk for contracting tuberculosis	As soon as possible	Calmette-Guérin bacillus (CGB)	0.1 ml given intradermally and divided into 2 sites over deltoid muscle

HBsAg, Hepatitis B surface antigen; *IM,* intramuscularly.
*As soon as possible.
†Pregnant mothers may provide passive immunity against pertussis if they receive Tdap between the 27th and 36th weeks of pregnancy.

HEPATITIS B

Prevention. Prenatal screening of women for hepatitis B surface antigen (HBsAg) is indicated and is cost effective. Use of active and passive immunization in infants born to HBsAg-positive mothers is indicated (Tables 22-3 and 22-4).[112] Use of active immunization for infants born to HBsAg-negative women is recommended at birth by the Advisory Committee on Immunization Practices. However, the CDC analyzed data from the 2006 National Immunization Survey (for the years 2003 to 2005), which showed that only 50.1% of newborns had hepatitis B vaccine by day 3 of life with a considerable geographic variation.[26]

Data Collection

History. Mothers who are HBsAg positive because of the chronic carrier state or acute disease before delivery may pass the infection to their infants at delivery.[5] Women at high risk include those of Asian, Pacific Island, or Alaskan Eskimo descent; women born in Haiti or sub-Saharan Africa; and those with a history of liver disease, IV drug abuse, or frequent exposure to blood in a medical-dental setting.

Signs and Symptoms. A neonate with hepatitis B is usually asymptomatic. Occasionally, infected infants demonstrate elevated liver enzymes or acute fulminating hepatitis.[112] Neonatal infection with subsequent chronic carriage has been implicated in the development of primary hepatocellular carcinoma later in life.

Laboratory Data. Most infants at risk for acquiring hepatitis from their mother are HBsAg negative at birth. Many untreated infants become HBsAg positive 4 to 12 weeks after birth and become lifelong asymptomatic carriers or develop hepatitis B.[112]

HEPATITIS C

Prevention. Neonates acquire hepatitis C virus (HCV) infection mostly through vertical transmission from the mother and rarely through transfusion of hepatitis C–contaminated blood products. Vertical transmission rates from the mother to the infant vary (approximately 5%), and risk factors associated with increased transmission are HCV viral load, coinfection with HIV, rupture of membranes more than 6 hours, and internal fetal monitoring.[33,90,106,107] Reducing viral load by maternal antiviral therapy, especially in HIV-coinfected women, and avoiding internal fetal monitoring are interventions that can reduce transmission but have not been evaluated. Breastfeeding is not associated with increased rates of transmission and is not contraindicated.[112] Screening of blood products for HCV is mandatory for prevention of transfusion-related HCV infection.

Data Collection

History. Approximately 1% to 2% of pregnant women in the United States are seropositive for HCV, but vertical transmission occurs only if the mother is HCV RNA positive at the time of delivery.[112] HCV RNA titers rise many weeks after birth in infants, indicating a perinatal acquisition rather than an intrauterine transmission.[33]

Signs and Symptoms. Neonates with perinatal acquisition of HCV infection are usually asymptomatic without jaundice and with normal or only mildly elevated liver transaminase levels.[107,118,140] Progression to chronic hepatitis is common and occurs in approximately 80% of infected infants. Liver biopsies in infants with perinatally acquired HCV during follow-up show evidence

of chronic inflammation. A small percentage (20%) of infants may spontaneously resolve their infection.[44]

Laboratory Data. The essential diagnostic feature is HCV RNA positivity on at least two occasions by PCR. Sensitivity of the PCR is 22% in infants younger than 1 month and 97% after 1 month of age.[40] Maternal antibodies may persist in the infant for 13 to 18 months and are not useful for diagnosis. Following liver transaminase levels may help monitor the course of hepatic inflammation.

Treatment. Ribavirin and interferon alfa are used in the treatment of adults. Small studies in children indicate efficacy of ribavirin with interferon alfa or pegylated interferon alfa combinations producing approximately 45% viral clearance rates.[61,149,150] However, only limited data exist for the use of ribavirin or interferons, and more research is needed.[71]

HERPES SIMPLEX (TYPES 1 AND 2) INFECTION

Prevention. The key to preventing herpes simplex is avoiding exposure. In the third trimester, use of maternal prophylaxis with antiviral agents for herpes decreases recurrence of maternal lesions and decreases the incidence of cesarean sections. However, there is insufficient evidence that this strategy prevents neonatal herpes.[70] Mothers with active lesions or in prodrome should have a cesarean section preferably within 4 to 6 hours of membrane rupture. Treatment with acyclovir should begin at the first sign of neonatal disease or when infants have been exposed to an active lesion.[5,112]

Communication is necessary between obstetric and neonatal staff to determine the status of a family with a history of herpes. Unnecessary restrictions should not be placed on postpartum mothers who are not actively infected.[5] Health professionals should employ all family-centered strategies used in their institutions with families unless such strategies are precluded by the need for the infant's treatment.

Data Collection

History. Disease caused by type 1 herpes simplex usually is spread by the oral route, whereas disease caused by type 2 herpes simplex is usually spread by the genital route.[112] Many mothers who transmit herpes simplex to their newborn infants are asymptomatic.[82] The risk to the infant from recurrent lesions is minimal.[52,112]

Signs and Symptoms. Infants with herpes simplex have a spectrum of illnesses ranging from localized skin lesions to generalized infections involving the liver, lungs, and CNS. This disseminated disease has high morbidity and mortality rates.[80,82,100]

Laboratory Data. A cytologic examination of the base of skin vesicles with a Giemsa stain (Tzanck test) may reveal characteristic but nonspecific giant cells and eosinophilic intranuclear inclusions. The virus may be readily identified on a tissue culture within 48 hours from the respiratory and genital tracts, blood, urine, and CSF.[100] Rapid viral diagnosis by direct fluorescent antibody tests is widely available.[112] Detection of virus in CSF by PCR assay is preferred, if available.[21] Although tests of paired serology such as complement fixation (CF) test, ELISA, and neutralization are available, they are of little value in an acute clinical situation.[112] Elevated liver transaminases and thrombocytopenia may indicate herpes infection.[18]

Treatment. Table 22-1 outlines the treatment of herpes simplex infection.

Parent Teaching. Families with herpes simplex require consistent and detailed teaching about prevention of transmission of herpes to the infant. Breastfeeding mothers can be reassured that they may continue to breastfeed as long as no lesions are on their breasts. Emphasis should be placed on the need for breastfeeding mothers to check their breasts for lesions.[5]

Parents with active herpes simplex should employ good handwashing technique while caring for their infants. Parents with oral herpes should avoid kissing their infants while lesions are open and draining.[112]

LISTERIA MONOCYTOGENES INFECTION

Prevention. Pregnant women should avoid unpasteurized dairy products (i.e., milk and cheese) to prevent *Listeria monocytogenes* infection.[42,114]

Data Collection. See Laboratory Data on p. 554.

Treatment. Table 22-1 outlines the treatment of *L. monocytogenes* infection.

Parent Teaching. See Early Onset Bacterial Disease, Parent Teaching on p. 555 and Parent Teaching on p. 562.

MYCOBACTERIUM TUBERCULOSIS INFECTION

Prevention. Mothers at risk for *Mycobacterium tuberculosis* infection may be identified with a tuberculin test during pregnancy. If the mother is a tuberculin converter (has had a positive skin test result within the past 2 years), a radiographic examination of the chest and lungs should be performed. If the mother has active tuberculosis, she should be treated with isoniazid plus rifampin and ethambutol for at least 9 months. Safety of pyrazinamide in pregnancy is not well established, and this drug is not used routinely in pregnant women. Pyridoxine (vitamin B_6) always should be given with isoniazid during pregnancy and breastfeeding because of the increased requirements for this vitamin. If the mother does not have active tuberculosis, household contacts should be screened. If the disease is identified in the mother or household contacts, the infant is at high risk for developing tuberculosis.[112]

Separate infants of mothers with active disease from the mother until the mother is not contagious (usually negative sputum). Treat high-risk infants with isoniazid (10 mg/kg/day) or a tuberculosis vaccine (Calmette-Guérin bacillus) (see Table 22-4).[5,112]

Data Collection

History. A strong history of maternal contact with tuberculosis favors the diagnosis. This is especially true in high-risk populations (Southeast Asians, American Indians, and families with a known cavitary disease). Mothers with HIV infection are at an increased risk for developing active tuberculosis.[112,137]

Signs and Symptoms. Mothers may be relatively asymptomatic or have signs and symptoms that are generalized (fever and weight loss) or localized to the respiratory tract.[112] A congenital infection is extremely rare.[5] Nonspecific signs and symptoms such as failure to thrive and unexplained hypothermia or hyperthermia are the most common manifestations in the neonatal period.

Laboratory Data. Acid-fast organisms found on smears of gastric aspirates, sputum, CSF, or infected tissues strongly suggest tuberculosis in the neonate. Isolating *M. tuberculosis* by culture is diagnostic and should be sought aggressively. The tuberculin test result usually is positive (greater than 10-mm induration) in active tuberculosis. However, a positive skin test result requires 3 to 12 weeks after infection to manifest itself, and the test result usually is negative in a neonate. A chest radiograph examination also usually yields a negative result in a neonate.[112]

Treatment. Because congenital tuberculosis is such a rare condition, optimal therapy has not been established. However, most recommendations suggest four-drug therapy (isoniazid, rifampin, pyrazinamide, and streptomycin or kanamycin).[112]

Parent Teaching. Infants who are treated with isoniazid or breastfed infants whose mothers are treated with isoniazid should receive pyridoxine supplementation.[112]

NEISSERIA GONORRHOEAE INFECTION

Prevention. Screening high-risk mothers before delivery may identify asymptomatic gonorrhea. Treating positive mothers before delivery or exposed infants at delivery is necessary.[112]

Administering silver nitrate, erythromycin, or tetracycline in the eyes is mandatory in all vaginal deliveries.[112]

Data Collection

History. Mothers with previous venereal disease are a high-risk group, because 80% of the infected women may be asymptomatic.

Signs and Symptoms. The predominant manifestation of gonorrhea is *ophthalmia neonatorum,* although a systemic bloodborne infection may rarely occur involving the joints, lungs, endocardium, and CNS. Conjunctivitis usually begins 2 to 5 days after birth. Eye prophylaxis minimizes but does not guarantee freedom from infection. Scalp abscess resulting from fetal monitoring has been reported.[112]

Laboratory Data. A Gram stain of purulent eye discharge revealing gram-negative intracellular diplococci is diagnostic. Culture confirmation using fermentation or fluorescence establishes the diagnosis of gonorrhea. The organism is labile, so specimens for culture should be taken to the laboratory and plated immediately. When gonorrhea is diagnosed, other sexually transmitted diseases may be present concomitantly (especially chlamydial infection).[112]

Treatment. Table 22-1 outlines the treatment of *Neisseria gonorrhoeae* infection.

VARICELLA

Prevention. Table 22-3 outlines prevention of infection.[112]

Data Collection

History. A history of varicella in the mother before conception virtually excludes the diagnosis. Varicella manifests in the mother with a fever, respiratory symptoms, and characteristic vesicular rash primarily on the trunk. If this occurs within 5 days of delivery, the newborn is at risk for infection.[112] Preventive measures should be instituted as soon as possible.[5] Acute perinatal varicella is frequently a devastating systemic disease. Nosocomially acquired transmission of varicella is a potentially significant problem for high-risk infants: premature infants born to susceptible mothers; infants who are severely premature regardless of maternal status; and immunocompromised patients of all ages (Table 22-5).

Signs and Symptoms. Congenital varicella is rare but has followed maternal varicella in the first trimester of pregnancy. Congenital manifestations include limb atrophy, skin scars, and CNS and eye abnormalities.[112]

Laboratory Data. The demonstration of multinucleated giant cells containing intranuclear inclusions in skin scrapings on Giemsa stain is nonspecific but helpful. Virus can be isolated from scrapings of vesicle base during the first 3 to 4 days of the eruption by direct fluorescent antibody test or isolation of virus in tissue culture.[24,27] Isolating the virus from the respiratory tract is difficult. A number of serologic tests such as the fluorescent antibody to membrane antigen test, immune adherence hemagglutination test, ELISA, and neutralization test are available but are not helpful in the acute clinical situation. CF serologic tests are relatively insensitive.[112]

EARLY-ONSET BACTERIAL DISEASE

Prevention. For GBS only, see p. 545.

Data Collection

History. Early-onset disease is almost always acquired perinatally and is discussed here. Late-onset disease is discussed under Postnatal Acquisition Late-Onset Bacterial Disease later in this chapter. Early-onset disease presents as a fulminant multisystem illness during the first days of life (less than 72 hours

TABLE 22-5								

INFECTION CONTROL MEASURES AND ISOLATION TECHNIQUES FOR SPECIFIC DISEASES

	RECOMMENDED PRECAUTIONS							
DISEASE/ ORGANISMS	WASH HANDS	PRIVATE ROOM OR COHORT	MASK	GOWN	GLOVE	INFECTIVE MATERIAL	DURATION OF ISOLATION/ PRECAUTION	COMMENTS
AIDS/HIV	X	D	No	(X)	(X)	Blood and body fluids	Duration of illness	Utmost care needed to avoid needle sticks
Adenovirus	X	X	No	(X)	(X)	Respiratory secretions and feces	Duration of hospitalization	During outbreaks, cohort patients suspected of having adenovirus infection
Conjunctivitis								
• Gonococcal (ophthalmia neonatorum)	X	X	No	No	(X)	Purulent exudates	Until 24 hr after initiation of effective therapy	
• Chlamydia	X	No	No	No	(X)	Purulent exudates	Duration of illness	
Coxsackievirus	X	D	No	(X)	(X)	Feces and respiratory secretions	For 7 days after onset of illness	
Cytomegalovirus	X	No	No	No	(X)	Urine and respiratory secretions	Counsel pregnant personnel	
Diarrhea	X	D	No	(X)	(X)	Feces	Duration of illness	Identify colonized or infected infants by culture; institute cohorting
Echovirus	X	D	No	(X)	(X)	Feces and respiratory secretions	For 7 days after onset of illness	
Gastroenteritis	X	X	No	(X)	(X)	Feces	Duration of illness	
Hepatitis — type A	X	D	No	(X)	(X)	Feces	For 7 days after onset of illness	Most contagious before symptoms
Hepatitis — type B	X	No	No	(X)	(X)	Blood and body fluids	Duration of positivity	Avoid needle sticks
Herpes simplex	X	X	No	(X)	(X)	Lesions, secretions, urine, and stool	Duration of illness	
Influenza A or B	X	X	No	(X)	(X)	Respiratory secretions	Duration of illness	Cohort patients suspected of having influenza during outbreak; staff should receive yearly influenza vaccine
Meningitis								
• Aseptic	X	D	No	(X)	(X)	Feces	Duration of illness	Cohort colonized or infected infants during a nursery outbreak
• Bacterial	X	No	No	No	No			

Continued

TABLE 22–5	INFECTION CONTROL MEASURES AND ISOLATION TECHNIQUES FOR SPECIFIC DISEASES — cont'd

	RECOMMENDED PRECAUTIONS							
DISEASE/ ORGANISMS	WASH HANDS	PRIVATE ROOM OR COHORT	MASK	GOWN	GLOVE	INFECTIVE MATERIAL	DURATION OF ISOLATION/ PRECAUTION	COMMENTS
Necrotizing entero-colitis	X	No	No	(X)	(X)	(?) Feces	Duration of illness	Cohort ill infants
Respiratory syncytial virus	X	X	X	(X)	(X)	Respiratory secretions	Duration of illness	Cohort suspected infants, especially premature infants, during outbreaks
Rubella	X	X	X	No	No	Respiratory secretions	Duration of hospitalization	Infants may shed virus for as long as 2 years; seronegative women should avoid contact
Staphylococcal disease (Staphylococcus aureus)	X	D	No	(X)	(X)	Purulent exudate	Duration of illness	
Streptococcal disease								
• Group A	X	D	No	(X)	(X)	Respiratory secretions	24 hr after initiation of effective therapy	
• Group B	X	D	No	(X)	(X)	Respiratory and genital secretions	Cohort ill and colonized infants during a nursery outbreak	
Syphilis	X	No	No	No	(X)	Lesion secretion and blood	24 hr after initiation of effective therapy	
Toxoplasmosis	X	No	No	No	No	None		
Varicella	X	X	X	X	X	Respiratory and lesion secretions	Until lesions are crusted	Neonates born to mothers with active chickenpox should be placed in isolation precautions at birth; persons who are not susceptible do not need to mask
Vancomycin-resistant organisms	X	X	No	X	X	Secretions	Duration of illness	

AIDS, Acquired immunodeficiency syndrome; *D,* desirable but optional; *HIV,* human immunodeficiency virus; *X,* recommended at all times; *(X),* recommended if soiling is likely or if touching infective materials.

of age). Significant risk factors for early-onset disease include prematurity, low birth weight, premature onset of labor, rupture of membranes for 18 hours or more, maternal intrapartum temperature higher than 38° C (100.4° F), and chorioamnionitis.[111,145] Bacteria responsible for early-onset disease are acquired from the birth canal before or during delivery and are listed in Box 22-2. Although the advent of intrapartum antibiotic prophylaxis for GBS infections has generally reduced early-onset disease of this pathogen, it has not been universally eliminated, and black

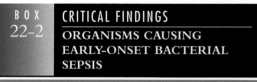

CRITICAL FINDINGS

BOX 22-2

ORGANISMS CAUSING EARLY-ONSET BACTERIAL SEPSIS

Common Organisms
Group B *Streptococcus*
Escherichia coli
Coagulase-negative *Staphylococcus*

Unusual Organisms
Staphylococcus aureus
Neisseria meningitidis
Streptococcus pneumoniae
Haemophilus influenzae (type B and nontypable)

Rare Organisms
Klebsiella pneumoniae
Pseudomonas aeruginosa
Enterobacter species
Serratia marcescens
Group A *Streptococcus*
Anaerobic species

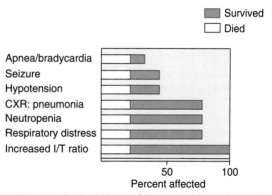

FIGURE 22-2 Clinical and laboratory findings in nine infants with signs and symptoms of early-onset group B streptococcal disease. *CXR,* Chest x-ray; *I/T,* ratio of immature to total neutrophils. (From Nelson SN, Merenstein GB, Pierce JR: Early onset group B streptococcal disease, *J Perinatol* 6:234, 1986.)

preterm infants remain at considerably greater risk than do white preterm infants and both black and white term infants.[23]

Also, since the practice of intrapartum prophylaxis began, a predominance of gram-negative organisms has been noted in infants weighing less than 1500 g at birth, and concern for this continued trend remains.[10,131] Gram-negative infections now account for more than half of the instances of early-onset sepsis.[132,134] Data from the National Institute of Child Health and Human Development (NICHD) Neonatal Research Network, which comprises 16 major neonatal units, showed an increase in *Escherichia coli* infections in very-low-birth-weight (VLBW) infants during the period 1998 to 2000 compared with 1991 to 1993 that persisted during the 2002 to 2003 period.[134] Data from the Norwegian National Cohort demonstrated that in infants born at less than 28 weeks' gestational age and with birth weight less than 1000 g, *E. coli* was the most common organism isolated on the first day of life.[120] Early-onset bacterial disease is associated with a high mortality rate and significant morbidity.[125,131,132]

Signs and Symptoms. Neonatal bacterial sepsis is characterized by systemic signs of infection associated with bacteremia. Meningitis in a neonate can be a sequela of bacteremia or can occur in 15% to 38% of neonates with negative blood culture.[9] In addition, bloodborne bacteria may localize in other tissues, causing focal disease. Both patterns of bacterial disease, early onset and late onset, have been associated with systemic infections during the neonatal period.[112,117]

In general, signs, particularly in early-onset disease, are nonspecific and nonlocalizing. Signs and symptoms may include temperature instability (hypothermia or hyperthermia), respiratory distress (apnea, cyanosis, and tachypnea), lethargy, feeding abnormalities (vomiting, increased residuals, and abdominal distention), jaundice (particularly increased direct fraction), seizures, or purpura (Figure 22-2).[117] Quantification of risk of early-onset neonatal sepsis using maternal risk factors and neonatal clinical examination may significantly decrease antibiotic use in neonates early after birth.[43]

Newborn Scale of Sepsis (SOS) is an objective, reliable, and validated scoring tool for the assessment of neonatal infection. By using both clinical indicators (e.g., color, perfusion, muscle tone, response to pain, respiratory distress and rate, temperature, and apnea) and laboratory findings (e.g., white blood cell count, ratio of immature to total neutrophils, platelet count, pH, and absolute neutrophil count), the health care provider assigns a score for each parameter. A score less than 10 indicates that the newborn does not have sepsis—a negative predictive value of 97%.[55] The SOS awaits testing in a large cohort of neonates.

Laboratory Data. Isolating bacteria from a nonpermissive site (blood, CSF, urine, closed body space) is the most valid method of establishing the diagnosis of bacterial sepsis.[151] Surface cultures (including ear and gastric aspirates) do not establish the presence of active systemic infection but merely indicate colonization. Bacterial antigens or endotoxins may be demonstrated in sera, CSF, urine, or body fluids by a variety of methods (counterimmunoelectrophoresis, latex agglutination, and limulus lysate tests). Such a demonstration is not totally definitive, nor does it allow the determination of the antibiotic sensitivity of the offending organism.[117] False-positive reactions may be caused by skin surface contamination or gastrointestinal absorption of antigen.[8] The CSF is examined in most infants suspected of sepsis, because meningitis is a frequent manifestation of sepsis in neonates, especially in symptomatic infants and infants with GBS sepsis and with late-onset disease (Table 22-6). It has been suggested that, because of the low yield and potential adverse effects from lumbar puncture, examination of CSF be deferred in asymptomatic infants being evaluated for maternal risk factors or respiratory distress.[48,73,117,127,147] The CSF is examined in most infants suspected of sepsis, because meningitis is difficult to exclude without a lumbar puncture and its diagnosis affects therapy and follow-up in a neonate.[117,131]

Several laboratory aids are used in assessing neonatal sepsis, but it must be realized that these tests are not sensitive or specific enough to influence clinical decisions on their own.[30,41,112] *Leukocyte indices* predict sepsis with sensitivities ranging from 17% to 90% and specificities from 31% to 100%.[30] *C-reactive protein (CRP)* is an acute-phase reactant synthesized in the liver in the first 6 to 8 hours of the infective process with a low sensitivity (60%) early in sepsis. However, serial CRP measurements at 24 and 48 hours improve sensitivity to 82% and 84% and specificity and positive predictive values range from 83% to 100%.[102] Negative predictive values for CRP are extremely high. Serial CRP patterns have been found to be useful to follow resolution of infection and guide antibiotic therapy.[37,51,78,144,148] CRP levels do not seem to be affected by gestational age and have better sensitivity and negative predictive values compared with leukocyte indices.[32,148] CRP response has been found to be better in gram-negative infections compared with infections with coagulase-negative *Staphylococcus*.[115,119] The use of CRP in neonatal sepsis has recently been reviewed.[69]

Procalcitonin, another acute-phase reactant, which rises within 4 hours of exposure to bacterial endotoxin, has a sensitivity and specificity ranging from 83% to 100%. The serum profile of procalcitonin has been claimed to be superior to that of CRP in the diagnosis of sepsis, after resolution of infection, and may differentiate between sepsis and

| | | | TABLE 22-6 | | | |

TABLE 22-6 NORMAL CEREBROSPINAL FLUID VALUES IN NEONATES*

	WHITE BLOOD CELLS	POLYMORPHONUCLEAR NEUTROPHILS	PROTEIN (mg/dl)	GLUCOSE (mg/dl)
Premature Infants				
Reported means	2-27		75-150	79-83
Reported ranges	0-112		31-292	64-106
Term Infants				
Reported means	3-5	2-3	47-67	51-55
Reported ranges	0-90	0-70	17-240	32-78

*Modified from Remington JS, Klein JO, editors: *Infectious diseases of the fetus and newborn infant,* ed 5, Philadelphia, 2001, Saunders. See also Mhanna MJ, Alesseh H, Gori A, et al: Cerebrospinal fluid values in very low birth weight infants with suspected sepsis at different ages, *Pediatr Crit Care Med* 9:294, 2008.

other inflammatory processes (e.g., trauma).[7,84,142] Procalcitonin may have sufficient diagnostic accuracy in differentiating invasive fungal infections from bacterial infections and uninfected individuals.[38]

Evaluation of a composite set of markers (e.g., CRP and interleukin-6[105]; CRP and leukocyte indices[59]) involving acute-phase reactants, leukocytes, and cytokines/chemokines may increase sensitivity and specificity in the diagnosis of sepsis. Serial measurements may be more useful, as is a combination of tests.[102] Radiographic examination of the chest and other specific areas indicated by clinical concerns may also be helpful.[117]

Several other nonspecific laboratory abnormalities may accompany neonatal sepsis, including hyperglycemia, hypoglycemia, and unexplained metabolic acidosis. Molecular techniques for diagnosis of infection are fast and reliable and may be very useful, especially in infants whose mothers have received intrapartum antibiotics. In a study of 548 paired neonatal blood samples that compared the utility of PCR for the bacterial *16S rRNA* gene with that of microbial culture by BACTEC 9240 instrument, sensitivity, specificity, positive predictive values, and negative predictive values were 96.0%, 99.4%, 88.9%, and 99.8%, respectively. This required a 9-hour turnaround time with blood volumes as little as 200 μL.[75] Real-time PCR assay targeting the highly conserved 380 bases of *16S rDNA* requires less than 4 hours with excellent agreement with blood culture results.[76] PCR with microarray hybridization not only detects bacteremia but also can identify the infecting organism rapidly and reliably.[128] It may be that using PCR assays with microarray hybridization will become the future for diagnosing bacteremia in an accurate and rapid way.

Treatment. Antibiotics are the cornerstone of the treatment for presumed or confirmed infections in neonates. The indiscriminate or inappropriate use of systemic antibiotics may cause undesirable side effects, favor the emergence of resistant strains of bacteria, and alter the normal flora of the newborn.[22] Adequate and appropriate specimens for culture should be obtained before antibiotic therapy is initiated. Emergence of antibiotic resistance in gram-negative organisms is a major clinical concern.[12] In the data from the NICHD Neonatal Research Network, 85% and 75% of early-onset *E. coli* infections were ampicillin resistant in the 1998 to 2000 and the 2002 to 2003 cohorts, respectively.[132,134] Plasmid-mediated extended-spectrum beta-lactamases (produced by *Klebsiella* spp., *E. coli,* and *Serratia*) that confer resistance to a variety of β-lactam agents (penicillins and cephalosporins) and chromosomally mediated AmP-C–type beta-lactamase (*Enterobacter* and *Citrobacter* spp.)–producing gram-negative organisms have been isolated from the NICU.[63,64,110] Exposure to third-generation cephalosporins (e.g., cefotaxime) and being a VLBW infant are noted risk factors for the acquisition of resistant organisms.

Broad-spectrum antibiotic coverage, usually with ampicillin and an aminoglycoside for early-onset sepsis, is commonly initiated pending culture and sensitivity results. Once causative organisms are identified and antibiotic sensitivities established, the most appropriate and least toxic antibiotic or antibiotic combination should be continued for an appropriate period by a suitable route. If adequate cultures are negative after a reasonable period (24 to 48 hours), antibiotic therapy may be discontinued in most situations.

Antibiotics are not the entire solution to treating the infected newborn.[47,53] Meticulous attention to the treatment of associated conditions, such as shock, hypoxemia, thermal abnormalities, electrolyte or acid-base imbalance, inadequate nutrition, anemia, or presence of pus or foreign bodies, may be as important as choosing the proper antibiotic. Further investigation is necessary before newer adjunctive therapies such as IV immunoglobulin and nonantibiotic therapies or preventive regimens can be recommended.[65,96,105,146] Table 22-1 provides guidelines for choosing the proper antibiotic for indicated conditions; Table 22-7 gives the proper dose, route, and frequency of administration of commonly used antibiotics in the newborn nursery. Table 22-8 describes the passage of antibiotics across the placenta, and Table 22-9 describes their passage into breastmilk.

Parent Teaching. Transplacental infection often results in fetal abnormality or death. Newborns who survive may have long-term sequelae such as developmental, neurologic, motor, sensory, growth, and physical abnormalities.

Before antibiotic use, the mortality rate from bacterial sepsis was 95% to 100%, but antibiotics and supportive care have reduced the mortality rate to less than 50%; however, survival is highly variable and depends on the organism and underlying or

TABLE 22-7	ANTIBIOTIC, ANTIVIRAL, AND ANTIFUNGAL AGENTS: DOSAGES FOR NEONATES

ANTIBIOTIC, ANTIVIRAL, OR ANTIFUNGAL	ROUTE	DAILY DOSAGES AND INTERVALS	
		0-7 DAYS OF AGE	MORE THAN 7 DAYS OF AGE
Acyclovir[†]	IV	20 mg/kg/dose q 8-12 hr depending on gestation and age	Same
Amikacin sulfate	IV, IM	7.5-10 mg/kg/dose q 12 hr depending on gestation and age	Same
Amoxicillin	PO	50 mg/kg/day divided q 12 hr	50 mg/kg/day divided q 8 hr
Amoxicillin/clavulanic acid	PO	Not recommended	30 mg/kg/day divided q 12 hr
Ampicillin			
• Meningitis	IV	100 mg/kg/day divided q 12 hr	150-200 mg/kg/day divided q 6-8 hr
• Other indications	IV, IM, PO	50 mg/kg/day divided q 12 hr	75 mg/kg/day divided q 8 hr
Azithromycin	IV, PO	5 mg/kg/day q 24 hr	10 mg/kg/day q 24 hr
Cefazolin*	IV, IM	50 mg/kg/day divided q 12 hr	50-75 mg/kg/day divided q 8-12 hr
Cefotaxime	IV, IM	100 mg/kg/day divided q 12 hr	150 mg/kg/day divided q 8 hr
Ceftazidime*	IV	100 mg/kg/day divided q 12 hr	150 mg/kg/day divided q 8 hr
Clindamycin	IV, PO	10-15 mg/kg/day divided q 8-12 hr	15-20 mg/kg/day divided q 6-8 hr
Erythromycin ethyl succinate (EES)	PO	20 mg/kg/day divided q 12 hr	30-40 mg/kg/day divided q 8 hr
Ganciclovir[†]	IV	6 mg/kg/dose q 12-24 hr depending on gestation and age	
Gentamicin	IV, IM	2.5 mg/kg/dose q 8-24 hr depending on gestation and age	Same
Meropenem*	IV	40 mg/kg/day divided q 12 hr	60 mg/kg/day divided q 8 hr (higher doses may be needed in meningitis)
Metronidazole	IV, PO	7.5-15 mg/kg/day divided q 12-24 hr	15-30 mg/kg/day divided q 12 hr
Nafcillin	IV	50-75 mg/kg/day divided q 8-12 hr	75-150 mg/kg/day divided q 6-8 hr
Nystatin[‡]	PO	400,000 units/day divided q 6 hr	Same
Penicillin G			
• Meningitis	IV	100,000-150,000 units/kg/day divided q 8-12 hr	200,000-225,000 units/kg/day divided q 6-8 hr
• Other indications	IV	50,000 units/kg/day divided q 12 hr	75,000 units/kg/day divided q 6-8 hr
Penicillin G, benzathine	IM	50,000 units/kg (1 dose only)	Same
Penicillin G, procaine	IM	50,000 units/kg/day once daily	Same
Pentamidine isethionate*	IV	4 mg/kg/day for 14 days (available from CDC, Atlanta, Georgia)	Same
Piperacillin/tazobactam	IV	100-200 mg/kg/day divided q 12 hr	300 mg/kg/day divided q 8 hr
Rifampin	IV, PO	10 mg/kg/day q 24 hr	Same
Ticarcillin	IV, IM	150-225 mg/kg/day divided q 8-12 hr	225-300 mg/kg/day divided q 6-8 hr

TABLE 22-7	ANTIBIOTIC, ANTIVIRAL, AND ANTIFUNGAL AGENTS: DOSAGES FOR NEONATES — cont'd		
ANTIBIOTIC, ANTIVIRAL, OR ANTIFUNGAL	**ROUTE**	**DAILY DOSAGES AND INTERVALS**	
		0-7 DAYS OF AGE	**MORE THAN 7 DAYS OF AGE**
Tobramycin	IV, IM	2.5 mg/kg/dose q 12-24 hr depending on gestation and age	2.5 mg/kg/dose q 8-18 hr
Trimethoprim/sulfamethoxazole (TMP/SMX)	IV, PO	10-20 mg/kg/day TMP and 50-100 mg/kg/day SMX	Same
Vancomycin	IV	15 mg/kg/dose q 12-24 hr depending on gestation and age	15 mg/kg/dose q 8-18 hr depending on gestation and age
Zidovudine[†]	IV	1.5 mg/kg/dose q 6-12 hr depending on gestation and age	Same
	PO	2 mg/kg/dose q 6-12 hr depending on gestation and age	Same

CDC, Centers for Disease Control and Prevention; *IM,* intramuscularly; *IV,* intravenously; *PO,* orally.
*Pharmacokinetics in newborns not well characterized. These drugs should be used with extra caution in neonates (pediatric infectious disease consultation recommended).
[†]Antiviral agent.
[‡]Antifungal agent.

TABLE 22-8	PASSAGE OF ANTIBIOTICS ACROSS THE PLACENTA*	
PERCENTAGE OF ANTIBIOTIC IN INDICATED CATEGORY		**ANTIBIOTIC**
Equal to serum concentration		Amoxicillin
		Ampicillin
		Carbenicillin
		Chloramphenicol
		Methicillin
		Nitrofurantoin
		Penicillin G
		Sulfonamides
50% of serum concentration		Aminoglycosides
10%-15% of serum concentration		Amikacin
		Cephalosporins
		Clindamycin
		Nafcillin
		Tobramycin
Negligible (<10% of serum concentration)		Dicloxacillin
		Erythromycin

*Several factors determine the degree of transfer of antibiotics across the placenta, including lipid solubility, degree of ionization, molecular weight, protein binding, placental maturation, and placental and fetal blood flow.

TABLE 22-9	PASSAGE OF ANTIBIOTICS INTO BREASTMILK*	
PERCENTAGE OF ANTIBIOTIC IN INDICATED CATEGORY		**ANTIBIOTIC**
Equal to serum concentration		Isoniazid
		Metronidazole
		Sulfonamides
		Trimethoprim
50% of serum concentration		Chloramphenicol
		Erythromycin
		Tetracyclines
<25% of serum concentration		Cefazolin
		Kanamycin
		Nitrofurantoin
		Oxacillin
		Penicillin G
		Penicillin V

*Data on concentrations of antibiotics in human breastmilk are sparse. Because most antibiotics are present in breastmilk in microgram amounts, they are normally not ingested by the infant in therapeutic amounts.

associated conditions. Debilitated infants (preterm and sick neonates) are at greater risk and have a higher incidence of morbidity and mortality than term healthy neonates. The most common complications of bacterial sepsis are meningitis and septic shock. The outcome is influenced by early recognition and vigorous treatment with appropriate antibiotics and supportive care.

POSTNATAL ACQUISITION LATE-ONSET BACTERIAL DISEASE

Prevention. The CDC defines *nosocomial* as all neonatal infections acquired in the intrapartum period or during hospitalization. Infants requiring the specialized care of NICUs are highly susceptible to infections. Prematurity, stress, immature immune systems, and complicated medical and surgical problems contribute to their increased susceptibility. In addition, most infants in the NICU require a variety of invasive diagnostic, therapeutic, and monitoring procedures; many of these procedures bypass natural physical barriers, which may allow colonization to occur and a nosocomial (late-onset) infection to develop.[54]

Central line–associated bloodstream infections (CLABSIs), also called catheter-related bloodstream infections, are the most frequent hospital-acquired infections and are of particular concern in the NICU because of the prevalence of indwelling catheter lines needed for fluids, nutrition, and medications. Infection occurs via the insertion site with migration of microorganisms along the catheter/catheter hub, seeding from another site of infection, and infusion of contaminated fluids.

Longer dwell times for catheters are also associated with increased CLABSIs. Rates of infection increase over the first 2 weeks and then remain elevated for the duration of the line. In the first 40 days from placement, coagulase-negative staphylococci are the most prevalent organisms. After 50 days the risk of gram-negative infection is increased.[87,93,104,115]

A systematic and multidisciplinary approach to reducing CLABSIs should be included in the infection control policies of every NICU. Evidence-based guidelines or "bundles" (of specific evidence-based interventions) are packaged together to reduce variability in insertion and catheter maintenance and have been shown to reduce CLABSIs. "Bundles" can be developed by individual NICUs or obtained through collaborative practice organizations. Strategies to prevent CLABSIs generally include (1) education for all health care providers, (2) need for adequate nurse staffing, (3) meticulous hand hygiene, (4) strict aseptic technique, (5) limitation of line manipulations, and (6) limitation on dwell time. For line placement, use of maximum sterile barriers (i.e., hat, mask, sterile gown and gloves) and a full sterile body drape is recommended. Other strategies include the use of ultrasound to limit placement attempts, avoiding the femoral vein for percutaneous placement, and proper disinfection of hubs, connectors, and injection ports.

Dressings should be changed when an occlusive dressing is used, every 2 days for gauze dressing, and when the dressing is loose, damp, or visibly soiled. Lines should be removed immediately when signs of infection or phlebitis are present. The need for line continuation should be evaluated daily and the line removed as soon as possible. A process for tracking CLABSIs is essential so that causes are identified and intervention quickly occurs when rates increase.[*]

Infection control principles and practices for the prevention of these nosocomial infections are outlined in Table 22-10. Table 22-5 outlines infection control measures and isolation techniques for specific diseases.[15,56,112,129]

Data Collection

History. Late-onset disease may occur as early as 3 days of age but is more common after the first week of life. Affected infants may have a history of obstetric complications, but they are less common than obstetric complications in early-onset disease. Bacteria responsible for late-onset sepsis and meningitis include those acquired from the maternal genital tract and organisms acquired after birth from human contact or from contaminated equipment or material (Box 22-3).[5] Gram-positive organisms predominate in late-onset sepsis, and gram-negative organisms account for about one third of late-onset cases of sepsis in VLBW infants.[133] Although prematurity remains the most significant factor, invasive procedures performed on a neonate, such as intubation, catheterization, and surgery, also increase the risk for bacterial infection.[53,85,133]

---

*References 49, 87, 93, 104, 115, 126.

| T A B L E 22-10 | INFECTION CONTROL PRINCIPLES AND PRACTICES TO PREVENT NOSOCOMIAL INFECTION |

PRINCIPLE	PRACTICE
Handwashing Handwashing is the most important procedure for controlling infection in the NICU.	1. Before each shift, wash hands, wrists, forearms, and elbows with antiseptic. Scrub hands with a brush or pad for 2-3 min and rinse thoroughly. Chlorhexidine, hexachlorophene, and iodophors are the preferred products. 2. Wash hands for 10-15 sec between infant contacts. Soap and water are adequate unless the infant is infected or contaminated objects have been handled. 3. Use an antiseptic for handwashing before surgical or similar invasive procedures. 4. Alcohol-based disinfectants are increasingly employed and are effective when used before and after patient contact.
Patient Placement Overcrowding in the NICU increases risk for cross-contamination.	1. Provide 4- to 6-ft intervals between infants.

Skin and Cord Care
The skin, its secretions, and its normal flora are natural defense mechanisms that protect against invading pathogens (see Chapter 19).
No single method of cord care has been identified to prevent colonization or limit disease.
	1. The American Academy of Pediatrics suggests using a dry technique:
	  a. Delay initial cleansing until temperature is stable. Manipulating an infant's skin must be minimized.
	  b. Use sterile cotton sponges and sterile water or mild soap to remove blood from face and perineal area.
	  c. Do not touch other areas unless they are grossly soiled.
	2. Local application of alcohol, triple dye, and various antimicrobial is currently used.

Medical Devices Medical devices facilitate infections by the following: 1. Bypassing normal defense mechanisms, providing direct access to blood and deep tissues 2. Supporting growth of microorganisms and becoming reservoirs from which bacteria can be transmitted with the device to another patient 3. Providing a "protected site" when placed in deeper tissue, so phagocytosis or defense mechanisms cannot eradicate the organisms 4. Using sterile medical devices that are occasionally contaminated from the manufacturer or central supply	1. Intravenous (IV) infusion devices predispose infants to phlebitis and bacteremia. Preventive measures include preparing the site with tincture of iodine (2% iodine in 70% alcohol), an iodophor, or 70% alcohol; anchoring the IV securely; performing site assessment and care every 24 hr (routine site care is not necessary with polyurethane dressing); rotating the IV site every 48-72 hr; changing the IV tubing every 24-48 hr on regular IVs; and discontinuing the IV at the first sign of complication. 2. Arterial lines predispose infants to bacteremia. Preventive measures include aseptically inserting the catheter using gloves, inspecting the site and performing site care every 24 hr, treating the catheter and stopcocks as sterile fields, and minimizing manipulation by drawing all blood specimens at the same time. 3. Intravascular pressure-monitoring systems predispose infants to septicemia. Preventive measures include replacing the flush solution every 24 hr, replacing the chamber dome, and replacing the tubing and continuous flow device (if used) at 48-hr intervals and between each patient. 4. Respiratory therapy devices increase the risk for contamination. Preventive measures include using aseptic technique during suctioning; dating opened solution for irrigation, humidification, and nebulization, and discarding after 24 hr; ensuring routine replacement and cleaning of all respiratory equipment, including Ambu bags, cascade nebulizers, endotracheal tube adaptors, and tubing; and checking sputum cultures and Gram stains every several days to assess the degree of colonization or infection in the intubated patient.

Continued

TABLE 22-10	INFECTION CONTROL PRINCIPLES AND PRACTICES TO PREVENT NOSOCOMIAL INFECTION—cont'd

PRINCIPLE	PRACTICE
Specimen Collection Improperly collected specimens cause infection at the site of collection or erroneous diagnosis, leading to the administration of the wrong antibiotic or delayed administration of the appropriate antibiotic.	1. Wash hands before collecting specimen. 2. Observe aseptic technique to reduce risk for infection and to avoid contamination of specimen. 3. Deliver specimens to the laboratory immediately. 4. Do not use femoral sticks.
Nursery Attire Personal clothing and unscrubbed skin areas of personnel should not touch infants.	1. Short-sleeved scrub gowns accommodate washing elbows. 2. Long-sleeved gowns should be worn and changed between handling of infected or potentially infected infants. 3. Sterile gowns are necessary for sterile procedures.

Employee Health
Transmission of disease among patients and employees can occur bidirectionally. Each NICU must establish reasonable guidelines for restriction of assignments based on the employee's potential to transmit disease and the potential risk for acquiring disease.
	1. Conditions that commonly restrict personnel from patient care in the NICU are skin lesions and draining wounds, acute respiratory infections, fever, gastroenteritis, active herpes simplex (oral, genital, or paronychial), and herpes zoster.
	2. Conditions that are transmitted from infants to personnel are the following:
	  a. Rubella: Obtain rubella titers from women of childbearing age; if a protective level is not present, they should be vaccinated.
	  b. Cytomegalovirus is a potential threat to pregnant women. Adherence to good infection control practices may reduce this threat.
	  c. Hepatitis B is usually not a major problem in the NICU, because host vaccine is available and may be considered for high-risk individuals (see Tables 22-3 and 22-4).
	  d. Use of gloves with body fluid contact will decrease the risk for transmission of hepatitis B virus and human immunodeficiency virus.

Cohorting Cohorting is an important infection control measure used primarily during outbreaks or epidemics in the NICU. The object of cohorting is to limit the number of contacts of one infant with other infants and personnel.	1. Group together infants born within the same time frame (usually 24-48 hr) or who are colonized or infected with the same pathogen. These infants should remain together until discharged. 2. Provide nursing care by personnel who do not care for other infants. 3. After all infants in cohort are discharged, clean the room before admittance of a new group of infants.

See References 56-58. *NICU,* Neonatal intensive care unit.

Signs and Symptoms. Similar to those of early-onset sepsis, signs and symptoms are nonspecific. Heart rate variability, the acceleration and deceleration of heart rate that occurs as a result of activity and neonatal states, has been researched as a sign of sepsis. Decreased heart rate variability (from baseline) and transient decelerations have been noted to occur up to 24 hours before symptoms of sepsis occur.[62,98] Therefore decreased heart rate variability is an early sign of late-onset sepsis.

Decreased baseline variability also occurs in systemic inflammatory response syndrome, necrotizing enterocolitis, intraventricular hemorrhage, and chronic lung disease. Medications also affect variability. Paralytics, anesthetics, and anticholinergics decrease variability, whereas dexamethasone improves variability.

As noninvasive screening tools for late-onset sepsis, algorithms that highlight changes in baseline heart rate variability have been developed. These algorithms are adjuncts to clinical assessment/observation and laboratory data in decision making regarding sepsis evaluation and need for empiric antibiotics. However, ongoing research is needed to determine if combining heart rate variability with the evaluation of other physiologic parameters improves accuracy as a predictive tool.[45,62,68,98]

Laboratory Data. A complete set of culture specimens should be obtained, but limitations are similar to those in early-onset infection.[48,127]

Treatment. Broad-spectrum antibiotic coverage, usually vancomycin and an aminoglycoside or a third-generation cephalosporin, is commonly initiated pending culture and sensitivity results. However, vancomycin resistance remains a potential problem in the care of sick neonates.[22,60,123] To minimize the development of these resistant organisms, the CDC has recommended prudent vancomycin use, education of medical personnel about the problem of vancomycin resistance, early detection and prompt reporting of organisms, and immediate implementation of appropriate infection control measures (see Table 22-10).

Complications. CLABSIs increase morbidity and mortality rates, length of stay, and cost of care.

FUNGAL INFECTION

Fungal infections have been a significant cause of neonatal morbidity and mortality.[72] Fungal infections are the second most common infection after 72 hours of life in infants weighing less than 1500 g.[133] *Candida* species are the most common. In extremely low-birth-weight (ELBW) infants, invasive *Candida* infections are associated with a mortality rate of approximately 30% and adverse neurodevelopmental outcomes in 50% of survivors.[11] In addition, they are usually seen in infants with congenital anomalies requiring surgery or infants who require multiple or prolonged vascular catheterization.

Prevention. Because these infants are often colonized at birth, strict adherence to aseptic technique when dealing with central catheters is essential. Use of broad-spectrum antibiotics (e.g., cephalosporins) and administration of histamine-2 (H2)–receptor blockers are significant risk factors, and their use should be minimized.

Data Collection

History. Prematurity (less than 32 weeks' gestation), Apgar score less than 5 at 5 minutes, shock, antibiotic therapy, parenteral nutrition for longer than 5 days, use of lipids for longer than 7 days, presence of a central catheter, length of stay in hospital longer than 7 days, use of H2 blockers, and intubation are risk factors for fungal infections.[124]

Signs and Symptoms. Signs and symptoms may be nonspecific, nonlocalizing, and difficult to differentiate from those of bacterial sepsis. Skin infections in high-risk infants, especially in VLBW infants, can become invasive and should be treated.[29]

Laboratory Data. Routine laboratory data, as may be collected based on clinical signs and symptoms, are rarely helpful in differentiating fungal from bacterial infection. A positive culture result from urine, blood, CSF, or a skin biopsy indicates systemic infection. Urine for analysis and culture, ophthalmologic examination, imaging of the brain by computed tomography scan or magnetic resonance imaging, echocardiogram for endocarditis, and renal ultrasound for fungal mycetomas are mandatory in disseminated fungal infections.[103]

TABLE 22-11	**ANTIFUNGAL THERAPY**	
DRUG	DOSAGE	COMMENTS
Amphotericin B	0.1-1 mg/kg/day IV; begin at 0.1 mg/kg and increase daily as tolerated	Nephrotoxic
Amphotericin B lipid complex	1-5 mg/kg/dose IV over 2 hr; begin at 1 mg/kg and increase daily as tolerated	Thrombocytopenia Anemia Hypokalemia
5-Fluorocytosine (5-FC)	50-100 mg/kg/day PO q 6 hr	Hepatotoxic Bone marrow suppression
Fluconazole	12 mg/kg IV loading dose; then 6 mg/kg per dose over 30 min every 24-72 hr depending on postnatal and gestational age	Liver toxicity

IV, Intravenously; *PO,* orally.

Treatment. Supportive care and removal of foci of infection (i.e., infected catheters or fungal mycetomas) are important. Antifungal therapy with amphotericin B is the mainstay of treatment for invasive fungal infections in the neonate.[109,112] For CNS candidiasis using monotherapy with amphotericin B, if the CSF does not become sterile within a few days or the neonate becomes more ill, 5-fluorocytosine (5-FC) is added. 5-FC has excellent CSF penetration and is reserved for use in combination with amphotericin B in neonates with CNS candidiasis[46] (Table 22-11).

Lipid formulations of amphotericin are available that are less toxic and may be the choice in infants who cannot tolerate standard amphotericin.[4] Fluconazole therapy may have efficacy similar to amphotericin but without the toxicity.[13,39] Intravenous fluconazole prophylaxis may help prevent invasive fungal infection in neonates and reduce mortality risk during hospital stay in neonates whose birth weight is less than 1500 g.[31,77] However, resistance to fluconazole remains a potentially serious concern.[13] In a meta-analysis of four trials of 536 VLBW infants that compared prophylactic fluconazole with placebo, fluconazole prophylaxis compared with placebo reduced invasive fungal infection (relative risk [RR] 0.23, 95% confidence interval [CI] 0.11 to 0.46) but without statistically significant difference in mortality rates before hospital discharge (RR 0.61, 95% CI 0.37 to 1.03).[31] There appeared to be no increased risk for the emergence of resistant *Candida* species with prophylactic fluconazole;

however, the follow-up periods were probably not sufficient to detect changes in the resistance pattern. Retrospective studies have reported conflicting results regarding the emergence of fluconazole-resistant *Candida* species. Recent evidence from the United States and Italy suggests that with commonly used fluconazole prophylaxis regimens in the NICU, emergence of resistance is an unlikely event but still warrants tracking.[16,66] In summary, fluconazole prophylaxis may be effective in reducing invasive fungal infections and mortality rates in high-risk patients (e.g., ELBW infants, neonates on multiple antibiotics, and in those neonatal units in which the baseline rate of systemic fungal infections is high).

PARENT TEACHING

Parents who have an infant with viral or bacterial infection require support and information about their infant's condition. Questions arise about treatment and prognosis, as well as possible long-range effects of the infection. Parents experience significant guilt feelings based on misperceptions about what role they had in causing the infection. Health care professionals should remain sensitive to the crisis that parents are experiencing and address the issues of etiology, as well as treatment and prognosis. Valid and factual data, as well as information about complications and long-term effects, should be shared with parents in a timely manner.

Controlling infection in the nursery is of prime importance but does not exclude parents from caring for their sick infant. Everyone must adhere to proper handwashing, gowning, and isolation techniques.[129] Educating the parents and siblings about the importance of these procedures, along with appropriate reminders, ensures cooperation. With proper precautions, there is no evidence of increased incidence of infection with parent and sibling visits.

All those entering the nursery must be screened for the presence of illness. Anyone (including staff) with a fever, respiratory symptoms (cough, runny nose, sore throat), gastrointestinal symptoms (nausea, vomiting, diarrhea), or skin lesions should not come in contact with the infant. People with communicable disease (e.g., varicella) or recent exposure to a communicable disease also should not come in contact with the

sick neonate.[15,129] Daily cord care should be demonstrated, and a demonstration by the parents should be observed before discharging the infant. *Every* parent should be taught the signs and symptoms of neonatal illness, because early recognition of signs and symptoms expedites prompt treatment. Parents must be taught to take axillary temperatures and to read a thermometer. They should be aware that both hypothermia and hyperthermia may be signs of neonatal illness.[15,129]

REFERENCES

For a full list of references, scan the QR code or visit http://booksite.elsevier.com/ 9780323320832.

23 RESPIRATORY DISEASES

SANDRA L. GARDNER, MARY ENZMAN HINES, AND MICHAEL NYP

Despite the marked improvement over the past years in the survival of premature newborns with respiratory distress, significant mortality and high morbidity rates persist. Much of the improvement in neonatal mortality has been the result of successful treatment and management of respiratory diseases in the neonate.

This chapter presents an overview of some of the common respiratory diseases, their treatments, and outcomes. General principles and concepts related to respiratory physiology, etiologic factors, and symptomatology are presented, followed by specific disease processes and their management.

GENERAL PHYSIOLOGY

Any discussion of general respiratory physiology must include some elements of anatomy and embryology and their significance to the clinician (Table 23-1).

Surface-active compounds such as phosphatidylcholine and phosphatidylglycerol stabilize the alveoli. Surface tension forces act on air-fluid interfaces, causing a water droplet to "bead up." The surface-active compound (e.g., soap added to a water droplet) reduces the surface tension and allows the droplet to spread out in a thin film. In the lung, surface tension forces tend to cause alveoli to collapse. A compound such as surfactant reduces surface tension and allows the alveoli to remain open.

However, the situation is more complicated than just described. Laplace detailed the magnitude of the pressure (p) exerted at the surface of an air-liquid interface as equaling twice the surface tension (st) divided by the radius (r) of curvature of the surface ($p = 2\ st \div r$). In the absence of surfactant, an alveolus with a small radius of curvature has a greater magnitude of pressure at its surface (tending to collapse it) than does an alveolus with a larger radius of curvature. Therefore smaller alveoli tend to collapse and empty contained gas into larger alveoli.

Surfactant modifies surface tension by decreasing surface tension when the radius of curvature is small and increasing surface tension when the radius of curvature is greater. An alveolus with a larger radius of curvature has a greater-than-expected pressure (tending to reduce its volume), and an alveolus with a smaller radius of curvature has less-than-expected pressure. Therefore the alveoli are stabilized at a uniform radius of curvature (uniform volume).

Surfactant provides a number of useful properties in addition to reducing surface tension, which increases lung compliance, provides alveolar stability, and decreases opening pressure. It also enhances alveolar fluid clearance, decreases precapillary tone, and plays a protective role for the epithelial cell surface. Surfactant is constantly being formed, stored, secreted, and recycled. Conditions that interfere with surfactant metabolism include acidemia, hypoxia, shock, overinflation, underinflation, pulmonary edema, mechanical ventilation, and hypercapnia. Surfactant production is delayed in infants of diabetic mothers (IDMs) of classes A, B, and C; infants with erythroblastosis fetalis; and infants who are the smaller of twins. Surfactant production is accelerated in the following:

- IDMs of classes D, F, and R
- Infants of heroin-addicted mothers
- Premature rupture of membranes of greater than 48 hours' duration
- Infants of mothers with hypertension

PURPLE type highlights content that is particularly applicable to clinical settings.

TABLE 23-1	LUNG DEVELOPMENT

STAGE AND MAJOR EVENTS	SIGNIFICANCE
Embryonic (Up to 5 Weeks)	
Single ventral outpocketing quickly divided into two lung buds. Mesenchyme surrounds endodermal lung buds, which continue to divide and extend into the mesenchyme.	Airways begin to differentiate.
Branching of the airways begins.	Branching anomalies (e.g., pulmonary agenesis and sequestered lobe) occur early in fetal life.
Pulmonary arteries invade lung tissue, following the airways, and divide as the airways divide. Pulmonary veins arise independently from the lung parenchyma and return to the left atrium, thus completing the pulmonary circuit.	
Pseudoglandular (5-16 Weeks)	
Progressive airway branching begins; bronchi and terminal bronchioles form.	All subdivisions that will form airways are complete by the sixteenth week.
Muscle fibers, elastic tissue, and early cartilage formation can be seen along the tracheobronchial tree. Mucous glands are found at 12 weeks and increase in number until 25-26 weeks, when cilia begin to develop.	
Diaphragm develops.	Herniation of the diaphragm occurs.
Canalicular (13-25 Weeks)	
Airway changes from glandular to tubular and increases in length and diameter.	Air-conducting portion (bronchi and terminal bronchioli) continues luminal development.
20 Weeks	
Fetal airways end in blind pouches lined with cuboid epithelium; a relatively large amount of interstitial mesenchyme is present; few pulmonary capillaries are present, and they are not closely associated with the respiratory epithelium.	
22-24 Weeks	
Rapid proliferation of the pulmonary capillary bed, an increase of the surface area of the respiratory epithelium, and formation of alveolar ducts and sacculi occur.	Development of gas exchange portion (the respiratory bronchi and alveolar ducts) begins; pulmonary vasculature develops most rapidly.
Respiratory epithelium contains cells that become differentiated into type I and type II pneumocytes.	
Type I pneumocytes produce an extremely thin squamous epithelial layer that lines the alveoli and fuses to the underlying capillary endothelial cells.	By the late fetal period, the resulting membrane between the alveoli and capillaries allows sufficient gas exchange to support independent life.
Type II pneumocytes (cuboid cells) are the site of surfactant synthesis and storage.	At 22 weeks, surface-active phospholipids (lecithin) can first be detected.
Terminal (24-40 Weeks)	
Lung differentiation: proliferation of the pulmonary vascular bed, creation of new respiratory units (alveolar ducts and alveoli), decrease in amount of mesenchyme, and fusion of the gas-exchange epithelium to the pulmonary capillary epithelium occur.	Before this time, the fetal lungs are incapable of supporting adequate gas exchange because of insufficient alveolar surface area and inadequate pulmonary vasculature.

TABLE 23-1	LUNG DEVELOPMENT—cont'd

STAGE AND MAJOR EVENTS	SIGNIFICANCE
34-36 Weeks Phosphatidylglycerol appears, and a dramatic increase in the principal surfactant compound phosphatidylcholine occurs.	Adequate amounts of surface-active material protect against the development of respiratory distress syndrome.
Alveolar (Postnatal Lung Development: Late Fetal Life to 8-10 Years of Age) At term, the number of airways is complete; there is sufficient respiratory surface for gaseous exchange, and the pulmonary capillary bed is sufficient to carry the gases that have been exchanged.	Although the infant is capable of sustaining respiratory effort and the lung is able to provide oxygenation and ventilation at birth, lung development is still incomplete.
Alveoli continue to increase in number, size, and shape; they enlarge and become deeper to maximize the exposed surface area for gas exchange.	Ongoing lung development implies that infants who have suffered severe lung disease at birth need not become lifelong pulmonary cripples.

- Infants subjected to maternal infection
- Infants suffering from placental insufficiency
- Infants affected by administration of corticosteroids
- Infants affected by abruption placentae

The fetal lung is filled with a volume of liquid (20 to 30 ml/kg) equal to the functional residual capacity. This fluid is not amniotic fluid but, rather, a liquid that has been produced in the lung and discharged through the larynx and mouth into the amniotic fluid. Lung fluid is continuously produced at a rate of approximately 2 to 4 ml/kg/hr.

The movement of lung fluid and its components (notably lecithin) into amniotic fluid, the lecithin-sphingomyelin (L/S) ratio has become a notable clinical tool. Noting a sharp increase in the L/S ratio, Gluck and Kulovich[157] found they could predict which infants were at risk for respiratory distress syndrome (RDS). In general, L/S ratios of more than 2:1 are not associated with RDS, whereas ratios of less than 2:1 are associated with it. Phosphatidylglycerol (PG), the second most common phospholipid in surfactant, appears at about 36 weeks' gestation and increases until term. The presence of PG is associated with a very low risk for RDS, whereas its absence is associated with the development of RDS. Unlike the L/S ratio, PG determination is valid in the presence of blood-contaminated amniotic fluid.

During vaginal delivery, approximately one third of the lung fluid may be removed during the thoracic "squeeze" as the infant passes through the birth canal; the remainder of the fluid is removed mainly by the pulmonary lymphatics, although pulmonary capillaries may play a role. After a cesarean section, all of the lung fluid will be removed by the pulmonary lymphatic system, capillaries, and reversal of the sodium and chloride pumps.

The *first breath of life,* a response to tactile, thermal, chemical, and mechanical stimuli, initiates respiratory effort. The fluid-filled lungs, surface forces, and tissue-sensitive forces are obstacles to the first breath. At birth, gas is substituted for liquid to expand the alveoli. After the alveoli are "opened" during the first few breaths, a film of surface-active material stabilizes the alveoli.

The first breath of life requires an opening pressure of 60 to 80 cm H_2O to overcome the effects of the surface tension of the air-liquid interface, particularly the small airways and alveoli. Thus on each subsequent breath, less pressure is necessary to allow for a similar increase in air volume in the lung. The effort of breathing is lessened with subsequent breaths.

GENERAL ETIOLOGIC FACTORS

Respiratory disease may be defined as a progressive impairment of the lungs to exchange gas at the alveolar level. Although the pathologic process causing respiratory distress in the neonate may occur in any portion of the respiratory system, the final common pathway in respiratory disease is impairment of gas exchange.

Prematurity is the single most common factor in the occurrence of RDS. Its incidence is inversely proportional to gestational age and occurs most frequently in infants of less than 1200 g and 30 weeks' gestation. RDS occurs in male infants twice as frequently as in female infants (2:1). The principal factor operating in the development of RDS in very premature infants is surfactant deficiency.

Multiple gestations increase the risk for respiratory disease related to lung maturity in the second, third, or more siblings. The second and subsequent infants may experience perinatal asphyxia, malpresentation, or mode of delivery (e.g., cesarean section) that contributes to respiratory disease. Grand multiparity is associated with increased risk for respiratory disease, particularly when other siblings have had RDS.

Prenatal maternal complications increase the risk for respiratory disease in the infant. Maternal illnesses such as cardiorespiratory disease, hypoxia, hemorrhage, shock, hypotension, or hypertension result in decreased uterine blood flow with subsequent hypoxia or ischemia at the placental level. Severe maternal anemia causes fetal cardiac depression and respiratory depression. Maternal diabetes may result in preterm delivery because of fetal and maternal indications. There is also a greater incidence of false-positive L/S ratios in diabetic populations. There has been a propensity of IDMs to develop RDS despite documentation of L/S ratios greater than 2:1. (A combination of an L/S ratio of 2:1 or greater and the presence of PG confirms fetal lung maturity.) Abnormal placental conditions (compressed umbilical cord caused by prolapse or breech delivery, placental disease such as infarcts or syphilis, or hemorrhage as a result of placenta previa or abruption placentae) affect oxygen transfer from mother to fetus and result in asphyxial insult to the developing fetal lung. Premature rupture of the membranes predisposes the fetus or newborn to the development of infections such as pneumonia, sepsis, or meningitis. Premature or prolonged rupture of the membranes not associated with neonatal infection accelerates fetal lung development and thereby lessens the incidence of RDS. Maternal toxemia and maternal drug addiction also hasten fetal lung maturation. Antenatal administration of glucocorticoids[281] results in less severe RDS and fewer doses of surfactant, fewer cases of patent ductus arteriosus (PDA) and intraventricular hemorrhage (IVH), and lower mortality rates.

Factors affecting the fetus during the birth process may lead to respiratory distress. Depression of the respiratory center can occur as a result of maternal medications that cross the placenta. An infant delivered shortly after analgesics, anesthetics, or magnesium sulfate is administered to the mother may have only minimal respiratory efforts at birth. Excessive uterine activity, usually as a result of oxytocin induction or augmentation of labor, may result in decreased uterine blood flow, late fetal heart deceleration, and respiratory depression in the infant at birth. Respiratory distress may be the result of direct trauma to the respiratory center or a cerebral hemorrhage in proximity to it. Fetal shock caused by difficult labor or dystocia, tight nuchal cord, cerebral hemorrhage, or hemorrhage from the fetal side of the placenta results in central nervous system (CNS) depression and hypoxia. Bleeding results in a generalized hypovolemic condition characterized by decreased oxygen-carrying capacity. Fetal or neonatal asphyxia and blood loss lead to progressive respiratory distress. Delivery by cesarean section prevents one third of the lung fluid from being expelled by the thoracic squeeze of vaginal birth. Thus after cesarean birth, all lung fluid must be absorbed through circulatory and lymphatic channels; therefore a greater incidence of transient tachypnea of the newborn may occur as the increased volume of retained fluid is absorbed.

The timing of cesarean section influences the incidence of RDS. Recent studies noting the increased risk of late preterm infants and RDS in elective cesarean sections are cited in Chapter 5.

Obstruction of the airway caused by aspiration of meconium or amniotic fluid occurs before birth, spontaneously at birth, or during resuscitative efforts. Although the lungs initially fill with air, subsequent atelectasis occurs as airway obstruction prevents further entrance of air. Conversely, a "ball-valve" or "air-trapping" effect may occur as air is allowed in but is unable to escape because of intermittent obstruction. The presence of amniotic debris, vernix, lanugo, and meconium in the respiratory tract increases the incidence and severity of pulmonary infection. Diaphragmatic paralysis occurs after phrenic nerve injury during birth (usually in a large-for-gestational-age [LGA] infant) and is often associated with brachial plexus injuries. The paradoxic movement of the paralyzed diaphragm during inspiration and expiration results in inadequate tidal volume and impaired gaseous exchange.

Existing neonatal conditions increase the risk for respiratory distress. Congenital defects that prevent transmission of the stimulus to or from the respiratory center, prevent normal respiratory effort, reduce gas-exchange surface area, or hamper the delivery of oxygen to the site of exchange will predispose the infant to respiratory embarrassment. Such defects include heart or great vessel anomalies, diaphragmatic hernia and hypoplastic lung, respiratory tract anomalies (e.g., choanal atresia or tracheoesophageal fistula), chest wall deformities, and CNS defects.

Diseases of the infant also can lead to respiratory distress. Hemolytic disease, such as ABO and Rh incompatibility, results in anemia and, if severe, in hypovolemic shock. Blood incompatibilities may cause respiratory distress by decreasing the oxygen-carrying capacity of the blood. Infections stress the body's systems, increase oxygen requirements, and contribute to an impairment of surfactant production. Chronic lung disease in the form of bronchopulmonary dysplasia (BPD) occurs in 17% to 54% of very-low-birth-weight (VLBW) infants.[185] Prolonged treatment of RDS may be necessitated by the severity of the disease but may increase the risk for developing chronic lung disease.

GENERAL PREVENTION

Antepartum

Prevention of respiratory disease begins with prevention of conditions that predispose to respiratory distress. These conditions that constitute "reproductive risks" have been identified and can be categorized as psychosocial, genetic, biophysical, or economic in nature. Once an individual is identified as being in a high-risk category, comprehensive prenatal care with immediate attention given to maternal complications that arise is crucial (see Chapter 2).

Intrapartum

Fetal well-being is assessed by using electronic monitoring of uterine activity, fetal heart rate, and fetal scalp blood sampling. Electronic fetal heart rate monitoring enables instantaneous fetal heart rate tracings that provide coincident correlation between uterine contractions and fetal response. These tools enable the practitioner to evaluate how well the fetus withstands the stresses of labor and to make decisions about the laboring course.

Fetal cardiac response to stress is unlike an older child's or adult's response to hypoxia, hypercapnia, and acidosis with tachycardia from sympathetic nervous system discharge. A fetus responds to these same stresses with an initial increase in heart rate. This is quickly followed by bradycardia from parasympathetic stimulation when the hypoxia, hypercapnia, and acidosis persist (see Chapter 2).

Postpartum

After delivery, an infant should be maintained in an environment that minimizes stress and thereby minimizes oxygen requirement. All infants, but particularly at-risk infants, should be maintained within the narrow parameter of physiologic homeostasis (as outlined in Unit Two, Support of the Neonate).

GENERAL DATA COLLECTION

Because the clinical manifestations of many neonatal illnesses include respiratory symptoms (cardiac, metabolic, neurologic, and hematologic), a systematic and thorough approach to data collection is essential in evaluating an infant in respiratory distress.

History

The perinatal history (antepartum, intrapartum, and postpartum) should be reviewed for risk factors (see Chapter 2).

Signs and Symptoms

Vital signs such as temperature, pulse, respiration, and blood pressure should be evaluated. Hypothermia and hyperthermia increase oxygen requirements by altering the basal metabolic rate. Hypotension often is associated with respiratory distress.

RESPIRATORY EXAMINATION

Respiratory effort is normally irregular in rate and depth and is chiefly abdominal, rather than thoracic, with a rate of 30 to 60 breaths/min. Bradypnea is characterized by a rate below 30 breaths/min that is regular (as opposed to periodic or apneic) and may be caused by an insult to the respiratory center of the CNS. Tachypnea, a rate of 60 breaths/min or greater after the first hour of life, is the earliest sign of respiratory (and often other) diseases. As a compensatory mechanism, tachypnea attempts to maintain alveolar ventilation and gaseous exchange. As a decompensatory mechanism, tachypnea increases oxygen demand, energy output, and the "work" of breathing.

Periodic respirations are cyclic respirations of apnea (5 to 10 seconds) and ventilation (10 to 15 seconds). The average respiratory rate is 30 to 40 breaths/min. Periodic breathing is a common occurrence in small preterm infants as a result of an immature CNS. Apnea is a nonbreathing episode lasting longer than 20 seconds and accompanied by physiologic alterations. The syndrome of apnea is discussed under Apnea later in this chapter.

Use of accessory muscles of respiration is indicative of a marked increase in the work of breathing. Retractions reflect the inward pull of the thin chest wall on inspiration. Retracting is best observed in relation to the sternum (substernal and suprasternal) and the intercostal, supracostal, and subcostal spaces. The increased negative intrathoracic pressure necessary to ventilate the stiff, noncompliant lung causes the chest wall to retract. This further compromises the lung's expansion. The degree of retraction is directly proportional to the severity of the disease.

Nasal flaring is a compensatory mechanism that attempts to take in more oxygen by increasing the size of the nares and thus decreasing the resistance (by as much as 40%) of the narrow airways. Grunting is forced expiration through a partially closed glottis. The audible grunt may be heard with or without the aid of a stethoscope. As a compensatory mechanism, grunting stabilizes the alveoli by increasing transpulmonary pressure and increases gaseous exchange by delaying expiration.[177]

Color is normally pink within the first 10 minutes of life. *Acrocyanosis,* which is peripheral cyanosis of the hands and feet in the first 24 hours of life, is normal. Pallor with poor peripheral circulation may indicate systemic hypotension. Ruddy, plethoric skin color may indicate hyperviscosity, polycythemia, or both as the cause of respiratory symptoms. However, the lack of a deep-red coloring does not rule out polycythemia or hyperviscosity.

Cyanosis, a late and serious sign, is a blue discoloration of the skin, nail beds, and mucous membranes. Differentiation between peripheral cyanosis (of hands and feet) and central cyanosis (of mucous membranes of mouth and generalized body cyanosis) is essential. Because a large decrease in Pao_2 may be tolerated without detectable cyanosis, the lack of cyanosis does not ensure a healthy infant. When hypoxemia reaches a level that produces frank cyanosis, the insufficiency is usually in advanced stages (see Chapter 8). Therefore cyanosis or its lack is not a reliable sign in neonates.

Symmetry of the newborn chest is characterized by a relatively round or barrel shape, because the anteroposterior diameter equals the transverse diameter. With prolonged respiratory distress, there is an increase in the anteroposterior diameter, so the neonate becomes *pigeon-chested.*

Auscultation of a newborn's chest includes comparing and contrasting one side with the other and noting the quality of breath sounds and the presence or absence of rales, rhonchi, or other abnormal sounds. Because of the relatively small size of the newborn's chest, it is hyperresonant, so breath sounds are widely transmitted. Therefore one cannot always rely on auscultation to detect pathologic conditions (e.g., pneumothorax). Percussion of the chest to determine the presence of air, fluid, or solids may not be useful in the neonate because of small chest size and hyperresonance. Palpation of the neonatal chest wall while the infant is crying may detect gross changes in sound transmission through the chest. Palpation of crepitus in the neck, around the clavicles, or on the chest wall suggests the complication of air leak.

NONRESPIRATORY EXAMINATION

Hypotonia is characterized by a froglike positioning and a lax, open mouth. Progressing from flexion to flaccidity indicates progression of hypoxia and exhaustion from the work of breathing. Cardiac and related findings such as a murmur, absence of pulses, bounding pulses, palmar or calf pulses, weight gain, hepatosplenomegaly, cyanosis, edema, bradycardia, or tachycardia indicate congestive heart failure or congenital heart defects. A scaphoid abdomen indicates a diaphragmatic hernia.

Laboratory Data

Because the clinical presentation of many respiratory and nonrespiratory diseases is the same, a chest x-ray examination may be the only way to differentiate cause and establish the proper diagnosis. X-ray evaluation helps eliminate congenital anomalies (e.g., diaphragmatic hernia with lung hypoplasia, masses, and obstruction) as the cause when acquired respiratory disease (e.g., RDS, transient tachypnea of the newborn, and pneumonia) is the cause of the distress. X-ray films confirm the presence of pneumothorax or other pulmonary air leaks.

Measurement of arterial blood gases is used to demonstrate alterations in oxygenation and acid-base balance and to differentiate between respiratory and metabolic components. Initial baseline values are followed by serial observations at least every 15 to 30 minutes after any change in therapy during the acute phase of illness. Pulse oximetry enables immediate evaluation of oxygenation status and is an adjunct to arterial blood gas sampling.[10] A *shunt study* may differentiate between lung origin and cardiac origin of respiratory distress. The symptoms of pulmonary disease (cyanosis and low PaO_2) are often alleviated with crying, increased FiO_2, or continuous positive airway pressure. If the same symptoms are cardiac in origin, they remain unchanged or worsen with these interventions. Administration of 100% FiO_2 for 10 minutes or longer may result in an increased PaO_2 (greater than 100 mm Hg), whereas in cardiac disease caused by right-to-left shunting, there is no change in PaO_2 after 100% FiO_2 administration. *CAUTION:* In the presence of severe lung disease with significant right-to-left shunting, cyanosis and PaO_2 may not be changed with 100% FiO_2.

The hematocrit value is used to rule out anemia or polycythemia as the cause of the respiratory distress. In anemia, inadequate oxygen content promotes tissue hypoxia. In polycythemia, increased viscosity and sludging of blood flow adversely affect tissue oxygenation.

The white blood cell count, differential, and C-reactive protein (CRP) (see Chapter 22) aid in diagnosing sepsis as the cause of distress. A blood culture is an invaluable aid when infection is suspected and should be obtained before antibiotic therapy is initiated. Blood glucose determination to rule out hypoglycemia as a cause is particularly important in IDMs, small-for-gestational-age (SGA) infants, LGA infants, and preterm appropriate-for-gestational-age (AGA) and late preterm infants. An electrocardiogram (ECG), echocardiogram, and cardiac catheterization are used to rule out cardiac abnormalities.

An electroencephalogram (EEG) and ultrasonographic examination of the brain help rule out CNS abnormalities. Serum electrolytes (calcium, sodium, and potassium) aid in eliminating metabolic aberration as the cause of the distress.

GENERAL TREATMENT STRATEGIES

Treatment of any condition should be directed at correction of its underlying cause. In meconium aspiration syndrome, the presence of meconium damages the neonatal lung. No therapeutic measure is available at present to augment the healing process. Therapy is thus directed at preventing or alleviating the consequences of neonatal lung diseases, such as hypoxemia and acidemia, allowing healing to take place and reducing the potential for iatrogenic complications.

Respiratory support is the hallmark of treatment of neonatal respiratory disease. Respiratory support involves increasing inspired oxygen tensions and providing ventilation if necessary.

Supplemental Oxygen

Oxygen is a *drug,* the most commonly used drug in neonatal care. Historically, the policy of unrestricted and unmonitored oxygen therapy was accompanied by potential harm (e.g., RDS, chronic lung disease [BPD/CLD], retinopathy of prematurity [ROP] (discussed in Chapter 31), PDA [see Patent Ductus Arteriosus later in this chapter], necrotizing enterocolitis [NEC] [discussed in Chapter 28], and IVH/periventricular leukomalacia, hypoxic-ischemic encephalopathy [PVL, HIE] [discussed in Chapter 26]) from oxygen free radicals without clear benefits.[17]

Free radicals are continuously produced in all cells as a byproduct of cell metabolism. Free radicals have positive effects in normal physiologic processes as follows: (1) biologic defense against bacteria, viruses, and cancer cells; (2) vasodilation; (3) neurotransmission; and (4) the up-regulation of some genes.[22] However, free radicals may also have harmful effects. Free radicals, highly reactive atomic molecules with unpaired electrons, regain their stability by quickly reacting with other molecules in proximity to obtain the molecules they need. Reaction with free radicals causes damage to these close molecules by changing their structure and function. To maintain homeostasis, the human body either uses or counters free radical activity with endogenous and exogenous antioxidants. Neonates, especially preterms, have maturational deficiencies in endogenous antioxidant systems, nutritional issues altering exogenous dietary intake of antioxidants, and diseases/conditions requiring interventions that preclude control of free radical–generating stimuli in their environment.[22] Therefore the neonatal period is an especially vulnerable time for free radical damage and injury.[347] The neonate, especially preterms and sick term infants, depend on care providers to use strategies that emphasize the prudent use of oxygen therapy (e.g., use of the minimum amount of oxygen to provide the desired therapeutic effect)[22,163,225,373] because the proper concentration of supplemental oxygen, especially for extremely preterm infants, remains to be established.[18,52,187,394]

When the neonate cannot maintain adequate oxygenation, supplemental oxygen must be provided. Because oxygen is a drug, it must be treated as such and given only for specific indications. Biochemical criteria (PaO_2 less than 60 mm Hg) and clinical criteria such as respiratory distress, central cyanosis, apnea, asphyxia, hypotonia, and low oxygen saturation are indications to prescribe oxygen. Institutional protocols for ordering, delivering, monitoring, and documenting oxygen therapy are recommended.[10]

Regardless of the mode of delivery (hood, nasal cannula or prongs, endotracheal tube, bag, or mask), safe and effective oxygen administration follows certain principles:

- No concentration of oxygen has been proved to be "safe." A concentration (e.g., 30%, 40%, 80%, 100%) that is therapeutic for one infant may be toxic for another. Oxygen blenders must be available wherever oxygen is being administered (e.g., delivery room, transition nursery, level I, II, or III nursery) so that delivery of different amounts of inspired oxygen concentration is possible.[22,163]

- To titrate inspired oxygen concentrations to the individual infant's need, arterial PO_2 should be measured and maintained in a normoxic state (PaO_2 between 60 and 80 mm Hg)[10]; both hypoxia and hyperoxia should be avoided.[227] Acutely ill neonates requiring supplemental oxygen therapy also should have blood pH and $PaCO_2$ measured.[10]

- To titrate inspired oxygen concentration to the individual neonate's need, oxygen saturation (using continuous noninvasive pulse oximetry [PO]) should be measured and maintained in the appropriate range for birth weight, gestational/chronologic age, and disease process wherever oxygen is being administered (e.g., delivery room, transition nursery, level I, II, or III nursery).[10,373] (See Oxygen Targeting later.)

- Oxygen administration without some form of continuous monitoring of the infant's oxygenation (e.g., arterial blood gases, pulse oximetry) is dangerous and not recommended.[10]

- Delivered oxygen should be humidified (30% to 40%), because dry gases are irritating to the airways and humidity decreases insensible water losses. To prevent respiratory therapy equipment from becoming a source of infection, humidifiers and tubing should be replaced per institutional and product protocol.

- Oxygen should be warmed (31° to 34° C [87.8° to 93.2° F]) so temperature at the delivery site is the same as the incubator temperature. Oxygen delivered by endotracheal tube should be warmed to core temperature (i.e., 36.5° to 37° C [97.7° to 98.6° F]).[163] This prevents cold stress and increased oxygen consumption from blowing cold air in the infant's face.[386]

- Oxygen concentration must be monitored by continuous or intermittent sampling (at least every hour) and recorded. In addition, hourly documentation of the following parameters should be recorded: (1) PO saturation values; (2) mode of oxygen delivery (e.g., hood, nasal cannula, continuous positive airway pressure [CPAP], ventilator); and (3) amount of oxygen being administered (e.g., FiO_2, liter flow/min).[10]

- Oxygen monitors and analyzers should be calibrated according to the manufacturer's recommendations.[10]
- A stable concentration of oxygen is necessary to maintain PaO_2 within desired normal limits. A sudden increase or decrease in oxygen concentration may result in a disproportionate increase or decrease in PaO_2 caused by vasodilation or vasoconstriction in response to oxygen.[386] Adjust FiO_2 in small increments (2% to 5%) to avoid hypoxia and/or hyperoxia. Adjustment of supplemental oxygen (particularly lowering FiO_2) must be done slowly to avoid the *flip-flop phenomenon*. Hypoxic insult initiates pulmonary vasoconstriction, which causes hypoperfusion and increased pulmonary vascular resistance. The infant should be weaned from supplemental oxygen cautiously.[386] Refer to Chapter 8 for a discussion of the "rule of seven," which states that the estimated percentage change in inspired oxygen is equal to the desired change in PaO_2 divided by 7.
- Observing color, respiratory effort, activity, and circulatory response and monitoring arterial oxygen concentration and/or oxygen saturation levels aid in determining the need for oxygen therapy and for appropriate adjustments.
- Clinical observations, FiO_2 concentrations, and time of adjustments must be described, documented, and reported.
- Oxygen concentration should be returned to previous levels if clinical observations of distress and inability to tolerate decreased levels of oxygen occur.

OXYGEN TARGETING FOR THE VLBW PRETERM INFANT

Because an infant who is hyperoxic (PaO_2 greater than 80 mm Hg)[407] clinically looks no different from an infant whose PaO_2 is normal, monitoring of oxygen saturations and partial pressure of oxygen with arterial blood gases is mandatory whenever oxygen is administered. Because PO gives immediate and continuous data, fewer PaO_2 values are obtained, so interpretation of PO readings and their relationship to PaO_2 values is critical. Because PO saturations higher than 92% can often be associated with hyperoxia (e.g., PaO_2 greater than 80 mm Hg),[407] observational[408] and

cohort[419] studies demonstrated a significant reduction in the incidence of ROP and BPD/CLD in preterms when their oxygen saturations were maintained in the lower (SpO_2 89% to 94%) rather than the higher range (SpO_2 96% to 99%). A systematic review and meta-analysis in 2011 found a 50% reduction in severe ROP and a 20% to 25% reduction in BPD/chronic lung disease when the lower rather than higher oxygen saturation range was used.[348] Two studies (i.e., STOP-ROP[405] and BOOST[18]) randomized preterm infants (several weeks after birth) to a lower or higher saturation range also found that higher saturations resulted in (1) more BPD/CLD, (2) no difference in the progression to threshold ROP, (3) more days on oxygen supplementation, and (4) a higher use of health care resources. However, larger randomized controlled trials (RCTs) of randomization soon after birth were needed.[16,349]

Five multicenter, multinational trials (i.e., SUPPORT,[394] three BOOST II trials,[52] and the COT trial[354]) randomized a total of 4911 premature infants, less than 28 weeks of gestation, to low (SpO_2 85% to 89%) or high (SpO_2 91% to 95%) ranges. Results of all five trials were systematically reviewed and a meta-analysis (the NEOPROM) performed to determine optimal oxygen saturation targets for preterm infants (mean gestational age of 26 weeks; mean birth weights of 820 to 850 g).[16,349] Combining data from all five studies showed (1) a lower mortality rate, a higher rate of severe ROP and BPD/CLD in the higher saturation groups, (2) a higher NEC rate in the lower saturation groups, and (3) IVH greater than or equal to 2 and PDA were evenly distributed between low and high saturation levels.[349] Combining data from all five studies, the lower oxygen saturation group's outcomes included (1) an increased mortality rate of 18% (including revised and nonrevised date) to 40% (using the revised algorithm), (2) a 26% reduction in severe ROP, (3) a 25% increase in NEC, and (4) no significant difference in BPD/CLD.[349] The higher death rate in the lower oxygen saturation group is attributed to an increased rate of intermittent hypoxemic episodes, even at 70 days after birth.[52,119]

Based on these studies, the systematic review, and meta-analysis, guidelines for oxygen targeting in preterm infants less than 28 weeks' gestational age recommend the following[349,396]:

- Target SpO_2 between 90% and 95%.

Maintaining ranges between 90% and 95% to avoid hypoxemia/hyperoxemia is an enormous challenge to care providers, especially neonatal nurses. During the use of lower oxygen saturation ranges, numerous studies showed various rates of success in keeping babies in the recommended ranges (e.g., 22% to 64%[171]). A more recent study of oxygen saturation targeting in preterms (less than 37 weeks'gestation) solely receiving CPAP found them to be in the target range for only 31% of the time.[249] For preterms 27 to 32 weeks'gestation there were 48 episodes per 24 hours of severe hyperoxia (SpO$_2$ greater than or equal to 98%) and 9 episodes per 24 hours of hypoxia (SpO$_2$ less than 80%). The fraction of inspired oxygen (FiO$_2$) concentration was adjusted between 16 and 41 times per day, with an average of 1 adjustment every hour. These researchers noted an increased frequency of prolonged hyperoxia when nurses were each caring for more than 1 neonate.[249] Factors influencing clinical decision making about oxygen titration include poor staffing, nursing shortage, and lack of knowledge about oxygen use.[199] New mechanical devices such as a closed-loop automatic control (CLAC) reduce nursing workload, improve oxygen administration, and automatically control FiO$_2$ to preterm infants receiving CPAP or mechanical ventilation.[173]

Fluctuations of PaO$_2$ (e.g., hypoxemia and hyperoxemia episodes) in the VLBW preterm may be a more significant risk factor than hyperoxia alone for the development of threshold ROP.[447] These episodes of hyperoxia and/or hypoxia may result from the underlying respiratory pathology or the result of care providers' interventions (e.g., positioning; suction; "chasing desaturations by increasing FiO$_2$"; surfactant administration).

DELIVERY METHODS

For instructions on the bag-and-mask resuscitation method, see Chapter 4. An oxygen hood is a clear plastic hood that fits over the infant's head to deliver a constant concentration of oxygen. If the infant has sufficient ventilation to maintain a normal arterial carbon dioxide tension, oxygenation by increased inspired oxygen tensions through an oxygen hood may be the only respiratory support that is necessary. This degree of support is particularly applicable in cases of mild RDS, transient tachypnea of the newborn (TTN), meconium aspiration, or neonatal pneumonia.

A blender system is the most reliable way to administer a fixed oxygen concentration via a hood. An appropriate-size hood should be used. If it is too large, the infant may slip out of the hood and FiO$_2$ may be diluted by leaks; if it is too small, pressure points may develop, especially around the neck. Another source of oxygen must be provided when the infant's head is removed from the hood because of feeding, being held, or suctioning. This secondary source may be set up from the blender source so that the infant's PaO$_2$ remains constant during suctioning or feedings. The infant may need increased FiO$_2$ from the secondary source, and this can be adjusted easily according to assessments made with pulse oximetry; these changes should be recorded.

For both home and hospital use, a nasal cannula is used to administer oxygen to the dependent infant who is developing social and motor skills:

- Choose the appropriate-size cannula for the infant—a cannula that is too large obstructs the nares, prevents air leak thus enabling an increase in CPAP, irritates the nasal mucosa, and is uncomfortable for the baby.[234]
- Position the cannula across the infant's upper lip. Secure it to the infant's face by first applying hydrocolloid barrier or transparent dressings directly to the infant's cheeks and taping the cannula to it to prevent skin irritation.
- Oxygen tubing should be long enough to provide opportunities for social and gross motor skill development.

CAUTION: Neonates are obligatory nasal breathers, so nasal obstruction (mucus or milk) will decrease the amount of oxygen actually received. Therefore nares should be suctioned as needed. Because the exact concentrations of oxygen delivered by cannula cannot be measured, flow rates are titrated by monitoring PaO$_2$ or pulse oximetry readings and by evaluating the clinical course.

Without adequate studies to establish safety and efficacy, many centers have adopted heated, humidified, high-flow (greater than 1 L/min) nasal cannula (HHHFNC) therapy as primary support for preterms with RDS, apnea of prematurity, and postextubation respiratory care, including weaning from nasal continuous positive airway pressure (NCPAP).[234,257,273,435] Use of nasal cannulas with oxygen rates above 0.5 L/min may result in inadvertent administration of continuous distending (positive) pressure, causing increased respiratory effort (i.e., tachypnea, retractions, thoracoabdominal asynchrony, exaggerated periodic breathing, and increased work of breathing.).[255] HHHFNC generates CPAP to the preterm airway that may be excessive given the conditions of (1) closed mouth, (2) tightly fitting nasal cannula (NC), (3) rate of flow, and (4) infant size (less than 1500 g).[234]

Commercial HHHFNC devices currently in use can achieve flow rates of 4 to 8 L/min.[144] Unlike CPAP devices that are equipped with a pressure gauge and a pop-off safety valve, HHHFNC devices do not have a direct measure of the pressure applied to the infant's airway or a pop-off valve to prevent the accumulation of excessive pressure; flow rates as high as 6 L/min have been used without measurement of the level of CPAP delivered.[144] Measurements of oral cavity pressures closely estimate the delivered CPAP of the HHHFNC devices; a recent study found similar pharyngeal pressures in two HHHFNC commercial devices.[83,234] CPAP generated with HHHFNC depends on flow rate and weight; the smallest infants with the highest flow rates and a completely closed mouth may achieve clinically significant and unpredictable levels of CPAP.[234,273,378,436]

Several small studies demonstrate improved ventilation and oxygenation with HHHFNC at flow rates above 2 L/min, comparable efficacy to use of NCPAP in preterms with RDS.[241,257,346,367] Care provider preference and perceived comfort (i.e., tolerance of the device by the preterm,[378] less nasal trauma,[81] parental preference,[226] similar noise levels as CPAP[332]) are cited reasons for use of HHHFNC rather than NCPAP.[257] A randomized, controlled study comparing HHHFNC with NCPAP for primary or postextubation respiratory support in neonates 28 to 42 weeks of gestation found no differences in need for intubation or supplemental oxygen, safety, rates of BPD/CLD- or discharge with oxygen.[446] As primary therapy for RDS, HHHFNC was recently compared with nasal intermittent positive-pressure ventilation (NIPPV) in preterms (less than 35 weeks' gestation and greater than 1000 g birth weight). There was no significant difference in the need for endotracheal intubation/ventilation or the rate of morbidities (i.e., pneumothorax, BPD, IVH, NEC, PDA, or nasal trauma) between the preterms randomized to the HHHFNC or the NIPPV treatment groups in this randomized pilot study.[235] Another study comparing the use of HHHFNC (e.g., up to 2.5 L/min) with NCPAP for treatment of apnea found that the HHHFNC was as effective as NCPAP.[378] *Note:* The use of HHHFNC for postextubation care is discussed under Weaning from the Ventilator later in this chapter.

However, a Cochrane review[435] (4 studies) and another review[257] (19 studies) of the evidence for use of HHHFNC in preterm infants both caution that the safety and efficacy HHHFNC has not been established. As an alternative to other noninvasive methods of respiratory support both reviews recommend large, randomized controlled trials that include long-term outcome follow-up. If used, HHHFNC should meet the following criteria: (1) only heated, humidified systems with flow rates greater than or equal to 2 L/min, using only maximum flow rates according to manufacturer's specifications; (2) choose nasal prong size that does not completely occlude the nares; and (3) set the flow rate based on infant's size: starting flow rate of 4 to 6 L/min in newly born preterm infants; use lower level (4 L/min) for preterms with birth weight less than 1000 g.[257]

Continuous Distending Pressure

Application of a continuous distending pressure (CDP) to the lungs increases functional residual capacity and PaO_2. Oxygenation is improved by decreasing intrapulmonary shunting and by improving the match of ventilation and perfusion. The application of CDP improves compliance of the lung and lessens the work of breathing.[164] Early application of CDP in preterms with RDS reduces the subsequent use of intermittent positive-pressure ventilation (IPPV) with its accompanying adverse effects.

In RDS, in which the functional residual capacity is reduced, increased respiratory oxygen tensions through an oxygen hood (oxyhood) may not be sufficient to maintain an adequate arterial oxygen tension. More invasive techniques may be necessary.

CPAP and continuous negative pressure (CNP) are two methods of delivery of CDP. If the infant cannot maintain a PaO_2 of 60 mm Hg in 0.6 FiO_2, a trial of CPAP through the nasal route is indicated. Initial levels of CPAP should be in the range of 4 to 5 cm H_2O. CPAP should be increased to 8 to 10 cm H_2O by 1- to 2-cm increments if necessary to raise the infant's PaO$_2$ (as measured by arterial blood gas determinations, noninvasive monitoring, or both).

Not all CPAP application techniques are equal. Neonates receiving "bubble" CPAP experience chest wall vibrations (similar to those seen in high-frequency ventilation [HFV]) that contribute to gaseous exchange. Two recent studies of the mechanics of bubble CPAP are important for information about maintenance of an adequately functioning system. Lung volume recruitment and breathing efficiency during bubble CPAP are influenced by the size and depth of submergence of the expiratory limb of a CPAP circuit, the diameter of the bubble generator bottle, and lung compliance.[444] Condensation in the exhalation limb of a patient circuit during bubble CPAP accumulates at the rate of 3.8 ml/hr.[448] When this condensation reaches volumes greater than 10 ml the oscillating fluid increases airway pressure and results in significant increases in mean tracheal pressure. These researchers recommend frequent (i.e., every 2 to 3 hours) emptying of the exhalation tube, continuous monitoring of pressure at the nasal airway interface, and using an adjustable pressure-relief valve in the circuit (set to 5 cm H$_2$O pressure above the desired mean pressure).[448]

Bubble CPAP reduces minute volume by 39% and respiratory rate by 7% compared with CPAP provided through a ventilator.[75] In one center, use of bubble CPAP from birth in 401- to 1000-g preterms has resulted in (1) fewer delivery room intubations, (2) fewer days on mechanical ventilation, (3) less use of postnatal steroids, (4) better weight gain, and (5) no increase in complications, including the incidence of CLD/BPD.[280] In an RCT, larger preterms (mean gestational age 36 weeks; mean birth weight 2900 g) with respiratory distress were treated with either supplemental oxygen in an oxygen hood or with bubble CPAP through nasal prongs.[57] Only 23% of the larger preterms who were treated with CPAP were transported to a higher-level neonatal intensive care unit (NICU) compared with 40% of the preterms who were treated with oxygen in a hood. Also, cost savings were realized and there was no increase in oxygen use or mortality rate. However, there was a clinically, not statistically, significant increase in the incidence of pneumothorax in the CPAP group; the 24-hour presence of a neonatal nurse practitioner or physician to relieve air leaks is mandatory with the use of CPAP.

More recent studies of bubble CPAP continue to demonstrate cost-effectiveness and better outcomes of preterms with RDS, including extremely low-birth-weight (ELBW) and VLBW preterms.[25,233,445] A 7-year retrospective review of respiratory outcomes in 633 VLBW infants found a significant reduction in BPD/CLD (43% lower chance), less mechanical ventilation, and fewer discharged with diuretics and supplemental oxygen after use of bubble CPAP.[148] A subset analysis of the outcomes of ELBW preterms receiving bubble CPAP found a faster extubation rate, fewer days of mechanical ventilation (more ELBW off mechanical ventilation at 1 week of age), less ROP, fewer PDA ligations and deaths, and an increase in low-grade IVHs.[148] Another study found a 27% improvement in survival with the use of bubble CPAP, especially in VLBW preterms, those with RDS, or those with sepsis.[213]

Large, multicenter RCTs of NCPAP starting at birth include the COIN trial,[272] the SUPPORT trial,[394] the VON Delivery Room Management trial,[129] the CURPAP,[344] Colombian Network,[335] and South American Neocosur Network[402] trials. The COIN trial[272] compared NCPAP with intubation and ventilation of 25 to 28 weeks' gestation preterms breathing spontaneously by 5 minutes of age with respiratory distress. Within the first 5 days of life, 46% of those randomized to NCPAP were intubated, at a median of 6.6 hours of life. Outcomes at 36 weeks were no different for either group in the combined outcome of death or oxygen dependence. A nonsignificant trend toward less CLD/BPD occurred in the more mature preterms, whereas there was a trend toward increased mortality rate in the less mature preterms randomized to NCPAP. Unlike other studies, only 77% of the infants randomized to intubation received surfactant and surfactant use was halved in the NCPAP group.[272] The SUPPORT trial compared immediate CPAP to intubation, surfactant, and mechanical ventilation in 24 to 27$^{6/7}$ weeks of gestation preterms and found fewer ventilator days, less postnatal steroid use, and no difference in air leaks, BPD/CLD, or death.[394] In the SUPPORT trial, the most immature (24 to 25 weeks' gestation) preterms benefited the most from the early initiation of NCPAP.[394] The CURPAP[344] and Colombian Network[335] trials demonstrated no difference in the rate of BPD/CLD with early CPAP versus prophylactic surfactant. From these data the American Academy of

T A B L E 23-2	CONTINUOUS POSITIVE AIRWAY PRESSURE	
INDICATIONS	**COMPLICATIONS**
Infant who breathes spontaneously yet has mild to moderate respiratory distress syndrome	Respiratory difficulty secondary to narrowing of the nasal passage with prongs, of the trachea with the presence of an endotracheal tube
Very-low-birth-weight infant with primary or secondary apnea	Pneumothorax and other air leaks
Support during weaning from mechanical ventilation	Nasal and/or septal irritation, trauma, deformity, obstruction[376a]; gastric and abdominal distention; perforation; infection (tracheal colonization on day 5 of NCPAP use also associated with longer need for respiratory support)[8]

Pediatrics (AAP) policy statement on respiratory support in preterm infants at birth recommends initiation of NCPAP at birth as an alternative to routine intubation and early surfactant therapy.[9] The policy also recommends combining early NCPAP with selective surfactant therapy in extremely preterm infants, which results in lower BPD/CLD and death rates compared with early/prophylactic surfactant therapy[9] (see also Surfactant Replacement Therapy and Box 23-9).

Alternate methods of delivering continuous distending pressure in neonates include biphasic NCPAP and nasal intermittent positive-pressure ventilation (NIPPV) (discussed under Weaning from the Ventilator). Biphasic CPAP delivers two alternating levels of distending pressure at specific rates independent of the neonate's own respiratory rate. Biphasic is similar to CPAP but possibly better at maintaining an appropriate functional residual capacity (FRC). One small, single-center study reported a reduction in length of respiratory support, oxygen exposure, and early discharge.[252] Even though biphasic CPAP delivery seems promising, specific volume drivers are required for its use, thus potentially limiting access.

Indications and complications in the use of CPAP are listed in Table 23-2. If the infant maintains ventilation as indicated by normal arterial carbon dioxide tension, no further respiratory support may be necessary. CPAP may be delivered by facemask, nasal pharyngeal tubes, nasal prongs, or endotracheal (ET) tube. Delivery of CPAP by nasal prongs is the most common method used; use of short binasal prongs is the most effective.[115] A study of preterms less than 31 weeks' gestation randomly assigned to nasal prongs or nasal mask for CPAP

found that the nasal mask was more effective at preventing complications of intubation and ventilation.[219] However, in much of the research literature, nasal prongs are compared with nasal pharyngeal tubes for administration of CPAP. Advantages to the use of nasal CPAP include the following[20,148,163,323]:

- Less invasive than endotracheal tube
- Decreased incidence, duration, and complications of intubation and mechanical ventilation
- Earlier extubation
- Decreased incidence and morbidity of BPD/CLD
- Improved oxygenation and decreased work of breathing
- Decreased need for surfactant and second doses of surfactant
- Reduced mortality rate

Disadvantages include (1) gaseous distention of the bowel or gastrointestinal (GI) perforation[150] (both are rare occurrences), (2) increased rate of pneumothorax,[57,272] (3) difficulties keeping prongs in the nose and maintaining patency, (4) infant agitation, and (5) alteration in appearance (dilation of the nares).[376a] CPAP is labor intensive for the neonatal nurse. Choosing the correct size of nasal prong is important to avoid movement and erosion of nasal tissue. Box 23-1 lists important aspects of care of the neonate on NCPAP to optimize safety and efficacy.

Criteria that indicate improvement on CPAP are listed in Box 23-2. Failure of CPAP is associated with (1) birth weight less than 1500 g, (2) gestational age 30 weeks or less, (3) "whiteout" chest x-ray, (4) Fio_2 50% or greater at 20 minutes of CPAP, and (5) positive end-expiratory pressure (PEEP) 5.5 cm H_2O or greater.[174] When the infant's

BOX 23-1	CARE OF INFANTS RECEIVING NCPAP TO OPTIMIZE SAFETY AND EFFICACY

Prongs

- Nasal prongs should fill the entire nares without distending or causing blanching of the nares
- Presence of a small space (at least 2 mm) between the nares and prong base
- Lateral straps are used to secure the prongs by providing gentle, equal tension
- Assess prongs and NCPAP device at least every hour to ensure proper positioning and functioning
- Remove NCPAP device q 2-4 hr to assess skin integrity (e.g., color, perfusion, pressure, excoriation) and massage nasal septum

Hat

- Use the appropriate-size hat to avoid prong movement; change hat size with neonatal head growth
- Position just above the eyebrows, with the back of the hat extending to the base of the neck, and completely covering the infant's ears
- Use ties on the hat to secure tubing, thus decreasing movement and/or upward pull of CPAP system

Nose

- Suction nares only PRN to maintain nasal patency
- Avoid deep nasal suctioning, unless absolutely necessary for individual infant
- Use a hydrocolloid dressing over the nose and philtrum to provide a barrier layer for skin protection

Mouth

- Place orogastric tube for decompression of the stomach
- Encourage closed mouth by use of pacifier and/or prone positioning

Comfort Measures

- Positioning prone, swaddled, or contained (to promote flexion) (see Chapter 13) decreases movement and pulling/dragging of the device on the nares
- Minimal handling and position change q 2-4 hr and/or with infant agitation
- Skin-to-skin care with parents (see Chapters 12 and 13)
- Pacifier, nonnutritive sucking, sucrose
- Environmental management — decrease light/noise (see Chapter 13)
- Use neonatal pain scale and administer pharmacologic sedation and/or pain relief (see Chapter 12)

Adapted from McCoskey L: Nursing care guidelines for prevention of nasal breakdown in neonates receiving nasal CPAP, *Adv Neonatal Care* 8:116, 2008; Squires AJ, Hyndman M: Prevention of nasal injuries secondary to NCPAP application in the ELBW infant, *Neonatal Netw* 28:13, 2009.
CPAP, Continuous positive airway pressure; *NCPAP,* nasal CPAP; *PRN,* as needed.

BOX 23-2	CRITICAL FINDINGS
	CRITERIA THAT INDICATE IMPROVEMENT ON CONTINUOUS POSITIVE AIRWAY PRESSURE

Blood Gases

- Decrease or stabilization of oxygen requirement Fio_2 ≤0.60 with Pao_2 >50 mm Hg or pulse oximetry >90%
- Maintenance of adequate ventilation
  - $Paco_2$ ≤50 to 60 mm Hg
  - pH 7.25-7.45

Clinical

- Decreased work of breathing — decreased respiratory rate, grunting, flaring, and retracting
- Improved lung volumes and appearance on chest x-ray films
- Improved patient comfort

Pao_2 is consistently over 70 mm Hg, inspired oxygen concentration or CDP may be lowered. Oxygen concentration is usually lowered in 5% to 10% increments to a level of 40% to 60%. CDP is lowered in increments of 1 cm H_2O to a level of 2 cm H_2O before discontinuation.[196] Results in weaning from NCPAP are seen when the pressure is lowered, then stopped, rather than removed for a number of hours during the day.[196] The infant may then be placed into an oxygen hood with the same Fio_2. Neonates should be monitored closely with pulse oximetry and arterial blood gases.

Pulmonary Hygiene

Pulmonary hygiene is normally maintained by ciliary activity, a covering of mucus, and narrowing and dilation of the bronchi with respiration and coughing. Anatomic and physiologic variations in the neonate alter these normal pulmonary mechanisms. The small airway of the neonate has a diameter that is four times smaller than that of the normal adult. Debris that causes only a moderate obstruction for the adult airway causes a disproportionately greater obstruction of the smaller airway of the neonate. Also, a neonate normally has an underdeveloped cough reflex. A sick neonate with insufficient respiratory effort and a weak or nonexistent cry has underventilated lungs. If a neonate who is attached to multiple life-support systems is cared for in the same position, secretions localize in the dependent pulmonary tree and predispose to hypostatic pneumonia.

Pulmonary hygiene consists of two major components: chest physiotherapy (CPT) and suctioning. The goals of pulmonary hygiene are the following:

- To maintain a patent airway by clearing secretions
- To promote optimal pulmonary oxygenation and ventilation
- To prevent pulmonary infection from accumulated secretions
- To facilitate removal of pulmonary debris by loosening and mobilizing secretions into the mainstem bronchi for suctioning

Pulmonary hygiene has been used as a treatment for intubated patients with conditions associated with atelectasis, increased secretions, and pulmonary debris (pneumonia, meconium aspiration, RDS, and BPD).

CHEST PHYSIOTHERAPY

CPT consists of positioning, percussion, and vibration. Postural changes use gravity to facilitate the movement of pulmonary debris from smaller to larger bronchi. Postural changes used with pediatric and adult respiratory patients have been used for neonatal CPT. However, most ill neonates, especially VLBW and ELBW infants, do not tolerate multiple positioning and repositioning. Periodic (every 2 to 4 hours with care) repositioning changes the ventilation-perfusion matching in dependent lung areas and improves oxygenation. Prone positioning improves lung mechanics and lung volumes and improves oxygenation (see Chapter 13).

Percussion of the chest wall creates a suction action that loosens secretions. Percussion should occur through gently tapping over the affected lung. In infants with BPD, rib fractures have been documented that resulted from vigorous percussion[319] and vibrator use.[441] Vibration of the neonate's chest may follow percussion. Even though vibration must be done on expiration to move secretions with the exhalation of air, this is very difficult to accomplish with the neonate's rapid, shallow breathing cycle.

Any manipulation of the sick neonate has the potential for decreasing oxygenation and precipitating hypoxia (see Chapter 13). During CPT, bradycardia, cyanosis, hypotonia, fighting, struggling, and alterations in oxygenation are signs of stress. There is also an increase in plasma epinephrine and norepinephrine levels with CPT and endotracheal suctioning; this stress response is decreased in sedated preterm infants.[165] CPT is no better than standard care for clearing secretions in ventilated neonates and is accompanied by hypoxia and increased oxygen requirements. Postextubation CPT has also shown no differences in preventing atelectasis, decreasing the number of apnea/bradycardia episodes, the need for reintubation, or the duration of supplemental oxygen.[24]

The most severe complications reportedly resulting from CPT are an increased risk for IVH (see Chapter 26) and cerebral encephalopathy. An increased incidence of severe intraventricular/periventricular hemorrhage has been reported in preterm infants treated with early CPT.[326] In 1992, a previously unrecognized and distinct pattern of severe, late-onset brain injury was reported in 15 neonates (24 to 32 weeks of gestational age; 600 to 1270 g birth weight). The pattern of brain injury was of extensive, dense, and cystic lesions involving the periphery of the brain bilaterally. This full-thickness cortical necrosis, called *encephaloclastic porencephaly,* resulted in 14 deaths and severe neurologic deficit in the only survivor.[96] This nursery changed its protocol to include holding the baby's head steady during CPT; no further cases of brain injury have occurred.[325]

Another study of 454 babies found 13 babies (24 to 27 weeks of gestational age; 680 to 1100 g birth weight) with lesions similar to the encephaloclastic porencephaly just described. The lesions in these infants were described as cystic with cortical and subcortical destruction, and peripheral rather than periventricular; they occurred between 2 and 3 weeks of life. These hemorrhagic infarcts are consistent with the pathologic changes in older infants from *shaken baby syndrome*.[228,229,340,437] The extremely immature brain of the VLBW infant may be particularly vulnerable to the shaking movements of CPT. Five of these infants died; seven of the eight surviving infants had handicaps (e.g., mild hemiplegia to severe spastic quadriplegia; cognitive delay) at 6 to 16 months of age. For longer than 3 years, no VLBW infant in this NICU has received CPT in the first month of life; no further cases of this brain injury have occurred.[86,175]

The techniques, efficacy, complications, outcomes, safety, and frequency of CPT have not been studied sufficiently.[192] Given the lack of data, the lack of clear evidence of benefit, and the concerns of safety for VLBW infants, recommendations include the following:

- Use CPT cautiously.
- Do not use CPT on VLBW infants in the first month of life.[175]
- Keep the infant's head steady during CPT.[325]
- CPT should be used only for definite indications when the infant is fit and able to tolerate the procedure.[325]
- CPT should never be done "routinely" but should be applied on an individual basis after careful and thorough assessment.[325]
- Percussion should be used only when secretions are not cleared by suction alone.[325]
- Use of CPT in the delivery room lacks evidence-based research.
- CPT should not be included in pulmonary hygiene until research clearly substantiates its benefits.[443]

SUCTIONING

Once secretions are loosened and mobilized, they must be removed through the nose, mouth, or trachea with suctioning.

Naso-oropharyngeal Suctioning. When an infant has no artificial airway, suctioning the naso-oropharynx serves two purposes: removing secretions and initiating a cough reflex that mobilizes secretions. With either a suction bulb or catheter, the infant is suctioned when secretions are produced. Providing an oxygen source during the procedure is necessary. Because stimulation of the nares causes reflex inspiration with possible inhalation of oropharyngeal contents, first the *mouth* and then the *nose* should be suctioned. The results should be documented.

CAUTION: Suctioning should be avoided for 30 minutes to 1 hour after feeding unless it is necessary to establish a patent airway. The catheter should be gently inserted upward and back into the nares, never forced. If the catheter is hard to pass or the nares seem blocked, this procedure should be abandoned to prevent swelling or trauma. Frequent nasal suction creates trauma and edema. The catheter may initiate vasovagal stimulation with alterations in heart rate[31] and/or resultant bradycardia.

Endotracheal Suctioning. An artificial airway prevents normal warming, humidifying, and cleansing of the air by the upper airway. The presence of the foreign body (the tube) also increases pulmonary secretions. To maintain a patent airway, sterile endotracheal suction should be performed on an individual basis, *never* on a routine basis (e.g., on a schedule of every 2, 3, or 4 hours).[13] Individual assessment criteria to establish that the infant "needs" suction are listed in Box 23-3. Knowledge of the infant's respiratory diagnosis suggests the need and the frequency of suction. The acute phase (first 72 hours) of RDS is a restrictive disease; few secretions are produced, so minimal suctioning (every 12 to 24 hours) is necessary. Studies have found no increase in occluded tubes when suction frequency was changed from every 6 to every 12 hours (during the first 72 hours of RDS)[439] and from every 4 to every 8 hours.[92] Disease processes noted for secretion production (e.g., the chronic phase of RDS, CLD/BPD, meconium aspiration syndrome, or pneumonia) may require early and frequent suctioning.

Endotracheal tube (ETT) suctioning is not an innocuous procedure. ETT suction is associated with numerous physiologic alterations and complications (Box 23-4). Hypoxia and changes in heart rate and blood pressure alter cerebral blood flow, increase intracranial pressure, and predispose the preterm to an increased risk for IVH (see Chapter 26). Pulse oximetry is a valuable tool in assessing oxygenation status during and after suctioning. The infant may be preoxygenated before suctioning, or if oxygen saturation falls (below 90%) during suctioning, the infant may be hyperventilated. *Preoxygenation* is the increase of Fio_2 above baseline concentration before ETT suction to prevent/reduce hypoxemia.[13] To avoid exposing the preterm to hyperoxic events that may predispose to ROP, the Fio_2 is increased by 10% to 20% above baseline when clinically

BOX 23-3	CRITICAL FINDINGS
	INDIVIDUAL ASSESSMENT CRITERIA FOR SUCTION

Evidence of Secretions
- Visible secretions in tube
- Audible coarse, wet, or decreased breath sounds
- Palpation of wet, coarse vibrations through chest wall

Alterations in Vital Signs
- Changes in respiratory pattern:
  - Increased work of breathing (retractions, grunting, flaring)
  - Tachypnea or apnea
- Change in cardiac pattern; tachycardia or bradycardia

Alterations in Neonatal State
- Increased agitation, irritability, restlessness
- Hypertonic or hypotonic
- Listless, lethargic

Alterations in Oxygenation and Ventilation
- Desaturations (<90%) or labile saturations on pulse oximeter
- Skin color changes — pale, dusky, cyanotic
- Changes in arterial blood gas values — increased P_{CO_2}, decreased Pa_{O_2}, respiratory acidosis
- Increased peak inspiratory pressure on mechanical ventilation and increased high-pressure alarms
- Decreased chest wall vibration with high-frequency ventilation (HFV)

BOX 23-4	PHYSIOLOGIC ALTERATIONS AND COMPLICATIONS ASSOCIATED WITH ENDOTRACHEAL TUBE SUCTION

- Hypoxia/hypoxemia[139,318]
  - Caused by disconnection from the ventilator and oxygen, as well as presence of suction catheter and application of negative pressure, which partially occludes the airway; handling during the procedure; desaturations on the PO
- Alterations in heart rate[31,139,331]
  - Bradycardia, dysrhythmias, and asystole are precipitated by hypoxemia
- Alterations in blood pressure
  - Hypertension/hypotension
- Alterations in cerebral blood flow[301a,331]
  - Changes in oxygenation, heart rate, and blood pressure increase cerebral blood flow, both during and after the procedure (late [6 minutes]/prolonged [25 minutes] elevations of CBF),[203a] and intracranial pressure, which increase the risk for intraventricular hemorrhage
- Increase in plasma epinephrine and norepinephrine levels[165]
- Tissue damage
  - Granuloma formation within airways; increased severity of CLD/BPD associated with colonization of lungs with gram-negative bacilli; lobar emphysema and atelectasis; bronchial stenosis
- Atelectasis
  - Marked increase in opening (inflation) pressures of the lungs; adequate lung recruitment and PEEP may prevent lung collapse and deterioration in arterial oxygenation; atelectasis
- Pneumothorax
  - From aggressively ventilating neonate above baseline pressures
- Infection
  - Airway colonization with gram-positive cocci and gram-negative bacilli by 2 weeks of life despite the method of suction
- Unplanned extubation

CBF, Cerebral blood flow; *CLD/BPD,* chronic lung disease/bronchopulmonary dysplasia; *PEEP,* positive end-expiratory pressure; *PO,* pulse oximetry.

indicated for an individual infant. For ELBW/VLBW infants, Fi_{O_2} increases may be from 2% to 5%. Using 100% oxygen only if it is clinically indicated for the individual infant prevents hyperoxia. *Hyperventilation* (e.g., increasing respiratory rate) with a bag or the manual breaths on the ventilator after each catheter pass minimizes hypoxia and contributes to shortened time of stabilization and recovery. More research is needed on the optimal timing of increasing the Fi_{O_2} and the amount of oxygen to use.[318]

Administration of intermittent doses of morphine during endotracheal suctioning has not been shown to reduce pain scores in ventilated preterms. In this same RCT, multisensory stimulation after suctioning also was not associated with reduced pain scores.[73] Comfort measures (e.g., nonnutritive sucking, sucrose, swaddling, facilitated tucking) are recommended during suction

to provide pain relief,[31,425] as well as to reduce bradycardia and desaturations (see Chapter 12).

Most of the physiologic alterations and complications of ETT suction are the result of decreases in PEEP, lung volume, and oxygen during disconnection of the ETT from the ventilator for use of the open suction procedure. Use of closed suction systems (e.g., an adapter to suction without disconnection from the ventilator) decreases associated hypoxemia and bradycardia by enabling oxygenation and ventilation to continue during suction.[92,442] However, a recent study found that closed suction interfered with ventilator function (i.e., substantial negative intratracheal pressure during suction; the potential for higher airway pressures and tidal volumes after suctioning).[223] Closed suction is associated with smaller decreases in cerebral oxygenation, smaller variations in cerebral blood volume, and related hemodynamic changes, particularly in ventilated preterms.[204,274] Use of a four-handed closed suction technique was recently found to have no advantages in baseline heart rate, oxygen saturation, or salivary cortisol levels.[85] However, in this randomized crossover design, four-handed suction was associated with fewer stress and more self-regulatory behaviors.[85] A small study comparing the effects of open versus closed suction for mechanically (conventional and high frequency) ventilated ELBW preterms ($n = 19$) found decreases in cerebral blood flow and heart rate during suction and return to baseline after suctioning ceased; both of these changes were independent of the kind of ventilation and the type of suction used.[331] Two more recent studies comparing open and closed suction had conflicting results: (1) no differences in an RCT of 39 neonates 34 weeks of gestational age or older,[299] and (2) a significant decrease in hypoxemia and drop in SpO_2 with a higher SpO_2, mean arterial Po_2, and mean oxygenation ratio after closed versus open suction.[311]

Closed suction removed secretions as effectively as open suction with no increase in the rate of bacterial airway colonization (with catheter change every 24 hours), suction frequency, reintubation, duration of mechanical ventilation, length of hospitalization, incidence of nosocomial pneumonia or sepsis, severity of BPD/CLD, or mortality rate in 175 low-birth-weight (LBW) infants.[91] Enclosure of the catheter in a clear sheath decreases the possibility of cross-contamination and environmental pollution of objects and personnel with bacterial and viral pathogens. Closed suction systems are easier to use, less time consuming, better tolerated by the neonate, cost-effective, and well accepted by neonatal nurses.[92] Closed suction improves short-term outcomes but needs more research to be recommended as the only method of ETT suction by Cochrane reviews,[403] but it is suggested by the American Association of Respiratory Care for neonates.[13] Closed ETT suction has been identified as "best practice" in reducing nosocomial sepsis in the NICU.[77]

The actual procedures used in closed and open suction are often not supported by research data. Table 23-3 outlines common suction techniques, research data, and recommendations to alter clinical practice.

Procedure for Closed Suction

Equipment to Be Prepared

- Inline suction catheter (changed daily)
- Sterile normal saline (without preservative)
- Suction canister and tubing (60 to 80 mm Hg negative pressure)

Procedure

- Unlock the inline suction catheter. Press suction control valve and check suction pressure.
- Place saline solution syringe on the proximal port of the adapter to irrigate the catheter before suction, place normal saline syringe or bullet at the distal port or adapter, and squeeze saline solution into the port while applying suction.
- Slide the catheter through the plastic cover down the endotracheal tube to the predetermined distance.
- Apply suction while withdrawing the catheter tip to the catheter window (the plastic cover will inflate from ventilation if the catheter is pulled back too far; the catheter will completely or partially occlude the ventilatory circuit if not pulled back far enough). Only one suction attempt should be made before the infant is again ventilated. Assess tolerance of the procedure by observing pulse oximeter and infant's color, heart rate, tone, and activity. Hyperventilate the lungs with appropriate Fio_2 for 6 to 8 breaths or until adequate oxygenation has been established.
- To irrigate the catheter after suction, place a normal saline syringe at the distal port adapter and squeeze saline solution into the port while simultaneously applying suction. Remove the saline solution and close the port when the catheter has been thoroughly rinsed.
- Rotate and lock the suction control cap to discontinue suction.
- Suction the nasopharynx and oropharynx as needed with a suction bulb or separate suction catheter and tubing. Do *not* disconnect the closed suction catheter from its suction line—this contaminates the setup for ETT suction.

TABLE 23-3	SUCTION PROCEDURE: RESEARCH BASIS AND RECOMMENDATIONS	

COMMON TECHNIQUES	RECOMMENDATIONS	RESEARCH DATA
Instillation of 0.25-0.5 ml sterile NS before suction *Purpose:* Mobilize and thin secretions; aid in catheter passage	Mucus is not miscible with saline solution so bolus saline does not thin or liquefy secretions[13]; vaporized or nebulized NS thins secretions.[13] Bolus saline accumulates at the end of the ETT; <20% of the saline solution is retrieved with suction, and remainder is absorbed by the body. Use of NS associated with increased hypoxia, deterioration of lung mechanics, and infection.[13] Maintenance of adequate humidification (100%) and warming oxygen to core temperature keep secretions loose and lubricate the ETT and the surrounding tissues. Routine use of NS instillation before suction should not be performed.[13]	*Closed suction:* Irrigate catheter before suction; place NS syringe at distal port adapter and squeeze saline solution into port while simultaneously applying suction. *Open suction:* Dip or moisten catheter tip in sterile NS or water-soluble jelly to facilitate sliding down the small-diameter ETT.
Head turned from side-to-side with suction *Purpose:* To advance catheter down contralateral bronchus	Suction causes fluctuations in cerebral blood flow, which increases ICP and the risk for intraventricular hemorrhage.[301a] Sharply turning head to the side occludes the jugular vein and increases ICP, which is at its lowest when the head is in the midline or slightly elevated.[301a]	*Turned head position:* Contraindicated because of data on increased ICP, jugular vein occlusion, and anatomic impossibility of passing catheter into bronchi using this strategy. Do not turn the infant's head during suction; keep head in midline for suction.
Catheter inserted until resistance (touching the carina) is met, withdrawn slightly; then suction applied	Application of negative pressure with suction and touching the bronchial mucosa with catheter cause irritation, tissue damage, and significant oxygen desaturations.[163]	Shallow suction does not touch the carina with the catheter tip[13,154]: Using the ETT markings and the length of the adapter, insert the catheter no more than 1 cm beyond the total distance (e.g., if the ETT is inserted 10 cm and the length of the adapter is 1.5 cm, the suction catheter should be inserted 11.5 cm to no farther than 12.5 cm).
Catheter is inserted and removed several times	One small study ($n = 16$) evaluated nurses' subjective reports of amount of secretions obtained with one and two suction passes; no difference was noted.	Limit number of catheter passes to the number needed to adequately remove secretions. Do not use up-and-down motion while removing the catheter, because this decreases oxygenation and promotes hypoxia and tissue damage. Only one suction attempt should be made before the neonate is again ventilated; every catheter passage is considered a suction event; occlude ETT with catheter for no longer than 5-10 sec.
Use as large a suction catheter as will easily go down the lumen of the ETT	Use suction catheter that occludes less than 70% of the lumen of the ETT.[13]	Impedance to gas flow occurs in an ETT when more than 70% of the lumen is occluded.[13]
No use of developmental care adjustments during the stressful procedure of suction	Body containment significantly decreases the magnitude of the preterm's response (e.g., pain, desaturations, and bradycardia) to suctioning.[139,425]	Use the developmental care technique of containment (swaddling or facilitated tucking), NNS, or sucrose during suction (see Chapters 12 and 13).

ETT, Endotracheal tube; *ICP,* intracranial pressure; *NNS,* nonnutritive sucking; *NS,* normal saline.

- Check respirator settings, including alarm system in "on" position. Check tube position to be sure the tracheal tube is not strained or bent.
- Note amount and type of secretions obtained.

Procedure for Open Suction

Equipment to Be Prepared

- Sterile suction catheter of appropriate size (discard after each suctioning)
- Sterile gloves
- Sterile normal saline solution (without preservative)
- Stethoscope
- Suction machine and tubing (60 to 80 mm Hg negative pressure)

Procedure.

- The sterile catheter and glove package are opened. Sterile normal saline solution (0.25 to 0.5 ml) is drawn up in a 1-ml syringe. The resuscitation bag is connected to oxygen, and the patency is checked so that, if the neonate becomes apneic or bradycardic during the procedure, resuscitation equipment is immediately available. If the infant is on a ventilator equipped with a bag, this may be used for resuscitation if necessary.
- Disconnect and dip the suction catheter in/ or wet the tip of the suction catheter with the sterile normal saline.
- Put gloves on and attach sterile catheter to suction tubing. With nondominant hand, disconnect ETT from ventilator.
- Gently pass catheter down endotracheal tube to premeasured length.
- Occlude suction hole in catheter and withdraw. Use continuous suction so that secretions are not "released" with intermittent suction. Only one suction attempt should be made before the infant is again ventilated. Assess tolerance of procedure by observing pulse oximeter and infant's color, heart rate, tone, and activity.
- Reconnect ETT to ventilator and hyperventilate with appropriate FiO_2 for 6 to 8 breaths or until adequate oxygenation has been established. Check ventilator settings including alarm system in "on" position. Check tube position to ensure that the tube is not bent or strained. Note amount and type of secretions obtained.

NOTE: When two persons are available for suction, one remains "sterile" and does the suctioning while the other detaches the ETT from the ventilator and hyperventilates the infant between suctionings.

Because ETT suctioning compromises the neonate's physiologic homeostasis, adequate recovery time is necessary after the procedure.[139] For ETT suction, an average of 4.4 minutes of recovery time is necessary (6 of 25 infants in one study never returned to baseline during the observation). Use of containment, such as facilitated tucking, has been shown to decrease pain response and improve oxygenation after suctioning.[425] These infants may need a significant rest period after suctioning before other aspects of care such as feeding are attempted.

Endotracheal Intubation

Endotracheal intubation may be accomplished by the orotracheal route or the nasotracheal route. An endotracheal tube diameter that approximates the diameter of the infant's fifth digit generally fits snugly into the trachea. To measure for an endotracheal tube, the distance from the oral orifice to midway between the glottis and carina may be calculated by multiplying the crown-heel length by 0.2. In an emergency, the distance from the lips to midway between the glottis and carina may be approximated by the *7-8-9-10 rule.* The distance is 7 cm in a 1-kg infant, 8 cm in a 2-kg infant, 9 cm in a 3-kg infant, and 10 cm in a 4-kg infant.

Premedication for intubation is recommended for any nonemergent intubation.[237] Intubation is a painful procedure associated with **unfavorable physiologic side effects such as bradycardia, desaturation, and increased blood pressure, intracranial pressure, and pulmonary pressure.** Increases in intracranial pressure in the ELBW infant are of particular concern because this population already is predisposed to IVH. Medications listed in Table 12-10 with rapid onset and short duration of action are ideal. The neonate should be pretreated for pain with an opiate such as fentanyl, remifentanil, or morphine. Midazolam may be used for additional sedation or to potentiate the effect of the opiate so smaller doses of each medication can be administered. Atropine, a vagolytic, increases the heart rate, blocks vagal response to placement of the laryngoscope blade/ETT, and minimizes oral secretions, allowing for easier visualization of the glottis and making securing of the ETT easier.[236]

The suggested dose of atropine for this use is 0.01 to 0.03 mg/kg/dose intravenously (IV) or intramuscularly (IM) over 1 minute with onset of action expected in 1 to 2 minutes.[236]

INTUBATION PROCEDURE

ETT placement must be immediately verified by auscultation and confirmed by a chest x-ray examination; ultrasound imaging may also be used for secondary confirmation. Findings on auscultation and what they suggest are listed in Table 23-4. End-tidal carbon dioxide ($ETCO_2$) detectors are available to immediately verify tube placement and have been tested in the delivery room and NICU.[21] In the presence of exhaled CO_2 (after six breaths), the $ETCO_2$ detector changes color from purple to yellow. The time necessary to detect proper ETT placement with these detectors is 4 to 12 seconds versus 0 to 90 seconds by clinical evaluation. This significantly faster time enables quicker extubation and reintubation if the ETT is in the esophagus.[21] Use of $ETCO_2$ detection devices to confirm proper ETT placement is recommended by the AAP in the Neonatal Resuscitation Program (NRP) Guidelines.[211] This device also is useful for ongoing assessment of ETT placement.[114] Other available devices are capnometry, with a numeric display, and capnography, with both a numeric and waveform display (see Chapter 7).[113]

For long-term stability, commercially available ETT anchors prevent accidental extubation. Some nurseries still prefer fixing tubes with tape or sutures.

TABLE 23-4	CHEST AUSCULTATION ABNORMALITIES AND UNDERLYING CAUSES
FINDING	**POSSIBLE CAUSE**
No air entry bilaterally	Air leak Plugged endotracheal tube
Diminished air entry	Air leak Endotracheal tube too high
Air entry over stomach	Unplanned extubation
Air entry unequal	Air leak Endotracheal tube too low
Cardiac point of maximum intensity shifted	Air leak with tension

EXTUBATION PROCEDURE

Assess the infant's condition by observing the heart rate, color, and respiratory rate and effort and by auscultating the chest. If the infant's condition is stable, proceed with extubation. Before extubating do not feed the infant or empty stomach contents to prevent vomiting. Neonates are obligatory nasal breathers; the nasopharynx also must be suctioned and patent for extubation.

Hyperinflate with deep breaths with the infant's head in the midline and remove the tube (1) on inflation (to provide adequate lung expansion and prevent atelectasis), (2) on expiration[164] (so that secretions that have accumulated around the tracheal tube are "blown away" on exhalation and tube removal), or (3) while suctioning (to remove secretions that have accumulated around the tube). Place the neonate in a warm, humidified oxygen hood at FiO_2 to keep pulse oximeter at 92% to 94%.

Reassess the infant's condition, especially for signs of increased work of breathing and distress. Document the tube removal and infant's tolerance to extubation. **Check arterial blood gases 15 to 20 minutes after extubation to assess oxygenation and ventilation status.** Perform a chest x-ray examination to document atelectasis or fully expanded lungs. Observe for complications of intubation (Table 23-5).

MECHANICAL VENTILATION

Mechanical ventilation is used in neonates to correct abnormalities in oxygenation ($\downarrow PaO_2$), alveolar ventilation ($\uparrow PaCO_2$), or respiratory effort (apnea, ineffectual respirations, or increased work of breathing). It may not be used to treat the primary disease but frequently is used to support the infant until the disease is treated or resolved (Box 23-5).

Ventilator Settings. To individualize assisted ventilation, knowledge of the ventilator capabilities is essential.

Intermittent Mandatory Ventilation. Most mechanical ventilators in common use today allow for intermittent mandatory ventilation (IMV). IMV provides a continuous flow of gas that is available to the infant during spontaneous respirations. Periodic occlusion of the system diverts gas under pressure to the infant. Because IMV provides for spontaneous and mechanical ventilation, only the amount of ventilatory assistance that is needed by the individual infant is provided.

TABLE 23-5	COMPLICATIONS OF ENDOTRACHEAL INTUBATION

COMPLICATIONS	COMMENTS
Immediate	
Malposition	
Too low	Usually in right mainstem bronchus; no or diminished breath sounds in left chest or upper right lobe; asymmetric chest movement; atelectasis (withdraw tube until breath sounds are heard bilaterally and equally).
Too high	Inadequate ventilation bilaterally; especially at lung bases.
Esophageal	Air movement auscultated in stomach with no or inadequate breath sounds.
Obstruction	
Plug	Partial—no change or diminished breath sounds audible.
	Complete—distant or no breath sounds audible.
Kinking of the Tube	
Head position	Flexion or extension of the head results in diminished or blocked airflow.
Perforation	
Vocal cords	
Trachea	
Pharynx	
Esophagus/gastric	
Pulmonary Hemorrhage	Rescue surfactant for respiratory failure accompanying pulmonary hemorrhage may be considered (see Box 23-9).
Infection	Colonization in the neonatal airway increases with the duration of intubation; presence of ETT longer than 72 hours is associated with colonization; this biofilm may contribute to the chondritis that precedes subglottic stenosis; MRSA tracheal infection causes subglottic stenosis. Late-onset sepsis is more common in VLBW infants with prolonged ventilation[390]; mechanical ventilation is a risk factor for nosocomial infection.
Air leak	ETT displacement (e.g., into the right mainstem bronchus or to the level of the carina) is a major factor in the development of air leaks.[285]
Increased intracranial pressure	Suctioning increases mean BP, which increases cerebral blood flow velocity and intracranial pressure, which increases the risk for IVH/PVL (see Box 23-4).
Postextubation	
Migratory lobar collapse	Prevent and treat with pulmonary hygiene.
Diffuse microatelectasis	In VLBW infants may be associated with apnea; treatable by pulmonary hygiene or nasal CPAP, or both.
Long-Term	
General	Vocal cord inflammation, stenosis, and eventual dysfunction; tracheobronchial fistula; subglottic stenosis; tracheal inflammation and stenosis; necrotizing tracheobronchitis; contributes to CLD/BPD.
Specific to the Type of Tube	
Orotracheal	Abnormal dentition; gingival and palatal erosion; palatal grooves.
Nasotracheal	Otitis media; erosion of alae nasi and nasal septum; nasal stenosis.

BP, Blood pressure; *CLD/BPD*, chronic lung disease/bronchopulmonary dysplasia; *CPAP*, continuous positive airway pressure; *ETT*, endotracheal tube; *IVH*, intraventricular hemorrhage; *MRSA*, methicillin-resistant *Staphylococcus aureus*; *PVL*, periventricular leukomalacia; *VLBW*, very-low-birth-weight.

<table>
<tr><td>

BOX 23-5

CRITICAL FINDING

SCRITERIA THAT QUALIFY NEWBORNS FOR ASSISTED VENTILATION

Blood Gases
- Severe hypoxemia (Pao_2 <50-60 mm Hg with Fio_2 ≥0.60 or Pao_2 <60 mm Hg with Fio_2 >0.40 in infant weighing <1250 g)
- Severe hypercapnia ($Paco_2$ >55-65 mm Hg with pH <7.20-7.25)

Clinical
- Apnea and bradycardia requiring resuscitation in infants with lung disease or unresponsive to CPAP or requiring theophylline therapy in preterm infants with normal lungs
- Inefficient respiratory effort, such as gasping respirations from asphyxia, narcosis, or primary cardiopulmonary disease
- Shock and asphyxia with hypoperfusion and hypotension
- RDS in infants weighing <1000 g, frequently making them incapable of maintaining ventilation

</td></tr>
</table>

CPAP, Continuous positive airway pressure; *RDS,* respiratory distress syndrome.

Using the noninvasive, nasal route to provide intermittent mandatory ventilation (NIPPV) as a primary ventilation strategy (rather than just for postextubation care) has become increasingly common.[156] A meta-analysis of 14 RCTs involving 1052 preterm and term neonates with RDS and apnea of prematurity compared NIPPV to NCPAP found the following benefits of NIPPV: (1) reduction in endotracheal tube ventilation, (2) increased rate of successful extubation, (3) lower mortality and BPD/CLD rates, and (4) fewer apneic episodes.[400] Two more recent studies, not included in the meta-analysis, showed benefits of NIPPV compared with NCPAP as a primary ventilation strategy. A total of 179 preterms and term infants with RDS were studied in an RCT that found fewer infants in NIPPV group required invasive ETT ventilation or required oxygen at discharge compared with the NCPAP group. In addition, more of the NIPPV-treated infants were feeding well and gaining weight at discharge.[366] An RCT of 40 infants with transient tachypnea of the newborn (TTN) found that nasal intermittent mandatory ventilation was well tolerated and as effective (i.e., similar duration of support, oxygen therapy, duration of TTN, and length of stay) as NCPAP.[114]

Continuous Distending Pressure. CDP is expressed in centimeters of water. CDP may be given without IMV (CPAP) or with it (PEEP). The effects of CDP include increased alveolar stability, increased functional residual capacity, decreased risk for atelectasis, increased intrathoracic pressure, and impeded passage of fluid from lung capillaries to alveolar spaces, aiding in the prevention or treatment of pulmonary edema. Effects of changes in PEEP depend on severity of lung disease and degree of lung inflation. High PEEP in the presence of relatively compliant lungs will cause overdistention, worsen Pao_2, and increase pulmonary vascular resistance. In addition, overdistention may increase the risk for barotrauma. However, the use of levels of PEEP that are too low contributes to hypoxia and pulmonary hypertension because of low lung volumes. Acute lung injury is actually worsened by the failure to recruit adequate lung volume by using insufficient PEEP.

Peak Inspiratory Pressure. Peak inspiratory pressure (PIP) is the maximum pressure measured during the delivery of gas (inspiration) during conventional mechanical ventilation. PIP reflects the effects of the amount of gas delivered to the lungs in a given breath (tidal volume: 4 to 6 ml/kg in preterms; 8 to 10 ml/kg in term infants) and the underlying mechanical properties of the lungs. For example, if the same PIP is used in neonates with severe RDS (with stiff, noncompliant lungs) as in neonates ventilated for apnea with minimal lung disease, the tidal volume will be much greater in the latter group. Recent studies suggest that overdistention of the lungs caused by excessive tidal volumes, and not pressure itself, worsens acute lung injury (so-called *volutrauma*). Thus adverse effects of high PIP depend on the degree of lung disease.

When questioning whether PIP or PEEP is more likely to cause air leaks, the answer is PIP. Both PIP and PEEP cause air leak if they are excessive and is influenced by the lung compliance of the infant. Evidence strongly suggests that lung injury results from excessive tidal volume (excessive PIP).[216] It would be difficult to overexpand the lungs with PEEP to the point of air leak. Too little PEEP is far more often the cause of air leak.[216]

Rate. The rate reflects how often a volume of gas in the system is delivered to the infant. It is expressed as breaths per minute. Too rapid a rate, especially with a poorly inflated lung, can cause lung injury caused by gas trapping ("inadvertent PEEP").

Inspiratory/Expiratory Ratio. The inspiration/expiration ratio (I/E ratio) reflects the relationship between time spent in inspiration and time spent in expiration. When the rate is 60 breaths/min and the total respiratory cycle is 1 second, an I/E ratio of 1:1 means 0.5 second is inspiration and 0.5 second is expiration. If the I/E ratio is 1:2 with a rate of 60 and the total respiratory cycle is 1 second, inspiration is 0.33 second and expiration is 0.66 second.

Prolonged inspiration may be associated with more efficient ventilation, optimal arterial oxygenation, a higher risk for air leak, and impeding venous return. Prolonged expiration also improves oxygenation, especially in air-trapping conditions (e.g., rapid-rate ventilation or airway disease).[53]

Mean Airway Pressure. Mean airway pressure (MAP) is the amount of pressure transmitted to the airway throughout an entire respiratory cycle.[53] *Any* change in ventilator settings affects the MAP. MAP is most affected by changes in PEEP, inspiratory time, or I/E ratio.[53] MAP is associated with optimal oxygenation ($\uparrow Pao_2$) and ventilation ($\downarrow Paco_2$) when pressures range between 6 and 14 cm H_2O.[53] When MAP exceeds 14 cm H_2O, there is a progressive deterioration of the blood gases ($\downarrow Pao_2$, $\uparrow Paco_2$).[53] The effects of any given level of MAP depend on the changes in mechanical properties of the lung caused by the primary disease. For example, high MAP may be needed to improve oxygenation in severe RDS or meconium aspiration syndrome, especially in term neonates. Low MAP in this setting causes sustained hypoxemia and atelectasis. In contrast, use of high MAP in neonates in the presence of minimal lung disease causes overdistention and deterioration of arterial blood gas tensions. In general, the goal of increasing MAP is to improve Pao_2 and usually is achieved by small increases in PEEP or prolongation of inspiratory time. Repeat chest x-ray examination and continuous monitoring of blood pressure and oxygenation (by pulse oximeter) help determine the optimal level of MAP.

Usual starting pressures for beginning ventilatory support are listed in Table 23-6. The inspired oxygen tension is adjusted to provide an adequate arterial oxygen tension. If the infant still has difficulty maintaining an adequate carbon dioxide tension, a faster rate or greater inspiratory pressure would be indicated. Table 23-7 lists the usual

TABLE 23-6	STARTING PRESSURES FOR BEGINNING VENTILATORY SUPPORT

PARAMETER	RANGE
Fio₂	At previous level or 10% higher than previously required concentration
PEEP	4-6 cm H₂0
PIP	16-20 cm H₂0
Rate	40-60
I/E ratio	1:1-1:2

I/E, Inspiration to expiration; *PEEP,* positive end-expiratory pressure; *PIP,* peak inspiratory pressure.

effects to be expected from changing specific ventilator settings.

To evaluate the efficacy of mechanical ventilation and any adjustments made with the system, continuous monitoring with pulse oximeters (see Chapters 7 and 8) must be maintained and/or blood gases obtained. During the acute phase of illness, blood gases should be obtained 15 to 30 minutes after beginning ventilatory support or after any change in settings, every 4 to 6 hours if no change is made in ventilator settings, and as needed based on the clinical condition of the infant.

Arterial blood gases should be maintained in the following range (see Chapter 8):
- Pao_2: 60 to 80 mm Hg
- $Paco_2$: 35 to 45 mm Hg
- pH: 7.35 to 7.45

Optimal arterial blood gas tensions are somewhat controversial. To decrease the risk for acute lung injury by minimizing lung overdistention and barotrauma, some investigators advocate strategies that target lower Pao_2 and higher $Paco_2$ ("permissive hypercapnia").[60,341] The risks and benefits of such strategies depend on the specific clinical setting. If excessive ventilator settings are necessary to lower $Paco_2$, allowing $Paco_2$ to rise (to 50 to 60 mm Hg) (as long as the pH is greater than 7.25) often is accepted in an attempt to avoid lung injury. In addition, because the goal of respiratory care is to optimize oxygen delivery to tissues, the effect of a given Pao_2 depends partly on cardiac function (see Chapter 24) and hemoglobin level (see Chapter 20). Accepting lower Pao_2 and O_2

TABLE 23-7	USUAL EFFECTS OF CHANGING CONVENTIONAL MECHANICAL VENTILATOR SETTINGS

	CAUSES			
INCREASING	PaO_2	$PaCO_2$	pH	COMPLICATIONS
FiO_2	↑	0	0	Oxygen toxicity (CLD/BPD, ROP); absorption atelectasis; FiO_2 may have no effect on oxygenation in the presence of severe R→L (right to left) shunt (PPHN), congenital heart disease, or marked intrapulmonary shunting as a result of severe parenchymal lung disease
CPAP/PEEP	↑	0/↑	0/↓	Hypoventilation with respiratory acidosis; decreased cardiac output with metabolic acidosis; air leaks
PIP	↑	↓	↑	Barotrauma with air leaks and CLD/BPD; respiratory alkalosis
Rate	↓	↓	↑	Respiratory alkalosis
I/E ratio (1:1-1:2)	↑	0	0	Increased intrapleural pressure; decreased venous return

CLD/BPD, Chronic lung disease/bronchopulmonary dysplasia; *CPAP,* continuous positive airway pressure; *I/E ratio,* inspiration to expiration ratio; *PEEP,* positive end-expiratory pressure; *PIP,* peak inspiratory pressure; *PPHN,* persistent pulmonary hypertension of the newborn; *ROP,* retinopathy of prematurity.

saturation may lead to worse outcomes in the setting of systemic hypotension and poor cardiac function (e.g., sepsis).

Recognizing that aggressive ventilator management (e.g., intubation, high PIP, high MAP) is associated with increased lung injury and CLD/BPD, gentler ventilator techniques and management have been developed and are being used. Many gentler strategies incorporate relinquishment of traditional ventilator controls (from the health care provider) to patient control of ventilator parameters. Facilitated by computer-assisted technology, newer types of ventilators are being used. Volume-targeted versus pressure-limited ventilation results in significant reductions in BPD/CLD, mortality risk, duration of ventilation, pneumothorax, hypocarbia, and the combined outcome of PVL or grade 3 to 4 IVH.[432]

Patient-Triggered Ventilation. Asynchrony between the infant's respiratory efforts and the ventilator is uncomfortable for the neonate and causes increased barotrauma, which contributes to lung injury (e.g., CLD/BPD). Altered cerebral blood flow may contribute to IVH. Patient-ventilator synchrony occurs when patient-triggered ventilation (PTV) responds to the neonate's signal representing spontaneous respiratory effort and delivers a mechanical breath, timed to the onset of inspiration. PTV has been demonstrated to do the following[120,305]:
- Decrease asynchrony
- Improve gaseous exchange (e.g., oxygenation and carbon dioxide elimination)
- Create respiratory support that is more synergistic with the neonate's respiratory efforts
- Increase comfort for the infant, thus reducing the need for use of sedatives, narcotics, and paralyzing medications
- Decrease the need for ventilatory support

Studies comparing PTV with conventional mechanical ventilation (CMV) have found no proven decrease in the following[36,44]:
- Incidence and severity of CLD/BPD
- Mortality rates
- Head ultrasound abnormalities

These studies did show an increased rate of pneumothorax, worsening arterial blood gas values, more frequent desaturations, and increased need for increased ventilatory support.[36,44]

Modes of PTV include the following:
- Synchronized intermittent mandatory ventilation (SIMV)
- Assist-control ventilation (ACV)—oxygenation, volume-guarantee ventilation (VGV), neurally adjusted ventilator assist (NAVA), and minute ventilation (V_{min})
- Pressure-support ventilation (PSV)

- Pressure-regulated volume control (PRVC)
- Proportional assist ventilation (PAV)

Synchronized Intermittent Mandatory Ventilation. SIMV, a commonly used form of PTV, delivers mechanical breaths at a fixed rate.[328] SIMV enables synchronization of ventilation breaths by sensing (through an airway or diaphragmatic sensor) the neonate's initiation of respiration and then triggering a mechanical breath. Synchronized ventilation prevents the generation of excessive pressure within the respiratory tract when infant exhalation coincides with mechanical ventilation. Use of SIMV is associated with a decrease in (1) oxygen need, (2) duration of ventilator therapy, (3) incidence of BPD, and (4) severity of IVH and is more comfortable for the infant.[45,305,328] Use of SIMV is also associated with fewer episodes of hypoxia and better oxygenation as a result of improved ventilation-perfusion and increased resting lung volume (functional residual capacity [FRC]) compared with IMV ventilation of VLBW infants.[145] Noninvasive ventilation strategies using SNIPPV as a primary mode of support for preterm infants with RDS shows similar results compared with bilevel NCPAP.[330]

Assist-Control Ventilation. Newer neonatal ventilators are equipped with computer technology with rapid digital feedback circuits. Computer-assisted control enables adjustments of FiO_2, PIP to control tidal volume, and ventilatory rate to control minute ventilation. ACV is used in preterms with RDS, infants with a strong respiratory drive, and infants who are not heavily sedated. ACV is also more comfortable for the infant but may result in difficulty weaning from the ventilator because of diaphragmatic muscle atrophy.[305] Small studies have reported that computer-assisted maintenance of target oxygen saturation is as effective as manual FiO_2 adjustments. Larger RCTs on safety and efficacy are warranted.

In volume-guarantee ventilation, a preset target tidal volume is maintained by the ventilator because the pressure limit varies inversely with lung compliance and the neonate's respiratory effort. Volume-targeted ventilation holds a significant advantage over pressure-targeted ventilation by delivering a physiologic tidal volume (about 4 to 5 ml/kg) potentially limiting excessive pressure and potential barotrauma. Historically measuring physiologic tidal volume in the smallest infants, the location of flow sensor,

and compensating for ET air leak had limited the utility of volume-targeted ventilation in the premature population. A recent Cochrane review of nine RCTs comparing volume-targeted ventilation to pressure-targeted ventilation found that volume-targeted ventilation resulted in a reduction of death, BPD/CLD, incidence of pneumothorax, days of ventilation, hypocarbia, and severe IVH/PVL.[432] Although the findings are promising, the ability to deliver measured/accurate volumes in the most extremely premature neonates remains limited by the sensitivity of the mechanical ventilation equipment to deliver measured tidal volume, location of flow sensor, and to compensate for ET air leak.

Several studies completed after the Cochrane review show benefit of volume-guarantee ventilation strategies. Combining volume-guarantee with assist-control ventilation in the acute phase of RDS and SIMV in the weaning process results in less variable tidal volumes, shorter duration of ventilation, and a significant improvement in the combined outcomes of mortality and BPD/CLD rates in VLBW infants.[127] Another RCT of volume-guarantee SIMV ventilation and surfactant therapy found a shorter duration of ventilation, as well as significantly fewer morbidities (i.e., ROP, BPD/CLD and IVH) in preterms with RDS.[170] Use of lower backup ventilation rates (i.e., 30 breaths/min rather than 50 breaths/min) enables greater triggering of ventilator inflations.[433] Certainly larger RCTs are necessary.

Neurally adjusted ventilator assist (NAVA) is a mode of ventilation that uses electromyographic (EMG) signaling from the diaphragm to match ventilator support to the infant's respiratory drive. EMG signaling from the diaphragm is acquired by electrodes embedded in a nasogastric tube and incorporated into a mechanical ventilator that converts the EMG signaling into a proportional assisted breath that is synchronized to infant-initiated breath. Diaphragm EMG activity is measured in magnitude (Edi signal). Ventilator support is adjusted by monitor Edi signal to optimize respiratory support. Early studies in neonates suggest improved patient ventilator interaction and synchrony with lower peak pressures.[37,56] Two recent studies compared NAVA to pressure-control ventilation[382] and to SIMV[245] in preterm infants and found that a lower PIP was required for adequate ventilation. Compared with pressure-control ventilation NAVA also required the use of lower FiO_2, lower respiratory rate to achieve a lower P_{CO_2}, and better compliance in five ventilated preterms less than 1500 g.[382]

Minute ventilation(i.e., the volume of gas moving in and out of the lungs over time, expressed in milliliters per kilogram per minute) is a successful predictor of readiness to wean, extubate, and establish optimal pulmonary mechanics.[153] Mandatory minute ventilation (MMV), a new ventilator mode in the NICU, provides mechanically generated breaths only if the neonate's spontaneous breathing does not meet a minimum level of minute ventilation (chosen by the health care provider). If the infant's spontaneous pressure-supported breaths exceed the minimum minute ventilation, no additional breaths are delivered by the ventilator. If the infant fails to meet the specified minute ventilation, intermittent mandatory breaths are delivered at the preset tidal volume. MMV enables the infant to control the rate, flow, and inspiratory time of the ventilator, which enhances synchrony and ensures a "backup" system to assume the work of breathing if the infant cannot maintain adequate minute ventilation.[169]

Pressure-Support Ventilation. PSV complements the infant's respiratory effort by triggering a mechanical breath, preset to a specific pressure. PSV decreases the work of breathing created by airway resistance (e.g., narrowed diameter of neonatal ETT) and ventilator circuit resistance. PSV also decreases work of breathing by assisting the activity of the infant's respiratory muscles. PSV is used alone (if the infant has effective respiratory drive) or in conjunction with SIMV. PSV is useful in chronic and acute situations, as well as weaning chronically ventilator-dependent infants. When PSV was compared with SIMV, preterms exhibited better respiratory function (e.g., lower respiratory rates and less work of breathing), so PSV is effective for fatigued or weaning infants.[298] Another study comparing two levels of PSV with SIMV found that PSV increased total minute ventilation, stabilized breathing for preterms less than 32 weeks' gestation, and may be a useful strategy to wean preterms from mechanical ventilation.[168]

Pressure-Regulated Volume Control. PRVC delivers four breaths and modifies the ventilator's pressure to attain the prescribed tidal volume; breaths are both volume and pressure regulated. Studies show conflicting results: (1) safe and a lower incidence of

air leaks and IVH[310] and (2) no benefit compared with SIMV in the treatment of RDS in preterm infants.[99]

Proportional-Assist Ventilation. In PAV, ventilator pressure increases in proportion to inspiratory volume (e.g., inspiratory flow varies to match the neonate's respiratory effort). Both volume and flow proportional assist relieve the neonate of both elastic (e.g., respiratory muscles) and resistive work of breathing. During PAV, the infant's breathing completely controls all variables of the ventilator breathing pattern through exceptionally fast computer-controlled feedback circuitry. In the initial trial using PAV in infants, lower MAP and transpulmonary pressure were used to effectively oxygenate and ventilate infants with mild to moderate respiratory insufficiency.[356] Respiratory rates were 50 to 80/min with a fast and shallow pattern and tidal volumes less than 5 ml/kg. A more recent RCT comparing PAV and PTV in ELBW preterms found that PAV safely maintained gaseous exchange at lower MAP compared with PTV. Although there were no adverse effects, the researchers concluded that backup conventional ventilation breaths must be provided during PAV to prevent apnea-related oxygen desaturations.[357]

High-Frequency Ventilation. Barotrauma/volutrauma is a major contributing factor to the development of chronic lung disease or death from progressive lung injury in newborns treated with conventional mechanical ventilation. The goal of HFV is to reduce barotrauma by the application of HFV early in the course of RDS or to reduce the progression of injury in infants who already have pulmonary interstitial emphysema, recurrent pneumothorax, or bronchopleural fistula. In addition to minimizing lung injury, the goal of HFV is to effectively enhance oxygenation over conventional ventilation.

HFV differs from conventional modes of ventilator support, using smaller tidal volumes (less than anatomic dead space) at supraphysiologic frequencies and allowing for generation of lower intrathoracic pressure. At high frequencies, the calculated tidal volume is less than dead space. Thus the physics of gas flow and exchange are different from the traditional teaching of lung mechanics and are related to augmented diffusion. Reduction in barotrauma occurs by allowing for ventilation with very small pressure amplitude around the mean airway pressure in the distal airway. Therefore at high frequencies (commonly 10 to 15 Hz), the peak inspiratory and expiratory pressures approach MAP (i.e., lower downstream pressures). Because of this effect, higher MAP can be used to improve oxygenation without worsening lung injury.

HFV can be achieved by jet ventilators, oscillators, or high-frequency flow interrupters. Jet ventilators and HFV deliver short bursts of high-flow gases directly into the proximal airway via a small cannula and have a passive exhalation cycle. This ventilatory mode usually is augmented with a backup rate by a conventional ventilator that gives sigh breaths. The frequency range of the HFJV is 240 to 660 breaths/min (4 to 11 Hz).[120]

Oscillators vibrate columns of air and have active exhalation cycles. The usual frequency is 600 to 900 breaths/min (10 to 15 Hz). Oscillators (high-frequency oscillatory ventilation [HFOV]) are used both as a rescue therapy when CMV is unsuccessful and electively as a primary mode of ventilation. The HFOV ventilator most commonly used is the SensorMedics 3100A, which uses a piston with a diaphragm to actively move gas into and out of the lung. Systematic reviews of early elective/rescue use of HFOV, compared with CMV, in preterm, late-preterm, and term infants found the following:

- No effect on mortality rate at 28 to 30 days of life or at term equivalent age[89]
- Inconsistent effect on BPD/CLD at term equivalent age across studies; overall reduction was of only borderline significance[89,179]
- Subgroup analysis of some trials show a decrease in BPD/CLD when[89]:
  - Lung protective strategies for CMV were not used
  - Randomization of preterms occurred at 2 to 6 hours of age
  - Inspiratory:expiratory (I:E) ratios of 1:2 used for HFOV
- More air leaks[89] versus no significant difference in air leaks[179]
- Short-term neurologic morbidity (found in some studies; not statistically significant)[89,179]
- Increased rates of IVH (grades 3 or 4) and PVL in two studies not using high volume strategy with HFOV[89]
- Overall reduction of ROP[89]
- Adverse long-term neurodevelopmental outcomes in one of five trials[89]

- No difference in days of ventilation or length of stay[179]
- No difference in risk of needing ECMO[179]

Reviewers concluded that there was no evidence that either elective or rescue HFOV offers advantages over CMV for acute or severe pulmonary dysfunction.[89,89,179]

According to the Vermont Oxford Database, one in every five LBW preterm infants receives HFOV during their NICU course, despite limited data supporting efficacy.[375] An RCT comparing HFOV and SIMV in preterms with RDS found better early oxygenation, reduction in oxygenation index, and shorter length of stay in the HFOV-treated group; survival and complication rates were similar.[370] A more recent study of HFOV versus CMV in pediatric (age 1 month to 18 years) respiratory failure found worse outcomes (i.e., length of ventilation, length of stay, mortality rate) in the HFOV group.[166] The researchers concluded that their study findings are similar to adult studies showing worse outcomes with HFOV.[166] One small (*n* = 19 preterms 30 weeks' gestation or less) retrospective cohort study of HFOV with low oscillatory frequency found benefits (i.e., improved oxygenation, reduced MAP, survival) in preterms with PIE.[377]

When HFOV was compared with PSV plus volume guarantee (VG), early use of HFOV treatment was associated with a reduction in lung inflammation in preterms less than 30 weeks' gestation[100]; another study found VG to result in lower inflammation markers than HFOV.[251] A more recent RCT of HFOV versus SIMV-PSV in 366 preterm infants with severe RDS found (1) significantly higher mortality and BPD/CLD rates in the SIMV-PSV group; (2) fewer days of mechanical ventilation and hospitalization, as well as less ROP and need for surfactant with HFOV; and (3) less moderate to severe neurologic disability at 18 months in the HFOV group.[393] Discordance in study findings may be attributed to (1) maturity/immaturity of preterm infants, (2) time to initiation of HFOV, (3) use of antenatal steroids, (4) use of surfactant replacement, (5) differences in techniques used (e.g., presence or absence of lung volume recruitment strategy), (6) level of MAP, (7) duration of use, and (8) variations in cerebral blood flow (CBF) secondary to changes in P_{CO_2}.[270] Some researchers recommend that CMV be the first choice in treatment of preterm infants with

RDS and HFOV be reserved for rescue therapy if CMV is unsuccessful.[270] Further research is needed to clarify which ventilator should be used initially.

Remember that the rate of carbon dioxide removal is determined by minute ventilation. Minute ventilation is the product of tidal volume and respiratory rate (TV × RR). In CMV, the tidal volume and rate can both be adjusted by increasing or decreasing the breaths per minute (rate) and by increasing or decreasing the PIP or PEEP for tidal volume (TV = PIP − PEEP). In HFV, the same minute ventilation equation holds true but the rate is set by breaths/min (hertz) and the tidal volume is determined by the amplitude (Box 23-6).

In HFOV, tidal volume is adjusted primarily by changing the amplitude setting. Amplitude is the amount of pressure oscillation that occurs around the MAP. Increasing the amplitude will increase the tidal volume and therefore decrease PCO_2. Conversely, decreasing the amplitude will decrease the tidal volume and therefore increase the PCO_2. Amplitude is initially set when chest rise is adequate and then slowly adjusted up or down in increments of one or two.

The respiratory rate in HFV is determined by the hertz setting. One hertz equals 60 breaths per minute. Therefore 10 Hertz equals 600 breaths/min. The rate is initially set between 10 and 15 Hz. There is a paradoxic effect of high-frequency breaths in the bronchi of the lungs so that when the hertz setting is increased, the PCO_2 increases. The opposite is also true. Whereas HFOV has an active expiration phase, HFJV has a passive expiration phase and therefore uses a low CMV backup rate to deliver intermittent sigh breaths to prevent air trapping and augment PCO_2 removal.

Oxygenation in CMV and HFV is determined by the FiO_2 and the MAP. With use of HFOV in the rescue mode, the MAP is initially set 1 to 2 cm H$_2$O above the previous CMV setting. Adjustments for oxygenation (MAP, FiO_2) and ventilation (amplitude, Hz) can be made independently and therefore can be done simultaneously (Table 23-8). Chest x-ray studies are helpful in determining optimal lung volume. As lung compliance improves, and it can improve quite rapidly after surfactant administration, there is a risk for overinflating the lungs with too much MAP.[421] This increase in MAP leads to an increase in intrathoracic pressure that may result in air leaks or IVH or may impede venous return, which can in turn lead to hypotension. MAP is generally slowly increased or decreased in increments of one or two. Chest x-ray studies, blood gases, and blood pressure should be monitored closely during HFV.

Synchronized mechanical ventilation, delivered as high-frequency positive-pressure ventilation (HFPPV), is another mode of oxygenation and ventilation in which positive airway pressure and spontaneous inspiration occur simultaneously. Adequate gas exchange should be achievable at lower peak airway pressures. HFPPV results in a reduction of air leaks and ventilator duration.

Inhaled Nitric Oxide. Vascular endothelial cells endogenously produce a potent vasodilator substance ("endothelium-derived relaxing factor"), later identified as nitric oxide. Nitric oxide (NO), delivered as a gas, causes potent, selective, and sustained pulmonary vasodilation in the perinatal pulmonary circulation.[221] The vasodilator response occurs as a result of inhaled nitric oxide (iNO) stimulation of soluble guanylate cyclase activity, increasing cyclic guanosine monophosphate (cGMP) in vascular smooth muscle and causing vasorelaxation. Selectivity of iNO for the pulmonary circulation is based on direct delivery of NO into the lung; because NO is avidly bound by hemoglobin in red blood cells and inactivated after metabolism to nitrite and nitrate, there are no direct effects on systemic arterial pressure.[221] Potential toxicities include decreased platelet aggregation, hemorrhage, and methemoglobinemia.

TABLE 23-8	CRITICAL FINDINGS
	COMPARISON OF VENTILATOR OPTIONS

	LOW O_2	HIGH O_2	LOW CO_2	HIGH CO_2
CMV/SIMV	Increase PEEP Increase PIP Increase Fio_2	Wean PIP Wean PEEP Wean Fio_2	Decrease rate Decrease TV	Increase rate Increase TV
HFOV	Increase MAP Increase Fio_2	Decrease MAP Decrease Fio_2	Decrease Amp Increase Hz	Increase Amp Decrease Hz
HFJV	Increase MAP Increase Fio_2	Decrease MAP Decrease Fio_2	Decrease Amp Increase Hz	Increase Amp Decrease Hz

Data from Donn SM, Sinha S: Invasive and noninvasive neonatal mechanical ventilation, *Respir Care* 48(4):426, 2003; Tarczy-Hornoch P, Mayock DE, Jones D, et al: Mechanical ventilators. Revised July 2008. Accessed October 3, 2009, from http://neonatal.peds.washington.edu/NICU-WEB/vents.

Amp, Amplitude; *CMV,* conventional mechanical ventilation; *Hz,* hertz; *HFJV,* high-frequency jet ventilation; *HFOV,* high-frequency oscillatory ventilation; *IMV,* intermittent mandatory ventilation; *MAP,* mean airway pressure; *PEEP,* positive end-expiratory pressure; *PIP,* peak inspiratory pressure; *SIMV,* synchronized intermittent mandatory ventilation; *TV,* tidal volume.

Inhaled NO has been approved by the U.S. Food and Drug Administration (FDA) for treatment of late-preterm (greater than 34 weeks of gestational age) and term neonates with persistent pulmonary hypertension of the newborn (PPHN)[221] (see Persistent Pulmonary Hypertension of the Newborn later in this chapter). Use of iNO in preterm infants (less than 34 weeks of gestational age) remains controversial, with a National Institutes of Health (NIH) consensus statement recommending against the routine use of iNO in preterms (less than 34 weeks of gestational age).[80]

Extracorporeal Membrane Oxygenation/Extracorporeal Life Support.
Extracorporeal membrane oxygenation/extracorporeal life support (ECMO/ECLS) is a modification of cardiopulmonary bypass that allows more prolonged therapy that is traditionally performed in the operating room for cardiac surgery.[140] ECMO/ECLS establishes a pulmonary bypass circuit, allowing gas exchange to occur outside of the lung by perfusion of blood through a membrane oxygenator. Blood is drawn from a catheter in the right internal jugular vein or right atrium, oxygenated as it crosses the membrane, and then returned to the patient via the right common carotid artery (venoarterial ECMO/ECLS) or the femoral vein (venovenous ECMO/ECLS). The pump produces a continuous, nonpulsatile flow through the membrane oxygenator as the patient is kept heparinized and continues to be ventilated at low pressures, rates,

and oxygen tensions. The goal of this therapy is to "buy time" for the severely injured lung to heal while attenuating ongoing lung injury by decreasing exposure to hyperoxia and barotrauma. Therapy can be continued for several days, until lung recovery appears sufficient to maintain adequate gas tension without ECMO/ECLS.

ECMO/ECLS therapy improves survival in term neonates with severe hypoxemic respiratory failure and PPHN. ECMO/ECLS is used as a treatment of last option when neonates are unresponsive to maximum conventional support. ECMO/ECLS criteria include the following[140]:

- Gestational age 34 weeks or older, weight 2000 g or more
- No more than 7 to 10 days of assisted ventilation
- Reversible lung disease
- No CNS or multisystem disease, no lethal congenital anomalies
- No intracranial hemorrhage above grade I or uncorrectable coagulopathy
- No cardiac disease (unless ECMO/ECLS is to be used for the preoperative/postoperative period for cardiac surgery)
- No severe asphyxia
- Failure of maximal medical management
- A ventilatory index (MAP × Rate) of 1500 or above or an oxygenation index (MAP × Fio_2 × 100/Pao_2) of 40 or more

Use of ECMO/ECLS for severe respiratory failure is beneficial in improving survival rates, especially in congenital diaphragmatic hernia, without increasing the risk for severe disability.[277] Conditions treated with ECMO/ECLS include meconium aspiration syndrome, congenital diaphragmatic hernia, sepsis, pneumonia, PPHN, and air leak syndromes.

In the past decade, the number of neonates being treated with ECMO/ECLS has declined by 40% to 50%.[383] Because ECMO/ECLS is invasive, labor intensive, and costly and involves risks associated with systemic anticoagulation (e.g., intracranial hemorrhage), alternative therapies (e.g., surfactant replacement, iNO, and HFV) are used initially and have reduced the need for ECMO.[283] These therapies have changed the population being treated with ECMO/ECLS, shortened length of stay, reduced costs, and raised concerns in delay of use of ECMO/ECLS. A study from the United Kingdom showed poor respiratory outcomes for infants older than 2 weeks when ECMO/ECLS was started and for infants needing ECMO/ECLS for respiratory distress syndrome.[36a] Considerable variability exists between centers, however, suggesting that the use of these techniques depends partly on the clinical strategy and other issues in patient management.

Complications of ECMO/ECLS depend on initial disease process, pre-ECMO/ECLS factors (e.g., asphyxia, coagulopathy, hypoventilation, hyperventilation), and type of ECMO/ECLS used (e.g., venoarterial vs. venovenous). The most common complications are hemorrhagic (e.g., intracranial [incidence 4.6%; survival 50%]) and nonhemorrhagic (e.g., infarctions [incidence 10.7%; survival 50%]) CNS insults. Neonates who develop intracranial hemorrhage are at highest risk for mortality and poor neurodevelopmental outcomes. There is a high (75%[295] to 81%[242]) survival rate with ECMO/ECLS in neonates with PPHN; survival for congenital diaphragmatic hernia is 51%.[295] Independent predictors of death in neonates with PPHN receiving ECMO/ECLS were prematurity, acidosis, profound hypoxemia, and use of ECMO for more than 7 days.[242]

Partial Liquid Ventilation. Although prenatal administration of steroidal agents, use of surfactant, and HFOV therapies have improved the clinical course of sick preterm newborns with respiratory failure, the morbidity of severe RDS persists. Based on 40 years of experimental (animal) studies, perfluorocarbon (PFC) liquids have been found to improve gaseous exchange, lung mechanics, and cardiopulmonary stability in various respiratory diseases.[95,162] PFC liquids are suitable for liquid ventilation because of their high solubility of respiratory gases, easy elimination by evaporation from the lungs, and lack of metabolism by the body.[162] Instillation of an FRC of PFC liquid into the lungs during gaseous ventilation constitutes partial liquid ventilation (PLV). The best ventilator management during PLV has not been determined and may differ with underlying lung pathology.[162]

PLV is applicable to the surfactant and structurally deficient preterm lung because it reduces or eliminates surface tension forces, optimizes lung recruitment, and reexpands atelectatic lung. In a term infant, PLV is applicable to structural lung disease (e.g., diaphragmatic hernia) or lung disease associated with airway debris (e.g., aspiration syndromes or pneumonia). A nonrandomized, nonblinded clinical study of 13 preterm infants with severe RDS who failed to improve with CMV showed improved oxygenation within 1 hour of initiation of PLV.[243] A case report of partial liquid ventilation accompanying HFV showed improved gas exchange with a decrease in oxygenation index.[265] In infants with respiratory failure, a combination of PLV, iNO, and surfactant may produce optimal response. The safety and efficacy of PLV are undergoing phase III trials in adults in the United States; trials are contemplated in infants and children in Europe.

WEANING FROM THE VENTILATOR

When the infant's condition improves, ventilatory support is slowly removed. Evidence of improvement includes biochemical, clinical, and pulmonary function parameters as follows:

- Arterial blood gases are stable and physiologic.
- Spontaneous respiratory efforts occur in addition to ventilator-generated respirations and if the infant is disconnected from the ventilator for suctioning.
- There is increased activity and muscle tone and progressively decreasing FiO_2 requirement.
- Pulmonary function studies (in LBW preterms with RDS) include (1) tidal volume values greater than 6 ml/kg, (2) minute ventilation greater than 309 ml/kg/min, (3) work of breathing less than 0.172 J/L, (4) dynamic compliance 1 ml/cm H_2O/kg or greater, and (5) airway resistance 176 cm H_2O/L/sec or less.[397]

Weaning an infant as soon as possible from intubation and the ventilator is associated with a decrease in the complications of intubation (see Table 23-5) and the incidence of CLD/BPD resulting from barotrauma, volutrauma, and oxygen toxicity.[20] With IMV, there is a gradual decrease in mechanical ventilation with a corresponding increase in spontaneous respiration. One ventilator setting at a time is changed, and arterial blood gases and pulse oximetry values are evaluated to determine the infant's response before another adjustment is made. Because each ventilator parameter has risks and benefits, each parameter must be evaluated before the decision is made as to which one will be lowered. Because high concentrations of oxygen are toxic to lungs and hyperoxia damages eyes, oxygen is usually lowered first to a level below 80% in 5% to 10% increments. PIP is lowered in 1- to 2-cm increments to a level of 16 to 18 cm H_2O, and respiratory rate is lowered in increments of 1 to 5 breaths/min until the infant has a rate of 15 to 20 breaths/min.

Failure of extubation results in a reintubation rate of 25% to 50% in ELBW/VLBW infants.[29,129,272,381,394] Nasal CPAP is effective in preventing extubation failure and decreasing CLD/BPD by preventing atelectasis, improving oxygenation, decreasing apnea/bradycardia, and improving thoracoabdominal motion synchrony, which indicates improved breathing strategy.[217] Using NCPAP pressures in the range of 7 to 9 cm H_2O, instead of 4 to 6 cm, has been shown to reduce extubation failure in an RCT of preterms with a birth weight of 500 to 1000 g and gestational age of 23 to 30 weeks.[58] Weaning an intubated neonate to ventilator CPAP increases the work of breathing associated with endotracheal tube resistance and dead space (e.g., breathing through a straw). A meta-analysis of three RCTs comparing use of ventilator CPAP with extubation to nasal CPAP showed a significant advantage (e.g., decreased the risk for reintubation and ventilation) for extubation to nasal CPAP, especially using nasal prongs.[109]

Despite the large body of evidence supporting NCPAP in prevention of extubation failure[110] and a lack of evidence supporting HHHFNC after extubation, there is increasing use of HHHFNC instead of NCPAP after extubation.[257] Older studies of HHHFNC compared with NCPAP have mixed results: (1) flow rates of 1.4 to 1.7 L/min resulted in more reintubations in the HHHFNC group, higher oxygen concentrations, and more apnea/bradycardia[59]; (2) no differences in extubation failure rates[190]; and (3) more failures of NCPAP than HHHFNC resulted in reintubation.[367] A study of 132 ventilated preterms (less than 32 weeks' gestation) randomized to NCPAP or HHHFNC after extubation found less nasal trauma and an extubation failure rate of 22% in the HHHFNC group versus 34% in the NCPAP group.[82] The largest multicenter trial compared the reintubation rates of 303 preterms (less than 32 weeks' gestation) randomized to HHHFNC or NCPAP after extubation.[258] Significantly less nasal trauma was noted, as well as a failure rate of 34.2% in the HHHFNC group and 25.8% in the NCPAP group and successful treatment of the HHHFNC failures with NCPAP. The researchers concluded that the efficacy of HHHFNC was similar and noninferior to NCPAP in very preterm infants after extubation.[258] Another RCT compared weaning from NCPAP to HHHFNC in a group of 60 preterms 28 weeks' gestation or older and found longer duration of respiratory support and exposure to oxygen in the HHHFNC group.[1]

Extubation directly to nasal CPAP has also been shown to be more effective than extubation directly to supplemental oxygen in a hood. A meta-analysis of six RCTs comparing nasal CPAP (by any method) with use of an oxygen hood after extubation found that nasal CPAP (1) decreases adverse clinical events (e.g., apnea, bradycardia, respiratory acidosis, hypoxia), (2) decreases the incidence of CLD/BPD, and (3) decreases the incidence of reintubation.[110] These positive effects increase when nasal prong CPAP is used, compared with nasopharyngeal CPAP, and the benefits are consistent across ranges of weight and gestational age.[110]

For weaning preterm infants from mechanical ventilation, prophylactic use of nasal CPAP (with nasal prongs) has been defined as the standard of care. However, variations in therapeutic methods and devices are associated with variations in outcomes. Although RCTs demonstrate a clear advantage of nasal prongs over nasopharyngeal administration, differences in design of nasal prongs may alter effectiveness. Use of binasal prongs is more effective than a single nasal prong in weaning ELBW infants from the ventilator.[116]

Various clinical strategies for initiation, management, and weaning of nasal CPAP are used. Use of nasal CPAP with the Aladdin/Infant Flow System (i.e., residual gas pressure is provided by the constant flow of gas) decreases the work of breathing by a more stable volume recruitment in the lungs and has been shown to facilitate extubation in VLBW infants compared with nasal pharyngeal CPAP.[94] Other studies show equal efficacy (e.g., no differences in apnea, bradycardia, or desaturation) when nasal prong CPAP is compared with nasal synchronized IMV[116] or nasal CPAP on a ventilator compared with the Infant Flow System.[381] A recent RCT comparison of bubble CPAP versus Infant Flow Driver CPAP for postextubation support found that use of bubble CPAP reduced the mean duration of CPAP use by 50% and in preterms ventilated for 14 days or less, there was a higher rate of successful extubation.[168]

If nasal CPAP fails, the nasal route may also be used to administer mechanical ventilation, which augments the effectiveness of NCPAP, reduces respiratory rate and the inspiratory work of breathing, improves rates of successful extubation, stimulates respiratory drive, increases ventilation, decreases $PaCO_2$ and is even being used as the initial method of respiratory support.[29,111] In multiple RCTs, both preterm infants (34 weeks of gestational age) and VLBW preterm infants extubated to synchronized nasal intermittent positive-pressure ventilation (SNIPPV) had a significantly higher success rate at 72 hours after extubation compared with an NCPAP group.[34,71,217,270] Even unsynchronized NIPPV use after extubation was superior to NCPAP in reducing reintubation, atelectasis after extubation, and mortality rate.[29,202]

Once adequate oxygenation and ventilation on CPAP alone have been maintained, the infant may be placed in an oxygen hood or on a nasal cannula. Oxygen should be adjusted by using targeted saturation ranges with pulse oximetry.

During the recovery phase of RDS (approximately 72 hours), changes in lung compliance occur rapidly. Hyperoxia, air leaks, increased intracranial pressure, and decreased cardiac output easily occur if high pressures and high oxygen concentrations are not decreased as rapidly as the lung is recovering.

Infants who are difficult or impossible to wean from the ventilator may have CLD/BPD, PDA, or CNS damage that affects the respiratory control center.

GENERAL COMPLICATIONS

Acute Complications

Acute and chronic complications are the result of the disease process, treatment, or both. Beginning with the least invasive therapy and progressing to more complicated ones only as needed accomplishes two goals: it individualizes therapy, and it minimizes the risk for complications. Continuous monitoring of the individual infant's progress is vital to decrease complications from the disease and from the interventions used to support the infant or treat the primary condition. Complications of respiratory diseases are listed in Box 23-7.

Sudden deterioration of the infant's condition is an emergency, and the cause must be found and corrected as soon as possible to minimize further damage. Causes of sudden deterioration are listed in Box 23-8.

RESPIRATORY

Management of an infant who has suddenly deteriorated begins with a visual inspection. The

---

BOX 23-7 | **COMPLICATIONS OF RESPIRATORY DISEASE**

1. Acute
a. Sudden deterioration of condition
b. Air leaks
c. Central nervous system
   Hypoxic-ischemic injury
   Increased intracranial pressure
   Hemorrhage
d. Cardiac
   Patent ductus arteriosus
   Decreased cardiac output
e. Infection
f. Bleeding diathesis
g. Tube
h. Pulmonary hemorrhage

2. Chronic
a. Oxygen toxicity and barotraumas (CLD/BPD)
b. Hyperoxia (retinopathy of prematurity)
c. Hypoxia
d. Tube

CLD/BPD, Chronic lung disease/bronchopulmonary dysplasia.

oxygen hood, CPAP, or ventilator must be properly connected and free of water. If all connections are intact, the infant must be disconnected from assisted ventilation and connected to a resuscitation bag (which is connected to an oxygen source and kept at the bedside). Manual ventilation matching pressure, rates, and FiO₂ to ventilator settings must be maintained. If the infant improves with these interventions, mechanical failure of the ventilator should be suspected. Assistance should be summoned to find the mechanical problem or replace the system. The infant's respiratory effort must be manually assisted until the problem is solved.

If the infant does not improve with manual ventilation, there is probably a problem with the tube. The infant's condition can be assessed by auscultating the chest for quality of breath sounds. Findings and what they suggest are listed in Table 23-9.

The ETT should be suctioned quickly. If there is no improvement in clinical condition or air entry, the tube should be replaced while supporting the infant with bag-and-mask ventilation. If the tube is too low, it can be repositioned by pulling it back 0.5 to 1 cm. If air entry and clinical condition improve with auscultation, the tube must be secured in the new position and a chest x-ray examination done to confirm tube placement. If assessment of the chest leads to suspicion of accidental extubation, the tube must be removed, ventilation with bag and mask administered, and reintubation performed. If the infant does not

improve with manual ventilation and the tube is in place, an air leak or IVH could be the cause.

Monitors and ventilators are equipped with alarm systems to warn care providers of sudden changes in the infant's condition or supportive systems. It is imperative that all alarm systems be maintained in the "on" position. Turning the alarms "off" during care for such procedures as suctioning and weighing creates the risk for forgetting to turn them on again. In a busy NICU, the compromised infant may not be visually noticed until the hypoxia is so severe that resuscitation is more difficult or impossible. Monitor parameters (both high and low alarm settings) must be individualized for each infant and recorded (see Chapter 7).

A sick neonate may experience a severe hypoxic insult when oxygen is too rapidly altered during caregiving procedures. Feeding, weighing, or turning without an alternative oxygen source may cause a sudden decrease in PaO₂, pulmonary vasoconstriction, hypoperfusion, and an iatrogenic worsening of the condition. Prolonged ETT suctioning (15 to 20 seconds) causes hypoxia and atelectasis. Care must be organized to conserve energy, minimize hypoxic insults, and maintain the infant in physiologic homeostasis. Alternative oxygen sources must be provided when the usual method of oxygen delivery is disrupted for giving care. Small alterations in FiO₂ prevent rapid increases or decreases in oxygen tension.

METABOLIC FACTORS

Hypoglycemia must never be overlooked as the cause of sudden collapse. Undetected infiltration

---

BOX 23-8	CAUSES OF SUDDEN DETERIORATION

1. Tube
   a. Accidental extubation
   b. Accidental disconnection
   c. Plug
2. Machine malfunction
   a. Ventilator or continuous positive airway pressure device
   b. Oxygen blender
   c. Tubing and connections
3. Alarm system "off"
4. Severe hypoxia
5. Metabolic factors
6. Air leak
7. Intraventricular hemorrhage

TABLE 23-9	CRITICAL FINDINGS — CHEST AUSCULTATION FOR ENDOTRACHEAL TUBE PLACEMENT	
FINDING	**CAUSE**	
No air entry bilaterally	Esophagus intubated; air leak	
Air entry over left upper abdominal quadrant	Esophagus intubated; air entry heard over stomach	
Diminished air entry	Endotracheal tube too high; air leak	
Air entry unequal; right chest better aerated than left chest	Endotracheal tube too low; down right mainstem bronchus	

or disconnection of intravenous fluids may cause a precipitous drop in blood glucose, with respiratory irregularity, apnea, or seizures. Quickly checking the blood glucose with a glucometer is always warranted. If low blood glucose is not the cause of the sudden deterioration, it may be a complication of the asphyxial episode. After the infant is stabilized, screening for hypoglycemia and providing adequate fluids and glucose are appropriate (see Chapter 15).

Hypothermia and overwhelming sepsis with their associated metabolic derangements may be the cause of sudden deterioration. Muted response to cold stress is a consequence of asphyxial insult, and cold stress must be avoided after the acute episode. A high level of suspicion for infection should accompany sudden deterioration (see Chapters 6 and 22).

AIR LEAKS

Physiology. When air dissects from an alveolus, it follows the tracheobronchial tree and may accumulate in the mediastinum (pneumomediastinum), in the pleural space (pneumothorax), in the space surrounding the heart (pneumopericardium), in the peritoneal cavity (pneumoperitoneum), or subcutaneously (subcutaneous emphysema). Air leaks are complications of respiratory diseases and treatment strategies. When air continues to accumulate, pressure builds in the pleural space, compresses the lung, and pushes the mediastinum toward the unaffected side and a tension pneumothorax results.

The free air released from ruptured alveoli may lead to *pulmonary interstitial emphysema* (PIE) (Figure 23-1). This free air intravasates into interstitial tissue and can compromise pulmonary vascular circulation and ventilation. Localized pulmonary interstitial emphysema sometimes resolves spontaneously. Frequently it can continue for weeks or even months. Use of HFV has improved the outcome of these infants.

Etiology. Infants at increased risk for the development of air leaks fall into three specific categories: healthy term neonates, neonates with pulmonary diseases, and neonates receiving positive-pressure support (CPAP and IMV).

Healthy term neonates generate pressures of 40 to 80 cm H_2O for their first breath of life. Therefore a spontaneous air leak is more common in the neonatal period (2% to 10%) than at any other time of life.

Pulmonary diseases such as RDS result in stiff, noncompliant lungs requiring higher pressures for alveolar ventilation. Aspiration syndromes

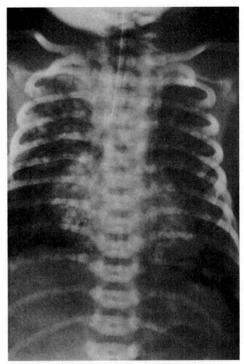

FIGURE 23-1 Pulmonary interstitial emphysema.

cause a ball-valve obstruction of debris with distal air trapping (meconium, milk, amniotic fluid, blood, and mucus). Hypoplastic lungs create a risk for air leaks because lung growth and development are abnormal and the lungs are stiff and noncompliant (diaphragmatic hernia and oligohydramnios syndrome). In either congenital lobar emphysema or PIE, alveolar rupture is associated with positive-pressure ventilation.

Positive-pressure ventilation, especially with excessive pressure, results in overdistention with alveolar rupture and air dissection. Air leaks occur in 16% to 36% of infants who are ventilated by CPAP or IMV or are resuscitated with a bag and mask or with an endotracheal tube and bag. ETT displacement is a major factor in the development of air leaks (see Table 23-5). Administration of surfactant lowers the levels of ventilatory support necessary to adequately ventilate the preterm infant's lungs and results in a reduced incidence of pneumothorax.

Prevention. Using the least amount of positive pressure to obtain physiologic results decreases the chances of air leaks. The incidence of pneumothorax is reduced in surfactant-treated prematures and with the use of HFV. Scrupulously clearing the airway before resuscitation and using pressure gauges on resuscitation equipment may prevent aspiration and the possibility of inadvertently using pressure that is too high. Vigilance in positioning, securing, and maintaining ETT position may significantly reduce the incidence of air leaks.[285] Air leaks alter systemic hemodynamics and are associated with the development of IVH (see Chapter 26). Rapid recognition of at-risk infants, recognition of clinical manifestations and diagnosis, and rapid emergency treatment improve survival and decrease the long-term sequelae of hypoxia and ischemia.

Data Collection

History. Pneumothorax or other air leaks should be suspected when any one of the following infants takes a sudden turn for the worse:

- A preterm infant with RDS either with or without positive-pressure support
- A term or postterm infant with meconium-stained amniotic fluid
- An infant with a chest radiograph showing interstitial or lobar emphysema
- An infant requiring resuscitation at birth
- An infant receiving CPAP or positive-pressure ventilation

Signs and Symptoms. Asymptomatic air leaks occur in term neonates; these frequently require no treatment and resolve spontaneously in 24 to 48 hours. Gradual onset of symptoms is characterized by increasing difficulty in ventilation, oxygenation, and perfusion. Early clinical manifestations may include restlessness and irritability, lethargy, tachypnea, and use of accessory muscles including grunting, flaring, and retractions. These subtle clinical changes may be unnoticed until the infant progresses to a sudden, profound collapse.

Sudden and severe deterioration in clinical course is characterized by the following:

- Profound generalized cyanosis
- Bradycardia
- Decrease in the height of the QRS complex on the monitor
- Air hunger including gasping and anxious facies
- Diminished or shifted breath sounds
- Chest asymmetry
- Diminished, shifted, or muffled cardiac sounds and point of maximal intensity (PMI)

- Severe hypotension and poor peripheral perfusion
- Easily palpable liver and spleen
- Subcutaneous emphysema
- Cardiorespiratory arrest

Laboratory Data. Arterial blood gas determinations reveal increasing hypoxemia ($\downarrow$PaO$_2$), increasing hypercapnia ($\uparrow$PaCO$_2$), and a persistent metabolic acidosis with gradual onset of symptoms. Transillumination of the chest with a fiber-optic probe may reveal hyperlucency of the affected side compared with the other side. A chest x-ray examination is the definitive diagnostic technique in air leaks. Because clinical manifestations of many other diseases may be similar to air leaks, the only way to be sure of the diagnosis is to perform a chest x-ray examination. Anteroposterior and lateral films must be obtained and a decubitus lateral x-ray film may be of value. X-ray findings in pneumothorax, the most common air leak, include the following:

- Increased lucency, overall increase in size, and flattened diaphragm on the affected side
- Widened intercostal spaces
- Decreased or absent pulmonary vascular markings
- Sharp contrast of the cardiac border and diaphragm (sharp edge sign)

Tension pneumothorax results in mediastinal shifts with decreased volume, increased opacity of opposite lung, and deviation of heart and trachea to the other side.

Treatment. An air leak is a surgical emergency of the chest. Tension within the chest cavity compromises lung excursion and cardiac output; without prompt treatment, the infant will not survive. Trained care providers must be available immediately to provide emergency management in any institution that provides positive-pressure ventilatory support.

Evacuation of trapped air to decrease tension and allow proper organ function is the goal of treatment. Pneumomediastinum rarely needs to be treated, but pneumopericardium often results in cardiac tamponade and requires needle aspiration or tube drainage. Pneumoperitoneum must be differentiated from a perforated viscus.

A suggested conservative treatment is endotracheal intubation of the unaffected lung. The tube is advanced 1 to 2 cm beyond the carina to occlude the involved lung. This procedure is difficult to perform if the left lung is involved. If the pulmonary interstitial emphysema is localized to one lung or lobe of the lung, differential ventilation or surgical removal of the lobe may be curative. Pneumothorax may be treated with needle aspiration of air. Tube thoracotomy with suction drainage is frequently necessary.

Use of fibrin glue to treat persistent pneumothorax has been reported, with resolution within 24 hours of treatment.[345] Complications included (1) bradycardia requiring manual ventilation, (2) significant hypercalcemia, (3) diaphragmatic paralysis, (4) contralateral pneumothorax, and (5) localized tissue necrosis.

Immediate Supportive Care. The head of the bed is elevated 30 to 40 degrees. This decreases the work of breathing by using gravity to localize the air in the upper chest and to push the abdominal organs downward away from the diaphragm.

Oxygen at 100% concentration is administered. The two goals for using 100% oxygen for immediate care are to improve oxygenation in a severely compromised infant and to increase by as much as sixfold the rate of absorption of the trapped air by means of a nitrogen washout technique.

CAUTION: Prolonged administration of 100% oxygen to treat an air leak in term infants has been used. Because of new understanding about the effects of oxidative stress from use of 100% oxygen, prolonged use for "nitrogen washout" should be used with caution (see Supplemental Oxygen earlier in this chapter). Exclusive use of 100% oxygen to treat trapped air is contraindicated in preterm infants because of the risk for developing retinopathy of prematurity and the length of time necessary to obtain complete resolution.

A severely compromised infant requires immediate emergency procedures. A diagnostic and therapeutic thoracentesis may be necessary in life-threatening situations in which there is not time to wait for x-ray examination.

Needle Aspiration. A scalp vein needle (23- to 25-gauge) or an Angiocath (24-gauge), a three-way stopcock, and a 10- to 20-ml syringe may be used for needle aspiration. The equipment is connected (syringe-stopcock-needle/Angiocath), the chest is aseptically prepared, and the needle is inserted into the third intercostal space in the anterior axillary line. A slight pop may be felt when the pleura is entered. Air is withdrawn into the syringe and evacuated into the room by turning the stopcock. This procedure is repeated until no more air can be aspirated or a chest tube can be placed.

Chest Tube. Chest tube thoracotomy is the definitive treatment for pneumothorax. The insertion of a chest tube is an invasive procedure that requires strict surgical technique, with each operator wearing a gown, gloves, mask, and cap. The infant should be appropriately positioned, restrained, provided with a sucrose pacifier, and monitored before the chest is prepared for asepsis. Ideally, the anterior chest wall should be prepared with a scrub solution for a minimum of 3 minutes. If a special tray is not available, a minor suture tray will usually contain the necessary instruments. Necessary equipment is as follows:

- Chest tube (8- to 12-Fr Argyle)
- Iodine or povidone-iodine (Betadine) scrub solution
- Gloves, gown, mask, hat
- Sterile drapes
- Syringes
- Sterile sponges (gauze)
- Medicine cups
- Lidocaine 1% without epinephrine
- Scalpel blades (no. 11 or 15)
- Hemostat (mosquito and Kelly clamps)
- Scissors
- Needle holder
- Sterile suture
- Sterile connectors (straight)
- Tubing
- Infant disposable underwater seal drainage system (two- or three-bottle or Pleur-evac system)
- Wall suction
- Sterile saline solution
- Tape, transparent dressing
- Chest tube clamp for emergency disconnection

The insertion site depends on the clinician's preference. In the lateral approach, the site is the fourth to sixth intercostal space on or lateral to the anterior axillary line. In the superior approach, the site is the second or third intercostal space on or just lateral to the midclavicular line (Figure 23-2). A case report of breast deformity, psychologic distress, and need for corrective surgery (in adolescent preterm girls) as a result of chest tube insertion for multiple pneumothoraces recommends a preventive strategy of using the anterior axillary line, maintaining a distance of 4 to 5 cm inferior to the nipple, and inserting the tube through the fifth or sixth intercostal space.[321]

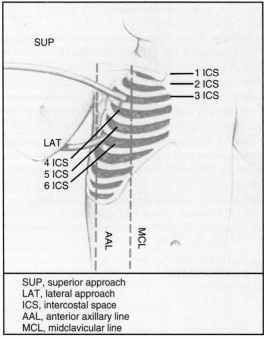

SUP

——1 ICS
——2 ICS
——3 ICS

LAT

4 ICS
5 ICS
6 ICS

AAL   MCL

SUP, superior approach
LAT, lateral approach
ICS, intercostal space
AAL, anterior axillary line
MCL, midclavicular line

FIGURE 23-2 Chest tube insertion site. (From Oellrich RG: Pneumothorax: chest tubes and the neonate, *MCN Am J Matern Child Nurs* 10:31, 1985.)

After infiltration of the area with 1% lidocaine for pain control, a small incision is made. A purse-string suture should be placed around the incision with ends left loose. A curved hemostat is inserted into the incision and opened. The catheter is advanced through the interspace and into the pleural space. The most frequent error by an inexperienced operator is applying too little force to enter the pleural cavity. The purse-string suture is tightened and tied and then tied to the chest tube. The tube is connected to the underwater drainage system, which may then be connected to a continuous suction device (10 to 20 cm H_2O is most commonly recommended). The tube should be secured with tape. An x-ray examination is used to confirm placement of the tube and evaluate the effectiveness of the therapy. After the procedure, attention to pain control with opioids and/or nonnarcotic analgesics is necessary (see Chapter 12).

Complications. In some instances, complications have arisen from the placement of chest tubes in neonates. These include hemorrhage, lung perforation, infarction, and phrenic nerve injury with eventration of the diaphragm. Clinical signs of eventration

(elevation of the diaphragm into the thoracic cavity) include a shift of the umbilicus upward and toward the affected side.[261]

Care of Chest Tube and Drainage System. The chest tube drainage system removes air and fluid material from the pleural space to restore negative pressure and expand the lung. Care providers must be familiar with the operation of the drainage system used in the nursery. The single-bottle water seal system drains air and fluid by gravity and blocks atmospheric air from being drawn into the pleural space. In addition to the water seal, the multiple-bottle systems allow suction to be applied to facilitate drainage and expansion. The Pleur-evac system is a single plastic unit divided into three chambers: the collection, water seal, and suction chambers.

Oscillation of fluid in the tube demonstrates effective communication between the pleural space and drainage bottle. In the small, sick infant, intrapleural pressure may cause only fluctuation in the tube at the chest wall. Fluctuation in either the tube or bottle should be observed. Fluctuation may cease as a result of fibrin or blood clots obstructing the tube, kinked or compressed tubing, or the suction apparatus not working properly. Milking and stripping the chest tube generally are unnecessary if only air is being removed. Presence of clots or debris may require gentle kneading of the tube. Milking and stripping generate tremendously high pressures that may entrap and damage the lung in the chest tube eyelets.

Bubbling in the drainage bottle indicates that air is being removed from the pleural space. Continuous bubbling may indicate an air leak in the system. To locate the source of the leak, the tube is momentarily clamped (beginning close to the chest and working toward the bottle) with a rubber-tipped hemostat. When the clamp is placed between the air leak and the water seal, the bubbling will stop. Patency of the tube, fluctuation, and bubbling should be observed and charted hourly.

Excessive or insufficient fluid in the drainage bottles may interfere with proper function of the drainage system. The bottle may have to be changed, or sterile saline may have to be added.

Frequent turning is important for maximum drainage and lung expansion. Proper stabilizing and positioning of the chest tube is necessary for function, comfort, and prevention of accidental removal. The tubing may be secured by encircling it with an adhesive tab, placing a safety pin through the tape (not the tube), and securing it to the bed. If the tube becomes dislodged, the opening should be covered with sterile gauze and pressure applied until the tube can be replaced.

When the infant is moved for such procedures as x-ray examination and weighing, the tube must be stabilized by holding it close to the chest. If the closed system is disturbed (e.g., because of a broken bottle), the tube should be clamped with a rubber-tipped hemostat that always should be kept at the bedside. The chest tube should be clamped for as short a time as possible. After necessary clamping, vital signs and clinical conditions should be closely monitored.

Bottles should be stabilized by being taped to an incubator or warmer so that they are not accidentally broken or picked up. The bottles must always be below the level of the infant's chest to prevent water from being pulled into the pleural space.

Removal of Chest Tubes. When bubbling has ceased for at least 24 hours and the chest x-ray films show no free air for 12 to 24 hours, the chest tube may be removed. Attention to pain relief during the removal process includes a sucrose pacifier and pharmacologic pain relief (see Chapter 12). Rapid, sterile removal of the tube is followed by application of a petrolatum gauze pressure dressing.

CENTRAL NERVOUS SYSTEM INSULT

Acute insult to the CNS may result in increased intracranial pressure, hemorrhage, or hypoxic-ischemic brain injury (see Chapter 26).

CARDIAC COMPLICATIONS

CDP or IMV may exert sufficient pressure on the pulmonary capillary bed to raise pulmonary artery pressure and interfere with cardiac output. The effect of CDP or IMV on the pulmonary vascular bed and cardiac output may be alleviated by lowering the PIP or PEEP, or both. At times, a fluid infusion to increase the intravascular volume may overcome the resistance to the pulmonary blood flow. The effect of MAP on cardiac output is difficult to monitor in most NICUs, because pulmonary artery or pulmonary wedge pressures are not routinely obtained. Until such time as these measurements are routinely obtained, the best CPAP is determined only on clinical grounds.

PDA is the most common cardiac complication in neonates with respiratory disease. Most often it is manifested by an increasing requirement or increased dependency on ventilatory support (see Chapter 24).

INFECTION AND BLEEDING

Procedures such as intubation expose the neonate to the risk for acquired (nosocomial) infection. Scrupulous attention must be given to technique when caring for respiratory equipment, and performing procedures such as sterile suctioning of the endotracheal tube minimizes the risks for infection. Handwashing before and after every contact with the neonate is the best method of preventing hospital-acquired infection in an already compromised, sick neonate. Neonates who are severely ill with respiratory disease may exhibit bleeding diathesis at birth or during the acute phase of their disease. Early recognition and treatment is important (see Chapter 20).

Chronic Complications

CHRONIC LUNG DISEASE/ BRONCHOPULMONARY DYSPLASIA

Despite improvements in neonatal respiratory care, the incidence of BPD/CLD continues to be high and is the direct result of the survival of extremely premature infants.[409] Survival of these extremely premature infants may be contributing to the static incidence of BPD/CLD reported by investigators. Several authors have reported an atypical type of BPD/CLD occurring in infants less than 1000 g at birth with mild or absent initial respiratory distress. A retrospective study of preterms with atypical BPD/CLD found that they (1) were born in hospital, (2) received natural surfactant therapy, (3) had fewer days of mechanical ventilation, and (4) were larger, more mature preterms.[296] The primary pathology of BPD/CLD is related to lung injury, it is in fact a multisystem disease, and most of the treatment is supportive.

BPD was first described by Northway and Rosan[288] as serial roentgenographic changes occurring in the lungs of premature infants who survived hyaline membrane disease (HMD). The clinical course of BPD is one of increasing respiratory distress and often is described as the chronic phase of RDS; CLD, a more inclusive term, occurs in a variety of conditions, including esophageal atresia, aspiration pneumonia, congenital heart disease, PDA, and meconium aspiration syndrome (MAS).

neonatal care have modified
...D as first described by North-
...n comparison with the infants
...ly neonates with BPD are far
...lower birth weights, and gen-
...e radiographic changes of cystic
...w BPD" is characterized by
...pment resulting from interfer-
ence with alveolarization and vascularization.[198]
VLBW neonates who require supplemental oxygen
at 28 to 30 days of life have BPD with further classification occurring at 36 weeks' postmenstrual age.[132]
Despite these changes, the incidence of chronic lung
disease in infants after NICU care remains a significant clinical problem, with an incidence of 13% to
35%.[426] Although atypical BPD/CLD is common in
preterms less than 1250 g, a recent retrospective study
found that the majority of preterms with BPD/CLD
still have classic BPD/CLD.[296]

The incidence of BPD/CLD varies among
NICUs because of variations in respiratory management associated with oxygen toxicity and
barotrauma and volutrauma. Although use of nasal
CPAP is associated with lower BPD/CLD rates,[20]
increased use of intubation, mechanical ventilation,
and high pressures (PIP and MAP) is associated with
increased BPD/CLD rates. When mechanical ventilation is used, the shorter the duration, the less often
BPD/CLD occurs.[62]

Pathophysiology. BPD/CLD is a disorder of primarily premature infants that is characterized by
respiratory distress and impaired gas exchange. The
pathogenesis of BPD/CLD is one of chronic and
constant and recurring lung injury, with ongoing
repair and healing of the injury. Chronic injury
and repair may in itself prolong the need for the
very factors that contribute to the development of
BPD/CLD: oxygen therapy and mechanical ventilation. In RDS, there is injury to the alveolar mucosa,
airway mucosa, serum exudation membranes, and
fibrin coagulation-forming hyaline membranes. If
sufficient hypoxia occurs with resultant damage,
the alveolar and airway epithelium and its basement
membrane will hemorrhage and round cell infiltration will begin. Cellular and noncellular debris fill
the alveoli and small airways. The obstruction causes
microatelectasis, and unobstructed airways become
hyperexpanded and emphysematous.

In the healing and repair process, type II alveolar
cells or their precursors multiply and differentiate

into type I pneumocytes, which provide alveolar
epithelium. Cells of the basal layer of the pseu-
dostratified, ciliated, columnar epithelium lining the
airways multiply and migrate to cover the injured
airway and rejuvenate the epithelium. During this
healing phase, the rapidly multiplying and differentiating transitional cells are squamous or cuboidal and
therefore appear "metaplastic." Epithelial metaplasia
is one of the characteristics of BPD.

As healing occurs, increased inspired oxygen tensions, barotrauma, and infection continue to injure
the cells that are taking part in the healing process.

Etiology. BPD/CLD is an iatrogenic disease caused
by oxygen toxicity and barotrauma resulting
from pressure ventilation. Even preterm infants
with mild respiratory distress in the first week of
life may develop BPD/CLD.[409] BPD/CLD is multifactorial, and prenatal predictors include prematurity (e.g., early gestational age and low birth weight)
and male gender.[180] Many studies have attempted
to identify biomarkers predictive of BPD/CLD,
including elevated placenta growth factor (P1GF)
level in cord blood at birth, higher trypsinogen-2
levels, and MMP/TIMP ratios.[63,134,414] However,
no current biomarker has been used routinely in
predicting risk of developing BPD/CLD. Plasma
concentration of soluble L-selectin (sL-selectin),
soluble E-selectin (sE-selectin), and soluble intercel-
lular adhesion molecule–1 may also be indicators for
treatment with dexamethasone. The arterial plasma
level of sL-selectin in infants who had RDS and did
not develop BPD/CLD was significantly decreased
when they were treated with dexamethasone.[27]

Oxygen Toxicity. BPD/CLD has been documented
in both long-term and short-term exposure to
oxygen at both low and high levels (greater
than 60% to 80%), as well as in infants treated
with mechanical ventilation without supplemental oxygen. As a result of these findings, many units
have instituted guidelines for oxygen use and monitoring of levels with pulse oximetry. Avoidance of
excessive oxygen exposure and careful attention
to oxygen saturations and arterial PaO_2 may help
reduce lung injury resulting from oxygen exposure.[164,347,408]

Barotrauma/Volutrauma. Development of BPD/CLD
is a result of barotrauma and volutrauma. BPD/
CLD has been described in infants who have received high PIPs and high PEEP[163] and neonates
with pneumothorax and PIE. A decrease in the

incidence of BPD/CLD has been noted when lower PIPs are used.[163] Although PIPs should be limited whenever possible, some infants with very noncompliant lungs require the use of high pressure for survival. Volutrauma (e.g., increased lung volume [stretch]) results in regional overdistention of lung units or airways, which may promote lung injury more than pressure itself. Using the smallest possible tidal volumes to inflate the lung avoids the overdistention and volutrauma that causes BPD/CLD.[163]

Use of surfactant therapy and newer ventilatory techniques[60,260,267] has decreased the pressures necessary to adequately oxygenate and ventilate the neonate's lungs, as well as resultant air leaks. A gentler ventilator strategy, "permissive hypercapnia" (e.g., accepting a $PaCO_2$ of 45 to 58 mm Hg) benefits the preterm by (1) use of lower PIP, MAP, rate, and tidal volume; (2) improving ventilation-perfusion matching; (3) decreasing days on ventilation, use of supplemental oxygen, and reintubation rates; (4) increasing oxygen availability at the tissue level; (5) increasing respiratory drive and decreasing apnea; (6) increasing cardiac output; and (7) decreasing BPD/CLD.[60,341]

Although alterations in $PaCO_2$ are associated with fluctuations in cerebral blood flow, in one study there was no difference in IVH and PVL, mortality, air leaks, ROP, or PDA compared with a control group.[260] Mild permissive hypercapnia may protect against cerebral hypoperfusion and subsequent PVL associated with hypocapnia; extreme hypercapnia, however, is associated with an increased risk for intraventricular hemorrhage.[328] Therefore large fluctuations of $PaCO_2$ values should be avoided, and further studies of the relationship between hypocarbia/hypercarbia and brain injury are needed. Even though mild permissive hypercapnia is safe and has modest benefit, the optimal $PaCO_2$ level has not been determined.

Use of HFV, HFV with surfactant replacement, and HFV with "high volume" technique are all associated with a decreased incidence of BPD/CLD (see High-Frequency Ventilation earlier in this chapter).

Patent Ductus Arteriosus. There is a high incidence of BPD among infants with PDA and congestive heart failure. The amount of oxygen and peak inspiratory pressure necessary to support a neonate through the pulmonary complications of PDA may result in damage from oxygen toxicity and barotrauma. The increased pulmonary blood flow that occurs may also contribute to pulmonary damage. Very preterm infants (less than 29 weeks' gestation) with a PDA have a higher mortality rate compared with preterms with a closed ductus (70.7% vs. 11.2%).[287] Because of these findings, medical closure of the ductus with indomethacin, ibuprofen, or surgical ligation is advocated (see Chapter 24) but has not affected the incidence of BPD.

Nutrition. SGA infants who were undernourished in utero have been shown to have an increased risk for BPD/CLD.[240] Inadequate nutrition caused by poor intake or increased nutritional requirements resulting in catabolism may potentiate the effects of oxygen and barotrauma on the neonatal lung. A retrospective review of the nutritional status of 30 preterms with BPD/CLD found that they received significantly less protein and calories (e.g., by 28 days of life, 98.63 kcal/kg/day instead of the recommended 120 kcal/kg/day for growth), resulting in a significant energy and protein deficit.[209] This undernutrition may be contributing to the development of BPD/CLD by altering the growth of immature lungs. Inadequate intake of antioxidants, trace elements, vitamins, and polyunsaturated fatty acids also may predispose the lung to injury. Optimizing nutritional support of infants at risk of BPD/CLD is an area of active research.

Fluids. BPD/CLD is common in preterms who have developed symptoms of fluid overload within the first few days of life. Fluid balance in a VLBW infant is complicated by huge insensible water loss and often intolerance for enteral feedings. Intake, output, and changes in weight must be closely monitored to calculate the fluid needs. Furthermore, clinical research indicates that careful restriction of water intake so that physiologic needs are met without allowing for significant dehydration is indicated. This practice also decreases the risk for PDA and NEC and might decrease the overall risk for death without significantly increasing the risk for adverse consequences.[39]

Family History of Asthma. Infants who develop BPD may have relatives with asthma who require periodic hospitalization. The lungs of these infants may be less tolerant of the insults of pulmonary disease, oxygen, pressure, and fluids.

Prematurity. Developmental immaturity is of principal importance in the etiologic picture of

BPD/CLD. Premature births alone may have a significant effect on pulmonary development, because prematurity results in differences in the development of small airways. As a result, premature infants are more susceptible to additional damage to the small airways from oxygen, ventilator pressure, fluids, and circulatory overload. As the survival rate of VLBW infants born at less than 28 weeks' gestation increases, the occurrence of BPD/CLD is increasing (e.g., the lower the gestational age, the higher the risk).[189] However, the current form of BPD/CLD is less severe, with fewer infants requiring tracheostomies and long-term ventilation therapy (6 months or more).[75]

Oxygen and Antioxidants. Oxygen accepts free electrons generated by oxidative metabolism within the cell and produces free radicals, molecules that are toxic to living cells or tissues.[347] Normally, antioxidants protect cells against free radicals, but this balance may be upset by increased free radical production or decreased antioxidant defense. A preterm neonate is deficient in antioxidants and thus more susceptible to lung damage from free radicals and oxidative stress.[28,75]

Inflammation. Oxygen radicals, barotrauma, infection, and other factors initiate the inflammatory process,[75] resulting in the infiltration of leukocytes, with release of other inflammatory mediators, resulting in pulmonary damage (e.g., decrease in capillary endothelial integrity, albumin leakage in the alveoli resulting in pulmonary edema). Neonates whose lungs are mechanically ventilated have increased pulmonary cytokine and phagocyte levels within 1 to 3 hours after the onset of mechanical ventilation.[75,416] Activated neutrophils release enzymes that directly destroy the elastin and collagen of the lung. Lung inflammation and injury predispose the lung to increased susceptibility to volutrauma and oxidant-induced lung injury.[75] This inflammatory cycle produces significant pulmonary injury during a critical period of rapid lung growth and development (24 to 40 weeks) (see Table 23-1). Increasingly, studies show that preterm infants exposed to antenatal inflammation and infection (e.g., chorioamnionitis) are at increased risk for developing BPD.[75,327] Postnatal nosocomial infection is associated with an increased risk for BPD/CLD.[390] Variation in nosocomial infection rates may be a factor in the variation in inter-NICU BPD/CLD rates.

Prevention. Potentially better practices to reduce the BPD/CLD in VLBW infants are listed in Box 23-9. Widespread use of antenatal steroids and surfactant administration has not reduced the rate of BPD/CLD or the NICU disparities in BPD/CLD rates. Use of surfactant does reduce the severity of BPD/CLD,[75] and use of a new synthetic surfactant recently has been shown to reduce the incidence

---

BOX 23-9

POTENTIALLY BETTER PRACTICES TO REDUCE THE INCIDENCE OF CLD/BPD IN THE VERY-LOW-BIRTH-WEIGHT PRETERM INFANT

- Use NCPAP in delivery room and as initial respiratory support as an alternative to routine intubation and early/prophylactic use of surfactant[9,315]
- Combine early NCPAP with selective surfactant therapy in extremely preterm infants[9,315]
- Avoid endotracheal intubation for mechanical ventilation[147,323]
- Use noninvasive mechanical ventilation strategies[29]
- Use of the antioxidant *vitamin A*
- Increased use of permissive hypercapnia[60]
- Decrease the incidence of sentinel events such as air leaks and unplanned extubations
- Minimize exposure in the delivery room to supplemental oxygen by titrating Fio_2 and monitoring oxygen saturations with PO
- Early closure of PDA, either medically or surgically
- Monitor and minimize tidal volumes on mechanically ventilated preterms
- Extubate from assisted ventilation as soon as possible[148,247]
- Use nasal bubble CPAP[148,247]
- Improve teamwork in the delivery room[247]
- Use Neopuff, instead of hand ventilation, to minimize overinflation of the preterm lung
- Provide consistent respiratory management and consistent ventilator weaning
- Provide blended Fio_2 in the delivery room and during transport to the NICU to minimize exposure to unnecessary levels of supplemental oxygen

Adapted from Geary C, Caskey M, Fonseca R, et al: Decreased incidence of bronchopulmonary dysplasia after early management changes, including surfactant and nasal continuous positive airway pressure treatment at delivery, lowered oxygen saturation goals, and early amino acid administration: a historical cohort study, *Pediatrics* 121:89, 2008; Payne NR, LaCorte M, Sun S, et al, and the Breathsavers Group: Evaluation and development of potentially better practices to reduce bronchopulmonary dysplasia in very low birth weight infants, *Pediatrics* 118:S65, 2006.

NICU, Neonatal intensive care unit; *PDA,* patent ductus arteriosus; *PO,* pulse oximeter.

of BPD/CLD.[276] A single course of antenatal steroid therapy decreases the incidence and severity of BPD/CLD.[281] Widespread use of both antenatal and postnatal steroid therapy has not improved the outcome in ELBW infants. Premature and full-term infants (with pneumonia or MAS) treated with surfactant replacement have a lower incidence of BPD/CLD because of (1) better ventilation and pressure distribution in the alveoli, (2) stabilization of the alveoli, (3) prevention of overdistention, and (4) decreased cytokines and inflammatory response.

Noninvasive respiratory support using NCPAP or mechanical ventilation using the nasal route reduces or eliminates the need for intubation and mechanical ventilation.[20,107,109,247] In an attempt to prevent reinjury and allow healing, inspired oxygen tensions should be kept as low as is reasonable to provide adequate arterial oxygen tension. Pressures on the ventilator should be reduced when possible to prevent barotrauma.

Use of inhaled nitric oxide in care of preterms with RDS remains controversial. A recent meta-analysis involving 12 trials showed no difference in death, development of BPD, or severe neurologic injury, but could not exclude a small reduction in the combined outcome of death and BPD/CLD with higher dose of iNO (20 ppm), used after 7 days of age[46] (see Treatment under Respiratory Distress Syndrome later in this chapter). iNO therapy appears to be safe from limited data and does not alter plasma biomarkers of oxidative stress in the preterm infant at risk for BPD/CLD.[28,413] Long-term pulmonary outcomes of preterm infants treated with iNO remain inconclusive and study results inconsistent.[383] One study suggested a reduction in bronchodilators, inhaled/systemic steroids, diuretics, and supplemental oxygen usage.[186] Two other studies showed no reduction in survival without brain injury or BPD[264] and no difference in functional residual capacity, wheezing, readmission rate, or use of respiratory medications.[190a] A systematic review of 14 RCTs, 7 follow-up studies, and 1 observational study found no reduction in mortality or BPD.[121]

In a multicenter trial, administration of vitamin A (e.g., 5000 international units IM three times a week for 4 weeks) to VLBW infants reduced the risk for BPD/CLD. Monitoring of serum levels (the desired range of plasma vitamin A concentrations is 30 to 60 mcg/dl; the desired plasma retinol-binding protein [RBP] concentration is greater than

25 mg/dl)[364] and assessment for manifestations of toxicity (e.g., lesions on skin/mucous membranes, bone and joint abnormalities, jaundice, hepatomegaly, and increased intracranial pressure) should accompany vitamin A administration.[364] Concurrent dexamethasone therapy increases serum blood levels of fat-soluble vitamins (e.g., A and E) independent of intake.[365] In another study, oral supplementation of vitamin A (e.g., 5000 IU/day for 28 days) in ELBW infants did not significantly alter the incidence of BPD/CLD.[427] Supplementing VLBW infants with vitamin A is associated with a reduction in death, oxygen requirement at 1 month of age, and oxygen requirement at 36 weeks' postmenstrual age in preterms less than 1000 g birth weight.[106] A recent retrospective analysis of use of vitamin A or vitamin A combined with iNO in preterms (750 to 999 g birth weight) found a reduction in BPD/CLD, BPD, and death.[149] In the most fragile preterms (500 to 749 g birth weight) the combination of vitamin A and iNO resulted in better neurocognitive outcomes at 1 year of age.[149]

Prevention of oxygen free radical injury to the pulmonary tree and CNS (e.g., CLD/BPD and IVH/PVL)[347] occurs with intratracheal injection of recombinant human CuZn superoxide dismutase (rhSOD). A significant decrease in markers of pulmonary inflammation occurred in rhSOD-treated preterm infants without short- or long-term abnormalities.[107]

Data Collection

History. A history of prematurity, moderate to severe RDS, intubation with oxygen and positive-pressure ventilation in the first week of life, inability to be weaned from the ventilator, and increasing oxygen requirement at the end of the first week of life are associated with BPD/CLD. Long-term features include tachypnea, rales, retractions, abnormal chest x-ray examination results, and the need for supplemental oxygen for more than 28 to 30 days of life or at 36 weeks of postmenstrual age.

Signs and Symptoms. Tachypnea, exercise intolerance (feeding and handling), oxygen dependence, and respiratory distress (retractions, nasal flaring, fine rales at the bases or throughout the lung fields) are associated with BPD/CLD.

Laboratory Data. X-ray findings (Figure 23-3) correlate with the stage of disease; however, the pathologic changes are often more severe than the chest x-ray findings indicate[288]:

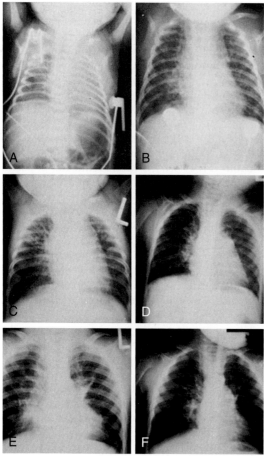

FIGURE 23-3 Serial chest x-ray films of premature infant with bronchopulmonary dysplasia over 2-year period. **A,** Newborn. **B,** Two months. **C,** Three months. **D,** One year. **E,** Two years. Infant's disease process was characterized by multiple hospitalizations for reactive airway disease and pulmonary hypertension. Note progressive lung disease characterized by hyperinflation and eventual clearing of infiltrate by 2 years of age **(F).**

- Stage I: Reticulogranular pattern and air bronchogram or RDS (first 3 days of life)
- Stage II: Coarse granular infiltrates that are dense enough to obscure the cardiac markings (first 3 to 10 days of life)
- Stage III: Multiple small cyst formation within the opaque lungs and visible cardiac borders (first 10 to 20 days of life)
- Stage IV: Irregular larger cyst formation that alternates with areas of increased density (after 28 days of life)

Mild hyperinflation as demonstrated on a chest x-ray film is a common finding in VLBW infants with BPD/CLD.

Cardiovascular changes include (1) right ventricular hypertrophy on ECG, (2) elevated right ventricular systolic time intervals or left ventricular and septal wall thickening on echocardiogram, or (3) elevated pulmonary vascular pressures and resistance at cardiac catheterization.

Treatment. The therapeutic goal is to reduce those factors that produce reinjury and to allow the lung to heal so that normal function can resume. This process may take weeks, months, or even years in severe lung injuries or in small infants under 1000 g.

Concurrent supportive therapies include (1) maintenance of adequate oxygenation and ventilation, (2) adequate nutrition and fluid restriction, (3) early PDA closure, and (4) pharmacologic management. Sufficient PIP should be used to prevent atelectasis while maintaining the lowest Fio_2 (if possible, 0.5 or lower) to maintain adequate oxygenation (i.e., Pao_2 60 to 80 mm Hg; O_2 saturation 90% to 95%). Weaning from mechanical ventilation is done slowly and may be facilitated by (1) use of SIMV that reduces the work of breathing, (2) use of methylxanthines before extubation, and (3) use of nasal CPAP after extubation.[20,109,110] Usually in BPD/CLD, the infant's ability to maintain ventilation develops before the ability to maintain adequate oxygenation. Often infants are discharged from the NICU on home oxygen therapy. Infants with BPD/CLD who require oxygen at a rate of 20 ml/kg/min or less and those who can maintain oxygen saturations of 92% or above after 40 minutes of breathing room air are ready to begin successful weaning from supplemental oxygen.[369]

Neonates with BPD/CLD have an increased resting metabolic expenditure as the major reason for growth failure, especially in the smallest, sickest infants.[239] These infants may require 150 to 200 kcal/kg/day to support adequate growth (i.e., 10 to 30 g/day weight gain). Without adequate protein or caloric intake, damaged pulmonary tissue cannot heal, and provision of appropriate nutrition to the neonate with BPD is essential (see Chapters 14 through 18).

Pharmacologic management of BPD/CLD includes the use of bronchodilators, steroids, and diuretics (Table 23-10). Inhaled and systemic

TABLE 23-10	PHARMACOLOGIC AGENTS USED IN TREATMENT OF CHRONIC LUNG DISEASE/BRONCHOPULMONARY DYSPLASIA	

DRUG	DOSAGE	COMMENTS
I. Bronchodilators		Further clinical trials are needed to assess the role of bronchodilators and diuretics in the treatment and prevention of CLD/BPD.[283a]
A. Inhaled		
1. Beta$_2$-agonists		
a. Albuterol (Proventil; Ventolin)	0.1 mg/kg up to 5 mg in 2 ml of NS solution q 4-6 hr Max dose: 0.5 ml or 2.5 mg/treatment; up to six treatments/24 hr Onset: 5-15 min Peak action: 30 min to 2 hr Duration: 3-4 hr	Drug of choice for bronchospasm—improves pulmonary resistance and lung compliance by bronchial smooth muscle relaxation; tachycardia, tremors, nausea and vomiting; can cause paradoxic bronchoconstriction, irritability. MDI dosage improves lung function as well as nebulization, is faster and more cost effective.
b. Terbutaline (Brethine)	0.03-0.3 mg/kg/day Onset: 5-30 min Duration: 3-4 hr	Same as for albuterol.
2. Histamine inhibitor (Cromolyn: 20 mg/2 ml solution for nebulizer)	**10-20 mg TID**	Prevents release of inflammatory mediators and reduces airway hypersensitivity; urticaria, rash, and throat irritation; dosage may need adjusting in patients with hepatic or renal dysfunction. A systematic review showed no significant evidence that cromolyn has a role in the treatment or prevention of CLD/BPD.[283b]
B. Systemic		
1. Methylxanthines		
a. Caffeine citrate	Loading: 20 mg/kg Maintenance: 5 mg/kg/day IV or PO Half-life: as long as 100 hr	Promotes weaning from low rates of ventilatory support by reduction of pulmonary resistance, improved lung compliance, and improved skeletal muscle and diaphragmatic contractility, has diuretic effect; excreted unchanged in urine; safer drug with fewer side effects than theophylline. Side effects rare but include tachycardia, diuresis, dysrhythmias, glucosuria, seizures, ketonuria, vomiting, hyperglycemia, jitteriness, hemorrhagic gastritis.
b. Theophylline (PO)	4-6 mg of active theophylline, which should produce a serum level of 10-20 mcg/ml Maintenance: calculated by rate of plasma clearance, usually 3-7 mg/kg/day q 12 hr Half-life: 30-40 hr	Metabolized to caffeine in the liver and excreted in urine; multisystem effect; CNS stimulant; increases respiratory rate, inspiratory drive, and surfactant production; increases GFR; increases heart rate, contractility, and output; decreases GI motility and increases GI secretions; increases glucose levels, ketonuria, and glycosuria; increases muscle contractility; increases catecholamine and insulin levels. Side effects: same as for caffeine citrate.
2. Beta$_2$-agonists a. Terbutaline	5 mcg/kg subcutaneously q 4-6 hr	Improves pulmonary mechanics; side effects same as for albuterol; adjunct to methylxanthines.
b. Albuterol	0.15 mg/kg/dose PO q 8 hr	Reduces pulmonary resistance; adjunct to methylxanthines; side effects same as albuterol.
II. Steroids		
A. Inhaled		

Continued

TABLE 23-10	PHARMACOLOGIC AGENTS USED IN TREATMENT OF CHRONIC LUNG DISEASE/BRONCHOPULMONARY DYSPLASIA—cont'd	
DRUG	**DOSAGE**	**COMMENTS**
1. Corticosteroids (dexamethasone [Decadron])	100 mcg/inhalation from MDI	30%-60% systemic bioavailability versus 53%-78% from oral intake; majority removed from lung within 20 min after administration; anatomic, physiologic, and pathophysiologic variations in the neonate, coupled with the aerosol delivery system and its use, influence the amount of drug actually administered and the aerosol's efficacy. Side effects: oral candidiasis, bronchospasm, and pituitary-adrenal suppression, tongue hypertrophy. No evidence that early (<2 weeks of age) administration to ventilated preterms is effective in reducing CLD/BPD.[363] No evidence of a difference in side effects or effectiveness in inhaled vs. systemic steroids.[361,367]
2. Glucocorticoids		
a. Flunisolide (Aerobid)	250 mcg/inhalation	Unknown stability—do not mix with other drugs; bronchospasm may result from buffers and/or preservatives.
b. Beclomethasone (Beconase; Vancenase)	42 mcg/inhalation	Side effects: same as for dexamethasone.
B. Systemic (corticosteroids— dexamethasone [Decadron])	0.5 mg/kg/day IV or PO q 12 hr for 3 days; decrease to 0.3 mg/kg/day for 3 days Taper 10%-20% q 3 days	Hyperglycemia; hypothalamic-pituitary-adrenal axis suppression; renal calcification; protein depletion and/or tissue catabolism (increase BUN; failure to gain weight); gastric irritation, perforation, bleeding; restlessness and/or irritability; myocardial hypertrophy; hypertension; increased risk for infection (see Box 23-10).
	Initial dose: 0.1-0.2 mg/kg/day for 3 days[197]	Use for ventilator-dependent infant at 14-28 days of age who is developing CLD/BPD to accomplish extubation.
	If extubated, taper dose over 3-6 days (total treatment 6-9 days) If unable to extubate after initial 3 days of therapy, discontinue therapy[197]	Lower dose for shorter treatment period. Avoids hyperglycemia and hypertension seen in the higher doses of longer duration.[197]

III. Diuretics

A. Furosemide (Lasix)	1-2 mg/kg/dose IV BID or 2-4 mg/ kg/dose PO BID Onset: 5 min IV; 1 hr PO Duration: 2-4 hr	Acute and chronic administration of furosemide in preterm infants >3 weeks of age with CLD/BPD improves lung compliance. Chronic administration of IV or PO furosemide also improves oxygenation. Routine or sustained use of systemic loop diuretics in infants with or developing CLD/BPD cannot be recommended based on current evidence.[388,389] Treatment of choice for fluid overload in CLD/BPD—decrease interstitial edema and PVR; daily or alternate-day administration improves pulmonary mechanics and facilitates weaning from ventilator. Side effects: metabolic acidosis, hypokalemia, hypocalcemia, hypochloremia, hyponatremia, renal calcifications, gallstones, ototoxicity, requires KCl supplementation. For preterms >3 weeks of age with CLD/BPD, administration of distal diuretics improves pulmonary compliance; chronic use improves oxygenation and lung compliance.[389] Acute and chronic administration of thiazides to preterms >3 weeks of age with BPD/CLD improves pulmonary mechanics and reduces the need for furosemide.[388]

TABLE 23-10	PHARMACOLOGIC AGENTS USED IN TREATMENT OF CHRONIC LUNG DISEASE/BRONCHOPULMONARY DYSPLASIA — cont'd

DRUG	DOSAGE	COMMENTS
B. Thiazide		
1. Chlorothiazide (Diuril)	5-20 mg/kg/dose IV or PO BID	Less potent than furosemide; promotes potassium and bicarbonate excretion with sodium and chloride; spares calcium given with spironolactone. Combination of thiazide and spironolactone results in improved lung mechanics and increased urine output. Side effects: electrolyte imbalance, hypercalcemia, hyperglycemia, decreased magnesium level, hypersensitivity, GI upset, glycosuria.
2. Hydrochlorothiazide (HydroDIURIL)	1-2 mg/kg/dose PO BID Onset: 1-2 hr Duration: 6-12 hr	Side effects: electrolyte imbalance, hypercalcemia, hyperglycemia, metabolic alkalosis, increased urinary losses of sodium, potassium, magnesium, chloride, phosphorus, and bicarbonate; spares calcium.
3. Spironolactone (Aldactone)	1.5 mg/kg/dose PO BID Onset: 2-3 days	Weak diuretic; causes increased sodium chloride and water loss; spares potassium. Side effects: irritability, lethargy, vomiting, diarrhea, rash.
4. Bumetanide (Bumex)	0.015 mg/kg/day up to 0.1 mg/kg/day PO	40 times the potency of furosemide; used in neonates and infants with CLD/BPD refractory to furosemide therapy. Side effects: same as for furosemide plus hypophosphatemia.

BID, Two times/day; *BUN,* blood urea nitrogen; *CLD/BPD,* chronic lung disease/bronchopulmonary dysplasia; *CNS,* central nervous system; *GFR,* glomerular filtration rate; *GI,* gastrointestinal; *IV,* intravenously; *KCl,* potassium chloride; *LOS,* length of stay; *MDI,* metered-dose inhaler; *NS,* normal saline; *PO,* per os, orally; *PVR,* pulmonary vascular resistance; *TID,* three times/day.

bronchodilators improve lung mechanics and gaseous exchange by relaxation of bronchial smooth muscle.[108] However, bronchodilators may fail to relieve airway obstruction because of relatively poor development of bronchial smooth muscle in preterm infants.

Methylxanthine therapy promotes weaning of infants with RDS from low rates of ventilatory support.[182] A meta-analysis of seven trials evaluating the prophylactic use of methylxanthine treatment for successful extubation observed a significant reduction in the incidence of failed extubation within the first week of life.[182] In addition at 18 to 21 months of age the preterms exposed to methylxanthine therapy had a lower rate of cerebral palsy, death, and major disability.[182]

Diuretics alone and diuretics combined with methylxanthines improve lung mechanics, clinical respiratory status, and ability to wean from mechanical ventilation (see Table 23-10). Aerosolized diuretics (e.g., a single dose of furosemide at 1 mg/kg) transiently improve lung mechanics in preterms older than 3 weeks with BPD/CLD. RCTs

are needed to evaluate the effects of aerosolized diuretics on oxygen dependence, mortality rates, duration of ventilator use, length of stay, and long-term outcomes.[55]

Steroids reduce lung inflammation and improve pulmonary function in severe RDS. Use of antenatal steroid (ANS) therapy is associated with (1) improved survival, (2) more rapid ventilator weaning because of decreased severity of RDS, (3) decreased need for supplemental oxygen (e.g., BPD/CLD), (4) lowered incidence of IVH and PDA, (5) no alteration of resting cortisol levels, and (6) a short-term (5-day) alteration in gene expression in leukocytes.[161,281,333,337,350] ANS is most effective when birth occurs within 7 days after a completed dose in preterms less than 33 weeks' gestation (especially in preterms of 24 to 29 weeks' gestation).[271,337] The incidence of RDS is not reduced in late preterms at 34 to 36 weeks' gestation.[205,317] Preterm infants exposed to a complete course of ANS have better lung compliance and intact neurodevelopment at 18 to 22 months compared with preterms exposed to an incomplete course or no ANS.[66,67] Even though antenatal steroids do not reduce the incidence of RDS in preterm infants 27 weeks' gestation or less, there is a significantly lower incidence of death or neurodevelopmental impairment at 18 to 22 months in preterms (i.e., 23 to 25 weeks' gestation) exposed to antenatal steroids.[61] Even the choice of which glucocorticoid to use antenatally may be significant. Betamethasone, rather than dexamethasone, is associated with reduced risk for neonatal death and trends toward risk reduction for other adverse neonatal outcomes (e.g., IVH, severe IVH, and ROP).[244,337]

The NIH consensus statement[281] discourages multiple courses of ANS because of (1) impaired head/fetal growth, in a dose-dependent manner[278,337]; (2) impaired brain development and behavior and psychomotor development; (3) increased incidence of IVH; (4) increased sepsis, mortality, and lung disease; (5) associated gastroesophageal reflux[70]; and (6) increased severity of ROP. The American College of Obstetricians and Gynecologists (ACOG) recommends a repeat course of ANS if the fetus is less than 34 weeks' gestation and the previous ANS course was more than 14 days ago.[14] Long-term effects of multiple ANS therapy are associated with increased cortisol activity in response to stress,[5] a non–statistically significant difference in the incidence of cerebral palsy (e.g., 2.9% in the repeated-doses group vs. 0.5% in the placebo group),[424] and a reduced risk of neurodevelopmental delay at 2 years of age due to a reduction in inflammation.[74]

Postnatal steroid use became widespread in the 1990s without properly conducted RCTs for safety and efficacy,[143] despite warnings from researchers in the 1970s about serious potential dangers. Steroid use has been enthusiastically accepted because of the dramatic, short-term improvements in respiratory status (e.g., facilitates extubation, more rapid ventilator weaning, reduces the risk for BPD/CLD and PDA).[46,122,125,126] Two large RCTs of postnatal steroid use were halted because of serious short-term complications—intestinal perforation, growth retardation, PVL, hyperglycemia, hypertension, and infection.[160,380] Adverse long-term outcomes are listed in Box 23-10. Adverse developmental outcomes are the result of the effects of steroids on the developing nervous system. Two meta-analyses caution that the short-term benefits of early (less than 7 days) and late (more than 7 days) postnatal steroids may not outweigh the actual or potential adverse effects.[125,126]

BOX 23-10   LONG-TERM ADVERSE EFFECTS OF STEROID USE

Slower Growth[380]
- Somatic and head/brain growth[297] (even into adolescence)[69]
- Arrested lung development caused by interference in pulmonary alveolarization and vascularization

"Neurotoxic" Substances[5,33]
- Further reduces size of cerebral and cerebellar[398] tissue/gray matter volume of premature brain[297] (effects lasting into adolescence)[69]
- Increased rate of cerebral palsy (CP)[123,440]
- Increased risk for CP significantly related to the total cumulative doses of dexamethasone[317a]
- Increased cognitive deficits at school age, children had lower scores on verbal or written language skills, math, perceptual organization, freedom from distractibility, and processing speed[440]
- Increased special education, poorer performance on neuropsychological tasks (i.e., alertness, visuomotor coordination, emotion recognition), poorer gross motor skills at 14-17 years of age[366,404]
- Increased severity of retinopathy of prematurity

Contributes to Long-Term
- Cardiovascular disease
- Immune system disorders/autoimmune diseases
- Renal calcifications
- Neurologic and behavioral deficits

The administration of inhaled corticosteroids to prevent or treat BPD/CLD in ventilated VLBW infants without exposing them to systemic steroids is an attractive alternative. However, meta-analyses of early (within the first 2 weeks of life)[363] and late (7 days of life or more)[293] prophylactic use of inhaled steroids show no evidence of benefit in ventilated or nonventilated preterms at increased risk for BPD/CLD. Inhaled steroids compared with systemic postnatal steroids found no efficacy in preventing[362] or treating[362] BPD/CLD. All of these meta-analyses conclude that inhaled steroids cannot be recommended and that more research is required.[293,362,363]

Historically, steroids have been "routinely" used with widely varying practices about type of medication (e.g., natural hormone [hydrocortisone] or synthetic hormones [dexamethasone; betamethasone]), dosage (e.g., standard or low dose), timing (e.g., early or late), and duration (e.g., weaning after 7 to 10 days or 42-day treatment).[143,197] Considered "routine practice," parents were rarely asked to give informed consent. Parents (in addition to health care providers)[32,380] must be honestly informed about the experimental nature of steroid use and its short-term and long-term complications, so that they are able to participate in giving or withholding their fully informed consent.[32,176] The DART Study of low-dose steroid use was halted because infants could not be recruited; fully informed parents concerned about risks to their infant refused permission to be part of the study.[123]

Based on the premise that very preterm infants have early adrenal insufficiency, early use of hydrocortisone therapy to decrease BPD/CLD has been studied in four RCTs.[51,302,428-430] In all four studies the hydrocortisone-treated preterms were favored with a significant increase in survival without BPD/CLD seen in two RCTs. The largest, multicenter, randomized trial to test early low-dose hydrocortisone therapy was halted because of an increase in spontaneous GI perforations in the treated preterms, especially those also receiving indomethacin.[428] Prophylaxis of early adrenal insufficiency decreased mortality rate and improved survival rate without BPD/CLD only in the chorioamnionitis-exposed preterms.[428] Another RCT of early administration (within the first 36 hours of life) of hydrocortisone to prevent BPD/CLD was terminated early because of the increased incidence of GI perforations and found lower rates of BPD/CLD.[302,303] The 18- to 22-month follow-up of the infants in both of these RCTs showed no difference in growth, no increase in cerebral palsy, and indicators of improved neurodevelopmental outcome in those treated with early, low-dose hydrocortisone.[303,430]

More recent studies of low-dose hydrocortisone have found that it is safer for the immature brain (i.e., no effect on cerebral tissue volume and no adverse neurodevelopmental outcomes) compared with dexamethasone.* Only one study demonstrated smaller brain volumes in the cerebellar, not the cerebral, regions with hydrocortisone use.[398] A single-center cohort study of 67 preterms receiving either betamethasone or hydrocortisone found that hydrocortisone was as effective as betamethasone in early extubation, without short-term adverse effects; long-term neurodevelopment,

however, was not studied.[42] However, low-dose hydrocortisone does not decrease the incidence of BPD/CLD or death.[124] A randomized multicenter trial of higher dose hydrocortisone's effect on the incidence of BPD/CLD, mortality, short-term pulmonary outcomes, adverse effects during NICU stay, and long-term neurodevelopmental outcomes (at 2 years' corrected age) is currently being conducted in Belgium and The Netherlands as the STOP-BPD study.[194,292]

After reviewing the short-term and long-term effects of systemic and inhaled corticosteroid use for the prevention and treatment of CLD/BPD in the VLBW infant, the AAP and Canadian Pediatric Society issued the first policy statement in 2006 about use of postnatal steroids.[11] Since the initial statement the use of postnatal steroids has declined.[197] The revised policy statement on use of postnatal corticosteroids to prevent or treat BPD recommends the following[12]:

- High-dose dexamethasone (0.5 mg/kg/day) cannot be recommended until RCTs show improved short- and long-term outcomes.
- Low-dose dexamethasone (less than 0.2 mg/kg/day) cannot be recommended because of insufficient evidence.
- Early hydrocortisone therapy (low dose: 1 mg/kg/day in the first 2 weeks of life) may be beneficial in a specific population of preterms (i.e., prenatal inflammation). However, hydrocortisone therapy cannot be recommended for all infants at risk for BPD because of insufficient evidence.
- High-dose hydrocortisone (3 to 6 mg/kg/day; started after the first week of postnatal age) cannot be recommended because of insufficient data.

The dose and duration of use of late postnatal corticosteroids should be minimized and reserved for preterms who cannot wean from the ventilator.[126,197] Table 23-10 gives a proposed (expert opinion rather than evidence-based) dosing regimen for low-dose, short-duration treatment with dexamethasone.[197]

Pulmonary hypertension complicates approximately 37% of BPD/CLD cases and results in a fourfold increase in mortality rate.[426] Use of phosphodiesterase inhibitors, such as sildenafil, to treat the pulmonary hypertension and pulmonary artery pressure of BPD/CLD is being studied. In a retrospective review 21 infants with BPD-associated pulmonary hypertension were treated with oral

---

*References 40, 194, 207, 215, 297, 320, 404, 430.

sildenafil to determine the effects of sildenafil on gas exchange.[290] Although sildenafil decreased pulmonary artery pressure, there was no corresponding improvement in gas exchange in the 48 hours after treatment. Chronic sildenafil therapy for BPD-associated pulmonary hypertension should be done cautiously, awaiting clinical studies and adequate evidence.[141,290,426]

Complications. Complications of CLD/BPD are most common in the smallest, sickest infants (Box 23-11).

Acute Respiratory Diseases

RESPIRATORY DISTRESS SYNDROME

Pathophysiology. RDS is a disease of immature lung anatomy and physiology. Anatomically, the preterm lung cannot support oxygenation and ventilation, because alveolar saccules are insufficiently developed, causing a deficient surface area for gas exchange. Also, the pulmonary capillary bed is deficient and the interstitial mesenchyme is present to a greater extent, increasing the distance between the alveolar and the endothelial cell membranes.

Physiologically, the volume of surfactant is insufficient to prevent collapse of unstable alveoli. Because the alveoli collapse with each breath, normal functional residual capacity (FRC) is not established. Because of alveolar collapse, oxygenation and ventilation are insufficient and each breath requires increased energy output.

Compliance is related to the volume achieved during a given application of pressure. Compliance of the lung is equal to the ratio of the change in volume to the change in pressure. The lung in RDS has low compliance (i.e., little change in volume is achieved with a relatively great application of pressure), thereby contributing to increased work of breathing. However, the chest wall of the neonate unfortunately is very compliant; a slight application of pressure results in a large change in volume. The infant may not be able to create enough inspiratory pressure to open the alveoli as the chest wall retracts and collapses about the relatively stiff lung. Thus in RDS, the diaphragm contracts, creating an inspiratory pressure that moves less volume into the lung than expected and simultaneously causes large sternal and intercostal retractions of the chest wall.

BOX 23-11 COMPLICATIONS OF CHRONIC LUNG DISEASE/BRONCHOPULMONARY DYSPLASIA

Increased Mortality
Increased Morbidity
Pulmonary
- *Acute:* pulmonary interstitial emphysema, air leaks, pulmonary hypertension, cyst formation
- *Chronic:* altered pulmonary function, pulmonary hypertension, respiratory infections, rehospitalizations, home oxygen

Cardiac
- Cor pulmonale and right-sided heart failure

Growth Restriction
- Somatic growth (weight)
- Head growth

Orthopedic
- Fractures, rickets

Neurodevelopmental Delay
- Cognitive impairment/impaired intelligence/increased need for special education services
- Cerebral palsy/delays in gross motor skills
- Behavior/attention/school problems
- Cerebral ventriculomegaly

Sensory Deficits
- Sensorineural hearing loss
- Increased severity (stage 3) retinopathy of prematurity

Gene Expression[307]
- Alteration of gene expression—nearly 10%

Long-Term Effects of Steroid Use
- See Box 23-10

The increased effort of these opposing forces usually results in hypoxemia and acidemia, which cause constriction of the pulmonary vascular (arterial) musculature, severely limiting pulmonary capillary blood flow. The integrity of pulmonary capillary blood flow is critical for the integrity of the alveolar epithelial membrane and the production of surfactant. Without adequate pulmonary capillary blood flow, the type II pneumocytes become deficient in the precursor material necessary for production of surfactant. Lack of surfactant production compounds the deficiency and leads to low compliance. These physiologic factors (surfactant deficiency and decreased lung compliance) promote increased work of breathing, fatigue, atelectasis, reduced FRC, and ventilation-perfusion (V/Q) mismatch.

In the fetus, pulmonary vascular resistance is high and pulmonary artery blood pressure is greater than systemic blood pressure, causing blood flow from the main pulmonary artery to travel through the open ductus arteriosus to the descending aorta. A second right-to-left shunt occurs across the foramen ovale in the fetus. The high pulmonary vascular resistance is "reactive" to the normal fetal "hypoxemia," because the pulmonary vascular resistance and the pulmonary artery blood pressure decrease as the PaO_2 of the neonate increases. At birth, the ductus arteriosus actively constricts in response to the increase in PaO_2 (PaO_2 greater than 50 mm Hg), eliminating blood flow across the ductus and completing the transition to neonatal circulation.

The fetal circulatory pattern may persist from birth or be initiated by a transient hypoxemic episode. In the instance of neonatal hypoxemia, the pulmonary vasculature "reacts" by vasoconstriction, raising pulmonary vascular resistance, and the ductus arteriosus "reacts" by relaxing, once again allowing blood flow from the pulmonary artery to the descending aorta, as normally occurs in the fetus. Pulmonary vascular resistance is increased with shunting through the ductus arteriosus. Fetal circulatory patterns are perpetuated by hypoxemia and acidemia and produce systemic hypoxemia that aggravates and perpetuates the condition.

Endothelial damage and alveolar necrosis aggravate the already existing surfactant deficiency. A cyclic deterioration is established, and hypoxia and acidosis persist unless treatment is initiated.

Microscopically, the events that occur in the lung include injury to and death of the alveolar epithelial cells and airway epithelial cells. This injury and death are followed by sloughing of the cells from the respiratory basement membrane, leaving the basement membrane denuded, followed by exudation of serum. Fibrin in the serum clots and hyaline membranes are formed, covering the denuded basement membranes in the airways and alveolar spaces.

If there is sufficient hypoxic damage to the cells and basement membranes, frank hemorrhage may fill the alveolar spaces. These factors decrease the total surface area of the gas exchange membrane. The end result is hypoxemia, acidemia, and increasing respiratory distress.

The entire sequence of events in RDS is related to the inability to maintain lung expansion and alveolar stability as a result of surfactant deficiency. RDS evolves from two interrelated problems: atelectasis and persistence of pulmonary hypertension (Figures 23-4 and 23-5).

Etiology. RDS occurs in infants born prematurely and is a consequence of immature lung anatomy and physiology. In premature or stressed infants, atelectasis from the collapse of the terminal alveoli resulting from lack of surfactant appears after the first few hours of life. In a premature infant, surfactant production is limited and stores are quickly depleted. Surfactant production may be further diminished by other unfavorable conditions such as high oxygen concentration, poor pulmonary drainage, excessive pulmonary hygiene, or effects of respirator management.

Data Collection

History. A history of prematurity, cesarean section, or asphyxial episodes may be seen in infants with RDS. In one study, elective cesarean section at "term" (i.e., 34 weeks' gestation or older) resulted in infants of 37 to 38 weeks' gestation being 120 times more likely to have surfactant deficiency requiring ventilatory support than those born at 39 to 41 weeks. Recommendations include only using delivery by elective induction or elective cesarean section at 39 weeks' gestation (see Chapter 5).

Physical Examination. Infants with RDS are often tachypneic and demonstrate grunting, nasal flaring, and chest retractions within the first few minutes to hours of life. Pallor or cyanosis also may be present. The trachea is midline, and the apical pulse is normal. Auscultation of the chest reveals decreased breath sounds and often rales. Many of these infants may be hypotensive with prolonged capillary refill.

Laboratory Data. Chest x-ray findings in RDS include (1) reduced lung volume, (2) air bronchograms, (3) reticulogranularity, and (4) lung opacification. Surfactant deficiency results

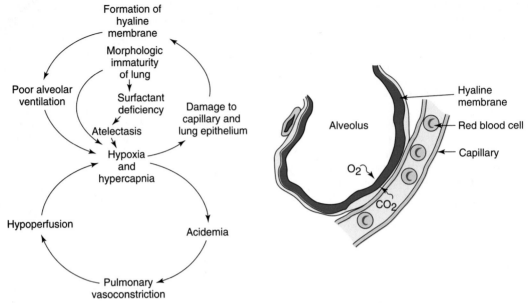

FIGURE 23-4 Interdependent relationship of factors involved in pathology of respiratory distress syndrome. (From Pierog SH, Ferrara A: *Medical care of the sick newborn,* ed 2, St Louis, 1976, Mosby.)

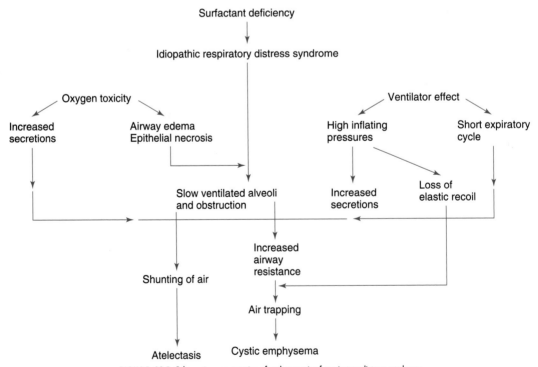

FIGURE 23-5 Schematic representation of pathogenesis of respiratory distress syndrome.

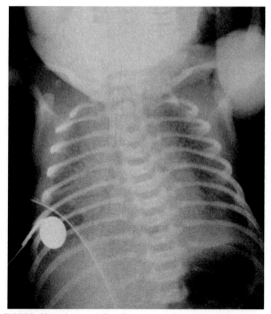

FIGURE 23-6 Chest x-ray film of a preterm infant (27 weeks' gestation) with respiratory distress syndrome. Note characteristic infiltrate pattern with air bronchograms.

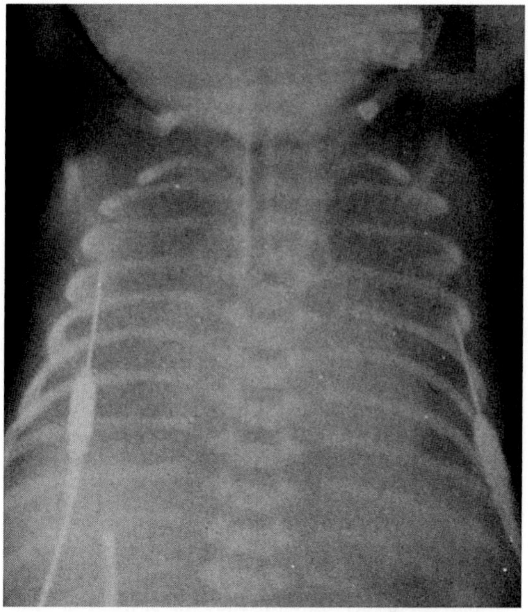

FIGURE 23-7 Chest x-ray film of a preterm infant (28 weeks' gestation) with severe respiratory distress syndrome. Note "whiteout" appearance.

in diffuse atelectasis, a reduction in lung volume, and decreased lung expansion as demonstrated on x-ray examination. Atelectasis increases lung density and results in visible outlines of air-filled bronchi (e.g., air bronchograms) against opaque lung tissue. Chest x-ray examination also reveals a ground-glass appearance that represents areas of atelectatic respiratory alveoli adjacent to expanded or even hyperexpanded respiratory units. This bilateral reticulogranular pattern is uniformly distributed throughout the lung fields and may also contain air bronchograms (Figure 23-6). Diffuse opacification caused by (1) nonexpanded alveoli with little or no terminal airway aeration, (2) pulmonary edema, or (3) pulmonary hemorrhage results in loss of visible heart borders, with a "whiteout" appearance on chest x-ray films (Figure 23-7). Lung ultrasound has been shown to have sensitivity (95.6%) and specificity (94.4%) in diagnosing both RDS and TTN.[423]

Arterial blood gases reveal hypoxemia and often acidemia that may be metabolic, respiratory, or a combination of both (see Chapter 8).

Prevention. A single course of antenatal steroids decreases the incidence and severity of RDS, comorbid conditions (e.g., NEC, intracranial hemorrhage, CLD), and mortality in infants of less than 32 weeks' gestation. Even a partial course appears to be beneficial.[281]

Prophylactic use of surfactant in animal studies is associated with more uniform and homogeneous distribution when administered to a fluid-filled lung.[358] Delayed surfactant administration (even by 15 minutes after the onset of assisted ventilation) may offset the benefits of surfactant.[358] Before the routine use of NCPAP initially after birth, prophylactic use of surfactant was associated with lower mortality rate, less air leak, and less BPD/CLD than rescue use of surfactant. After routine use of NCPAP, the benefits of prophylactic surfactant were no longer demonstrated.[336,394]

Treatment

Surfactant Replacement Therapy. Because surfactant deficiency is the primary abnormality of RDS, the development of an effective clinical strategy for administering exogenous surface-active material to premature infants was the focus of research efforts for many years. Administration of surfactant leads to the following[374,387,421]:

- Reduction in surface tension
- Dramatic and rapid improvement in gas exchange
- Decreased need for high levels of supplemental oxygen and ventilatory support
- Less barotrauma
- Improved chest x-ray findings because of improved lung compliance and lung volume

The use of lower levels of ventilatory support decreases the mortality rate and the incidence of pneumothorax. However, surfactant administration does not fully correct lung abnormalities of the VLBW infant with RDS.[212]

Optimal clinical strategies—the type of surfactant to use, the timing and method of administration, and the number of doses—affect surfactant safety and efficacy.[374,387] Several studies have documented the safety and efficacy of INSURE (i.e., INtubation, early SURfactant therapy, followed by Extubation to nasal CPAP) in preterms of varying gestational ages.[151,335,387] Prophylactic surfactant and rapid extubation to NCPAP is associated with a higher risk of mortality and BPD/CLD compared with early NCPAP and selective surfactant use.[129,336] Therefore there is no benefit of the INSURE strategy when early NCPAP is used[129,336] as recommended in the AAP respiratory support and surfactant therapy guidelines.[9,315]

Numerous studies comparing surfactants have documented more rapid improvement in respiratory status, decreased incidence of pneumothorax, lower mortality rates, improved survival, and less ROP and CLD/BPD with natural than with synthetic surfactant.[136] Use of animal-derived surfactants entails the risks of infection, immunogenicity, proinflammatory mediators, and variability of concentration of active ingredients in different aliquots. A next-generation synthetic surfactant, lucinactant, has been developed and is as safe and effective as the natural surfactants without the potential risks (Table 23-11). This synthetic surfactant contains a peptide, sinapultide, that mimics surfactant protein B (SP-B) and its effects on lung tissue. An RCT of lucinactant use in infants with acute hypoxic respiratory failure found that it was safe, improved oxygenation, and reduced the need for retreatment.[406] Outcomes of preterms treated with synthetic versus natural surfactant are equivalent.[276,306]

Various methods of surfactant administration have been studied, with bolus injection improving the homogeneous distribution of surfactant in lungs compared with slow injection or ultrasonic nebulization. Instilling surfactant, without endotracheal intubation, through a fine catheter inserted into the trachea of spontaneously breathing preterms on CPAP has been shown to reduce the number of mechanical ventilator days, without an effect on other neonatal outcomes in some studies and lower rates of IVH, death, PVL, BPD/CLD, and ROP in other studies.[102,159,206,225]

Aerosolized surfactant therapy may prevent the need for intubation. Pilot studies showing clinical efficacy despite low total administered dose, enhanced pulmonary distribution, and cost-effectiveness need to be confirmed in RCTs.[3,309] In addition, optimal delivery route (i.e., mask, nasal prongs, nasolaryngeal or nasopharyngeal), dose and redosing intervals need to be determined.[309] Laryngeal mask surfactant administration to preterms with established RDS is associated with a reduction in oxygen requirements; adequately powered trials are necessary to determine laryngeal mask safety and efficacy.[2] There is a potential for the new synthetic surfactant (i.e., lucinactant) to be available in a formulation for nasal or nasopharyngeal aerosolization or nebulization, thus avoiding intubation and mechanical ventilation.

Rapid bolus injection has been associated with alteration in CBF (which may increase the risk for IVH).[351] A study of bolus administration showed no alteration in CBF (with careful attention to FiO$_2$ and pressures); however, alterations in CBF were related to changes in mean systolic blood pressure.[289] Repeated doses of surfactant increase survival, decrease mortality, and decrease incidence of pneumothorax.[374] Long-term outcome studies of preterm infants who have received surfactant therapy show no significant effects on the rates of neurologic, developmental, behavioral, medical, or educational outcomes.[315]

Methods of resuscitation, types of ventilators (NCPAP vs. CMV vs. HFOV),[387] and ventilation style[387] (e.g., as few as six large tidal volume breaths in a surfactant-deficient lung causes lung injury)[195] also contribute to lung injury resulting in BPD/CLD. Use of noninvasive ventilation strategies benefits the preterm lung. The first study of SNIPPV as the primary method of respiratory

TABLE 23-11 SURFACTANT REPLACEMENT THERAPY

DRUG/SOURCE	INDICATIONS	ADMINISTRATION AND DOSAGE	ADVERSE EVENTS
Beractant* (Survanta) Exogenous surfactant from bovine lung extract	Prophylaxis and treatment ("rescue") of RDS in preterm infants; significantly reduces the incidence of RDS, mortality, and air leak complications[376] Prophylaxis: In preterm infants <1250 g BW or with evidence of surfactant deficiency, give as soon as possible, preferably within 15 min of birth Rescue: To treat infants with RDS confirmed by x-ray examination and requiring mechanical ventilation, given within the first 12 hours after birth[315]	Administration: For intratracheal administration only; instillation through a 5-Fr end-hole catheter inserted into the infant's ETT and/or via a thin catheter during spontaneous breathing or on NCPAP[102,103,159,206,225] above the infant's carina; each dose is 100 mg of phospholipids/kg BW (4 ml/kg; 100 mg/kg); four doses can be administered in the first 48 hr of life; give doses no more frequently than every 12 hr (unless surfactant is being inactivated by blood, meconium, or an infectious process[315]); repeat doses are based on the infant's BW	The most commonly reported adverse experiences are associated with the dosage procedure: transient bradycardia, oxygen desaturation, alterations in BP, drug reflux
Poractant alpha* (Curosurf) Modified porcine-derived minced lung extract	Prophylaxis and treatment ("rescue") of RDS in preterm infants	For *intratracheal* administration, see above Dosage: *Initial dose:* 2.5 ml/kg divided into aliquots *Subsequent dose:* Up to two doses of 1.25 ml/kg/dose given 12 hr apart, if needed Meta-analysis of 200 mg/kg of poractant versus 100 mg/kg of beractant found reduction in mortality rate with higher dose of poractant[368]	As for beractant
Calfactant* (Infasurf) Natural surfactant extracted from calf lung lavage	Prophylaxis and treatment ("rescue") of RDS in preterm infants	Administration: For *intratracheal* administration, see above Dosage: *Initial dose:* 3 ml/kg (105 mg/kg) divided into two aliquots *Subsequent dose:* Up to three doses of 3 ml/kg/dose given 12 hr apart, if needed	As for beractant
Lucinactant (Surfaxin) Synthetic surfactant containing a peptide, sinapultide, that mimics surfactant protein B (SP-B)[278]	Prophylaxis and treatment ("rescue") of RDS in preterm infants	For *intratracheal* administration, see procedure for beractant Dosage: *Initial dose:* 5.8 ml/kg (175 mg/kg) dosing q 6 hr based on clinical response Gels when stored at 4° C; requires up to 15 min of warming at 44° C in a heating block to liquefy; rapidly cools to body temperature when removed from heating block	As for beractant

BP, Blood pressure; *BW*, birth weight; *C*, centigrade; *ETT*, endotracheal tube; *RDS*, respiratory distress syndrome.

*Use of bovine and porcine products may be objectionable to persons of Jewish, Islamic, and/or Hindu beliefs; informed consent from parents is essential.

BOX 23-12	RECOMMENDATIONS FOR SURFACTANT REPLACEMENT THERAPY[315]

- Initiate NCPAP at birth as an alternative to routine intubation and early/prophylactic surfactant therapy.[9]
- Combine early NCPAP with selective surfactant therapy in extremely preterm infants.[9]
- Preterm infants <30 weeks' gestation who require mechanical ventilation for severe RDS should be given surfactant after initial stabilization.
- Rescue surfactant may be considered when respiratory failure is due to secondary surfactant deficiency occurring with meconium aspiration syndrome, sepsis, pneumonia, or pulmonary hemorrhage.
- Nursery and transport professionals with experience in administering surfactant and managing multisystem illness should care for preterm and term neonates receiving surfactant.
- Providers inexperienced with surfactant administration and managing multisystem illness should wait for transport team to arrive.

BOX 23-13	TREATMENT FOR RESPIRATORY DISTRESS SYNDROME

1. Reducing hypoxemia (see General Treatment Strategies in this chapter and in Chapter 8)
   a. Maintain in thermoneutral environment (see Chapter 6)
   b. Maintain blood pressure and hematocrit (see Chapters 5 and 20)
   c. Decrease stimuli from the neonatal intensive care environment (see Chapter 13)
   d. Recognize and relieve pain or agitation (see Chapter 12)
2. Correcting acidemia (see Chapter 8)
3. Increase the functional residual capacity (see General Treatment Strategies)
   a. Maintain appropriate temperature (see Chapter 6)
   b. Monitor vital signs and arterial blood gases (see Chapters 7 and 8)
   c. Provide appropriate fluid, electrolytes, glucose, and calories (see Unit Three)
   d. Observe for complications of disease and treatments (see General Complications)
4. Monitoring for complications (see Acute Complications and Chronic Complications under General Complications)
5. Care for parents (see Chapters 29, 30, and 32)
6. Prepare for discharge and follow-up care (see Chapter 31)

support for RDS compared the outcomes of 600- to 1250-g preterms who were randomized to CMV or SNIPPV after their initial dose of surfactant.[46] Only 20% of the preterms receiving SNIPPV versus 52% receiving CMV had the primary outcome of BPD/CLD/death with no difference in the groups on mental/psychomotor indices.[47] Two more recent studies showed benefits of NIPPV compared with NCPAP: (1) reduced need for and duration of invasive mechanical ventilation and incidence of BPD[324] and (2) an equal rate of survival to 36 weeks' postmenstrual age without BPD/CLD.[224] Other outcomes, such as air leaks, NEC, length of respiratory support, and time to full enteral feedings, also did not differ between the groups.[224]

Recommendations for surfactant replacement therapy for RDS are outlined in Box 23-12. Surfactant preparations are commercially available as (1) organic solvent extract of minced bovine lung, (2) artificial or synthetic surfactant, (3) modified porcine-derived minced lung extract, and (4) natural surfactant extracted from calf lung by lavage. Table 23-11 summarizes the commercially available products for surfactant replacement. Other treatment is directed toward the indications in Box 23-13.

Inositol Therapy. Inositol, an essential nutrient, promotes maturation of several components of surfactant. A systematic review of inositol supplementation for RDS found significant reductions in (1) CLD/BPD, (2) mortality, (3) ROP, and (4) grade III to grade IV IVH with no increase in sepsis or NEC.[193] A multicenter RCT to confirm these findings is recommended.[193]

Inhaled Nitric Oxide Therapy. Inhaled nitric oxide (iNO) therapy not only is a selective pulmonary vasodilator but also improves oxygenation by redirecting blood from poorly aerated (atelectatic) and diseased lung (with RDS) regions to better aerated distal air spaces.[221] Early RCTs of iNO in late preterm infants found improved oxygenation, decreased need for mechanical ventilation, improved survival without increase in IVH, and a trend toward a decrease in CLD/BPD.[282] Several studies of preterms with moderate RDS demonstrated that iNO reduced the combined endpoint of death and CLD.[222,355] However, more recent meta-analyses,[15,35] NIH Consensus panel,[80] and AAP clinical report[236] on use of iNO in preterm infants found no improvement in (1) survival of preterms with respiratory failure, (2) incidence of BPD/CLD, (3) severe IVH, (4) neurodevelopmental outcomes,[130,392] or (5) pulmonary outcomes.[236] Therefore inhaled nitric oxide is not recommended for use in preterm infants (see Table 23-17).

PULMONARY INSUFFICIENCY OF THE NEWBORN

Pulmonary insufficiency continues to be a diagnosis used in term newborns demonstrating respiratory symptoms soon after delivery. This condition was first described as the insufficiency of gas exchange commonly caused by atelectasis of the lung, congenital abnormalities, and in infants with aspiration syndrome.[43] Additionally, another group of respiratory diseases caused by the development of hyaline membranes were described as HMD[57] and later referred to as RDS. With HMD/RDS, the neonate is generally observed to be normal with good respiratory effort for up to several hours after delivery, when progressive dyspnea occurs, and is predominantly a disease of the term infant. Respiratory distress is a major cause of death in early neonatal life.

Pathophysiology. This is a condition of term infants and consists of the insufficiency of gas exchange secondary to atelectasis, congenital anomalies, or aspiration syndrome.

Etiology. These infants are often term or near term and born with adequate respiratory effort. Within minutes to a few hours after delivery they decline, requiring supplemental oxygen support.

Data Collection
History. Near or term infants who usually start with normal Apgar scores and then decline within minutes to a few hours after delivery.

Physical Examination. Evidence for respiratory distress, including tachypnea, mild retractions, grunting, and flaring, may be seen. Cyanosis in room air also may be present.

Laboratory Data. Mild hypoxemia (requiring less than 40% oxygen) and mild acidemia are usually present.

Treatment. In general, support of the neonate with pulmonary insufficiency requires only the provision of sufficient supplemental oxygen to maintain an arterial oxygen tension of more than 70 to 80 mm Hg and maintenance of usual supportive neonatal care. These infants are often discharged on low-flow oxygen until respiratory status improves.

TRANSIENT TACHYPNEA OF THE NEWBORN (RESPIRATORY DISTRESS SYNDROME TYPE 2)

Pathophysiology. TTN is the result of delayed reabsorption of normal lung fluid, and thus an alternative name is *wet lung syndrome,* or *RDS type 2.* Lung fluid accumulates in the peribronchiolar lymphatics and the bronchovascular spaces. Thus TTN is an "obstructive" lung disease, whereas RDS is a "restrictive" lung disease. Abnormalities in lung function of neonates with TTN include high total ventilation, high breathing frequency, low tidal volume, high dead space, prolonged nitrogen clearance, and low dynamic compliance. Reabsorption of lung fluid occurs by the following: (1) lung liquid production slows; (2) pulmonary epithelium changes from chloride-secreting to sodium-absorbing barrier; (3) air intake at birth shifts fluid from alveoli to interstitium and perivascular spaces; and (4) a higher protein content and osmotic pressure of blood/lymph facilitates flow of lung fluid.

Etiology. TTN generally occurs in term or late-preterm infants with a history of cesarean section (especially elective section in the late-preterm infant—see Chapter 5), low Apgar scores, pulmonary artery hypertension, poor left ventricular function, lower umbilical artery pH (less than 7.25), and precipitous delivery.[26,117,214] In these situations, there is a lack of the gradual compression of the chest that eliminates some fluid during a normal vaginal delivery. Accumulation of interstitial fluid interferes with the forces that hold the bronchioli open, causing collapse and air trapping. In term infants with TTN decreased surfactant function may also contribute to TTN, as well as a prolonged course.[256]

Data Collection
History. Term or late-preterm male infants with a history of cesarean section, precipitous delivery, prenatal exposure to methamphetamine, or other abnormalities of labor and transition are predisposed to TTN.[117] Onset is usually 2 to 6 hours after birth. At initial presentation TTN has a similar presentation as pneumonia. However, the presence of perinatal infectious agents is more common in pneumonia and the course of pneumonia is for a longer period of time and with more support (i.e., oxygen and ventilation).[93]

Physical Examination. Evidence for respiratory distress, including tachypnea, mild retractions, grunting, and flaring, may be seen. Cyanosis in room air also may be present.

Laboratory Data. Mild hypoxemia (requiring less than 40% oxygen) and mild acidemia are usually present. A significant degree of hypoxemia or acidemia tends to constrict the pulmonary vasculature and aggravate the problem. Lower umbilical cord levels of cortisol, adrenocorticotropic hormone, and free triiodothyronine, as well as a higher epinephrine level, have been found in neonates developing TTN who were delivered by cesarean section.[19]

Chest x-ray examination reveals hyperexpansion with streaky infiltrates radiating from the hilum. These infiltrates are thought to represent interstitial fluid along the bronchovascular spaces. Air trapping causes the appearance of mild to moderate hyperaeration or inflation on the chest radiograph. Visible fluid in the pulmonary fissures and cardiomegaly also may be seen on chest radiograph.

Use of lung sonography in infants with TTN shows a difference in echogenicity between the upper and lower lung fields—specifically the presence of comet-tail artifacts ("double lung point") in the inferior lung fields.[90] Lung ultrasound shows a high sensitivity (95.6%) and specificity (96.5%) in diagnosing TTN and RDS.[423]

Treatment. In general, support of the neonate with TTN requires only provision of sufficient supplemental oxygen to maintain an arterial oxygen tension of more than 70 to 80 mm Hg and maintenance of usual supportive neonatal care. Usually little more than general support is necessary while the normal absorption of lung fluid through the lymphatics takes place. As the lung fluid clears, both the x-ray abnormalities and clinical presentation resolve within 72 hours. Use of the nasal route for CPAP or mechanical ventilation is well tolerated and effective.[114,128]

Although diuretic agents have been advocated, a recent Cochrane systematic review found no benefit and recommends against use of oral or intravenous furosemide for treatment of TTN.[210] Use of empiric antibiotics in infants with TTN who do not have risk factors for infection is not warranted.[342,431] Mild fluid restriction was found in a recent pilot study to decrease the duration of respiratory support, the length of stay, and hospital costs.[391] One small study of 40 neonates with TTN found a shorter duration of supplemental oxygen and use of empiric antibiotics with inhaled albuterol therapy, with no adverse effects.[220]

Complications. TTN is independently and significantly associated with the development of childhood wheezing and asthma, especially in male infants.[50,248]

MECONIUM ASPIRATION SYNDROME

Pathophysiology. Before meconium aspiration can occur, meconium must find its way into the amniotic fluid. A hypoxic event before birth stimulates intestinal peristalsis and relaxation of the anal sphincter. Colonic peristalsis ensues, resulting in the expelling of meconium into the amniotic fluid and, in severe cases, gasping in utero that leads to meconium aspiration. Respirations after birth draw meconium first into major airways and subsequently into the smaller airways, causing obstruction, atelectasis, air trapping, and pneumothorax. Meconium can also cause chemical pneumonitis and inactivation of surfactant, further impairing gas exchange and potentiating barotrauma. This condition occurs more often in term or postterm infants when a hypoxic episode is experienced in utero.[420] These movements open the glottis so that meconium flows into the oropharynx and on into the lung. Thus the pathophysiology of lung disease in meconium aspiration syndrome (MAS) is related to the mechanisms causing fetal stress, as well as the direct adverse effects of meconium in the lung. MAS is a common reason for lung disease in neonates.

Etiology. Meconium aspiration produces disease by several mechanisms: (1) meconium physically obstructs the glottis, trachea, or any number of smaller airways, resulting in atelectasis, air trapping, alveolar collapse, and ventilation–perfusion mismatching; (2) it promotes an inflammatory response known as *chemical pneumonitis;* (3) it contains increased levels of secreted phospholipase A_2 that promote inflammation[338]; (4) it inhibits surfactant function; and (5) it increases pulmonary vascular resistance, caused by asphyxial episodes, resulting in increased right-to-left shunting and the development of PPHN (Figure 23-8).[152] Of the 8% to 19% of infants born through meconium-stained amniotic fluid, 2% to 33% develop MAS.[152] A more recent population-based study from France found the rate of

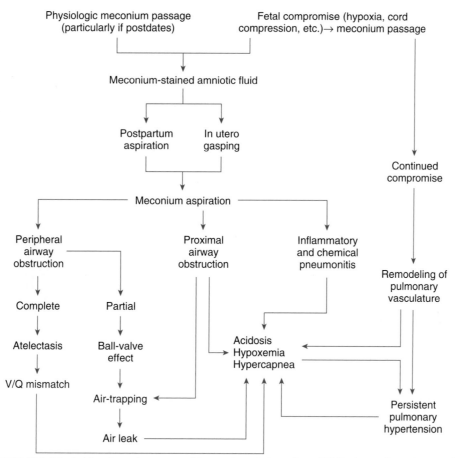

FIGURE 23-8 Pathophysiology of meconium passage and the meconium aspiration syndrome. *V/Q,* Ventilation-perfusion. (From Wiswell T, Bent R: Meconium staining and the meconium aspiration syndrome: unresolved issues, *Pediatr Clin North Am* 40[5]:957, 1993.)

infants born through meconium-stained fluid to be 7.93%, with severe MAS occurring in 0.067% of the overall population.[146]

Prevention. Before an infant is born, meconium aspiration may be prevented by early recognition of the compromised fetus, elective induction for pregnancy at greater than or equal to 41 weeks' gestation, aggressive management of abnormal fetal heart rate patterns, and fewer infants with low Apgar scores.[395] Amnioinfusion does not reduce the risk for moderate-to-severe MAS or perinatal death and is not recommended to prevent MAS.[189]

A large multicenter (i.e., 12-hospital) RCT of intrapartum oropharyngeal or nasopharyngeal suctioning for term infants born through meconium-stained amniotic fluid showed no significant difference in the incidence of MAS (e.g., 4% for both the suction and the no-suction group), the need for mechanical ventilation, mortality rate, duration of oxygen use, days of ventilation, and length of stay.[418] The study conclusion, that routine suctioning does not prevent MAS, has resulted in revision of present recommendations for care of these infants (see Chapter 4). Routine tracheal suction is recommended *only* for depressed infants (e.g., nonvigorous infants with depressed tone and respirations and/or heart rate less than 100 beats/min) and those with respiratory symptoms.[418,420] An interdisciplinary health care team for "rapid response" prepared and credentialed (e.g., NRP) for management of the neonate born through meconium-stained amniotic fluid, coupled with interdisciplinary postnatal assessment, observation, and prompt treatment, is recommended for prevention of MAS and its associated morbidity and mortality risks.[49]

Use of orogastric suctioning and chest physiotherapy to prevent MAS is not supported by evidence from any studies.

Data Collection

History. A history of asphyxia, intrauterine growth restriction (IUGR), postterm delivery, meconium-stained amniotic fluid, thick meconium, nonreassuring fetal heart tracing, fetal tachycardia, low Apgar scores (less than or equal to 3 at 1 minute; less than 5 at 5 minutes), and African American race may be present.[146,188,371,379] There is a positive association between chorioamnionitis or infection and the passage of meconium at term gestation.[412] Maternal risk factors associated with placental insufficiency (e.g., hypertension, pregnancy-induced hypertension, chronic respiratory/cardiovascular disease, diabetes, IUGR, heavy cigarette smoking, drug use, and postterm pregnancy) may also lead to fetal asphyxia and meconium passage.[434]

Physical Examination. Tachypnea, rales, and cyanosis are seen in mild cases. Respiratory distress occurs in 33.4% of infants born through meconium-stained amniotic fluid and 25.9% are MAS.[371] Respiratory distress occurs within 12 hours in 97.9% and is severe in 21.7% of cases.[371] In moderately severe cases, grunting, retractions, and nasal flaring also may be seen. In severe cases, the infant is asphyxiated and severely depressed at birth. There is profound cyanosis and pallor, irregular gasping respirations, and an increased anteroposterior diameter of the chest (a barrel chest) as a result of gas trapping and alveolar overdistention.

Laboratory Data. The chest x-ray examination shows marked air trapping, hyperexpansion, and hyperinflation. There are bilateral, diffuse, coarse, patchy infiltrates (Figure 23-9). Complete occlusion by debris results in atelectatic areas. Air leaks are frequently seen. Pleural effusion may occur as a result of the inflammatory process in the lung. Cardiomegaly may be present; this results from intrauterine asphyxia or cardiac hypoxia.

Severe hypoxemia and hypercapnia as a result of ventilation-perfusion mismatching

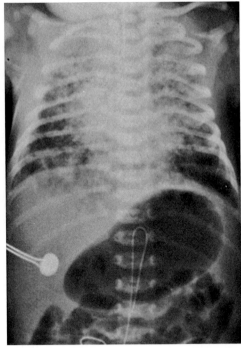

FIGURE 23-9 Chest x-ray film of infant with meconium aspiration. Note diffuse infiltrates.

and right-to-left shunting caused by pulmonary hypertension are present. Severe acidosis usually is combined respiratory and metabolic acidosis. Infants with MAS have elevated serum cytokines and chemokines.[291]

A small study ($n = 15$) using spectrophotometric analysis of umbilical cords found significantly higher absorption peaks in cords of infants with meconium-stained amniotic fluid and MAS.[415] The researchers concluded that this technology may be useful in identifying infants with MAS and meconium-stained fluid.

Treatment. Hypoxemia is the major problem in meconium aspiration, and treatment should be directed at improving oxygenation. Mildly affected infants will frequently require only warmed, humidified oxygen by hood. Increasing severity of meconium aspiration will require increased levels of intervention. About 30% to 50% of infants with MAS require CPAP or mechanical ventilation.[102] Some infants respond to CPAP (4 to 6 cm H_2O), but others require full ventilator support. Because these infants are usually term or

TABLE 23-12	DRUGS FOR PARALYZATION	
DRUG	**DOSAGE**	**COMMENTS**
Pancuronium (Pavulon)	0.1 mg/kg IV push (0.04-0.15 mg/kg) q 1-2 hr based on duration of paralysis Onset: 1-2 min	*Indications:* paralysis for mechanical ventilation to improve oxygenation/ventilation; reduce barotrauma and alteration in cerebral blood flow Although paralyzed, neonate still feels pain—analgesia necessary for painful procedures and to accompany paralysis (see Chapter 12) *Adverse effects:* corneal drying (lubricate eyes); tachycardia; increased salivation; blood pressure changes (hypotension and hypertension) Reversed by: Neostigmine: 0.04-0.08 mg/kg IV Atropine: 0.02 mg/kg
Vecuronium	0.1 mg/kg IV push (0.03-0.15 mg/kg) q 1-2 hr based on duration of paralysis Onset: 1-2 min	*Indications:* same as above *Adverse effects:* corneal drying (lubricate eyes); decreases in heart rate and blood pressure when used with narcotics; special sensitivity in preterms (that diminishes with age); duration of effect prolonged in preterms *Reversed by:* same as above

postterm, they resist assisted ventilation and may require paralyzation (Table 23-12), sedation, and/or analgesia (see Chapter 12) to ventilate and oxygenate the lungs adequately. With paralysis, these infants may require rapid rates, high peak inspiratory pressure, and PEEP for adequate oxygenation and ventilation. Even though the majority of MAS infants are able to be treated with CPAP and CMV, use of other treatment modalities (e.g., HFV, iNO, ECMO/ECLS) may become necessary with accompanying PPHN and severe respiratory failure.[102]

Meconium in the lung inhibits surfactant function in a dose-dependent manner. To decrease surfactant inactivation in MAS, the following is recommended: (1) aspirate meconium from the airway and lungs to decrease the amount that interacts with surfactant in the alveoli, (2) provide surfactant replacement at a sufficient dose to replace inactivated endogenous surfactant and repeat as necessary, and (3) combine surfactant replacement with antiinflammatory drugs to reduce meconium-induced inflammation.[268,269] Studies of surfactant replacement to infants with MAS suggest improvement in some neonates with severe respiratory failure and MAS. Improved oxygenation/ventilation, decreased severity of respiratory compromise, no increase in air leaks, and less use of ECMO have been observed in

some studies.[136] Variable study results of surfactant use in MAS may result from timing, type, amount, and method of surfactant administration. Animal studies of surfactant replacement in MAS show that a combination of glucocorticoid and surfactant therapies improved gaseous exchange and was longer-lasting than surfactant alone[266] and that a synthetic surfactant is as efficient as porcine surfactant in treating MAS.[343]

Surfactant lavage has been shown to result in (1) improved oxygenation/ventilation and pulmonary function measurements (e.g., increased lung compliance and decrease in airway resistance), (2) earlier weaning from assisted ventilation, (3) need for less oxygen, (4) less mortality and use of ECMO, and (5) more rapid weaning of mean airway pressure.[72,104,231] Recovery of lung lavage fluid is associated with lower MAP at 24 hours and shorter duration of respiratory support and should be a priority in the lavage procedure.[105] Complications of lung lavage include hypoxemia (transient or severe) and no alterations in heart rate and blood pressure or systemic hypotension.[104] A systematic review of studies of lavage with diluted surfactant found some benefit in the composite outcomes of death or use of ECMO; more studies are needed.[172] Surfactant lavage remains an experimental therapy.

Mucosal irritation and increased mucosal secretion hamper respiratory and mucociliary clearance efforts. Frequent pulmonary hygiene (every 2 to 3 hours) may help alleviate this problem.

As with any sick infant, close attention must be given to physiologic support and homeostasis. (See General Treatment Strategies earlier in this chapter; see also Chapters 6, 7, and 8 and Unit Three.)

Complications. Use of new treatments has decreased the mortality rate to less than 5%.[420] Persistent pulmonary hypertension frequently complicates MAS, potentiates the difficulties in oxygenation, and contributes to a large portion of the mortality associated with MAS.[152] Air leaks are complications of both the disease (ball-valve obstruction causing air trapping) and the treatment. Infants with MAS are at increased risk for adverse neurologic outcomes (e.g., CP and global delays)[38] and long-term pulmonary problems (e.g., increased airway reactivity, abnormal pulmonary function).[449] A recent study found elevated aspartate aminotransferase levels in infants with MAS at birth who eventually have poor neurodevelopmental outcomes.[68] These researchers recommend early intervention to improve the neurodevelopmental outcomes of those MAS infants with high levels of aspartate aminotransferase at birth.[68]

NEONATAL PNEUMONIA

Neonatal pneumonia occurs perinatally or postnatally in about 1% of term neonates and 10% of preterm neonates, and may be as high as 28% for ventilated ELBW infants in the NICU.[41] Neonates requiring prolonged hospitalization in the NICU are at risk for developing pneumonia from nosocomially acquired organisms. The organisms most often causing neonatal pneumonia are mainly group B streptococci and gram-negative organisms (e.g., *Escherichia coli, Klebsiella, Pseudomonas,* and *Serratia marcescens*) but also include *Staphylococcus aureus, Staphylococcus epidermidis, Streptococcus pneumoniae,* and *Candida.* Less commonly acquired viral infections include herpes, cytomegalovirus, varicella–zoster, and syphilis. Community-acquired viral infections also occur in the NICU setting and include respiratory syncytial virus, enterovirus, adenovirus, and parainfluenza virus infections (Table 23-13).[41]

Pathophysiology. In bacterial pneumonia, alveoli are often more edematous and inflamed than in viral infections. Protein-rich fluid may partially or completely fill the alveoli. This is often followed by an influx of polymorphonuclear leukocytes and red blood cells. Macrophages enter the alveoli and remove intraalveolar debris, restoring normal lung functioning.[75] *S. aureus* and *Klebsiella* organisms often cause severe damage to alveoli and often destroy lung tissue by causing necrosis of the septum between the alveoli. In some cases, abscesses form.

Viruses and *Mycoplasma* organisms also may be acquired transplacentally, during the delivery, or postnatally. Viral and mycoplasmal pneumonias commonly involve the bronchi and peribronchial interstitium more often than the alveoli. Viral and mycoplasmal organisms cause loss of epithelial ciliary appendages and sloughing into the airways. This results in stasis of mucus and secretions and bronchial obstruction with atelectasis. A secondary inflammatory response is characterized by mononuclear infiltration into the submucosa and perivascular areas causing narrowing of the airway lumen. Another response to this inflammatory process is smooth muscle constriction, which leads to increased airway obstruction and bronchospasm. In severe cases of viral and mycoplasmal infection, the inflammatory process involves the alveoli.

Fungal infections, the most common being *Candida* infection, may be acquired in utero, during the birth process, or in the postnatal period. Congenitally acquired pneumonia can be diffuse resulting from the inflammatory process at birth. *Candida* often invades the pharynx and larynx and may produce a thick layer of hyphae that lines the upper and lower respiratory tract. Ulceration of the pharynx, larynx, and the lower respiratory tract can occur.

Etiology. Predisposing factors that lead to the development of neonatal infections and pneumonia include, in part, the immaturity of the immune system, colonization of the mother's genital and vaginal tracts with pathogens, amnionitis, prolonged rupture of membranes, prematurity requiring intubation and assisted ventilation, and nosocomial infections acquired in the NICU.[41] Bacterial pneumonia can be secondary to the spread of pathogens from the mother to the baby in utero.[93] Pneumonia acquired in utero often leads to stillbirth and premature delivery.

Neonates who require NICU care are at particularly high risk for colonization of their upper respiratory tract with pathogenic organisms and

T A B L E 23-13	ETIOLOGIC FACTORS AND CHEST X-RAY FINDINGS IN NEONATAL PNEUMONIA

CAUSATIVE AGENT	CHEST X-RAY FINDINGS
Bacterial	
Group B beta-hemolytic streptococci (GBS)	Diffuse reticulogranular pattern, opacity ("whiteout"), patchy infiltrates, and pleural effusion
Streptococcus pneumoniae	Patchy infiltrates (lobar), pleural effusion
Staphylococcus aureus	Diffuse infiltrates; pneumatocele
Methicillin-resistant *Staphylococcus aureus* (MRSA)	Diffuse infiltrates; abscess formation
Staphylococcus epidermidis	Hazy lung fields; infiltrates
Listeria monocytogenes	Bilateral patchy infiltrates
Escherichia coli	Lobular consolidation; pneumatocele
Klebsiella	Bilateral consolidation; lung abscess, pneumatocele
Pseudomonas and *Serratia*	Parenchymal consolidation (patchy or basilar); pneumatocele
Haemophilus influenzae	Nonspecific; x-ray findings similar to those of GBS (above) or respiratory distress syndrome
Viral	
Herpes virus	Perihilar infiltrates; streaky, lobar consolidation; pleural effusion (late onset)
Cytomegalovirus	Nonspecific, perihilar streaking; hazy lung fields; infiltrates; opacification
Rubella virus	Interstitial infiltrates; hazy lung fields
Respiratory syncytial virus	Hyperexpansion; patchy consolidation
Adenovirus, enterovirus	Hyperexpansion; patchy consolidation
Fungal	
Candida albicans	Diffuse granularity; coarse infiltrates; opacification
Mycoplasma	
Ureaplasma urealyticum	Fine reticular pattern progressing to opacification and consolidation
Mycoplasma hominis	Diffuse reticular pattern, opacity, and pleural effusion
Other	
Treponema pallidum (syphilis)	Diffuse opacification; consolidation
Chlamydia trachomatis	Hyperinflation; streaky infiltrates
Pneumocystis jiroveci (formerly *carinii*)	Diffuse haziness; granularity; opacity

Modified from Carey B, Trotter C: Neonatal pneumonia, *Neonatal Netw* 19:46, 2000.

the passage of pathogens from caregivers or contaminated equipment.[65] *Ventilator-associated pneumonia* (VAP), a nosocomial-acquired infection in a neonate who has been ventilated for longer than 48 hours, occurs from 1.4 to 7 episodes per 1000 ventilator-days in developed countries to 16 to 89 episodes per 1000 ventilator-days in developing countries.[65] Risk factors for VAP include (1) prematurity, (2) LBW/VLBW/ELBW, (3) reintubation, and (4) prolonged duration of mechanical ventilation.[23,41,65,399] Most causative agents of VAP are gram-negative bacteria (i.e., *E. coli*, *Klebsiella*, and *Pseudomonas*), followed by gram-positive organisms (i.e., *S. aureus*) and fungi (i.e., candida).[4,23,64]

Prevention. Prevention begins with identifying mothers at risk for infection (e.g., group B *Streptococcus* [GBS], herpes, chlamydial infection, syphilis, gonorrhea); early management of infections with antibiotic therapy; meticulous equipment disinfection and hand hygiene practices (handwashing/alcohol-based hand sanitizers) by health care providers in the NICU[334]; and restricting the entry of *anyone* with respiratory infections into the NICU (see Chapter 22).

Rapid extubation and use of noninvasive ventilator strategies prevents and reduces the incidence of VAP.[65,284] Prophylactic use of probiotics prevents sepsis in the NICU[259] and may also prevent neonatal VAP.[65] An RCT of 60 intubated infants (half in supine position and the other half in side-lying) investigated whether positioning would decrease VAP. Despite no significant difference in the number of positive tracheal cultures after 2 days, after 5 days, cultures were positive in 87% of the supine versus 30% of the side-lying group.[7] In developing countries, initiation of multidimensional infection control strategies has resulted in reduction of VAP rates.[339,451] There is no evidence to support interventions used in adults (e.g., head-of-bed elevation and oral care) as preventive of VAP in neonates.[65]

Data Collection

History. The clinical presentation of neonatal pneumonia varies, depending on the infecting organism and the incidence of acquisition. Acute respiratory distress is frequently seen in intrauterine and intrapartally acquired secondary infections. Neonates with pneumonia often have a history of low Apgar scores, temperature instability, and poor tone and activity. The clinical signs and symptoms of pneumonia are similar to those of respiratory distress, TTN (RDS type II)/retained lung fluid, or sepsis. Late-acquired pneumonia may have a gradual or abrupt onset, depending on the organism. Infants with chlamydial pneumonia frequently present with a characteristic staccato cough.

Physical Examination. The infant with pneumonia often presents with respiratory distress (e.g., tachypnea, low pulse oximetry readings, respiratory deterioration, apnea, temperature instability, hypoglycemia). The signs and symptoms of pneumonia often are nonspecific and difficult to differentiate from other neonatal respiratory problems without the aid of chest x-ray evaluation. VAP results in an increase in the volume and character of secretions (i.e., purulent mucus) suctioned from the ETT.[64,65] Many NICU infants with viral respiratory tract infections are asymptomatic.[41]

Laboratory Data. The appearance of pneumonia varies depending on the duration of infection, cause of the pneumonia, and presence of underlying respiratory disease (e.g., RDS, BPD). Serial x-ray films are more valuable than one isolated x-ray examination in making the diagnosis and following the course of the disease. Infiltration patterns on chest x-ray films include lobar consolidation; patchy alveolar infiltrates; hilar and peribronchial infiltrates; reticulogranular, nodular, or miliary infiltrates; and hazy or opaque lungs (see Table 23-13). Lung ultrasound has been shown to be a reliable diagnostic tool in neonatal pneumonia.[253]

Tracheal aspiration and blood culture also are useful tools in identifying the organisms of pneumonia. A workup for sepsis is often part of the diagnostic evaluation for these neonates (see Chapter 22).

Treatment. Treatment of neonatal pneumonia includes supportive care (e.g., thermoregulation, nutrition, oxygenation, ventilation if necessary, and parenteral support). If the causative agent is bacterial, antibiotic therapy must be instituted after a sepsis workup; if viral, an antiviral agent is considered; if fungal, an antifungal agent is used (see Chapter 22). Neonatal pneumonia may be accompanied by surfactant inactivation; use of rescue surfactant for respiratory failure accompanying neonatal pneumonia may be considered (see Box 23-12). Early use of surfactant in pneumonia is associated with lower risk of mortality and use of ECMO.[231]

Complications. The mortality rate for perinatally acquired pneumonia is variable but has been estimated at 20%, with a higher mortality rate (50%) for postnatally acquired pneumonia. In a recent review of perinatally acquired neonatal infections, the overall mortality rate for pneumonia was 10%.[65] The decline in mortality rate is the result of perinatal antibiotic use. VAP in the NICU results in longer length of stay, higher cost, and higher mortality rate.[65]

PERSISTENT PULMONARY HYPERTENSION OF THE NEWBORN

PPHN manifests as severe pulmonary hypertension with pulmonary artery pressure elevation to levels equal to systemic pressure or higher and large right-to-left shunts through the foramen ovale and the ductus arteriosus. PPHN manifests early in life: 77% of cases are diagnosed in the first 24 hours of life, 93% in the first 48 hours, and 97% by 72 hours of age. The incidence of PPHN is 2 to 6 in 1000 live births and complicates one third of infants with moderate to severe CLD/BPD.[383]

Pathophysiology. Once the placental blood source is severed, adequate oxygenation of the newborn depends on inflation of the lungs, closure of the fetal shunts, a decrease in pulmonary vascular resistance, and an increase in pulmonary blood flow (an eight-fold to tenfold increase at the first breath). Normally, pulmonary vascular resistance decreases with the first breath of life. When it remains high, successful transition from fetal to neonatal circulation is impaired. In an infant manifesting PPHN, high pulmonary vascular resistance and pulmonary hypertension impede pulmonary blood flow. Factors that increase and decrease pulmonary vascular resistance are listed in Table 23-14.

Increased PVR leads to hypoxemia, acidemia, hypercarbia, and eventually lactic acidosis. The pulmonary arterioles respond to this process with further constriction, promoting an additional decrease in blood flow; thus a cyclic pattern is established.[383] Pulmonary vascular resistance also maintains higher right-sided pressures in the heart that equal or exceed systemic pressures, resulting in right-to-left shunting, which is characteristic of PPHN. PPHN also produces direct and indirect effects on myocardial function. A combination of pressure alterations, hypoxia, and acidemia leads to a cyclic pattern of decreased cardiac output, decreased pulmonary blood flow, and further vasoconstriction (Figure 23-10).

Etiology. Pulmonary vascular resistance (PVR) remains high after birth because of underdevelopment, maldevelopment, or maladaptation of pulmonary vasculature (Table 23-15). In utero, development of increased vascular smooth muscle or perinatal factors that cause or contribute to vasospasm are thought to be prime mechanisms of PPHN. Independent predictors of pulmonary hypertension in the preterm infant include (1) low Apgar scores, (2) preterm premature rupture of membranes (PPROM), (3) oligohydramnios, (4) pulmonary hypoplasia, and (5) sepsis.[238]

TABLE 23-14	FACTORS THAT ALTER PULMONARY VASCULAR RESISTANCE (PVR)	
LOWERS PVR	**INCREASES PVR**
Endogenous mediators and mechanisms:	Endogenous mediators and mechanisms:
Oxygen	Hypoxia
Nitric oxide	Acidosis
PGI_2, PGE_2, PGD_2	Endothelin-1
Adenosine, ATP, magnesium	Leukotrienes
Bradykinin	Thromboxanes
Atrial natriuretic factor	Platelet-activating factor
Alkalosis	Ca^{2+} channel activation
K^+ channel activation	Alpha-adrenergic stimulation
Histamine	$PGF_{2\alpha}$
Vagal nerve stimulation	
Acetylcholine	
Beta-adrenergic stimulation	
Mechanical factors:	Mechanical factors
Lung infection	Overinflation or underinflation
Vascular cell structural changes	Excessive muscularization, vascular remodeling
Interstitial fluid and pressure changes	Altered mechanical properties of smooth muscle
Shear stress	Pulmonary hypoplasia
	Alveolar capillary dysplasia
	Pulmonary thromboemboli
	Main pulmonary artery distention
	Ventricular dysfunction, venous hypertension

From Kinsella J, Abman S: Recent developments in the pathophysiology and treatment of PPHN, *J Pediatr* 126:855, 1995.
ATP, Adenosine triphosphate; *$PGF_{2\alpha}$,* prostaglandin $F_{2\alpha}$; *PGI_2, PGE_2, PGD_2,* prostaglandins I_2, E_2, and D_2; *PVR,* pulmonary vascular resistance.

Prevention. Prevention of PPHN includes minimizing intrauterine and perinatal risk factors when possible, maintaining postnatal physiologic homeostasis, and detecting and correcting any underlying abnormality.

Data Collection

History. In addition to the risk factors listed in Table 23-15, maternal tobacco use, maternal obesity, premature rupture of membranes, maternal lack of private or use of public insurance, cesarean delivery, late-preterm or postterm birth, LGA

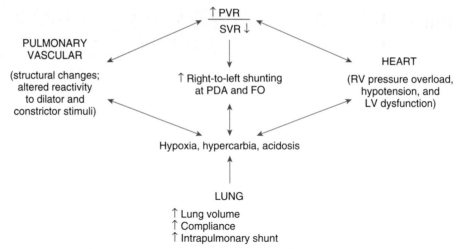

FIGURE 23-10 Cardiopulmonary interactions in persistent pulmonary hypertension of the newborn. *FO,* Foramen ovale; *LV,* left ventricle; *PDA,* patent ductus arteriosus; *PVR,* pulmonary vascular resistance; *RV,* right ventricle; *SVR,* systemic vascular resistance. (From Kinsella J, Abman S: Recent developments in the pathophysiology and treatment of PPHN, *J Pediatr* 126:855, 1995.)

infant, race (black, Asian), maternal diabetes, and maternal asthma are associated with an increased risk for PPHN.[184]

There are two major considerations in the history of these infants: (1) the recognition of major disease processes or syndromes that are highly associated with pulmonary hypertension and (2) the timing of the onset of cyanosis and the deterioration of the infant.

Physical Examination. The initial clinical presentation is usually a late-preterm (34 weeks' gestational age or greater), term, or postterm infant with worsening cyanosis within the first 24 hours of life. Tachypnea is a common finding and, when accompanied by retractions, is indicative of decreased pulmonary compliance. Cyanosis may be either intense at birth or progressively worsen in association with increased right-to-left shunting.

Despite increasing FiO_2, the infant continues to have low PaO_2 (hypoxemia) as a result of right-to-left shunting. Milder cases of PPHN feature minimal tachypnea and cyanosis, frequently associated with stress from crying or feeding. Severe cases are characterized by marked cyanosis, tachypnea, low systemic blood pressure, and decreased peripheral perfusion.

Increased pulmonary artery pressure results in the following signs:
- Pulmonic systolic ejection clicks
- A second heart sound that is single, loud, or narrowly split with a loud pulmonary component
- A prominent right ventricular impulse that is visible or palpable at the lower left sternal border
- A soft systolic murmur in the pulmonary area

Laboratory Data. The laboratory evaluation of an infant with suspected PPHN should include a complete blood count (CBC) with differential, platelet count, chest x-ray examination, and serum glucose, calcium, electrolytes, and arterial blood gas determinations. The CBC is used to detect anemia, which could contribute to systemic hypertension; detect polycythemia, which could lead to increased pulmonary vascular resistance; and detect an infectious process such as group B streptococcal sepsis or pneumonia.

Arterial blood gases demonstrate acidosis, hypoxia, and increased $PaCO_2$. If blood gas specimens are obtained simultaneously in the right radial artery (preductal) and the descending aorta (postductal), the right-to-left shunt can be documented (preductal PaO_2 greater than postductal). Simultaneous preductal and postductal pulse oximetry or transcutaneous oxygen measurements may also be useful in the diagnosis. Other diagnostic tests are outlined in Table 23-16.

The most common chest x-ray findings associated with PPHN include the following:
- Prominent main pulmonary artery segment
- Mild to moderate cardiomegaly
- Variable pulmonary vasculature (increased, decreased, or normal)

TABLE 23-15	CRITICAL FINDINGS ETIOLOGIC FACTORS IN PERSISTENT PULMONARY HYPERTENSION OF THE NEWBORN

DEVELOPMENTAL PROCESS	PATHOPHYSIOLOGY	ASSOCIATED CONDITIONS
Underdevelopment, a decreased number of pulmonary vessels	Interruption in lung development, resulting in shunting of blood because of fewer pulmonary vessels and less area for gaseous exchange	Pulmonary hypoplasia (e.g., diaphragmatic hernia, premature rupture of membranes, oligohydramnios, Potter syndrome)
Maldevelopment, abnormally developed pulmonary vessels	Hypertrophy of musculature and extension into nonmuscularized arteries resulting in smaller lumen size, which increases PVR	Intrauterine asphyxia/hypoxia, MAS, and maternal smoking Intrauterine fetal ductus arteriosus closure increases pulmonary blood flow Congenital heart defects that result in abnormal pulmonary vessel formation (TAPVR, pulmonary vein stenosis)
Maladaptation (from intrauterine to extrauterine life) as a result of transient or persistent vasoconstriction	Results in remodeling and abnormal muscularization of small pulmonary arteries Results in pulmonary vasospasm and vascular remodeling	Hypoxia/acidosis/asphyxia Asphyxia may result in persistent vasospasm Pulmonary parenchymal disease (RDS, MAS, pneumonia, TTN, surfactant protein B deficiency)
	Pulmonary vasospasm and decreased cardiac output resulting from release of endotoxins and reaction to systemic inflammatory response	Bacterial sepsis Prenatal pulmonary hypertension (e.g., fetal systemic hypertension or premature closure of the ductus arteriosus) associated with maternal ingestion of NSAIDs (e.g., ibuprofen, naproxen, indomethacin), salicylates, phenytoin, lithium, prostaglandin inhibitors, or SSRIs (absolute risk <1%)[218,294]
	Prevents normal circulatory transition at delivery	Delayed or ineffective resuscitation, narcosis, other central nervous system depression, hypothermia, hypotension
	Potentiation of vasoconstriction	Hypothermia, hypoglycemia, hypocalcemia, acidosis, hypoxia, myocardial dysfunction, and ischemia
	Functional obstruction of pulmonary vascular bed	Polycythemia, hyperviscosity

Data from VanMarter L: Persistent pulmonary hypertension of the newborn. In Cloherty J, Stark A, editors: *Manual of neonatal care*, ed 4, Philadelphia, 1998, Lippincott-Raven; Weardon M, Hansen T: Persistent pulmonary hypertension of the newborn. In Hansen T, Cooper T, Weisman L, editors: *Contemporary diagnosis and management of neonatal respiratory diseases*, ed 2, Newton, Pa, 1998, Handbook of Health Care; Steinhorn RH: Diagnosis and treatment of pulmonary hypertension in infancy, *Early Hum Dev* 89:865, 2013.

MAS, Meconium aspiration syndrome; *NSAIDs*, nonsteroidal antiinflammatory drugs; *PVR*, pulmonary vascular resistance; *RDS*, respiratory distress syndrome; *SSRI*, selective serotonin reuptake inhibitors; *TAPVR*, total anomalous pulmonary venous return; *TTN*, transient tachypnea of the newborn.

- Signs of left ventricular dysfunction that include pulmonary venous congestion and cardiomegaly

The ECG is usually normal but may demonstrate right ventricular hypertrophy, evidence of pulmonary hypertension, and signs of myocardial ischemia. Echocardiography is essential in (1) evaluating cardiac structures, (2) ruling out cyanotic cardiac lesions, (3) diagnosing the right-to-left shunting at the foramen ovale and/or ductus arteriosus, (4) estimating pulmonary artery pressure, (5) determining therapy, and (6) evaluating response to therapy.[221]

Treatment. Historically, treatment of PPHN included hyperventilation, IV infusions (e.g., systemic vasodilators, sedatives, narcotics, paralysis, alkali, and inotropes), surfactant administration, high–frequency ventilation, and ultimately ECMO/ECLS as a last resort, and in limited neonatal centers. These treatments were widely used without RCTs to test safety and efficacy, and none of these treatments improved survival in infants with PPHN.

Treatment of PPHN focuses on preventing or intervening in the development of the cyclic pattern illustrated in Figure 23-10. Goals of current therapy include (1) treating associated pathology (e.g., antibiotics for sepsis/pneumonia; partial exchange transfusion for polycythemia/hyperviscosity; volume expanders), (2) providing adequate oxygenation, (3) reducing PVR by pulmonary vasodilation that improves pulmonary blood flow, (4) increasing and maintaining systemic vascular resistance (SVR) (e.g., systemic blood pressure), and (5) preventing right-to-left shunting by decreasing PVR and increasing SVR. Pulmonary blood flow should increase if PVR is decreased or if SVR is increased.[383,384]

Adequate Oxygenation. Maintaining adequate oxygenation is a prime goal of care of infants with PPHN; alterations in "routine" care and handling

are essential. Because handling a sick newborn for *any* reason causes a fall in PaO_2, the benefits of handling for routine care such as changing linens, weighing, suctioning, and taking vital signs must be balanced against the risk for iatrogenic hypoxia. PaO_2 variations in the newborn are as follows[98,138]:

- At rest: ±15 mm Hg variation
- While crying: ↓PaO_2 by as much as 50 mm Hg
- With routine care: ↓PaO_2 by as much as 30 mm Hg

Maintaining organized, coordinated care and minimizing disturbances are therefore very important. Keeping the infant calm is important because severe hypoxia accompanies crying. Using pacifiers and decreasing noxious stimuli (e.g., invasive procedures) keep struggling and crying to a minimum. Continuously monitoring vital signs, blood pressure, and pulse oximetry decreases the need for physical manipulation and disturbance. These large, vigorous infants require sedation and analgesia (see Chapter 12) or paralysis (see Table 23-12) to promote effective oxygenation and ventilation and decrease air leaks.

Ventilation Therapy. Use of conventional mechanical ventilation to produce hypocarbia (↓$PaCO_2$) and respiratory alkalosis is no longer used due to the effects resulting from (1) adverse neurologic sequelae (e.g., CP and cystic PVL); (2) exposure of the lung to barotrauma/volutrauma, CLD/BPD, and air leaks; (3) the increased risk of sensorineural hearing loss; and (4) no improvement in the clinical outcomes of PPHN.[101,395]

HFV, both oscillator and jet, is used to treat PPHN. Use of HFOV optimizes lung inflation and oxygenation, improves ventilation, and achieves respiratory alkalosis. HFOV is an effective rescue treatment for some neonates meeting ECMO/ECLS criteria who were unresponsive to CMV.[78] A discussion of the combination of HFOV and inhaled nitric oxide follows. A Cochrane review of the use of HFJV compared with CMV in preterms with severe pulmonary dysfunction found no difference in mortality rates or adverse events in a small study done before widespread use of early surfactant or antenatal steroids.[201]

Inhaled Nitric Oxide (iNO). Endogenous NO production dilates the fetal pulmonary vascular bed and is essential in decreasing PVR after birth.[84] Because endogenous production of NO in the pulmonary

T A B L E 23-16	DIAGNOSTIC TESTS FOR PERSISTENT PULMONARY HYPERTENSION OF THE NEWBORN (PPHN)	
TEST	**USE**
Hyperoxia test	If PO_2 does not increase in 100% oxygen, a right-to-left shunt is demonstrated (may be secondary to either PPHN or congenital heart defect)
Comparison of preductal and postductal arterial PaO_2	Demonstrates ductal shunting; if negative, it does not rule out PPHN; most infants with congenital heart disease have no ductal shunting
Contrast echocardiography "bubble echo"	Demonstrates foramen ovale shunting but should be present in most cases of PPHN
Hyperoxia-hyperventilation	Most definite test; if PO_2 <50 mm Hg prehyperventilation and rises above 100 mm Hg is almost always PPHN

From Duara S, Gewitz MH, Fox WW: Use of mechanical ventilation for clinical management of persistent pulmonary hypertension of the newborn, *Clin Perinatol* 11:641, 1984.

vasculature of neonates with PPHN is reduced, treatment with iNO is beneficial because iNO is a selective pulmonary vasodilator (e.g., decreases pulmonary hypertension and increases oxygenation without reducing systemic blood pressure).[221] Early clinical studies of iNO demonstrated brief exposure actually improved oxygenation and lowered pulmonary artery pressure. RCTs from multicenters have confirmed that prolonged iNO treatment for PPHN (1) results in sustained improvement of oxygenation,[142,282] (2) decreases the need for ECMO/ECLS treatment,[282] (3) is an adjunct to CMV,[282] and (4) combined therapy (e.g., iNO, HFOV) is more effective than either therapy alone. The Neonatal Inhaled Nitric Oxide Study Group (NINOSG)[283] found that iNO had no effect on mortality rate, length of stay, number of days of ventilatory support, incidence of air leak, CLD/BPD, IVH/PVL, seizures, and pulmonary and GI

hemorrhages. Use of iNO for PPHN is associated with severe coagulopathies.[401] The effectiveness of iNO depends on (1) the initial degree of pulmonary vasoconstriction and hypoxemia, (2) the severity of parenchymal lung disease, and (3) the recruitment of adequate lung volume/inflation that decreases intrapulmonary shunting and improves iNO delivery to the pulmonary system.[221] In the ECMO/ECLS population, iNO use has increased from 0% to 24%.

Inhaled NO is an effective treatment for PPHN but "should be considered a part of the overall clinical strategy that cautiously manages parenchymal lung disease, cardiac performance, and systemic hemodynamics."[221] Inhaled NO has been approved by the U.S. Food and Drug Administration for treatment of near-term (greater than 34 weeks' gestational age) and term neonates with PPHN. Recommendations for use of iNO are listed in Table 23-17. Use of iNO in moderate

TABLE 23-17 RECOMMENDATIONS FOR USE OF INHALED NITRIC OXIDE (iNO)

RECOMMENDATION	RESEARCH BASIS
Gestational Age	
≥34 weeks' gestation	Clinical trials,[78a,282] Canadian Pediatric Society,[300] and FDA approval support use of iNO in late-preterm/term newborns.[221]
≤34 weeks' gestation	Clinical data do not support use of iNO for early routine, early rescue, or later rescue therapy in preterm infants.[15,35,80,236]
Postnatal Age	
Within the first week of life; postnatal age alone should not define the duration of therapy when prolonged therapy could be beneficial	Clinical trials support iNO use within the first week of life; may also be used as adjunct therapy after ECMO/ECLS treatment.
Severity of Illness	
Oxygenation index (OI) = (MAP × Fio_2 × 100 ÷ Pao_2) >25 with echocardiographic evidence of extrapulmonary right-to-left shunting	Mean OI in multicenter trials was 40. Earlier use of iNO at lower OI (15-25) has not resulted in reduction of mortality, ECMO/ECLS use, or outcomes.[232,384] Delayed use (OI >40) increases length of supplemental oxygen use.[158]
Dose	
Initial: 20 ppm in term newborns with PPHN Brief exposure to 40-80 ppm is safe Sustained treatment with 80 ppm increases the risk for methemoglobinemia	Increasing dose to 40-80 ppm does not improve response to 20 ppm. Initial treatment with low dose (1-2 ppm) does not compromise responses to higher doses (10-20 ppm); a majority of low doses require dose increases. The lowest effective starting dose has not been determined.
Duration	
Typically <5 days	Longer usage may be necessary in pulmonary hypoplasia. For therapy >5 days, other causes of pulmonary hypertension should be investigated.

Continued

TABLE 23-17	RECOMMENDATIONS FOR USE OF INHALED NITRIC OXIDE (iNO) — cont'd

RECOMMENDATION	RESEARCH BASIS
Weaning and Discontinuation Differing approaches toward weaning have been studied with few differences in outcomes until iNO is discontinued: After 4 hours at 20 ppm, iNO reduced to 6 ppm without change in oxygenation iNO decreased by 20% increments in stepwise fashion to dose of 1 ppm before discontinuation	Withdrawal of iNO can be associated with life-threatening elevations in PVR, profound oxygen desaturation, and systemic hypotension because of decreased cardiac output. Dose-response relationship between iNO given and a drop in Pao_2. A decrease in iNO to 1 ppm before discontinuation minimizes decrease in Pao_2, and compensatory changes in Fio_2 and ventilator parameters are unnecessary.
Ventilator Management High-frequency oscillatory ventilation (HFOV) With significant parenchymal lung disease	Inadequate lung inflation results in less response to iNO therapy. Combination of HFOV and iNO results in best improvement in oxygenation because of improved lung inflation during HFOV that augments response to iNO by reducing intrapulmonary shunting and improving iNO delivery to pulmonary circulation.
Without significant parenchymal lung disease	Combination of HFOV and iNO and iNO alone are more effective than HFOV alone.
Congenital Diaphragmatic Hernia Routine use in CDH not recommended	CDH infants are poor responders to iNO. Limited to CDH infants with suprasystemic PVR (after establishing optimal lung inflation and echocardiography determination of adequate LV function).
Late pulmonary hypertension in CDH infants	Late pulmonary hypertension is clinically evident when PVR becomes suprasystemic with right-to-left venoarterial admixture across the FO and/or ductus arteriosus measured on echocardiography.
Use in ECMO/ECLS Centers Use to stabilize before cannulation for ECMO Use of iNO has not adversely affected outcome by delaying ECMO	Lower mortality rate for iNO-treated group than for infants not treated with iNO.[76] iNO treatment associated with improved short-term pulmonary outcomes,[78a] and decreased ECMO use is not associated with increased late-term morbidity.[76,283]
Use in Non-ECMO/ECLS Centers and Transport with iNO If progressive deterioration in oxygenation occurs in centers without ECMO/ECLS, transport to ECMO/ECLS center without interruption of iNO therapy must be accomplished	Withdrawal of iNO to transport to an ECMO/ECLS center may result in acute and life-threatening deterioration.

Modified from Kinsella JP: Inhaled nitric oxide in the term neonate, *Early Hum Dev* 84:709, 2008. Data from Kinsella JP: Inhaled nitric oxide in the term neonate, *Early Hum Dev* 84:709, 2008. *CDH,* Congenital diaphragmatic hernia; *CLD/BPD,* chronic lung disease/bronchopulmonary dysplasia; *ECMO/ECLS,* extracorporeal membrane oxygenation/extracorporeal life support; *FDA,* Food and Drug Administration; *FO,* foramen ovale; *IVH,* intraventricular hemorrhage; *LV,* left ventricular; *NIH,* National Institutes of Health; *PPHN,* persistent pulmonary hypertension of the newborn; *PVR,* pulmonary vascular resistance.

PPHN improves oxygenation,[155] decreases the amount of ventilation needed, and prevents progression to severe PPHN. A retrospective study comparing the use of HFOV and HFJV with iNO found similar short-term effects of decreasing the need for ECMO and improving oxygenation and ventilation of infants with PPHN regardless of which type of ventilator was used.[79] A recent case report of iNO administration through a nasal cannula precluded the use of mechanical ventilation in a spontaneously breathing term infant with PPHN.[279]

Use of HFOV and iNO to treat PPHN has decreased the number of neonates meeting ECMO/ECLS criteria who subsequently require

TABLE 23-18	VASOPRESSOR RESPONSE IN THE NEONATE

DRUG DOSE	DISADVANTAGE
Dopamine	
<4 mcg/kg/min: renal vasodilation, mesenteric and cerebral vasodilation (effects unknown) plus increase in cardiac output	May decrease systemic arterial pressure
5-20 mcg/kg/min: increase in cardiac output depending on myocardial norepinephrine	Loss of renal and mesenteric perfusion
>20 mcg/kg/min: systemic arterial pressure increases more than pulmonary artery pressure	Cardiac output may decrease Myocardial oxygen consumption increases Marked increase in left ventricular afterload Dysrhythmias noted
Dobutamine	
10 mcg/kg/min: increases cardiac contractility directly; cardiac output increases depending on myocardial catecholamine stores	No selective renal or mesenteric vasodilation Tends to increase skeletal blood flow at the expense of viscera Increase in pulmonary artery pressure
Isoproterenol	
0.05-1 mcg/kg/min: lowers pulmonary vascular resistance in pulmonary hypotensive and vascular disease in child and adult; lowers hypoxemia-induced pulmonary vascular resistance in animal models	Dysrhythmias No specific vasodilation effects
Nitroprusside	
0.4-5 mcg/kg/min: cardiac output increases because of decreased left ventricular afterload; systemic vascular resistance (indicated by blood pressure) decreases because of decreased left ventricular afterload	Systemic vascular resistance remains constant if CO_2 increases

Modified from Drummond W: The use of cardiotonic therapy in the management of infants with PPHN, *Clin Perinatol* 11:715, 1984.

ECMO/ECLS treatment, has shortened length of hospital stay, and has decreased costs.

Pharmacologic Therapy. Surfactant replacement therapy is used when significant parenchymal lung disease (e.g., MAS) is the cause of PPHN. Secondary surfactant deficiency also may exist in PPHN. Surfactant replacement in the early phase of PPHN significantly decreases the need for ECMO/ECLS in term newborns without increasing the risk for complications.[236] In term and late-preterm infants with hypoxic respiratory failure, early use of surfactant and iNO improves outcomes (less mortality and ECMO use).[231]

Use of inotropic support (e.g., vasopressors) (Table 23-18) increases SVR, which decreases right-to-left shunting through the foramen ovale and ductus arteriosus. Cardiac output, cardiac contractility, and systemic blood pressure are all increased. A small study of newborns (n = 18) treated with iNO for PPHN (but with symptoms of circulatory failure [despite adequate fluids]) showed that IV norepinephrine improved lung function by decreasing the ratio between pulmonary and systemic artery pressures and improving cardiac performance.[411]

Systemic vasodilators (e.g., tolazoline, sodium nitroprusside, prostaglandin E$_1$) have been used to decrease PVR. These medications have resulted in variable and unpredictable results and are associated with systemic hypotension, the need for volume expansion and fluid resuscitation, and an inability to achieve and maintain pulmonary vasodilation. When vasodilators are infused in dosages sufficient to decrease pulmonary hypertension, there is increased venous admixture as a result of right-to-left shunting of venous blood and pulmonary ventilation-perfusion mismatch. Because of these adverse effects, use of systemic vasodilators is no longer recommended.

From 40% to 50% of neonates do not respond to iNO therapy, so alternatives and synergistic agents are used for pulmonary vasodilation. The reason for nonresponse to iNO is unknown, but a recent retrospective review found that infants receiving iNO with blood group A were poorer responders than those with B or O blood groups.[135] In poor or partial response to iNO, the need for ECMO is able to be predicted after 72 hours of iNO therapy.[417]

Phosphodiesterase inhibitors are used as an alternative, as a supplement, or for weaning from iNO

in PPHN[262,263,275,384,385] (Table 23-19). In term and late preterm neonates with PPHN who are nonresponders or have a suboptimal response to iNO, use of IV milrinone results in improved clinical and ECMO changes.[262,263] Intravenous (IV) milrinone improves oxygenation without compromising systemic blood pressure.[262,263] Use of sildenafil (1) is as effective as iNO in improving pulmonary vasodilation, (2) assists weaning from iNO, (3) improves oxygenation, (4) may or may not decrease systemic blood pressure, (5) improves cardiac output, (6) is more effective when used together with iNO than either used separately, and (7) is safe, effective, and well tolerated with chronic use.[30,286,359,383,385] A recent trial of oral sildenafil and inhaled iloprost to treat 47 term neonates with PPHN found the iloprost to be effective, safe,

TABLE 23-19 PHOSPHODIESTRASE INHIBITOR THERAPY FOR PPHN

DRUG	DOSE	COMMENTS
Milrinone[263,316]	Loading dose: 50-75 mcg/kg over 60 min Maintenance dose: 0.33-0.99 mcg/kg/min for 24-72 hr Half-life: 4.1 hr Duration: 24-42 hr	Improves oxygenation (increased Pao$_2$) Reduces Fio$_2$ Decreases oxygen index, MAP, and iNO dose Lowers inotrope score Improves base deficit and plasma lactate levels Monitor: blood pressure for transient systolic hypotension; heart and respiratory rate and rhythm; assess COP; fluid/electrolytes and renal function; platelet counts for thrombocytopenia Used in suboptimal or nonresponders to iNO ECHO: Lowers PA pressure Better right-to-left ventricular function Less right-to-left shunting
Sildenafil*[359]	0.3-1 mg/kg/dose per OG tube every 6-12 hr Peak concentration: 30-120 min Bioavailability: 40% Loading dose: 0.4 mg/kg continuous IV over 3 hr[385] Maintenance dose: 1.5 mg/kg/day continuous IV infusion[385]	Pulmonary vasodilation as an alternate, supplement, or weaning agent from iNO. Concentrated in the presence of erythromycin, cimetidine, amlodipine Adverse effects: systemic hypotension, blood pressure lability, worsening oxygenation (decreased Pao$_2$)

ECHO, Echocardiogram; Fio$_2$, fraction of inspired oxygen concentration; iNO, inhaled nitric oxide; MAP, mean airway pressure; OG, orogastric; PA, pulmonary artery; PPHN, persistent pulmonary hypertension of the newborn.

*FDA issued a warning against the use of sildenafil for the treatment of pediatric pulmonary hypertension because of the higher risk of death with higher (3-6 mg/kg/day) versus lower doses (from US Food and Drug Administration. Revatio (sildenafil): drug safety communication—recommendation against use in children. Silver Spring, Md, 2012, US Food and Drug Administration. Accessed July 2, 2014); FDA issued a clarification of the 2012 warning stating that use of sildenafil in children may be warranted when the benefits outweigh the risks, when other treatment options are limited, and when use of sildenafil can be closely monitored. (From US Food and Drug Administration: Revatio (sildenafil): drug safety communication—FDA clarifies warning about pediatric use for pulmonary arterial hypertension. Silver Spring, Md, 2014, US Food and Drug Administration. Accessed July 2, 2014.)

inexpensive, and without hypotension as a side effect in the treated infants.[203] RCTs are needed to establish the safety, efficacy, side effects, and outcomes of sildenafil and milrinone use in PPHN; until then, use is experimental.[30,262,286,359,383]

Complications. Follow-up at 18 to 24 months of age of the neonates in the NINOSG trial found no increase in neurodevelopmental or behavioral abnormality; the children in the control group experienced a higher incidence of seizures after discharge than did the iNO-treated group.[283] Two other studies also showed no increase in adverse neurodevelopmental or pulmonary outcomes as a result of treatment with iNO and avoidance of ECMO treatment.[76,250] Other studies found high rates of neurodevelopmental impairment at 18 months of age[232] and a lower incidence of respiratory morbidity (26%) compared with the respiratory morbidity after ECMO treatment (37%) or CMV (56%).[191]

A recent follow-up study of 85 children (at 5 to 11 years of age) who had been treated for PPHN compared with a matched reference group found (1) sensorineural hearing loss (11%), (2) increase in chronic health problems (42% vs. 17%), (3) use of bronchodilators (21% vs. 8%), and (4) increased use of remedial education (19% vs. 5%).[137] Survivors of PPHN may have significant pulmonary and neurodevelopmental impairment whether treated with conventional methods or with ECMO/ECLS and should have long-term follow-up.

APNEA

Pathophysiology. The two major control mechanisms that regulate pulmonary ventilation are the neural and chemical systems. The cerebral cortex and brainstem are the governing agents for the neural control system, which regulates respiratory rate and rhythm. The peripheral components of this system are found in the upper airway and lung. The chemical control center is found in the medulla and is sensitive to changes in $Paco_2$. The peripheral portion of the chemical system lies in the carotid and aortic vessels and is sensitive to changes in $Paco_2$. Alveolar ventilation is controlled by the chemical system, and this system is the principal defense against hypoxia. Neonates have a unique response to hypoxemia and carbon dioxide retention. Unlike adults, who have sustained increase in ventilation to hypoxemia, infants have a brief period of increased ventilation followed by respiratory depression.

Carbon dioxide responsiveness is less developed in the preterm infant, which may be the result of decreased sensitivity in the chemical center or mechanical factors that prevent an increase in ventilation. Apnea is the cessation of breathing for 20 seconds or longer or cessation of breathing for 15 seconds with cyanosis and/or bradycardia. Apnea of prematurity or primary apnea is not associated with other specific disease entities. The younger the gestational age, the greater is the incidence of apnea, so at least 85% of preterms less than 34 weeks' gestation have apnea of prematurity.[353] Apnea and bradycardia episodes usually begin within the first week after birth and spontaneously resolve at 36 weeks of postmenstrual age.[308] In infants born at 27 weeks' gestation or earlier, 58% to 60% have persistent apnea at 36 weeks' postconceptual age.[133] Apnea may be associated with hypoxemia, neuronal immaturity, sleep, catecholamine deficiency, and respiratory muscle fatigue.

Etiology. Causes of apnea in the premature are characterized as *central apnea* (absence of breathing effort), *obstructive apnea* (breathing efforts occur but the airway is blocked), or, most commonly, *mixed apnea* (an initial central apnea followed by obstruction of the airway).[296] Various conditions may cause apnea in the premature infant by producing hypoxia and/or altering the sensitivity of peripheral or central chemoreceptors (Table 23-20). Neuronal immaturity is a plausible cause for apnea because respiratory efforts are more unstable at younger gestational ages. The decreased response appears to be the result of a general lack of dendritic formation and limited synaptic connections, thereby decreasing the excitatory drive. Another hypothesis is that apneic episodes are manifestations of synaptic disorders that occur without a motor component. Such phenomena have been confirmed on EEG. Infants depend on alternating excitation and inhibition to establish rhythmic breathing; therefore imbalances (e.g., hypoxia, hypoglycemia, hypocalcemia) may cause respiratory arrest.

Apnea is more frequent during sleep and especially during rapid eye movement (REM) or active sleep in both term and preterm infants.[410] Apnea associated with sleep becomes more significant in that premature infants, particularly those of less than 32 weeks' gestation, spend 80% of their time asleep. Equally significant is the time spent in REM sleep, the predominant sleep state of premature infants. Apnea is uncommon in non-REM

TABLE 23-20	CAUSES OF APNEA IN THE PREMATURE INFANT	

CAUSE	SPECIFICS
Infection	Pneumonia, sepsis, meningitis
Respiratory distress	Immaturity of respiratory development, RDS, airway obstruction, CPAP application, postextubation, congenital anomalies of the upper airways
Cardiovascular disorders	Patent ductus arteriosus, congestive heart failure
Gastrointestinal disorders	Vomiting, necrotizing enterocolitis, deglutition syncope
Central nervous system disorders	Depressant drugs, intraventricular hemorrhage, seizure, elevated bilirubin levels, bilirubin encephalopathy/kernicterus, infection, tumors/ischemia
Metabolic disorders	Hypoglycemia, hypocalcemia, hyponatremia/hypernatremia
Environmental	Rapid increase of environmental temperature, hypothermia, vigorous suctioning, feeding, stooling, stretching/movement; fatigue/stress, prenatal exposure to maternal cigarette smoking, position, sleep state (e.g., active vs. quiet) Pain* First immunization (DTP/IPV/Hib): increase in apnea, bradycardia, and desaturations within 72 hours of immunizations
Hematopoietic	Polycythemia, anemia

DTP, Diphtheria-tetanus-pertussis; *CPAP,* continuous positive airway pressure; *Hib,* Haemophilus influenzae type B; *IPV,* inactivated polio virus; *RDS,* respiratory distress syndrome.
*Oral sucrose relieves pain but does not decrease apnea and bradycardia.[208]

sleep, but periodic breathing may be observed. The effects of REM sleep are inhibition of spinal motor neurons, increase in brain activity causing increasing eye movements and muscular twitching, and changes in brain temperature and cerebral blood flow and CNS arousal, shown by EEG changes.

A premature infant has a more compliant chest cage and less compliant lungs, resulting in greater respiratory workload. Respiratory muscle fatigue occurs easily in the absence of fatigue-resistant fibers.

Secondary apnea may be associated with a particular disease entity or in response to special procedures. Many disorders leading to secondary apnea may exert their influence through hypoxemia and subsequent respiratory center depression.

The majority of cases of secondary apnea arise from four conditions. In RDS, apnea is related to the degree of parenchymal disease and may result from muscle fatigue. With CNS hemorrhage and seizures, apnea arises from asphyxia with subsequent hypoxemia and respiratory center depression or actual brain injury. Apnea is related to central depression in sepsis. In addition, carbon dioxide retention and hypoxemia associated with the left-to-right shunting of a PDA may cause apnea.

Iatrogenic causes of apnea include increased environmental temperature, sudden increases in environmental temperature, vagal response to suctioning of the nasopharynx or to a gavage tube, vomiting, and obstruction of the airway. Reflex apnea occurs when foreign material (milk or secretions) is present in the oropharynx. This laryngeal chemoreflex is protective in that it prevents inhalation of the substance into the airway and has been documented in preterm and hospitalized infants. Obstruction may occur from improper neck positioning or aspiration.

Cerebral blood flow (CBF) velocity decreases with apnea and bradycardia[301] and is directly correlated with the severity of bradycardia,[322] and an increase in CBF may occur on recovery.[254] Decreased oxygen saturation also correlates with the duration of apnea, regardless of type. Obstructive apnea is associated with significantly greater maximum fall in cerebral blood volume than central or mixed apneic episodes. Because alteration of CBF may cause or exacerbate IVH, obstruction of upper airways with resultant apneic episodes should be prevented.

Prevention. All infants assessed as being at high risk for apneic spells should be carefully monitored for at least 10 to 12 days. Impedance apnea monitors do not distinguish normal respiratory efforts from gasping movements associated with obstruction. Both heart and respiratory rates should be monitored. Alarm systems should be used at all times. A qualified observer is essential.

Apneic episodes are frequently associated with alterations in heart rate and oxygen saturation—the degree of these changes is related to the duration of apnea. Apnea generally precedes a drop in heart rate and oxygen desaturation. Changes in oxygen saturation are distinct from heart rate changes, so the desaturation cannot be predicted from changes in heart rate patterns. Because episodes of apnea and bradycardia are associated with a decrease in CBF and because oxygen desaturation (as little as 5% to 10%) is associated with alteration of cerebral circulation,[254] oxygen saturation monitoring should accompany cardiorespiratory monitoring (both in-hospital and home monitoring).

Pulse oximetry monitors may detect hypoxemic conditions that may lead to apneic spells. In a premature infant younger than 32 weeks' gestation, this type of apnea is common. Care should be organized to decrease stressful, hypoxic episodes.

Apneic episodes may be prevented or decreased by several means. Reducing environmental stress by providing adequate rest has resulted in a faster rate of decline in apneic episodes.[409a] Gentle tactile stimulation alone has been shown to be effective in decreasing and preventing apneic spells in most premature infants. Noxious stimuli such as shaking or banging on the incubator should be avoided. If tactile stimulus is ineffective and temporary bag-and-mask ventilation is necessary, attention should be paid to preventing undue pressure on the lower chin and neck so that the airway remains open. Bagging that is too vigorous also may stimulate pulmonary stretch receptors and induce apnea; therefore it should be avoided. Waterbed flotation may decrease the frequency of apnea but generally does not completely eliminate it. Systematic reviews have concluded that (1) prophylactic use of kinesthetic stimulation (e.g., waterbed, oscillating mattress) to reduce apnea or bradycardia cannot be recommended,[181] (2) prophylactic use of methylxanthine for prevention of apnea is not supported by data,[182] and (3) prophylactic use of methylxanthines increases the chances of successful extubation of preterm infants within 1 week.[178]

Increased environmental temperature and sudden changes in temperature have resulted in apneic episodes; prevention includes maintaining the environmental temperature at the lower end of the normal spectrum, particularly if an apneic episode already has occurred. Incubator temperature may require a 0.5° to 1.0° C (1° to 2° F) decrease to counter the problem. The frequency of apnea during active sleep is influenced by temperature: more apnea occurs in a warmer environment, whereas apnea is less frequent in cooler conditions.[410] Phototherapy may provide sufficient radiant energy to increase an infant's temperature and contribute to the incidence of apnea. Care should be taken to avoid sudden changes in temperature. An infant should not be placed on a cold scale; he or she should be placed in a prewarmed incubator or bed. Oxygen should be warmed and humidified before administration.

Careful attention must be paid to prevent airway obstruction. Small neck rolls under the neck and shoulders have been used to decrease neck flexion and prevent airway obstruction when in the supine position. Prone positioning improves lung mechanics and oxygenation; however, with increasing gestation age (greater than 32 weeks), the sudden infant death syndrome precautions of supine position for sleep need to be followed (see Chapter 13). A study comparing supine with prone positioning of preterm infants ($n = 21$) found no clinically significant increase in acid gastroesophageal reflux (GER) or obstructive apnea episodes associated with GER in asymptomatic convalescent preterms.[48] Close monitoring should be done during procedures such as lumbar puncture in which accidental airway obstruction may occur.

A recent RCT using olfactory stimulation with vanillin compared with no intervention was conducted in 36 preterm infants less than 2500 g at 2 days of age.[131] Compared with no intervention, the preterms exposed to a saturated vanillin solution had a significantly lower (3.1-fold) incidence of apnea, as well as arterial oxygen saturation and heart rates, during the study. In addition to more research the study authors speculated that vanillin might also be used to treat apnea of prematurity.[131]

Data Collection. Evaluation of apnea should include studies to rule out treatable causes.

History. Evaluation of the prenatal and birth history may give a clue to the causes and also provide a basis for further study.

Physical Examination. A thorough physical and neurologic examination rules out grossly apparent abnormalities. Observation and documentation of apneic and bradycardic episodes and any relationship to precipitating factors help differentiate primary from secondary apnea. A continuous, computerized analysis system to document apnea, bradycardia, and desaturation is more reliable in accurately capturing episodes.[422]

Laboratory Data. A CBC and CRP assay assess for infection and anemia as causes of apnea. Measurements of serum glucose, calcium, phosphate, magnesium, sodium, potassium, and chloride levels assess metabolic causes. Arterial blood gas measurements assess hypoxemia and metabolic and respiratory contributions to apnea. Blood, urine, and cerebrospinal fluid (CSF) cultures rule out sepsis as the cause of apnea. The CSF culture usually is performed only when other signs and symptoms of infection are present. Chest x-ray examinations assess cardiac and respiratory causes. The examinations may also rule out aspiration of gastric contents caused by vomiting or gastroesophageal reflux. Ultrasonographic examination of the head and an EEG may be used to rule out IVH or other neurologic causes of apnea.

Treatment. Treatment of secondary apnea is aimed at the diagnosis and management of the specific causes. In the treatment of primary apnea (apnea of prematurity), initial efforts should begin with the least invasive intervention possible. Gentle tactile stimulation is frequently successful, especially with early recognition and intervention. When infants do not immediately respond to external stimuli, bag-and-mask ventilation must be initiated. Generally, an FiO_2 approximating that used before the spell but not exceeding a 10% increase will alleviate hypoxemia and avoid marked elevations in the arterial PaO_2. The use of pulse oximetry monitoring allows closer evaluation of PaO_2 fluctuation and helps prevent complications of oxygen toxicity. Elevation in ambient oxygen concentrations, although decreasing the frequency of apnea, causes prolongation of apnea spells.

Apnea responds to low-pressure (3 to 5 cm H_2O) nasal CPAP.[313] Mechanical ventilation may be necessary if the infant fails to respond to lesser measures and continues to have repeated and prolonged apneic episodes. It also may be necessary in extremely immature, unstable, or debilitated infants. Mechanical ventilation for apnea may be administered with nasal prongs or nasotracheal tube to avoid intubation. Synchronized nasal intermittent positive-pressure ventilation (SNIPPV) is useful in augmenting the beneficial effects of nasal CPAP in preterms with frequent or severe apnea.[246]

Methylxanthines (e.g., caffeine, theophylline, aminophylline) are used to treat apnea of prematurity (Table 23-21). They are used only in

TABLE 23-21	METHYLXANTHINES USED TO TREAT APNEA OF PREMATURITY		
DRUG	DOSAGE	THERAPEUTIC LEVELS	SIDE EFFECTS
Caffeine citrate	Route: PO Loading: 20-40 mg/kg Maintenance: 5-8 mg/kg/day administered 24 hr after the loading dose Route: IV Dose: Cafcit 20 mg/ml Administer IV over 15-30 min to avoid cardiac dysrhythmias Half-life: 3-4 days with a range of 40-230 hours; inversely related to gestational age and postconceptual age[200]	Afterload: 8-14 mcg/mL Maintenance: 5-25 mcg/ml Toxic: >40-50 mcg/ml	Administer orally with feedings: administer in morning so infant's sleep pattern is less disrupted than evening administration Tachycardia (withhold dose if >180/min), dysrhythmias, diuresis, glucosuria, ketonuria, hyperglycemia, jitteriness, seizures, vomiting, hemorrhagic gastritis, NEC
Theophylline	Route: PO Loading: 4-6 mg/kg Maintenance: 1.5 mg/kg q 8 hr to 3 mg/kg q 12 hr IV: Aminophylline 4-6 mg/kg over 30 min	5-15 mcg/ml, although levels of 3-4 mcg/ml have been shown to be effective in decreasing apnea	See above IV theophylline delays gastric emptying in VLBW infants Aminophylline is effective in preventing apnea that is associated with prostaglandin E_1 (PGE_1) injection in infants with ductal-dependent lesions[248a]

Data from Young T, Magnum B: Neofax 2008, Raleigh, NC, 2008, Acorn Publishing.
IV, Intravenous; *NEC,* necrotizing enterocolitis; *PO,* per os, by mouth; *VLBW,* very-low-birth-weight.

primary apnea (i.e., when pathologic causes have been eliminated). Methylxanthines are potent cardiac, respiratory, and CNS stimulants and smooth muscle relaxers.[112] The effect on decreasing the frequency of apnea is related to central stimulation rather than to changes in pulmonary function. Caffeine citrate is considered the drug of choice because (1) administration is once a day; (2) there is an earlier onset of action; (3) it has a wide therapeutic range, requiring fewer serum blood level evaluations; (4) there is no alteration of CBF; and (5) there are fewer side effects than with theophylline.[183] Methylxanthines reduce the frequency of apnea and are associated with a decrease in the use of mechanical ventilation.[178,182,183] A large (*n* = 2006 preterms with birth weight of 500 to 1250 g) multisite, international RCT of caffeine use for apnea of prematurity found that caffeine (1) reduced the incidence of CLD/BPD (36% in the treated group vs. 47% in the placebo group), (2) reduced the use of positive airway pressure by 1 week, and (3) temporarily (in the first 2 weeks of the study) reduced weight gain.[352] A recent RCT determined the frequency of intermittent hypoxia after caffeine therapy was discontinued and whether extended use of caffeine (to 40 weeks' postmenstrual age) reduced intermittent hypoxia with apneic episodes.[329] Extended use of caffeine reduced intermittent hypoxia (PO less than 90%) by 47% for preterms of 35 to 39 weeks' postmenstrual age.[329]

Theophylline has been shown to significantly decrease CBF velocity. A recent RCT comparing theophylline with inhalation of (0.8%) CO_2 to treat apnea of prematurity found equal efficacy in decreasing the number and duration of apneic episodes, with fewer side effects, and no alteration of CBF with the inhalation therapy.[6]

Although gastroesophageal reflux is frequent in preterm infants because of lower esophageal sphincter relaxation, recent studies do not find an association between predischarge apnea and reflux.* Reflux events are unrelated to apneic events; apneic events are not a frequent marker of reflux, and when there is a temporal association, there is no effect on apnea duration, desaturation, or bradycardia.[118] Another study measured cardiorespiratory and GER event rates during prefeeding and postfeeding intervals and found that the frequency, height, and pH of GER are significantly altered

---

* References 48, 118, 230, 304, 312, 314.

by feedings in preterms but that apnea, bradycardia, and desaturations were not more prevalent after feeding.[372]

Medications to improve gastric emptying (e.g., metoclopramide) have been used to treat reflux and decrease apnea secondary to reflux, although a relationship between gastric emptying and reflux in preterm infants has not been supported by research.[230,304,312,314] Antireflux medications have not been found to decrease the incidence of apnea and bradycardia in preterms, so their efficacy requires testing. Because a large proportion of preterm infants have abnormally high degrees of esophageal acid, administration of acid-reducing agents (e.g., ranitidine, omeprazole) may be beneficial, and these have fewer side effects and drug interactions.

Complications. Side effects of xanthines include gastric irritation, hyperactivity (restlessness, irritability, wakefulness), myocardial stimulation (tachycardia, hypotension), and increased urinary output.

The prognosis for apnea arising from an underlying cause depends on the outcome of the disease process itself. The prognosis for apnea is generally good in infants who are otherwise well and healthy and for whom the apnea is not prolonged. Delayed resolution of apnea (greater than 36 weeks' postmenstrual age) and increased frequency and duration of episodes are associated with an increased risk for neurodevelopmental disturbance at 13 months' postconceptual age.[308] Long-term follow-up of the preterms in the randomized multicenter trial of caffeine use for apnea of prematurity study found improved rates of survival without neurodevelopmental disability, reduced incidence of cerebral palsy, and reduced BPD/CLD at 18 to 21 months of age among the caffeine-treated group.[353] Prompt recognition and intervention decrease the possibility of severe complications from hypoxia.

PARENT TEACHING

Parental attachment to an infant with respiratory disease is especially difficult. It is made more difficult if the infant is also premature. Normal interaction is curtailed by the infant's condition and appearance, the environment, and the parent's reaction to these factors. An infant who is in an oxygen hood or receiving ventilation therapy to the lungs

BOX 23-14	PARENT TEACHING IMPORTANT ASPECTS FOR PARENTS OF INFANTS WITH RESPIRATORY DISEASE

- Individualize parent teaching and evaluate parental readiness to care for an infant with ongoing respiratory care needs (e.g., home oxygen, tracheostomy, or ventilator care).
- Involve and teach parents care of their infant throughout hospitalization.
- Provide parents with written instructions for home care (e.g., tracheostomy care; suction; gastrostomy tube [g-tube] care).
- Provide parents with written instructions about all medications (dose, route of administration, side effects).
- Teach parents how to feed their infant, and encourage frequent feeding opportunities; teach parents how to feed with alternative feeding methods such as gastrostomy tube.
- Teach parents and other care providers how to perform cardiopulmonary resuscitation.
- Instruct parents in use of apnea monitors and other equipment for home use.
- Instruct parents to notify emergency personnel about their infant; posting emergency phone numbers.
- Instruct parents about the importance of follow-up care.

may give inadequate cues to arouse parental attachment and instead may arouse feelings of grief and loss (see Unit Six).

The goal of discharge planning is the best possible outcome with the least family disruption. Evaluation of parental readiness to care for their infant is essential to effective teaching and learning (Box 23-14). Physical surroundings and preparations for the infant are assessed when possible by a home visit. Parental concerns at bringing home an infant with special care needs must be assessed and discussed. The parents learn to be comfortable in handling and caring for their infant gradually throughout hospitalization. A specially designated or decorated room is used for family visiting and caregiving. Before discharge, the mother and/or father spends the night caring for the infant. Positive reinforcement and praise from the professional staff should be freely given to parents who attend classes and successfully master the tasks of caregiving for their infant.

Special equipment such as oxygen tanks, nasal cannulas, a ventilator, and suction equipment for home use must be acquired before discharge. Sources, mode of delivery, and use of equipment must all be taught to parents before discharge. Pulmonary hygiene for infants with prolonged difficulty in handling secretions also must be taught. Written protocols and instructions should be provided to parents whenever possible. Parents must be informed of dosage, route of administration, side effects, and planned duration of use of all medications.

Fluid and nutritional status is very important to any infant with a chronic condition and nutritional information for parents is necessary. Infants with tachypnea (CLD/BPD) often have difficulty with coordinating suck and swallow. Often smaller, more frequent feedings are necessary with use of supplemental oxygen. Alternative feeding methods such as gavage or gastrostomy feeding may be necessary to safely provide enough calories with a minimum of work.

Apnea is especially distressing to parents because of their fears of recurrence once the infant goes home. If apnea is related to an underlying disease, treatment of the cause should result in resolution of the apneic episodes. Parents can be assured reliably that recurrence is unlikely unless the disease recurs. With apnea of prematurity, assurance can be offered that infants do grow into a regular ventilatory pattern as their respiratory center matures and that all means to protect the infant will be used until that time. Also, the parents can be assured that the infant will not go home until he or she is ready and the parents are adequately prepared to handle situations that may arise.

Before an infant needing a home monitoring system is discharged from the hospital, the parents must be given adequate support and instruction. Classes on the use of the apnea monitors must include demonstration of the equipment and return demonstrations. Minor equipment checks and repairs should be mastered before discharge.

Support by the primary care providers after discharge is essential. Parents must have telephone numbers of the medical facility and personnel they can call 24 hours a day in case of problems or equipment failure.

Anticipatory support includes discussion of potential stress factors related to having an infant on a monitor and oxygen at home: sibling rivalries, marital stresses, scheduling problems, potential problems with babysitters, and the parents' own fears of the situation.[450] An apnea monitor in the home may provoke anxiety despite discussion and instruction. When infants are discharged with apnea monitors, there is a marked increase in maternal fatigue 1 month after discharge compared with a similar group discharged without monitors.[438] Increased fatigue interferes with activities of daily living and ability to parent and increases caregiver stress.[438] Interventions to alleviate fatigue after discharge may include spousal support, household help, child care for siblings, and opportunities for increasing sleep.

The parents of every infant who has apneic episodes or serious respiratory disease must be taught CPR. This set of skills is learned over the course of time by reading written materials and seeing and returning the demonstration. Learning CPR cannot be done on the day of discharge but, rather, must be a staged process of individual and class instruction. Supplying instructional pamphlets written just for parents aids in initial learning and provides a quick reference. If other family members or babysitters will provide child care during work or evening hours, they too must be able to resuscitate the infant.

Other emergency actions for which parents must be prepared include clearing the infant's airway, calling for help (having emergency phone numbers easily accessible), planning for an alternative communication source (e.g., neighbor's phone), and notifying the community rescue squad of the infant's presence in the home.

Parents must be taught how to recognize signs of illness or significant deterioration in the condition of their infant. In addition to information about special care needs, parents need information about normal newborn care. Developing realistic expectations and positive parenting skills is as important to these parents as to all new parents.

For the parents of an infant with special respiratory problems, the importance of continuous follow-up care must be emphasized. Follow-up visits should coincide with developmental stages, the natural course of the disease, and expected complications of the disease.

The parents whose child has special respiratory needs must learn a myriad of involved technical information. The primary care provider (frequently the primary nurse) is responsible for organizing, teaching, coordinating, and documenting the information. This nurse is also responsible for ensuring that the parents have not only been taught but in fact understand these concepts.

REFERENCES

For a full list of references, scan the QR code or visit http://booksite.elsevier.com/9780323320832.

24 CARDIOVASCULAR DISEASES AND SURGICAL INTERVENTIONS

TARA SWANSON AND LORI ERICKSON

Congenital heart disease (CHD) is the most common life-threatening birth defect encountered in the neonatal intensive care unit (NICU). Although the incidence of these conditions has remained constant at approximately 1% of all infants born in the United States, the methods of diagnosis and treatment have undergone tremendous change over the past several decades.[28,76] It is the responsibility of the practitioner to recognize the presence of CHD and to provide accurate diagnosis and treatment. This chapter reviews the anatomy and physiology of the fetal and neonatal circulations, the pathophysiology of congenital heart disease, and the most current evidence-based treatments.

CONGENITAL HEART DISEASE: OVERVIEW

History

In 1892, Dr. William Osler wrote that congenital heart disease was of "limited clinical interest as in a large proportion of cases the anomaly is not compatible with life, and in others, nothing can be done to remedy the defect or even relieve the symptoms."[11] Dr. Maude Abbott, along with Dr. Helen Taussig and Dr. Alfred Blalock, suggested surgery to help these "blue babies."[74] This opened up the field of surgical treatment for cyanotic malformations of the heart. In 1938 Dr. Robert Gross was the first to successfully ligate a patent ductus arteriosus (PDA) in a 7-year-old girl at Boston's Children's Hospital. The first successful adult heart transplant in the United States was done at Stanford University by Dr. Norman Shumway in 1968.[9] Remarkable progress has been made in the assessment and treatment of congenital heart disease in the subsequent decades. This is the direct result of advances in pediatric and fetal cardiology, cardiac surgery, neonatology, and neonatal intensive care nursing.

Incidence

Each year, approximately 36,000 babies born in the United States are diagnosed with congenital heart disease.[2] Highly sensitive echocardiography has led to the detection of more trivial forms of congenital heart disease such as tiny ventricular septal defects. This inclusion has led to the higher incidence figures in recent years. The incidence of moderate to severe structural congenital heart defects in liveborn infants is 6 to 8 per 1000 live births.[11] Of these infants, approximately 3 per 1000 live births will have *critical congenital heart disease* (CCHD) that results in death or requires cardiac surgery or cardiac catheterizations during the first year of life.[27,52] Advances in diagnostic imaging, cardiac surgery, and neonatal intensive care have led to significant decreases in mortality rates. Infants with cardiac lesions that were once considered fatal are now surviving into adulthood.

Embryology

The heart is one of the earliest differentiating and functioning organs. In human embryos, the heart begins to beat at about 22 to 23 days of life and begins to effectively pump blood in the fourth week of life. The heart develops from the

---

PURPLE type highlights content that is particularly applicable to clinical settings.

cardiogenic mesoderm and begins as a primitive heart tube. During the first few weeks of life, this primitive heart tube receives blood from three different venous systems (cardinal, vitelline, and umbilical) and supplies blood to six paired aortic arches. These veins and aortic arches must each regress or mature and the primitive heart tube must undergo a complex process of looping, shifting, and septating to result in a normal heart with normal venous and arterial communications. Cardiac development is almost complete by week 6 of gestation, which may be before a pregnancy is even recognized.

Alterations in normal cardiac embryology result in a nonviable circulation (which leads to spontaneous fetal demise) or the abnormal but viable congenital heart diseases we see postnatally. Some cardiac lesions are viable in the setting of fetal circulation with a patent foramen ovale (PFO) and patent ductus arteriosus (PDA), but are not viable if these fetal connections close. These congenital heart lesions require lifesaving treatment soon after birth, so a diagnosis must be made prenatally or within hours after birth to prevent cardiovascular collapse and death.

Physiology

The physiologic changes that occur during the transition from intrauterine to extrauterine life have been well documented. To develop a clear understanding of the various congenital heart defects, knowledge of the basic principles of fetal circulation must be established.

FETAL CIRCULATION

Fetal circulation relies on the placenta for gas exchange, whereas postnatal circulation uses the lungs for gas exchange (Figure 24-1). Highly oxygenated blood from the mother enters the fetal circulation through the vein in the umbilical cord. This blood enters the inferior vena cava via the ductus venosus. Blood from the inferior vena cava enters the right atrium (RA). Most of this blood is directed through the *foramen ovale* (a special fetal opening between the left and right atria) and into the left atrium (LA). Blood then passes through the mitral valve into the left ventricle (LV) and then through the aortic valve into the aorta. From the aorta, blood is first sent to the coronary arteries and brachiocephalic vessels. This results in perfusion of the brain, the upper extremities, and the heart with the most

highly oxygenated fetal blood. Only a small percentage of this blood will travel further in the aorta to supply the rest of the body. After oxygen has been removed by the organs of the upper body, the blood returns to the right atrium through the superior vena cava. Some of the blood entering the right atrium stays on the right side of the heart, traveling through the tricuspid valve, right ventricle (RV), and pulmonic valve to eventually flow into the pulmonary artery.

Fetal lungs are not used for breathing. The work of exchanging oxygen and carbon dioxide is performed by the placenta. Because of high pulmonary vascular resistance (PVR), fetal circulation shunts most of the blood away from the lungs. Blood is shunted from the pulmonary artery to the aorta through a connecting fetal blood vessel called the *ductus arteriosus*.[58] Blood traveling through the ductus arteriosus has low oxygen content. This blood supplies the lower portion of the fetal body before returning to the placenta through the two umbilical arteries. Blood then enters the placental circulation and is resaturated.

TRANSITION FROM PRENATAL TO POSTNATAL CIRCULATION

In utero, systemic vascular resistance (SVR) is low, primarily because of low resistance in the placenta. Conversely, the PVR is high, with the constricted and hypertrophied pulmonary arterioles being relatively resistant to blood flow.

Both the labor process and the first few breaths of life begin the termination of fetal circulation and the transition to newborn circulation. At birth, the placenta is removed from the circulation, thereby greatly increasing the SVR. The first few breaths inflate the lungs for the first time and also increase the oxygen content in the neonatal blood. Both of these changes cause a decrease in PVR, which leads to increased pulmonary blood flow.

The *patent ductus arteriosus* (PDA) is extremely sensitive to oxygen levels in the blood. As the neonatal Pao_2 rises, this fetal connection between the aorta and the pulmonary artery (PDA) is no longer needed and begins to close. Constriction of the PDA leads to functional closure of this vessel within the first few days of life. Permanent, fibrotic closure of the PDA usually occurs weeks to months after birth. As the PVR drops and PDA closes, circulation to the lungs

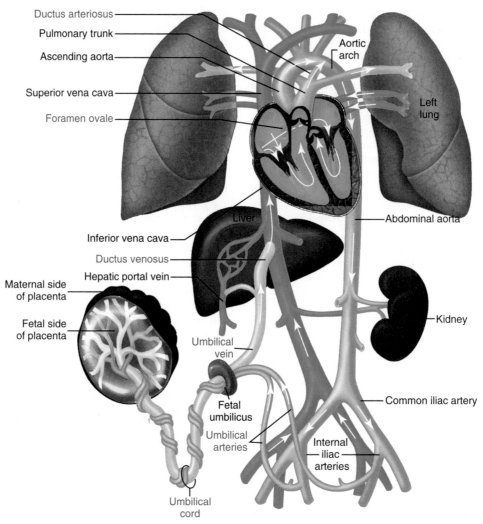

FIGURE 24-1 Fetal circulation. *LA*, Left atrium; *LV*, left ventricle; *RA*, right atrium; *RV*, right ventricle. (Modified from Patton KT, Thibodeau GA: *Anatomy and physiology*, ed 7, St Louis, 2010, Mosby.)

increases, resulting in increased blood return to the left atrium. This increased pressure in the left atrium causes the foramen ovale to close. Anatomic closure of the foramen ovale can take months to years. Finally, with the clamping of the umbilical cord, umbilical venous flow ceases and the ductus venosus begins to close, with anatomic closure taking approximately 1 to 2 weeks.[58]

Once these changes occur, the newborn's circulation resembles that of an adult (Figure 24-2). Deoxygenated blood returns to the heart by the inferior and superior venae cavae and enters the right atrium, right ventricle, pulmonary artery, and pulmonary circulation where oxygen and carbon dioxide are exchanged. Oxygenated blood then returns to the heart through the pulmonary venous system and enters the left atrium, left ventricle, and ultimately the aorta and systemic arterial system. However, PVR and pressures in the right ventricle and pulmonary system remain elevated in the neonate because of the hypertrophy of the pulmonary vessels. This hypertrophy slowly resolves so that PVR and right heart pressures decrease to lower levels between 1 and 2 months of age.

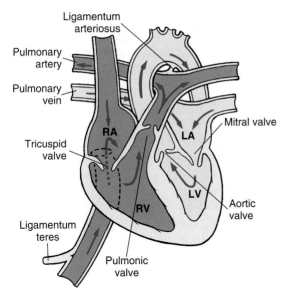

Ligamentum arteriosus

Pulmonary artery

Pulmonary vein

RA

Tricuspid valve

Ligamentum teres

Pulmonic valve

RV

LV

LA

Mitral valve

Aortic valve

FIGURE 24-2 Postnatal circulation. (Modified from Hockenberry MJ, Wilson D: *Wong's essentials of pediatric nursing*, ed 8, St Louis, 2009, Mosby.)

Etiology

In most cases, the cause(s) of abnormal cardiac development is unknown. Traditionally, the etiology of congenital heart defects has been viewed as multifactorial, involving a complex interaction between genetic and environmental factors. Some maternal factors contribute to the risk for CHD. For example, women with pregestational diabetes or women with excessive alcohol consumption are at increased risk for having an infant with a heart defect. Maternal phenylketonuria, maternal systemic lupus erythematosus, or maternal infections also increase the risk of congenital heart disease for offspring. We now recognize that use of assisted reproductive technology also results in increased risk for a heart defect in fetuses conceived by these methods.*

However, most congenital heart disease occurs in the absence of any identifiable maternal risk factors, so most mothers should be reassured that they did not cause their child's malformation. Table 24-1 lists the most common maternal and familial risk factors for cardiac malformations. Box 24-1 lists fetal risk factors associated with an

*References 5, 35, 42, 59, 62, 63.

increased incidence of cardiac defects that should be referred for evaluation by a fetal cardiologist.[15]

Recent studies suggest that the single greatest risk factor for congenital heart defects is genetic. Table 24-2 shows the most common genetic abnormalities associated with congenital heart defects. Children with chromosomal abnormalities such as trisomy 13, trisomy 18, and trisomy 21 often have significant congenital heart disease. At the individual gene level, there are well-established single-gene mutations that cause heart disease, such as mutations in *NOTCH-1* that cause aortic valve disease.[37] Smaller genetic abnormalities such as deletions, duplications, and rearrangements can also be closely associated with high risk of structural heart disease. For example, 1p36 deletion syndrome is a microdeletion with up to 71% of patients having a structural abnormality.[6] With rapid advances in genetic testing capabilities such as robust microarray testing and extremely rapid genome sequencing, new genetic causes of abnormal cardiac development are being identified daily.[73]

PRENATAL DIAGNOSIS

Because of the widespread use of antenatal ultrasound, it is increasingly common for the fetus to be diagnosed with congenital heart disease. Fetal echocardiography has proven to be a valid, reliable, and accurate tool in the prenatal diagnosis of CHD.[14] A recommended timing for a fetal echocardiogram is between 18 to 20 weeks of gestation, although detailed cardiac evaluation and accurate congenital heart disease diagnoses can be made as early as 12 weeks' gestation.[48] Studies have shown that prenatal diagnosis of congenital heart disease can improve patient outcomes and survival after birth.[21,37] Born at or near a hospital with pediatric cardiothoracic surgery services has also been shown to reduce neonatal morbidity and mortality rates.[49] Some neonates with extremely critical congenital heart disease require cardiac intervention within the first minutes to hours of life; these children have little chance of survival unless their heart disease is identified prenatally and their postnatal care providers are prepared and capable of delivering emergency treatment in the delivery room.

Unfortunately, less than half of children with congenital heart disease receive a prenatal diagnosis.[45] Even when routine prenatal ultrasound screening is performed during the pregnancy, one study showed that only 39% of congenital heart

TABLE 24-1	**MOST COMMON MATERNAL AND FAMILIAL RISK FACTORS ASSOCIATED WITH CHD**	
	ASSOCIATED RISK, % LIVE BIRTHS	TIMING FOR FETAL EVALUATION AND COMMENTS
Maternal Factors		
Pregestational DM or DM noted in the first trimester	3-5	18-22 weeks for fetal echocardiogram; DM can be associated with numerous cardiac defects and ventricular hypertrophy in the third trimester with poorly controlled DM
Phenylketonuria	12-14	18-22 weeks for fetal echocardiogram
Lupus or Sjögren's syndrome if SSA/SSB autoantibody positive	1-5	16 weeks initially then frequently if heart block identified Maternal hypothyroidism or vitamin D deficiency may also increase risk
Maternal infections	1-2	18-22 weeks for fetal echocardiogram. Maternal rubella has been associated with CHD; parvovirus, coxsackievirus, adenovirus, and cytomegalovirus have been associated with fetal myocarditis
Teratogens: medication exposures	1-2	
Anticonvulsants	1.8	18-22 weeks for fetal echocardiogram
Lithium	<2	18-22 weeks for fetal echocardiogram
ACE inhibitors	2.9	18-22 weeks for fetal echocardiogram
Retinoic acids	8-20	18-22 weeks for fetal echocardiogram
Vitamin A (>10,000 IU retinol/day)	1.8	18-22 weeks for fetal echocardiogram
SSRIs	1-2	18-22 weeks for fetal echocardiogram, reports of associated risk for RVOT lesions
NSAIDs	1%-2% structural defects 5%-50% for ductal constriction	18-22 weeks for fetal echocardiogram With daily use rule out ductal constriction after exposure
Maternal and Family History		
Use of assisted reproductive technology	1.1-3.3	18-22 weeks for fetal echocardiogram Both IVF and IVF with ICSI seem to carry risk for CHD
Maternal structural cardiac disease	3-7 (all) 10-14 (atrial ventricular septal defects) 13-18 (aortic stenosis) <3 (TOF, d-TGA)	18-22 weeks for fetal echocardiogram
Paternal structural cardiac disease	2-3	18-22 weeks for fetal echocardiogram
Sibling with structural disease	3 Up to 8% for hypoplastic left heart syndrome	18-22 weeks for fetal echocardiogram
Second- and third-degree relatives with CHD	1-2	18-22 weeks for fetal echocardiogram

ACE, Angiotensin-converting enzyme; *CHD,* congenital heart disease; *DM,* diabetes mellitus; *d-TGA,* d-transposition of the great arteries; *ICSI,* intracytoplasmic sperm injection; *IVF,* in vitro fertilization; *NSAIDs,* nonsteroidal antiinflammatory drugs; *RVOT,* right ventricular outflow tract; *SSRIs,* selective serotonin reuptake inhibitors; *TOF,* tetralogy of Fallot.

disease is detected.[56] Thus access to medical care is not the only barrier to prenatal detection of heart lesions. Better screening methods are required along with referral for detailed fetal echocardiogram for any child at increased risk of having heart disease (see Box 24-1).[15] Even in the most experienced hands, fetal echocardiography is limited by technical and fetal factors that make some cardiac diagnoses impossible to detect before birth. Box 24-2 lists CHDs that are often undetected by prenatal ultrasound evaluation.

Extracardiac anomalies should prompt referral for intense cardiac evaluation because there is a high incidence of heart disease in children with even one other organ abnormality.[66] Conversely, children prenatally diagnosed with a congenital heart lesion should have detailed evaluation of extracardiac structures to rule out associated anomalies.

Data Collection

HISTORY

A detailed family history should be obtained because a parent or sibling with congenital heart disease increases the likelihood of CHD for a child.[15] Pregnancy details such as viral exposure during pregnancy (rubella, coxsackievirus B, and enteroviruses), maternal medications, and maternal ingestion of alcohol or illegal substances should be evaluated. Labor and delivery complications should be carefully examined for risk factors that could affect the cardiovascular system. For example, intrauterine hypoxia and perinatal hypoxia are risk factors for the development of myocardial dysfunction or persistent pulmonary hypertension of the newborn (PPHN).

CLINICAL PRESENTATION OF INFANTS WITH SEVERE CARDIAC DISEASE

Congenital heart disease is often not suspected until after birth when a newborn presents with one or more signs or symptoms (Box 24-3).[75] Timing of presentation of signs or symptoms depends on

BOX 24-1	FETAL RISK FACTORS FOR CONGENITAL HEART DISEASE THAT SHOULD BE REFERRED FOR FETAL ECHOCARDIOGRAM BY A FETAL/PEDIATRIC CARDIOLOGIST

Fetal Factors
- Suspected cardiac abnormality on obstetric ultrasound
- Rhythm abnormalities: tachycardia, bradycardia, complete heart block, irregular rhythm
- Identified noncardiac abnormality: central nervous, respiratory, gastrointestinal, genitourinary, musculoskeletal
- Known or suspected chromosomal abnormality
- Increased nuchal translucency on obstetric ultrasound
- Abnormality of umbilical cord, placenta, or intraabdominal venous anatomy
- Monochorionic twinning
- Hydrops fetalis

TABLE 24-2	CHROMOSOMAL ABERRATIONS EVIDENT IN NEONATAL PERIOD THAT ARE ASSOCIATED WITH CONGENITAL HEART DISEASE			
POPULATION	INCIDENCE OF CONGENITAL HEART DISEASE (%)	MOST COMMON LESIONS		
		1	2	3
Trisomy 21 syndrome	50	Ventricular septal defect, endocardial cushion defect	Atrial septal defect	Patent ductus arteriosus
Trisomy 18 syndrome	99+	Ventricular septal defect	Patent ductus arteriosus	Pulmonary stenosis
Trisomy 13 syndrome	90	Ventricular septal defect	Patent ductus arteriosus	Dextrocardia
Turner syndrome	35	Coarctation of the aorta	Aortic stenosis	Atrial septal defect
22q deletion syndrome (DiGeorge syndrome)	50	Interrupted aortic arch	Truncus arteriosus	Tetralogy of Fallot

<table>
<tr><td>

BOX 24-2   **CARDIAC LESIONS OFTEN UNDETECTED BY FETAL ECHOCARDIOGRAPHY**

- Small ventricular septal defect (VSD)
- Atrial septal defect (ASD)
- Persistent patent ductus arteriosus (PDA)
- Total or partial anomalous pulmonary venous return (TAPVR/ PAPVR)
- Mild aortic or pulmonary stenosis
- Coarctation of the aorta

</td></tr>
</table>

BOX 24-3   **CRITICAL FINDINGS**
SEVERE CARDIAC DISEASE

- Cyanosis
- Respiratory distress
- Congestive heart failure
- Diminished cardiac output
- Abnormal cardiac rhythm
- Cardiac murmurs

severity of the defect and alterations in cardiovascular physiology during transitional circulation (i.e., closure of the ductus arteriosus and the fall in PVR). Despite the presence of many heterogeneous forms of heart disease, a limited number of signs and symptoms present in the neonate.

Murmurs. Heart murmurs are a common finding in neonates and can be normal. Closure of the PDA causes a murmur, so all neonates who go through normal cardiac transition will have a murmur briefly as the ductus arteriosus closes. Although cardiac murmurs in the neonatal period do not necessarily indicate heart disease, they must be carefully evaluated. The absence of a murmur does not exclude severe life-threatening cardiac anomalies.

Pathologic murmurs tend to appear at characteristic ages. Murmurs associated with semilunar valve stenosis and atrioventricular valve insufficiency tend to be noted very shortly after birth. In contrast, murmurs caused by left-to-right shunt lesions (PDA, VSD) may not be heard until the second to fourth week of life. The age of the neonate when the murmur is first noted gives an important clue about the nature of the cardiac defect. The timing of the murmur during the cardiac cycle is important; diastolic murmurs are almost never innocent. The intensity (loudness), quality (harsh, vibratory), location, and radiation of the murmur can all be used to help make a diagnosis.

Cyanosis. Cyanosis (a bluish discoloration of the skin, nail beds, and mucous membranes) is one of the most common presenting signs of congenital heart disease in the neonate. Cyanosis occurs with congenital heart disease when deoxygenated venous blood abnormally shunts "right to left" within the heart and then enters the systemic arterial system again (without going through the lungs to pick up oxygen). Depending on the underlying skin complexion, clinically apparent cyanosis is usually not visible until there is more than 3 g/dl of desaturated hemoglobin in the arterial system.[20] Cyanosis depends on both the severity of hypoxemia (which determines the percent of oxygen saturation) and the hemoglobin concentration. True central cyanosis should be differentiated from acrocyanosis (blueness of the hands and feet only), which is a normal finding in the neonate.

Cyanosis in the newborn must be differentiated between cardiac and noncardiac causes. Primary lung disease (see Chapter 23) is a common cause of labile cyanosis due to persistent pulmonary hypertension.[24] Central nervous system abnormalities can also cause hypoxia and result in cyanosis. Clinical cyanosis can occur without hypoxemia in a neonate with *methemoglobinemia* and *polycythemia.*

The *hyperoxia test* is beneficial in differentiating respiratory disease from cyanotic heart disease. This test is a sensitive and specific tool in the initial evaluation of the neonate with suspected congenital heart disease and is used to investigate the possibility of a fixed (intracardiac) right-to-left shunt. The hyperoxia test is performed by obtaining arterial blood gas measurements (preferably from the right radial artery) when the infant is in room air and then after the infant has been in 100% oxygen for 5 to 10 minutes. If the Pao_2 is greater than 150 mm Hg, the presence of a right-to-left shunt and congenital heart disease as the cause of cyanosis is unlikely.[72]

Pulse oximetry screening is a simple and effective screening tool that has recently become mandated by many individual states in the United States

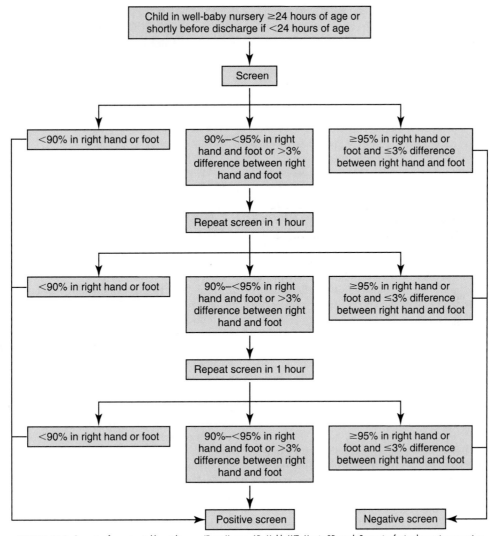

FIGURE 24-3 Screening for congenital heart disease. (From Kemper AR, Mahle WT, Martin GR, et al: Strategies for implementing screening for critical congenital heart disease, *Pediatrics* 128:e1-8, 2011.)

to screen for *critical congenital heart disease* (CCHD). Routine pulse oximetry is performed in asymptomatic newborns after 24 hours of life but before hospital discharge (see Chapter 31).[43,44] Utilization of routine pulse oximetry screening has found that infants with CCHD may have low percentage of oxygen saturation before other clinical symptoms are noted (Figure 24-3).[36] Pulse oximetry completed after 24 hours of age has been shown to have a high sensitivity (76.5%) and specificity (99.9%) and a low false-positive rate (0.05%).[53]

Oxygen saturation (SpO_2) less than 92% and SpO_2 differences greater than 10% from preductal to postductal can be indicators of ductal-dependent cardiac disease.[24] Although all hypoxia found with pulse oximetry screening may not be caused by CHD (as noted with the false-positive results), infants with significant noncardiac hypoxia likely require NICU care.

Respiratory Distress. Most infants with cyanosis from CHD do not have respiratory distress (e.g., tachypnea, intercostal retractions, grunting, nasal flaring). Often the degree of cyanosis is not proportional to the degree of respiratory distress evaluated from the physical and chest x-ray examinations. If a cardiac lesion is present that allows a fixed right-to-left shunt, increasing inspired oxygen will have little effect on the arterial blood gases. However, if the cyanosis is caused by a diffusion defect in the lungs (pulmonary disorder), the degree of cyanosis often decreases with increasing inspired oxygen.

Respiratory distress most often occurs with congenital heart disease when the lungs become too "wet." This occurs when too much blood is pumped to the lungs (pulmonary overcirculation) or when the lung circulation cannot drain well due to pulmonary vein or left heart abnormalities. When there is too much blood in the lung circulation, fluid leaks into the lung tissues and causes pulmonary edema. This can affect the lungs' ability to exchange oxygen and carbon dioxide, and it is difficult for lungs to expand when they are stiff due to excessive fluid. Signs and symptoms of respiratory distress include tachypnea, retractions, nasal flaring, head bobbing, and abdominal breathing. A chest x-ray identifies cardiomegaly and pulmonary edema, although it cannot determine whether the pulmonary edema is due to primary lung disease or a congenital heart lesion.

Congestive Heart Failure. Congestive heart failure (CHF) occurs when the heart cannot meet the metabolic demands of the tissues. Signs and symptoms of CHF reflect decreased cardiac output and decreased tissue perfusion. In the early stages, the neonate may be tachypneic and tachycardic with an increased respiratory effort, diaphoresis, hepatomegaly, and delayed capillary refill. If severe, CHF may present acutely with cardiorespiratory collapse, particularly with obstructive defects. In less severe cases, feeding difficulties and growth failure occur if the CHF persists long term. Edema caused by CHF is rarely seen in neonates. Birth asphyxia and anemia must also be considered as causes of CHF in neonates.

The common symptoms associated with CHF (Box 24-4) can be understood using the physiologic principles previously outlined.

Tachycardia. The heart attempts to compensate for the decrease in cardiac output (CO) by increasing either the heart rate (HR) or the stroke

BOX 24-4	CRITICAL FINDINGS
	CONGESTIVE HEART FAILURE

- Tachycardia
- Cardiac enlargement
- Tachypnea
- Gallop rhythm
- Decreased peripheral pulses and skin mottling in the extremities
- Decreased urine output and edema
- Diaphoresis
- Hepatomegaly
- Hypotension
- Decreased activity
- Failure to thrive and feeding problems
- Diminished cardiac output

volume (SV) (CO = HR × SV). Because the neonatal myocardium has fewer contractile elements and is poorly innervated by the sympathetic nervous system, capacity to increase stroke volume is limited. Therefore neonatal increases in cardiac output are achieved mainly by increasing the heart rate. In the sick neonate, a fast heart rate must be inspected closely to be certain it is a sinus tachycardia rather than an arrhythmia.

Cardiac Enlargement. Hypertrophy and dilation of the heart occur in response to a pressure or volume overload. This is referred to as *cardiomegaly*. This enlargement is evident on chest x-ray examination.

Gallop Rhythm. The gallop rhythm is an abnormal filling sound that can be present with congestive heart failure. It is heard as a triple rhythm on auscultation.

Decreased Peripheral Pulses/Poor Capillary Refill. Decreased cardiac output results in a compensatory redistribution of blood flow to vital tissues. Peripheral tissue perfusion is decreased, which results in decreased peripheral pulses and poor capillary refill. A decrease in peripheral perfusion is often subtle, but is an alarming sign of declining cardiac output and impending cardiovascular collapse. Capillary refill and peripheral pulses are essential to monitor in the child at risk for decreased cardiac output.

Decreased Urine Output and Edema. Decreased renal perfusion results in decreased glomerular filtration. The body interprets this as a decrease in intravascular volume and begins to initiate compensatory mechanisms such as vasoconstriction and retention of fluid and sodium. Neonates manifest this as weight gain and periorbital edema. Poor urine output can be a sign of poor central perfusion and, as such, urine output should be monitored closely.

Diaphoresis. Congestive heart failure leads to an increase in metabolic rate and increased activity of the autonomic nervous system, resulting in diaphoresis. This is representative of the increased workload of the heart in failure. In neonates, this is most concerning during feedings or other periods of increased metabolic demands.

Hepatomegaly. The right ventricle in congestive heart failure is less compliant and does not adequately empty. This leads to elevated pressures in the right atrium, central venous system, and hepatic system. *Hepatomegaly* results from hepatic venous congestion and is an easily evaluated sign of systemic venous overload.

Decreased Activity and Exercise Intolerance. The decreased perfusion to peripheral tissues and the increased energy needed by the heart in failure leaves little energy for activities such as feeding and crying. The infant in heart failure may sleep more than other infants.

Failure to Thrive/Feeding Difficulties. The basal metabolic rate is increased in neonates with congestive heart failure, and cardiac inefficiencies due to a congenital heart lesion cause the heart to work harder and thus require more energy. However, tachypnea and easy fatigability compromise the infant's ability to feed. Poor growth and failure to thrive occurs from the mismatch between above-normal caloric needs and below-normal ability to eat. Significant feeding support is often necessary. Most infants require higher calorie formula or expressed breastmilk supplemented with high-calorie additives. Nasogastric (NG) or gastrostomy (G) feeding tubes may be required when caloric intake requirements cannot be met with oral feeding. Supplemental feeding tubes also decrease the amount of work required to feed, so they can be beneficial to help augment the caloric intake and decrease the caloric needs of an infant. Cardiac nutrition and dietary support are vital for infants with CHD and heart failure.

Dysrhythmias. Abnormalities of the cardiac rhythm and murmurs are discussed individually later.

CARDIAC EXAMINATION

See Specific Conditions later in this chapter.

LABORATORY DATA

Blood Pressure/Four-Extremity Blood Pressure. Adequate blood pressure is vital to deliver enough blood to the body. Hypotension is an alarming sign that may suggest worsening cardiac function and poor cardiac output. An ill neonate may first show signs of peripheral vasoconstriction and poor perfusion, maneuvers that will maintain normal central blood pressure at the expense of peripheral tissue perfusion. Neonates at risk for decreased cardiac output should have blood pressure evaluated frequently, as well as frequent monitoring of capillary refill and peripheral pulses.

The measurement of blood pressure should be taken in both arms and both legs. A systolic pressure that is more than 10 mm Hg higher in the right upper extremity compared with the lower body is abnormal and suggests coarctation of the aorta, aortic arch hypoplasia, or interrupted aortic arch. However, this is a highly specific test with low sensitivity; the lack of systolic blood pressure gradient does not conclusively rule out aortic arch abnormalities. After an aortic arch anomaly has been ruled out, routine blood pressure monitoring may be performed in a single extremity.

Chest X-ray Examination. Frontal and lateral views (if possible) of the chest should be obtained. In neonates, the size of the heart may be difficult to determine because of the overlying thymus. Chest x-ray examination may be normal even in the presence of life-threatening CHD. However, the degree of pulmonary vascularity helps define the type of CHD present and is characterized as being increased, normal, or decreased. Pulmonary edema can also be assessed and can suggest pulmonary overcirculation or pulmonary venous congestion. The heart size should be evaluated and the cardiac silhouette can suggest which cardiac chamber may be enlarged.

Near-Infrared Spectroscopy. Near-infrared spectroscopy (NIRS) is a helpful, noninvasive tool to monitor cerebral and splanchnic oxygen saturations and can be used to infer details about regional hemodynamics in the critically ill newborn. Downtrends in values may be an early indicator of low cardiac output before other clinical signs are noted. NIRS monitoring is especially helpful for left-sided obstructive lesions such as hypoplastic left heart syndrome and coarctation of the aorta to monitor for early clinical indicators of low cardiac output.[29]

Arterial Blood Gases. The $Paco_2$ in cardiac disease is often normal, unless primary pulmonary disease is also present. In congestive heart failure and low cardiac output, metabolic acidosis may be present. Frequent monitoring of blood gases may be necessary with CCHD that is ductal dependent to assess cardiac output and peripheral tissue perfusion. In general, the acid-base balance should be monitored closely in neonates with critical congenital heart disease.

Venous Blood Gases. Venous, capillary, and arterial blood gases can be used to assess acid-base status and guide ventilator and respiratory support. Mixed central venous saturations can provide important information about cardiac output and tissue oxygenation.[71]

Lactic Acid. Lactic acid production increases when there is poor tissue perfusion. An increased lactic acid level can indicate low cardiac output or insufficient systemic perfusion.

Basal Metabolic Panel (BMP). Electrolyte and renal function evaluation should be normal. With low cardiac output, poor renal perfusion may lead to decreased renal function. Renal function should be closely monitored, including blood urea nitrogen (BUN) and creatinine levels.

Hypoglycemia is not a primary effect of CHD, but it can result from poor feeding, genetic abnormalities associated with CHD, or medications used to treat the infant. Glucose level should be closely monitored and neonates should be maintained in a normal glycemic state.

Use of diuretics for congestive heart failure can lead to electrolyte imbalances. Neonates taking diuretics may require electrolyte monitoring and supplementation to maintain normal balance. Sodium, potassium, and chloride depletions are most commonly noted with prolonged diuretic use.

Complete Blood Count (CBC). Significant anemia decreases the blood's oxygen-carrying capacity, increases the cardiac workload, and worsens hypoxemia in neonates with CHD. Desired hemoglobin level may be altered based on the infant's age and hypoxia, because polycythemia is an expected and potentially helpful response to chronic cyanosis. Elevation of white blood cell count is not expected with CHD and, if present, should prompt assessment for possible infection. Platelet levels should be normal in neonates with CHD.

Brain-Natriuretic Peptide (BNP). Although levels may vary in individual cardiac defects, following trends for BNP or NT-Pro BNP levels may help to predict clinical outcomes and degree of cardiac stress. These values are not reliable in the first few days of life as an indicator of CHD alone but can be used in the preoperative and postoperative management of simple and complex CHD.[19]

Electrocardiogram. Neonatal electrocardiogram (ECG) is most useful for evaluating cardiac dysrhythmias and less useful for evaluating structural heart disease. An abnormal ECG can help define the type of structural heart disease, but frequently a newborn ECG is "normal for age" despite significant structural defects (e.g., transposition of the great arteries). Some structural heart defects are associated with abnormal development of the conduction system. An ECG is essential to evaluate conduction system abnormalities, including sinus node dysfunction, heart block, or accessory pathways.

Echocardiogram. The echocardiogram is indispensable in the diagnosis of congenital heart disease. Two-dimensional echocardiography can define cardiac anatomy and can assess cardiac physiology by estimating pressures and gradients and evaluating cardiac function.[47] Supplemented with Doppler and color Doppler, the echocardiogram has become the primary diagnostic tool in pediatric cardiology. During the procedure, close monitoring is recommended with attention to vital signs, respiratory status, and temperature.

Noninvasive transthoracic echocardiogram is the most commonly used approach. Three-dimensional echocardiograms that offer real-time three-dimensional imaging have improved significantly and are becoming more clinically useful, especially for evaluating valve anatomy and function. Transesophageal echocardiography (TEE) is almost never used for infants outside of the operating room, but this imaging modality is routinely used for cardiac evaluation in the operating room immediately before and after surgical repair.

Computed Tomography. Sixty-four–slice multidimensional computed tomography (64-MDCT) can image some thoracic regions beyond the scope of an echocardiogram and can help define the spatial relationship and distance between thoracic structures when planning surgery. Computed tomography (CT) currently requires significantly shorter scan times compared with cardiac magnetic resonance imaging,[67] so sedation is not usually required. This benefit can be substantial when evaluating a sick, unstable neonate. CT exposes the infant to radiation, but newer technologies and protocols are now applied to keep the radiation dosing as low as possible.[12]

Magnetic Resonance Imaging. Like CT, magnetic resonance imaging (MRI) offers three-dimensional reconstruction and high-resolution images of the heart and great vessels. MRI is of particular use in evaluating extracardiac vascular abnormalities, such as arch anomalies, vascular rings, and pulmonary arteriovenous anomalies. MRI provides high spatial resolution, excellent soft-tissue definition, and a large field of view, and it does not expose the patient to radiation. However, an hour or two may be required to perform the test, so sedation is often required and this may be contraindicated for an unstable patient. In addition, MRI is expensive.[25]

General Treatment Strategy

Optimal management of infants with heart disease requires specialized expertise. Infants require close monitoring for hypoxia, hypoglycemia, acidosis, congestive heart failure, and poor peripheral perfusion.

The infant must be kept in an incubator or radiant heat warmer in which body temperature is maintained while color changes (pallor and increased cyanosis) may be observed. A cardiorespiratory monitor is necessary for continuous cardiac monitoring to detect bradycardia, tachycardia, and dysrhythmias. Monitoring of oxygen saturations is mandatory to determine adequacy of pulmonary blood flow and/or increased need for supplemental oxygen. Respiratory effort should be frequently assessed for tachypnea, shallow breathing, apnea, retractions, grunting, abdominal breathing, head bobbing, and nasal flaring. Urine output, peripheral pulses, and

blood pressures, NIRS, and capillary refill should be monitored closely. Other signs of CHF should be documented, such as diaphoresis, hepatomegaly, decreased activity level, and poor feeding behavior.

MANAGEMENT OF CONGESTIVE HEART FAILURE

The medical management of congestive heart failure (CHF) attempts to reverse the outlined process and helps the heart compensate with increased cardiac output. Maintaining the balance of pulmonary blood flow and systemic blood flow is the primary concept that is used to treat CHF in neonates.

If CHF is due to a ductal-dependent cardiac lesion, prostaglandin infusion should be used after consultation with pediatric cardiology. If signs of low cardiac output are present, small-volume fluid boluses may be needed to increase preload to improve systemic blood flow. Continuous inotrope or vasoactive infusion may be needed with significant CHF and CCHD.

Digoxin acts primarily as a positive inotropic (improves contractility) agent (Box 24-5). This drug should be used with caution if acidosis, myocarditis, or obstructive lesions (e.g., tetralogy of Fallot, subvalvular pulmonary stenosis, asymmetric septal hypertrophy) are present. Diuretics such as furosemide (Table 24-3) decrease total body water (which is increased as a result of CHF), and they effectively decrease pulmonary edema, which helps to decrease work of breathing. Medications that reduce afterload such as captopril, enalapril, and milrinone may be used to reduce the systemic blood pressure and encourage systemic perfusion. Chronic fluid restriction and low-salt diets are not commonly used in newborns or infants with CHF.

Infants with CHF often have difficulty feeding. They may have trouble sucking, swallowing, and breathing simultaneously. They may have to rest frequently during a feeding, thus prolonging feeding times, and they may fall asleep exhausted before adequate caloric intake is achieved. Caloric requirements are higher in infants with CHD, thus the use of higher-caloric formulas may be necessary. Adequate nutrition must be ensured by the following:

- Observing the infant's ability to nipple feed (a soft, free-flowing nipple offers the least resistance to sucking and helps the infant

BOX 24-5	DIGOXIN DOSAGES AND COMMON SIDE EFFECTS

Digitalizing Schedule

Preterm Infant PO route: 20-30 mcg/kg total dose* **Term Infant** PO route: 25-35 mcg/kg total dose*	Total dose is usually divided into three doses giving one half, then one fourth, then one fourth of the total dose q 8 hr. Check electrocardiogram rhythm strip for rate, PR interval, and dysrhythmias before each dose. Doses based on lean body weight and normal renal function for age.

Maintenance Schedule

Preterm Infant PO route: 5-7.5 mcg/ kg/day* **Term Infant** PO route: 6-10 mcg/kg/day	Total dose should be divided BID. Allow 12-24 hr between last digitalizing and first maintenance doses. It takes about 6 days to "digitalize" a patient with maintenance doses alone. The sign of digitalis effect is usually prolongation of the PR interval. The first sign of digitalis toxicity is usually vomiting, dysrhythmia, or bradycardia. Drugs such as quinidine, amiodarone, and diuretics predispose to digoxin toxicity. The clearance of digoxin is directly related to renal function. Dosage must be reduced in patients with impaired renal function.

Data from Lexicomp Online: Digoxin, accessed June 22, 2014.[40]
BID, Twice daily.
*Intravenous (IV) dose is 75% of oral (PO) dose.

conserve energy) and, if necessary, using alternative feeding methods (i.e., gavage or continuous nasogastric drip) if the infant is sucking poorly
- Providing adequate calories for growth, including higher-calorie formula or expressed breastmilk supplemented with a high-calorie additive
- Anticipating the infant's hunger and offering feedings before the infant uses energy by crying
- Positioning the infant in a semierect position for feeding

- Maintaining oral feedings at 15 to 20 minutes to minimize overexertion for the neonate
- Burping the infant after every half ounce consumed to help minimize vomiting
- Weighing the infant daily to check for appropriate weight gain

Before discharge from the nursery, the infant should be feeding well and gaining weight appropriately.

Many infants gain weight very slowly because of their cardiac defects. Poor nutrition has been associated with infection risk, increased hospital stay, and mortality risk after cardiac surgery. However, adequate growth can be achieved with the use of fortified formula or breastmilk, NG tube, and possible G-tube supplementing basic oral feedings. Frequent monitoring of weight gain is necessary. Cardiac nutrition experts and cardiology providers can work together to promote nutrition with standardized feeding guidelines in the high-risk cardiac population.[3]

The family of an infant in CHF needs support and teaching. Explanation of the term *congestive heart failure* should be given early because it is a frightening term for parents. The phrase "heart failure" is often interpreted as "heart attack" or "cardiac arrest." Parents must understand that saying an infant is in heart failure does not imply that the infant's heart will stop beating. Describing heart failure as a condition in which the heart struggles to pump enough blood to meet all the needs of the body can help decrease anxiety for the family.

SPECIFIC CONDITIONS

Patent Ductus Arteriosus

PHYSIOLOGY

The ductus arteriosus is a normal pathway in the fetal circulatory system and allows blood from the right ventricle and pulmonary arterial system to flow into the descending aorta for ultimate delivery to the placenta (Figure 24-4). After birth, as a result of a decrease in the pressure of the pulmonary circulation and an increase in the pressure of the aorta, the blood flow through a PDA is predominantly from the aorta to the pulmonary artery (left-to-right shunt). Functionally, the *patent ductus arteriosus* (PDA) closes within a few hours

TABLE 24-3 CARDIAC DRUGS

DRUG	ROUTE	DOSE	ONSET OF ACTION	COMMENTS
Adenosine	IV	0.05-0.1 mg/kg, increase by 0.05-0.1 mg/kg for nonresponsive SVT	Seconds	Slows the spontaneous heart rate and prolongs the PR interval; may cause transient complete heart block and hypotension; half-life is only 9.3 seconds so its effects quickly dissipates
Amiodarone	IV PO	10-15 mg/kg/day in 1-2 divided doses 2.5-10 mg/kg/day daily maintenance dose	Hours 2-3 days	Should only be used with a pediatric cardiologist and electrophysiology consultation Hypotension, abnormal liver function, and abnormal thyroid function can occur
Atropine	IV	0.01-0.03 mg/kg/dose PRN (max 0.4 mg)	Seconds	May cause tachycardia, urinary retention, or hyperthermia
	ETT	Give 2-3 times the IV dose followed by NS flush	Minutes	May cause tachycardia
Calcium chloride (10% solution)	IV	10-20 mg/kg/ dose q 4-6 min PRN for hypocalcemia	Minutes	Slow infusion; must be IV; potentiates digoxin, bradycardia
Calcium gluconate (10% solution)	IV	200-800 mg/kg/day divided in 4 doses for hypocalcemia	Minutes	Slow infusion (over 10-30 min); must be IV; potentiates digoxin, bradycardia/dysrhythmias
Captopril (Capoten)	PO	Preterm and postnatal age <7 days: Initial dose: 0.01 mg/kg/dose q 8-12 hr Titrate: up to max 0.5 mg/kg/dose Term neonates >7 days: Initial dose: 0.05-0.1 mg/kg/day Titrate: up to 0.5 mg/kg/dose in 1-4 divided doses	15 min +	Hypotension, tachycardia, increased BUN and serum creatinine, hypercalcemia
Chlorothiazide (Diuril)	IV PO	5-10 mg/kg/day in 2 doses 20-40 mg/kg/day in 2 divided doses	15 min 2 hours	Hypotension, electrolyte disturbances
Dobutamine (Dobutrex)	IV	2-15 mcg/kg/min	Minutes	Do not use if IHSS or tetralogy of Fallot, may cause ventricular ectopy, tachycardia, or hypertension Incompatible with alkaline solutions
Dopamine (Intropin)	IV	1-15 mcg/kg/min	Minutes	Tachydysrhythmia, vasoconstriction, gangrene of extremities, anginal pain, and palpitations can occur; inactivated in alkaline solution
Enalapril	PO	0.1 mg/kg/day in 1-2 divided doses, increase to max of 0.5 mg/kg/day	Hours	Monitor for hypotension with initiation and dosage changes
Epinephrine (1:10,000)	IV/ETT	0.1-0.3 ml/kg/dose (max 5 ml/dose) q 3-5 min PRN	Seconds	May cause tachycardia, dysrhythmias, or hypertension; not effective if acidosis is present
Esmolol (Brevibloc)	IV	*Initial dose:* 50-75 mcg/kg/min Continuous infusion: titrate 50-200 mcg/kg/min	Minutes	May cause bradycardia, hypotension, bronchoconstriction
Flecainide	PO	1-3 mg/kg/day in 3 divided doses	Hours	May cause ECG changes and hypotension
Furosemide (Lasix)	IV PO	1-2 mg/kg/dose 1-4 mg/kg/dose	5-15 min 30-60 min	May cause metabolic alkalosis and hypokalemia; monitor electrolytes — may need KCl supplementation; renal calcification

Continued

TABLE 24-3   CARDIAC DRUGS—cont'd

DRUG	ROUTE	DOSE	ONSET OF ACTION	COMMENTS
Ibuprofen lysine (NeoProfen)	IV	10 mg/kg first dose; then 5 mg/kg second and third dose (q 24 hr)	Most effective in first 3 days of life	Monitor urine output and creatinine levels; discontinue drug if dramatic decrease in urine output Significantly fewer adverse effects (compared with indomethacin) on renal and mesenteric blood flow; less oliguria and increase in serum creatinine levels
Indomethacin (Indocin)	IV	0.1-0.2 mg/kg/dose; may be repeated q 8 hr for a total of 3 doses		Less effective if administered after 7 days of age; probably will have no effect after 14 days Monitor urine output and creatinine levels; discontinue drug if dramatic decrease in urine output Contraindications: severe renal impairment, active bleeding in the CNS or GI tract, and NEC
Isoproterenol (Isuprel)	IV	0.05-2 mcg/kg/min	30-60 seconds	May cause tachycardia/ventricular tachydysrhythmia; may also cause subendocardial ischemia
Lidocaine (Xylocaine)	IV	*IV bolus:* 1-2 mg/kg *IV drip:* 20-50 mcg/kg/min		May cause dysrhythmia, CNS agitation or depression
Milrinone (Primacor)	IV	*Loading:* 50 mcg/kg over 15 min *Maint.:* 0.25-1 mcg/kg/min	5-15 minutes	May cause ventricular dysrhythmias, ventricular fibrillation, or hypotension
Nitroprusside (Nipride)	IV	0.2-4 mcg/kg/min (protect from light; change solution q 4 hr)	Within 2 minutes	May cause hypotension and reflex tachycardia; may cause thiocyanate toxicity, especially if decreased renal function is present
Procainamide (Pronestyl)	IV	*Loading:* 7-10 mg/kg/dose over 5 min (max 100 mg) *Maint.:* IV 20-80 mcg/kg/min	1-5 min	May cause hypotension or lupus-like syndrome
Propranolol (Inderal)	PO	Dysrhythmias: 0.25 mg/kg/dose TID-QID (max daily dose 5 mg/kg/day)	30-60 min	May severely decrease cardiac output
Prostaglandin E₁ (Prostin VR)	IV	*Initial dose:* 0.02-0.1 mcg/kg/min cont. IV infusion *Maint.:* 0.01-0.05 mcg/kg/min cont. IV infusion	30 min	May cause apnea, fever, or hypotension
Sotalol	PO	*Initial dose:* 1 mg/kg/dose q 12 hr Increase gradually as needed every 3-5 days until stable rhythm is maintained *Maximum dose:* 4 mg/kg/dose q 12 hr		Antiarrhythmic used to treat refractory ventricular and supraventricular tachyarrhythmias Proarrhythmia effects in first days of treatment; cardiorespiratory monitoring essential
Spironolactone (Aldactone)	PO	1-2 mg/kg/day	3-5 days	Hyperkalemia, drowsiness, GI upset

Data from Miller-Hoover SR: Pediatric and neonatal cardiovascular pharmacology, *Pediatr Nurs* 29(2):105, 2003; Lexicomp Online Medication Reference: Accessed June 22, 2014.[41]
Standard Concentrations: Each institution's concentration may vary; NOT to exceed maximum concentration per pharmacy reference manuals. Neonatal Drug Guidelines. Updated May 7, 2002.
BID, Twice daily; *BP,* blood pressure; *BUN,* blood urea nitrogen; *CNS,* central nervous system; *ETT,* endotracheal tube; *GI,* gastrointestinal; *IHSS,* idiopathic hypertrophic subaortic stenosis; *IV,* intravenous; *IM,* intramuscular; *KCl,* potassium chloride; *kg,* kilograms; *Maint.,* maintenance; *max,* maximum; *mcg,* micrograms; *mg,* milligrams; *min,* minutes; *NEC,* necrotizing enterocolitis; *NS,* normal saline; *PO,* per os, by mouth; *PRN,* as needed; *q,* every; *QID,* four times a day; *SVT,* supraventricular tachycardia; *TID,* three times a day.

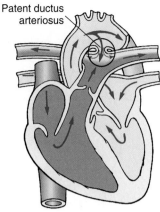

Patent ductus arteriosus

FIGURE 24-4 Patent ductus arteriosus. (Modified from Hockenberry MJ, Wilson D: *Wong's essentials of pediatric nursing*, ed 8, St Louis, 2009, Mosby.)

to several days after birth, but this closure is often delayed in premature infants. The hemodynamic changes and the resultant clinical manifestations of a PDA depend on the magnitude of the pulmonary vascular resistance and the size of the ductal lumen.

DATA COLLECTION

History. Preterm birth, respiratory distress, inability to wean from a ventilator, labile blood pressures, feeding difficulties, necrotizing enterocolitis (NEC), intracranial hemorrhage, and increased oxygen (Fio$_2$) demand can all accompany a PDA.

Physical Findings. Increased flow to the pulmonary circulation often results in increased pulmonary edema and work of breathing.

Cyanosis. Generally, cyanosis is not present in an isolated PDA because the predominant shunt is from left to right. Oxygen saturation monitoring should be normal values.

Heart Sounds. Infants with a PDA may have an audible murmur as a result of the left-to-right shunting through the ductus during systole. A grade I to III systolic murmur is best heard at the upper left sternal border with radiation to the left axilla and faintly to the back. Although this murmur occasionally may spill into diastole, the classical continuous machinery-like murmur is an unusual occurrence in the newborn period. It is often helpful to briefly disconnect the newborn from the ventilator before auscultation. There are cases of large PDAs in which no murmur is audible.

Pulses. With a rapid upstroke and wide pulse pressure, the peripheral pulses are bounding. Assessment of the pulses should include palpation of brachial, plantar, and femoral pulses. The presence of an easily palpated, hyperdynamic pulse in these areas suggests the presence of an aortic run-off lesion, which is most commonly a PDA.

Congestive Heart Failure. With a volume overload of the left ventricle, the infant may show signs of congestive heart failure and pulmonary edema (see Congestive Heart Failure earlier in this chapter).

Laboratory Data

Arterial Blood Gases. Arterial blood gas values are usually normal. A large PDA in a premature neonate may prevent adequate systemic blood flow and acidosis may result.

BMP. Electrolyte abnormalities may occur with use of diuretics to manage pulmonary congestion. Close monitoring to maintain normal electrolytes should be used. Renal function should be monitored during medical treatment closure of PDA.

Chest X-ray Examination. Chest x-ray examination is normal in small shunts. Cardiomegaly is present with increased pulmonary vascularity in large shunts. Pulmonary edema is present with CHF.

Brain Natriuretic Peptide. BNP values of greater than 123 to 300 ng/L have been reported with a hemodynamically significant PDA requiring intervention.[31]

Electrocardiogram. The ECG may be normal, demonstrate left ventricular hypertrophy, or demonstrate combined ventricular hypertrophy.

Echocardiogram. Direct imaging is the preferred method both to diagnose patency and to determine the significance of the ductus arteriosus. An echocardiogram should be performed before medical or surgical closure of the PDA to rule out a ductal-dependent lesion or other associated anomalies. Color-flow Doppler mapping allows visualization of the PDA and aids in determining the size and direction of the shunt across the PDA (i.e., left to right, right to left, bidirectional).

Cardiac Catheterization. Cardiac catheterization is usually not necessary for diagnosis. However, coil or device closure of a PDA by cardiac catheterization is highly successful later in infancy or childhood. In a clinically symptomatic preterm infant with a moderate to large PDA, medical or surgical closure is preferred.

TREATMENT

Medical Management. Asymptomatic infants with PDAs generally do not require medical management or surgical ligation. These infants should be monitored for evidence of CHF, failure to thrive, increasing oxygen requirement, or other complications.

Fluid restriction, watchful waiting, and ventilator support are frequently used as management strategies. However, severely symptomatic infants require ductal closure by either pharmacologic management or surgical ductal ligation. Indomethacin was first reported in the 1970s and became first-line therapy for the treatment of persistent PDAs, and ibuprofen lysine has been shown to be effective.[52] Table 24-3 has indomethacin and ibuprofen lysine doses, contraindications, and side effects. Urine output and creatinine levels should be closely monitored with both medications. If urine output decreases dramatically, the drug should be discontinued.

Surgical Treatment. Although surgical ligation of the ductus arteriosus through a lateral thoracotomy incision is a low-risk procedure when performed by an experienced surgical team, this should be reserved for those infants who cannot tolerate or have failed pharmacologic intervention. Questions have been raised about the long-term effects of surgical PDA closure in extremely low-birth-weight infants and the relationship between ligation and bronchopulmonary dysplasia (BPD), severe retinopathy of prematurity (ROP), and neurosensory impairment.[30]

COMPLICATIONS AND RESIDUAL EFFECTS

Complications and residual effects, although rare, include recanalization, recurrent laryngeal or phrenic nerve palsies, and false aneurysms. The surgical mortality rate in the neonatal period is generally less than 1%.

PROGNOSIS AND FOLLOW-UP

Asymptomatic infants have an excellent prognosis, although follow-up is necessary. If the ductus arteriosus remains patent beyond infancy, closure by interventional cardiac catheterization may be recommended. Symptomatic infants with PDA generally experience failure to thrive, continued CHF, increased oxygen requirements with resultant BPD, or pulmonary infections.

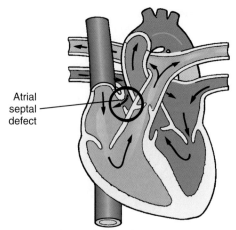

FIGURE 24-5 Atrial septal defect. (Modified from Hockenberry MJ, Wilson D: *Wong's essentials of pediatric nursing,* ed 8, St Louis, 2009, Mosby).

Patent Foramen Ovale

A patent foramen ovale (PFO) is a communication in the atrial septum between the left and right atrium. Unlike an atrial septal defect, this is a flap-like opening with no deficiency of tissue. A PFO is needed before birth to allow blood to flow from the right atrium to the left atrium. After birth, left atrial pressure exceeds right atrial pressure and the flap opening shuts. A trivial left-to-right shunt often persists until permanent anatomic closure is completed. More than 20% of adults have a persistent PFO, but this rarely has clinical consequences.[26]

A PFO is considered a normal finding and requires no treatment or cardiology follow-up.

Atrial Septal Defect

PHYSIOLOGY

An atrial septal defect (ASD) may occur as an isolated anomaly or as part of a more complex cardiac disease. Only isolated ASDs are discussed in this section.

ASDs are common congenital heart lesions that are challenging to diagnose (Figure 24-5). Prenatal diagnosis of an ASD rarely occurs because a natural atrial septal communication (patent foramen ovale) is always present before birth. Neonates with atrial septal defects are generally asymptomatic, so diagnosis often does not occur until later in life.

Three types of ASDs exist and are classified by location. A *secundum atrial septal defect* is most common and is located in the central portion of the atrial septum. A *primum atrial septal defect* is located close to the mitral and tricuspid valves and is often associated with a cleft mitral valve or atrioventricular septal defect. A *sinus venosus defect* is not a defect in the atrial septum, but it is often classified as an ASD due to its similar effects on the heart; this defect can be associated with partial anomalous pulmonary venous return. Secundum ASDs can spontaneously close in the first few years of life, but primum ASDs and sinus venosus defects always require surgical closure.

DATA COLLECTION
Physical Findings
Cyanosis. An isolated ASD does not cause cyanosis because the predominant shunt is from left atrium to right atrium. Oxygen saturation monitoring should be normal values.

Heart Sounds. Abnormal heart sounds are not usually appreciated during infancy. In older children, fixed splitting of S_2 can be appreciated due to delayed closure of the pulmonary valve. S_1 is normal. Flow across the ASD does not create a murmur. However, when left-to-right atrial level shunting is large, excessive flow across the pulmonary valve can create a systolic, ejection-type murmur that is indistinguishable from the murmur of mild pulmonary stenosis. Less commonly, excessive flow across the tricuspid valve can cause a low-pitched "diastolic rumble."

Congestive Heart Failure. Congestive heart failure does not occur, even in the presence of a large ASD.

Laboratory Data
Arterial Blood Gases. Arterial blood gas values are normal.

Venous Blood Gases. Venous blood gas values are normal.

BMP. No major electrolyte abnormalities or renal dysfunction should be present related to an ASD.

Chest X-ray Examination. A chest x-ray examination is normal. Later in life, right-sided heart dilation and cardiomegaly may be present.

Electrocardiogram. The ECG in an infant with an ASD is usually normal. As right-sided heart dilation occurs over the first few years of life, right atrial enlargement and right ventricular enlargement may be detected by ECG.

Echocardiogram. Two-dimensional echocardiogram is diagnostic and can demonstrate number, size, and location of atrial septal defects. Right-sided heart enlargement may also be appreciated in older infants and children.

Cardiac Catheterization. A diagnostic cardiac catheterization is not necessary. (See Treatment section for discussion of interventional cardiac catheterization.)

TREATMENT
Medical Management. Medical management is not necessary because ASDs do not cause significant symptoms during childhood.

Cardiac Catheterization (Device Closure). Device closure of a secundum ASD by interventional cardiac catheterization is often possible. This involves placing a device across the defect to plug the hole. Device closure is contraindicated if there are insufficient rims around the defect; the device must sandwich the atrial septum around the entire defect to avoid embolization of the device. Less commonly, device closure cannot be performed because the child's atria are too small to accommodate the appropriately sized device or the ASD is larger than commercially available devices. This procedure is rarely performed in infants or toddlers. Procedural risks are very low, but embolization of the device and erosion of the device through the heart are rare adverse events that can be life-threatening.

Surgical Treatment. Surgical treatment of an ASD is necessary for primum ASDs, sinus venosus defects, or secundum ASDs that cannot be closed by cardiac catheterization intervention. Surgery for isolated defects is rarely performed during infancy or toddler years. Either primary suture closure or patch closure of the defect is performed through a median sternotomy incision.

COMPLICATIONS AND RESIDUAL EFFECTS
Complications or residual effects rarely occur but may include a persistent shunt (residual ASD) or rhythm abnormalities.

PROGNOSIS AND FOLLOW-UP
Eighty percent of secundum ASDs measuring 8 mm or less will close spontaneously within the first 2 years of life.[57] If spontaneous closure occurs, cardiology follow-up is not required. After surgical

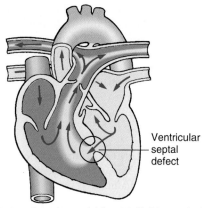

FIGURE 24-6 Ventricular septal defect. (Modified from Hockenberry MJ, Wilson D: *Wong's essentials of pediatric nursing,* ed 8, St Louis, 2009, Mosby.)

or device closure of an ASD, long-term cardiology follow-up is recommended.

Ventricular Septal Defect

PHYSIOLOGY

A ventricular septal defect (VSD) may occur as an isolated anomaly or as part of a more complex cardiac lesion. Only isolated VSDs are discussed in this section. VSDs are the most common congenital heart defect. VSDs can be located in various portions of the ventricular septum and are classified according to their anatomic position (Figure 24-6). The VSD types each have clinically important differences, such as the likelihood of spontaneous closure, possibility of affecting neighboring valve function, or complications that can develop with or without surgical repair.

In addition to VSD type, the size of the defect also has an important role in clinical symptoms and treatment. A small VSD allows only a small amount of blood to shunt from the high-pressure left ventricle to the lower-pressure right ventricle. This small amount of left-to-right shunting is not enough to be clinically important or cause symptoms. Conversely, a large VSD allows a large amount of left-to-right shunting. Highly oxygenated blood returning from the lungs is shunted across the defect and back out to the lungs again. This pulmonary overcirculation results in CHF, pulmonary edema, respiratory distress, and failure to thrive.

Although the size of the VSD is of critical importance, the pulmonary vascular resistance (PVR) also plays a role in how much blood shunts left to right across the ventricular septum. PVR is nearly systemic immediately after birth, so minimal blood travels across even a large defect. With minimal shunting, there are minimal symptoms and a minimal murmur. PVR usually rapidly falls in the first several days of life, and then continues to fall more gradually over the next few months. As PVR declines, more blood is shunted across the VSD and symptoms gradually increase. Premature infants tend to have lower pulmonary vascular resistance at birth, allowing greater left-to-right shunting, and therefore may be symptomatic. Infants with severe lung disease (e.g., RDS, BPD, pneumonia) may have elevated PVR and therefore minimal left-to-right shunting.

DATA COLLECTION
Physical Findings
Cyanosis. Infants with isolated VSDs are rarely cyanotic. As pulmonary vascular resistance falls, oxygen saturation greater than 80% to 85% may be accepted with cardiology consultation to reduce pulmonary congestion.

Heart Sounds. Most infants with VSDs have a heart murmur. The time when this murmur is first audible depends on the PVR and the size of the defect. The murmur is typically a grade II to III/VI harsh systolic murmur heard best at the lower left sternal border. A diastolic flow rumble at the apex indicates a large left-to-right shunt.

Congestive Heart Failure. Congestive heart failure is unusual in the neonate with an isolated small VSD. A child with a moderate to large VSD will have increasing symptoms of CHF over the first few months of life as the PVR drops (see Congestive Heart Failure earlier in this chapter).

Laboratory Data
Arterial Blood Gases. Arterial blood gas values are normal.

BMP. Electrolytes are normal. If diuretics are used to treat CHF symptoms, electrolytes should be monitored and electrolyte supplementation may be required.

Chest X-ray Examination. A chest x-ray examination shows a normal to increased heart size with increased pulmonary blood flow.

Electrocardiogram. The ECG in an infant with a VSD is usually normal but may demonstrate left or biventricular hypertrophy.

Echocardiogram. A two-dimensional echocardiogram can accurately diagnose even the smallest VSDs noninvasively. The use of color-flow studies is particularly advantageous in identifying the presence of multiple VSDs and the direction of blood flow across a VSD.

Cardiac Catheterization. Cardiac catheterization is not necessary for diagnosis. Cardiac catheterization for intervention and device closure may be possible in older children and adults, depending on the type of VSD and associated cardiac issues.

TREATMENT

Medical Management. Medical management of CHF associated with VSDs includes digoxin, diuretics, afterload reducers, and caloric supplementation (see Congestive Heart Failure earlier in this chapter). Failure to thrive despite maximum medical treatment is an indication for surgical repair of the defect.

Surgical Treatment. Surgical treatment of a VSD consists of either suture closure or patching (using most commonly a synthetic material such as Dacron). The surgical approach is through a median sternotomy incision. The defect is approached through the right atrium and tricuspid valve, thereby avoiding a right ventriculotomy.

If the infant is small (less than 2 kg) or if multiple muscular VSDs are present, it may be necessary to perform a palliative procedure called *pulmonary artery banding* to decrease pulmonary blood flow until the infant is older and can undergo debanding and closure of the VSDs. With improvements in surgical technique and technology, VSD closure can be performed safely and effectively in the younger pediatric population.[38]

COMPLICATIONS AND RESIDUAL EFFECTS

Complications or residual effects may include (1) a persistent shunt (residual VSD), (2) conduction abnormalities (right bundle-branch block and third-degree heart block), and (3) aortic or tricuspid insufficiency (less than 1%). The mortality rate from surgical repair of an isolated VSD is less than 1%,[23] although surgical correction in the neonatal period is rare and associated with higher mortality rate.

PROGNOSIS AND FOLLOW-UP

Depending on the anatomic type, approximately 50% of small VSDs may close spontaneously in

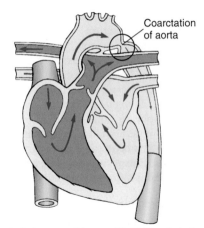

FIGURE 24-7 Coarctation of the aorta. (Modified from Hockenberry MJ, Wilson D: *Wong's essentials of pediatric nursing,* ed 8, St Louis, 2009, Mosby.)

the first months of life. After spontaneous closure, complications have rarely been reported, and routine outpatient cardiology follow-up is generally not necessary. After surgical repair, long-term cardiology follow-up is recommended. If a large left-to-right shunt is persistent after 12 to 24 months of age, the child is susceptible to the development of irreversible and life-limiting pulmonary vascular disease (Eisenmenger syndrome).

Coarctation of the Aorta

PHYSIOLOGY

Coarctation of the aorta is a localized constriction of the aorta that usually occurs at the junction of the transverse aortic arch and the descending aorta in the vicinity of the ductus arteriosus (Figure 24-7). However, coarctation can occur anywhere in the aorta from above the aortic valve to the abdominal aorta. The precise location of the coarctation and the presence or absence of associated anomalies affect the clinical presentation. Associated anomalies include PDA, VSD, and bicuspid aortic valve (50%). Coarctation is one of the more common congenial heart defects, accounting for approximately 7% of cardiac lesions.[17] Coarctation is observed in approximately 10% of infants with Turner syndrome.[16]

Coarctation of the aorta may only develop postnatally when the ductus arteriosus closes and causes constriction of the aortic periductal tissue. As such, coarctation of the aorta is difficult to diagnose before birth. Neonates who had a fetal echocardiogram concerning for coarctation development may require a "coarctation watch" for the first few days after birth. This involves very close bedside monitoring of lower extremity pulses, four-extremity blood pressures, urine output, and other measures of fetal well-being until post-natal echocardiogram confirms that the ductus arteriosus is completely closed. Untreated infants with severe coarctation often have a rapidly deteriorating clinical course that can progress to death unless prostaglandin infusion is started.

DATA COLLECTION

Physical Findings. In utero, the majority of systemic blood flow to the lower body is via the ductus arteriosus. After ductal closure, the neonate with coarctation becomes critically ill because the left ventricle cannot pump the entire cardiac output past a significant point of obstruction. Newborns with critical coarctation of the aorta will have signs and symptoms of CHF and low cardiac output. Severe coarctation of the aorta is a medical and surgical emergency.

Cyanosis. Generally, cyanosis is not present in the newborn with isolated coarctation of the aorta, but an oxygen saturation difference may be found between the upper and lower extremities. Goal saturations should be greater than 92% unless another heart defect is noted.

Heart Sounds. A cardiac murmur may or may not be heard in isolated, severe coarctation of the aorta. If other cardiac defects are present, however, a murmur may be heard. A soft grade I to II/VI systolic murmur may be present at the left sternal border, radiating to the left axilla and to the back. A murmur heard only in the back is strongly suggestive of coarctation. A gallop rhythm sometimes is present and is associated with CHF. The murmurs of associated anomalies, however, usually are dominant.

Pulses and Blood Pressure. The blood pressure proximal to the area of obstruction is higher than the blood pressure distal to the area of obstruction. The most consistent physical finding in infants with critical coarctation of the aorta is a higher systolic blood pressure (greater than 10 mm Hg) in the right upper extremity than in the lower extremities. This blood pressure must be measured with the appropriate-size cuff. In addition, pulses are easily palpable in one or both upper extremities

but are difficult to palpate or are absent in the lower extremities. As mentioned earlier, pulses should be carefully evaluated in all extremities and blood pressures obtained in both arms and both legs.

Congestive Heart Failure. CHF is a common finding in infants with severe coarctation and is the result of pressure overload on the left ventricle (see Congestive Heart Failure earlier in this chapter).

Laboratory Data

Arterial Blood Gases. Arterial blood gas values are normal until PDA closure causes severely decreased lower body perfusion. Metabolic acidosis due to peripheral tissue hypoxia then occurs.

Chest X-ray Examination. Cardiomegaly may be seen on the radiograph. Pulmonary vascularity is normal unless associated anomalies are present.

Near-Infrared Spectroscopy (NIRS). Systemic NIRS monitoring can help monitor for signs of low cardiac output.

Electrocardiogram. Right ventricular hypertrophy is frequently present. Left ventricular hypertrophy or combined ventricular hypertrophy is rarely seen in the newborn period. The ECG may be normal.

Echocardiogram. The area of coarctation can be visualized using two-dimensional techniques and color-flow mapping. However, interpretation of the findings may be difficult if a PDA is present.

Cardiac Catheterization. Cardiac catheterization is rarely necessary. Cardiac catheterization for balloon angioplasty of the coarctation is rarely performed because the results are usually only temporary for neonates.

TREATMENT

Medical Management. Medical management consists of continuous intravenous infusion of prostaglandin E_1 (PGE_1) to keep the ductus arteriosus open, dopamine and/or dobutamine for inotropic support, and correction of metabolic acidosis, hypoglycemia, and anemia. CHF should be treated immediately and aggressively for stabilization before surgery. Intractable CHF, acidosis, oliguria, and hypertension are indications for corrective surgery as soon as possible. (See General Treatment Strategy under Congenital Heart Disease earlier in this chapter.) Since the introduction of PGE_1, emergency surgical repair is rarely necessary.

Surgical Treatment. The most common surgical procedure is resection of the coarctation with end-to-end anastomosis.[39] The area of the coarctation is resected and the ends of the aorta reanastomosed. Coarctation repair is performed through a lateral thoracotomy incision and is highly successful in relieving coarctation and providing for future growth of the aorta.

COMPLICATIONS AND RESIDUAL EFFECTS

Before surgery, significant lower body ischemia puts neonates affected with this CHD at risk for NEC. After surgery, complications and residual effects include residual coarctation, persistent hypertension, chylothorax, phrenic nerve injury, and diaphragm paralysis. The overall operative mortality rate is low at less than 1%, but is increased for low-weight infants less than 2.5 kg.[17] A higher mortality rate may apply if the neonate is medically unstable before surgery, weighs less than 2.5 kg, or there are significant associated cardiac lesions.[69]

PROGNOSIS AND FOLLOW-UP

Infants with mild coarctation require minimal care initially. If these patients are medically managed, close follow-up is mandatory with repair likely at a later date. Infants with severe coarctation require prompt medical and surgical treatment. If this therapy is instituted early, the prognosis generally is favorable.

After surgical repair, frequent follow-up is necessary to ensure adequate coarctation repair. Cardiac catheterization may be necessary several months to years after the surgical procedure is completed if recoarctation occurs. Balloon dilation and stent placement can be performed for recoarctation. In adulthood, patients must continue to be monitored by a cardiologist for complications such as systemic hypertension and aneurysm formation at the coarctation site.

Critical Aortic Stenosis

PHYSIOLOGY

Obstruction of the left ventricular outlet may occur below the aortic valve, at the aortic valve, or above the aortic valve (subvalvular, valvular, or supravalvular aortic stenosis) (Figure 24-8). Valvular aortic stenosis is the most common type and is discussed here. Critical aortic stenosis is present if adequate blood supply to the body cannot get through the severely stenotic valve. In critical aortic stenosis, right-to-left shunting through the PDA helps

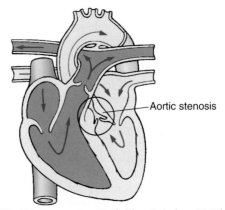

FIGURE 24-8 Aortic stenosis. (Modified from Hockenberry MJ, Wilson D: *Wong's essentials of pediatric nursing*, ed 8, St Louis, 2009, Mosby.)

supply blood to the body; with PDA closure, low cardiac output occurs and can be fatal.

DATA COLLECTION

Physical Findings. Although most infants with aortic stenosis are asymptomatic in the neonatal period, a neonate with critical or severe aortic stenosis needs emergent treatment. As the PDA closes, the infant with critical aortic stenosis will develop pale gray, cool skin with decreased perfusion and peripheral pulses.

Cyanosis. Cyanosis is generally not present in isolated valvular aortic stenosis. Oxygen saturation should be normal if the aortic stenosis defect is isolated.

Heart Sounds. A grade II to IV/VI harsh systolic murmur is typically heard at the upper right sternal border, radiating to the upper left sternal border and faintly to the neck. An ejection click may be heard at the apex. A suprasternal notch thrill is sometimes palpable.

Congestive Heart Failure. Infants with critical aortic stenosis may have CHF caused by a pressure overload of the left ventricle (see Congestive Heart Failure earlier in this chapter).

Laboratory Data

Arterial Blood Gases. Arterial blood gas values are generally normal unless metabolic acidosis develops due to low cardiac output.

Venous Blood Gases. Venous blood gas values are generally normal but mixed venous gas values may be helpful in ensuring adequate cardiac output is being met.

Lactic Acid. Increased lactic acid level can be a sign of low cardiac output and should be monitored frequently.

Chest X-ray Examination. A chest x-ray examination shows cardiomegaly with normal pulmonary vascularity.

Electrocardiogram. The ECG may be normal or demonstrate left ventricular hypertrophy. There is poor correlation between an electrocardiographic abnormality and the degree of aortic stenosis.

Echocardiogram. The aortic valve is usually thickened and appears to open abnormally on an echocardiogram. Doppler interrogation can accurately estimate the systolic pressure gradient from the left ventricle to the ascending aorta and identify the level or levels of obstruction.

NIRS. Systemic NIRS monitoring can be helpful for monitoring for signs of downtrends possibly indicating low cardiac output.

Cardiac Catheterization. Cardiac catheterization is not required for diagnosis.

TREATMENT

Medical Management. Medical management consists of continuous intravenous infusion of PGE_1 to keep the ductus arteriosus open, dopamine and/or dobutamine for inotropic support, and correction of metabolic acidosis, hypoglycemia, and anemia. CHF should be treated immediately and aggressively for stabilization before cardiac catheterization intervention. Intractable CHF, acidosis, and oliguria are indications for cardiac catheterization as soon as possible for critical aortic stenosis in the newborn (see General Treatment Strategy earlier in this chapter).

Cardiac Catheterization. Cardiac catheterization is performed to balloon dilate the aortic valve and improve aortic valve opening. Dilation of the aortic valve often results in damage to the valve leaflets, resulting in valve regurgitation. Care must be taken to balance the desired improvement in aortic valve opening with the detrimental effect on aortic valve closing. Subsequent cardiac catheterizations for balloon valvuloplasty are often required during infancy and early childhood.

Surgical Treatment. Initial treatment with surgical aortic valvotomy is rarely required because balloon dilation of the valve in the cardiac catheterization laboratory is highly successful. However, repeated balloon valvuloplasties often result in significant aortic regurgitation, which can only be definitively treated with surgery. Newborns with critical or severe aortic stenosis most often require surgical valve repair or replacement later in life.

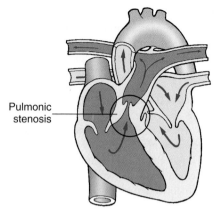

FIGURE 24-9 Pulmonic stenosis. (Modified from Hockenberry MJ, Wilson D: *Wong's essentials of pediatric nursing,* ed 8, St Louis, 2009, Mosby.)

COMPLICATIONS AND RESIDUAL EFFECTS

Complications and residual effects include aortic insufficiency and residual aortic stenosis. The mortality rate from aortic balloon valvuloplasty is low and can be done safely even in premature infants weighing less than 2 kg. The newborn with critical obstruction has the highest risk.

PROGNOSIS AND FOLLOW-UP

All patients with critical aortic stenosis require lifelong follow-up. Further surgical or catheter intervention is almost always necessary.

Critical Pulmonary Stenosis

PHYSIOLOGY

In critical pulmonary stenosis, the flow to the pulmonary artery from the right ventricle is obstructed. The obstruction may occur below the valve in the infundibular area, at the valve, or above the valve (subvalvular, valvular, or supravalvular). In valvular stenosis, the orifice of the pulmonary valve is markedly narrowed (Figure 24-9). The pulmonary artery distal to this area of stenosis may be dilated. The right ventricle is subjected to a marked increase in pressure and becomes hypertrophied.

DATA COLLECTION
Physical Findings
Cyanosis. Cyanosis is generally not present in an isolated lesion but may occur in the presence of a right-to-left atrial shunt. Goal oxygen saturations are often greater than 85% due to decreased pulmonary blood flow.

Heart Sounds. A harsh grade II to III/VI systolic murmur is heard in the upper left sternal border, radiating to both axillae and faintly to the back. A murmur of tricuspid insufficiency (soft, systolic murmur at the lower left sternal border) may be heard. An ejection click also may be heard at the left sternal border.

Congestive Heart Failure. The infant with critical pulmonary stenosis typically has signs and symptoms of right-sided CHF resulting from excessive pressure overload (see Congestive Heart Failure earlier in this chapter).

Laboratory Data

Arterial Blood Gases. Arterial blood gas values generally are normal unless there is an atrial right-to-left shunt.

Venous Blood Gases. Venous blood gas values generally are normal.

Chest X-ray Examination. The chest x-ray examination may be normal but usually demonstrates cardiomegaly with normal or decreased pulmonary vascularity.

Electrocardiogram. The ECG may be normal or demonstrate right ventricular hypertrophy.

Echocardiogram. Two-dimensional echocardiogram is diagnostic. Doppler interrogation and color-flow mapping can accurately estimate the systolic pressure gradient from the right ventricle to the pulmonary artery and identify the level or levels of obstruction.

Cardiac Catheterization. Cardiac catheterization is not required for diagnosis.

TREATMENT

Medical Management. PGE_1 has been used successfully to maintain the patency of the ductus arteriosus, thereby allowing adequate pulmonary blood flow until balloon dilation is performed. Oxygen saturations should be monitored as a sign of adequate pulmonary blood flow through the ductus arteriosus before the cardiac catheterization procedure.

Cardiac Catheterization. Catheter balloon valvuloplasty is the treatment of choice for this defect. Successful balloon valvuloplasty is associated with excellent clinical results, although subsequent balloon dilation procedures may be necessary later in life. Pulmonary regurgitation often results from balloon valvuloplasty, but this rarely requires surgical pulmonary valve repair or replacement later in life.

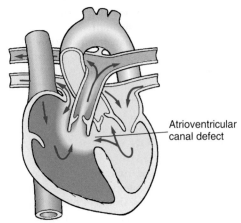

FIGURE 24-10 Atrioventricular (endocardial cushion) defect. (Modified from Hockenberry MJ, Wilson D: *Wong's essentials of pediatric nursing,* ed 8, St Louis, 2009, Mosby.)

Surgical Treatment. Surgical pulmonary valvotomy is rarely required because balloon dilation of the valve via cardiac catheterization procedure is highly successful.

COMPLICATIONS AND RESIDUAL EFFECTS

Complications and residual effects include pulmonary insufficiency and residual pulmonary stenosis. The mortality rate for pulmonary balloon valvuloplasty is low, even in premature infants weighing less than 2 kg.

PROGNOSIS AND FOLLOW-UP

All patients with pulmonary stenosis require lifelong follow-up. Repeated catheterization procedures may be performed during infancy and childhood to treat residual or recurrent obstruction. Long-term prognosis is good.

Atrioventricular Septal Defect, Endocardial Cushion Defect (Atrioventricular Canal)

PHYSIOLOGY

An atrioventricular canal defect occurs when the endocardial cushions that form the central crux of the heart do not form normally. This can result in an atrial septal defect, a ventricular septal defect, and one common atrioventricular valve (which should have separated into the tricuspid and mitral valves) (Figure 24-10). Nearly 70% of infants with complete balanced atrioventricular canal have trisomy 21 (Down syndrome).

These infants usually have a left-to-right shunt at both the atrial and ventricular levels. AV valve insufficiency also may be present. The symptomatology depends on the degree of shunting at the atrial and ventricular levels and the amount of AV valve insufficiency present.

DATA COLLECTION
Physical Findings
Cyanosis. There may be mild cyanosis, particularly in the immediate neonatal period before the pulmonary vascular resistance has fallen. Goal oxygen saturations should be greater than 75% on room air.

Heart Sounds. Often there is no murmur in the neonatal period. If AV valve insufficiency is present, a blowing, holosystolic murmur best heard at the apex with radiation to the left axilla may be appreciated.

Congestive Heart Failure. During the first few weeks of life, there are usually minimal cardiac symptoms due to elevated PVR. As the PVR falls, increasing left-to-right shunting causes infants to have increasing CHF symptoms. AV valve insufficiency may also contribute to ventricular volume overload and may exacerbate the CHF (see Congestive Heart Failure earlier in this chapter). A minority of patients with trisomy 21 have persistent pulmonary hypertension and do not develop CHF symptoms. Oxygen saturations greater than 75% should be accepted because oxygen supplementation can be detrimental and cause CHF through pulmonary overcirculation.

Laboratory Data
Arterial Blood Gases. The $Paco_2$ may be elevated if there is severe AV valve insufficiency and pulmonary edema. The pH and Pao_2 are usually normal.

BMP. Electrolytes are normal. With diuretic use for CHF symptoms, electrolytes should be monitored and replaced as necessary.

CBC. Anemia may cause increased cyanosis and should be monitored in this cardiac defect. Inversely, chronic cyanosis may cause polycythemia.

Chest X-ray Examination. The heart size may be normal or increased. The pulmonary vascularity is generally increased.

Electrocardiogram. An ECG with a left axis deviation, counterclockwise loop in the frontal plane, and superior axis suggests AV septal defect.

Echocardiogram. A two-dimensional echocardiogram with Doppler and color-flow mapping is diagnostic and demonstrates the ASD, VSD, common AV valve, and degree of AV valve insufficiency.

Cardiac Catheterization. Cardiac catheterization is generally not required.

TREATMENT
Medical Management. Medical management of CHF includes diuretics, digoxin, and afterload reducers and caloric supplementation. Failure to thrive despite maximum medical treatment is an indication for surgical repair of the defect (see Congestive Heart Failure earlier in this chapter).

Surgical Treatment. Surgical repair is necessary. However, most centers do not perform surgery during the neonatal period. Waiting until a few months of age has benefits, such as allowing the PVR to drop and allowing the child to grow bigger and stronger. The surgical procedure is performed through a median sternotomy incision and involves patch closure of the ASD and VSD and separation of the common atrioventricular valve into a mitral and tricuspid valve.

COMPLICATIONS AND RESIDUAL EFFECTS
Complications and residual effects include (1) persistent shunt (residual ASD or VSD), (2) mitral regurgitation, (3) tricuspid regurgitation, (4) left ventricular outflow tract obstruction, (5) conduction abnormalities (including third-degree heart block), and (6) dysrhythmias.

PROGNOSIS AND FOLLOW-UP
The prognosis after surgical repair is generally good and future surgeries or cardiac interventions are rarely required. The prognosis is less favorable if early surgical repair was required, pulmonary hypertension persists after surgery, or surgical complications occur. Significant residual defects (shunt or AV valve regurgitation) may require subsequent surgical repair.

Ebstein's Anomaly

PHYSIOLOGY
Ebstein's anomaly is an uncommon but important anatomic heart defect.[26,54] Anatomically, there is a downward displacement of the tricuspid valve into

the body of the right ventricle. The resultant right ventricular cavity is smaller than normal and cardiac output from the right ventricle to the pulmonary artery is usually decreased. Low right ventricular output in the neonate can improve with time as the PVR drops.

Right ventricular output is also dependent on the degree of regurgitation through the dysplastic tricuspid valve. Children with minimal tricuspid regurgitation generally have minimal symptoms and clinically do well. However, when severe tricuspid regurgitation is present, the right ventricle can only eject a trivial amount of antegrade flow into the pulmonary arteries. These neonates rely on the PDA to supply pulmonary blood flow and thus require prostaglandins to survive. Infants with severe tricuspid regurgitation have significant shunting of deoxygenated blood from the right atrium into the left atrium through the foramen ovale, causing cyanosis.

DATA COLLECTION
Physical Findings
Cyanosis. Varying degrees of cyanosis are present, depending on the amount of right-to-left shunting at the foramen ovale and the amount of blood that enters the pulmonary circulation by the right ventricle. In severe cases, the amount of pulmonary blood flow is markedly decreased, and these infants may be deeply cyanotic. Goal oxygen saturations should be greater than 75% and should be continuously monitored to ensure adequate pulmonary blood flow.

Heart Sounds. The second heart sound, S_2, is normal in the mildly affected infant, but the pulmonary component of S_2 may be diminished or inaudible in severely affected patients. The holosystolic murmur of tricuspid regurgitation is usually present and varies from a grade I/VI to a grade V/VI. Diastolic murmurs and triple or quadruple rhythms can also be heard.

Congestive Heart Failure. Newborns with significant tricuspid regurgitation have CHF resulting from volume overload (see Congestive Heart Failure earlier in this chapter).

Laboratory Data
Arterial Blood Gases. The PaO_2 may be normal to very low, depending on the amount of shunting at the atrial level. PaO_2 values in the low 20s are not uncommon.

Lactic Acid. Lactic acid levels should be normal. Elevated lactic acid levels can suggest a state of low cardiac output.

Chest X-ray Examination. The chest x-ray examination shows cardiomegaly with decreased pulmonary vascularity. Massive cardiomegaly generally indicates severe tricuspid insufficiency.

NIRS. NIRS monitoring is helpful to assess cerebral and splanchnic blood flow. Depression in NIRS can be a red flag for worsening cardiac output.

Electrocardiogram. An ECG shows abnormal P waves and can demonstrate various degrees of heart block. The QRS complex generally has a right bundle-branch block pattern. *Wolff-Parkinson-White* (WPW) (preexcitation) syndrome is frequently present, and dysrhythmias such as supraventricular tachycardia are common.

Echocardiogram. A two-dimensional echocardiogram is diagnostic. Doppler interrogation and color-flow mapping are very useful in evaluating the degree of tricuspid insufficiency, the amount of antegrade blood flow through the pulmonary valve, and shunting at the atrial level.

Cardiac Catheterization. This procedure is not generally performed unless a question about the differential diagnosis exists (to rule out pulmonary atresia).

TREATMENT
Medical Management. Medical management is aimed at supporting the neonate through the initial period of transitional circulation. Because of elevated PVR, pulmonary blood flow may be severely limited with profound hypoxemia and acidosis. PGE_1 may be required to maintain a patent ductus arteriosus. Providing a high level of supplemental oxygen, inhaled nitric oxide, and maintaining a mild respiratory alkalosis may help decrease PVR and promote antegrade pulmonary blood flow. Sildenafil may also be helpful to reduce right ventricular afterload and improve forward flow of blood across the pulmonary valve.[1]

Ebstein's anomaly is often associated with WPW syndrome and supraventricular tachycardia. Arrhythmia medications may be necessary to control rhythm abnormalities.

Surgical Treatment. Surgical treatment for Ebstein's anomaly is controversial and generally reserved for the severely symptomatic patient. The procedure, performed through a median sternotomy incision, involves repositioning the tricuspid valve and an annuloplasty to improve the competency of the valve. In addition, plication of the atrialized ventricle is performed. Replacing the tricuspid valve may be necessary. In severe cases, a *Blalock-Taussig shunt* (BT shunt) is placed to provide pulmonary blood flow if prostaglandin infusion cannot be removed without causing severe cyanosis. This may lead a patient fully or partially down the single ventricle pathway with bidirectional *Glenn* and *Fontan* subsequent surgeries.

COMPLICATIONS AND RESIDUAL EFFECTS

Ebstein's anomaly can be associated with pulmonary hypoplasia because the massively enlarged right heart in utero can prevent normal pulmonary development. Other complications include tricuspid insufficiency and dysrhythmias.

PROGNOSIS AND FOLLOW-UP

The prognosis for mild Ebstein's anomaly is favorable. Infants with severe Ebstein's anomaly may improve as the PVR decreases and right ventricular output increases. Although surgery has been used successfully in the more severe forms of Ebstein's anomaly, the prognosis is less favorable in patients requiring surgical intervention. The prognosis for neonates presenting with profound cyanosis caused by Ebstein's anomaly is grave. Long-term cardiology follow-up is necessary, and visits may be more frequent if arrhythmias are persistent.

Persistent Pulmonary Hypertension in the Newborn

PHYSIOLOGY

Infants with abnormally elevated PVR have persistent pulmonary hypertension of the newborn (PPHN) or persistent fetal circulation. These infants are generally hypoxic and acidotic but usually do not have severe pulmonary parenchymal disease or underlying cardiac disease. These infants have a right–to–left shunt at the ductal and atrial levels.

DATA COLLECTION

History. PPHN is usually associated with severe antepartum or peripartum conditions that involve hypoxia reflected by low Apgar scores (see Chapter 23). These infants are generally term or late preterm and are symptomatic within the first hours after birth. Associated findings may include polycythemia, hypoglycemia, or an anatomic abnormality such as congenital diaphragmatic hernia.

Physical Findings

Cyanosis. The milder cases of PPHN have minimal transient tachypnea and cyanosis associated with stress (crying or feeding). Severe cases demonstrate marked cyanosis, tachypnea, acidosis, and decreased peripheral perfusion.

Heart Sounds. A loud pulmonary component of S_2 and occasionally the systolic ejection murmur of tricuspid regurgitation are heard.

Congestive Heart Failure. Infants with PPHN may have CHF because of pressure overload of the right ventricle (see Congestive Heart Failure earlier in this chapter).

Laboratory Data

Arterial Blood Gases. Arterial blood gas values demonstrate acidosis, hypoxia, and increased $Paco_2$. If a blood gas measurement is obtained simultaneously from the right radial artery (preductal) and from the descending aorta with an umbilical artery catheter (postductal), the right-to-left shunt at the ductal level can be documented. If blood gas measurements are repeated after intubation and pharmacologic intervention (see Treatment earlier in this chapter), the degree of hypoxia is often reduced.

Pulse Oximetry. Simultaneous preductal and postductal transcutaneous oxygen measurements may also be used.

Chest X-ray Examination. The chest x-ray examination demonstrates mild to moderate cardiomegaly with normal pulmonary vascular markings. The lung fields may be clear.

Electrocardiogram. The ECG frequently is normal but may demonstrate right ventricular hypertrophy.

Echocardiogram. An echocardiogram is helpful to rule out a cyanotic cardiac lesion. Evaluating the right ventricular and pulmonary artery pressures by Doppler interrogation and the degree of right-to-left shunting at the atrial and ductal levels is also helpful.

Cardiac Catheterization. Cardiac catheterization usually is not performed.

TREATMENT

Medical Management. See Chapter 23.

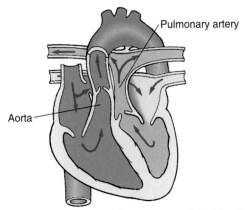

Pulmonary artery

Aorta

FIGURE 24-11 D-transposition of the great arteries. (Modified from Hockenberry MJ, Wilson D: *Wong's essentials of pediatric nursing*, ed 8, St Louis, 2009, Mosby.)

D-Transposition of the Great Arteries

PHYSIOLOGY

D-transposition of the great arteries (Figure 24-11) is one of the most common forms of serious heart disease. The aorta arises from the right ventricle, receives unoxygenated systemic venous blood, and returns this blood to the systemic arterial circulation. The pulmonary artery arises from the left ventricle, receives oxygenated pulmonary venous blood, and returns this blood to the pulmonary circulation. This creates a situation of "parallel circulations," which requires shunting of blood at the atrial and PDA levels for survival. Some patients with transposition have an associated VSD, which also allows for mixing between the parallel systemic and pulmonary circulations. The d-transposition anomaly can occur by itself or can be associated with other cardiac defects (e.g., pulmonary stenosis).

DATA COLLECTION

History. Transposition of the great arteries is more prevalent in males and is typically found in infants who are full term. The etiology of this congenital heart lesion is not well understood. Genetic defects are rarely associated, extracardiac anomalies are rarely present, and the pathogenesis is thought to be different from other conotruncal abnormalities.[70]

Physical Findings. The major physiologic abnormalities in d-transposition of the great arteries are an

oxygen deficiency in the tissues and excessive workload of the right and left ventricles. The only mixing of oxygenated and unoxygenated blood occurs in the presence of associated lesions (e.g., patent foramen ovale, ASD, VSD, PDA). The extent of the mixing depends on the number, size, and position of the anatomic communications, the pressure differential between the two systems, and changes in the systemic and pulmonary vascular resistances.

Cyanosis. These infants are usually cyanotic within the first hours of life, leading to their early diagnosis. Cyanosis is present in varying degrees, depending on the amount of intracardiac mixing present. Cyanosis may be mild if the mixing occurs through a significant VSD or PDA. Cyanosis is profound with intact ventricular septum or a closing PDA. Oxygen therapy will be of limited benefit. Only a certain amount of oxygenated blood can reach the systemic circulation, and administration of additional oxygen does not improve this situation. An emergency cardiac catheterization procedure to enlarge the interatrial communication may be lifesaving. Enlargement of the atrial communication is done by balloon septostomy (Rashkind procedure) and is performed to improve mixing between the two parallel circulations.

Cyanosis is exacerbated by neonatal stressors (crying, feeding, or exposure to cold temperatures). If the Pao_2, measured at rest in room air, is not greater than 35 mm Hg or if persistent metabolic acidosis is present, inadequate intracardiac mixing should be suspected.

Oxygenation monitoring by pulse oximetry should reveal saturations greater than 75% due to a complete mixing lesion. Oxygen and ventilation support should be given to maintain this level of saturation.

Heart Sounds. The aorta arises from the anterior (right) ventricle, and the closure of the aortic valve is easily heard. The S_2 is single with an increased intensity. Murmurs, if present, are usually those of associated lesions.

Congestive Heart Failure. Congestive heart failure is usually not present.

Laboratory Data

Arterial Blood Gases. In neonates with transposition of the great arteries and an intact ventricular septum, a very low Pao_2 (15 to 20 mm Hg) with normal $Paco_2$ and mild metabolic acidosis are often seen.

Lactic Acid. Lactic acid levels should be normal if adequate intracardiac mixing is present preoperatively.

BMP. Electrolytes should be normal. Following renal function to ensure adequate preload and hydration can be important for ensuring hemodynamic stability with this mixing lesion.

CBC. Anemia can worsen hypoxemia with mixing cardiac lesions. Intermittent evaluation of hemoglobin and hematocrit should be performed, and aiming for a higher baseline is clinically helpful.

Chest X-ray Examination. The chest x-ray examination may be normal or demonstrate either decreased or increased pulmonary vascularity. The cardiac silhouette may assume the shape of an "egg on a string." However, this finding is not diagnostic.

Electrocardiogram. The ECG may be normal or demonstrate right ventricular hypertrophy.

Echocardiogram. The echocardiogram is diagnostic. Special attention is directed at the size of the ASD, size of the PDA, associated lesions, and coronary arteries.

NIRS. NIRS monitoring is used to assess cardiac output and is especially helpful in the setting of a critical mixing lesion.

Cardiac Catheterization. Cardiac catheterization may be necessary to perform a balloon atrial septostomy to improve intraatrial mixing and to delineate the coronary artery anatomy, if not evaluated completely by transthoracic echocardiogram.

TREATMENT

Medical Management. Serial venous and arterial pH measurements should be obtained to rule out the presence of a persistent metabolic acidosis that would suggest inadequate intracardiac mixing. PGE_1 infusion is used to maintain ductal patency.

Surgical Treatment. The *arterial switch procedure* is the treatment for d-transposition of the great arteries. This procedure, performed through a median sternotomy incision, involves transection of the main pulmonary artery and the aorta above the respective valves.[65] The pulmonary artery is anastomosed to the right ventricle and the aorta is anastomosed to the left ventricle (the aortic valve becomes a functional pulmonary valve and the pulmonary valve becomes a functional aortic valve). The coronary arteries are resected with a button of surrounding tissue and reanastomosed to the supravalvular area of the ascending aorta.[55] Additional defects are also

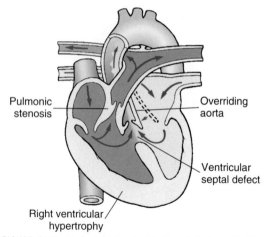

FIGURE 24-12 Tetralogy of Fallot. (Modified from Hockenberry MJ, Wilson D: *Wong's essentials of pediatric nursing*, ed 8, St Louis, 2009, Mosby.)

repaired, including closure of atrial or ventricular defects and ligation of the PDA. Surgery is usually performed in the first week of life.

COMPLICATIONS AND RESIDUAL EFFECTS

Complications and residual effects of the arterial switch procedure include (1) dysrhythmias, (2) myocardial ischemia and infarction, and (3) aortic or pulmonary supravalvular stenosis.

PROGNOSIS AND FOLLOW-UP

After successful arterial switch operation, long-term prognosis is good. Lifetime cardiology follow-up is mandatory.

Tetralogy of Fallot

PHYSIOLOGY

Tetralogy of Fallot is the most common cyanotic congenital heart defect (Figure 24-12). The four components of tetralogy of Fallot are a VSD, an overriding of the ascending aorta, obstruction of the right ventricular outflow tract, and right ventricular hypertrophy. Although these patients have a large VSD, they traditionally do not have symptoms of CHF because their pulmonary circulation is protected from overcirculation by the right ventricular outflow tract obstruction.

The degree of right ventricular outflow tract obstruction can vary significantly. A minority of children have too much pulmonary blood flow due to minimal right ventricular outflow tract obstruction. CHF will develop over time, much like a child with a simple large VSD (see Ventricular Septal Defect earlier in this chapter). A child with minimal right ventricular outflow tract obstruction is sometimes called a "pink tet" and will not be cyanotic. On the other end of the spectrum, a child with severe right ventricular outflow tract obstruction may have too little pulmonary blood flow. In this case the ductus arteriosus may be vital to augment blood flow to the lungs and the child may need prostaglandins and neonatal surgery. Most children fall somewhere in the middle of the spectrum and have sufficient pulmonary blood flow but no CHF symptoms.

DATA COLLECTION

Physical Findings. Symptomatology in these infants relates to the degree of right ventricular outflow tract obstruction. Newborns that are symptomatic usually have severe right ventricular outflow tract obstruction.

Cyanosis. The predominant intracardiac shunt is usually right to left; therefore, most infants with tetralogy of Fallot are cyanotic. Varying degrees of cyanosis are present, depending on the amount of right-to-left intracardiac shunting and the amount of blood that enters the pulmonary circulation by the right ventricle. In severe cases, pulmonary blood flow is markedly decreased and these infants are deeply cyanotic. However, if the right ventricular outflow obstruction is only mild or moderate, the intracardiac shunt can be left to right and the infant will not be cyanotic.

Infants with tetralogy of Fallot are at risk for hypercyanotic (or "tet") spells. These spells consist of severe and intractable cyanosis, irritability, pallor, tachypnea, flaccidity, and possibly loss of consciousness. These spells are thought to be secondary to a transient increase in the obstruction of the right ventricular outflow tract, resulting in minimal or no pulmonary blood flow. See Medical Management later for treatment. True hypercyanotic spells rarely occur, but one significant spell should prompt early surgery as they can be life-threatening.

Baseline oxygen saturations should be obtained before discharge from the neonatal intensive care unit. Oxygenation monitoring at home may be used if baseline oxygen saturations are 75% to 85% or if a BT shunt is placed before discharge.

Heart Sounds. A grade II to IV/VI harsh systolic murmur at the mid to upper left sternal border is usually present but is diminished or absent during a hypercyanotic spell. The S_2 is usually loud and single (representing aortic closure).

Congestive Heart Failure. CHF is uncommon in tetralogy of Fallot. In rare "pink tet" cases, as described earlier, clinical symptoms will resemble a simple large VSD and CHF will develop over time.

Laboratory Data

Arterial Blood Gases. The $Paco_2$ and pH are normal. The Pao_2 is normal if the pulmonary stenosis is mild and there is little right-to-left shunting at the ventricular level. If the pulmonary stenosis is more severe, the amount of right-to-left shunting is substantial and the Pao_2 will be low.

CBC. Anemia can worsen hypoxemia with mixing cardiac lesions. Intermittent evaluation of hemoglobin and hematocrit should be performed and aiming for a higher baseline is clinically helpful.

Chest X-ray Examination. The classic chest x-ray examination shows the shape of a boot with a normal-size heart. However, the classic chest x-ray pattern described is not common in the newborn. Pulmonary vascularity is either normal or decreased.

Electrocardiogram. The ECG demonstrates right ventricular hypertrophy.

Echocardiogram. An echocardiogram is diagnostic. Doppler interrogation helps define the degree and level of pulmonary stenosis. Color-flow mapping can help delineate the size of the VSD and direction of blood flow across the atrial and ventricular septums.

Cardiac Catheterization. Cardiac catheterization is not generally required.

TREATMENT

Medical Management. Immediate medical management is not generally required. Most infants with tetralogy of Fallot are stable and require no interventions or medications. Neonates with severe right ventricular outflow tract obstruction may require PGE_1 infusion to keep the ductus arteriosus open.

Medical management of hypercyanotic (or "tet") spells includes knee-chest positioning, oxygen, morphine, and fluid boluses. If at home parents should be instructed to calm the infant quickly and bring the infant's knees to his or her chest. A beta blocker (propranolol) and systemic vasopressor may also be tried. Rarely, emergent surgery is needed when medical management is insufficient.

Surgical Treatment. Total correction of tetralogy of Fallot involves intracardiac repair with patch closure of the large VSD and relief of the right ventricular outflow obstruction performed through a median sternotomy incision. Often a patch across the pulmonary valve annulus is necessary. Contraindications include small size of the infant, anomalous left anterior descending coronary artery, and hypoplastic pulmonary arteries.

Total surgical repair of tetralogy of Fallot is not usually carried out in the neonatal period. Surgery is usually performed electively within the first year of life.[33,34] If surgical intervention in infancy is warranted (i.e., the infant is severely hypoxic because of inadequate pulmonary blood flow), a systemic-to-pulmonary shunt (BT shunt) is performed to provide adequate pulmonary blood flow until complete surgical repair at a later date.

COMPLICATIONS AND RESIDUAL EFFECTS

Surgical repair of tetralogy of Fallot often requires a patch across the pulmonary valve annulus. This makes the pulmonary valve dysfunctional and leaves the child with no functional valve in the pulmonary position. "Free" pulmonary regurgitation can be tolerated for decades with minimal symptoms, but right ventricular dilation gradually occurs and right ventricular function can eventually be affected.[34] Pulmonary valve replacement is being performed earlier in life (teenage years), and advancements are moving toward performing pulmonary valve replacements by a cardiac catheterization procedure and tissue bioengineered valves that may one day grow with the patient.

PROGNOSIS AND FOLLOW-UP

Prognosis after surgical repair is good, although most children are left without a pulmonary valve. Severe pulmonary regurgitation can cause functional limitations on activities of daily living for some patients, and the right ventricular dilation secondary to severe pulmonary regurgitation can lead to ventricular arrhythmias and sudden death. Long-term follow-up after corrective surgery is necessary, and most children require a future surgery or intervention for pulmonary valve replacement.[61]

Pulmonary Atresia with Intact Ventricular Septum

PHYSIOLOGY

Pulmonary atresia is characterized by complete agenesis of the pulmonary valve. This lesion produces severe signs or symptoms soon after birth and is not compatible with life unless there is an associated interatrial communication and an additional pathway of entry for blood into the pulmonary circulation (through a PDA or collateral blood flow). Because flow to the lungs may depend on a PDA, death may occur when this structure closes. The right ventricle is usually hypoplastic but may be normal or dilated, depending on the degree of tricuspid insufficiency present. The presence of sinusoidal connections between the right ventricle and the coronary arteries is associated with poorer long-term survival.[11]

DATA COLLECTION
Physical Findings

Cyanosis. Cyanosis is always present due to reduced pulmonary blood flow and atrial right-to-left shunting. Acceptable oxygen saturations are greater than 75% on room air when on PGE_1 infusion.

Heart Sounds. The S_2 is single, and a soft systolic murmur may be heard as a result of either the PDA or tricuspid insufficiency.

Congestive Heart Failure. CHF is not present unless there is significant tricuspid insufficiency (see Congestive Heart Failure earlier in this chapter).

Laboratory Data

Arterial Blood Gases. The pH and $PacO_2$ are usually within normal range. The PaO_2 is usually very low (20 to 30 mm Hg) unless there is a large shunt at the ductal or bronchial collateral level. In some cases, the amount of pulmonary blood flow is insufficient, causing a low pH due to metabolic acidosis.

CBC. Anemia can worsen hypoxemia with mixing cardiac lesions. Intermittent evaluation of hemoglobin and hematocrit should be performed, and aiming for a higher baseline is clinically helpful.

Chest X-ray Examination. Heart size is normal unless tricuspid insufficiency causes cardiomegaly. Pulmonary vascularity is either decreased or normal, depending on the amount of shunting through the PDA or collateral blood flow.

NIRS. NIRS monitoring can be helpful for monitoring in the immediate stabilization period, especially if the defect was not prenatally diagnosed.

Electrocardiogram. The ECG is usually normal but may demonstrate left ventricular hypertrophy.

Echocardiogram. Two-dimensional echocardiogram is diagnostic. Color-flow mapping can suggest the presence of coronary artery sinusoids.

Cardiac Catheterization. Cardiac catheterization may be performed if intervention to open the pulmonary valve is possible. Catheter intervention on the pulmonary valve is not possible if right-ventricle–dependent coronary sinusoids are present or if the pulmonary valve annulus is extremely small. Balloon atrial septostomy may be performed at the time of catheterization but is rarely needed.

TREATMENT

Medical Management. PGE$_1$ is used to maintain patency of the ductus arteriosus until surgical intervention (see General Treatment Strategy earlier in this chapter).

Surgical Treatment. In most medical centers, a systemic-to-pulmonary shunt such as the Blalock–Taussig operation is performed. In cases where the right ventricle and tricuspid valve are not severely hypoplastic, a pulmonary valvotomy or right ventricular outflow tract reconstruction may also be performed in addition to a shunt. This establishes an open pathway through the atretic valve area between the pulmonary artery and the right ventricle and establishes blood flow through the right ventricle and pulmonary artery to promote growth of the right heart. The pulmonary valvotomy and pulmonary outflow patch procedures are performed through a median sternotomy incision.

COMPLICATIONS AND RESIDUAL EFFECTS

Complications and residual effects of the Blalock-Taussig operation include CHF from a large shunt, inadequate pulmonary blood flow due to a too small shunt or a shunt stenosis, a reduction in functional health status and exercise tolerance,[33] and sudden death due to sudden shunt obstruction. The mortality rate in infants is 25% or higher as children went through long-term surgical and medical follow-up.[4]

PROGNOSIS AND FOLLOW-UP

Pulmonary atresia is fatal without surgical intervention. The size and function of the right ventricle

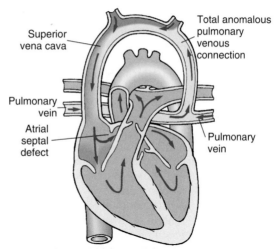

FIGURE 24-13 Total anomalous pulmonary venous return. (Modified from Hockenberry MJ, Wilson D: *Wong's essentials of pediatric nursing*, ed 8, St Louis, 2009, Mosby.)

and tricuspid valve determine if a child can eventually have a two-ventricle repair (where the right side of the heart functions independently and performs its normal job) or end up with single-ventricle physiology (where the right side of the heart is functionless and the left side of the heart does all the work) or something in the middle. Long-term prognosis depends on original anatomy and the surgeries performed.[1] Multiple surgeries and long-term cardiac follow-up are always necessary.

Total Anomalous Pulmonary Venous Return

PHYSIOLOGY

Total anomalous pulmonary venous return (TAPVR) occurs when all the pulmonary veins do not drain normally into the left atrium. Instead, the pulmonary veins drain into an abnormal vein (or veins) connecting to the systemic venous system (SVC, IVC, or coronary sinus). The systemic veins drain to the right atrium, so the oxygenated pulmonary venous blood ends up on the right side of the heart. The presence of an ASD is necessary to sustain life. The four main varieties of TAPVR are as follows:

- Supracardiac (most common) (Figure 24-13), in which the four veins join behind the heart, travel superiorly, and the drainage is to the superior vena cava

- Infracardiac, in which the four veins join behind the heart, pass inferiorly through the diaphragm, and connect to the portal venous system or inferior vena cava
- Intracardiac, in which the pulmonary veins drain into the coronary sinus or directly into the right atrium
- Mixed, in which at least two of the above types of anomalous pulmonary drainage occur in the same child (for example, right pulmonary veins return to the superior vena cava and left pulmonary veins drain to the coronary sinus)

Each of the various types of anomalous drainage can occur with or without obstruction along the pulmonary venous pathway. The presence or absence of obstruction profoundly affects the clinical course. Because all pulmonary venous return (oxygenated blood) ultimately enters the right atrium (as opposed to the left atrium), a right-to-left shunt at the atrial level is necessary to sustain life.

DATA COLLECTION
Physical Findings
Cyanosis. Infants with TAPVR are frequently cyanotic with saturations less than 80% or lower if obstructed venous return is present. Obstructed TAPVR causes pulmonary venous congestion, which leads to reduced pulmonary blood flow and pulmonary edema, both of which also contribute to cyanosis.

Heart Sounds. Murmurs are rarely heard in infants with TAPVR.

Congestive Heart Failure. Infants with unobstructed TAPVR usually show signs of CHF resulting from volume overload of the right ventricle (see Congestive Heart Failure earlier in this chapter). Infants with obstructed TAPVR have pulmonary venous congestion that can be life-threatening.

Laboratory Data
Arterial Blood Gases. The pH and $PaCO_2$ are usually normal. The PaO_2 is usually low, but may be within the normal range if there is a large amount of pulmonary blood flow (always associated with severe congestive heart failure). If pulmonary venous obstruction is present, pulmonary blood flow is reduced and the PaO_2 is low.

Chest X-ray Examination. If the TAPVR is obstructed, the chest x-ray examination will demonstrate pulmonary venous congestion without cardiomegaly.

If the TAPVR is unobstructed, the chest x-ray examination will demonstrate a marked increase in pulmonary vascularity and cardiomegaly.

Electrocardiogram. An ECG may demonstrate right axis deviation, right ventricular hypertrophy, and right atrial enlargement.

Echocardiogram. TAPVR is easily diagnosed by echocardiogram. In two-dimensional imaging, an extravascular structure is seen behind the small left atrium. Color-flow mapping is helpful to trace the abnormal pulmonary venous connection to the superior vena cava, coronary sinus, inferior vena cava, or mixed locations. The right-to-left shunting across the atrial septum can also be demonstrated.

Cardiac Catheterization. Cardiac catheterization is not usually required.

TREATMENT
Medical Management. Obstructed TAPVR is a surgical emergency. Nonobstructed TAPVR is usually stable enough to await elective surgery and rarely requires medical management.

Surgical Treatment. Surgical correction of TAPVR depends on the variety. Supracardiac and infracardiac varieties require surgical reimplantation of the common vein into the left atrium. Intracardiac TAPVR can usually be surgically repaired by realigning the atrial septum during closure of the ASD and directing the anomalous veins to the left atrial side.[27] All repairs are performed through a median sternotomy incision.

COMPLICATIONS AND RESIDUAL EFFECTS
Complications and residual effects include pulmonary venous obstruction and dysrhythmias. The mortality rate varies from 10% to 25% in infancy.[32]

PROGNOSIS AND FOLLOW-UP
Infants with nonobstructed TAPVR generally do well if the lesion is recognized early and early corrective surgery is performed. The prognosis for obstructed TAPVR is less favorable despite early surgical intervention.

Tricuspid Atresia

PHYSIOLOGY
In tricuspid atresia, there is complete agenesis of the tricuspid valve with no direct communication

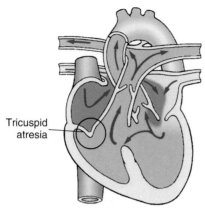

Tricuspid atresia

FIGURE 24-14 Tricuspid atresia. (Modified from Hockenberry MJ, Wilson D: *Wong's essentials of pediatric nursing*, ed 8, St Louis, 2009, Mosby.)

between the right atrium and right ventricle. Systemic venous blood entering the right atrium is shunted through a patent foramen ovale or ASD into the left atrium. If a large VSD is present, the right ventricle and pulmonary arteries may be normal in size. If the ventricular septum is intact but a large PDA is present, the right ventricular cavity may be hypoplastic and the pulmonary arteries are usually slightly decreased or normal in size (Figure 24-14). About 30% to 50% of these infants will have transposition of the great arteries and other associated anomalies such as coarctation of the aorta.[68]

DATA COLLECTION
Physical Findings
Cyanosis. Cyanosis is always present, although the degree of cyanosis varies. Newborns will have marked cyanosis if the pulmonary blood flow is compromised. Oxygen saturations should be greater than 75% due to complete mixing of the oxygenated and deoxygenated blood within the heart.

Heart Sounds. Murmurs of associated shunts or lesions (VSD, PDA, and pulmonary stenosis) may be present.

Congestive Heart Failure. CHF may be present with a large shunt (PDA or VSD) (see Congestive Heart Failure earlier in this chapter).

Laboratory Data
Arterial Blood Gases. The pH and $PaCO_2$ usually are normal. The PaO_2 may vary from near normal if there is a large VSD or PDA to extremely low if there is limited shunting into the pulmonary system.

CBC. Anemia can worsen hypoxemia with mixing cardiac lesions. Intermittent evaluation of hemoglobin and hematocrit should be performed and aiming for a higher baseline is clinically helpful.

Chest X-ray Examination. A chest x-ray examination may show a normal heart size or cardiomegaly. Pulmonary vascularity may be normal, decreased, or increased, depending on the amount of pulmonary blood flow.

Electrocardiogram. An ECG usually demonstrates left axis deviation with a counterclockwise loop, a superior axis in the frontal plane, and left ventricular electrical dominance.

Echocardiogram. Absence of the tricuspid valve is diagnostic of tricuspid atresia. Color-flow mapping can identify the right-to-left shunt at the atrial level and the presence of a VSD, PDA, or valve stenosis.

Cardiac Catheterization. Cardiac catheterization is rarely required unless balloon atrial septostomy is necessary to improve intraatrial mixing.

TREATMENT
Medical Management. Immediate medical management is aimed primarily at maintaining adequate pulmonary blood flow. In the usual case of severely limited pulmonary blood flow, PGE_1 infusion maintains pulmonary perfusion via the ductus arteriosus.

Surgical Treatment. Complete repair of this heart defect is not possible because mitral and tricuspid valves are necessary to achieve a two-ventricle circulation. Instead, the single-ventricle palliative surgeries are necessary to allow the single left ventricle to perform all the work of the heart. This palliative route may start with a systemic-to-pulmonary shunt (such as the Blalock-Taussig operation) if there is insufficient pulmonary blood flow, a pulmonary artery band placement if there is excessive pulmonary blood flow, or no surgery if there is a balanced circulation. Two subsequent staged surgeries are required called the *bidirectional Glenn* and *Fontan* procedures. Any associated defects are also repaired.

COMPLICATIONS AND RESIDUAL EFFECTS
If a BT shunt is required for pulmonary blood flow, interstage complications can include shunt occlusion

and possible sudden death. Long-term single ventricle complications and residual effects include heart failure, chronic pleural effusions, renal or liver failure, persistent shunts, conduit obstruction, dysrhythmia, plastic bronchitis, and protein-losing enteropathy.[64] Survival through all three palliative surgeries depends on institutional experience and specifics of each individual case, but is generally up to 85% with a single left ventricle anatomy.[13]

PROGNOSIS AND FOLLOW-UP

The short-term prognosis for tricuspid atresia is guarded. Longer term, it is not known how long children can live with only a single ventricle performing all the work of the heart. Heart transplantation may eventually be performed. Long-term cardiology follow-up is a necessity.

Truncus Arteriosus

PHYSIOLOGY

Truncus arteriosus is characterized by one great artery arising from the left and right ventricles, overriding a VSD. This common artery has one valve and gives rise to (in order) the coronary arteries, the pulmonary arteries, and the brachiocephalic arteries. A second semilunar valve is not present. A coexisting VSD is present in more than 98% of cases. Truncus arteriosus is classified into three types, depending on the origins of the pulmonary arteries:

1. Type I—a short, main pulmonary artery arises from the common trunk that bifurcates into the right and left pulmonary arteries
2. Type II—the right and left pulmonary arteries arise directly from the posterior surface of the common trunk
3. Type III—the right and left pulmonary arteries arise directly from the lateral walls of the common trunk (Figure 24-15)

In truncus arteriosus, the common trunk receives a mixture of unoxygenated blood from the right ventricle and oxygenated blood from the left ventricle. Blood flow to the lungs varies with the type of truncus but is usually increased and at systemic level pressure.

The ductus arteriosus is usually absent. A right aortic arch may be present. Extracardiac anomalies are present in 20% to 40% of cases, and 35% to 40% of neonates with truncus arteriosus have 22q11 deletion syndrome.[15]

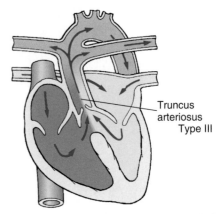

Truncus arteriosus Type III

FIGURE 24-15 Truncus arteriosus type III. (Modified from Hockenberry MJ, Wilson D: *Wong's essentials of pediatric nursing*, ed 8, St Louis, 2009, Mosby.)

DATA COLLECTION
Physical Findings

Cyanosis. Cyanosis may be present at birth but varies in intensity according to the amount of pulmonary blood flow. Minimal cyanosis indicates adequate pulmonary blood flow.

Heart Sounds. The first heart sound, S_1, is normal, but the S_2 is single and loud because of the single valve of the common trunk. A loud systolic ejection click is frequently heard.

A loud pansystolic murmur maximal at the lower left sternal border that radiates to the entire precordium is commonly heard. A middiastolic rumble may be present. If the truncal valve is insufficient, a blowing diastolic murmur may be heard. A wide pulse pressure is often present.

Congestive Heart Failure. The presence of CHF depends on the amount of pulmonary blood flow. Persistently high pulmonary arteriolar resistance in the first few weeks of life limits excessive pulmonary blood flow, and CHF may not be present until the PVR drops. However, if the truncal valve has significant stenosis or regurgitation, CHF develops earlier due to pressure or volume overload (see Congestive Heart Failure earlier in this chapter).

Laboratory Data

Arterial Blood Gases. The pH and $PaCO_2$ are usually normal. PaO_2 may be near normal if there is adequate pulmonary blood flow (usually associated with severe CHF).

CBC. Anemia can worsen hypoxemia with mixing cardiac lesions. Intermittent evaluation of hemoglobin and hematocrit should be performed, and aiming for a higher baseline is clinically helpful.

Chest X-ray Examination. Cardiomegaly, displaced pulmonary arteries, and increased vascular markings are typical findings on the chest x-ray examination.

Electrocardiogram. Combined ventricular hypertrophy is most often seen on an ECG. Left atrial enlargement is also commonly found.

Echocardiogram. A two-dimensional echocardiogram is diagnostic. Particular attention is paid to the number of truncal valve leaflets, the presence of truncal valve insufficiency or stenosis, and location of the bilateral branch pulmonary arteries.

Cardiac Catheterization. A cardiac catheterization is rarely necessary.

TREATMENT

Medical Management. Medical management of these infants consists of stabilizing and treating CHF when present. Calcium should be closely monitored because of the possibility of 22q11 deletion syndrome.

Surgical Treatment. Repair of truncus arteriosus consists of separating the pulmonary arteries from the common trunk, closing the VSD with a patch, and inserting a right ventricular–to–pulmonary artery valve conduit. The use of homograft conduits for repair of truncus arteriosus is common. Total repair of truncus arteriosus is performed through a median sternotomy incision.

COMPLICATIONS AND RESIDUAL EFFECTS

Complications and side effects include pulmonary vascular disease, residual shunts, truncal valve insufficiency, and conduit obstruction. The mortality rate is 10% to 30% dependent on the anatomy and severity of truncal valve abnormality.

PROGNOSIS AND FOLLOW-UP

The longer-term outcome depends on the competency of the truncal valve. Severe truncal valve regurgitation or stenosis after truncus arteriosus repair is not well tolerated and may require reintervention.[10] Associated extracardiac anomalies or genetic abnormalities also significantly affect prognosis. Lifelong follow-up is always required.

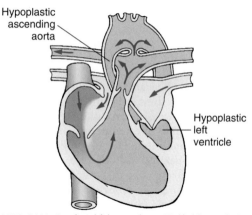

FIGURE 24-16 Hypoplastic left heart syndrome. (Modified from Hockenberry MJ, Wilson D: *Wong's essentials of pediatric nursing*, ed 8, St Louis, 2009, Mosby.)

Hypoplastic Left Heart Syndrome

PHYSIOLOGY

Hypoplastic left heart syndrome (HLHS) represents a clinical spectrum that includes severe coarctation of the aorta, severe aortic valve stenosis or atresia, and severe mitral valve stenosis or atresia (Figure 24-16). The left ventricle and ascending aorta are hypoplastic. Blood flow to the body is dependent on right-to-left shunting through the PDA. Ductal closure results in poor systemic perfusion and death. An atrial septal communication is also required to allow oxygenated pulmonary venous blood to shunt from left atrium into the right atrium; a restrictive atrial septal defect can be life-threatening and require emergent cardiac catheterization intervention.

DATA COLLECTION

Physical Findings

Cyanosis. These infants are cyanotic, with a goal oxygen saturation in the 75% to 85% range. Blood flow to the lungs and systemically is in a delicate balance, so too much blood flow to the lungs results in poor systemic perfusion. This results in high oxygen saturations, but marked poor perfusion, vasoconstriction, poor urine output, and CHF. Too little blood flow to the lungs through the PDA can cause pulmonary undercirculation and low oxygen saturations.

Heart Sounds. A nonspecific systolic murmur is heard in some infants with hypoplastic left heart syndrome. A single S_1 and S_2 may be appreciated.

Congestive Heart Failure. CHF is present as a result of right ventricular volume and pressure overload (see Congestive Heart Failure earlier in this chapter).

Laboratory Data

Arterial Blood Gases. The arterial blood gas may represent the single best indicator of hemodynamic stability. Low arterial saturation (75% to 80%) with normal pH indicates an acceptable balance of systemic and pulmonary blood flow with adequate peripheral perfusion. Elevated oxygen saturation (greater than 90%) with acidosis represents significantly increased pulmonary and decreased systemic flow.

CBC. Anemia can worsen hypoxemia with mixing cardiac lesions. Intermittent evaluation of hemoglobin and hematocrit should be performed, and aiming for a higher baseline is clinically helpful.

BNP. BNP values may be helpful to differentiate respiratory or cardiac instability in neonates with HLHS. Values should be followed for trends rather than individual markers.

Chest X-ray Examination. Cardiomegaly with increased pulmonary vascularity and pulmonary edema is seen on the x-ray examination.

Electrocardiogram. An ECG frequently demonstrates right axis deviation and right ventricular hypertrophy. However, the ECG may be normal.

Echocardiogram. An echocardiogram is diagnostic with a small left ventricular cavity and ascending aorta, mitral and aortic valve atresia or hypoplasia, and a dilated right ventricle. Adequate atrial septal defect, patent ductus arteriosus, myocardial function, and degree of tricuspid regurgitation are essential parts of the echocardiogram.

NIRS Monitoring. NIRS monitoring is recommended to evaluate cerebral and systemic perfusion and monitor for low cardiac output.

Cardiac Catheterization. Cardiac catheterization carries a high risk in infants with hypoplastic left heart syndrome and is usually not necessary unless the atrial septal defect is not adequate for intraatrial mixing. A balloon atrial septostomy and atrial septal stent placement can be performed if necessary.

TREATMENT

Medical Management. Pharmacologic maintenance of ductal patency with PGE$_1$ with continuous infusion is required. Institutional practices vary, but the goal is a balanced pulmonary and systemic circulation by the use of volume expansion, inotropic support,

and intubation. Maneuvers such as hypoventilation to increase PVR and redirect cardiac output to the body have been used. This may be a sign that cardiac surgery is necessary in an urgent manner due to inability to balance systemic and pulmonary circulation.

Surgical Treatment. Palliative cardiac surgeries are required for survival and occur over the first few years of life.[18] The *Norwood procedure* is performed initially, consisting of enlargement of the atrial septal defect, ligation of the PDA, Damus-Kaye-Stansel (DKS) anastomosis of the pulmonary artery to the ascending aorta, aortic arch reconstruction, and creation of an aortopulmonary shunt (BT shunt) to provide pulmonary blood flow. Some centers use a hybrid approach with a PDA stent and bilateral pulmonary artery bands as a stage I palliation.[8,22] In the second stage, a *bidirectional Glenn* (anastomosis between the superior vena cava and the pulmonary arteries) is performed and the aortopulmonary shunt is removed; this is usually performed at 5 to 9 months of age. The final stage is the *Fontan procedure,* which connects the inferior vena cava to the pulmonary arteries; this is generally done at 3 to 5 years of age.[18] Cardiac transplantation is an alternative surgical option, although infant donor hearts are rarely available. In some centers, the Norwood procedure is performed as a bridge to transplantation, allowing the infant to survive until a donor heart is available.

PROGNOSIS AND FOLLOW-UP

The longer-term outcome is variable and depends on associated factors such as a restrictive atrial septum, lung disease, genetic syndromes, and extracardiac anomalies. Turner syndrome, trisomy 13, trisomy 18, Holt-Oram, Smith-Lemli-Optiz, partial trisomy 9, Jacobsen syndrome, and many others have been associated with HLHS. Since 2008 there has been an increased focus on improving interstage mortality after discharge from stage I Norwood (BT shunt) to stage II Norwood (Glenn), but this is still a high-risk time for infants with HLHS. Current expectations are that up to 65% to 70% of newborns born today will survive all three palliative surgical procedures, but longer-term survival is not easily achieved.[13]

Heart Transplantation in Infants

For infants born with cardiomyopathy or uncorrectable congenital heart disease, heart transplantation may offer the only chance of long-term

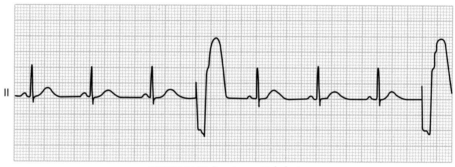

FIGURE 24-17 Premature ventricular beats.

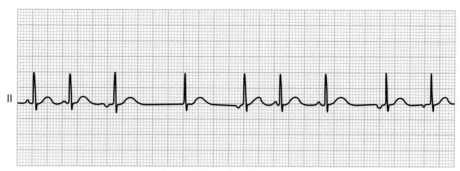

FIGURE 24-18 Wandering atrial pacemaker with junctional escape (fourth complex).

survival. Heart transplantation in infancy is severely limited by donor availability. There is a scarcity of donor hearts in this age and size group, so many infants on transplant lists die waiting for donors. It is also important that families understand that heart transplantation requires lifelong medications, cardiac biopsies, hospitalizations for rejection of the organ or suspected infection (in the setting of the immunosuppression required after transplantation), and likely retransplantation in the future.

Dysrhythmias

When evaluating an infant with a dysrhythmia, it is essential to assess simultaneously the electrophysiology and hemodynamic status. A neonate with poor perfusion and hypotension should first be treated for shock. A 12-lead ECG can then be done for definitive diagnosis of the type of dysrhythmia. When analyzing the ECG for the mechanism of dysrhythmia, a notation should be made in three main areas: (1) atrial and ventricular rates, (2) rhythm, and (3) QRS morphology.

PHYSIOLOGY

The development of the cardiac conduction system continues after birth with a steady increase in the sympathetic innervation of the heart. This accounts for the observed heart rate variability and the high frequency of benign dysrhythmias in the newborn. Premature ventricular beats (Figure 24-17), premature atrial beats, brief episodes of ectopic atrial rhythms, wandering atrial pacemakers (Figure 24-18), and even brief episodes of sinus arrest are all frequently seen in the newborn period. The majority of these dysrhythmias do not require immediate treatment; however, if they persist, the presence of congenital heart disease, sepsis, drug toxicity, persistent hypoxia, adrenal insufficiency, disorders of electrolyte and acid–base balance, hypoglycemia, and hypocalcemia should be considered.

All cardiac tissue is capable of generating a spontaneous depolarization. However, the sinoatrial (SA) node, atrioventricular (AV) node, and His–Purkinje system consist of specialized conductive tissue with rapid spontaneous depolarization. The SA node is the normal pacemaker of the heart because it has

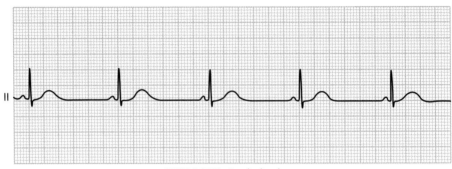

FIGURE 24-19 Sinus bradycardia.

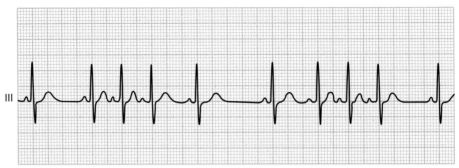

FIGURE 24-20 Sinus dysrhythmia.

the fastest rate of spontaneous depolarization. If, however, the spontaneous depolarization of the SA node is delayed or slower than normal, an escape rhythm is generated by either the AV node or His-Purkinje system (these rhythms are called *nodal escape* or *ventricular escape,* respectively). Dysrhythmias also can originate from an automatic "ectopic" pacemaker located anywhere in the heart. These ectopic pacemakers become more active in the presence of hypoxia, acidosis, digoxin toxicity, abnormal sympathetic nervous system stimulation, increased wall tension (CHF), or altered electrolyte balance.

Drug therapy for dysrhythmias is based on the ability of certain medications to alter the electrophysiologic properties of cardiac tissue. One class of antidysrhythmic drugs directly increases the automaticity of certain cardiac fibers. Examples of such drugs are procainamide and lidocaine (see Table 24-3). Other drugs directly or indirectly affect the autonomic nervous system activity. Propranolol is a beta-adrenergic blocker and works in this fashion.

BENIGN DYSRHYTHMIAS: SINUS BRADYCARDIA, SINUS TACHYCARDIA, AND SINUS DYSRHYTHMIA

Of normal premature infants, up to 40% have brief episodes of sinus bradycardia (Figure 24-19), sinus tachycardia, or sinus dysrhythmia (Figure 24-20) that are benign and require no treatment. Healthy premature and term infants may have heart rates that range from 90 to 200 beats/min. Sustained heart rates (longer than 15 seconds) above or below this range should be evaluated with a 12-lead ECG and rhythm strip. The bedside monitor display is often contaminated with artifact that makes accurate interpretation of dysrhythmias impossible. A 12-lead ECG provides necessary information that cannot be obtained from the bedside monitor alone.

SUPRAVENTRICULAR TACHYCARDIA

Supraventricular tachycardia (SVT) (Figure 24-21) is the most common tachydysrhythmia in the newborn period. SVT can result from dual AV nodal pathways, rapid conduction through an accessory

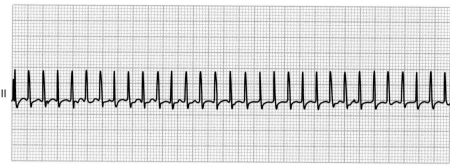

FIGURE 24-21 Supraventricular tachycardia.

bundle (WPW syndrome), or the existence of an ectopic atrial pacemaker. SVT is occasionally associated with specific heart diseases, such as Ebstein's anomaly of the tricuspid valve, cardiomyopathy, or myocarditis. These lesions are present in up to 25% of infants with SVT and should be excluded with appropriate evaluation, an echocardiogram.

Criteria for SVT include (1) persistent ventricular rate over 200 to 220 beats/min, (2) a fixed and regular R-R interval, and (3) little variability in heart rate with various activities (e.g., crying, feeding, apnea). The QRS complexes are most often narrow-complex and P waves may be absent. Newborns with SVT often have a history of restlessness, tachypnea, irritability, and poor feeding. These symptoms may start abruptly with SVT initiation or may develop after 12 to 24 hours of SVT as ventricular function worsens. Without treatment, prolonged SVT can result in cardiovascular collapse and death.

Treatment. Various maneuvers may be used to attempt to convert the infant to normal sinus rhythm (NSR). Vagal maneuvers such as carotid occlusion and ocular compression should *never* be used. However, stimulation of the diving reflex using an ice bag applied to the infant's face may be attempted and is the first line of treatment in the hemodynamically stable neonate with SVT. Caution must be used with this procedure to ensure adequate ventilation for the infant. Adenosine, a purinergic agonist, is an especially effective antidysrhythmic drug for treatment of SVT (see Table 24-3). Adenosine slows the sinus rate and produces transient AV block, which can interrupt some types of SVT. Adenosine must be administered as a rapid bolus through an intravenous line

to be effective, so venous access must be available to use this medication. Overdrive atrial pacing has been successful in converting SVT to NSR. However, direct-current (DC) cardioversion (1 to 2 watt-seconds/kg) is the most effective and rapid therapy and is the treatment of choice for a hemodynamically unstable neonate with SVT. The defibrillator must always be in the synchronous mode. If cardioversion is successful, maintenance drug therapy should be initiated with the consultation of pediatric cardiology.

For infants without WPW syndrome, digoxin or propranolol is often used for initial maintenance therapy. Digoxin should not be used in WPW syndrome, so this disorder should be ruled out before digoxin is used. Propranolol can be used for infants with SVT caused by WPW syndrome in the absence of CHF. Beta-blocking agents may inhibit circulating catecholamines, which are needed for the maintenance of adequate cardiac output in the face of CHF. In premature infants, propranolol may cause apnea and hypoglycemia. Esmolol is another beta-blocking agent that can be administered intravenously for SVT (see Table 24-3).

If the SVT fails to convert using the methods outlined previously, other drugs such as amiodarone, flecainide, or procainamide may be necessary. After conversion to NSR, maintenance drug therapy should be continued for 6 to 12 months or longer based on pediatric electrophysiology recommendations. Relapses during the first 48 hours are common (70%) and should be anticipated.

Fetal SVT is uncommon but, when present, can be associated with severe CHF and hydrops fetalis. Fetal SVT requires aggressive management, including conversion with maternally administered digoxin, flecainide, sotalol, or other antiarrhythmic

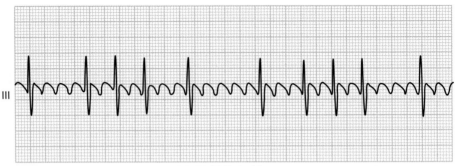

FIGURE 24-22 Atrial flutter.

medication. A favorable outcome usually can be expected for fetal SVT. Failure to control the fetal SVT in the presence of fetal hydrops is an indication for delivery if the fetus is of viable gestational age. The likelihood of SVT becoming a persistent problem after birth and cardioversion depends on the type and etiology of the fetal SVT.

ATRIAL FLUTTER AND FIBRILLATION

The presence of atrial flutter (Figure 24-22) is often suggestive of a serious organic heart disease (endocardial fibroelastosis, Ebstein's anomaly of the tricuspid valve, or complex heart defect). Atrial flutter is diagnosed when (1) the atrial rate is greater than 220 beats/min; (2) the P waves are very regular; and (3) there is a characteristic saw-tooth pattern, indicating a flutter wave. The ventricular rate will vary depending on the degree of AV block present. Atrial fibrillation is extremely rare and almost always indicates a serious organic heart disease. The prognosis for atrial flutter and fibrillation tends to be less favorable than those of SVTs caused by an accessory pathway or ectopic atrial pacemaker. However, some cases of atrial flutter have been found in infants receiving broad-spectrum antimicrobials or those with an intracardiac catheter causing mechanical irritation of the right atrium.[51] Atrial flutter is more difficult to treat in utero, more likely to be associated with structural heart defects, and more likely to develop hydrops fetalis.

Treatment. The treatment of atrial flutter or fibrillation is DC cardioversion or overdrive atrial pacing with pediatric electrophysiology consultation. In many cases, the neonate with atrial flutter will require a single cardioversion and then not require medication therapy to prevent further episodes. However, maintenance therapy with an antidysrhythmic medication may be indicated and initiated by an electrophysiology specialist.

VENTRICULAR TACHYCARDIA

Ventricular tachycardia is relatively rare and is usually seen with severe medical illnesses such as hypoxemia, shock, electrolyte disturbances, and digoxin toxicity. Ventricular tachycardia is recognized by its characteristic wide QRS complexes, although it can be difficult to differentiate ventricular tachycardia from a supraventricular tachycardia with aberrant ventricular conduction. A wide-complex tachycardia should always be assumed to be ventricular tachycardia until proven otherwise. The presence of ventricular tachycardia is always alarming because the etiology is rarely benign, it can abruptly start and cause rapid hemodynamic instability and clinical deterioration, and it can be challenging to treat.

Treatment. Ventricular tachycardia is best treated with immediate DC cardioversion. Lidocaine may be used as a bolus (1 to 2 mg/kg intravenously) or as a continuous intravenous infusion of 20 to 30 mcg/kg/min. After conversion, maintenance therapy should be initiated using propranolol, lidocaine, procainamide, or amiodarone (see Table 24-3).

COMPLETE ATRIOVENTRICULAR BLOCK

In complete heart block, the SA node functions normally and sends out a depolarization impulse to the atria, but the AV node is dysfunctional and does not transmit this signal to the ventricles. As the ventricles receive no signal to depolarize from the atria, they depolarize on their own but at a much slower rate than the atrial rate. The result is that atrial and ventricular depolarizations are completely independent of each other. The ECG demonstrates P waves at a normal heart rate for age, but QRS complexes that occur at a much slower rate and are completely dissociated from the P waves.

Complete heart block can be seen in infants with specific structural cardiac defects, myocarditis, or endocardial fibroelastosis. There is a strong association between congenital heart block and maternal collagen diseases such as systemic lupus erythematosus. Often these mothers have no signs or symptoms of lupus, but laboratory confirmation is often possible.

Treatment. No treatment is immediately required unless the neonate is hemodynamically unstable due to significant ventricular bradycardia. Cardiac output is directly dependent on the ventricular rate; isoproterenol may be used temporarily to increase the ventricular rate until a pacemaker is placed. If the ventricular rate is consistently below 55 beats/min, signs or symptoms of low cardiac output, or an associated congenital heart defect, pacemaker placement is indicated. In most cases, the pacemaker will be set to listen to the child's normal SA node activity and will transmit these depolarization signals to the ventricles (the normal role of an AV node).

SICK SINUS SYNDROME

Sick sinus syndrome (SSS) is a broad term used to describe dysrhythmias resulting from abnormal sinus node function and includes a wide array of brady-dysrhythmias, including sinus bradycardia, sinus pause/arrest, sinoatrial exit block, and slow escape rhythms, including junctional bradycardia. Although most commonly acquired during surgical repair for CHD (because of the proximity to the sinus node), SSS may also be found congenitally in the neonatal period. Mutations in the cardiac sodium channel gene *SCN5A* can result in congenital SSS.[76] Treatment of SSS requires pacemaker placement, but treatment is not always indicated.

PARENT TEACHING

The diagnosis of CHD in their child—whether given prenatally or postnatally—is a frightening experience and causes much distress to parents.

> **BOX 24-6**
>
> **PARENT TEACHING**
> **KEY POINTS FOR PARENTS OF NEWBORNS WITH HEART DISEASE**
>
> - Refer to a pediatric facility experienced with infants with heart disease.
> - Reassure and support family for understanding that "this is not their fault."
> - Explain all tubes, monitors, and equipment to decrease anxiety.
> - Help parents accept and understand their infant's diagnosis.
> - Encourage parental bonding with their infant and participation in care.
> - Detail home care, including medications, signs and symptoms, and when to call physician.
> - Encourage normal activity.
> - Explain the necessity of subacute bacterial endocarditis protection.
> - Supply parents with resource information—booklets, brochures, Internet resources.

Parents may grieve over the loss of the healthy newborn they had anticipated and experience shock, denial, guilt, anger, despair, or confusion.[20] Comprehensive teaching, reassurance, and support are essential for the well-being of both the infant and the family (Box 24-6).

If the diagnosis of CHD is made prenatally by fetal echocardiography, parent education begins before the birth of the infant. Expectant parents should be referred to a pediatric facility experienced in providing complex medical and surgical care for infants with CHD. Arrangements should be made for parents to meet with key members of the medical and surgical team and tour the intensive care units. A multidisciplinary approach with providers and support staff from cardiology, cardiac surgery, the intensive care team, social work, chaplaincy, genetic counseling, and the palliative care team should be used.

Understanding the heart defect aids in decreasing anxiety, as well as allowing parents to provide good care for their child. Explain the infant's heart defect to the parents. Draw or show a picture of the heart defect, explaining the normal circulation of the heart in simple terms and how their infant's heart differs from normal. This explanation should be repeated often for parental understanding and retention. Careful explanation of all tubes, monitors, equipment, and procedures in the nursery also helps decrease parental anxiety.

Heart defects are not visible lesions. Infants with CHD can appear quite normal and healthy. It may be difficult for some parents to accept that their infant has a cardiac defect. In addition, parents are under great emotional and sometimes physical stress (from labor and delivery), which decreases their ability to hear new information and retain details. Patience and repetition of information is important.

Some parents may initially be unable to respond to their newborn with a heart defect. Health care providers should facilitate bonding by encouraging interaction with the infant and enabling parents to participate in their infant's care. Parental participation enables opportunities for parents to practice under the guidance of professionals and enables professional assessment of parental competencies. Parents should be encouraged to assist with diaper changes, positioning, and oral care, and provide comfort measures even during the critical phase of illness. During the postoperative and convalescent phase of hospitalization, parents should assume more of the infant's care, such as feeding, care of the incision, and medication administration. Before discharge, parents should be encouraged to room with and completely care for their infant, with nursing assistance available as needed. Parents must feel comfortable caring for their infant and must demonstrate their ability to do so before discharge from the hospital.

Teaching home care of the infant before discharge should be detailed and include medications, signs to observe, and guidelines for care. It is critical that these be written instructions that can be referred to often. All medications should be explained in detail, including their purpose, action, and administration. Parents should be made aware of the potential adverse effects (side effects) of all of their infant's medications. Parents should be observed giving medications in the nursery before the infant is discharged. Parents should be instructed to telephone their physician if the infant demonstrates red flags such as (1) any behavior or bodily change that worries parents; (2) fevers; (3) poor weight gain; (4) increased work of breathing or stopping to breathe during feeds; (4) feeding difficulty, increased sweating during feeds, or excessive spitting up; (5) new or changed vomiting or diarrhea for a 12- to 24-hour period; (6) decreased activity level

or irritability; (7) low oxygen saturations if home monitoring was prescribed; or (8) low number of wet diapers in a day.[50] Provide information about the infant's prognosis, follow-up care, and anticipatory guidance about special growth and development considerations.

Cyanotic heart disease is particularly disturbing to parents because their infant's skin color is "blue." Parents should be cautioned that their infant will appear blue, especially around the mouth, mucous membranes, hands, and feet, and that the blueness will increase with activity such as crying, feeding, and bowel movements. Single-ventricle anatomy after the first stage of surgery requires that the discharged infant be followed closely with oxygen saturation checks twice a day or more, and parents should understand their child's expected oxygen saturation and how to contact their primary cardiac team for changes and concerns.

Normal Newborn Care and Maintenance

Many parents will develop a narrow, disease-oriented focus. Emphasize to parents that their infant should be treated as normally as possible. It is often difficult for first-time parents to differentiate "normal baby problems" from cardiac-related problems. It is important to have open communication among the family, primary care provider, and cardiologist. Parents should be encouraged to call medical personnel as needed for support, answers to questions, and reassurance. Support groups can also provide information, empathy, and practical tips to parents caring for children with CHD.

The trip home should occur in an appropriate car seat, and a car seat screen is recommended to ensure oxygen saturations are maintained while restrained. Infection prevention strategies, such as handwashing before handling the infant, avoiding ill contacts, and avoiding large crowds, are especially important to teach parents. Discharge planning should include normal newborn procedures if possible, including standard pediatric immunizations, hearing screen, and circumcision if permitted by the cardiac team. If there is a medical reason to delay these procedures, this should be discussed with parents and future plans for these procedures should be made.

Infectious Endocarditis Protection

Infants with congenital heart disease are at increased risk for developing adverse outcomes associated with infectious endocarditis (IE), also known as bacterial endocarditis (BE). The American Heart Association's Endocarditis Committee extensively reviewed published studies and found no conclusive evidence to link dental, gastrointestinal, or genitourinary tract procedures with the development of IE in most patients with congenital heart defects.[7] Antibiotic prophylaxis with dental procedures is recommended only for patients with cardiac conditions (e.g., prosthetic valves, previous endocarditis, cardiac transplant) associated with the highest risk for adverse outcomes from endocarditis. Antibiotic prophylaxis is also recommended for the following categories of CHD: (1) unrepaired cyanotic CHD; (2) completely repaired CHD with prosthetic material; and (3) repaired CHD with residual defects adjacent to prosthetic material.[7] Parents are encouraged to speak with their pediatric cardiologist regarding any questions related to IE antibiotic prophylaxis.

Activity

Normal newborn activity is encouraged after discharge. There are no activity restrictions for infants with heart disease because infants "self-limit" according to their capacity. However, special precautions may be indicated for handling the infant. Parents should avoid picking the infant up under the arms until the sternal wound and underlying structures are healed. If discharge occurs soon after surgery, there may also be special instructions for bathing the infant.

Supporting Ongoing Development

Infants with CHD are at risk for neurodevelopmental disorders, disability, or developmental delay for a number of reasons, including that the incidence of brain abnormalities is higher in children with CHD than in the general population. Inform parents about their infant's increased risk for developmental delay, review normal developmental milestones, and provide pragmatic strategies to maximize infant development. These may include simple interventions such as prone placement ("tummy time") after sternotomy has healed and continued oral stimulation if G-tube is required. Referral to early intervention programs and cardiac neurodevelopmental clinics for developmental surveillance, screening, and evaluation throughout childhood may allow for later academic, behavioral, psychosocial, and adaptive functioning to maximize the child's potential development.[46]

Parenting an infant with CHD requires coping, adaptation, and evolution—from diagnosis to discharge from the hospital and through caretaking and parenting at home. Parents have reported feelings of posttraumatic stress associated with caring for infants with the most complex single-ventricle anatomies.[60] Consultation with a mental health professional may enable the family to recognize and build on strengths that will help them cope with this enormous challenge.

FUTURE RESEARCH

Improvements in the diagnosis, understanding, and treatment of CHD have drastically reduced the morbidity and mortality rates associated with these defects. Children with critical congenital heart disease that was once considered fatal are now living into adulthood, thanks to innovations in cardiac surgery, cardiology, anesthesia, intensive care, and nursing practices. However, we still have much to discover. The etiology of congenital heart disease is still poorly understood or completely unknown. Cardiac genetic research is focusing on similar cardiac anatomy and how genetic involvement may play into the development of CHD, but without an understanding of true CHD etiology, prevention of CHD is almost impossible. Future developments are needed to promote earlier and widespread prenatal detection of CHD, as well as improvements on current fetal catheter and surgical interventions to intervene on defective cardiac development during fetal life. Advanced screening methods are also necessary to promote early postnatal detection of CHD and avoid the morbidity and mortality risks that can occur at home from undiagnosed CHD.

Medical, catheter-based, and surgical treatments for CHD continue to exponentially advance. Clinical practice guidelines are increasingly being used to standardize care and evaluate best practices.[50] Valve replacement without surgery is a rapidly developing reality, and the development of a tissue-engineered valve that will grow with a child is expected in the near future. Although we have much left to learn, the future is exciting and will bring improved care and health for children with congenital heart disease.

REFERENCES

For a full list of references, scan the QR code or visit http://booksite.elsevier.com/ 9780323320832.

25

NEONATAL NEPHROLOGY

MELISSA A. CADNAPAPHORNCHAI, MARY BIRKEL SCHOENBEIN, ROSANNE WOLOSCHUK,

DANIELLE E. SORANNO, AND JACINTO A. HERNÁNDEZ

In utero, the fetal kidney is not necessary for toxin removal or fluid and electrolyte homeostasis; rather, the placenta performs these functions. By contributing to amniotic fluid, the fetal kidney instead has an essential role in the normal development of the fetus. After birth, as the infant adapts to the external milieu, the kidney gradually assumes its role as regulator of fluid and electrolyte homeostasis. At birth, renal function changes dramatically, complicating clinical assessment. Assessment of renal function is an even greater challenge in the premature infant. The more complicated an organ is in its development, the more subject it is to maldevelopment. In this aspect, the kidney outranks most other organs. Abnormalities of the genitourinary system constitute up to 30% of all anomalies diagnosed prenatally.[127,169] Some anomalies may be readily apparent in the neonatal period, whereas others remain undiagnosed until later life.

Although renal disease can clearly affect the health of the newborn, it may also contribute to lifelong renal pathology. Congenital renal dysplasia, renal obstructive disorders, and cystic diseases account for a substantial percentage of patients with end-stage renal failure. Furthermore, a growing body of data supports a link between prenatal and neonatal events and later hypertension and renal insufficiency in adolescents and adult.[17,100,101]

NORMAL DEVELOPMENT

Anatomic Development of the Kidney

The mammalian embryo progressively develops three sets of excretory organs, all of which might be termed the "embryonic kidney."[169] The pronephros and mesonephros regress in the human but induce the metanephros, which is the direct precursor of the adult kidney (Figure 25-1). The pronephros, a solid mass of cells along the nephrogenic cord, is located at the cervical level at approximately 3 weeks' gestation. Degeneration of the pronephros begins soon after its formation, and regression has completely occurred by week 5. The pronephros has no excretory function but plays an important role in the formation of the mesonephros. The primitive ureter of the pronephros forms the *wolffian, or mesonephric, duct* via fusion of the pronephric tubular buds. The mesonephric duct then induces the formation of the second kidney, *the mesonephros,* at approximately 4 weeks' gestation. The mesonephros develops from the nephrogenic cord and forms 40 pairs of thin-walled tubules and glomeruli with excretory function. Portions of the mesonephric duct system are retained in the male fetus and form the *ducts of the epididymis, the ductus deferens, and the ejaculatory duct.* The remainder of the mesonephric duct system in the male infant has degenerated by the fourth month of gestation as the metanephric kidney develops. In the female, near-complete degeneration has occurred by the third month of gestation.

The *metanephros* appears at 4½ to 5 weeks' gestation. The metanephric kidney is the product of a series of inductive interactions between the metanephric mesenchyme and epithelial ureteric bud. Initially, the ureteric bud grows from the mesonephric duct into the mesenchymal portion of the urogenital ridge; concomitantly, the metanephric mesenchyme changes, becoming histologically distinct from the surrounding tissue. When the metanephric mesenchyme and ureteric bud make contact,

---

PURPLE type highlights content that is particularly applicable to clinical settings.

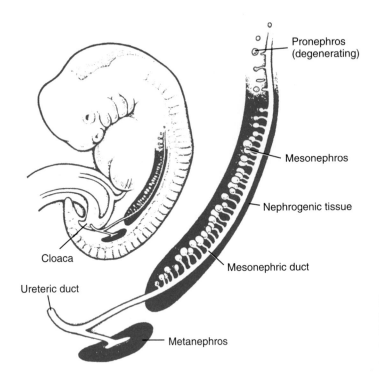

FIGURE 25-1 Schematic representation of overlapping stages in embryogenesis of human kidney. See text for detailed description. (From Holliday MA: Developmental abnormalities of the kidney in children, *Hosp Pract* 13:101, 1978. www.informahealthcare.com)

a condensation of cells begins along the surface of the bud. These cells are the beginnings of pretubular aggregates that undergo mesenchymal-to-epithelial transformation to become the segmented nephron. The condensed mesenchyme is also thought to produce a number of stem cells, which remain undifferentiated and proliferative. These cells serve to maintain a supply of precursor cells until the completion of nephron development. Thus, the epithelial portion of the adult kidney is derived from both the metanephric mesenchyme, via the stem cells ultimately responsible for individual nephron formation, and the ureteric bud, whose migration and division determine the pattern of formation of the urinary collecting system via its pretubular aggregates. The ureteric bud migrates to the most caudal end of the nephrogenic cord and finally to the lumbar region by week 8 of gestation. The ureteric bud also rotates 90 degrees medially along the longitudinal axis. Abnormalities in ascent or rotation can lead to pelvic kidneys, horseshoe kidneys, or crossed fused ectopia. Because of the complex interaction of metanephric mesenchyme and ureteric bud, anomalies of the kidney often accompany anomalies of the collecting system.

Congenital anomalies of the kidney and urinary tract (CAKUT) are a family of diseases with a diverse anatomic spectrum of kidney anomalies (agenesis, hypo/dysplasia, multicystic kidney dysplasia) and ureteropelvic anomalies (duplex collecting system, megaureter, vesicoureteral reflux, posterior urethral valves).[134,166] CAKUT commonly cause progressive chronic kidney disease and constitute the most frequent cause of end-stage kidney disease and renal replacement therapy in childhood.

Nephrogenesis is the process of nephron formation via growth and differentiation of multiple cell types and leads to formation of the overall renal architecture. The process begins in the renal cortex closest to the medulla (juxtamedullary nephrons) and proceeds in a dichotomous branching centrifugal pattern with the outermost (superficial cortical) nephrons forming last. There are multiple phases of growth and structural reorganization after the interactions between the metanephric mesenchyme and the ureteric bud. The formation of the collecting system is controlled by the branching pattern of the ureteric bud, and this occurs at the same time as the formation of functional nephron units.

Four progressive phases of nephrogenesis occur, during which the nephron proceeds through several intermediate forms. By the fourth stage, there is a definitive glomerulus with highly differentiated visceral and parietal epithelial cells. The vascular system development occurs in concert with nephron formation. The surrounding major vessels and neural ganglia grow into the metanephros to complete the remaining cell types, and vessel architecture is similar to the newborn kidney by 15 weeks of gestation.

Physiologic Development of the Kidney

Although newborn kidneys are usually described as "immature," they are perfectly suited to their usual responsibilities.[28,119] During the latter part of gestation, their primary role is maintenance of amniotic fluid volume. This requires a large volume of urine with a relatively high concentration of sodium. Thus, fetal urine output is on the order of 10 ml/kg/hr of sodium-rich urine. Fetal fractional excretion of sodium (FENa; i.e., the fraction of sodium in glomerular filtrate that appears in urine) is especially high, approximately 15%. This compares to less than 1% in a growing infant born after a full-term pregnancy.

The next major responsibility of the newborn kidney occurs during the first week of life. Fetuses have a large amount of extracellular fluid (ECF) compared with older children and adults. ECF as a percentage of body weight progressively diminishes throughout gestation, at approximately 65% of body weight at 26 weeks of gestation, 40% at full-term, and 25% by 1 year of age. Most of the postnatal reduction occurs in the first week of life and is the primary reason that body weight may decrease by up to 10% in breastfed term infants and even more in premature infants. The healthy newborn kidney can handle this challenge without difficulty. Finally, in subsequent weeks, the kidney must retain the electrolytes needed for growth and the production of dilute urine to accommodate the large water load presented by breast milk. Growth itself is a powerful homeostatic ally. A substantial portion of carbohydrates, electrolytes, and nitrogenous wastes from protein absorbed from breast milk are never presented to the kidney for excretion but are instead incorporated into the growing body.

Only when the otherwise healthy neonatal kidney has to cope with unexpected derangements of water, electrolyte, or acid–base status secondary to premature birth or illness does its relative lack of ability to concentrate urine, excrete sodium and potassium loads, conserve sodium (in preterm infants), and regulate acid–base status become problematic. In older children and adults, normal kidneys can correct for substantial errors in clinical judgment in water and electrolyte administration or creation and/or correction of acid–base abnormalities. This is not so with neonatal kidneys, especially in smaller preterm infants.

With that in mind, it is helpful to review specific aspects of neonatal renal development and function.

Nephron Development

The process of forming the adult complement of approximately 600,000 (range 250,000 to 2,000,000) nephrons in each kidney is complete by 34 to 35 weeks' gestational age (GA).[*] Development proceeds in centrifugal fashion, with juxtamedullary nephrons developing first and superficial cortical nephrons last. In general, nephron development continues after birth in premature infants but at a slower rate than during gestation; thus, preterm infants are at higher risk for decreased nephron number compared with term infants (Figure 25-2). Importantly, infants with intrauterine growth restriction and those born with extremely low birth weight may never achieve a normal number of nephrons. Thus, compromised renal function and elevated blood pressures have been reported in long-term follow-up of small preterm or intrauterine growth-restricted infants.[101]

Glomerular Filtration Rate

Glomerular filtration rate (GFR) is the rate at which filtrate of renal plasma appears in proximal renal tubules.[1,9,145,154,161] For the fetus, the placenta serves to maintain fluid and electrolyte composition and clearance of metabolic wastes. Thus, renal arterial blood flow is approximately 5% of fetal cardiac output, compared with 25% in later life. This rapid increase in blood flow correlates with an increase in GFR from approximately 20 to 60 ml/min/1.73 m^2 by 6 months of age (see Figure 25-2). GFR continues to improve over the first 2 years of life, typically reaching adult norms (when corrected for body surface area) by about 19 months of age.

---

*References 41, 48, 63, 83, 136, 138.

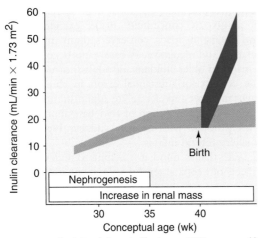

FIGURE 25-2 Correlation of glomerular filtration rate (GFR) as measured by inulin clearance and postconceptual age. Note marked increase in GFR postnatally. However, this increase in GFR does not occur after 40 weeks unless birth occurs. If birth occurs before nephrogenesis is complete (usually at 35 weeks), this increase will not occur until 34 to 35 weeks' postmenstrual age. (From Guignard JP: Neonatal nephrology. In Holliday MA, Barratt TM, Vernier RL, editors: *Pediatric nephrology*, ed 2, Baltimore, 1987, Williams & Wilkins.)

Tubular Function

Urine flow depends on both GFR and tubular reabsorption.[45,75,129] Oliguria is ordinarily defined as urine output of less than 1 ml/kg/hr. However, urine output may transiently decrease immediately after birth to less than 1 ml/kg/hr because tubular reabsorption of water increases due to an increase in fetal antidiuretic hormone (ADH) during labor. Nevertheless, 50% of full-term infants void by 12 hours, 92% by 24 hours, and 99% by 48 hours of life. Causes for prolonged failure to void include true or perceived decreased effective circulating volume, primary renal dysfunction, and obstruction to urine flow. After transient oliguria/anuria, urine flow rate increases as the newborn excretes the physiologically expanded fetal extracellular fluid volume as described earlier.

The newborn has limited capacity to concentrate urine. Several factors account for this observation. The concentration of osmotically active solutes in the urine is low during the first few weeks of life in association with high water and low protein content of breast milk and infant formulas, and ingested protein is preferentially used for growth rather than urea synthesis. Neonates also demonstrate resistance to ADH with decreased expression of collecting duct aquaporin-2 water channels, which normally enhance tubular water reabsorption. These factors result in increased risk of intravascular volume depletion when fluid intake is limited. High protein diets or urea supplementation can increase urinary urea excretion in newborn infants, thus enhancing urinary concentrating ability.

Proximal Tubular Function

The proximal tubule is responsible for reabsorbing glucose, amino acids, and most of the bicarbonate, sodium chloride, uric acid, and water in glomerular filtrate.[15,37,63,148] In smaller preterm infants, tubular transport mechanisms are insufficient to prevent spillage of each of these in varying degrees.

SODIUM

Physiologic diuresis in the first week of life is accompanied by physiologic natriuresis. The kidney is then responsible for conserving sufficient dietary sodium for growth.[79] This is a challenge for preterm infants (Figure 25-3), who often require extra sodium intake to compensate for obligatory sodium wastage. Conversely, in the presence of a sodium load (e.g., from administration of large amounts of sodium), the neonatal kidney cannot compensate with a rapid increase in fractional excretion of sodium. The result is edema and possibly circulatory overload.

POTASSIUM

The kidney is an important site for regulation of potassium balance.[74,139] In the adult, it is responsible for maintaining zero balance. In contrast, to sustain the neonate, the kidney must maintain positive potassium balance. In this context, it is less surprising that mechanisms for potassium excretion are underdeveloped at birth. Serum potassium concentrations tend to be high in neonates (5.5 to 6 mEq/L). The levels are not of pathologic significance and perhaps play a role in supporting growth.

ACID–BASE BALANCE

By adult standards, serum bicarbonate concentrations are low in full-term newborns (19 to 21 mEq/L) and even lower in premature infants (16 to 20 mEq/L).[128,132] Lower serum bicarbonate concentrations reflect limited ability to cope with the acid load from high protein intake and acid generated by formation of new bone.

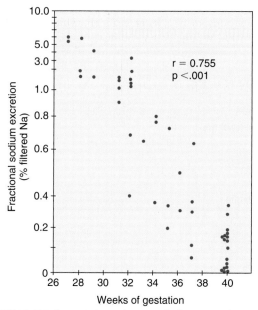

FIGURE 25-3 Decrease in fractional excretion of sodium occurs with increasing postconceptual age. *Na,* sodium. (From Siegel S, Oh W: Renal function as a marker of human fetal maturation, *Acta Paediatr Scand* 65:481, 1976.)

The capacity of the neonatal proximal tubule to reabsorb filtered bicarbonate is one third that of an adult. Proximal tubular bicarbonate reabsorption is further compromised if ECF is overexpanded with crystalloid solutions; because proximal tubular sodium and bicarbonate reabsorption are closely linked, bicarbonate is wasted as sodium reabsorption decreases to rid the body of excess sodium chloride. The capacities of the collecting duct to secrete hydrogen ions and of the proximal tubule to make ammonium to buffer secreted hydrogen ion are also limited. The net result is limited capacity to correct metabolic acidosis. This limitation is particularly evident in the setting of pathologic metabolic acidosis as may be seen in acute kidney injury. However, the ability to achieve minimal urine pH values is usually intact. That is, if serum bicarbonate is low enough (e.g., 14 to 15 mEq/L), the kidney can completely reabsorb the smaller amount of filtered bicarbonate and achieve a urine pH of 5. Serum bicarbonate concentrations increase to adult levels of 24 to 26 mEq/L by the end of the first year.

URIC ACID

Serum uric acid concentrations are elevated in the newborn because production from nucleotide breakdown is increased just after birth, especially in premature infants.[151,157] This is accompanied by increased uric acid excretion. High urinary uric acid concentrations may leave pink or red uric acid crystals in the diaper, which are often mistaken for blood. A microscopic urinalysis is helpful to exclude true hematuria in this setting.

CLINICAL ASSESSMENT OF RENAL DISEASE IN THE NEONATE

History

A complete family history of renal disease or syndromes that involve the kidneys is important to obtain. Prenatal exposures to maternal infection, drugs, toxins, or medications are risk factors for neonatal renal disease. Paternal smoking and advanced age may also be associated with an increased risk for urinary tract anomalies.

The quantity of amniotic fluid is an indicator of fetal renal function because fetal urination is responsible for most of the amniotic fluid volume beginning in the second trimester of pregnancy. Normally, amniotic fluid volume increases during gestation, peaking at 34 weeks' gestation. Any fetal renal condition associated with significant impairment in function with markedly diminished urine output can be associated with oligohydramnios. With worsening oligo/anhydramnios, a Potter sequence can be observed, in which the fetus develops pulmonary hypoplasia, flattened nose, recessed chin, low-set ears, and limb compression.[125,126] Severe urinary concentrating defects (e.g., diabetes insipidus and Bartter syndrome) may be associated with polyhydramnios.

A review of the perinatal history should identify risk factors for renal ischemia. Special attention to the composition of administered parenteral fluids can help to identify iatrogenic contributions to fluid/electrolyte derangements. Several potentially nephrotoxic medications are commonly used in the neonatal period including diuretics, aminoglycosides, and nonsteroidal antiinflammatory drugs (NSAIDs).

Signs and Symptoms

Physical findings that are indicators of genitourinary tract abnormalities are outlined in Table 25-1. Although lower urinary tract and renal anomalies are

TABLE 25-1   PERINATAL INDICATORS SUGGESTIVE OF ABNORMALITIES OF THE GENITOURINARY TRACT

FINDING	SUSPECTED ABNORMALITY
Oligohydramnios	Any congenital renal lesion associated with significant impairment in function
Polyhydramnios	Diabetes insipidus, Bartter syndrome
Enlarged placenta (>25% of infant birth weight) or >10-fold increase in maternal serum AFP	Congenital nephrotic syndrome — Finnish type
Velamentous insertion of umbilical cord	Increased congenital anomalies
Asphyxia neonatorum	Acute tubular or cortical necrosis
PHYSICAL EXAMINATION	
Hypertension	See text
SKIN	
Hemangioma	Hemangioma of kidney or bladder
Edema	Congenital nephrotic syndrome
Adenoma sebaceum	Tuberous sclerosis (angiomyolipomata, renal artery stenosis)
HEAD	
Encephalocele	Meckel-Gruber syndrome (polycystic kidneys)
Cleft lip and palate	Urinary tract anomalies
Macroglossia	Beckwith-Wiedemann syndrome (nephromegaly, cysts, structural urinary tract anomalies, nephrocalcinosis); Johanson-Blizzard syndrome (hydronephrosis, dysplasia); orofacial-digital syndrome (renal cystic disease)
EYES	
Phakoma	Tuberous sclerosis
Retinitis pigmentosa	Nephronophthisis/renal ciliopathy
Cataracts	Lowe syndrome, WAGR, congenital rubella
Aniridia	WAGR
EARS	
Low-set or malformed	Increased risk for renal abnormalities, Potter syndrome/sequence
Ear tags	Branchio-oto-renal (BOR) syndrome
Preauricular pits	Structural renal disease
SKELETON	
Hemihypertrophy	Wilms' tumor
Spina bifida	Neurogenic bladder
Arthrogryposis	Potter syndrome/sequence
Dysplastic nails	Nail patella syndrome
Vertebral anomalies	VATER/VACTERL syndrome
Polydactyly	Meckel-Gruber; renal ciliopathies
Limb anomalies	VACTERL syndrome

TABLE 25-1	PERINATAL INDICATORS SUGGESTIVE OF ABNORMALITIES OF THE GENITOURINARY TRACT—cont'd

FINDING	SUSPECTED ABNORMALITY
CARDIAC	
Congenital heart disease	Increased risk for renal abnormalities in association with multiple syndromes
ABDOMEN	
Absence of abdominal musculature	Prune-belly syndrome
Single umbilical artery	Increased congenital anomalies of the urinary tract
Umbilical discharge	Patent urachus
Abdominal mass	See Table 25-5
Hepatomegaly	Storage diseases, Beckwith-Wiedemann; Zellweger syndrome
PULMONARY	
Spontaneous pneumothorax	Oligohydramnios, Potter sequence
Pulmonary hypoplasia	Oligohydramnios, Potter sequence
GENITOURINARY — MALE	
Undescended testes	Prune-belly syndrome, Noonan syndrome, Lawrence-Moon-Biedl syndrome, Denys-Drash syndrome
Congenital absence of vas deferens	Renal agenesis or ectopia
Hypospadias	Increase in renal anomalies
Abnormal urinary stream	Bladder dysfunction or urethral outlet obstruction
GENITOURINARY — FEMALE	
Enlarged clitoris	Adrenogenital syndrome
Cystic mass in urethral region	Ectopic ureterocele, paraurethral cyst
Abnormal urinary stream or dribbling	Bladder dysfunction, urethral obstruction, urethral vaginal fistula
Common cloaca	Urinary tract abnormalities, obstructive uropathy
URINALYSIS	
	See text
RECTAL	
Abnormal anal sphincter tone	Neurogenic bladder dysfunction
Dilated prostatic urethra	Posterior urethral valves, prune-belly syndrome
Masses	Tumor, polycystic kidney disease, hydronephrosis, multicystic kidney disease
Anal atresia	VATER/VACTERL syndrome

Modified from Retek AB: Genitourinary problems in children, *Hosp Pract* 11:133, 1976.

AFP, alpha-fetoprotein; *WAGR,* Wilms tumor, aniridia, genitourinary anomalies, retardation; *VATER/VACTERL,* vertebral defects, imperforate anus, cardiac disease, tracheoesophageal fistula, and limb anomalies.

seldom the presenting feature of chromosomal disorders, they frequently form part of a multisystem malformation syndrome caused by chromosomal anomalies. Renal disorders seen with chromosomal disturbance can include fused kidneys, duplication defects, renal agenesis or hypoplasia, hydronephrosis and hydroureter, renal dysplasia or cystic disease, hypospadias, micropenis, and cryptorchidism. The overall pattern of malformation with individual chromosomal disorders is usually sufficient for diagnosis; however, variation can be seen from one individual to another, even for patients with aneuploidy. Although certain renal anomalies are characteristic of certain chromosomal disorders, no one renal malformation is unique to any particular chromosomal disorder. Detailed description of chromosomal disorders associated with renal anomalies can be found elsewhere.[85]

Laboratory Data

SERUM CREATININE CONCENTRATION

Serum creatinine concentration is generally used to monitor renal function in the newborn. Cystatin C has been proposed as an alternative and possibly more accurate marker of renal function, but results may not be immediately available at all institutions, and normative data are often lacking.[1] Serum creatinine is elevated at birth, reflecting maternal renal function, but rapidly declines to a stable level around 0.4 mg/dl by 1 to 2 weeks of age in the term infant. In the otherwise normal very premature infant, there is a transient increase in serum creatinine (due to tubular reabsorption of creatinine) with a peak around day 4 of life, followed by a progressive decrease to normal neonatal values within 3 to 4 weeks of birth. In general, the more premature the infant, the higher the serum creatinine and the longer it takes to normalize.

Under ideal steady-state conditions (which are not always met by the ill neonate), serum creatinine concentrations should provide an accurate indirect indication of GFR, thus eliminating the need for timed urine collection or nuclear GFR scans. Creatinine is produced at a relatively constant rate. In a steady state, creatinine excretion in urine is equal to creatinine production and likewise constant. The equation for estimation of GFR with serum creatinine is as follows[142,143]:

$$\text{Estimated GFR } \left(\text{ml / min / 1.73 m}^2\right) = 0.413 \times$$
$$\text{height (cm) / serum creatinine (mg / dl)}$$

Serum creatinine concentration is thus equal to a constant divided by GFR. Therefore, a true increase in creatinine concentration from 0.4 to 0.5 mg/dl, indicates a reduction in GFR of 20%. As a general guideline, rising or stable serial serum creatinine concentrations, or an isolated value exceeding 0.5 mg/dl after 1 week of age indicate renal dysfunction.

URINALYSIS
Specific Gravity. Urine specific gravity is a measure of the concentration of solutes in the urine, specifically the ratio of urine density compared with water density. Specific gravity in term infants ranges from <1.005 to 1.020. Specific gravity has been shown to have good correlation with urine osmolality in neonates although the relationship of these variables is somewhat different than in adults, likely due to decreased neonatal renal tubular reabsorption of low-molecular-weight proteins and other small molecules.[96] It is, however, useful as an indicator of the ability of the kidney to concentrate and dilute. It can be altered by the presence of glucose, protein, and urinary contrast agents. In such cases, osmolality must be measured directly.

Glucosuria. Trace quantities of glucose may be found occasionally in term infants and more frequently in premature infants. Even minor elevations of plasma glucose concentrations may cause glucosuria. Large glucose loads may cause osmotic diuresis.

Urinary pH. Urinary pH is typically around 6, although most neonates can achieve a urine pH of 5. Urine pH is frequently 7 or greater with distal tubular acidification defects.

Hematuria. A positive dipstick test for blood can be seen with hematuria, hemoglobinuria from hemolysis, or myoglobinuria from muscle breakdown, usually from perinatal asphyxia. Thus, a microscopic urinalysis is necessary to confirm the presence of true hematuria, which is defined as >5 red blood cells (RBCs)/high power field (hpf). Hematuria may occur if kidneys are traumatized during delivery, especially with an enlarged kidney (e.g., polycystic kidney disease or large hydronephrotic kidney). Hematuria is also common in perinatal asphyxia. Other conditions associated with hematuria include renal vein or artery thrombosis, urinary tract infection, bladder trauma from catheterization, renal artery emboli (especially from umbilical artery catheters), renal cortical necrosis, hypercalciuria, and rarely coagulopathies. Factitious hematuria may occur as a result of blood from circumcision, perineal irritation, uterine bleeding caused by withdrawal from maternal hormones, and uric acid crystals. If hematuria is persistent, it should be evaluated with microscopic examination, consideration of urine culture, evaluation of urine protein and calcium excretion, assessment of GFR, and an anatomic evaluation of the kidneys.

Pyuria. Pyuria is common in newborns, especially females. Pyuria may indicate infection, and a urine culture should be obtained if clinically indicated. However, pyuria also may indicate noninfectious renal injury. Interstitial nephritis is distinctly uncommon in the neonatal period.

Proteinuria. A positive dipstick test for protein indicates the amino groups of proteins. Although convenient, dipstick testing is subject to limitations. Because albumin and low-molecular-weight proteins give positive results, dipstick testing cannot fully distinguish between glomerular and tubular proteinuria. An alkaline urine (pH of ~8) may give a false-positive result as can prolonged immersion of the strip and the presence of detergents in the urine. The dipstick provides a qualitative assessment of proteinuria, which must be further confirmed by quantification of protein. Because 24-hour urine collection is cumbersome in neonates, a random urine protein creatinine ratio (normal <0.5 mg/mg) may be helpful clinically.

IMAGING STUDIES

Fetal ultrasound can provide (1) estimation of amniotic fluid volume; (2) information on the appearance, size, and echogenicity of kidneys; and (3) evidence of collecting system dilation. Prenatal ultrasonography can define anatomy but does not accurately predict function. Mild dilation does not necessarily denote obstruction, whereas more severe dilation and reduced amniotic fluid volume are more likely to signify obstruction and compromised renal function. The more severe the dilation (>7 mm after 32 weeks of gestation), the more likely the infant has urinary tract pathology. The later in pregnancy that dilation is found, the more likely hydronephrosis will be confirmed postnatally. Although fetal ultrasound is helpful to detect renal anomalies, a confirmatory postnatal ultrasound is imperative.

Nuclear renal scans (Tc99m-MAG3 [mercaptoacetyltriglycine] or Tc99m-DTPA [diethylene triamine pentaacetic acid]) are most useful to examine differential renal flow and function but are of limited value when GFR is low, due to limited filtration of tracer. A *voiding cystourethrogram* (VCUG) can exclude vesicoureteral reflux and detect posterior urethral valves, bladder diverticula, and urinary tract fistulae. *Computed tomography (CT)* or *magnetic resonance imaging (MRI)* may be indicated in select cases when further anatomic definition is needed, but this is rare in the neonate outside of tumor evaluation.

ACUTE KIDNEY INJURY

Pathophysiology

Acute kidney injury (AKI) in the newborn is a relatively common problem. Although the precise incidence and prevalence of acute kidney injury in the neonatal intensive care unit (NICU) is unknown, several studies have shown an incidence between 6% and 24%.[7,38,88,152] *AKI* is characterized by the sudden deterioration of the kidney's baseline function and is usually characterized by a decrease in GFR with associated increase in the blood concentration of creatinine and nitrogenous waste products, and by the inability of the kidney to appropriately regulate fluid and electrolyte homeostasis.

As noted previously, any rising serum creatinine from initial baseline, or a serum creatinine greater than 1.5 mg/dl with normal maternal function, should be investigated. Decreased urine output is not a constant feature of AKI, which can also be associated with normal or increased urine output.

Etiology

There are many causes of acute kidney injury in the newborn (Box 25-1). It is helpful to classify these etiologies as prenatal, intrinsic renal, and postrenal (obstructive). The preponderance of factors causing AKI in the newborn is prerenal in nature (e.g., hypoxia, hypovolemia, hypotension).

In prerenal failure, renal function is diminished because of decreased renal perfusion and the kidney is intrinsically normal. Renal hypoperfusion can result from a true decrease in intravascular volume (e.g., hemorrhage, dehydration) or from decreased effective circulating volume (e.g., congestive heart failure, cardiac tamponade, third

BOX 25-1 ETIOLOGY OF ACUTE KIDNEY INJURY IN NEWBORNS

Prerenal Failure

Decreased Intravascular Volume

- Dehydration/intravascular volume depletion
- Gastrointestinal losses
- Hemorrhage
- Salt-wasting renal or adrenal disease
- Diabetes insipidus

Decreased Effective Circulating Volume

- Congestive heart failure
- Pericarditis
- Cardiac tamponade
- Third space losses (sepsis, traumatized tissue, liver failure, nephrotic syndrome)

Intrinsic Renal Disease

Acute Tubular Necrosis

- Ischemic/hypoxic insults
- Drug induced
  - Aminoglycosides
  - Intravascular contrast
  - Nonsteroidal antiinflammatory drugs
  - Amphotericin
- Pigment nephropathy
- Rhabdomyolysis/myoglobinuria
- Hemoglobinuria
- Vascular lesions
  - Renal artery thrombosis
  - Renal venous thrombosis
- Infectious causes
  - Pyelonephritis in a solitary kidney

Obstruction (Postrenal)

- Obstruction in a solitary kidney
- Bilateral ureteral obstruction
- Urethral obstruction

Adapted from Andreoli SP: Acute renal failure in the newborn, *Sem Perinatol* 28:112, 2004.

space losses). Timely correction of the underlying disturbance and restoration of normal perfusion will return renal function to normal. Alternatively, profound and prolonged hypoperfusion can lead to acute tubular necrosis (ATN) and even cortical necrosis. However, the evolution of prerenal failure to intrinsic renal failure is not sudden, and a number of compensatory mechanisms work together to maintain renal perfusion when it is otherwise compromised.[7]

Intrinsic renal failure includes tubular and vascular lesions. Glomerulonephritis and interstitial nephritis are exceedingly uncommon in the neonate. There are a number of intrinsic renal parenchymal diseases that cause renal failure in the newborn period but are more appropriately considered chronic in nature and are thus considered later in this chapter. Asphyxia is the most common cause of ATN in the term neonate (65%), both oliguric and nonoliguric.[124] In the premature infant, sepsis is the second most common cause (35%). Patients with congenital heart disease appear to be especially vulnerable to tubular necrosis after cardiac catheterization and cardiac surgery.

Nephrotoxin-induced tubular injury in newborns is also commonly associated with the administration of aminoglycoside antibiotics, NSAIDs, intravascular contrast media, or amphotericin B. Aminoglycosides are one of the most common causes of drug-induced nephrotoxicity in neonates. Pharmacokinetic monitoring can achieve desired concentrations (peak 6 to 8 mcg/ml and trough <2 mcg/ml) and reduce risk.[93,160] Although gentamicin-induced renal toxicity was recently confirmed in the neonatal kidney independent of peak and trough serum levels, the long-term effects of neonatal aminoglycoside exposure on renal development are not well established.[64,172] The nephrotoxicity induced by aminoglycosides typically manifests clinically as nonoliguric renal failure, with a slow rise in serum creatinine and a hypo-osmolar urine developing after several days of treatment. Aminoglycoside nephrotoxicity is believed to be secondary to a small percentage of retained drug within the kidney's proximal epithelial cells.[98] Initial tubular alterations include proteinuria, hypo-osmotic urine, and increases in blood urea nitrogen (BUN) and creatinine reflecting a decrease in GFR. More severe injury is evident with tubular wasting of potassium, magnesium, calcium, bicarbonate, and glucose. Ototoxicity is the second main adverse effect of aminoglycosides and, in contrast to nephrotoxicity, is irreversible.[146]

Since the 1970s, premature infants with symptomatic patent ductus arteriosus (PDA) have been treated with indomethacin, a nonspecific prostaglandin inhibitor. Indomethacin, as well as other NSAIDs, has been shown to have various side effects including hemodynamic changes in cerebral, mesenteric, and renal circulations.[110] The renal side effects seen with indomethacin appear to be related to three phenomena: (1) intrauterine cyclooxygenase (COX) inhibition may induce renal dysplasia and dysgenesis and alter renal maturation by slowing glomerular maturation, (2) oligohydramnios may be the end result of fetal indomethacin exposure with concomitant decline in renal blood flow and glomerular filtration, and (3) indomethacin given for closure of PDA may induce and exacerbate renal failure by changing the balance of cortical juxtamedullary nephron perfusion. The fragile balance of vasoconstrictor (angiotensin II, endothelin) and vasodilatory (atrial natriuretic peptide, nitric oxide, prostaglandins, kallikrein-kinin) forces is now altered in favor of vasoconstriction and further reduction of the already low GFR. For preterm infants and newborns, the administration of NSAIDs should be done with care and frequent monitoring of renal function, even though these changes often are reversible.[4] When a change or decline in GFR is noted (e.g., plasma creatinine increase), then the administration of NSAIDs should be halted. Patients at higher risk include those with persistent patent ductus arteriosus, intravascular volume depletion, and simultaneous administration of other nephrotoxic drugs. The combined use of furosemide and indomethacin does not improve outcome. There are currently no human studies on the effect of selective COX inhibitors on PDA closure.

Diuretics can contribute to acute tubular necrosis in association with intravascular volume depletion. Pigment nephropathy due to hemoglobinuria or myoglobinuria is rare in the newborn but can occur. Hemoglobinuria can be seen in particular with hemolysis associated with extracorporeal membrane oxygenation.

The recovery of renal function in ATN depends on the nature and duration of exposure to the underlying events that precipitated the injury. The time to recovery is quite variable (few days to several weeks). Return of renal function may be accompanied by a polyuric phase with excessive urine output. During this phase, close attention to fluid and electrolyte balance is important to ensure adequate fluid support to promote recovery and prevent additional renal damage, which could result from intravascular volume depletion with subsequent prerenal insult.

Vascular lesions include renal artery thrombosis and renal vein thrombosis. These conditions can occur in association with an underlying thrombophilia or may be precipitated by significant intravascular volume depletion. Symptoms may include flank mass, microscopic or gross hematuria, oliguria, hypertension, and thrombocytopenia. AKI is observed when disease is bilateral, or unilateral in a solitary kidney.

Postrenal failure: A variety of obstructive lesions can be associated with AKI in the newborn. Renal insufficiency is observed when there is functional or anatomic obstruction of both kidneys (e.g., bilateral ureteropelvic or ureterovesical junction obstruction, bladder outlet obstruction) or obstruction of a solitary kidney.

Diagnosis

The diagnosis of AKI in the newborn is not an easy one because oliguria is not a consistent finding and serum creatinine is often an unreliable predictor of glomerular filtration in neonates. Variable definitions for AKI exist in the literature. However, serum creatinine values consistently above the 99th percentile, prolonged oliguria, or failure to achieve a diuresis are all clinically relevant.

Urine osmolality (UOsm), urine sodium concentration (UNa), and fractional excretion of sodium (FENa) have been proposed as tools to help differentiate prerenal failure from ATN. This differentiation is based on the premise that the tubules are working appropriately in prerenal failure and therefore can conserve salt and water, whereas in ATN, the injured tubules cannot conserve sodium appropriately. However, and of importance, because the renal tubules in newborns and premature infants are relatively immature, the distinction between prerenal failure and ATN is not as clear-cut as in older children. In the newborn, values suggestive of prerenal failure include urine osmolality (UOsm) greater than 350 mOsm/L, urine sodium (UNa) less than 20 to 30 mEq/L, and FENa of less than 3%. Alternatively, values suggestive of ATN are UOsm less than 350 mOsm/L, UNa greater than 30 to 40 mEq/L, and FENa greater than 4% to 5%. Note that these values vary according to gestational age and maturity, and there is increased overlap of

TABLE 25-2	ETIOLOGY OF ACUTE KIDNEY INJURY IN THE NEONATE				
	URINARY INDICES IN ACUTE KIDNEY INJURY				
	UNa(mEq/L)	FENa (%)	RFI	U/P_{cre}	U/P_{osm}
Prerenal	31.4 ± 19.5	0.95 ± 0.55	1.29 ± 0.82	29.2 ± 15.6	>1.3
Intrinsic renal and postrenal	63.4 ± 34.7	4.25 ± 2.2	11.6 ± 9.6	9.6 ± 3.6	>1

Cre, creatinine (mg/dl); *FENa*, fractional excretion of sodium; *Osm*, osmolarity (mOsm/L); *P*, plasma concentration; *RFI*, renal failure index (U_{Na} × P/U creatinine); *U*, urine concentration.
Adapted from Mathews OP, Jones AS, James E, et al: Neonatal renal failure: usefulness of diagnostic indices, *Pediatrics* 65:57, 1980.

values with increasing prematurity.[39] Therefore, it is important to recognize the limitations of these indices in the assessment of renal failure in the newborn period (Table 25-2).

A renal ultrasound examination should be performed in all neonates with AKI to assess for possible urinary tract obstruction, renal vascular thrombosis, and congenital renal abnormalities causing chronic renal disease.

Prevention

The prevention of AKI in the preterm and term infant is complicated. Nonetheless, the following are some general recommendations:
- Minimization of perinatal asphyxia
- Avoidance of maternal and infant angiotensin-converting enzyme (ACE) inhibitor use
- Aggressive management of hypoxemia, hypovolemia, hypotension, acidosis, and hypothermia
- Early detection and treatment of infection
- Judicious use of agents with vasoactive or nephrotoxic properties that can exacerbate renal injury (e.g., diuretics, aminoglycosides, NSAIDs)

Management and Treatment

Once the diagnosis of AKI has been established, management of metabolic derangements needs to be initiated promptly including consideration of fluid balance, electrolyte status, acid–base balance, and nutrition, as well as initiation of renal replacement therapy when appropriate.

Maintenance of Intravascular Volume

Prerenal causes require improved perfusion of the kidney by restoring intravascular volume, cardiac output, and blood pressure to normal. In the setting of appropriate cardiac function, fluid challenge of 10 ml/kg of body weight of crystalloid for small preterm infants and up to 20 ml/kg of body weight for term infants should be attempted. In selected cases, colloid or inotropic support may be preferred. Accurate measurement of central venous pressure (CVP) may be helpful to target euvolemia.

If restoration of intravascular volume to the euvolemic state does not improve urine output, diuretic therapy may be helpful to enhance urine output. Although the conversion of oliguric to non-oliguric AKI has not been shown to alter the course of the AKI,[32] increased urine output can ease management by allowing for increased fluid intake in the form of vital medications and nutrition. When using diuretics in newborns with AKI, potential risks and benefits need to be considered. Excessive diuresis can induce intravascular volume depletion and exacerbate ATN. Loop diuretics are generally used as primary agents. Most diuretics need to be filtered before reaching their therapeutic target in the tubular lumen. Therefore, in the setting of diminished GFR, higher doses of loop diuretics (e.g., furosemide 3 to 5 mg/kg intravenously) may be required to achieve appropriate tubular fluid concentrations. Mannitol should be avoided in neonates, especially premature infants, because of its hyperosmolarity and increased risk for intraventricular hemorrhage.

The use of "renal" dose dopamine or fenoldopam to improve renal perfusion after an ischemic insult has been proposed. However, there is little evidence that these medications decrease the need for dialysis or improve survival in neonates.[61,135,171]

ELECTROLYTE AND ACID–BASE DISTURBANCES

Mild hyponatremia is common in AKI and usually the result of fluid overload with dilutional hyponatremia. This level of hyponatremia responds well to fluid restriction or free water removal by dialytic therapy. In severe cases (serum sodium <120 mEq/L), there is a greater risk for seizures and correction to a sodium level of approximately 125 mEq/L with hypertonic saline should be considered.

Hyperkalemia is a common and potentially life-threatening complication. The risk for disturbances of the cardiac rhythm secondary to hyperkalemia increases with the presence of acidosis and hypocalcemia. Severe hyperkalemia requires prompt therapy with sodium bicarbonate, intravenous glucose and insulin, and intravenous calcium gluconate. It is important to remember, however, that maneuvers to decrease total body potassium content, such as loop diuretics or cation exchange resins, are essential because other available measures simply provide cardiac protection (calcium) or shift potassium intracellularly without removing potassium from the body. However, the use of cation exchange resins has been associated with necrotizing enterocolitis in preterm infants.[137,170] Refractory hyperkalemia is an indication for dialysis.

Hypocalcemia and metabolic acidosis are common in AKI. Severe metabolic acidosis can be treated with intravenous or oral sodium bicarbonate, oral sodium citrate solutions, and/or dialysis therapy. When treating acidosis, it is important to consider the serum ionized calcium level. Rapid correction of acidosis will decrease the ionized calcium concentration and thus may precipitate tetany and/or seizures. Finally, hyperphosphatemia is a common electrolyte abnormality noted during AKI. Hyperphosphatemia should be treated with dietary phosphorus restriction and with oral calcium carbonate with goal serum phosphorus concentration less than 6.5 to 7 mg/dl. Hyperphosphatemia is rarely an indication in itself for dialysis.

In many instances, AKI is associated with marked catabolism, and malnutrition can develop rapidly, leading to delayed recovery from AKI. Proper nutrition is essential in the management of the newborn with AKI.

RENAL REPLACEMENT THERAPY

Renal replacement therapy is indicated for fluid overload, metabolic acidosis, or hyperkalemia that are refractory to medical management; symptomatic uremia, which is unusual in the neonate; hyperammonemia refractory to medical management; and drug or toxin overdose. Options for dialysis therapy in neonates include hemodialysis (HD), continuous renal replacement therapy (CRRT), or peritoneal dialysis (PD). All dialytic therapies rely on the principles of diffusion (movement of solute from higher to lower concentration) and convection/ultrafiltration (bulk movement of solute in association with fluid removal). The optimal modality for any given neonate will be determined by goals of therapy, hemodynamic stability, comorbid conditions, anticoagulation risk, and institutional preferences as outlined next.

Hemodialysis. In hemodialysis, blood is removed from the neonate via a central hemodialysis catheter and flows across an appropriate size artificial filter (dialyzer) while dialysate of the preferred composition travels countercurrent (in the opposite direction to blood) across the filter. In this manner, solutes diffuse from higher to lower concentration, such that urea, creatinine, potassium, ammonia, dialyzable drugs and toxins, among other substances, are removed from the patient while bicarbonate diffuses into the patient's blood. The countercurrent flow of dialysate optimizes the diffusion gradient for solute removal. A transmembrane pressure is applied to the filter to induce fluid removal at the targeted rate. The fluid that is removed contains solutes in a concentration equivalent to plasma. The blood is then returned to the neonate. A typical hemodialysis session lasts 2 to 4 hours but may be more prolonged if needed (e.g., for toxin or ammonia removal). An anticoagulant, most commonly heparin, is provided to prevent circuit clotting, particularly given the low blood flow rates used for neonates, with adjustment to target the goal activated clotting time. The advantage of hemodialysis is that solute and fluid abnormalities can be rapidly corrected. Disadvantages include the need for vascular access (usually a 7-Fr double lumen venous hemodialysis catheter), continuous skilled nursing support during the procedure, and systemic anticoagulation, which increases the risk of bleeding complications including intraventricular hemorrhage in premature infants. Most neonates will also require a blood prime of the circuit because of the relatively large extracorporeal circuit volume.

Continuous Renal Replacement Therapy (CRRT). Over the past several years, CRRT has become increasingly popular in the treatment of AKI (Figure 25-4). The therapy consists of several variations of diffusion and convection, which all result in net solute clearance and fluid removal from blood. The procedure itself is similar to hemodialysis, but the therapy is provided on a continuous basis (e.g., 24 hours per day). Thus, CRRT allows for an overall slower rate of solute and fluid removal, which may be better tolerated in hemodynamically unstable patients. Ongoing dialytic support may also be valuable in toxin/drug overdose in which prolonged clearance is needed or the toxin/drug is associated with rebound of plasma levels, as the support can be aggressive initially and

then decreased but maintained over time. Disadvantages of CRRT include the need for continuous vascular access and anticoagulation. In many NICUs, the bedside intensive care nurse operates the CRRT machine while providing care for the neonate, so the personnel support is less intensive than with hemodialysis. Anticoagulation can be systemic (e.g., heparin) or regional (e.g., citrate, which anticoagulates the blood as it leaves the patient and enters the circuit with calcium provided as blood reenters the patient to reverse the anticoagulation). In recent years, improvements in the technologies of CRRT have made it more suitable for use in neonates, and most centers in North America can provide CRRT routinely for acute neonatal dialysis. However, filter sets (dialyzer and tubing) specific to the size of the neonate are not yet available for most CRRT systems in the United States, leading to the current need for blood prime of each new circuit.

Peritoneal Dialysis. Acute *peritoneal dialysis* (PD) is a major modality of therapy for acute and

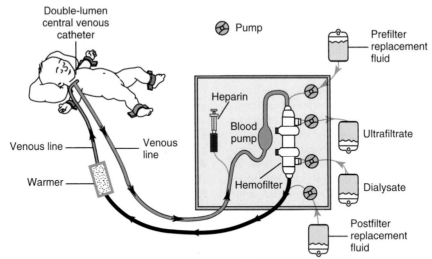

FIGURE 25-4 Continuous renal replacement therapy (CRRT) in the newborn. A typical setup is shown in the figure. Blood is pumped from the patient through a central line across a hemofilter (artificial kidney) at a rate of 5 to 10 ml/kg/min (minimum 30 ml/min). A constant anticoagulant infusion (shown here as heparin) is maintained to prevent circuit clotting. Dialysate can be administered countercurrent (in the direction opposite to blood flow) across the hemofilter (continuous venovenous hemodialysis [CVVHD]); replacement fluid can be administered pre- or post-hemofilter (continuous venovenous hemofiltration [CVVH]); or both dialysate and replacement fluid can be used (continuous venovenous hemodiafiltration [CVVHDF]). The amount of ultrafiltrate (fluid removed) is regulated according to individualized need and tolerance. The discarded ultrafiltrate contains fluid and solutes/toxins; thus, these are removed from the patient's circulation. Before the blood is returned to the patient, it is passed through a blood warmer to prevent hypothermia. With most commercially available CRRT systems, the total volume of the circuit exceeds 10% of the neonate's blood volume so a blood prime of the circuit is required. Individual therapy goals and institutional preference affect the choice of vascular access, modality (CVVHD vs. CVVH vs. CVVHDF), anticoagulant, and flow rates.

chronic kidney failure in the neonate, particularly when vascular access is difficult to maintain. PD works by the processes of diffusion and ultrafiltration using the peritoneal membrane as a filter. For this therapy, an acute or chronic peritoneal dialysis catheter is placed into the peritoneum. The best results are usually obtained with a well-secured "permanent" peritoneal dialysis catheter that is surgically placed in the operating room by an experienced pediatric surgeon. The preferred catheter is a curled silastic Tenckhoff catheter with one or two cuffs that adhere locally to immobilize the interior portion of the catheter. Dialysis fluid (dialysate) is infused into the peritoneal space, either via a machine or manually, and allowed to "dwell" for a designated time. During the dwell phase, particles move from high concentration to low concentration (diffusion). The composition of the dialysate, which contains electrolytes and dextrose, is altered via this exchange of solutes between the dialysate and the peritoneal capillaries that perfuse the peritoneal lining. For example, high concentrations of urea and creatinine are filtered from the blood into the dialysate, which contains no urea or creatinine. Alternatively, the high concentration of bicarbonate diffuses from the dialysate into the blood, thus helping to counter metabolic acidosis. The concentration of dextrose in the dialysate, which is markedly higher than the serum glucose concentration, creates an osmotic load that stimulates movement of fluid from the blood into the dialysate (ultrafiltration). The dialysate is then drained and discarded, and the cycle repeats. Advantages of PD include that it is relatively easy to perform, does not require anticoagulation, and is well tolerated in hemodynamically unstable neonates. However, a peritoneal dialysis catheter cannot be placed in children with major intraabdominal disease (postsurgical, gastroschisis, necrotizing enterocolitis, etc.). Because of the nature of the procedure, the correction of solute and fluid abnormalities occurs at a slower rate than by HD or CRRT, and fluid removal cannot be precisely controlled due to variation in individual peritoneal membrane transport characteristics. The initial fill volume is generally around 20 ml/kg progressing to 40 ml/kg for chronic dialysis; occasionally even this small initial volume is poorly tolerated in the setting of severe respiratory failure. There is also the potential for peritonitis.

Outcome and Prognosis

In the newborn infant, the prognosis and recovery from acute kidney injury highly depends on the underlying etiology of the AKI. Factors that are associated with increased mortality include multiorgan failure, hypotension, need for vasopressors, hemodynamic instability, and need for mechanical ventilation and dialysis.[7]

In general, newborns who require more than 1 month of dialysis support for AKI are considered to have end-stage renal disease (ESRD). Newborns who recover from AKI but have suffered substantial loss of nephrons as may occur in cortical necrosis, hypoxic/ischemic injury, and nephrotoxic injury are at significant risk for late development of progressive chronic kidney disease long after the initial insult.[8,67,104] Those who required dialysis for renal failure, particularly if a prolonged course, are of particular concern. This risk of chronic kidney disease is also anticipated to be higher in preterm infants who have not completed nephrogenesis and in intrauterine growth–restricted neonates who often have decreased nephron mass.[100,101] Therefore, newborns with AKI should have lifelong monitoring of their renal function, blood pressure, and urinalysis. Typically, the late development of chronic kidney disease will first become apparent with the development of hypertension, proteinuria, and eventually an elevated BUN and creatinine. The lack of renal reserve may not be apparent until puberty or later.

INTRINSIC RENAL PARENCHYMAL ABNORMALITIES

Several congenital renal abnormalities can be classified by the amount of tissue, differentiation of tissue, and position of the kidneys.

Renal Agenesis

Congenital absence or agenesis of renal tissue can occur unilaterally or bilaterally. Unilateral renal agenesis is seen more frequently (~1:3000 live births)[121] and may manifest as a solitary kidney with eventual enlargement caused by compensatory hypertrophy. The condition appears to be more common in males and infants of African American or diabetic mothers.[121] Unilateral agenesis has also been associated with Turner, Poland, and VATER syndromes. In unilateral agenesis, patients are often asymptomatic and are diagnosed inadvertently on imaging or based on the significant association with malformations of the lower genitourinary tract. In newborns with a known solitary kidney, a VCUG should be obtained to exclude vesicoureteral reflux.[167] Renal dysplasia may rarely occur in the remaining kidney; thus compensatory hypertrophy of the remaining kidney is an encouraging sign. There is no need for long-term follow-up if a solitary kidney without additional involvement is found. Restriction from participation in contact sports based on the solitary kidney does not appear to be warranted.[68,69]

Bilateral renal agenesis, also known as *Potter disease,*[125] is seen rarely, with an incidence of 1 per 4000 births. In bilateral renal agenesis, the majority of affected infants are male and small for gestational age with a history of maternal oligo/anhydramnios. The characteristic facial features accompanying Potter syndrome include wide-set eyes, flattened nose, receding chin, and large, low-set ears with little cartilage. Other associated malformations can include pulmonary hypoplasia, hydrocephalus, meningocele, multiple skeletal anomalies, and imperforate anus. In the absence of fetal intervention, the fetus is typically stillborn or dies within hours of birth due to pulmonary hypoplasia.

Renal Hypoplasia

Renal hypoplasia is a deficiency in the amount of renal tissue and is expressed as an abnormally small kidney. Histologically, the kidney structure is otherwise normal. However, the decreased nephron mass is often insufficient to maintain normal GFR throughout the child's life. The condition is apparent by ultrasound with variably echogenic kidneys, which are small for body size and do not grow at the expected rate with serial ultrasound.

Renal Dysplasia

Abnormalities in renal tissue differentiation are most commonly expressed as dysplastic kidneys. Renal dysplasia is a failure of the metanephric tissue to mature appropriately. Monogenic causes include mutations in individual genes, such as TCF2/hepatocyte nuclear factor 1ss (HNF1beta),

PAX2, and uroplakins, but there are also recent reports of children with compound heterozygote mutations in several renal/urinary tract developmental genes.[134,168] The result is a persistence of immature structures and a decrease in normal functioning renal tissue. Renal dysplasia may be seen in one or both kidneys and can involve the entire kidney, segments of the kidney, or microscopic foci of a kidney. Dysplasia is often expressed as cyst formation. The extent of dysplasia will determine the risk of chronic kidney disease and need for eventual renal replacement therapy.

MULTICYSTIC DYSPLASTIC KIDNEY (MCDK)

MCDKs are nonfunctional and therefore bilateral disease is not compatible with life. Unilateral MCDK is both the most common cystic lesion of the neonatal kidney and one of the most frequently palpated abdominal masses in the newborn. MCDK is usually sporadic, but some familial and syndromic cases have been reported. MCDK is slightly more common in males and on the left side.[5,141] Usually the ureter is absent, atretic, or stenotic. No orifice is found in the bladder. Such kidneys are enlarged and diffusely cystic with histopathology showing nests of cartilage and mesenchymal mantles surrounding primitive tubules. A nuclear renal scan shows no flow or function of the MCDK. Renal function and structure may be normal in the remaining kidney of infants with unilateral MCDK; however, approximately one-third of patients can be shown to have abnormalities of the contralateral kidney, most commonly vesicoureteral reflux, ureteropelvic junction (UPJ) obstruction, or dysplasia.[141] Therefore, a VCUG should be performed on every patient with consideration of a nuclear renal scan to exclude obstruction in the setting of hydronephrosis with a normal VCUG. There is an increased risk of chronic hypertension, proteinuria, and chronic kidney disease in patients with contralateral abnormalities.[105] Such kidneys generally involute with time so a conservative approach is recommended.[46] The risk of malignancy in the MCDK has been shown to be negligible.[46] Rarely, the MCDK impacts nutrition because of its large size in the small preterm infant.

POLYCYSTIC KIDNEY DISEASE

Polycystic kidney disease (PKD) may present as one of two types in the infant: (1) autosomal recessive polycystic kidney disease (ARPKD) or (2) autosomal dominant polycystic kidney disease (ADPKD).

Autosomal Recessive Polycystic Kidney Disease.

Autosomal recessive polycystic kidney disease (ARPKD) manifests with varied severity, but it is always bilateral. The kidneys are enlarged with a proliferation of renal tubules and dilated collecting tubules. These are not true "cysts" but ectatic dilations of the collecting tubules, and the kidney has a reniform shape. Various combinations of cystic renal disease and hepatic disease occur in ARPKD, with liver disease including congenital hepatic fibrosis due to ductal plate malformation with eventual hepatosplenomegaly and complications of portal hypertension, or nonobstructive dilation of intrahepatic bile ducts *(Caroli disease)* with high risk of recurrent cholangitis. Prenatal ultrasound frequently shows bilaterally enlarged echogenic kidneys often associated with oligohydramnios. Significant hypertension, nephromegaly, pulmonary hypoplasia, and renal insufficiency may be evident in the affected neonate.[70] However, a subset of patients manifest primarily liver disease and may not be diagnosed until adulthood.[72] Nonetheless, ARPKD will eventually progress to ESRD. The condition is transmitted in an autosomal recessive manner so there may be a history in siblings of ARPKD or family history of miscarriage or early infant death. Evaluation includes assessment of renal function and blood pressure. The postnatal abdominal ultrasound typically shows enlarged bilateral kidneys with decreased corticomedullary differentiation. Liver abnormalities may be evident in the neonatal period but more commonly become apparent over time. Current treatment consists of supportive management including control of hypertension and complications of chronic kidney disease. ACE inhibitors are frequently the preferred antihypertensive agent although there is no evidence to support the superiority of this class of medications, and their use should be limited with GFR less than 30 ml/min/1.73 m^2 and in preterm infants before completion of nephrogenesis. Renal replacement therapy including kidney transplantation with or without liver transplantation is typically required in later life. The vast majority of children presenting with significant clinical manifestations in the neonatal period will reach ESRD in early to mid-childhood.

Autosomal Dominant Polycystic Kidney Disease.

Autosomal dominant polycystic kidney disease (ADPKD) involves cyst formation in any portion of the nephron and Bowman's space. The condition is associated with progressive development of renal macrocysts leading to compression of normal renal parenchyma and progression to ESRD at an average age of 60 years. Cysts also develop in other visceral organs including the liver, pancreas, and spleen with increasing age. There is a strong association between ADPKD and cerebral artery aneurysms.[20,21] ADPKD may be evident on prenatal ultrasound with enlarged echogenic and/or cystic kidneys, only rarely accompanied by oligohydramnios. In contrast to ARPKD, increased corticomedullary differentiation has been observed. However, it can be difficult to distinguish ADPKD from ARPKD by prenatal or early infancy ultrasound. The family history and sonographic evaluation of both parents can be helpful in this regard although the spontaneous mutation rate for ADPKD approaches 15%. Many children who are diagnosed by prenatal ultrasound demonstrate improvement in sonographic findings over the first 1 to 2 years of life and likely would not have otherwise been diagnosed on clinical grounds for several years. However, a small subset of children with "very early onset" ADPKD present within 18 months of birth with hypertension, gross hematuria, abnormal renal function, or other symptoms.[53,147] This group appears to show early progression of renal insufficiency. Management includes routine monitoring of blood pressure with consideration of ACE inhibitor treatment when blood pressure exceeds the 75th percentile for age, sex, and height. ACE inhibitors in this setting have been shown to prevent the decline in renal function and the increase in left ventricular mass index associated with ADPKD. Recently pravastatin has been shown to slow progression of structural kidney disease in affected children and young adults ages 8 to 22 years[29]; however, this has not been studied in younger children.

RENAL VEIN THROMBOSIS

Renal vein thrombosis (RVT) can be an acute life-threatening condition or insidious in onset.[25,47,95] RVT is associated with conditions that cause intravascular volume depletion and decreased oxygenation within the kidney. Perinatal associations with neonatal RVT include maternal diabetes, toxemia, maternal thiazide therapy, polycythemia, placental insufficiency, birth asphyxia, prematurity, respiratory distress syndrome (RDS), and sepsis. Angiography has also been associated with RVT. Thrombosis most often occurs in the smaller renal veins rather than in the main renal vein. The involved kidney may enlarge secondary to obstruction to blood flow and forms a palpable flank mass. Other clinical signs and symptoms may include gross or microscopic hematuria, decreased urine output, anemia, and thrombocytopenia (<75,000). Family history of thrombophilia should be reviewed, and evaluation pursued in appropriate settings. Management includes treatment of the underlying illness, maintenance of appropriate intravascular volume, and consideration of anticoagulation. Administration of anticoagulants remains controversial for RVT. The effects of heparin-based anticoagulation and thrombolytic therapy on the long-term renal function of affected patients has yielded conflicting results.[25] Surgical excision of the thrombus is not usually necessary. Renal tubular dysfunction is often observed after recovery from RVT. Long-term follow-up may be needed to assess renal growth and function.

HYDRONEPHROSIS

Etiology and Associated Findings

The collecting system of the kidney is composed of the ureter, pelvis, and calyces, all of which function as a system for removing urine from the kidney. Hydronephrosis, one of the most common causes of abdominal mass in the newborn, involves dilation of the pelvis and calyces, most often as a result of congenital obstruction.[18,108] The impaired drainage of urine from severe or chronic obstruction during renal development may induce dysplastic and cystic changes that further impair kidney development and function.

The most common ureteral site of obstruction is at the ureteropelvic junction (UPJ). The ultrasound demonstrates ballooning of the renal pelvis with a normal appearance of the ureter and bladder. Obstruction at the ureterovesical junction (UVJ), also known as *primary megaureter,* occurs more often in the male infant. UVJ obstruction more frequently affects the left ureter. The ultrasound demonstrates hydroureteronephrosis with a normal

appearing bladder. Affected patients with UPJ or UVJ obstruction are usually asymptomatic unless obstruction is bilateral. Rarely recurrent vomiting, particularly after fluid intake, or abdominal discomfort may be evident. A nuclear renal scan is helpful to diagnosis both UPJ and UVJ obstruction. Definitive surgical repair can be undertaken in both conditions. In the case of UVJ obstruction, the stenotic segment can be removed and the ureter reimplanted into the bladder.

Posterior urethral valves (PUVs) are the major cause of urethral obstruction in males.[111] Affected males show renal insufficiency and diminished urine output due to bladder outlet obstruction. Complications include poor growth and urinary tract infection. In some cases, the enlarged bladder or hydronephrotic kidney(s) can be palpated. The ultrasound typically shows an enlarged thick-walled bladder with varying degrees of hydroureteronephrosis and renal dysplasia. A VCUG is the definitive diagnostic study, highlighting the trabeculated bladder and a dilated posterior urethra. In some cases, the valve leaflets are evident as lucencies; if leaflets are not apparent, prominence of the posterior urethra distally over the bulbar urethra may be noted. The anterior urethra is typically underfilled, and voiding is incomplete. Associated vesicoureteral reflux is also evident by VCUG. Bladder decompression is indicated until surgical repair of PUV is undertaken, and any secondary features of chronic kidney disease should be addressed. Postobstructive diuresis may occur with decompression, so careful attention to volume status is required. Tubular dysfunction with renal tubular acidosis or pseudohypoaldosteronism is frequent. Definitive surgical repair includes transurethral fulguration of the valves. In preterm infants who are too small for a transurethral approach, an indwelling urethral catheter or suprapubic tube may be left in place, or less commonly a vesicostomy created, awaiting somatic growth. Many affected males have chronic bladder dysfunction, and recent studies suggest a guarded long-term prognosis for renal function in later life, even in those who appear to do well clinically in childhood.[31,76]

Prune-belly syndrome, also known as *Eagle-Barrett syndrome,* is a less common cause of functional obstruction and dilation of the pelvis and calyces with an incidence approaching 1:50,000. There is a strong male predominance. This triad of anomalies includes (1) absence or hypoplasia of the abdominal wall muscles, (2) bilateral cryptorchidism, and (3) urinary tract abnormality. The loose, shriveled abdomen is responsible for the "prune belly" appearance, which diminishes with age and rarely requires surgical correction. Renal dysplasia is usually seen in prune-belly syndrome and may range from mild to severe involvement. The enlarged bladder may be seen in conjunction with a patent urachus draining urine. A VCUG demonstrates a hypoplastic prostatic urethra, no evidence of PUV, and variable degrees of vesicoureteral reflux. Management includes ensuring appropriate drainage of urine, addressing any complications of chronic kidney disease, and eventual orchiopexy.

Vesicoureteral reflux is further discussed in the section on urinary tract infection.

Treatment

Mild to moderate unilateral obstruction does not require immediate treatment, assuming the other kidney is normal. Close follow-up is indicated for monitoring of kidney growth, and significant obstruction should be addressed with surgical intervention when feasible. Fetal intervention can be offered for significant bilateral disease with decreased amniotic fluid, depending on the gestational age of the fetus and severity of hydronephrosis. However, surgical intervention in utero is controversial and center-dependent, and the morbidity of this therapy is high. Although there is selection bias, in many fetal intervention cases, ESRD is reached in early childhood.

HYPERTENSION

Systemic hypertension is an important clinical problem in neonates. Although the reported incidence in all neonates is low, ranging from 0.2% to 3%,[56,149,164] hypertension is more commonly observed in premature and other newborns cared for in the NICU, particularly those with chronic lung disease and/or a history of umbilical artery catheterization.[16,57,144] Hypertension in the neonate is often asymptomatic, although rarely marked hypertension is present and can be associated with severe sequelae such as congestive heart failure or intracranial hemorrhage.

Diagnosis

The gold standard for assessment of blood pressure (BP) in neonates is direct measurement by intraarterial analysis of the pulse pressure wave form.[42] In contrast to older children, there is good correlation between umbilical artery and peripheral artery catheter BPs in neonates.[27] Indirect measurement of BP by palpation or auscultation is not recommended for routine assessment in the NICU setting, and sonographic Doppler assessment has largely been replaced by oscillometric measurement.[99,114] It is important to note, however, that the latter procedure is based on detection of pressure oscillations within the artery; therefore, this method determines the mean arterial pressure and then uses an algorithm specific to each manufacturer to establish systolic and diastolic BP values. There is generally good correlation between oscillometric and umbilical or radial artery BP in neonates and young children.[122] However, there are important limitations of this methodology. Few studies have compared specific oscillometric BP monitors to direct arterial measurements in neonates, and these have shown variable accuracy depending on the size of the infant,[40] with increased frequency of oscillometric methods to overread BP compared with direct measurement.[118]

It is also critical to consider the state of the infant at the time of BP assessment. Significant BP variations are observed with the neonate's level of activity, position, and particularly during feeding.[73] A standardized protocol for conditions of BP assessment in neonates has been proposed,[117] including measurement of the right upper arm BP by an oscillometric device with the infant in a prone or supine position, 1.5 hours after feeding or medical intervention, using an appropriate size cuff with width to arm circumference ratio in the range of 0.45 to 0.55. The BP is to be obtained on three successive readings at 2-minute intervals after a 15-minute period of rest after cuff placement with the infant in an asleep or quiet-awake state. This protocol has yet to be widely adopted.

Normal values for BP have been developed by body weight and postnatal age[50] (Figure 25-5). Studies in term and preterm infants show that BP increases with both gestational and postconceptional age as well as birth weight.[89,90,174] Systolic and diastolic BP have been shown to increase

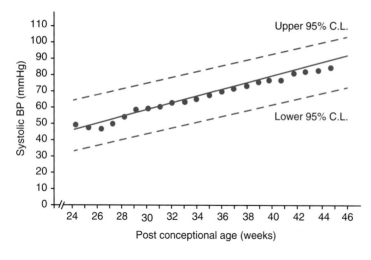

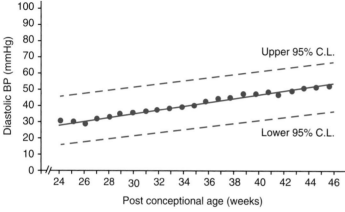

FIGURE 25-5 Linear regression of mean systolic (upper panel) and diastolic (lower panel) blood pressure (BP) by postconceptional age in weeks, with 95% confidence limits (CL, upper and lower dashed lines). (From Zubrow AB, Hulman S, Kushner H, Falkner B, and the Philadelphia Neonatal Blood Pressure Study Group: Determinants of blood pressure in infants admitted to neonatal intensive care units: a prospective multicenter study, *J Perinatol* 15:470, 1995.)

about 2 mm Hg/day over the first 5 days of life. The rate of increase then slows to 0.25 mm Hg/day for systolic and 0.15 mm Hg/day for diastolic BP over the next 3 months.[174] Preterm infants born at 28 to 31 weeks' gestation have been shown to have a more rapid rise in BP over the first 2 to 3 weeks compared with infants born at later gestational age.[90] BP reaches a steady value for the first year of life by 2 to 3 months of age. Age-specific percentiles for normal BP for boys and girls from birth to 12 months have been published.[113] How the percentile ranking for an infant's BP will track into later childhood or adulthood is still unclear although associations between late childhood or adolescent BP and adult BP clearly exist.[10,36,86,156] Normal values for BPs in neonates after 2 weeks of age are shown in Table 25-3 and during infancy are shown in Figure 25-6.

Etiology

The causes of hypertension can be seen in Box 25-2. All infants with hypertension require appropriate evaluation looking for a specific etiology. The most common etiologies of systemic hypertension in neonates include renovascular and renal parenchymal diseases. Up to 9% of neonates with umbilical artery catheters (UAC) develop hypertension. UAC-associated thromboembolism affecting the aorta and/or the renal arteries was initially described in the 1970s[115] and can occur even in the absence of demonstrable thrombi. Not surprisingly, longer duration of UAC placement is associated with higher risk of thrombus formation.[24] Although high UAC placement is associated with fewer ischemic events such as necrotizing entero-colitis, the frequency of hypertension does not

TABLE 25-3	ESTIMATED BLOOD PRESSURE VALUES AFTER 2 WEEKS OF AGE IN INFANTS FROM 26 TO 44 WEEKS' POSTCONCEPTIONAL AGE		
POSTCONCEPTIONAL AGE (weeks)	50TH PERCENTILE	95TH PERCENTILE	99TH PERCENTILE
44			
SBP	88	105	110
DBP	50	68	73
MAP	63	80	85
42			
SBP	85	98	102
DBP	50	65	70
MAP	62	76	81
40			
SBP	80	95	100
DBP	50	65	70
MAP	60	75	80
38			
SBP	77	92	97
DBP	50	65	70
MAP	59	74	79
36			
SBP	72	87	92
DBP	50	65	70
MAP	57	72	77
34			
SBP	70	85	90
DBP	40	55	60
MAP	50	65	70
32			
SBP	68	83	88
DBP	40	55	60
MAP	49	64	69
30			
SBP	65	80	85
DBP	40	55	60
MAP	48	65	68

Continued

TABLE 25-3	ESTIMATED BLOOD PRESSURE VALUES AFTER 2 WEEKS OF AGE IN INFANTS FROM 26 TO 44 WEEKS' POSTCONCEPTIONAL AGE — cont'd		
POSTCONCEPTIONAL AGE (weeks)	50TH PERCENTILE	95TH PERCENTILE	99TH PERCENTILE
28			
SBP	60	75	80
DBP	38	50	54
MAP	45	58	63
26			
SBP	55	72	77
DBP	30	50	56
MAP	38	57	63

From Dionne JM, Abitbol CL, Flynn JT: Hypertension in infancy: diagnosis, management and outcome. *Pediatr Nephrol* 27:22, 2012.
DBP, Diastolic blood pressure; *MAP,* mean arterial pressure; *SBP,* systolic blood pressure.

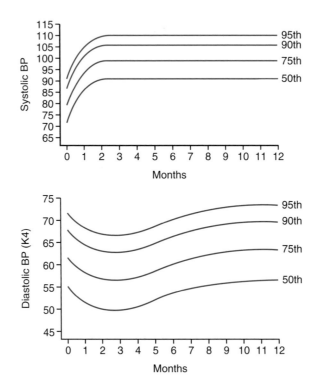

90th Percentile												
Systolic BP	87	101	106	106	106	106	106	105	105	105	105	105	105
Diastolic BP	68	66	63	63	63	66	66	67	68	68	69	69	69
Height (cm)	51	59	63	66	66	70	72	73	74	76	77	78	80
Weight (kg)	4	4	5	5	6	7	8	9	9	10	10	11	11

FIGURE 25-6 Age-specific percentiles for blood pressure in the first year of life in boys (A) and girls (B). (From Report of the Second Task Force on Blood Pressure Control in Children—1987. Task Force on Blood Pressure Control in Children. National Heart, Lung, and Blood Institute, Bethesda, Maryland, *Pediatrics* 79:5, 1987.)

Continued

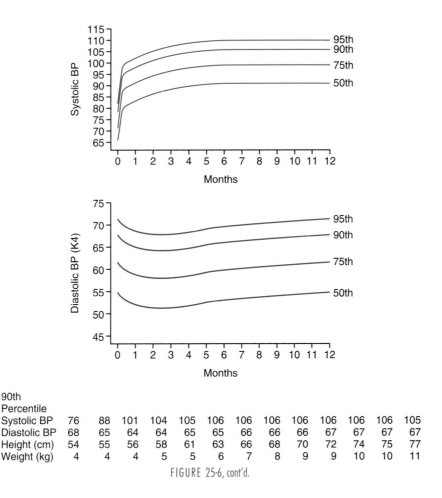

90th Percentile												
Systolic BP	76	88	101	104	105	106	106	106	106	106	106	106	105
Diastolic BP	68	65	64	64	65	65	66	66	66	67	67	67	67
Height (cm)	54	55	56	58	61	63	66	68	70	72	74	75	77
Weight (kg)	4	4	4	5	5	6	7	8	9	9	10	10	11

B

FIGURE 25-6, cont'd.

differ between high and low placement.[11] Thus, it has been proposed that UAC-related hypertension is related to thrombus formation associated with endothelial disruption at the time of catheter placement. Renal vein thrombosis is discussed earlier in this chapter and can be associated with severe and prolonged hypertension. Fibromuscular dysplasia can be seen in infancy and is typically associated with branch vessel disease rather than main renal artery disease.[158] Mechanical compression of one or both renal arteries by tumor, abdominal mass, or a hydronephrotic kidney can induce renovascular hypertension.

Polycystic kidney disease, both autosomal recessive and less commonly autosomal dominant, can be associated with neonatal hypertension. Urinary tract obstruction can also be

associated with hypertension in the absence of renal artery compression. Hypertension is commonly seen in acute tubular or cortical necrosis due to fluid overload or hyperreninemia. Hypertension may be more prominent in the recovery phase of ATN.

Abman et al. first described hypertension associated with bronchopulmonary dysplasia (BPD) in the mid-1980s[3] with an incidence of hypertension upon discharge of 43% in infants with BPD compared with 4.5% without BPD. Importantly, more than half of the infants with BPD who developed hypertension did not demonstrate elevated BP until after hospital discharge, emphasizing the importance of routine BP assessment in follow-up of NICU graduates. The mechanism underlying BPD-associated hypertension is not known although chronic

| BOX 25-2 | ETIOLOGY OF HYPERTENSION IN THE NEONATE |

Vascular

- Thromboembolism
- Renal artery stenosis
- Coarctation of the aorta
- Hypoplastic abdominal aorta (midaortic coarctation)
- Renal vein thrombosis
- Renal artery compression
- Congenital rubella infection
- Idiopathic arterial calcification

Renal Parenchymal Disease

- Congenital
  - Polycystic kidney disease (autosomal dominant or recessive)
  - Multicystic dysplastic kidney (rare)
  - Renal hypo/dysplasia (rare)
  - Tuberous sclerosis
  - Urinary tract obstruction
- Acquired
  - Acute tubular necrosis
  - Renal cortical necrosis
  - Hemolytic-uremic syndrome (rare)
  - Urinary tract obstruction
  - Reflux nephropathy

Neoplasia

- Wilms tumor
- Neuroblastoma
- Bronchopulmonary dysplasia

Endocrine

- Adrenogenital syndrome
- Cushing disease
- Hyperaldosteronism
- Thyrotoxicosis
- Pseudohypoaldosteronism type II (Gordon syndrome)

Other

- Closure of abdominal wall defects (compartment syndrome)
- Fluid overload
- Hypercalcemia
- Increased intracranial pressure
- Medications
  - Phenylephrine
  - Corticosteroids
  - Theophylline/caffeine
  - Deoxycorticosterone
  - Vitamin D intoxication (hypercalcemia)
  - ACTH
  - Maternal cocaine or heroin use
- Adrenal hemorrhage
- Extracorporeal membrane oxygenation

From Dionne JM, Abitbol CL, Flynn JT: Hypertension in infancy: diagnosis, management and outcome, *Pediatr Nephrol* 27:17, 2012.

hypoxemia and hypercarbia are known to induce diminished nitric oxide production and increased endothelial inflammation and vascular dysfunction in older children with obstructive sleep apnea.[114] BPD-associated hypertension is correlated with greater need for diuretic and bronchodilator use[2] consistent with the concept that the risk is higher with more severe chronic lung disease. Aortic coarctation can be associated with hypertension both before repair and with postoperative stenosis, which can develop over a period of years. Monogenic hypertension is rare in the neonate. Numerous medications can induce systemic hypertension in the neonate. Maternal cocaine or heroin use may affect the developing kidney, resulting in increased risk of hypertension.[44,81] Tumors are rarely seen in the neonatal period but can cause direct compression of one or both renal arteries, urinary tract obstruction, or production of hormones that elevated blood pressure. Hypertension is commonly seen in neonates requiring extracorporeal membrane oxygenation. The underlying mechanisms are not clear.[23]

Data Collection

HISTORY

A detailed history of prematurity and associated comorbidities including chronic lung disease or intracranial hemorrhage is indicated. A history of UAC placement is important. It is important to review the medication history for specific contributors. The family history should be reviewed for early-onset hypertension, although monogenic hypertension is rare and often not evident within the first days of life.

SIGNS AND SYMPTOMS

Most neonates with systemic hypertension are asymptomatic. Congestive heart failure, renal dysfunction, or hypertensive retinopathy can occasionally be seen with severe hypertension. Nonspecific symptoms may be evident, including feeding difficulty, lethargy, irritability, failure to thrive, or seizures. The general appearance of the infant including any dysmorphic features should be assessed. A careful abdominal examination may demonstrate a mass suggestive of either a hydronephrotic or polycystic kidney or tumor. Abnormal genitalia suggest congenital adrenal hyperplasia. Femoral pulses should be assessed and BP measurements taken in all extremities to exclude coarctation of the aorta.

LABORATORY DATA

Laboratory evaluation should include review of electrolytes (e.g., hypokalemic metabolic alkalosis in monogenic hypertension/mineralocorticoid excess), renal function, serum calcium, and urinalysis. If proteinuria is present it can be quantified. Assessment of serum cortisol, thyroid function tests, or serum aldosterone may be appropriate in select cases. Plasma renin activity is not recommended as a routine test in evaluation of neonatal hypertension but may be helpful in the setting of specific electrolyte abnormalities.[57] Levels are typically elevated in infancy, particularly in premature infants,[12] and peripheral plasma renin does not necessarily correlate with intrarenal pathology. Plasma renin can also be affected by medications such as caffeine and other methylxanthines as well as diuretics and ACE inhibitors.

All neonates with hypertension should have a Doppler renal ultrasound. Such imaging is valuable to evaluate renal anatomy, exclude renal vein or artery thrombosis, and look for aortic and renal artery thrombi. Color-flow Doppler can be used to exclude renal artery stenosis, although sensitivity and specificity vary with the experience of the ultrasonographer. Magnetic resonance angiography (MRA) or CT with contrast add information about the anatomy of larger vessels, but neither is typically sufficient to diagnose intrarenal branch stenosis. In such cases, classic contrast angiography may be helpful. However, the neonate's size and the potential for

intervention should be considered before ordering these examinations. Even when intrarenal pathology is evident, definitive intervention may need to be delayed awaiting somatic growth. Echocardiogram or VCUG may be appropriate in select cases.

Treatment

Initial steps in management should include correction of any iatrogenic causes, treatment of hypoxemia in BPD, and hormone replacement as appropriate in endocrine disorders. Any underlying disorders should be appropriately treated (e.g., urinary tract obstruction should be relieved). There is general agreement that neonatal hypertension should be treated with medications if blood pressure exceeds the 99th percentile.[42,57,58]

There are few controlled trials of antihypertensive medications in neonates. Therefore, treatment relies on case-series data, older clinical trials, expert opinion, and personal experience. Drugs and dosages commonly used in the neonate are shown in Table 25-4. In infants with acute severe hypertension, especially with systemic symptoms, continuous intravenous infusion of antihypertensive medication is indicated to provide sustained control without rapid fluctuations in blood pressure, which can contribute to cerebral ischemia or hemorrhage particularly in premature infants. Continuous infusions of several antihypertensive medications have been successfully used in neonates, including nicardipine, esmolol, sodium nitroprusside, and labetalol.[42,106,109] In such situations, continuous monitoring via an indwelling arterial catheter is most appropriate. Intermittent intravenous therapy with hydralazine or labetalol may be useful in neonates who cannot take oral antihypertensives. Of note, intravenous enalaprilat is not recommended in neonates because of the wide published range for appropriate dosing and risk of prolonged severe hypotension and acute kidney injury.[42] Oral antihypertensive medications commonly used in neonates include longer-acting dihydropyridine calcium channel blockers, vasodilators such as minoxidil or hydralazine, or beta blockers. Short-acting nifedipine has fallen out of favor for management of hypertension because of potential for rapid change in BP. Beta blockers should be avoided in chronic lung disease. Diuretics may have a role in control of BP, particularly in children with underlying BPD, who may have pulmonary benefit from these medications. The ACE inhibitor captopril

TABLE 25-4	RECOMMENDED DOSES FOR SELECTED ANTIHYPERTENSIVE AGENTS FOR TREATMENT OF HYPERTENSIVE NEONATES				

CLASS	DRUG	ROUTE	DOSE	INTERVAL	COMMENTS
ACE inhibitors	Captopril	Oral	0.01-0.05 mg/kg/dose, max 2 mg/kg/day	TID	First dose can cause rapid drop in BP, especially if receiving diuretics
	Lisinopril	Oral	0.07-0.6 mg/kg/day	QD	
α- and β-Antagonists	Labetalol	Oral	0.5-1 mg/kg/dose; max 10 mg/kg/day	BID-TID	BPD relative contraindication
		IV	0.2-1 mg/kg/dose; 0.25-3 mg/kg/hr	Q4-6 hr; infusion	
	Carvedilol	Oral	0.1-0.5 mg/kg/dose	BID	
β-Antagonists	Esmolol	IV	100-500 mcg/kg/min	Infusion	Ultra short acting; monitor heart rate; avoid in BPD
	Propranolol	Oral	0.5-1 mg/kg/dose; max 8-10 mg/kg/day	TID	
Calcium channel blockers	Amlodipine	Oral	0.05-0.3 mg/kg/dose; max 0.6 mg/kg/day	QD	All may cause reflex tachycardia
	Isradipine	Oral	0.05-0.15 mg/kg/dose; max 0.8 mg/kg/day	QID	
	Nicardipine	IV	1-4 mcg/kg/min	Infusion	
Central α-agonist	Clonidine	Oral	5-10 mcg/kg/day; max 25 mcg/kg/day	TID	May cause mild sedation
Diuretics	Chlorothiazide	Oral	5-15 mg/kg/dose	BID	Monitor electrolytes
	Hydrochlorothiazide	Oral	1-3 mg/kg/dose	QD	
	Spironolactone	Oral	0.5-1.5 mg/kg/dose	QD-BID	
Vasodilators	Hydralazine	Oral	0.25-1 mg/kg/dose; max 7.5 mg/kg/day	TID-QID	Tachycardia, fluid retention
		IV	0.15-0.6 mg/kg/dose	TID-QID	
	Minoxidil	Oral	0.1-0.2 mg/kg/dose	BID-TID	Tachycardia, fluid retention, hypertrichosis
	Nitroprusside	IV	0.5-10 mcg/kg/min	Infusion	Risk for thiocyanate toxicity with prolonged use (> 72 hr) or kidney failure

From Dionne JM, Abitbol CL, Flynn JT: Hypertension in infancy: diagnosis, management and outcome, *Pediatr Nephrol* 27:22, 2012.
ACE, Angiotensin-converting enzyme; *BID*, twice a day; *BPD*, bronchopulmonary dysplasia; *IV*, intravenous; *kg*, kilogram; *mcg*, microgram; *mg*, milligram; *PO*, per os, orally; *Q*, every; *Q*, once daily; *QID*, four times a day; *TID*, three times a day. For ACE inhibitors, only captopril and lisinopril are U.S. Food and Drug Administration approved in infancy.

is one of the few medications that has been studied in neonatal hypertension. However, caution is indicated because it can induce an exaggerated drop in BP in premature infants. Moreover, the renin-angiotensin system is critical for normal nephron development. ACE inhibitors or angiotensin receptor blockers should not be given until nephrogenesis is complete, with some recommending avoidance through 44 weeks' postconceptional age.

Surgical intervention may be appropriate in selected cases, such as ureteropelvic junction obstruction, tumor, and aortic coarctation.

Outcome

The long-term prognosis for neonatal hypertension appears to be good in many cases although comprehensive studies into adulthood are limited in availability. Most infants with UAC-related hypertension demonstrate resolution of hypertension over time.[60] It is common to see a need for increasing antihypertensive doses for some months with somatic growth followed by stable BP, with infants "outgrowing" the antihypertensive dose. Whether such infants are at risk for hypertension in later life is not known. Certainly there is concern that prematurity/intrauterine growth restriction are associated with decreased nephron mass, which may increase risk for hypertension and/or early renal insufficiency later in life. Children with intrinsic renal disease or renal vein thrombosis may require more long-term antihypertensive therapy. Neonates clearly represent a high-risk group for early hypertension as well as development of hypertension in later childhood and adulthood. Thus, routine follow-up of BP from the neonatal period on is recommended.[114]

ABDOMINAL MASSES

Abdominal masses in neonates reflect a wide spectrum of pathologies, ranging from small lesions found incidentally, to large ones occupying the entire peritoneal cavity; from unilocular cysts to complex solid cysts; from lesions that can cause significant morbidity and mortality, to entities that may be safely observed.[34,51,65,92] This spectrum is further broadened by the variety of organs that can give rise to such masses.

In the era of almost universal prenatal ultrasound, many such masses are identified, and some are even treated, before delivery. Others are discovered during the course of a thorough routine examination of the neonate. Although most of these babies are otherwise healthy, such a finding is disturbing to new parents. It is incumbent on the infant's physician to determine the nature of the mass in a timely, safe, and cost-effective manner.

Just over 50% of abdominal masses present during the newborn period are of renal origin.[34,51,65] The literature offers no consistent data on frequency of abdominal masses in infants, but there is general agreement about the urgent need to comprehensively evaluate these infants to establish an accurate diagnosis and to plan appropriate intervention.

TABLE 25-5	NEONATAL ABDOMINAL MASSES	
TYPE OF MASS	**PERCENT OF TOTAL**	
RENAL MASSES		
Hydronephrosis	55	
Multicystic dysplastic kidney		
Polycystic kidney disease		
Mesoblastic nephroma		
Renal ectopia		
Renal vein thrombosis		
Nephroblastomatosis		
Wilms tumor		
GENITAL MASSES		
Hydrometrocolpos	15	
Ovarian cyst		
GASTROINTESTINAL MASSES		
Duplication	15	
Volvulus		
Complicated meconium ileus		
Mesenteric-omental cyst		
"Pseudocyst" proximal to atresia		
NONRENAL RETROPERITONEAL MASSES		
Adrenal hemorrhage	10	
Neuroblastoma		
Teratoma		
HEPATOSPLENOBILIARY MASSES		
Hemangioendothelioma	5	
Hepatoblastoma		
Hepatic cyst		
Splenic hematoma or cyst		
Choledochal cyst		
Hydrops of gallbladder		

Adapted from Kirks DR, Merten DF, Grossman H, et al: Diagnostic imaging of pediatric abdominal masses: an overview, *Radiol Clin North Am* 19:527, 1981.

Etiology

The differential diagnosis in the infant with abdominal mass is shown in Table 25-5. The workup of most abdominal masses requires only a thorough physical examination and specific goal-oriented studies. Usually, the location of the mass is a helpful clue to the possible organ involved and the most likely diagnosis:

1. Flank: The most common cause of flank mass is renal in origin, including hydronephrosis, multicystic dysplastic kidney, polycystic kidney disease, or renal artery or vein thrombosis. Other flank masses of importance include solid tumors of the kidney, such as the *benign congenital mesoblastic nephroma,* and *Wilms tumor.* Wilms tumor occurs at a rate of 8 to 9 per 100,000 per year in the United States with two-thirds of patients presenting in the first 3 to 6 months of life. The tumor is described as firm, smooth, and confluent with the kidney. Both kidneys are involved in 10% of cases. Juxtarenal lesions include neuroblastoma, adrenal hemorrhage, bronchogenic cyst, and infradiaphragmatic (extralobar) pulmonary sequestration.

2. Right upper quadrant (RUQ): Most RUQ masses arise from the liver and biliary tract. In fact, the classic presentation of the most frequent benign hepatic tumor, *infantile hepatic hemangioma (hemangioendothelioma),* is a palpable RUQ mass. Other masses in this region include the benign mesenchymal hamartomas, hepatoblastoma (the only significant primary hepatic malignancy in neonates), and choledochal cysts.

3. Left upper quadrant (LUQ): Splenic cysts or hematomas are rarely observed in infancy.

4. Midabdominal: Midabdominal masses usually involve the intestine. Duplications of the gastrointestinal (GI) tract can occur anywhere from esophagus to anus and are usually cystic or less commonly tubular. They are typically present as an asymptomatic palpable mass but may also cause pain, intestinal obstruction, GI bleeding, or even volvulus. Other midabdominal masses include intestinal lymphatic malformations, meconium pseudocyst, and omphalomesenteric remnants. Failure of the vitelline duct to fully resorb can result in a variety of related entities, including *Meckel diverticulum* and omphalomesenteric sinus, cyst, or fistula.

5. Pelvic: A residual pelvic mass after voiding in a female infant may represent an enlarged vagina (hydrocolpos) or uterus (hydrometrocolpos). Such findings indicate a need for further examination of the perineum and vaginal introitus. Other pelvic masses include ovarian masses, urachal cysts, and teratomas. Cystic ovarian tumors are more common than solid ones, and the majority of them are benign; however, cystic ovarian masses require further investigation as malignancies have been reported.

Physical Examination

The infant should be in the supine position for abdominal examination. Inspection of the abdomen before manual exploration enables the examiner to see a mass that may be missed with a tense abdomen. The shape of the abdomen should be noted along with the position of the umbilicus and the presence of any hernias. Bimanual palpation using the flat surface of the fingers while supporting the infant's flank with the other hand facilitates exploration of the abdomen during deep palpation. Characteristics of the mass including location, size, shape, texture, mobility, and tenderness should be documented. The differentiation between solid and cystic masses can be difficult on physical examination. Percussion may outline the suspected area, and transillumination is sometimes helpful.

If gastric distention or intestinal obstruction is suspected, a nasogastric tube is inserted and air and fluid evacuated. If there is a question of urinary retention, the infant should be reexamined after placement of a urinary catheter or after inducing voiding with a Credé maneuver. Rectal examination, applied judiciously, may provide useful information, particularly for pelvic masses. Clues to the nature of the lesion may be external or distant to the mass.

Signs and Symptoms

Many abdominal masses are asymptomatic in neonates but can be detected by thorough physical examination. Renal masses may be associated with hypertension or abnormal renal function. If not detected by prenatal ultrasound, autosomal recessive polycystic kidney disease commonly presents with bilateral nephromegaly perceived to be abdominal masses. Liver masses are occasionally associated with evidence of hepatobiliary obstruction or liver dysfunction. A large mass may affect the infant's ability to feed successfully, particularly the preterm infant.

Laboratory Data

Assessment of hepatobiliary and renal function may be helpful. However, radiographic imaging is usually the next step. Plain films can provide a surprising amount of information, such as organomegaly, calcifications in a number of tumors or, displacement of the intestines as a subtle clue to the presence and sometimes the nature of a mass. Ultrasound is perhaps the most important tool in the assessment of abdominal mass in the neonate. Ultrasound is noninvasive, accessible for bedside studies, radiation-free, painless, and can provide detailed information on the location, nature, and vascularity of the mass and adjacent structures. Doppler sonography is particularly helpful to assess flow in the setting of the multicystic dysplastic kidney and renal artery or vein thrombosis. When ultrasound is not definitive, it may provide clues that help to determine the next appropriate studies. Renal scintigraphy can be helpful to differentiate a nonfunctioning multicystic dysplastic kidney from a hydronephrotic or cystic dysplastic kidney but is not frequently needed for this purpose. A voiding cystourethrogram is the method of choice to diagnose vesicoureteral reflux, which can be associated with significant hydroureteronephrosis and/or bladder outlet obstruction. CT or MRI is occasionally indicated, especially in evaluation of the origin and extent of tumors.

Treatment and Prognosis

Treatment and prognosis are dependent on the nature of the underlying lesion. Specific renal lesions have been reviewed previously in this chapter. Wilms tumor generally has an excellent prognosis with treatment, which often includes surgical removal of the tumor, irradiation, and chemotherapy. The prognosis in malignant neuroblastoma is related to the site of the primary tumor, histologic appearance of the tumor, staging of the disease, and age of the patient. Significant hydronephrosis may be associated with chronic issues with glomerular or tubular dysfunction.

RENAL TUBULAR DISORDERS

Although most of the renal tubular disorders are congenital, many do not manifest clinically during the newborn period.[33] However, in sick infants admitted to the intensive care unit, these tubular abnormalities can lead to severe and frequently life-threatening electrolyte disorders and fluid depletion.

Etiology

The term *renal tubulopathy* encompasses a wide variety of conditions. Proximal tubular defects can include proximal (type II) renal tubular acidosis (RTA), which can be an isolated phenomenon, or can occur in the setting of generalized proximal tubular dysfunction *(Fanconi syndrome)*. Isolated proximal RTA rarely causes major difficulties in the neonatal period although normal anion gap hyperchloremic metabolic acidosis and failure to thrive may be evident in later infancy; the condition often spontaneously resolves in early childhood. In contrast, Fanconi syndrome, which is characterized by proximal RTA, aminoaciduria, phosphaturia, hyperuricosuria, and glycosuria, can be associated with several underlying genetic and metabolic diseases, including cystinosis, Lowe (oculocerebrorenal) syndrome, tyrosinemia, galactosemia, hereditary fructose intolerance, and a variety of mitochondrial cytopathies.

Bartter syndrome is a tubulopathy of the loop of Henle, which in its classic form is characterized by maternal polyhydramnios, premature birth, perinatal salt wasting, chronic polyuria and polydipsia, hypokalemic metabolic alkalosis, and nephrocalcinosis. The metabolic findings are akin to treatment with a loop diuretic. Specific mutations in the distal tubule contribute to *Liddle syndrome* (hypertension with hyporeninemic hypokalemic metabolic alkalosis), pseudohypoaldosteronism type 1 (recurrent episodes of life-threatening hyperkalemia associated with aldosterone resistance), pseudohypoaldosteronism type 2 (*Gordon syndrome;* hypertension with hyperkalemic metabolic acidosis).

Distal (type 1) RTA can be attributed to a variety of defects in the distal tubule that impair acidification of the urine, resulting in normal anion gap hyperchloremic acidosis with high urine pH with clinical features including failure to thrive and nephrocalcinosis. Autosomal recessive distal RTA can be associated with progressive sensorineural deafness. Obstruction of the urinary tract, which is frequently diagnosed prenatally, is commonly associated with renal tubular acidosis (RTA), particularly the hyperkalemic type (type IV). Defects of the vasopressin V2 receptor or aquaporin-2 water channels in the collecting duct result in *nephrogenic diabetes insipidus* (NDI) with clinical features including polyhydramnios, impaired urinary concentrating ability, polyuria and polydipsia, neonatal failure to thrive, and high risk for recurrent dehydration with hypernatremia/hyperosmolality. V2 receptor mutations are inherited in an X-linked manner, whereas aquaporin-2 mutations are usually autosomal recessive or dominant in nature.

Given the inherited nature of many tubulopathies, review of the family history can be helpful, particularly with respect to the health of siblings.

Treatment and Complications

Although many tubular disorders are not clinically evident at birth, the clinician should keep a high index of suspicion in those infants with prenatal diagnosis of urologic abnormalities or serious abnormalities in water and electrolyte metabolism. Treatment depends on the underlying condition but often requires replacement of the electrolytes or minerals that are lost in the urine. Therapies specific to several tubulopathies do exist but are beyond the scope of this chapter to review in detail. It is important to note, however, that early evaluation and treatment of renal tubular disorders may prevent catastrophic complications such as life-threatening episodes of dehydration and delayed growth and development.

URINARY TRACT INFECTION

Urinary tract infections (UTIs) affect approximately 1% of full-term infants and 3% of premature infants. Male infants are affected 5 times more frequently than females.[13,19,77] *Vesicoureteral reflux* (VUR) is a common radiographic finding in infants. Primary reflux is seen in abnormalities of the ureterovesical junction, ureteral duplication, and ureterocele. Secondary VUR is associated with PUV, neurogenic bladder, and other causes of bladder outlet obstruction. In addition to causing significant acute illness, UTIs can also lead to long-term renal sequelae such as scarring with resultant hypertension, decreased functioning renal mass, glomerular hyperfiltration, and/or chronic kidney disease.

Etiology

Abnormalities of the urinary tract are responsible for a large number of UTIs in the neonate. Whether the infection is more commonly spread in an ascending or hematogenous matter is not clear but certainly identification of VUR should prompt evaluation for potential secondary etiologies. Reflux is graded on a four- or five-point scale depending on the rating system utilized, with grade IV to V denoting VUR into the kidney with massive hydroureteronephrosis with tortuosity of the ureter.

Maternal urinary infections also have been associated with neonatal UTI. Symptomatic manifestations include abnormal weight loss during the first days of life, decreased feeding, dehydration, irritability, lethargy, cyanosis, jaundice, and septicemia. In some cases, the affected kidneys are palpable. Infected infants also may be asymptomatic.

Data Collection

Evaluation of a neonate with suspected UTI includes immediate urine and blood cultures and a complete blood count (CBC). The optimum method of obtaining urine for culture is suprapubic aspiration of the bladder or catheterization. Catheterization may not be recommended in the neonate if there is concern for urethral stricture, which is more commonly observed in males. Urine obtained in a urine bag should not be used for cultures because it is easily contaminated. With diagnosis of UTI, radiographic evaluation, including ultrasound and VCUG, should be undertaken to rule out anatomic abnormality. A recent study in infants suggests that the timing of VCUG does not affect the presence or severity of observed VUR after UTI[43]; however, given the potential risks, the urine should be sterile before obtaining the VCUG. Some have advocated obtaining the VCUG as soon as sterile urine is documented due to risk of loss to follow-up. Renal scintigraphy can be useful to document the presence and/or extent of renal scarring; however, this is rarely needed in the newborn period.

Treatment

Pyuria (10 to 15 white blood cells [WBCs] per hpf) can be observed in the neonate normally. Treatment for UTI is indicated when an organism is cultured from the urine. However, a low threshold for antibiotic treatment awaiting culture results may be needed, particularly when other concerning symptoms are present. Any growth in a urine specimen obtained by suprapubic aspiration should be considered to represent an infection if the procedure was cleanly performed. Any aspiration of bowel contents must affect the interpretation of culture results. Traditional antibiotic coverage consists of both ampicillin and an aminoglycoside pending culture results. The advent of third-generation cephalosporins has allowed for excellent gram-negative coverage without the nephrotoxicity of the aminoglycosides. *Escherichia coli* is the organism most often implicated in neonatal UTIs, followed by *Klebsiella*. Sulfonamides are contraindicated in the neonate because of their potential to complicate hyperbilirubinemia.

Antibiotic therapy should continue for 10 to 14 days, with a follow-up urine culture 3 days after therapy is discontinued. Many practitioners recommend antibiotic prophylaxis until significant reflux or anatomic abnormality is ruled out. The value of prophylactic antibiotics for prevention of reflux nephropathy in the setting of documented VUR remains controversial. The potential benefits need to be weighed against risks, knowing that neonates and young infants with acute UTI may present with more vague or nonspecific symptoms compared with older children.

NEUROGENIC BLADDER

Neurogenic bladder is an anatomic interruption of the micturition reflex normally triggered by a full bladder.[14,62,163] The bladder may be flaccid and unable to empty urine or spastic, hyperreflexive, and unable to store urine. Infants with lumbosacral spinal malformations commonly have neurogenic bladder. Lower motor neuron deficit causes bladder atony, and upper motor neuron deficit can cause spasticity.

Signs and Symptoms

Often there is a mixed presentation of symptoms. The flaccid bladder requires aggressive intervention in the neonate. Diagnosis begins immediately at the bedside when the newborn has no apparent voiding stream or the urine flow rate falls below expectations

without other explanations. Further clarification of the diagnosis can be made by VCUG and cystometric studies. If there is concern for bladder dysfunction, renal function should be assessed as obstruction can lead to obstructive nephropathy.

Treatment

Surgical intervention may be indicated in the neonate with neurogenic bladder with associated obstruction, especially in the setting of severe VUR or recurrent UTI. The urologist creates a vesicostomy to allow the free flow of urine into diapers.

Complications

Early diagnosis and intervention for infants with neurogenic bladder can decrease the risks of future complications. Long-term complications of neurogenic bladder include recurrent UTI and vesicoureteral reflux, obstructive uropathy, and associated electrolyte imbalances. Obstructive nephropathy is a leading cause of chronic kidney disease in children and can result in ESRD with resultant dialysis or transplant dependence.

NEPHROCALCINOSIS AND NEPHROLITHIASIS

Nephrocalcinosis and nephrolithiasis are common in infants, particularly those who are preterm or who have had a prolonged NICU course.[35,82,91,112] Studies suggest that nephrocalcinosis/lithiasis may affect 30% to 60% of preterm infants, with increasing risk at lower birth weight and earlier gestational age. Loop diuretics such as furosemide, which increase urinary calcium excretion, appear to be major contributors to these findings. Additional risk factors include relative hypercalcemia in late gestation, low urinary citrate excretion, and renal ischemia or use of nephrotoxic drugs, which can enhance intrarenal deposition of calcium phosphate or oxalate crystals in the setting of tubular injury. Specific conditions associated with nephrocalcinosis include William syndrome, which can be associated with chronic hypercalcemia[97]; neonatal primary hyperparathyroidism; distal renal tubular acidosis; primary hyperoxaluria; and neonatal Bartter syndrome. Thiazide diuretics can be used for treatment of renal calcium deposition due to their hypocalciuric effect. Potassium citrate may also be helpful in the setting of documented hypocitraturia but has not been shown to prevent the development of nephrocalcinosis when given on a prophylactic basis to preterm infants.[140] Adequate hydration is generally important in the approach to stone disease; however, this goal should not supersede appropriate nutrition. Whether nephrocalcinosis confers long-term risk for poor renal function and growth in this population remains controversial[91,123] because the prematurity-associated decrease in nephron mass is a confounding factor.

CHRONIC RENAL FAILURE

With advances in fetal therapeutic intervention and neonatal care, the number of infants requiring chronic dialysis is rising. Such therapy is accompanied by unique ethical dilemmas because many providers continue to view neonatal dialysis as optional rather than obligatory therapy due to the associated high medical, financial, and psychosocial burdens placed on family and society, as well as uncertainties about long-term outcomes.[94,173] These ethical concerns are certain to increase in complexity with advances in fetal urologic surgery and the ability of serial amnioport infusion to prevent death from pulmonary hypoplasia in oligohydramnios, even with complete absence of kidneys.[22] It is therefore important to educate parents as comprehensively as possible regarding the anticipated course and complications for neonates in whom chronic dialysis is indicated. Management of these complex neonates requires a multidisciplinary team of pediatric specialists, including the neonatologist, nephrologist, urologist, transplant surgeon, dialysis nurse, renal dietitian, and social worker.

Renal Replacement Therapy in Neonatal ESRD

The goal of dialysis is to permit appropriate growth and health maintenance in infants until they are suitable candidates for kidney transplantation. Hemodialysis (HD) or peritoneal dialysis (PD) can be offered on a chronic basis to support infants with ESRD, with peritoneal dialysis preferred at most institutions. Although neonates and infants can tolerate HD routinely, functioning

vascular access and intradialytic anticoagulation are required. Moreover, because of the large-volume component of nutrition as well as the metabolic rate in infancy, most infants will require chronic HD 5 to 7 days per week, in contrast to older children and adults who require HD three times per week. Families who do not reside within convenient distance of a pediatric hemodialysis center must relocate for such therapy. These factors obviously have major psychosocial and financial implications for the family.

Peritoneal dialysis (PD) is often technically easier to accomplish in the small child and can be performed by the family within the home setting; the home caregiver(s) are trained to provide continuous cycling peritoneal dialysis for a 10- to 12-hour treatment on a nightly basis under the supervision of a pediatric nephrology program. Thus, PD is the most common choice for renal replacement therapy in small children.[6,165] Contraindications to chronic PD include documented loss of peritoneal function; extensive intraabdominal adhesions that limit dialysate flow, the latter seen most commonly in children who have required major or recurrent intraabdominal surgery; uncorrectable mechanical defects that prevent effective PD or increase the risk of infection (e.g., omphalocele, gastroschisis, diaphragmatic hernia, bladder exstrophy); and absence of a social support system to perform PD within the home. Although technically challenging, long-term PD has been performed in very low-birth-weight infants with birth weight as low as 930 grams.[49,131] Despite continued improvement in the availability of infant catheters and dialysis tubing, chronic PD remains extremely time-consuming, challenging, and demanding for the infant, the family, and medical personnel.

Dialysis in the small child is routinely considered to be a bridge to kidney transplantation. Kidney transplantation is rarely performed with recipient body weight less than 7 to 8 kg, and many programs prefer a minimum body weight of 10 kg to minimize technical and other complications because the majority of donor kidneys are obtained from adults. En bloc or single kidney transplants from infant donors have historically been associated with increased risk of major complications and are thus currently avoided by most pediatric transplant programs. The average 5-year patient survival rate is approximately 75% for children initiating dialysis before 1 year of age.[6,107] However, worsened survival is observed in children who begin dialysis before 3 months of age (hazard ratio fourfold higher) compared with those between 1 to 2 years of age.[6] These cohorts of ESRD children have similar median age at transplant, likely due to the current standards for recipient body weight as described earlier; thus, the time awaiting transplant is more prolonged with decreasing age at dialysis initiation. The median survival of a kidney allograft in the current era is 10 to 12 years.[159] Therefore, neonates with ESRD can anticipate multiple kidney transplants with interval periods of dialysis during their lifetime. Because of antigen sensitization, it is unusual to receive more than three allografts for any individual patient. Although little is known regarding the life expectancy of neonates with ESRD, all-cause mortality rates in children receiving maintenance dialysis are at least 30 times higher than the general pediatric population, with even higher relative risks in very young children.[107] Thus, the decision to embark on chronic renal replacement therapy in the neonate requires careful consideration and discussion with the family. With these considerations, we now turn to particular concerns in the management of ESRD in neonates and young infants.

Management of ESRD in Neonates and Infants

Neonates and infants who require chronic dialysis experience the same complications of chronic renal failure that are observed in older children and adults, including anemia of chronic disease, secondary hyperparathyroidism, chronic acidosis, hypertension, and iron and vitamin D deficiency. However, certain aspects of ESRD are unique to childhood and of particular concern with onset of ESRD during infancy, including altered nutrition, impaired somatic growth, and impaired neurocognitive development.

NUTRITION AND GROWTH

Appropriate nutrition is a critical aspect of ESRD management during infancy. Multiple factors contribute to growth failure in infants with chronic kidney disease, including anorexia; nausea and vomiting; gastroesophageal reflux, which can be exacerbated by abdominal distention from indwelling dialysate during peritoneal dialysis; altered gastrointestinal motility, including delayed gastric emptying, which can be associated with the use of calorically dense formulas; the need for fluid and electrolyte restriction; salt-wasting nephropathy, renal osteodystrophy;

chronic anemia; and developmental abnormalities that affect the mechanics of oral intake. Nutritional intake has the greatest influence on growth during the infancy phase. Although oral feeding is desired and supported, enteral feedings will be necessary in the vast majority of cases to meet protein and caloric requirements sufficient to promote somatic growth and neurocognitive development in the setting of renal failure.[162,175] *Gastrostomy tubes* are usually preferred to nasogastric tubes given the anticipated lengthy duration of support. The timing of gastrostomy placement is important because there is a high risk of infection, including fungal peritonitis, as well as loss of peritoneal membrane function with gastrostomy placement in children already receiving PD. Fundoplication may be required and can be performed concurrently; in our experience, symptoms of gastroesophageal reflux often increase once PD is started because of the pressure associated with increasing volumes of intraabdominal dialysate. Placement of feeding tubes also supports successful administration of the numerous medications that these infants routinely require. Tube feedings that are administered as supplements to oral intake can be provided either as daytime bolus feeds given in intervals that mimic usual infant feeding patterns or as continuous nightly infusions at rates that are regulated by a feeding pump.

Energy Intake. There is no evidence to suggest that children with chronic renal failure require increased energy compared with healthy children of the same age. The recommended goal for energy intake is 100% of the estimated energy requirement for chronologic age and sex, adjusted for physical activity level and body size, with a balance of carbohydrate, saturated and unsaturated fat, and protein similar to infant formula (36% to 56% carbohydrate, 40% to 54% fat, 7% to 12% protein).[87] Low-birth-weight infants and children with established growth delay will require supplemental calories to support catch-up growth. Glucose absorption from peritoneal dialysate can be significant, providing an additional 10 to 20 kcal/kg/day[102] and should be estimated in children with greater than expected weight gains.

Protein Intake. Protein goals, calculated in grams/kg ideal body weight, vary by stage of chronic kidney disease (CKD). Protein goals for children on peritoneal dialysis are set at dietary reference intake (DRI) plus 0.15 to 0.3 g/kg/d to compensate for dialysate-related protein and amino acid losses. It is important to consider the type of protein as well because whey protein is more bioavailable than casein, and evidence suggests that whey protein may promote more rapid gastric emptying.[59] Compared with casein predominant formulas, whey predominant formulas also have lower aluminum content.[116]

Milk Intake. Additional caloric or protein supplements may be added as appropriate. The patient's renal limitations and gastrointestinal tolerance will guide which infant formula to use. Breast milk is low in potassium and phosphorus and thus is often well tolerated by neonates with ESRD. Alternatively, specialized formulas for chronic kidney insufficiency that are low in potassium and phosphorus content are available for infants, older children, and adults (Table 25-6). Similac PM 60/40 (Ross Abbott) and Goodstart Gentle (Gerber) are both appropriate first choices for infants with kidney failure. Concentration of formula is often necessary to achieve adequate intake of energy, protein, and other nutrients within accepted volumes.

FLUID AND ELECTROLYTE REQUIREMENTS

Fluid and electrolyte requirements for neonates with kidney failure vary widely depending on the underlying kidney disease, degree of kidney failure, and mode of renal replacement therapy. *Anuric or oliguric* children require fluid and sodium restriction. In contrast, children with *polyuric renal failure,* as is often seen with congenital obstructive uropathy, may require sodium and fluid supplementation. Parekh et al. demonstrated improved growth of children with polyuric, salt-wasting renal insufficiency when they received 180 to 240 ml/kg/d of dilute (0.3 to 0.5 kcal/ml) formula that contained sodium supplementation on the order of 2 to 4 mEq/100 ml formula.[120] Neonates undergoing peritoneal dialysis may demonstrate significant sodium loss through the dialysate, necessitating sodium supplementation.[133,155] Restriction of dietary potassium intake may be indicated in some neonates. When adequate nutrition is limited by potassium intake, breast milk and formula can be treated with sodium polystyrene to decrease the potassium content before feeding.[26,155] Diluted adult renal formulas can also be provided,[78] but the effect

on infants of adult formulas is not known, and thus it may be prudent to use infant formulas in those under 1 year of age.[59]

CALCIUM AND PHOSPHORUS

Normal serum calcium and phosphorus levels are higher in infants compared with older children, and age-specific norms should be targeted to optimize bone health. Calcium intake from nutritive sources and phosphorus binders should be 100% to 200% of DRI for age and gender, and phosphorus intake should be decreased if secondary hyperparathyroidism is present, with or without hyperphosphatemia.[87] If an older infant still receiving breast milk presents with hyperphosphatemia, the breast milk can be treated with a phosphorus binder to effect phosphate reduction.[52,130]

Vitamins. It is recommended that children with CKD meet 100% of DRI for B vitamins; folic acid; vitamins C, A, E, K; and copper and zinc. If this cannot be achieved through dietary intake alone or if there is clinical evidence of a deficiency, supplementation of these nutrients up to DRI is indicated. Additionally, it is suggested that children on dialysis receive supplemental water-soluble vitamins to replace dialysate-related losses.[87] Several commercial renal multivitamin formulations are available, including a liquid that can be easily dosed and added to breast milk or formulas.

Infant Growth. Half of adult height is realized by 2 years of age and during this phase a child may experience a loss in growth potential that cannot be recovered. ESRD is associated with linear growth failure due to relative resistance to growth hormone (GH). Such resistance is multifactorial in nature but includes reduced density of GH receptors in target organs and reduced levels of free insulin-like growth factor (IGF)-1 due to increased inhibitory IGF-binding proteins.[103] Growth hormone therapy is essential in pediatric ESRD to attain a normal adult height[54,55] and is often started in the toddler or early school age years. Although recombinant human growth hormone has not been fully investigated in infants, recent studies suggest that growth hormone treatment in infancy is generally well tolerated and may be useful as an adjunct for children who continue to grow poorly despite optimization of dialysis therapy and nutrition.

TABLE 25-6	INFANT FORMULAS AND MODULAR SUPPLEMENTS IN RENAL FAILURE

	FORMULA (per 100 ml)						
	Breast milk	Similac PM 60/40	Goodstart Gentle	Similac Advance	Suplena	Nepro	Renalcal
Energy (kcal)	67-77	68	68	68	180	180	200
MACRONUTRIENT DISTRIBUTION (% TOTAL CALORIES)							
CHO	36	41	46	43	42	34	58
Protein	4	9	9	8	10	18	7
Fat	41	50	46	49	48	48	35
CHO (g)	6.9-7.5	6.9	7.8	7.3	19.6	16	29
Protein (g)	0.85-1.25	1.6	1.5	1.4	4.5	8.1	3.4
Fat (g)	3.5-4.3	3.8	3.4	3.65	9.6	9.6	8.2
Sodium (mmol)	0.69-0.96	0.7	0.8	0.7	3.5	4.6	0.3
Potassium (mmol)	1.26-1.44	1.5	1.9	1.8	2.9	2.7	0.2
Calcium (mg)	25.4-30.6	38	45	53	105	105	6
Phosphorus (mg)	11.8-16.2	19	26	28	72	72	10
Iron (mg)	0.02-0.04	0.15	1	1.2	1.9	1.9	—

	MODULARS			
	Beneprotein	Microlipid	MCT oil	Duocal
Formulation	Powder	Liquid	Liquid	Powder
Per unit measure	7 g/21 ml	15 ml	15 ml	100 g
Energy (kcal)	25	68	115	492
MACRONUTRIENT DISTRIBUTION (% TOTAL CALORIES)				
Protein	100	0	0	0
Fat	0	100	100	41
CHO (g)	0	0	0	73
Protein (g)	6	0	0	0
Fat (g)	0	7.5	14	22.3
Sodium (mmol)	0.43			<0.87
Potassium (mmol)	0.9			<0.13
Calcium (mg)	30			<5
Phosphorus (mg)	15			<5
Iron (mg)				

Adapted from Foster BJ, McCauley L, Mak RH: Nutrition in infants and very young children with chronic kidney disease, *Pediatr Nephrol* 27:1432, 2012.
CHO, Carbohydrate; *MCT*, medium-chain triglyceride.
Similac PM 60/40, Similac Advance, Suplena, and Nepro are produced by Ross Abbott Nutrition. Goodstart Gentle is produced by Gerber. Renalcal is produced by Nestle Nutrition. Polycose is produced by Ross Abbott Nutrition; Beneprotein, Microlipid, and MCT oil are produced by Nestle Nutrition. Duocal is produced by Nutricia.

The nutritional management of infants with kidney disease is complex. It is recommended that the growth parameters of infants with moderate CKD be monitored twice as frequently as those of healthy infants and those of children with severe CKD with even greater frequency.[87] Frequent assessment is necessary to ensure that timely and effective nutrition intervention and support can be offered to pave the way for the best possible outcomes. For this reason, it is imperative that a skilled pediatric renal dietitian guide the multidisciplinary team in the nutrition plan for this population.

Neurocognitive Development

Emerging evidence suggests that neurocognitive deficits are common in children with ESRD. A recent cross-sectional study of children with moderate to severe chronic renal insufficiency demonstrated that approximately one-third of participants scored at least one standard deviation below the mean on measures of intelligence quotient, academic achievement, attention regulation, or executive functioning.[80] A more recent but small study in children initiating dialysis before 16 months of age showed significant deficits in intellectual and metacognitive functioning compared with sibling controls.[84] Fewer months on dialysis and younger age at transplant were associated with better outcomes. Although limited data are available at this time, these results have important implications for long-term educational and occupation outcomes and support the need for early intervention services for affected infants.

NURSING CARE OF THE NEONATE WITH RENAL FAILURE

Clinical and Metabolic Assessment

Nurses play a critical role in assessing and managing the neonate with renal failure.[66,71,150,153] Changes in the neonate including decreased urine output, weight gain, and electrolyte imbalance can signal concern for acute renal failure. Symptoms of fluid overload include generalized edema in the face, extremities, and abdomen, increased work of breathing, and increases in blood pressure and weight.

Because electrolyte abnormalities are common in renal failure, nurses should note these values and report them, as well as anticipate clinical signs and symptoms that will follow. *Hyponatremia* often indicates excess intravascular volume due to fluid retention in the setting of renal failure; however, some neonates have salt-losing nephropathy, which leads to hyponatremia and dehydration. Treatment for low sodium concentration may therefore include fluid restriction or replacement of sodium depending on the underlying mechanism. *Hyperkalemia* can result in a medical emergency if not appropriately monitored and treated. Treatment includes restriction of potassium intake in formula and parenteral fluids and discontinuation or alteration of medications known to contribute to high serum potassium concentrations. Measures to shift potassium intracellularly, such as intravenous sodium bicarbonate or insulin and glucose, will temporarily decrease the plasma potassium concentration, but more definitive removal of potassium from the body through the urinary (potassium-wasting diuretics) or GI (cation exchange resins) tracts is warranted. The *electrocardiogram* should be monitored closely because hyperkalemia can lead to ventricular arrhythmias. Intravenous calcium can stabilize the myocardium to help minimize the effect of hyperkalemia on cardiac rhythm. Low serum bicarbonate concentrations are often observed in renal failure because the kidney is instrumental in maintaining acid–base balance in the blood.

Assessment and Management of Peritoneal Dialysis

PD is the dialysis treatment of choice for the neonatal patient. The process of PD is described in detail earlier in this chapter. Regulation of electrolyte and fluid balance must be closely monitored by following serum electrolytes and by close documentation of intake and output and daily weight. These measures provide critical data for clinical management because fluid removal by PD is inexact, being affected by multiple factors including the dextrose concentration of the dialysate and individual peritoneal membrane transport characteristics. PD relies on an intact abdomen for success. Therefore, occasionally hemodialysis is indicated in infants or small children who have abdominal defects or surgery that prevents use of the abdomen for PD.

Nurses have an essential role when dialysis is initiated. The nephrologist determines the type of dialysate including any additives that may be required such as heparin or electrolytes. The fill volumes are based on the weight of the infant and usually start at 10 to 20 ml/kg with an eventual goal of 40 ml/kg. These small initial volumes are necessary to prevent leakage of the newly placed catheter and to "stretch" the peritoneal cavity gradually for comfort. Neonates typically start with continuous manual PD, which is a closed system connected to warmed dialysis solution bags that fill the peritoneum by gravity from a premeasured Volutrol. The fluid dwells in the abdomen for the designated time prescribed by the nephrologist and then is drained from the abdomen by gravity into a drainage system by turning a stopcock. Accurate measurement of the drained fluid is crucial, performed by subtracting the fluid that was infused and recording the difference as the net output. The bedside nurse will perform the manual dialysis, which can be a tedious but life-sustaining job. The nurse must also monitor the abdomen with particular attention to the dressing of the PD catheter to ensure that no leakage of dialysate is occurring along the catheter tract or at any postlaparoscopy sites. The risk for leaks can be decreased by delaying use of the catheter after placement; however, this is not always clinically possible. When the infant is bigger and can tolerate a fill volume of at least 100 ml, the dialysis can be delivered by an automated peritoneal dialysis machine. The machine can be programmed to deliver the prescribed amount of dialysate, allow the fluid to dwell, and automatically drain the abdomen for the designated time. Trained dialysis nurses typically are involved at this point to manage the setup of the machine.

Complications that can occur with peritoneal dialysis include the following:

1. *Infection:* Infection of the exit site and/or peritonitis (infection of the peritoneal lining) can occur if strict attention to aseptic technique is not followed. Weekly dressing changes over the exit site using sterile technique are recommended until the catheter site is healed, which can take 2 to 6 weeks. More frequent dressing changes should be performed if drainage is excessive or the dressing becomes soiled or wet. The risk of infection is significantly higher in the presence of leak. Application of a topical antibiotic cream or ointment at the time of the weekly dressing change is recommended. Immobilization of the catheter below the

dressing to restrict movement is helpful to prevent trauma to the insertion site. Daily tubing changes for manual dialysis setup should be performed with sterile technique for connection of bags and tubing. Once the infant is on an automated dialysis machine, trained dialysis staff performs daily bag and tubing changes. Assessment of the quality of the PD effluent during drain cycles is necessary to detect any signs of peritonitis. Fever and abdominal pain are also indicators of possible peritonitis. If the effluent appears cloudy or fibrin is present, a culture of the fluid is necessary to exclude peritonitis. The PD fluid should be sent for cell count and differential, Gram stain, and culture. Antibiotics may need to be administered pending culture results. The nephrologist may prescribe intraperitoneal antibiotics to be directly added to the bags of dialysate; these antibiotics are systemically absorbed and are dosed to reach blood concentrations similar to those obtained with intravenous administration.

2. *Inflow/outflow problems:* Inflow and outflow problems may occur while performing PD either manually or via the automated dialysis machine. Accurate measurement of the dialysate is done with each manual exchange. If problems occur with inflow, check lines for closed clamps or kinks. Attempt to reposition the patient to encourage better flow. Manual dialysis relies on gravity, so ensure the patient is positioned higher than the drainage system. Good inflow but poor outflow can signal migration of the PD catheter tip, blockage of the catheter tip by omentum, or constipation. Notify the nephrology team of the problem. An abdominal x-ray can be helpful to detect the presence of stool and determine the location of the catheter. Correction of the problem may be as simple as evacuating stool and as complicated as returning to the operating room for catheter revision. In any event, if the problem is not corrected, dialysis cannot continue. The success of the dialysis treatment depends on a functioning catheter.

3. *Potential fluid overload or dehydration:* Accurate measurement of the inflow and outflow of each exchange is essential when determining fluid balance. Check weights before

and after the dialysis treatments and review intake and output measurements to assure fluid balance. Frequent monitoring of vital signs to detect any changes in heart rate or blood pressure will help to determine signs of dehydration or fluid overload. Symptoms of dehydration including poor skin turgor, sunken eyes and fontanel, delayed capillary refill, hypotension, tachycardia, and weight loss signal excessive fluid removal with the current dialysis plan. Signs of fluid overload include generalized or increasing edema, rapid weight gain, increasing blood pressure, and potentially respiratory distress. The physician should be notified of any of these discrepancies so that adjustments can be made to the dialysis plan.

4. *Hernias:* Hernias are a complication of PD. Umbilical and inguinal hernias are the most common and can occur due to the increased intraabdominal pressure from the dialysate load. Decreasing the fill volume until hernia repair can be performed, as well as immediately postoperatively, is recommended to diminish stress in this area.

Renal failure and its treatment in the neonate with PD require competent nursing assessment and accurate documentation of vital signs, weight, and intake/output. The chronic nature of dialysis at this young age can be stressful on the family. Spousal tension, sibling neglect, and financial stress are common. The family's success in managing the infant's dialysis and nutritional needs requires the support of all members of the multidisciplinary care team. The successful growth and development over the coming years needs to be the goal of all team members to ensure eventual renal transplant and hopes for a long, healthy life.

REFERENCES

For a full list of references, scan the QR code or visit http://booksite.elsevier.com/9780323320832.

26 NEUROLOGIC DISORDERS

JULIE A. PARSONS, ALAN R. SEAY, AND MONA JACOBSON

The developing nervous system provides ongoing challenges for researchers and clinicians. Investigations continue in a wide variety of areas, yet basic mechanisms for a pathophysiologic understanding of common events such as neonatal seizures and intraventricular hemorrhages (IVHs) remains unclear.

Improved neonatal care in recent years has not significantly reduced neurologic sequelae. Whether this is a reflection of survival of sicker and more immature infants is difficult to assess. Primary neurologic disease and secondary neurologic complications from such common conditions as cardiopulmonary disease, metabolic derangements, shock, infection, and coagulopathies still represent major problems encountered in every intensive care nursery. Serious congenital nervous system anomalies still appear with regularity, although in small numbers.

This chapter deals with selected topics in neonatal neurology including: congenital malformations, trauma, seizures, hypoxic-ischemic encephalopathy, hypotonia, stroke, and IVH.

CONGENITAL MALFORMATIONS

Physiology, Etiologic Factors, and Clinical Features

Congenital malformations of the nervous system occur when the usual sequence of maturation and development is interrupted (Table 26-1).[5,65] These malformations are present at birth, and the etiology is multifactorial and sometimes unclear. Although strictly destructive lesions (e.g., hydranencephaly resulting from bilateral carotid artery occlusion) are separate from primary failures of morphogenesis, both may be included in the broad category of congenital malformations. The distinction between the two types lies in an understanding of the causes.

Understanding congenital malformations requires an appreciation of the normal embryologic sequence.[65] The clinical and pathologic identification of normal and abnormal structures makes it possible to determine the timing of the insult or development failure. Once timing is established, an appropriate search for the cause can be made.

Neural Tube Defects

The incidence in the United States of neural tube defects (NTDs) is approximately 1 to 2 in 1000 births (Box 26-1).[68] Although the prevalence of NTDs has decreased, they are one of the most common congenital anomalies contributing to morbidity and mortality in neonates.[45] Changes in vertebral, vascular, meningeal, and dermal structures are typically found along with the defects. The more common types of NTDs include anencephaly, encephalocele, myelomeningocele, and occult spina bifida.[10] Genetic and environmental factors play a role in the development of NTDs. Familial incidence also plays a role; when one family member is affected, the risk increases by 2% to 3% in subsequent offspring and doubles if two or more family members are affected.[10] Cytogenic abnormalities are found in approximately 2% to 16% of neonates

---

PURPLE type highlights content that is particularly applicable to clinical settings.

TABLE 26-1	CENTRAL NERVOUS SYSTEM DEVELOPMENT AND RELATED DEFECTS	
MATURATIONAL PROCESS	**TIME**	**ASSOCIATED DEFECTS**
Neural tube defects (dorsal induction, neurulation)	3-4 weeks	Craniorachischisis Anencephaly Myeloschisis Encephalocele Myelomeningocele Chiari malformation
Prosencephalic development[90]	2-3 months	Cyclopia Holoprosencephaly Arrhinencephaly Septo-optic dysplasia Agenesis of corpus callosum Agenesis of septum pellucidum
Proliferation	2-4 months	Microcephaly Megalencephaly Neurocutaneous syndromes (?)
Migration[90]	3-5 months	Schizencephaly Lissencephaly Pachygyria (macrogyria) Microgyria (polymicrogyria) Neuronal heterotopias
Neuronal organization and functional organization	6 months	Down syndrome (?) Mental retardation (?) Genetic epilepsy (?)
Myelination[90]	2nd trimester[90]	Anoxic/ischemic damage

BOX 26-1	CRITICAL FINDINGS **NEURAL TUBE DEFECTS**

- As many as 50% or more of neural tube defects (NTDs) are preventable.
- Two-thirds of American women fail to ingest an adequate amount of folic acid, and enriched grain products supply only one-fourth of daily need.
- All women of childbearing age should consume **400 mcg** of folic acid daily even when not planning to become pregnant.
- **At increased risk:** women with a previous NTD pregnancy. For these women, the recommended dose of folic acid is **increased to 4 mg daily.** It should be taken at least 1 month before conception.
- **Sources:** Dietary supplements, enriched grain products, and consumption of foods with folic acid content (citrus fruit, beans, leafy greens).
- The Centers for Disease Control and Prevention, the American Academy of Pediatrics, and the March of Dimes have all recommended an increase in the amount of folic acid used to fortify grain products from 140 to 350 mcg per 100 g of grain.
- Inadequate education of women continues to be a problem.

who have an isolated NTD.[56] Teratogen exposure has also been linked to NTDs.[65] A prepregnancy history of diabetes, specific drugs (especially anticonvulsants and sulfonamide drugs), and maternal hyperthermia secondary to using a hot tub or sauna have been identified as risk factors.[29] Recently, prepregnancy maternal obesity also has been linked to an increased risk.[93]

The major environmental factor linked to NTDs is a dietary level of folic acid.[49] Folic acid supplements before and during pregnancy have been cited as substantially lowering the incidence of these NTDs. The U.S. Public Health Service issued a recommendation that women of childbearing years consume 400 mcg of folic acid each day to prevent NTDs. The American Academy of Pediatrics (AAP)

also supports this recommendation.[17,28,49,65] Such an intake can be achieved by dietary supplementation of folate, adding folic acid to U.S. enriched grain products (e.g., bread, flour), and consuming foods containing folic acid (e.g., citrus fruit, beans, leafy greens). The Food and Drug Administration (FDA) required all enriched grain products to be fortified with folic acid by 1998.[12,28] Despite this, it has been reported by the Centers for Disease Control and Prevention (CDC) that two-thirds of American women fail to ingest an adequate amount of folic acid.[17] It has been argued that the amount of folic acid supplementation in grain products may be inadequate, supplying only about one-fourth of daily need.[66] Noting the 26% decrease in the incidence of NTDs after the FDA required 140 mcg folic acid per 100 g of grain, the March of Dimes recommended an increase in the level of folic acid fortification.[58,92] Others, including the CDC and American Academy of Pediatrics, concur with this recommendation to increase the requirement to 350 mcg folic acid per 100 g of grain.[14]

A Cochrane review concluded that supplementation with folate provides "a strong protective effect against neural tube defects."[55] Recommendations were made to increase availability of information about folate. Another recommendation was to advise women with a previous NTD pregnancy of the increased risk for future pregnancy and to provide them with folate supplementation.[55] For these women, the recommended dosage of folic acid is increased to 4 mg daily, which should be taken for at least 1 month before conception.[12,28,32] Unfortunately, not enough providers who care for women of childbearing age are counseling them about the importance of folic acid consumption or the appropriate amount to take.[32] Mothers who take antiepileptic drugs are also at particularly high risk for having babies with NTDs.[97] It should not be expected that improved consumption of folic acid will completely prevent NTDs because of multifactorial etiologic factors such as the environment and genetics.

At the end of the first embryonic week, the primitive streak is present on the rostral surface of the embryo. A second streak, the notochordal process, develops alongside the primitive streak. The notochord is responsible for the induction of both the neural plate and the neurenteric canal. Cells proliferate along the lateral margin of the neural plate to form the neural folds around the central neural groove.[90]

Cells at the apex of the neural folds make up the neural crest. Schwann cells, pia-arachnoid cells, sensory ganglia, melanocytes, and various secretory cells arise from the neural crest. The neural folds meet and fuse with the rostral (anterior) and caudal (posterior) ends (neuropore), closing by approximately the end of the fourth embryonic week.[90]

Failure of development at this stage results in the defects of neurulation (or dorsal induction). The most severe of these defects is craniorachischisis, in which there is significant malformation of the brain (as in anencephaly), absence of the posterior skull, and an open spine along the full length of the spinal cord. Only a few affected embryos survive to early fetal stages.[90]

Anencephaly is similar to craniorachischisis without the spinal defect. There is essentially no normal brain tissue above the brainstem and thalami, and parts of those structures are malformed. Onset is thought to occur before 24 days' gestation. About one-fourth of the fetuses survive into the neonatal period, but three-fourths are stillborn. The majority of anencephalic infants die within the first week of life without intensive care.[90]

Myeloschisis involves the failure of the posterior neural tube to close. There is no well-defined sac protruding from the defect.[15]

Encephaloceles are caused by a limited failure of closure at the rostral (head) end of the neural tube.

Extensions of meninges or brain tissue through the skull may occur on the ventral or rostral surface.[90]

Myelomeningoceles (or the more limited meningoceles) are a limited form of myeloschisis with failure of closure at the caudal (tail) end of the neural tube. With meningocele, the meninges protrude through the vertebrae and are contained within a sack. The spinal cord and nerve roots are generally in normal position, which improves the outcomes for these children. Unfortunately, myelomeningoceles, the more common defect, results in protrusion of both meninges and spinal cord through the opening in the spinal column. Neurologic deficits occur below the level of the protrusion.[56,77,86] Chiari malformations are typically included in this category. Chiari I malformation, with herniation of the cerebellar tonsils into the foramen magnum, is not associated with spina bifida and is usually not symptomatic in childhood. Chiari II malformations, however, are often seen in conjunction with myelomeningocele, and involve the brainstem and cerebellum. In Chiari II malformations the cerebellar vermis is pulled down through the foramen magnum, and the brainstem is elongated. Because the fourth ventricle is typically partially herniated into the cervical canal, hydrocephalus is common. Dilation of ventricles often occurs without increased head circumference or clinical symptoms of increased intracranial pressure in this group of infants; therefore, serial ultrasound scans should be performed with a fast sequence T2-weighted magnetic resonance imaging (MRI) when surgical intervention is being considered. Symptoms of brainstem involvement such as central apnea or vocal cord paralysis may be present. Any defect in which the spinal or cranial contents are "open" to the outside, such as myelomeningocele or encephalocele, are associated with an elevation of alpha-fetoprotein (AFP) in the amniotic fluid. This is important in prenatal diagnosis.[90]

Segmentation Defects

After formation and closure of the neural tube, the development of different regions of the brain begins to occur. Between 10 and 13 weeks' postconception, the division of the brain into hemispheres, formation of the ventricular system, and formation of the major gyral patterns all occur[68] and are all part of this period of development. Major areas of the brain, including the cerebellum, basal ganglia, brainstem nuclei, thalamus, and hypothalamus, form at this time.[90] Defects of segmentation and cleavage occur during this phase of neural development. For unknown reasons, defects of segmentation and cleavage are far less common than defects of neurulation. Because these malformations involve abnormalities of ventral induction rather than dorsal induction (e.g., neurulation), the face, eyes, nose, mouth, and hair are also involved. When any of these brain malformations are suspected or when features suggestive of them are seen, careful examination of the hair, eyes, ears, mouth, and nose may reveal other related anomalies.

Holoprosencephaly is characterized by a single midline lateral ventricle, incomplete or absent interhemispheric fissure, absent olfactory system, midfacial clefts, and hypotelorism (abnormally decreased space between the eyes). The most severe form of holoprosencephaly is cyclopia (a single fused midline eye) and supraorbital nasal structure. At times, the nasal structure and eye are absent. An intermediate form is cebocephaly, which includes ocular hypotelorism and a flat nose with single nostril.[90]

Migration and Cortical Organizational Defects

The remaining development of the brain takes more than twice as long as previously described development and includes cellular proliferation, migration, organization, and myelination. Cells that later form the cerebral cortex begin in the germinal matrix (near the caudate nucleus around the lateral ventricles). These cells then migrate in a radial fashion to their final positions near the surface of the brain. Abnormalities of cellular migration result in collections of gray matter in unusual places (heterotopias), abnormal gyri and sulci, abnormal spaces in the brain, and clinical signs of gray matter dysfunction. Frequently, these clinical problems are not apparent in the newborn period.

Microcephaly means "small brain" and is manifested as a head circumference measuring greater than two standard deviations below average for infants at that gestational age.[29] Microcephaly may be (1) genetic (dominant, recessive, sex-linked) or chromosomal (translocation [see Chapter 27]), (2) caused by teratogens (cocaine, alcohol), (3) caused by infection (rubella, cytomegalovirus), or (4) of unknown cause. Occasionally, there is a paucity of germinal matrix cells or they fail to adequately migrate, resulting in a brain cortex with a decreased number of neuronal cells.[90]

In *lissencephaly,* the brain is smooth in appearance, having little or no gyri (convolutions). An important fact is that the normal fetal brain is smooth early in gestation with convolutions forming throughout gestation, creating the sulci and gyri seen in term infants. Lissencephaly is a cortical migrational abnormality, resulting in agyria, pachygyria, and other issues in term infants.

Although not generally present at birth, poor head growth resulting in microcephaly usually occurs within the first year in type I lissencephaly. Neonatal seizures may also occur, but seizures are more commonly present at 6 to 12 months of age. A general phenotype is marked by hollowing at both temples, a small jaw, and generalized hypotonia. *Miller-Dieker syndrome* is a genetic form of type I lissencephaly due to a microdeletion of 17p13.3. The characteristics are narrow forehead, long philtrum, upturned nose, retrognathia, retinal hypervascularization, and digital abnormalities. In type II lissencephaly, macrocephaly is generally present at birth or develops soon afterward. Retinal, cerebellar, and muscular abnormalities always are present.[64] Other clinical features of lissencephaly include hypotonia, feeding problems, and decreased movement sometimes presenting with arthrogryposis in the newborn. Abnormalities on the electroencephalogram (EEG) are noted. Later, significant intellectual disability and severe spasticity may be noted and death may occur.[90]

Additional Defects

Cerebellar malformations are quite varied. Most often, at least a portion of the cerebellum is preserved, but total absence is possible. Hemispheric aplasia or vermian aplasia is seen, and familial forms have been reported. *Dandy-Walker cyst* is another complex malformation involving the cerebellum in which the fourth ventricle is dilated into a cystic structure. The foramina of Magendie and Luschka are atretic, and hydrocephalus results. The cerebellum is small and displaced upward. Associated anomalies include heterotopias, agenesis of the corpus callosum, aqueductal stenosis, and syringomyelia. Causation is unknown. The differential diagnosis includes an arachnoid cyst of the posterior fossa. In the case of an arachnoid cyst, the fourth ventricle is not part of the malformation and is normal, although it may be displaced.[90]

Clinical features of Dandy-Walker cyst include progressive hydrocephalus, enlargement of the occipital shelf and posterior part of the skull, and clinical symptoms of increased intracranial pressure.[90] Symptoms may be absent in the newborn period. Malformations in other organ systems such as renal and cardiac are frequently associated.

Craniosynostosis is the abnormally early closure (fusion) of the bones of the skull. The cause of this malformation is unknown. The premature closure of sutures may involve one or multiple sutures, with resulting deformity of the skull. Various skull shapes such as plagiocephaly, brachycephaly, scaphocephaly, and trigonocephaly may result depending on which sutures are prematurely fused.[90]

Craniosynostosis should be suspected in the presence of microcephaly or misshapen head. Appropriate evaluation requires a clinical assessment with palpation of the sutures to determine whether they are overriding or fused, x-ray films of the skull and a computed tomography (CT) scan to define which of the sutures are stenosed and whether there might be an associated brain malformation or hydrocephalus.[90] Craniosynostosis should be differentiated from positional deformities occurring from an infant lying in one position for a prolonged period of time. A classic example is dolichocephaly (narrow and elongated shape) seen in premature infants.

Hydrocephalus may occur as a result of various etiologies. Hydrocephalus results when the normal flow of cerebrospinal fluid (CSF) is obstructed. This may be the result of an atretic portion of the ventricular system, blockage from the outside, inflammation within the ventricular system causing a permanent blockage, or, rarely, overproduction of CSF. An inherited X-linked form of hydrocephalus exists. Intrauterine infection is another cause. Hydrocephalus may be associated with many of the malformations described previously.[56,90]

Data Collection

The diagnosis of malformations of the central nervous system (CNS) may be quite obvious (as in anencephaly) or more subtle. Careful examination of all newborns results in the identification of most malformations. At times, the diagnosis is suspected not based on examination findings but because of an accompanying sign, such as seizures.[10] Prenatal diagnosis of congenital malformations of the nervous system can be made using imaging studies. Ultrasonographic examination (an abdominal ultrasound scan of the mother) or fetal MRI, which is now available at many large centers, provides an opportunity to identify certain malformations by viewing the fetus during development. Hydrocephalus, encephaloceles, myelomeningoceles, cerebellar malformations, hemorrhage and stroke, and anencephaly may be identified prenatally.

Determination of alpha-fetoprotein (AFP) levels in the amniotic fluid and maternal serum allows the identification of anencephaly and open myelomeningoceles. A nonenclosed nervous system is associated with a significant rise in AFP in the amniotic fluid. Amniocentesis provides the amniotic fluid necessary for this determination. Testing of maternal serum for AFP is also an option and at some centers may be used along with ultrasonography or fetal MRI for diagnosis, allowing amniocentesis to be omitted.[90] Clinical signs and symptoms have been described for each individual nervous system malformation presented earlier in this chapter.

Treatment

Limited treatment is available for congenital malformations of the nervous system. A variety of strategies are available for reducing secondary complications or providing earlier management to handle these complications more efficiently.

The greatest efforts and accomplishments have been made for infants with congenital malformations who might be expected to have productive lives. When secondary complications are managed appropriately, the majority of children with myelomeningoceles are ambulatory (total or partial) and continent of urine.[90]

Myelomeningocele generally is surgically repaired as soon as possible (within 24 to 48 hours).[10,56,77,90] Prevention of infection is paramount. In addition to sterile technique, prophylactic antibiotics have been shown to be beneficial.[90] Trauma to the area should be avoided by keeping the infant in the prone position and maintaining sterile gauze moistened with warm, sterile normal saline. Tape should be avoided.[10,56,75] Preventing fecal contamination is vital. Several authors recommend the use of a sterile, plastic drape fastened above the anus but below the lesion to keep fecal material isolated from the site.[56,75] Latex

BOX 26-2 POSTOPERATIVE VENTRICULOPERITONEAL SHUNT CARE

- Positioning:
  - Place infant on unaffected side (may position on shunt side with "doughnut" over operative site once incision has healed). Keep head of bed flat (15-30 degrees) to prevent too-rapid fluid loss.
  - Support head carefully when moving infant.
  - Turn every 2 hr from unaffected side of head to back.
- Shunt site:
  - Use strict aseptic technique when changing dressing.
  - Pump shunt if and only as directed by neurosurgeon.
  - Observe for fluid leakage around pump.
- Observe and document all intake and output. Watch for symptoms of excessive drainage of cerebrospinal fluid:
  - Sunken fontanel
  - Increased urine output
  - Increased sodium loss
- Observe, document, and report any seizure activity or paresis.
- Observe for signs of ileus:
  - Abdominal distention (serially measure abdominal girth)
  - Absence of bowel sounds
  - Loss of gastric content by emesis or through orogastric tube
- Perform range-of-motion exercises on all extremities.

- Observe and assess for symptoms of increased intracranial pressure (shunt failure):
  - Increasing head circumference (measure head daily)
  - Full or tense fontanel
  - Sutures palpably more separated
  - High-pitched, shrill cry
  - Irritability and/or sleeplessness
  - Vomiting
  - Poor feeding
  - Nystagmus
  - Sunset sign of eyes
  - Shiny scalp with distended vessels
  - Hypotonia and/or hypertonia
- Observe and assess for signs of infection:
  - Redness or drainage at shunt site
  - Hypothermia and/or hyperthermia
  - Lethargy and/or irritability
  - Poor feeding and/or poor weight gain
  - Pallor
- Parent teaching:
  - Demonstrate and receive return demonstration of drug administration.
  - Teach parents side effects of medications.
  - Document on neonatal intensive care unit's routine discharge teaching checklist with routine care.

precautions also should be initiated because these infants have an increased propensity for developing sensitivity to latex.[10]

In addition, spina bifida has been repaired in utero at early gestational age. Such repairs have risks for both mother and fetus but have resulted in reported significant drops in the number of infants developing hydrocephalus that would require a postnatal ventriculoperitoneal shunt.[27] The National Institutes of Health (NIH) sponsored Management of Myelomeningocele Study (MOMS) trial was a multicenter, prospective, randomized controlled trial comparing prenatal surgery with standard neonatal treatment. The study demonstrated that surgery before 26 weeks' gestation decreased the need for ventriculoperitoneal shunts, decrease hindbrain herniation, and preserved neurologic function. However, there were complications of premature delivery and some maternal complications as well. MOMS II study will continue to follow the cohort of 183

babies to monitor neurologic and cognitive function as well as bowel and bladder function to determine whether benefit is sustained.[23]

Some of the malformations are lethal soon after birth (anencephaly), limiting management options to comfort measures and family support (see Chapter 32). When appropriate, genetic counseling should be requested. For other malformations, treatment requires management of symptoms such as seizures, signs of increased intracranial pressure, and infection. A consult to neurosurgery and neurology is indicated. Other helpful consults may include physical therapy, infectious disease, urology, and orthopedics.[54] For hydrocephalus, shunting may become necessary (Boxes 26-2 and 26-3, and Figure 26-1).[90]

Generally, skull deformity is present in infants with craniosynostosis. It is prudent to consider the presence of craniosynostosis in any infant with a small head. If present, total craniosynostosis, or premature fusion of all the sutures should be treated surgically.[56]

BOX 26-3	PARENT TEACHING

WOLFSON CHILDREN'S HOSPITAL PARENT HANDOUT: NEWBORN VENTRICULOPERITONEAL SHUNT (FOR USE WITH VENTRICULOPERITONEAL SHUNT TEACHING CHECKLIST)

Purpose of Ventriculoperitoneal Shunt

- Ventricles are compartment-like spaces that are located in the normal brain. Spinal fluid forms daily in these ventricles. This clear fluid flows out over the brain and down around the spinal cord. Spinal fluid helps cushion the brain from injury, keeps the brain moist, and carries away waste products.
- Hydrocephalus is a condition in which an abnormally large amount of spinal fluid builds up in your baby's ventricles and usually is caused by a blockage in the spinal fluid path. Because the ventricles continue to make spinal fluid daily, a buildup of fluid occurs when it cannot escape. This excess fluid can cause pressure on the brain and result in permanent damage to the brain unless it is properly treated.
- The purpose and function of your baby's VP shunt is to allow the excess spinal fluid to drain through a tube from the ventricle into the abdomen, where it is absorbed.

Pathway of the Ventriculoperitoneal Shunt (see Figure 26-1)

- A small incision is made on the scalp, and the tube is passed through the skull and into the ventricle. Located under the skin, the tube passes behind the ear, down the side of the neck, and continues to the abdomen, where a second incision is made to put the end of the tube into the abdominal cavity. A third incision is sometimes needed in the neck area with some babies.
- The scalp incision will be hidden as your baby's hair grows. You will see and feel the shunt tubing (like a large vein under the skin), but it is barely noticeable after the baby gains weight.

Signs and Symptoms of Shunt Infection

- The shunt is at risk for infection because it is a foreign object located inside the body. You will have to watch for these signs of shunt infection and report them **immediately** to your doctor:
  - Temperature of 101° F or higher
  - Swelling, redness, or drainage along the pathway of the shunt tube
  - Lethargy or irritability (change in behavior)
  - Loss of appetite or poor feeding

Signs and Symptoms of Shunt Failure/Increased Intracranial Pressure

- The spinal fluid contains proteins and chemicals that may build up and block off the shunt. It is also possible for tissue within the brain or abdomen to block the shunt or for the shunt device itself to fail. This shunt failure (malfunction) means that the spinal fluid will once again build up and result in pressure on the brain and possible irreversible damage. Therefore it is very important for you to watch for the signs of increased pressure in the brain that occurs with shunt failure and report them to your doctor immediately:
- Lethargy or sleepiness
- Unusual irritability, fussiness, or excessive crying
- Repeated vomiting
- Poor feeding
- Bulging soft spot when baby is sitting up quietly
- Shrill, high-pitched cry
- Eyes that look downward
- Increase in spaces between the bones of the skull
- Seizures/posturing

Reason and Importance of Prompt Treatment of Health Problems

- Prompt treatment of your baby's health problems (e.g., ear infections, skin infections) is important to prevent infections spreading to the shunt. It is also vital to seek medical care for signs of shunt infection or failure as noted.

Importance of Close Medical Follow-up

- Your baby will have to be followed up by a neurosurgeon and your pediatrician after being discharged. Bring the baby to every follow-up appointment so that your baby's head can be measured and physical condition can be evaluated. Your baby will also go to the Developmental Evaluation Clinic where a specialist in baby development can examine him or her. If development problems occur, this will ensure early diagnosis and treatment.

Care of the Shunt

- You can handle, cuddle, and play with your baby like any baby. Your baby also can sleep in any position after the initial postoperative period.

BOX 26-3

PARENT TEACHING — cont'd

WOLFSON CHILDREN'S HOSPITAL PARENT HANDOUT: NEWBORN VENTRICULOPERITONEAL SHUNT (FOR USE WITH VENTRICULOPERITONEAL SHUNT TEACHING CHECKLIST)

**BAPTIST MEDICAL CENTER
WOLFSON CHILDREN'S HOSPITAL**
JACKSONVILLE, FLORIDA

Wolfson Children's HOSPITAL
at Baptist Medical Center

VENTRICULOPERITONEAL (VP) SHUNT TEACHING CHECKLIST

GOAL/SKILL	NURSING (Date and Initials)		CARE GIVER #1	CARE GIVER #2	CARE GIVER #3
1. Verbalizes understanding of reason for VP shunt.	H - "An Introduction to Hydrocephalus"	☐			
2. Identifies the pathway of the VP shunt and the shunt's function.	H - "Ventriculoperitoneal Shunt" (Newborn)	☐			
	H - "Hydrocephalus and Shunts" (For infants with Cordis Shunts)	☐			
	H - "Your Valve System for Hydrocephalus" (For Cordis Valve System Shunts)	☐			
	H - "Just Like Any Other Little Beagle"	☐			
	V - "Just Like Any Other Little Beagle"	☐			
3. Lists signs and symptoms of shunt infection and emergent need to notify MD.					
4. Lists signs and symptoms of shunt failure and emergent need to notify MD.					
5. Discuss the reason and importance of prompt treatment of health problems.					
6. Verbalizes understanding of importance of close medical follow-up.					

SIGNATURE/INITIAL		TEACHING CODES	PARENT SIGNATURE(S)
		L - Lecture/Discussion	
		D - Demonstration (or return demo)	
		U - Verbalizes Understanding	
		R - Reinforced Teaching	
		V - Video	PATIENT LABEL
		H - Handout	
		E - Equipment	

20-207 Rev 5/96

Courtesy Baptist Medical Center, Wolfson Children's Hospital, Jacksonville, Fla.

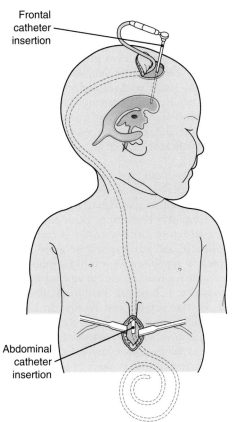

Frontal catheter insertion

Abdominal catheter insertion

FIGURE 26-1 Ventricular peritoneal shunt. (From Rengachary SS, Ellenbogen RG: *Principles of neurosurgery*, ed 2, Edinburgh, 2005, Mosby Ltd.)

The management of congenital hydrocephalus consists primarily of early shunting as soon after birth as possible. Fetal surgery for placement of a ventriculoamniotic shunt has been proposed, but an improvement in outcomes compared with surgery after birth is uncertain. In addition, hydrocephalus in a fetus is often associated with serious developmental abnormalities that may increase morbidity and mortality.[90]

In Volpe's series, outcome was variable and the procedures were not as reliable as hoped. It was not always possible to distinguish true hydrocephalus from ventriculomegaly without increased pressure. Shunting soon after birth often produces a far better outcome than would be assumed with minimal motor deficit and only a mild to moderate deficit in intellect.[90]

Monitoring of pregnancies with fetal ultrasound allows the detection of congenital hydrocephalus.

Induction of lung maturation with steroids has been suggested to allow a preterm delivery (with a smaller head) without excessive pulmonary complications. In this way, a permanent shunt can be placed sooner than with term delivery.[90]

Complications

Many of the expected complications were dealt with previously in the sections describing the malformations and their associated problems. It is difficult to separate true complications from problems resulting from the malformation. For example, hydrocephalus develops in many infants with myelomeningocele and may be present at birth.[10,77] Other complications or associated problems of myelomeningocele include bowel and bladder incontinence, meningitis, urinary tract infections, and paralysis.[56]

Malformations carry with them altered anatomy and physiology that is reflected in abnormal function. Common comorbidities include seizures, intellectual disability, sensorimotor abnormalities, disturbances in primary sensory function such as vision and hearing, orthopedic problems, and vegetative functions.[90]

Associated problems encountered are ordinarily explained on the basis of the malformation and the anatomy involved. Often midline defects in the brain (particularly at the base of the brain) result in clinical problems involving the hypothalamus and the hypothalamic-pituitary axis. This dysfunction may manifest itself in impaired temperature regulation, thyroid abnormalities, diabetes insipidus, and adrenal insufficiency. When absence of the septum pellucidum is diagnosed, the optic nerves should be evaluated to rule out septo-optic dysplasia, which is frequently associated with hypothalamic and electrolyte abnormalities.

Involvement of the cortex causes seizures, cognitive deficits, and sensorimotor problems. White matter damage can cause spasticity. If the brainstem is involved in the malformation (e.g., Chiari or Dandy-Walker malformations), apnea, deafness, sleep disturbance, oculomotor disturbances, and problems with sucking and swallowing may be seen. Spinal cord lesions cause quadriplegia or paraplegia. Genitourinary problems and, to a lesser extent, gastrointestinal problems also are seen.

Most of the complications occur after the newborn period. In many circumstances, the problem is already present but functional expression such as impaired ambulation, intellectual disability or deafness, is lacking. In the infant's follow-up examinations, careful attention must be given to problems likely to develop or intensify with age. When a specific malformation is diagnosed, it is necessary to become familiar with potential sequelae, not only to anticipate problems as they appear but also to lessen any secondary damage that might occur if the diagnoses go unrecognized.

Parent Teaching

Parents of an infant born with congenital malformations are faced with a stressful event that may develop into a major life transition. Parents, especially mothers, report feelings of guilt and self-blame, although they may not initially share these feelings with hospital staff. After the birth of a malformed child, they go through stages of grief (see Chapters 29 and 30): shock or denial, anger, bargaining, depression, and acceptance. Some authors question whether full acceptance occurs for the family of the handicapped child because of return of grief and sorrow each time a developmental milestone is missed or the child experiences illness.[61,75]

Social support received from hospital personnel, family, and friends can help parents feel less stressed and more able to cope with the illness of their infant. The ability of the staff to accurately anticipate and assess parental feelings and concerns can be invaluable when assisting families through this difficult time. Parents should be encouraged to verbalize their feelings and fears in a supportive environment. Reassurances, when appropriate, should be provided (e.g., parents were not responsible for the congenital malformation; it is normal for the mother to experience [or at least report] more fears than her husband). The ultimate goal of intervention is to reduce stress, assist families to confront fears, improve coping, and facilitate the bonding process.[61]

Infants with congenital malformations present such a complex variety of problems that parent teaching and emotional support need to begin as early as possible. With improved surveillance such as ultrasound and fetal MRI, parents often know from the time of birth or earlier that a major problem exists. In other circumstances, the anomaly is detected only after appropriate studies are performed.

When the infant is not viable, care should be directed at meeting the emotional needs of the family. Every effort should be made to give family members positive experiences and memories by encouraging early parental holding of the infant and, whenever possible, participation with care (see Chapter 30). Anticipatory counseling from social services and chaplain staff can help the family during grieving, and with funeral arrangements. If there are also questions about etiologic factors and genetics, these questions should be dealt with according to the family's wishes (see Chapter 27).

If serious handicaps are anticipated and the infant is expected to survive, the parents should be encouraged to participate in the care of the infant from the beginning. Both adjustment and specific aspects of care within the circumstance will be enhanced and learning will be more effective if parents are supported. A multidisciplinary team approach to parent education and support allows individualized hospital resources for specific needs of the patient and family. In addition to medical, nursing, social service, and chaplain involvement, team members can be drawn from psychology, developmental specialists, physical therapy/occupational therapy, and other services based on specific needs and circumstances. Parent teaching and support must be individualized according to the anomaly. When available, support groups, integrative discharge planning, and specialized clinics can help with postdischarge care and parent education.

Parent teaching for mothers and fathers of infants with congenital anomalies should (1) be started early, (2) involve the parents in the care of the infant, (3) use the resources of the hospital and community for specialized help, and (4) continue after the infant has gone home from the hospital or dies.[61]

BIRTH INJURIES

Physiology and Etiology

Birth injuries (birth traumas) are the direct result of difficulties encountered during the delivery process. These may be minor injuries without expected sequelae or the direct cause of death in the neonatal period. Classification of birth injuries usually is etiologic (predisposing factors or mechanisms of injury) or anatomic. An anatomic classification is used in this discussion to illustrate commonly encountered problems (Table 26-2).

TABLE 26-2 ANATOMIC CLASSIFICATION OF BIRTH INJURIES

SITE OF INJURY	TYPE OF INJURY
Scalp	Caput succedaneum
	Cephalhematoma
	Subgaleal hemorrhage
Skull	Linear fracture
	Depressed fracture
	Occipital osteodiastasis
Intracranial	Epidural hematoma
	Subdural hematoma (laceration of falx, tentorium, or superficial veins)
	Subarachnoid hemorrhage
	Cerebral contusion
	Cerebellar contusion
	Intracerebellar hematoma
Spinal cord (cervical)	Vertebral artery injury
	Intraspinal hemorrhage
	Spinal cord transection or injury
Plexus injuries	Erb's palsy
	Klumpke's paralysis
	Total (mixed) brachial plexus injury
	Horner syndrome
	Diaphragmatic paralysis
	Lumbosacral plexus injury
Cranial and peripheral nerve injuries	Radial nerve palsy/nerve injuries
	Medial nerve palsy
	Sciatic nerve palsy
	Laryngeal nerve palsy
	Diaphragmatic paralysis
	Facial nerve palsy

The timing of birth injuries can be used to identify and describe causes. Etiologic classification of birth injuries includes uterine injury (antenatal), fetal monitoring procedures, abnormal or difficult presentations or methods of delivery, and multifactorial injuries. It should be recognized that an injury might have multiple causations. Thus, a cephalhematoma could be the result of forceps delivery, vacuum extraction, or routine vaginal delivery. A variety of specific predisposing factors increase the risk for birth injury, as follows:

- Macrosomia
- Cephalopelvic disproportion
- Uterine abnormalities
- Dystocia

- Prematurity
- Prolonged or precipitous labor
- Breech presentation/abnormal lie
- Instrumented delivery: forceps/vacuum
- Rotation of fetus
- Version and extraction
- Handling after delivery

Multiple factors often are present. When multiple predisposing factors are present, a single underlying maternal disease often links them. A common example is that of a premature, macrosomic fetus with a diabetic mother in whom labor is not progressing properly.

The common factors that are present in deliveries complicated by birth injuries are as follows:

- Unusual progress of labor
- Unusual size or shape of the fetus (large for gestational age or hydrocephalus)
- Problems encountered during delivery (dystocia or forceps application)
- Unusual or unexpected presentations (breech or unexpected twin)

The maternal history must always be explored for an underlying disease process or condition that might increase the risk of a birth injury.

Prevention

Careful attention to risk factors and the appropriate planning of delivery should reduce the incidence of birth injuries to a minimum. Transabdominal and transvaginal ultrasonography facilitates awareness of macrosomia, hydrocephalus, and unusual presentations before delivery. Particular pregnancies then may be delivered by controlled elective cesarean section to avoid significant birth injury. Care must be taken to avoid substituting a procedure of greater risk. A small percentage of significant birth injuries cannot be anticipated until the specific circumstances are encountered during delivery. Emergency cesarean delivery may provide last-minute salvage, but in these circumstances, the injury may be truly unavoidable.

SPECIFIC BIRTH INJURIES

Injuries to the Scalp

The three commonly encountered forms of extracranial scalp injuries are caput succedaneum,

BOX 26-4	CRITICAL FINDINGS
	EXTRACRANIAL HEMORRHAGE

There are three common forms of extracranial hemorrhage but with different etiology and clinical assessment findings, as follows.

1. Caput succedaneum
   a. *Etiology:* Trauma to scalp (usually vertex vaginal delivery) results in hemorrhagic edema superficial to the aponeurosis of the scalp.
   b. *Findings:* Soft, pitting edema that crosses suture lines.
2. Cephalhematoma
   a. *Etiology:* Mechanical trauma; most common in primiparous women, with delivery using forceps or in vacuum-assisted deliveries.
   b. *Findings:* Firm, tense collection of blood confined by the sutures. Area often increases in size after delivery. No significant blood loss. Blood collects beneath the periosteum (subperiosteal).
   c. *Warning:* Associated with linear skull fracture in up to 25% of the cases.
3. Subgaleal hemorrhage
   a. *Etiology:* Forces that compress and then drag head through pelvic outlet.
   b. *Findings:* Firm swelling that crosses suture lines and is fluctuant to palpation. Blood collection is under the aponeurosis (connective tissue connecting the occipital and frontal muscles). Bleeding (swelling) may continue after birth and dissect along tissue planes into the neck.
   c. *Warning:* Acute blood loss may occur. Presenting symptom may be shock.

Monitor VS for signs of shock:
   Elevated HR
   Decreasing BP
Monitor baby for signs of shock:
   Pallor
   Delayed capillary refill time
   Diminished tone
   Respiratory distress
Transfusion may be necessary: type and cross-match.
Serial Hct should be followed.
Elevated bilirubin is a common complication as a byproduct of broken-down red blood cells.

BP, Blood pressure; *Hct,* hematocrit; *HR,* heart rate; *VS,* vital signs.

cephalhematoma, and subgaleal hemorrhage and are distinguished not only in clinical manifestations but also in pathophysiology (Box 26-4).[90] These three extracranial scalp injuries are included with neurologic birth injuries, not because they have associated neurologic problems, but because the family or health care providers often raise the question of possible neurologic involvement.

PHYSIOLOGY AND ETIOLOGY

Caput succedaneum is caused by trauma to the scalp, usually during a routine vertex vaginal delivery. The caput is the result of hemorrhagic edema superficial to the periosteum of the scalp. Therefore, spread of the edema is not restricted to suture lines and is soft and pitting because of its superficial location.[56,90]

Cephalhematoma is a subperiosteal collection of blood that is confined by the skull sutures. The incidence is 1% to 2% of all live births. The cause is nearly always mechanical trauma, and its occurrence is more common in primiparous women and in forceps or vacuum-assisted delivery. Males are generally more likely to be affected than females. It is associated with an underlying linear skull fracture in up to 25% of cases. The firm, tense collection of blood frequently increases in size after birth, but significant blood loss does not occur.[10,56,90]

Forces that compress and drag the head through the pelvic outlet are associated with *subgaleal hemorrhage.* Significant acute blood loss can occur with shock as the presenting symptom. Bleeding may continue after birth with enlargement of the accumulated blood and dissection of the blood along tissue planes into the neck. Such a hemorrhage carries the greatest potential for complications, but fortunately it is the least common form of birth injury to the scalp.[53,56,90]

DATA COLLECTION

With caput succedaneum, physical examination reveals soft, pitting edema that is diffuse and crosses suture lines. Laboratory tests are not needed.[56,90]

Cephalhematomas may occur anywhere but are most commonly found in the parietal area on one side. Because the location of the blood is subperiosteal, the blood is confined by suture lines. Symptoms are normally absent. A skull fracture underlying the cephalhematoma is present in 10% to 25% of affected infants. X-ray examination of the skull defines the fracture. Rare complications include infection, osteomyelitis, hyperbilirubinemia, meningitis, and late-onset anemia.[56,90]

Because the subgaleal collection of blood is under the aponeurosis (connective tissue connecting the occipital and frontal muscles) and superficial to the periosteum, subgaleal hemorrhage crosses suture lines. Extravasated blood progresses down to the nape of the neck from the scalp, may result in a protruding ear and is firm but fluctuant to palpation. Vital signs should be carefully monitored for symptoms of shock. Serial measurements of head circumference should be documented. Pallor, delayed capillary refill time, diminished tone, respiratory distress, elevated heart rate, or decreasing blood pressure should be observed for and treated promptly. Transfusion may be necessary. The hematocrit should be serially followed, and bilirubin levels should be determined during recovery.[56,90]

TREATMENT

Usually, no treatment is necessary for caput or cephalhematoma. In subgaleal hemorrhage, treatment of blood loss and shock may be necessary. During resolution, the breakdown of the blood may cause hyperbilirubinemia requiring treatment (see Chapter 21).[56,90]

PARENT TEACHING

Parents of an infant with a cephalhematoma should be instructed that the cephalhematoma may enlarge but that they should not be concerned unless localized changes occur, suggesting secondary infection (erythema, induration, or drainage). This lesion should not be drained and may be evident for 6 to 8 weeks. A small calcification may remain after reabsorption of hemorrhage. The hemorrhage can be significant enough to cause hyperbilirubinemia or (rarely) anemia. Outpatient evaluation of bilirubin levels and hematocrit may be needed in some cases.

Parents of an infant with caput succedaneum should understand that the swelling is outside of the cavity of the brain and will usually reabsorb within 48 hours.[56] Careful preparation of the parents for the acute side effects of subgaleal hemorrhage is important. Parents should be warned of the possibility of swelling and discoloration of the face, head, and neck. The purpose of serial hematocrit and bilirubin checks should be explained. Parents can expect 2 to 3 weeks for the swelling to resolve.[56]

Skull Fractures

Three forms of skull fracture should be identified and differentiated: linear fractures, depressed fractures, and occipital osteodiastasis.[56,90]

PHYSIOLOGY AND ETIOLOGY

Linear skull fracture (a nondepressed fracture) is the most common type of skull fracture. The result

of compression of the skull during delivery, a linear skull fracture most often has no associated injuries and causes no symptoms. Bleeding may be seen extracranially (common) or intracranially (rare). Intracranial bleeding causes symptoms referable to the bleeding rather than to the fracture itself.[56,90]

The typical depressed skull fracture is of the "ping-pong" type, an indentation without loss of bony continuity. When forceps are used during delivery, the direct cause of injury may result but is often without complications or sequelae. When neurologic signs are present, direct cerebral injury, intracranial bleeding, or free bone fragments should be suspected.[56,90]

Occipital osteodiastasis, a separation of the cartilaginous joint between the squamous and lateral portion of the occipital bone, occurs during traumatic breech deliveries. This injury results in a posterior fossa subdural hemorrhage that is associated with laceration of the cerebellum. Because of the increased morbidity to the neonate, the American College of Obstetricians and Gynecologists recommends cesarean delivery rather than planned vaginal birth for term breech singletons.[2] In 2002, 87% of full-term breech singletons were delivered by cesarean delivery, and thus occipital osteodiastasis is uncommon.[59]

DATA COLLECTION

A linear skull fracture usually produces no signs or symptoms unless intracranial bleeding has occurred. Skull x-ray films most frequently demonstrate a parietal fracture. A depressed skull fracture may be noted by presence of a visible depression or a palpable "ping-pong" fracture in the parietal or temporal area. No other signs and symptoms are present unless intracranial bleeding or focal irritation of the cortex causes them. Evaluation with a skull x-ray examination or CT scan is necessary to delineate the type of fracture and to identify complications.

TREATMENT

No treatment is necessary for a linear skull fracture. Treatment of a depressed skull fracture varies. If free bone fragments or clots are identified, neurosurgical intervention is necessary. More conservative approaches are indicated when no complications or neurologic symptoms are present. Noninvasive treatments such as vacuum extractors and breast pumps have been used with success to raise the depressed bone segment.[90]

COMPLICATIONS

With a linear skull fracture, the single complication to be aware of is a "growing" skull fracture. A dural tear may allow leptomeninges to extrude into the fracture site, setting up the possibility of a leptomeningeal cyst. As the cyst enlarges, the edges of the fracture may fail to fuse and even spread apart, giving the appearance of a "growing" fracture. Palpation and x-ray examination demonstrate the lesion. Surgical correction may be necessary to ensure healing and prevent further complications. With a depressed skull fracture, intracranial bleeding and direct cerebral injury with seizures or residual neurologic deficit are rare.

PARENT TEACHING

Parents should be instructed to have the fracture site monitored for several months to ensure that reunion of the bone has taken place. Patients will require no other aftercare unless neurosurgical intervention was necessary or complications developed.

Intracranial Birth Injuries

Three major forms of intracranial bleeding occur: epidural hematoma, subdural hemorrhage, and subarachnoid hemorrhage (Box 26-5). Added to these are cerebellar hemorrhages, cerebellar contusions, and cerebral contusions. Each has its own particular set of signs and symptoms, complications, and sequelae. necrosis are seen. Shearing forces may cause trauma and is covered separately in this chapter.

BOX 26-5

CRITICAL FINDINGS

INTRACRANIAL BIRTH INJURIES

1. Epidural hematoma
   a. *Occurrence:* Rare.
   b. *Location:* Bleeding occurs into the epidural space. Blood is located between the inner area of skull bone and the periosteum.
   c. *Pathophysiology:* Most (not all) with history of traumatic labor or delivery.
   d. *Clinical findings:*
      • Increased intracranial pressure (swollen fontanel).
      • Seizures may occur.
   e. *Associated problems:* Almost always accompanied by a linear skull fracture.
2. Subdural hemorrhage
   a. *Occurrence:* More common in term infants than in preterm.
   b. *Location:* Bleeding is produced from tear of cerebral vein or sinus, which is often accompanied by a tear in the dura. Exact location of the hematoma depends on the location of the bleeding source.[90]
      • Laceration of the tentorium
      • Laceration of the falx
      • Laceration of the superficial cerebral vein
      • Occipital osteodiastasis
   c. *Pathophysiology:*
      • Debate as to whether its presence indicates birth trauma. Volpe indicates that most cases result from trauma.[90]
      • Linked to maternal use of aspirin and maternal ingestion of phenobarbital.
   d. *Clinical findings:* Neurologically abnormal at birth, if massive bleed:
      • Seizures
      • Stupor or coma

   • Skew deviation of eyes
   • Pupil changes: unequal pupils, poorly responsive pupils, fixed and dilated pupils
   • Nuchal rigidity
   • Apnea and bradycardia
   • Signs of increased intracranial pressure
   e. *Associated problems:* Risk for herniation with lumbar puncture.
3. Subarachnoid hemorrhage
   a. *Occurrence:* Most common type of neonatal intracranial hemorrhage.
   b. *Location:* Blood is within the subarachnoid space but not because of extension from other areas. Small hemorrhages are more common than large ones. Source believed to be small vascular channels.[90]
   c. *Pathophysiology:*
      • Term: Usually caused by trauma
      • Preterm: Usually caused by hypoxia
   d. *Clinical findings:*
      • Most common: Minimal or no symptoms
      • Seizures (especially with term infants): "Well baby with seizures"
      • Apnea (especially with preterm infants)
      • For massive bleed (rare): Sudden and marked deterioration; death
   e. *Associated problems:*
      • Usually none for infants without significant trauma or hypoxia.
      • After major bleed:
        Hydrocephalus (most common sequela)
        Neurologic residual
        Death

PHYSIOLOGY AND ETIOLOGY

An *epidural hematoma* is pathophysiologically difficult to form in newborns resulting from a relatively thick dura. When present, it is almost always accompanied by a linear skull fracture across the middle meningeal artery.

Subdural hemorrhage is more common in term infants than in preterm infants, and occurs from trauma tearing veins and venous sinuses. Although some assume its presence represents birth trauma, several authors indicate that this is not necessarily the case.[56,90] Subdural hemorrhage has been linked with maternal use of aspirin and also to maternal ingestion of phenobarbital.[64] Four major pathologic entities are defined: (1) laceration of the tentorium, (2) laceration of the falx, (3) laceration of the superficial cerebral vein, and (4) occipital osteodiastasis. Tentorial laceration causes a posterior fossa clot with compression of the brainstem. The straight sinus, vein of Galen, lateral sinus, and infratentorial veins may be involved. Laceration of the falx is caused by rupture of the inferior sagittal sinus. The laceration usually occurs at the junction of the tentorium and the falx, and the clot appears in the longitudinal cerebral fissure over the corpus callosum. Laceration of superficial cerebral veins causes subdural bleeding over the convexity of the brain. Subarachnoid bleeding or contusion of the brain also may be present.[57,90]

A subarachnoid hemorrhage is the most common type of neonatal intracranial hemorrhage. In term infants, trauma is the most common cause, whereas in preterm infants, hypoxia is more often the cause. Small hemorrhages are more common than massive ones and usually result from venous bleeding. Underlying contusion may be present.[7,57,90]

Cerebral contusions are uncommon as an isolated event. Focal blunt trauma is necessary to produce a contusion. Pathologically, focal areas of hemorrhage and necrosis are seen. Shearing forces may cause slit-like tears in the white matter.

Cerebellar contusion and *intracerebellar hemorrhage* are uncommon events usually seen in association with occipital osteodiastasis and infratentorial subdural hemorrhage. These are catastrophic events and most often result in the death of the patient.

DATA COLLECTION

For epidural hemorrhage, the signs and symptoms may be diffuse (increased intracranial pressure with a bulging fontanel) and may include focal or lateralizing seizures, eye deviation, and hemiplegia syndromes. Laboratory tests should include x-ray examination to look for fractures and CT scan or MRI to identify bleeding.

Infants with subdural hemorrhage are often neurologically abnormal at birth. Tentorial lacerations and laceration of the falx tend to produce brainstem signs caused by pressure. These signs include skew deviation of the eyes, unequal pupils, apnea, or coma. Nuchal rigidity and opisthotonus are signs of progressive herniation. Signs and symptoms of subdural hemorrhage from laceration of the superficial cerebral veins are variable. Small clots may produce no identifiable dysfunction. Typical signs are those of focal or lateralized cerebral dysfunction, although increased intracranial pressure may occur. CT scans or cranial MRI including views of the posterior fossa should be obtained immediately when a subdural hemorrhage is suspected. Lumbar puncture is not used as a diagnostic tool because of the risk for herniation.[90]

With subarachnoid hemorrhage, underlying contusion may cause focal neurologic signs. Often no significant increase in intracranial pressure is found acutely. Irritability and a depressed level of consciousness may persist. Seizures are common in term infants, whereas apnea is common in preterm infants. Diagnosis generally is made with CT scan. If a lumbar puncture is performed, it is generally done for another reason (e.g., meningitis workup) and shows elevated red blood cells (RBCs) and protein.[7,57,90] For infants without serious injury from trauma or hypoxia, the prognosis is good.[90] Focal signs predominate in cerebral contusions.

TREATMENT

Surgical evacuation of epidural and subdural clots may be necessary as emergency procedures. Subdural taps may be useful in the symptomatic infant with subdural bleeding from laceration of superficial cerebral veins. In the presence of coagulation defects, prompt intervention may require platelets, vitamin K, or replacement therapy for deficient coagulation factors.[7,57,90] Many infants with intracranial bleeding may require treatment for seizures.[57,90]

COMPLICATIONS

The complications of epidural hemorrhage range from none to permanent neurologic deficits with or without seizures. Sequelae of subdural hemorrhage occur in 20% to 25% of affected infants. The most common sequelae are focal neurologic signs. Seizures and hydrocephalus are seen less often. Hydrocephalus is the major potential complication of subarachnoid hemorrhage, and directly alters outcome.[90]

PARENT TEACHING

Because long-term outcome is variable and may be abnormal even in infants who appear normal at discharge from the nursery, parent teaching must be individualized. Emphasize the need for appropriate follow-up and intervention. Referral to available support groups is usually beneficial.

Spinal Cord Injuries

PHYSIOLOGY AND ETIOLOGY

Injuries to the spinal cord (usually the cervical portion) are seen most often in complicated breech deliveries. Before cesarean deliveries were routinely performed for breech delivery, fatal attempts to deliver vaginally were often associated with intraspinal hemorrhage. Breech presentation in conjunction with a hyperextended head is the most dangerous situation and is worsened by fetal depression. Traction, rotation, and torsion cause mechanical strain on the vertebral column. Cephalic deliveries are not entirely safe because of the difference in mechanical forces; a different clinical picture is seen with a higher-level lesion.[36,90]

DATA COLLECTION

Clinical manifestations depend on the severity and location of the injury. Clinical syndromes include stillbirth or rapid neonatal death, respiratory failure, and spinal shock syndrome. High cervical cord injuries are more likely to cause stillbirths or rapid death of the neonate. Lower lesions cause an acute cord syndrome. Common signs of spinal shock include flaccid extremities (may involve just the lower extremities if the cervical cord is spared); a sensory level, diaphragmatic breathing, paralyzed abdominal movements, atonic anal sphincter, and distended bladder. Useful laboratory tests include MRI or CT scan of the spine and somatosensory-evoked potentials (i.e., the response of peripheral nerves to electrical stimulation) to help determine the extent and site of the lesion. The differential diagnosis includes dysraphism, neuromuscular disease, and cord tumors.[36,90]

COMPLICATIONS

After the acute phase, chronic lesions include cysts, vascular occlusions, adhesions, and necrosis of the spinal cord. Flaccid or spastic quadriplegia is expected. Some infants with spinal cord injuries are ventilator dependent, and bowel and bladder problems continue.

PARENT TEACHING

Parents should understand fully the implications of severe injury to the spinal cord. Recovery is frequently minimal to nonexistent. Continued specialized care may be necessary, including ventilator therapy. The overwhelming implications for the family cannot be emphasized strongly enough.

An individualized multidisciplinary team approach to discharge planning is vital to parental confidence and a timely discharge. The problems of both patient and family are complex and not limited to medical concerns. A successful discharge is unlikely unless family emotional, financial, and educational concerns are addressed early in the planning process. The timely assessment of needs and involvement of supportive agencies allow resolution of problems well before the projected discharge date. Such assistance should include early family referral to available federal programs for financial aid (e.g., Supplemental Security Income [SSI]) and assistance with patient transportation to their multiple outpatient follow-up appointments. Early assessment of equipment needs and home nursing requirements is also of primary importance and should include a determination of the availability of these resources in the community, parent acceptance of their use, and whether the home can accommodate them (i.e., adequate electrical system and space).

Plexus Injuries

PHYSIOLOGY AND ETIOLOGY

Plexus injuries occur more commonly than cord injuries and result from lateral traction on the shoulder[81] (vertex deliveries) or the head (breech deliveries).[90] Risk factors include large infant, fetal depression, breech delivery, and a variety of obstetric factors.[25,56,90] Any factor resulting in a difficult vaginal delivery of the baby can increase the risk for injury (e.g., prolonged second stage of labor, placenta previa).[25,85] A study of 35,796 infants (54 with brachial plexus injury) concluded that brachial plexus injury is not predictable before delivery.[24] Some authors note the preventability of some risk factors.[90] Estimates of the incidence of brachial plexus injuries range from 0.5 to 2 per 1000 live births.[90] Extremely mild cases often have undetectable findings and may remain unidentified.

Pathologic changes range from edema and hemorrhage of the nerve sheath to actual avulsion of the nerve root from the spinal cord. Of the reported cases of plexus injuries, 90% involve the cervical nerve 5 (C5) to C7 nerve roots and are classified as *Erb's palsy*.[36,90] In a small minority of cases, the C4 nerve root is also affected. The site of injury in Erb's palsy is Erb's point where C5 and C6 nerve roots join to form the upper trunk of the brachial plexus. The shoulder and upper arm are involved, and the biceps reflex is decreased. When C4 is involved, diaphragmatic dysfunction is present.

Total brachial plexus palsy occurs in 8% to 9% of the cases. Plexus involvement is diffuse (cervical 5 [C5] to thoracic nerve 1 [T1] and occasionally C4). The upper and lower arm and hand are involved. Biceps and triceps reflexes are decreased.[36,90] When T1 is involved, the sympathetic fibers become affected with an ipsilateral *Horner syndrome* (ptosis, anhidrosis, and miosis) and possible delay in pigmentation of the iris.

Klumpke's palsy rarely occurs in the newborn period and involves only the distal upper extremity (lower arm and hand), whereas the muscles in the proximal extremity are normal. The lower part of the plexus, C8 to T1, is involved. Triceps reflex is decreased. When both distal and proximal weakness occur, it should be classified as total plexus palsy.[25,90]

DATA COLLECTION

Signs of brachial plexus palsies vary somewhat, most often because of the overlap of pure clinical syndromes. Shoulder and arm findings are characteristic of a true Erb's palsy. Involvement of the hand and fingers is seen in total forms or Klumpke's palsy. Table 26-3 lists the specific spinal cord levels involved, as well as their various functions that might be assessed.

Evaluation of diaphragmatic function by x-ray examination is at times necessary. Spinal cord MRI may be necessary to identify nerve root avulsion, which generally should be suspected when recovery does not occur. Electromyography often shows abnormalities early in the course of the injury, suggesting that the process actually may have begun in

T A B L E 26-3	BRACHIAL PLEXUS EXAMINATION: DISTINGUISHING FEATURES
PART EXAMINED	**SPINAL LEVEL**
Diaphragm movement (downward)	C4 (C3-5)
Deltoid muscle	C5
Spinatus muscle	C5
Biceps muscle	C5-6
Brachioradialis muscle	C5-6
Supinator of arm	C5-6
Biceps tendon reflex	C5-6
Wrist extensors	C6-7
Long extensor of the digits	C6-7
Triceps tendon reflex	C6-7
Wrist flexor	C7-8, T1
Finger flexors	C7-8, T1
Dilator of iris (sympathetic chain, Horner syndrome)	T1
Eyelid elevator (full elevation) (same as above condition)	T1
Moro reflex (shoulder abduction)	C5
Moro reflex (hand motion)	C8-T1
Palmar grasp	C8-T1

C, Cervical; T, thoracic.

the last weeks of pregnancy rather than at the time of delivery.[90]

TREATMENT

Treatment includes passive range-of-motion exercises followed by a gradual increase of activity to the affected limb. Initially, treatment may include immobilization for 1 to 5 days, followed by gentle passive range-of-motion exercises to prevent contractures. Finger and wrist splints also may be necessary.[90] For infants failing to achieve sufficient functional recovery by 3 months of age, referral to a clinic specializing in brachial plexus injury should be considered. Rarely, nerve graft surgery of the injured nerve root is necessary.[25,90]

COMPLICATIONS

Associated trauma may occur and should be carefully investigated. Common associated injuries include clavicle fracture, shoulder dislocation, cord injury, facial nerve injury, and humeral fracture. Full recovery of plexus function was seen in 88% to 92% of cases in the first year of life during the National Collaborative Perinatal Study.[48]

PARENT TEACHING

Parents should be taught passive range-of-motion exercises to encourage the infant's mobility and prevent contractures. Instructions should begin before discharge from the hospital. Usually a neonatal nurse or occupational or physical therapist gives the instructions.

Parents may equate the presence of a brachial plexus injury with poor obstetric care. This is often not the case. The awareness of early changes on electromyography should be used to help families understand that the factors causing injury to the plexus begin before the onset of labor.

Cranial and Peripheral Nerve Injuries

Median nerve injuries usually are postnatal and result from brachial and radial artery punctures. Sciatic nerve injury may be a result of inferior gluteal artery spasm (umbilical artery line drug instillation). Recovery is variable.

Median nerve palsy is manifested by decreased pincer grasp, decreased thumb strength, and the continuous fixed position of the fourth finger. *Radial nerve damage* usually is seen in conjunction with a humeral fracture. Prolonged labor is normally present. Congenital amniotic bands may also be causative. Recovery takes place over weeks to months. Radial nerve palsy is manifested by wrist drop (decreased finger and wrist extension) and normal grasp.

Laryngeal nerve palsy may be seen in conjunction with facial or diaphragmatic paralysis. If the paralysis is unilateral, a hoarse cry may be heard. Bilateral involvement causes breathing to be difficult and the vocal cords to remain closed in the midline. In these cases, it is essential to rule out intrinsic brainstem disease. Often the presence of other brainstem related abnormalities such as oculomotor problems, apnea, or facial palsy helps clarify this. Both brainstem auditory and somatosensory evoked potentials may help rule out brainstem involvement.

Laryngeal nerve palsy is manifested by difficulty in swallowing (superior branch), difficulty in breathing (bilateral), and difficulty in vocalizing (recurrent branch). Also, the head is held high

and fixed laterally with slight rotation. Severe cases may require tracheotomy and assisted feedings by gavage or gastrostomy tube.[90]

Diaphragmatic paralysis is most often seen in association with plexus injuries (80% to 90% have an associated plexus injury) and has the same etiology. Some series involving unilateral paralysis have a mortality rate of 10% to 20%. Most patients recover fully in 6 to 12 months. Although fewer than 10% of patients have bilateral diaphragmatic paralysis, the mortality rate for these patients is almost 50%. Treatment has consisted of using rocking beds, electric pacing of the diaphragm, continuous positive airway pressure (CPAP), respirators, or plication. Because diaphragmatic paralysis may occur in other conditions such as a myotonic dystrophy, attention to the differential diagnosis is important, particularly when an associated brachial plexus problem is not present.[90]

Diaphragmatic paralysis is demonstrated by respiratory difficulty in the first few hours of life. X-ray film shows elevation of the hemidiaphragm with paradoxic movement that may disappear on positive end-expiratory pressure (PEEP) or CPAP.[36,90]

Facial palsy may be part of intrinsic brainstem disease (see previous discussion of laryngeal nerve palsy), prenatal compression, trauma, malformation of the nerve itself, or other conditions such as Möbius syndrome or myotonic dystrophy. When it is traumatic in origin, facial palsy is thought to be caused by the position of the face on the sacral promontory at the exit of the nerve from the stylomastoid foramen.[90] Normally, both the upper (temporofacial) and lower (cervicofacial) branches are involved. Facial palsy is seen on the left side in 75% of cases. Features include a widened palpebral fissure, flat nasolabial fold, and decreased facial expression. Most infants completely recover within 3 weeks, although some infants continue to have deficits months later.[90] Known complications (from lack of total resolution) include contractures and synkinesis. Cosmetic surgical procedures occasionally are necessary but often are delayed for years.

PARENT TEACHING

Infants with facial palsy may require the use of artificial tears if unable to completely close the eye on the involved side. Occasionally it may be necessary to tape the eye to prevent injury to the cornea. Parents also should be taught to expect some drooling of formula from the corner of the mouth during breast or bottle feedings.

Most infants with laryngeal nerve palsy recover in the first 6 to 12 months of life. Symptoms initially require supplemental parent education and support. An infant's risk for aspiration necessitates careful feeding and appropriate response if choking occurs. Additional education for gavage feedings, a tracheotomy, or an apnea monitor may be necessary for the parents of a few infants. The teaching requirements for the infant with diaphragmatic paralysis must also be tailored to meet the individual needs and circumstances of the infant and family.

HYPOTONIA

Hypotonia is a common presenting symptom in the newborn. It is important to distinguish between hypotonia and muscle weakness. The majority of infants with hypotonia have a cause centered in the central nervous system. In these cases, hypotonia is more prominent than weakness. Hypotonia might be due to a congenital encephalopathy (hypoxic-ischemic encephalopathy being the most common), intracranial hemorrhage, a congenital brain malformation, or metabolic disorder. Causes of motor weakness may involve cranial nerve motor nuclei (as in Mobius syndrome), anterior horn cells (as in spinal muscular atrophy), spinal cord injury (causing severe weakness), peripheral nerves, the neuromuscular junction (neonatal myasthenia gravis), or muscle itself (myotonic dystrophy, congenital myopathy, muscular dystrophy).[90]

Data Collection

A cranial MRI is performed to evaluate for a central nervous system cause for hypotonia. If this is normal, investigation then turns to other causes. A creatine kinase (CK) level that is quite elevated may determine a dystrophic process, with breakdown in muscle fibers. The CK is modestly elevated for a few days after vaginal birth. An aldolase level rarely adds additional information and is not necessary. A lumbar puncture can be performed to look for elevated cerebrospinal fluid protein seen in demyelinating syndromes. Genetic testing for myotonic dystrophy and spinal muscular atrophy are readily available and should be performed if clinically indicated. When myotonic dystrophy

is suspected, both parents should be examined for myotonia, which can be helpful in diagnosing their infant with the same disorder. An electromyogram (EMG) and nerve conduction study (NCS) can be performed to help determine whether weakness is due to a nerve or muscle problem. EMGs are difficult in newborns and require a skilled examiner. A muscle biopsy can be performed if absolutely necessary, although many times it is more helpful when the infant is older. Muscle is typically sampled from the quadriceps muscle.[90]

Parent Teaching

Parent teaching will depend on the infant's diagnosis. In general, infants who have a neuromuscular disorder have respiratory and feeding issues. These infants may need ventilatory assistance and nasogastric or gastrostomy tube feedings. Physical and occupational therapy should be involved to help with positioning and recommending equipment for the family at home. In the case of a genetic disorder such as myotonic dystrophy or spinal muscular atrophy, genetic counseling should be provided to the family.

NEONATAL SEIZURES

Seizures are among the most frequent clinical signs, though occasionally the only sign, of central nervous system dysfunction in neonates. The occurrence of neonatal seizures should prompt an immediate search for the underlying etiology as well as an overall assessment of associated medical disorders. Depending on the clinical history, suspected etiology, and seizure frequency, use of antiepileptic medications may be indicated in addition to correcting any underlying metabolic disturbances.

The overall incidence of neonatal seizures is difficult to ascertain, in part because the incidence varies in relation to gestational age and birth weight. For infants weighing less than 1500 g, the seizure frequency is 57.5 per 1000, whereas it is 2.8 per 1000 for infants weighing 2500 to 3999 g.[51] Seizures occur more frequently during the neonatal period than at any other period of life.[19,20,33,52]

Neonates with seizures are at increased risk of having or developing other neurologic deficits, developmental impairments, and an increased risk of death.[37,98] Early and aggressive seizure management improves the infant's neurologic and developmental outcome.[90] The occurrence of neonatal seizures may also predispose the child to later cognitive and behavioral complications as well as epilepsy.[19,20,52]

Recognition and treatment of neonatal seizures and their underlying etiology are critical to improving the child's short and long-term outcomes. Seizures are commonly related to significant general medical disorders, which may also require specific treatment. Untreated neonatal seizures may interfere with supportive therapies such as assisted ventilation and nutrition. Experimental data suggest that repetitive or prolonged seizures may cause brain injury and contribute to an adverse clinical outcome.[19,20,38,62,82]

Epileptic seizures are the result of excessive synchronous electrical discharges from neurons within the CNS.[74] Neonatal seizures should be viewed not as a specific disease entity, but as a symptom. Seizures may be associated with many disorders that directly or indirectly affect the brain by altering its electro-chemical stability. Intracranial processes that may result in neonatal seizures include meningitis, intracranial hemorrhage (subdural, intraventricular, primary subarachnoid), ischemic cerebral infarction (stroke), encephalitis, and congenital cerebral neoplasms.

Seizures also occur secondary to systemic or metabolic disturbances including hypoglycemia, hypoxia-ischemia, hypocalcemia, hypomagnesemia, hyponatremia, drug intoxications, drug withdrawal, and inborn errors of metabolism. A link between intrapartum fever and unexplained seizure activity in term infants also has been reported in the literature.[95] Presence of fever increased the likelihood of seizure activity by four times normal even when the presence of an infection was not confirmed.[54]

Clinically, seizures are characterized by a paroxysmal alteration in neurologic functions, including behavioral, motor, or autonomic functions. These clinical signs may or may not be accompanied by electrical abnormalities detectable by scalp EEG recordings. Clinical presentation of seizures in neonates differs considerably from the well-organized seizure activity seen in older children and adults.[26,90] Incomplete neurophysiologic development of the premature infant results in even less organized seizure activity than that seen in the term infant.

Etiology and Data Collection

Neonatal seizures may be caused by a variety of acute and chronic disorders of the brain. Table 26-4 lists the general groups of causes of neonatal seizures. A detailed history of perinatal problems often narrows the differential diagnosis to one or two likely causes. Acute, reversible, or treatable metabolic disorders that can cause seizures need to be investigated quickly. Blood glucose should be checked immediately in the neonatal intensive care unit with a glucometer, and also in the laboratory, because hypoglycemia is a dangerous but treatable cause of seizures (Table 26-5).

Lumbar puncture should be done to diagnose or exclude bacterial meningitis, another dangerous but treatable cause of seizures. Sepsis should never be overlooked as a potential cause of seizures because the responsible infectious agent may directly invade the CNS. Systemic infections may also cause seizures through complications such as shock, coagulopathy, impaired oxygenation, and multisystem organ failure. When the cerebrospinal fluid (CSF) is examined, not only should the changes associated with infection be identified but also evidence of bleeding (RBCs) or cell destruction (protein) may be detected.

Neuroimaging studies are performed to detect underlying structural lesions. If the infant's clinical status allows safe transport to radiology, MRI or CT imaging can be done. If the infant cannot be transported safely, cranial ultrasound (CUS) imaging can be done at the bedside. CUS can detect IVH, periventricular white matter injury, hydrocephalus, and other structural lesions related to seizures.

The infant's clinical history may be the best tool available to the clinician for identifying the etiology. Physical examination may provide further clues to the diagnosis. Blood should be drawn for assessment of arterial blood gases, electrolytes, glucose, calcium, and magnesium.

Appropriate cultures must be obtained of blood, urine, pharyngeal and tracheal aspirates, and CSF. The CSF should be examined for red and white cells, protein concentration, glucose concentration, and Gram stain. In addition, viral cultures and polymerase chain reaction tests may be ordered.

In addition to its initial contribution to identifying the etiology of seizures, cranial ultrasound imaging can be used to monitor the evolution of IVH and hydrocephalus. With ultrasound imaging the infant is not exposed to radiation, and there are

TABLE 26-4	**COMMON CAUSES OF NEONATAL SEIZURES**
CLASSIFICATION	CAUSES
Acute metabolic conditions (assess blood gases, pH, HCO_3^-, Na, K, Ca, Mg, glucose, blood urea nitrogen)	Hypocalcemia Hypoglycemia, hyperglycemia Hypomagnesemia Pyridoxine dependency or deficiency Hyponatremia, hypernatremia
Inherited metabolic conditions (acidosis is common; assess blood amino acids, blood lactate and pyruvate, blood ammonia $[NH_3]$ galactose, and urine amino and organic acids)	Maple syrup urine disease Nonketotic hyperglycemia Hyperprolinemia Hyperglycinemia Galactosemia Urea cycle abnormalities Organic acidemias
Infections (12% of cases; assess CSF; culture blood, CSF; polymerase chain reaction assay in CSF; imaging)	Viral encephalitis, herpes or enterovirus infection Congenital infections Bacterial meningitis Sepsis Brain abscess Septic venous thrombosis
Intracranial hemorrhage (15% of cases; assess imaging; CSF examination)	Subdural hematoma Cerebral contusion Subarachnoid hemorrhage Epidural hemorrhage Intraventricular hemorrhage (premature)
Hypoxic ischemia (0-3 days) most common (60%) Cerebral infarction Congenital malformations Neonatal drug withdrawal (see Chapter 11) (e.g., opiates) Local anesthetic intoxication Kernicterus Specific nongenetic syndromes Benign familial neonatal seizures Idiopathic (in only 10%, no cause is found)	

CSF, Cerebrospinal fluid.

no known immediate or long-term risks or complications. CUS may be repeated as often as needed and has the advantage of being performed at the infant's bedside.

Clinical Seizure Types

The use of continuous EEG video recordings and continuous amplitude-integrated EEG recordings allows for a more accurate diagnosis of subtle behaviors, apneic and bradycardic spells, and other jerks and movements commonly seen in preterm newborns and suspected of being epileptic seizure activity.[13,19,20] Some of these events may be confirmed as epileptic seizures, whereas others will not be associated with an EEG electrical seizure pattern.

Seizures result from abnormal, excessive electrical discharge or depolarization of cortical neurons. They are manifestations of an underlying disorder rather than being an isolated disorder. As a paroxysmal alteration of neurologic function, these behavioral, motor, or autonomic clinical phenomena are associated with EEG electrical seizure activity. In neonates, there are also paroxysmal, stereotyped clinical phenomena that are not consistently correlated with EEG electrical seizure activity, as determined by scalp recordings. An increasing body of evidence, however, indicates that epileptic activity can occur at subcortical levels, which is not detectable by surface, EEG recordings.[90] Table 26-6 lists the classification of clinical seizure types and usual EEG findings. Many neonatal, electrical seizures identified by EEG are not accompanied by any motor or behavioral clinical activity, a phenomenon referred to as subclinical seizure activity or electroclinical dissociation.

Focal clonic and multifocal clonic seizures are the most likely types of seizure activity to be associated with an electrocerebral, seizure pattern on EEG. Eye blinking, a type of clonic manifestation, or nystagmus may be seen as the only outward manifestation of a seizure. Focal clonic seizures are important manifestations of cerebral infarction and stroke in the neonate. Apnea accompanied by electrical seizure activity has been seen as an ictal manifestation, most commonly in full-term infants. Apneic episodes in the premature population, however, are most often not epileptic events and are not associated with epileptiform EEG patterns.

The lack of continuous EEG monitoring in most neonatal units makes accurate identification

TABLE 26–5	DRUG THERAPY FOR NEONATAL SEIZURES[90]

DRUG	DOSE	COMMENTS
Glucose	10% solution 2 ml/kg bolus IV if hypoglycemic. *Maintenance:* as high as 8 mg/kg/min IV (see Chapter 15).	Treat if hypoglycemic with glucose meter testing (e.g., Accu-Chek; One Touch II).
Phenobarbital (drug of choice for neonatal seizures)	*Loading:* 20 mg/kg IV given slowly over 10-15 min; additional 5 mg/kg can be given 1 hour after dose to maximum of 40 mg/kg total for refractory seizures.	*Therapeutic level:* 15-40 mcg/ml (obtain levels any time); respiratory depressant; incompatible with other drugs in solution.
	Maintenance: 3-4 mg/kg/24 hr in 2 divided doses beginning no earlier than 12 hours after last loading dose.	Maintain adequate oxygenation and ventilation.
Fosphenytoin (Cerebyx) preferred over phenytoin* (added if seizures not controlled by phenobarbital alone)	Fosphenytoin dose is expressed in PE; fosphenytoin 1 mg PE = phenytoin 1 mg. *Loading:* 15-20 mg PE/kg IM or IV† given slowly over minimum of 10 min. Flush IV with normal saline before and after.	*Fosphenytoin advantages:* high water solubility; pH value closer to neutral; faster, safe rate of administration; safe to give IM; absence of tissue injury with IV infusion; easy to prepare in IV solution. *Therapeutic level:* measure trough serum phenytoin (not fosphenytoin) 48 hr after IV loading dose; 10-20 mcg/ml desirable level.
	Maintenance: 4-8 mg PE/kg/24 hr IM or IV slow push (see above for dilution); infuse no faster than 1.5 mg/kg/min. Flush IV before/after with NS. Maintenance should be initiated 24 hr after loading dose. Term infants greater than 1 wk of age may need up to 8 mg PE/kg/dose every 8-12 hr.	Monitor blood pressure closely during infusion; can be given with lorazepam or phenobarbital at terminal injection site. Safety with newborns still not clearly established; use with caution in infants with hyperbilirubinemia.
Phenytoin used instead of Cerebyx to control seizures that are not controlled by phenobarbital alone	Loading: 15-20 mg/kg IV infusion over at least 30 min (no more rapidly than 0.5 mg/kg/min). Flush with NS before and after giving. **Never give IM.** **Never give in central lines.** *Maintenance:* 4-8 mg/kg/24 hr‡ IV slow push (no more rapidly than 0.5 mg/kg/min) or by mouth (PO). Flush with NS before and after. Absorption erratic with PO route. Term infants greater than 1 week of age may need up to 8 mg/kg/dose every 8-12 hr.	Phenytoin disadvantages: incompatible with glucose and all other drugs; cannot be given IM (crystallizes in the muscle); rapid administration can result in bradycardia, dysrhythmias, hypotension. The pH of IV solution is 12, which is irritating to veins. Extravasation may result in tissue necrosis. *Therapeutic level:* measure trough level 48 hr after loading dose. Serum level 6-15 mcg/ml initially and 10-20 mcg/ml after the first few weeks.
Pyridoxine (vitamin B$_6$) as indicated	50-100 mg IV push or IM.	Used to diagnose and treat seizures resulting from pyridoxine (vitamin B$_6$ deficiency). Monitor EEG while giving. Protect from light. Diagnostic when seizures cease within minutes and the EEG normalizes within minutes or hours.

TABLE 26-5	DRUG THERAPY FOR NEONATAL SEIZURES—cont'd	
DRUG	DOSE	COMMENTS
Lorazepam (Ativan) for seizures uncontrolled by phenobarbital and fosphenytoin (or phenytoin if used)	0.05-0.1 mg/kg IV slow push over several min.	Enters brain rapidly; onset of action in less than 5 min. Monitor for respiratory depression. Monitor IV site for phlebitis or extravasation. Safer to use than diazepam (Valium), which is contraindicated for use in the newborn.
ADDITIONAL THERAPY AS INDICATED:		
Calcium gluconate, 5% solution Magnesium sulfate, 50% solution IV antibiotics (bacterial infection; see Chapter 22) Acyclovir (herpes; see Chapter 22)		

EEG, Electroencephalogram; *IM,* intramuscularly; *IV,* intravenously; *mcg,* micrograms; *NS,* normal saline; *PE,* phenytoin equivalents.
*Appears to be preferred, although safety has not been clearly established.
†Must be diluted in NS or D$_5$W to a concentration of 1.5 to 25 mg PE/ml for IV use.
‡Volpe cites 3 to 4 mg/kg/24 hr IV in divided doses every 12 hr, starting 12 hr after loading dose.[90]

TABLE 26-6	CRITICAL FINDINGS	
	TRADITIONAL CATEGORIZATION OF NEONATAL SEIZURES[90]	
CLASSIFICATION/TYPES	CLINICAL MANIFESTATIONS	DEFINITION/DESCRIPTION
Clonic • Focal clonic • Multifocal clonic	• Rhythmic jerks (1-3/sec) • Rate slows during seizure • + EEG seizure activity	• Focal: well-localized to a body part • Multifocal: several body parts jerking simultaneously or in migrating order
Tonic • Focal tonic • Generalized tonic	• Characterized by posturing • Focal: + EEG seizure activity • Generalized: usually no EEG seizure activity	• Focal: continued posturing of limb or a posturing (asymmetric) of trunk or neck • Generalized: extension of lower limbs with either upper limb extension (looks like decerebrate posturing) or upper limb flexion (looks like decorticate posturing)
Myoclonic • Focal myoclonic • Generalized myoclonic	• Faster jerking than in clonic seizures • Flexor muscles (limbs) involved • Focal: usually no EEG seizure activity • Generalized: + EEG seizure activity	• Focal: flexor jerking of upper limbs • Generalized: bilateral jerking of upper extremities; sometimes lower limbs are involved; often single or irregular jerks
Subtle (more common in the premature infant)	• Abnormal behavioral, autonomic, or motor activities that do not result from the other three seizure classifications • + EEG seizure activity with only some of the seizure activities	• Ocular: nystagmus, horizontal or vertical deviation of eyes, staring episodes, eyelid flutter or blinking • Facial: repetitive sucking, mouth movements, tongue protrusion, chewing, drooling • Limb: bicycling, swimming movements, "boxing" or "hooking" motions, stepping • Apnea: only 2% result from seizures • Autonomic or vasomotor changes

EEG, Electroencephalogram.

TABLE 26-7	CRITICAL FINDINGS SEIZURES VERSUS JITTERINESS		
CLINICAL OBSERVATIONS		SEIZURE	JITTERINESS
Ocular abnormalities (eye deviations or staring)		Yes	No
Gentle restraint of the involved body part halts the activity		No	Yes
Activity is easily elicited with stimulation (e.g., voice, motions)		No	Yes
Dominant movement is a slower clonic jerking having both fast and slow elements		Yes	No
Tremor in which the amplitude and rate of the alternating movements are equal		No	Yes
Autonomic changes are present (e.g., apnea, tachycardia, elevated blood pressure, pupil changes, increased salivation)		Yes	No

of seizures difficult. The best EEG-clinical correlation can be made by obtaining an EEG during a period of the suspected seizure activity. As discussed previously, however, there is evidence that deep-seated epileptic discharges may be present but not detectable by scalp EEG recordings.

A commonly used classification of neonatal seizures is presented in Table 26-6. The classification of neonatal seizures is distinct from the International Classification of Seizures applicable to seizures in older children and adults. Seizures are more subtle and more difficult to recognize in neonates than in older infants and children. Further compounding the difficulty of diagnosis are conditions that mimic epileptic neonatal seizures, such as neonatal jitteriness (Table 26-7).

Episodes characterized as tonic and subtle are the most likely types to be seen in premature infants. Tonic episodes are quite commonly associated with IVH. Clonic and multifocal clonic seizures are more common in term infants. Neonatal seizures may result from metabolic causes, such as nonketotic hyperglycemia or urea cycle disorders, some of which require specific metabolic therapies to prevent clinical deterioration[39,72] (see Table 26-6). Generalized myoclonic seizures in preterm neonates are associated with high mortality and poor prognosis in survivors.[76]

Prevention

Many neonatal seizures can be successfully prevented through careful attention to possible metabolic changes expected on the basis of the infant's condition. Hypoglycemia, hypocalcemia,

hypomagnesemia, and often hypoxia can be anticipated and controlled. Those infants born with brain malformations or brain injuries or who develop neonatal infections, intracranial hemorrhages, or strokes can be observed carefully for the early occurrence of seizures and treated promptly.

Treatment

The initial treatment of neonatal seizures involves stopping seizure activity with a loading dose of an antiepileptic medication, preventing further seizures with maintenance doses of medication, minimizing side effects of seizure therapy, and correcting underlying treatable conditions.

The first goal is stopping repetitive or prolonged seizures. Frequently recurring and prolonged or persistent seizures may result in injurious metabolic changes in the brain and also lead to cardiorespiratory difficulty. Seizures are associated with increased energy consumption by neurons, which may interfere with cerebral perfusion and adequate oxygenation. Although the neonatal brain appears to be less sensitive to seizure-induced injury than the adult brain, repeated seizures may nevertheless be detrimental to the developing nervous system.[38]

The most commonly used drugs for control of neonatal seizures are phenobarbital and fosphenytoin (see Table 26-5), although other medications such as lorazepam, midazolam, topiramate, and levetiracetam are being evaluated and used with increasing frequency.[11,19-21] When the administration of a single drug fails to result in seizure control, a second or third antiepileptic medication is indicated. Both phenobarbital and fosphenytoin are given initially as an intravenous loading dose of 20 mg/kg, which produces a therapeutic blood concentration in most infants. Subsequent to the loading dose, maintenance doses of phenobarbital can be continued using doses typically between 3 and 5 mg/kg/day, orally or intravenously. Because the half-life of phenobarbital in neonates is 40 hours or more, monitoring blood levels regularly can be helpful in guiding dosing frequency and in avoiding dose-related, systemic side effects and neurotoxicity. If seizures are not controlled with phenobarbital alone, other medications should be considered. The duration of prophylactic antiepileptic therapy is based on the severity and frequency of seizures as well as the presence of other neurologic impairments. A common approach is to treat with antiepileptic medications for several weeks or months after the child is discharged from the neonatal nursery, and then reassess the need for continued therapy.[34]

The identification and correction of underlying treatable conditions will assist in seizure management. Empiric administration of glucose, calcium, and pyridoxine may be considered, particularly for frequently recurring seizures or seizures refractory to antiepileptic medications. For seizures that remain refractory to usual therapy, genetic testing may be considered to determine whether the infant has an identifiable gene mutation related to neonatal or early infantile seizures, such as mutations affecting sodium channels, potassium channels, or gamma-aminobutyric acid (GABA) receptors.[9,22,83] Knowing that such a mutation is present may assist in selecting antiepileptic drugs that will be most beneficial or in avoiding drugs that might worsen seizure activity.

Complications and Outcome

It is difficult to separate potential deleterious effects of seizures from those of the underlying cause. Some of the metabolic disorders, such as hypocalcemia, are relatively benign conditions that once corrected allow full recovery without complications. In contrast, seizures related to cerebral malformations, hypoxic-ischemic injury, stroke, IVH, or meningitis are likely to persist and evolve into epilepsy.[37] Those infants who have an abnormal neurologic examination or who have severely abnormal EEG patterns, such as burst-suppression

or diffuse very low voltage, are likely to have seizures that persist into later childhood and beyond.[76]

Parent Teaching

Parents need to know what seizures are and what may be the cause of seizures in their infant. Accurate information should address the specific concerns of each parent. Appropriate first aid measures should be discussed to ensure that the parents have a clear understanding of how their child is being treated in the nursery and how parents will need to manage seizures should they occur after the infant goes home. Parents need to know the significance of tests (e.g., EEG and brain imaging tests), the limitations of these tests and how future tests will be used to monitor the child's condition. Parents also need information about the different types of seizures that can occur during early infancy. While the child is still in the nursery, the parents need to be educated on how to recognize and document seizure activity (Box 26-6). Handouts written in a clear simple style are useful when parents are learning to care for an infant with seizures. Handouts should be available in a variety of languages to meet the needs of a diverse population.

While the infant is in the hospital, the parents should become involved in the daily care including administering medications. In the hospital, parents can be coached and encouraged by the nursing staff. During this time, the parents can also be informed about local and national parent support groups and organizations designed to assist and support families after their infant is discharged from the hospital.

HYPOXIC-ISCHEMIC ENCEPHALOPATHY

Pathophysiology

The combination of hypoxia and ischemia is a common cause of brain injury in both term and preterm neonates. *Hypoxemia* refers to low levels of oxygen in the blood and potentially in brain tissue. *Ischemia* refers to a reduction in cerebral perfusion. *Asphyxia* is impaired exchange of oxygen and carbon dioxide across the respiratory organ (placenta before birth, lungs after birth) resulting

BOX 26-6

PARENT TEACHING

SEIZURE DISORDER FAMILY TEACHING CHECKLIST

BAPTIST MEDICAL CENTER
WOLFSON CHILDREN'S HOSPITAL
JACKSONVILLE, FLORIDA

Wolfson Children's HOSPITAL at Baptist Medical Center

SEIZURE DISORDER FAMILY TEACHING CHECKLIST

GOAL/SKILL	PRESENTATION/ NURSE DEMONSTRATION DATE AND INITIAL	CARE GIVER/ PATIENT DEMONSTRATION DATE AND INITIAL	CARE GIVER/ PATIENT DEMONSTRATION DATE AND INITIAL	COMMENTS/ HANDOUTS DATE AND INITIAL
1. Verbalizes understanding of seizure pathophysiology.				Handouts given:
2. Describes signs that indicate a seizure.				
3. Lists important observations to make during a seizure.				"Seizure Recognition"
4. Describes care of a child during a seizure.				
5. Identifies child's a. medication, dosage and schedule b. side effects of anticonvulsants c. consequences of non-compliance d. correct administration of medication				Medication _____ Dosage _____ Schedule _____ Medication handout given _____
6. Verbalizes how to seek emergency assistance from home.				
7. Identifies resources for families with a child with a seizure disorder.				
VIDEOS FOR PARENTS (Date that care giver/ patient views)	_____ "How Medications Work" _____ "Understanding Seizure Disorders"			

Courtesy Wolfson Children's Hospital, Jacksonville, Fla, 1996.

in comorbidities, low levels of circulating oxygen, and high levels of carbon dioxide. When comparing hypoxemia and ischemia, ischemia is more devastating because there is impaired delivery of oxygen and glucose to cerebral tissue and impaired removal of lactate and other neurotoxic byproducts of cellular metabolism.[40]

Brain injury due to hypoxemia and ischemia occurs in two phases.[50,88,89,94] Tissue is first injured directly by the initial lack of oxygen and blood flow that leads to a decrease in high-energy phosphate compounds and acidosis. During the second phase, reperfusion injury occurs 8 to 16 hours after oxygenation and perfusion has been restored. This second period of injury relates to a secondary decrease in high-energy phosphate compounds. During this secondary phase, metabolic derangements develop that lead to further brain injury as a result of elevation in tissue glutamate levels, release of neurotoxic cytokines, inflammation, impairment of mitochondrial function, and generation of free radicals. The period between the primary phase of injury and the secondary phase is the *therapeutic window* for potential neuro-protective interventions.

Etiology

Impaired placental or pulmonary function (i.e., asphyxia) is a common, but rarely the only, cause of HIE. HIE occurs in approximately one to two neonates per 1000 live births with about one-third of these neonates demonstrating significant neurologic sequelae.[64] About 20% of cases are related to antepartum events, such as maternal hypertension, maternal diabetes, or intrauterine growth restriction. About 35% are related to intrapartum events, including placental abruption, cord prolapse, or traumatic delivery; and about 10% are related to postnatal cardiopulmonary failure. In approximately 35% of cases, there are combinations of antepartum and intrapartum difficulties.

Guidelines have been published by the American Academy of Pediatrics and the American College of Obstetrics and Gynecology regarding criteria needed to attribute neurologic injury to intrapartum HIE[1]:

1. Metabolic acidosis is severe with pH <7.0 and base deficit ≥12 mmol/L.
2. The neonate (34 weeks' gestation or later) should have displayed a significant, moderate to severe encephalopathy during the neonatal period.
3. For CP to be attributed, it should either be spastic quadriplegia or dyskinetic type.

Other potential causes of neonatal encephalopathy (meningitis, encephalitis, genetic conditions, or thrombophilic disorders) should have been excluded. In addition to these major criteria, the task force considered the following to be suggestive of timing to the intrapartum period: (1) a sentinel hypoxic event occurring immediately before or during labor; (2) a sudden and sustained fetal bradycardia or absence of fetal heart rate variability in the presence of persistent, late, or variable decelerations, usually after a hypoxic sentinel event when the pattern was previously normal; (3) Apgar scores of 0 to 3 at 5 minutes or more after birth; (4) multisystem involvement with an onset within 72 hours of birth; and (5) the presence of evidence of acute, nonfocal cerebral abnormality shown on an early imaging study.

Prevention

Preventing HIE requires the early anticipation, avoidance, and early treatment of those conditions (antepartum, intrapartum, or immediate postpartum) that lead to impaired oxygen delivery and blood flow to the brain. For example, the early detection and treatment of chorioamnionitis may reduce the risk of cerebral injury related to circulating cytokines. Postpartum cardiopulmonary support is essential to reducing the risk of CNS injury. Keeping blood glucose levels normal is important because both high and low levels may be deleterious in the setting of HIE.

Data Collection

HISTORY

The diagnosis of HIE depends in part on a detailed history of the antepartum, intrapartum, and postpartum events, as well as a thorough physical examination. Infants may have a history of intrauterine distress evidenced by abnormal fetal heart rate patterns or sudden cessation of movements. The infant may be depressed at birth or have low Apgar scores that persist beyond 5 or 10 minutes. Multiorgan damage may be evident, and there are signs of a significant encephalopathy.

SIGNS AND SYMPTOMS

The diagnosis of HIE may also be supported by physical findings indicative of encephalopathy[63] (Table 26-8). HIE is also suspected when seizures occur within the first 12 hours after birth.

LABORATORY DATA

Laboratory information often reflects multisystem dysfunction including altered electrolyte concentrations, elevated hepatocellular enzymes, altered liver function tests, abnormal renal function tests, and abnormal coagulation studies. Blood gases may provide evidence of hypoxemia, hypercarbia, and either metabolic or respiratory acidosis, or both. The ECG may be indicative of hypoxic-ischemic cardiac injury. CSF studies may provide evidence of infection or subarachnoid hemorrhage. Chest x-ray studies may show evidence of pulmonary dysfunction and immaturity. An EEG will assist in the diagnosis of seizures and the assessment of the neonatal encephalopathy.[19,20,78,79] Burst-suppression patterns, isoelectric patterns, and very low EEG amplitude all indicate severe CNS dysfunction and are associated with poor prognosis. MRI provides valuable information regarding the nature, distribution, and extent of CNS injury and regarding specific patterns of injury that correlate highly with hypoxic-ischemic injury.[91] MRI scan can also provide valuable sequential monitoring of specific injuries and their evolution.[18]

Treatment

Treatment is focused largely on general supportive care including the following: support of ventilation; maintenance of normal blood pressure; temperature regulation; maintenance of normal glucose, calcium, and electrolyte levels; and control of seizures.

In addition to general supportive measures, the use of moderate hypothermia has become standard treatment during the past few years.* *Head cooling* or *whole-body cooling* techniques have been used (Box 26-7). Inducing modest hypothermia provides neuroprotection of injured CNS cells and also provides a method to control cerebral edema. The use of hypothermia has been shown to improve outcome of neonates with HIE, including lowering the rate of

---

*References 4, 13, 35, 41, 80, 81.

T A B L E 26-8	CRITICAL FINDINGS STAGES OF HYPOXIC-ISCHEMIC ENCEPHALOPATHY AND NEUROLOGIC ASSESSMENT[63,78,91]	

STAGE	NEUROLOGIC ASSESSMENT
Stage I: Mild encephalopathy	Hyperalert, with normal tone and activity, exaggerated response to stimulation, reactive pupils, no seizure activity
Stage II: Moderate encephalopathy	Hypotonic, weak suck, constricted but reactive pupils; periodic breathing or apnea Development of seizure activity or lethargy indicates deteriorated status
Stage III: Severe encephalopathy	Stupor or coma, absent reflexes, pupils nonreactive, no spontaneous activity, requires mechanical ventilation

neurodevelopmental disability. Complications of cooling procedures include disorders of cardiac rate and rhythm, hypotension, thrombocytopenia, coagulopathy, renal dysfunction, and subcutaneous fat necrosis. Procedural details of these cooling methods are beyond the scope of this chapter. Other neuroprotective strategies being investigated include the use of free-radical scavengers, antiinflammatory agents, neurotrophic factors, antagonists of excitotoxic amino acids, and implantation of stem cells.[31,43,64]

Complications

Neonates who suffer HIE have an increased mortality rate, with up to 20% to 50% dying in the neonatal period. Long-term neurologic complications include epilepsy, hyperactivity, spasticity, movement disorders, dystonia, ataxia, hearing loss, visual loss, and intellectual and cognitive impairments.[64,69]

INTRAVENTRICULAR HEMORRHAGE

IVH is a major problem in preterm infants with a large percentage of these infants developing neurodevelopmental complications. With recent

BOX 26-7	CRITERIA FOR NEONATAL COOLING FOR HIE

Screening Inclusion Criteria

- Postmenstrual age ≥36 weeks
- Admitted ≤6 hours of age with a diagnosis of encephalopathy
- pH ≤7 or base deficit >16 mmol/L on cord blood or blood gas within first hour of life (for head cooling)
- pH 7.01-7.15 and base deficit 10-15.9 mmol/L in the first hour of life (for whole body cooling)
- If no blood gas available in the first hour, there also must be:
  - Evidence of an acute perinatal event, **or**
  - 10-minute Apgar score <5 **or**
  - Assisted ventilation (PPV or CPAP) initiated at birth and continued for a minimum of 10 minutes

Inclusion Criteria

- Seizure activity present
- Diagnosis of moderate or severe encephalopathy, which includes any one of the following:
  - Lethargy
  - Decreased tone (may have normal peripheral tone but have central hypotonia), abnormal tendon reflexes, myoclonus, weak suck, abnormal Moro reflex
  - Any evidence of seizures
  - Abnormal breathing
  - Moderate to severe EEG amplitude reduction (lower margin <5 microvolts and/or upper margin <10 microvolts) on a 20-minute aEEG or evidence of seizures

Exclusion Criteria

- >6 hours of age
- Severe intrauterine growth restriction (<1.8 kg)
- Major congenital anomaly
- Head trauma resulting in severe intracranial hemorrhage (head cooling)
- Prophylactic high-dose anticonvulsants (head cooling)
- Parents do not grant consent
- Inability to initiate cooling by 6 hours of age

Data from Gluckman PD, Wyatt JS, Azzopardi D, et al: Selective head cooling with mild systemic hypothermia after neonatal encephalopathy: multicenter randomized trial, *Lancet* 365:663, 2005; Higgins RD, Tonse NKR, Perlman J, et al: Hypothermia and perinatal asphyxia: executive summary of the National Institute of Child Health and Human Development workshop, *J Pediatr* 148:2, 170, 2006; and Shankaran S, Laptook AR, Ehrenkranz RA, et al: Whole-body hypothermia for neonates with hypoxic-ischemic encephalopathy, *N Engl J Med* 353:1574, 2005.

aEEG, Amplitude-integrated electroencephalogram; *CPAP,* continuous positive airway pressure; *EEG,* electroencephalogram; *HIE,* hypoxic-ischemic encephalopathy; *PPV,* positive-pressure ventilation.

medical advances and the increased survival of premature infants, IVH continues to be a significant issue for neonates.[8] IVH is found in 20% to 25% of preterm infants with incidence higher in those with very low birth weight.[8,60] IVH mainly occurs in infants less than 32 weeks' gestation with the incidence increasing with decreasing gestational age.[60] The incidence of IVH in term infants is approximately 3.5%, making IVH both an uncommon and unanticipated diagnosis in this group.

Physiology

Although the bleeding is regularly spoken of as *intraventricular* and *intracranial hemorrhage,* these terms do not accurately reflect its causes. Highly vascularized areas, which have relatively fragile and poorly supported blood vessels, are the source of bleeding. In premature infants, the *germinal matrix,* in the subependymal area adjacent to the caudate nucleus, is the primary site of bleeding[6,90] (Figure 26-2).

The extent of bleeding generally predicts the likelihood of complications and sequelae. Bleeding may be confined to the germinal matrix or the choroid plexus, or it may enter the ventricular system. When filled under pressure, the ventricular system may dilate. Blood may also extravasate out into the brain parenchyma.

There are several classification schemes to assess the degree of bleeding or the amount of blood present. Volpe listed three grades of germinal matrix IVH using ultrasound scanning to identify the presence and extent of blood in the germinal matrix and lateral ventricles (Table 26-9). A "separate notation" is made for the existence of "periventricular hemorrhage infarction or of other parenchymal lesions." He clarified the use of this separate notation by noting that these abnormalities are not usually the result of simple "extension" of matrix or IVH hemorrhage into "normal brain parenchyma."[90]

An older classification system grades germinal matrix hemorrhages based on CT scans (Figure 26-3) is not used as frequently today. Because both grading systems are still cited in the literature, both are included here.

0—No bleeding
I—Germinal matrix only
II—Germinal matrix with blood in the ventricles

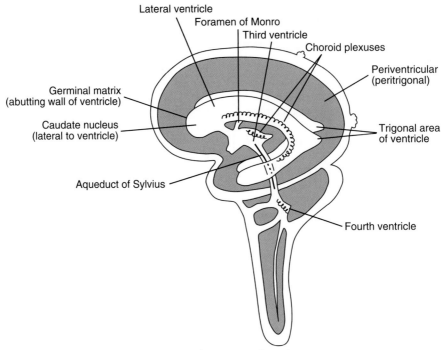

FIGURE 26-2 Central nervous system/ventricular system.

T A B L E 26-9	GRADING OF SEVERITY OF GERMINAL MATRIX—INTRAVENTRICULAR HEMORRHAGE BY ULTRASOUND SCAN
SEVERITY	**DESCRIPTION**
Grade I	Germinal matrix hemorrhage with no or minimal intraventricular hemorrhage (10% of ventricular area on parasagittal view)
Grade II	Intraventricular hemorrhage (10%-50% of ventricular area on parasagittal view)
Grade III	Intraventricular hemorrhage (>50% of ventricular area on parasagittal view; usually distends lateral ventricle)
Separate notation	Periventricular echodensity (location and extent)

From Volpe JJ: *Neurology of the newborn*, ed 5, Philadelphia, 2008, Saunders.

III—Germinal matrix with blood in the ventricles and hydrocephalus (ventricular dilation)

IV—Intraventricular and parenchymal bleeding (other than germinal matrix)

Etiology

The etiologic factors identified in infants who have experienced IVH are multiple and can be divided into prenatal, neonatal, and postnatal factors. These include asphyxia, severe respiratory distress, pneumothorax, hypoglycemia, shock, acidosis, blood transfusions, seizures, and rapid volume expansion (Box 26-8). What appears to be the common factor underlying the pathologic condition is a fluctuation/alteration in cerebral blood flow that causes the numerous and thin-walled blood vessels in the germinal matrix to bleed.[8,60,90] Recently genetic factors have been implicated in development of IVH. Mutations of genes that can predispose to thrombophilia and collagen formation have been found to be

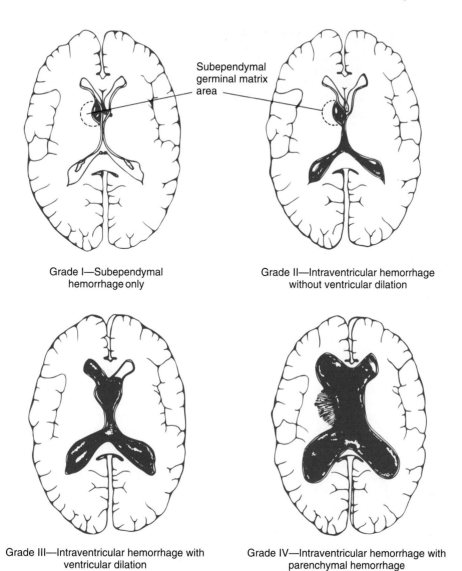

Grade I—Subependymal
hemorrhage only

Grade II—Intraventricular hemorrhage
without ventricular dilation

Grade III—Intraventricular hemorrhage with
ventricular dilation

Grade IV—Intraventricular hemorrhage with
parenchymal hemorrhage

FIGURE 26-3 Periventricular-intraventricular hemorrhage, grades I to IV. (From Rozmus C: Periventricular-intraventricular hemorrhage in the newborn, *Matern Child Nurs* 17:79, 1992.)

involved in IVH.[6,8,60] Intraventricular bleeding tends to occur in the first few hours or days of life.

Profound physiologic changes normally seen after birth coupled with multiple problems (primarily cardiorespiratory) typically experienced by the premature infant make intraventricular bleeding common. The degree to which the aggressive management of premature newborns has a role in the development of bleeding cannot be accurately assessed. Generally sicker infants both require more intervention and have a greater likelihood of bleeding.

Data Collection

HISTORY

Because premature infants, particularly those weighing less than 1500 g, tend to have multiple problems, it is not surprising that the clinical presentation of IVH may range from subtle (or even undetectable) to catastrophic.[6]

BOX
26-8

CRITICAL FINDINGS

FACTORS THAT PREDISPOSE THE PREMATURE INFANT TO INTRAVENTRICULAR HEMORRHAGE

Prematurity
- Birth weight <1500 g
- Less than 34 weeks' gestation

Asphyxia (see Chapters 4 and 8)
- Before, during, after birth

Respiratory (see Chapters 8 and 23)
- Idiopathic respiratory distress syndrome
- Hypoxia
- Positive-pressure ventilation
- Pneumothorax
- Apnea

Cardiovascular (see Chapter 4)
- Rapid volume expansion
- Elevated venous pressure
- Elevated or lowered arterial pressure (shock, transfusions)

Hematologic (see Chapter 20)
- Hyperosmolarity
- Coagulation disorders
- Hyperviscosity

Metabolic (see Chapters 8, 14, and 15)
- Hypoglycemia/hyperglycemia
- Hypernatremia/hyponatremia
- Metabolic acidosis
- Rapid pH shifts

Miscellaneous
- Hypothermia (see Chapter 6)
- Acetylsalicylic acid ingestion by mother
- Neonatal pain (see Chapter 12)
- Neonatal environmental stressors (see Chapter 13)

Modified from Gardner S, Hagedorn M: Physiologic sequelae of prematurity: the nurse practitioner's role. VIII. Neurologic conditions, *J Pediatr Nurs* 6:265, 1992.

SIGNS AND SYMPTOMS

Common signs of germinal matrix hemorrhage include apnea, hypotension, drop in hematocrit, seizures, flaccidity, areflexia, full fontanel, tonic posturing, and oculomotor disturbances.[8]

LABORATORY DATA

When intracranial bleeding is suspected, appropriate studies of intracranial structures should be performed as soon as possible. For IVH, ultrasonography is the study of choice.[90] The American Academy of Neurology practice parameter recommends screening of all neonates less than 30 weeks of gestation. The first ultrasound should be done between 7 and 14 days looking for IVH and the second ultrasound at 36 to 40 weeks' postmenstrual age to look for CNS lesion.[60] Additional follow-up imaging using MRI is indicated because MRI is better at detecting white matter changes, cysts, and bleeding lesions.[60]

Prevention

Strategies to prevent IVH have focused on both prenatal and postnatal interventions. Prenatal interventions such as preventing preterm delivery, maternal transport to a regional neonatal center, and prenatal glucocorticoids have been shown to be helpful in prevention of IVH.[8] Other pharmacologic agents studied including vitamin K, phenobarbital, and magnesium sulfate have unproven benefit.[6,8]

Postnatal pharmacologic treatment of IVH shows varying success in the literature. Agents studied include phenobarbital, Pavulon, vitamin E, ethamsylate, indomethacin, ibuprofen, and recombinant factor VIIa.[6,8,60] None of these have good data to support routine use. Postnatal prophylactic use of phenobarbital in preterm infants to prevent IVH has been one of the most widely studied therapies. However, because phenobarbital results in a greater requirement for mechanical ventilation, it is not recommended for use in postnatal prophylactic prevention of IVH.[6,8,60,90]

Treatment

The primary treatment of IVH is supportive care. Ventilatory support, maintenance of oxygenation, regulation of acid–base balance, suppression of seizures, and treatment of any attendant coagulopathy are all extremely important in reducing mortality and morbidity.[8] However, the role that successful management has in the amelioration or prevention of complications is unclear.

Complications

The complications from IVH relate to the underlying causes and the extent of bleeding. Massive bleeding with dilation of the ventricular system is much more likely to cause an acute change in brain function, with increased intracranial pressure, brainstem abnormalities, and apnea. Milder degrees of hemorrhage may be asymptomatic or associated with seizure-like events, changes in muscle tone, or apnea.

When bleeding extends into the parenchyma, porencephaly may result from liquefactive necrosis or ischemia-induced encephalomalacia. Follow-up structural brain studies may show hypodense areas in which blood was present; later they may show areas of porencephaly.[60]

Other complications of IVH are *posthemorrhagic hydrocephalus* (PHH) and *periventricular leukomalacia* (PVL).[8,84] Evidence of posthemorrhagic hydrocephalus should be investigated in all survivors of germinal matrix hemorrhage. CT scanning or ultrasonography to assess ventricular size should be used because clinical signs alone are not reliable.[90]

With the hope of avoiding the necessity of placing a shunt, some attempts at control of the hydrocephalus have been made. Various studies have evaluated intraventricular streptokinase, lumbar or ventricular punctures and drainage/irrigation/fibrinolytic therapy with no interventions being effective.[60]

The majority of infants with IVH suffer neurologic complications. In general the sickest and smallest neonates tend to have the most complications. There is a clear correlation between the grade of bleed and the likelihood of significant neurologic complications. Over 50% of preterm children with a grade 3 to 4 IVH will have significant cognitive deficits with 75% of these children requiring special education.[84] Even those with lower-grade bleeds have been shown to have psychiatric and behavioral issues.[8] The influence of other factors on neurologic outcome may be more significant than that of the actual bleed itself. Hypoxia, hypoperfusion, and other conditions known to damage the developing nervous system cannot easily be separated as individual factors affecting outcome.

Parent Teaching

Parents of an infant with IVH should be involved with their infant's care plan. The rationale for a minimal handling protocol needs to be explained. Encouraging parents to participate in setting "timeout" and "touch me" times will facilitate their ability to visit and assist with care. During visits, they should be encouraged to recognize signs of overstimulation and become knowledgeable about the appropriate interventions to take to calm their infant.

The infant with IVH has both short- and long-term problems of varying degrees. If acute hemorrhage resolves without ongoing problems, possible complications such as hydrocephalus may still occur. Teaching parents to measure head circumference and alerting them to the signs of increased intracranial pressure such as poor feeding, posturing, eye movement difficulties, full fontanel, and lethargy enable them to participate more fully in the medical follow-up (see Box 26-3).

Parents must understand the risk for long-term neurologic sequelae. Despite the difficulty of predicting sequelae with any degree of certainty, parents should understand that mental and motor handicaps, delays in the acquisition of milestones, seizures, and problems associated with hydrocephalus and potential shunt placement may occur.[90] Specific preparation for these potential problems begins in the nursery, with more education as needed in follow-up visits. Prompt and appropriate referral to medical specialists and supportive services is important in both inpatient and outpatient settings. Parents may find support and information from national and state organizations (see "Parent Resources for Neurologic Disorders" at the end of the chapter).

PEDIATRIC STROKE

Pathophysiology

Stroke in the newborn period is defined as a group of heterogeneous conditions in which there is (1) focal disruption of cerebral blood flow secondary to arterial or cerebral venous thrombosis or embolization, (2) between 28 weeks of fetal life through the

28th postnatal day, and (3) confirmed by neuroimaging or neuropathologic studies.[73] Perinatal stroke can be further divided into three subtypes: perinatal arterial stroke (PAS), cerebral sinovenous thrombosis (CSVT), or perinatal hemorrhagic stroke (PHS).[30,46]

The most common stroke, PAS, affects both term and preterm infants with an estimated incidence of 1 in 2300 to 5000 births.[46,71,73] The most common site for PAS is the left middle cerebral artery.[71] Some studies have also noted male newborns affected slightly more often than females.[87]

CSVT is less common than PAS with an incidence ranging from 40 per 100,000 live births per year.[96] As with PAS, there is a male predominance with CSVT.[96] CSVT is diagnosed as "the presence of a thrombus in a cranial venous sinus, a large deep brain vein or a smaller cortical or deep vein with partial or complete occlusion."[30] PHS is the least common type of stroke in neonates with a prevalence of 6.2 per 100,000 live births.[3] There are limited studies looking at etiology, complications, and long-term outcomes from PHS.

Etiology

The mechanisms that lead to PAS are varied and multifactorial.[73] Causes can be divided into emboli that are cardiac in origin, cerebral vessel disorders, and stasis of blood flow leading to thrombosis. In more than half of newborns with PAS, a coagulation disorder has been identified, with thromboemboli being the most common cause.[46,87] Newborns are especially at high risk for these emboli because of placental changes at delivery. Neonatal cardiac anatomy allows venous clots to cross the patent foramen ovale and right to left shunts also occur in cardiac disorders.[87] PHS occurs as a hemorrhagic transformation of arterial or venous infarction, from intraparenchymal hemorrhage due to vascular abnormalities, bleeding diatheses, or unknown etiology.[3,16]

Prevention

Because PAS is multifactorial, one preventive strategy alone is not effective. Preventing any maternal risk factor (i.e., smoking, adequate weight control, and using compression stockings during periods of immobility) in women with a clotting disorder is advisable.[70] Because dehydration is a risk factor for thrombosis, attention to fluid intake during labor is indicated.[46,70]

Data Collection

HISTORY

There are numerous risk factors for PAS with no single factor as the main etiology. Risk factors may include maternal and placental disorders, perinatal asphyxia, blood disorders, cardiac disorders, infections, trauma, and drugs.[30,46,71] CSVT is also multifactorial with antepartal, intrapartal and postpartal influences. Pregnancy factors include preeclampsia, chorioamnionitis, and gestational diabetes.[42,87] Delivery risk factors include fetal distress and birth asphyxia. The normal process of birth leading to head molding and overlapping of sutures may compress the dural sinus causing clot formation.[42,87] Postdelivery dehydration, sepsis, cardiac defects, and meningitis also may play a role.[42,87] Neonates receiving extracorporeal membrane oxygenation are at risk for CSVT because of disturbed jugular vein flow due to cannulation. The role of prothrombotic abnormalities in the development of CSVT in neonates is unclear. Recent studies have identified predictive risk factors for hemorrhagic stroke to be fetal distress and postmaturity of the neonate.[3,16] In addition congenital heart disease was also a factor in another study.[16]

SIGNS AND SYMPTOMS

Most infants with PAS present normally at birth with symptoms developing after the first day of life. Because many newborns do not show signs of focal deficits, a high index of suspicion in at-risk neonates is warranted. Twenty-five percent of neonates with a stroke have systemic illness.[45] Seizures, on the side opposite the infarction, are the most common presentation of neonatal stroke and occurring in 70% to 90% of cases.[46,87] As with PAS, neonates with CSVT present in the first day after birth to the first week of life.[42] Seizures are the most common presentation of CSVT. Lethargy, irritability, poor feeding, apnea, and jitteriness are also common.[42,87] Neonates with PHS present similarly to the other stroke subtypes: seizures, apnea, respiratory distress, fever, and poor feeding are common. Diagnosis is based on CT or MRI or magnetic resonance antiography (MRA)/V.

LABORATORY DATA

Imaging is indicated for diagnosis of neonatal stroke. MRI, using diffusion-weighted sequences, is the imaging mode of choice for PAS, CVST, and PHS.[45,46,73] MRI detects thrombi and infarcted areas. Ultrasound is less useful in diagnosing PAS, and CT scan can miss small or early infarcts. CT detects hemorrhage in PHS. For CVST, Doppler flow ultrasound demonstrates decreased flow.[44,87] Pediatric stroke consensus guidelines also recommend noninvasive vascular imaging to diagnose previously undetected vessel abnormalities.[45] Neonatal seizures require an EEG and laboratory workup for the etiology of seizures: complete blood count, CSF, cultures and glucose, calcium, and electrolytes. Coagulation studies are indicated with a family history of coagulopathy.[71] Multifocal infarcts seen on MRI or an abnormal cardiac examination (i.e., murmur) require echocardiogram for congenital cardiac anomaly. Evaluation of the placenta is helpful in discerning sources of thromboemboli and systemic vascular abnormalities.[71,73]

MR venography is needed to evaluate for the presence of a thrombus. Doppler flow ultrasound can support a diagnosis by demonstrating absent or decreased flow.[44,87] Additional workup will depend on clinical presentation and can include laboratory testing, lumbar puncture, EEG, and echocardiography.

Treatment

Management of PAS is supportive and directed at treating any underlying condition. Maintenance of normal hydration, electrolytes, and glucose, oxygen, and pH levels are indicated.[46,87] Seizures are treated acutely with seizure medication, although most newborns do not need to be discharged on seizure medication. PAS is not routinely treated with aspirin or anticoagulation.[45,87] A congenital cardiac defect as the cause of the PAS may require treatment with antiplatelet agents or anticoagulation (i.e., heparin or low-molecular-weight heparin [LMWH]) with the consultation of pediatric cardiology.[45,47,87] If a genetic thrombophilia is diagnosed, pediatric hematology guides treatment with antiplatelet or anticoagulation agents. Treatment of CSVT focuses on treatment of the underlying cause for thrombus formation. Antithrombotic therapy consists of the use of heparin or LMWH in neonates without significant intracranial hemorrhage, followed by LMWH for 6 to 12 additional weeks.[67] If hemorrhage is present, radiology monitoring of the thrombus (at days 5 and 7) is followed by treatment with anticoagulation but only if the thrombus increases in size.[67]

This treatment regimen is in contrast to the American Heart Association Stroke Council guideline that recommends treatment only if there is increased size of the thrombus.[42,96] Most studies have found significant variability in anticoagulation use, and more research is needed.

Complications

The main complication of PAS is hemiplegic cerebral palsy, which occurs in 20% to 80% of children.[46,73,87] There is also ongoing risk of seizures, which occur in 15% to 40% of children with PAS.[46,73] Deficits in cognition, language, vision, and behavior are common and become evident in childhood.[46,47,73] A normal or mildly abnormal neonatal neurologic examination is not predictive of future complications because of the plasticity of newborn brains and their greater ability to recover from injuries.[47] Neonates with CSVT have a high incidence of significant neurologic complications. Neurologic deficits include epilepsy, cerebral palsy, and cognitive impairments.[96] Because there are few studies of PHS, long-term complications are difficult to determine. A recent study did indicate that almost half of PHS survivors had short-term neurologic deficit.[16]

Parent Teaching

For a newborn diagnosed with any type perinatal stroke, parental education focuses on dealing with complications and associated conditions. Neonates with seizures are given antiseizure medications and may be discharged having weaned from them or still taking the medications.[45] Parents need to learn to recognize seizures in their infant, to safely administer medications, and know the side effects of all medications. Seizure medications may cause drowsiness/sleepiness, and parents need to know whom to contact if they are concerned about their infant's behavior.

Parents should be encouraged to use the services of multidisciplinary teams for their infant's rehabilitation needs.[47] Encouraging parents to begin early intervention services after discharge helps to lessen motor deficits. If no risk factors are identified, parents need to be reassured that the potential for recurrence of perinatal stroke is less than 1%.[47] If there is an identified cardiac or underlying abnormality, then recurrence risk is higher. A small subset of newborns with underlying cardiac or hematologic risk factors will go home on antiplatelet or anticoagulant medication. These parents need to learn to dose these medications properly and know their side effects. Parents should be aware that stroke morbidity lasts a lifetime, but their child's quality of life can be good because of the plasticity of the newborn brain.[47]

REFERENCES

For a full list of references, scan the QR code or visit http://booksite.elsevier.com/9780323320832.

27 GENETIC DISORDERS, MALFORMATIONS, AND INBORN ERRORS OF METABOLISM

ANNE L. MATTHEWS AND NATHANIEL H. ROBIN

A neonate born with a malformation, a genetic syndrome, or an acute metabolic disorder presents a management challenge for the neonatal intensive care unit (NICU) staff. If these conditions are not suspected and diagnosed in a critically ill neonate, an appropriate course of action might not be taken. Thus, a specific diagnosis becomes imperative. An accurate diagnosis provides the staff with information about the cause of the condition, points the way toward appropriate treatment, and indicates the prognosis so that the most appropriate care of the infant can be initiated. Moreover, the broader issues of providing supportive care and counseling for the affected infant's family can be addressed.

Genetic evaluation is a complex process that requires expertise in differentiating normal variations from abnormal findings and knowledge of the principles of embryology and dysmorphology to provide an accurate diagnosis. Skills in obtaining detailed information of prenatal and family histories may be equally important.

The field of genomics and genetic medicine has witnessed an explosion of new knowledge, much of which was generated by the efforts of the Human Genome Project.[13] Advances in understanding of the genetic basis of development and function as well as the interaction of genes and the environment, continue to provide new insights into human health.

This chapter presents a concise overview of the major categories of genetic disorders and the appropriate techniques to establish specific diagnoses. For an excellent review and detailed explanation of concepts, terminology, and specific genetic mechanisms, refer to *Thompson and Thompson Genetics in Medicine.*[40] See Box 27-1 for a comprehensive list of terms.

GENETIC PRINCIPLES

Genes

A *gene* is a segment of a deoxyribonucleic acid (DNA) molecule that codes for the synthesis of a single polypeptide and contains the hereditary information needed for development or function. DNA, which allows the storing, duplicating, and processing of hereditary information, consists of two long strands twisted around each other to form a double helix. Each strand of DNA is composed of four nucleotides: guanine (G), adenine (A), thymine (T), and cytosine (C). The specific order of the nucleotides determines the precise information that will be encoded at that site. Genes can (1) regulate other genes by turning them "on" or "off"; (2) specify the exact structure of proteins, which then control the activities of the cells; and (3) specify ribonucleic acid (RNA), which is necessary for protein synthesis.

Chromosomes

Genes are packed in linear order on chromosomes. *Chromosomes* are found in the nuclei of cells. In humans, normal somatic cells contain 46 chromosomes (diploid number), of which

---

PURPLE type highlights content that is particularly applicable to clinical settings.

GLOSSARY

Acrocentric chromosome A chromosome with the centromere near the end of the chromosome.

Allele One of a pair or series of alternate forms of a gene at the same locus.

Aneuploid Any chromosome number that is not an exact multiple of the haploid set.

Autosome A chromosome that is not a sex chromosome.

Centromere The primary constriction of a chromosome in which the long and the short arms meet.

Chromatid After replication of a chromosome, two subunits attached by the centromere can be seen; each is called a *chromatid,* and after separation, each becomes a chromosome of a daughter cell.

Chromosomes The microscopic structures in the cell nucleus composed of DNA and proteins that contain the genes.

Congenital Present at birth.

Dermatoglyphics The dermal ridge patterns on the digits, palms, and soles.

Diploid Two copies of all chromosomes; the number of chromosomes normally present in somatic cells. In humans, this is 46 and is sometimes symbolized as *2N.*

Dominant A gene (allele) that is expressed clinically in the heterozygous state. In a dominant disorder, the mutant allele overshadows the normal allele.

Dysmorphic Morphologic abnormality, often a minor physical finding that may or may not have any cosmetic or functional significance and is present in less than 4% of the newborn population.

Fluorescence in situ hybridization (FISH) Molecular cytogenetic method for detection of microdeletions of chromosomes.

Gamete Mature reproductive cell, the egg or the sperm, containing the haploid number of chromosomes.

Gene The functional unit of heredity.

Genotype A person's genetic constitution.

Haploid One copy of all chromosomes; the number of chromosomes present in the gamete; in humans this is 23 and can be symbolized as *N.*

Hemizygous The condition in which only one copy of a gene is normally present, so its effect is expressed because there is no counterpart gene present (e.g., the genes on the X or Y chromosome of the male).

Heterozygote An individual who has two different alleles at a given locus of two homologous chromosomes.

Homologous chromosomes Members of the same chromosome pair; normally they have the same number and arrangement of genes.

Homozygote An individual who has two identical alleles at a given locus of two homologous chromosomes.

Karyotype The standard pictorial arrangement of chromosome pairs, numbered according to centromere position and length.

Locus The position or place that a gene occupies on a chromosome.

Malformation A primary structural defect that results from a localized error of morphogenesis; abnormal development.

Metacentric chromosome Chromosome with the centromere in the center of the chromosome.

Monosomy Absence of one chromosome of one pair.

Mosaicism Presence in the same individual of two or more different chromosomal constitutions.

Mutation A heritable alteration in the genetic material.

Nondisjunction Failure of two homologous chromosomes to separate equally during cell division into two daughter cells, resulting in abnormal chromosome numbers in gametes or somatic cells.

Phenotype The observable expression of traits either physically or biochemically.

Recessive A gene (allele) that is expressed clinically in the homozygous state. In a recessive disorder, both genes at a given locus must be abnormal to manifest the disorder.

Sex chromosomes The X and Y chromosomes.

Syndrome Recognizable pattern of multiple malformations that occur together and have the same cause.

Transcription The process by which complementary messenger RNA is synthesized from a DNA template.

Translation The process through which the amino acids in a given polypeptide are synthesized from the messenger RNA template.

Translocation Transfer of all or part of a chromosome to another location (i.e., on the same or another chromosome) after chromosome breakage.

Trisomy The presence of three homologous chromosomes rather than the normal two.

X-linked A gene located on an X chromosome.

Zygote A fertilized egg that develops into an embryo.

---

44 are termed *autosomes* and 2 are *sex chromosomes.* Females have two X chromosomes (XX), and males have an X and a Y chromosome (XY). Gametes—eggs or sperm—contain 23 chromosomes (haploid number). In the zygote and somatic cells, chromosomes are paired (homologs). In each pair, one homolog is maternal and the other is paternal in origin. Each chromosomal pair has unique morphologic characteristics that allow it to be distinguished from other chromosomes, such as size, position of the centromere, and the unique banding pattern that is demonstrated by special staining techniques (Figure 27-1).[19] To pass on the genetic information to daughter cells, the chromosomes must replicate and then divide correctly. Somatic cells undergo *mitosis,* in which

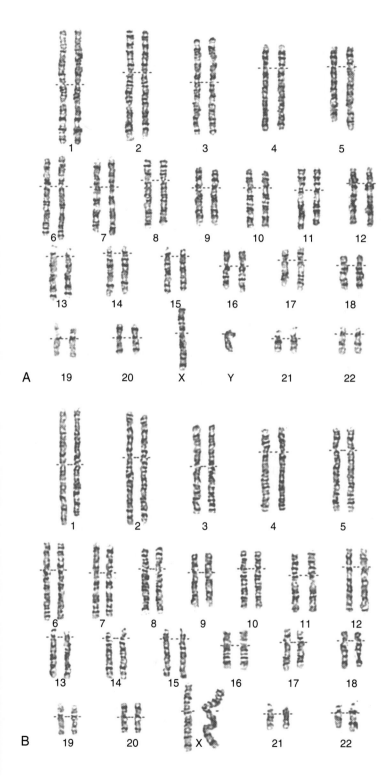

FIGURE 27-1 **A,** Normal male karyotype. **B,** Normal female karyotype. Each karyotype contains 46 chromosomes (44 autosomes and 2 sex chromosomes: XY, male; XX, female). The autosomes are numbered from 1 to 22. Note banding pattern, unique for each chromosomal pair. (Courtesy Dr. Loris McGavran, PhD, Cytogenics Laboratory at the University of Colorado at Denver and Health Sciences Center, Denver.)

cells replicate and then divide chromosomal material into two genetically identical daughter cells with 46 chromosomes each. In gametes, the process is known as *meiosis,* which is different from mitotic division in that daughter cells contain the haploid number of chromosomes (23) and crossing over or recombination between two homologs occurs, thus facilitating genetic variation in offspring.[40]

An individual's chromosome constitution can be determined by examining dividing body cells under certain laboratory conditions from any accessible tissue such as blood lymphocytes or skin fibroblasts. The resulting *karyotype* (see Figure 27-1), or pictorial arrangement, demonstrates the number and structure of that individual's chromosomes.

ETIOLOGY

Malformations and genetic disorders caused wholly or partly by genetic factors can be categorized into four major areas: (1) chromosomal disorders caused by numeric or structural abnormalities of chromosomes; (2) single-gene or Mendelian disorders, which are secondary to single-gene mutations; (3) complex or multifactorial disorders resulting from interaction of genes and environmental influences; and (4) abnormalities caused by environmental exposures of the fetus during development.

More recently, better understanding of molecular processes has allowed the identification of additional genetic mechanisms contributing to genetic disorders: germline mosaicism, genomic imprinting, and uniparental disomy.

Chromosomal Disorders

Chromosomal abnormalities are relatively common. Approximately 0.5% to 0.7% of all live newborns have a chromosomal abnormality, and 4% to 7% of perinatal deaths result from a chromosomal abnormality. Moreover, it is estimated that at least 50% of all recognized first-trimester miscarriages are caused by a chromosomal aberration.[18] Current cytogenetic techniques, such as high-resolution banding, fluorescence in situ hybridization (FISH), and microarray-based comparative genomic hybridization (array-CGH), have increased the detection rate of chromosomal aberrations. Submicroscopic deletions, duplications, or other abnormal rearrangements of chromosome material that may not have been identified a few years previously are now being detected in children with congenital malformations or intellectual disability.

Chromosomal aberrations should be suspected in any of the following situations:
- Small for gestational age for weight, length, or head circumference
- Presence of one or more congenital malformations
- Presence of dysmorphic features
- Neurologic or neuromuscular dysfunction
- Family history of multiple miscarriages or siblings with intellectual disability or birth defects along with one or more of the previous other situations listed here

Chromosomal abnormalities can be classified into two major categories: (1) abnormalities of chromosome number (aneuploidy), in which there is an extra or missing chromosome and (2) abnormalities of chromosome structure that result in the loss or duplication of part of the chromosomal material. Abnormalities of autosomes usually have more significant deleterious effects on the development of the infant than those seen with sex chromosome abnormalities.

ABNORMALITIES OF CHROMOSOME NUMBER

Numeric chromosomal abnormalities occur as a result of nondisjunction in which aberrant segregation leads to loss or gain of one or more chromosomes. Nondisjunction can occur during either meiosis or mitosis, resulting in an abnormal gamete (egg or sperm) or abnormal somatic cell, respectively (Figure 27-2). Fertilization of an aneuploid gamete by a normal gamete produces a zygote with an extra chromosome *(trisomy)* or missing chromosome *(monosomy)*. Aneuploidy in somatic cells results in *chromosomal mosaicism* (i.e., the presence of some cells with the normal number of chromosomes and other cells with an abnormal number of chromosomes) (Figure 27-3). Although nondisjunction may affect any chromosomal pair, the most commonly recognized trisomies in liveborn infants are trisomy 21 (Down syndrome), trisomy 18 (Edward syndrome), and trisomy 13 (Patau syndrome). Conversely, trisomy 16 has been found exclusively in spontaneous abortions.[18]

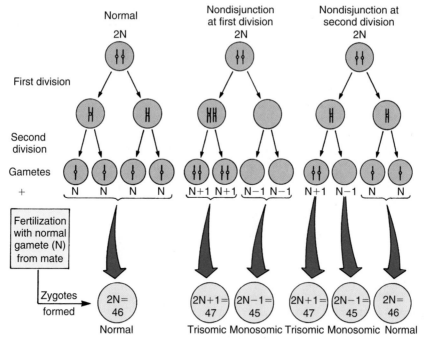

FIGURE 27-2 Nondisjunction. During formation of gametes, errors of nondisjunction can occur during either first or second meiotic division.

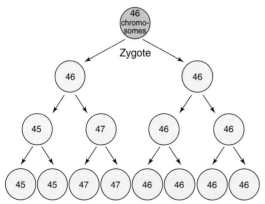

FIGURE 27-3 Mosaicism. Nondisjunction occurring after fertilization and zygote formation results in some cells containing the normal 46-chromosome complement and other cells having an abnormal number of chromosomes.

The most common monosomy is 45,X, Turner syndrome. As a rule, numeric chromosomal abnormalities are associated with intrauterine growth restriction (IUGR), dysmorphic features, malformations, and intellectual disability. Physical abnormalities may be milder or absent in the newborn with mosaicism.

ABNORMALITIES OF CHROMOSOME STRUCTURE

Structural abnormalities have been described in all chromosomes. These include deletions, translocations, duplications, and inversions (Figure 27-4). A *deletion* is a loss of chromosome material and results in partial monosomy for the chromosome involved. Loss of material from the end of a chromosome is known as a *terminal deletion,* as seen in 5p-, or cri du chat syndrome. An *interstitial deletion* involves a loss of chromosomal material that does not include the ends of the chromosome. A terminal deletion of both arms of a chromosome may result in reattachment of the remaining arms, leading to a formation of a ring chromosome. The presence of additional chromosome material results in *duplication* or partial trisomy of a chromosome. *Translocation* is the detachment of a chromosome segment from its normal location and its attachment to another chromosome. The translocation is balanced if the cell contains two complete copies of all chromosomal material, although in different order. In an unbalanced translocation, the rearrangement results in partial trisomy or monosomy.

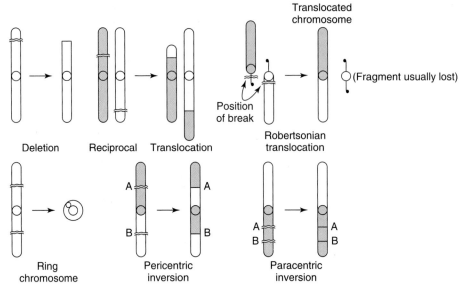

FIGURE 27-4 Schematic example of structural chromosomal abnormalities. (From Hathaway WE, Groothius J, Hay W, editors: *Current pediatric diagnosis and treatment,* ed 10, Norwalk, Conn, 1991, Appleton & Lange.)

Translocations can be reciprocal or Robertsonian. A reciprocal translocation involves exchange of segments between two chromosomes (e.g., part of the short arm of chromosome 4 trades a place with a part of chromosome 10). Robertsonian translocations involve two acrocentric chromosomes fused at their centromeres. The most common Robertsonian translocation is formed between chromosomes 14 and 21.[22]

Inversions are the result of a double break in a single chromosome and reinsertion of the chromosomal material that has been inverted. Inversions are either pericentric (including the centromere) or paracentric (without the centromere). The most common inversion is a small pericentric inversion of chromosome 9, which is considered to be a normal variant, found in approximately 1% of the general population.[40] All other inversions may produce gametes that result in an individual with an unbalanced rearrangement (i.e., having both a duplication and a deletion of some chromosome material, such as that seen in recombinant 8 syndrome).

MICRODELETIONS AND SYNDROMES

At times, structural chromosomal abnormalities are submicroscopic and therefore cannot be detected by conventional cytogenetic techniques. FISH is a molecular cytogenetic method that facilitates the detection of microdeletions. FISH uses segments of fluorescently labeled DNA called *probes,* constructed so that each probe can attach only to a specific segment of a chromosome, which then will be fluorescent during a microscopic visualization. In the case of a deletion of that chromosome segment, the probe cannot attach to the chromosome; thus the fluorescent segment is missing from the deleted segment of that chromosome.[50]

The most recent advance being used to detect very small submicroscopic deletions and duplications is *comparative genomic hybridization* (array-CGH).[15] This technology blends molecular techniques with cytogenetics and allows the genome to be scanned at a higher resolution than conventional techniques. DNA from a patient sample and DNA from a control sample are differentially labeled, mixed in equal proportions, and hybridized to DNA substrates fixed on an array platform (i.e., bacterial artificial chromosomes [BACs] or oligonucleotides [short segments of DNA usually 8–50 base pairs]). This technique can measure the difference between two different DNA samples in copy number (dosage) of a particular segment of DNA. Thus microscopic gains and losses from a patient sample can be quantified.[15]

Microdeletions result in phenotypic abnormalities. A number of well-recognized microdeletion syndromes may be suspected in the NICU. *Prader-Willi syndrome,* caused by an interstitial deletion of chromosome 15 (q11q13), usually manifests in a newborn as severe hypotonia, feeding difficulties, and micropenis or hypoplastic labia.[9] *Williams syndrome* is caused by an interstitial deletion or mutation of the elastin gene (ELN) on the long arm of chromosome 7 (7q11).[38] The condition is often first seen in an affected newborn in the postterm period; the infant is small for family size. There may be a congenital heart defect, in particular, supravalvular aortic stenosis or peripheral pulmonic stenosis; hypotonia; failure to thrive with gastroesophageal reflux; poor suck and swallow; and vomiting and irritability or colic. Infantile hypercalcemia is seen in approximately 20% of these infants. Subtle dysmorphic facial features may be noted in the newborn.[38]

One of the most commonly seen microdeletion syndromes is 22q11.2 deletion syndrome (22q11DS), which is characterized by cleft palate or velopharyngeal insufficiency, hypernasal speech, learning disabilities, conotruncal heart defects, and characteristic facies. 22q11DS actually represents one of a spectrum of clinical disorders all known to be caused by a deletion in chromosome 22q11 (del22q11). These include *velocardiofacial syndrome* (VCFS; palatal anomalies, congenital heart disease, characteristic facial features, and developmental delay or learning difficulties), *DiGeorge syndrome* (DGS; conotruncal heart defect, hypocalcemia, and thymic hypoplasia), and *conotruncal anomaly face syndrome* (CTAF; conotruncal heart defects and typical facies). In addition, del22q11DS has been found in 11% to 16% of cases of nonsyndromic congenital conotruncal heart disease and has been reported to present as apparently isolated neonatal hypocalcemia or learning problems.[14] Overall, del22q11DS has an estimated incidence of 1 in 2000 to 4000 newborns. The availability of molecular cytogenetic testing by FISH and chromosomal microarray (CMA) has led to appreciation of both the high incidence of the del22q11DS, as well as the increasing variety of clinical presentations that can be seen even within a single family.[34,35]

In the newborn period, the characteristic facial features are seldom obvious. However, most affected individuals manifest some of these findings by early childhood. Most prominent is the nose, which is described as long, with a "built up nasal bridge,

squared off nasal root, and bulbous nasal tip."[46] The eyes appear narrow and slitlike, the mala (cheeks) are flat, and the jaw is recessed. The ears usually are small and in some way abnormally formed. There may be an overt cleft of the secondary palate, a bifurcated uvula, a subtle submucosal cleft, or cleft lip with or without cleft palate. Other nonstructural palatal abnormalities can be seen, most commonly velopharyngeal insufficiency. In an older child or adult, this presents as hypernasal speech; in a newborn, one sees excessive nasal regurgitation. Congenital heart disease (CHD) is seen in 74% of del22q11DS patients. The type of CHD is fairly specific and includes those lesions classified as "conotruncal heart defects" (truncus arteriosus, interrupted aortic arch, tetralogy of Fallot, left-sided aortic arch, vascular rings, and some types of ventricular septal defects [VSDs]). Additional nonspecific findings include abundant scalp hair, hypospadias, renal abnormalities that can include renal agenesis, tortuous retinal vessels, ectopic/aberrant/unilateral absence of carotid and vertebral artery, microcephaly, and microdontia (there are 166 findings to date).[46]

Developmental delay, learning disabilities, or mental retardation is common and quite variable. Behavioral and psychiatric problems are common but underappreciated findings in VCFS. These individuals have a characteristic personality, marked by a flattened affect and abnormal social interaction, ranging from being intermittently withdrawn to socially precocious. A host of other psychiatric diagnoses have been seen in patients with 22q11DS.

More than 95% of cases of 22q11DS are deleted for a 2.54-Mb region of chromosome 22 encompassing approximately 40 genes including the *TBX1* gene.[35] Point mutations in *TBX1* have also been found when no deletion was identified.[55] Although 93% of cases are de novo, it is important to obtain family histories and examine parents for subtle features of the syndrome as approximately 7% of infants have inherited the abnormality from a parent.[35]

CLINICAL EXAMPLES OF CHROMOSOMAL ABNORMALITIES

Down Syndrome. Down syndrome has an incidence of approximately 1 in 600 live births. Approximately 95% of cases are caused by nondisjunction involving chromosome 21, 4% are caused by a translocation, and 1% are mosaic. Down syndrome may manifest with marked hypotonia; a number of major malformations, most commonly congenital heart defects, duodenal atresia, and tracheoesophageal fistula; and a characteristic pattern of dysmorphic features. The classic phenotype seen in Down syndrome includes a flattened occiput, midfacial hypoplasia, depressed nasal bridge, upward-slanting palpebral fissures, epicanthic folds, grayish speckling of the iris (Brushfield spots), micrognathia, excess nuchal skin, single palmar creases (simian creases), single flexion creases and in-curving of the fifth fingers (clinodactyly), and increased distance between the first and second toes (Figure 27-5).

In full-term infants with the classic phenotype of Down syndrome, the clinical diagnosis is usually not difficult. However, it is imperative that cytogenetic studies be done to confirm the diagnosis and to differentiate a nondisjunctional trisomy from a translocation. This distinction has important implications for recurrence risks (see discussion in "Prevention" section). In premature infants, the classic facial phenotype is frequently missing, making clinical diagnosis more difficult. The presence of an atrioventricular (AV) canal or duodenal atresia with minor malformations, such as abnormal dermatoglyphics, should alert the clinician to the possibility of Down syndrome.

Trisomy 18. Trisomy 18 has an incidence of 1 in 6000 live births. The major phenotypic features include prenatal growth restriction, complex cardiac malformations, abnormal muscle tone, microcephaly, prominent occiput, short sternum, low-set and malformed ears, corneal opacities, micrognathia, peculiar hand posturing with the second and fifth digits overlapping the third and fourth, hypoplasia of fingernails, abnormal dermatoglyphics, prominent calcanei, and deep plantar furrows between the first and second toes (Figure 27-6). The prognosis is poor, and the majority of infants with trisomy 18 die within the first few months of life. Those who survive into childhood are profoundly intellectually disabled.

Trisomy 13. Trisomy 13 is seen in approximately 1 in 15,000 live births. Phenotypic features include prenatal and postnatal growth restriction, microcephaly, sloping forehead, coloboma of the iris, microphthalmia or anophthalmia, low-set or malformed ears,

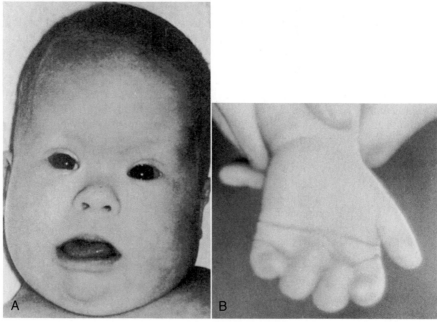

FIGURE 27-5 Infant with Down syndrome. **A,** Note midface hypoplasia, epicanthic folds, and depressed nasal bridge. **B,** Single palmar crease. (**A** from Cohen MM: *The child with multiple birth defects,* ed 2, New York, 1997, Raven Press. **B** courtesy Dr. Eva Sujansky, Genetic Services at The Children's Hospital, Denver, Colo.)

cleft lip and palate, postaxial polydactyly, and abnormal palmar creases and dermatoglyphics (Figure 27-7). Internal abnormalities may include a number of central nervous system (CNS) malformations, such as holoprosencephaly, cardiac malformations, omphalocele, renal malformations, and urogenital abnormalities such as cryptorchidism in males and uterine malformations in females. The prognosis is extremely poor for these infants, with most dying within the first few months of life.

Turner Syndrome. The only monosomy to be seen in live births is that of Turner syndrome—females with a 45,X karyotype. In addition, it is the only numeric abnormality of the sex chromosome that may be identifiable at birth. Turner syndrome has an incidence of 1 in 5000 female births.[44] Clinical features that may be evident in the newborn period are a short, webbed neck or redundant skin on the back of the neck and marked lymphedema of the dorsum of the hands and feet (Figure 27-8). Congenital heart defects are seen in approximately half of the patients, with 30% having a coarctation of the aorta. Renal anomalies may also be present.[23] Prognosis is usually excellent but depends on the presence and severity of the congenital heart defect. Intelligence is normal; however, some females with Turner syndrome have been noted to have problems with spatial perception or fine motor abilities.[44]

Cri du Chat. *Cri du chat,* or "cat cry" syndrome, is the result of loss of the terminal end of the short arm of chromosome 5 (5p-). The name of the syndrome reflects the unusual catlike, weak cry these infants have in the neonatal period. These infants are usually small for gestational age, hypotonic, and microcephalic and may have ocular hypertelorism, epicanthic folds, downward slant of the palpebral fissures,

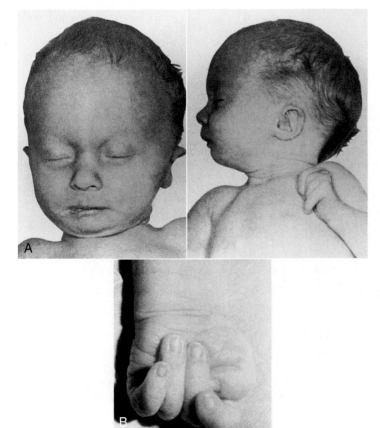

FIGURE 27-6 Infant with trisomy 18. **A,** Typical facies with small chin, abnormal pinna, and prominent occiput. **B,** Typical hand posturing with overlapping fingers. (From Paerregaard P, Mikkelsen M, Froland A, et al: Trisomy no. 17–18: report of two cases, *Acta Pathol Microbiol Scand* 67:479, 1966.)

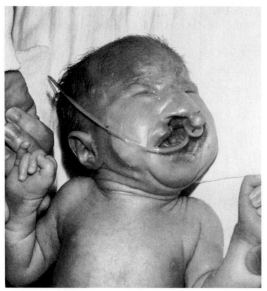

FIGURE 27-7 Infant with trisomy 13. Facial clefts and microcephaly; abnormal positioning of the hands. (From Hathaway WE, Groothuis J, Hay W, editors: *Current pediatric diagnoses and treatment,* ed 10, Norwalk, Conn, 1991, Appleton & Lange.)

low-set ears, and micrognathia. They are significantly intellectually disabled.

San Luis Valley Syndrome. *Recombinant 8* or the *San Luis Valley syndrome,* named for the area in which many of these individuals were first identified, is an example of an unbalanced pericentric inversion with both duplication and a deletion of chromosome 8 material.[48] The pericentric inversion of chromosome 8 found in a parent and other relatives of a child with recombinant 8 syndrome have no phenotypic consequence because it is a balanced rearrangement. However, a carrier is at risk for producing unbalanced gametes during meiosis. In recombinant 8 syndrome, there is a deletion of chromosomal material of the short arm of chromosome 8 and a duplication of chromosome material of the long arm of 8. The phenotype is characterized by unusual facial features, including a wide face, depressed nasal bridge, hypertelorism, down-slanting palpebral fissures, upturned nose, long philtrum, low-set and malformed ears, cleft lip or cleft palate, congenital heart disease, and renal abnormalities.[48]

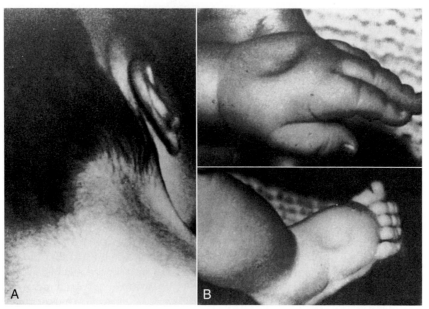

FIGURE 27-8 Female infant with Turner syndrome. **A,** Webbed neck with low posterior hairline. **B,** Lymphedema of the dorsal surfaces of the hands and feet. (From Knuppel R, Drukker JD, editors: *High risk pregnancy: a team approach,* Philadelphia, 1988, Saunders.)

PREVENTION

The identification of chromosomal abnormalities in the newborn is important, not only for management issues about the infant but also because of the recurrence risks the abnormality carries for the family. In general, numeric chromosomal abnormalities carry low recurrence risks (approximately 1%–2%).[18] In the presence of structural abnormalities, recurrence risks depend on whether one of the parents carries a balanced rearrangement. If parental chromosomes are normal, the recurrence risk is minimal. However, if a parent carries a balanced chromosomal rearrangement, the recurrence risk is significantly increased. The exact risk figure varies with the nature of the specific chromosomal rearrangement and, in some cases, the sex of the carrier parent. In either situation, prenatal diagnosis for chromosome analysis is available for parents and families concerned about recurrence risk.

Single-Gene Disorders

McKusick's online catalog of Mendelian inherited disorders currently lists more than 21,000 entries with approximately 7000 single-gene disorders with known patterns of inheritance.[41] Many of these disorders are singularly rare; however, collectively, they affect about 1% of the population. Single-gene disorders are the result of either a single or double dose of an abnormal gene. Single-gene disorders are classified as autosomal dominant, autosomal recessive, X-linked dominant, and X-linked recessive. Humans have two copies of each gene located at identical places (gene loci) on homologous chromosomes. In a single-gene disorder, an abnormal or mutated allele (an alternate form of a gene) is found on one or both members of a pair of chromosomes.[40] Individuals with identical alleles at a particular locus are homozygous for the gene. Individuals with different alleles are heterozygous for the gene. Because males have only one X chromosome and most genes located on the Y chromosome do not correspond to those located on the X, males are hemizygous for the genes on the X chromosome. Abnormal genes located on one of the 44 autosomes are the cause of autosomal disorders: disease-causing genes located on the X chromosome are the cause of X-linked disorders. Disorders are *dominant* when the phenotype is expressed in the presence of only one copy of the mutated gene.

In *recessive disorders,* the phenotype is expressed only when both chromosomes carry the mutated gene.

AUTOSOMAL DOMINANT DISORDERS

Autosomal dominant disorders are ones in which the disorder is expressed in the heterozygous state. Major characteristics include the following: (1) multiple generations are affected (i.e., an infant would have an affected parent); (2) both males and females are affected, and both sexes can transmit the disorder to their offspring (i.e., male-to-male transmission can occur); (3) there is a 50% risk for each offspring to inherit the gene from an affected parent; and (4) individuals who do not have the gene cannot transmit the disorder to their offspring.

A negative family history does not rule out the presence of an autosomal dominant disorder. Possible explanations for a negative family history are the following: (1) the infant's disorder is a result of a new mutation; (2) a parent has a very mild expression of the disorder and may not have been previously diagnosed; (3) nonpaternity; (4) decreased penetrance (i.e., not all individuals with the gene have phenotypic abnormalities, i.e., skipped generation); and (5) germline mosaicism for the mutation (see the "Nontraditional Inheritance" section).

Dominant disorders that may be seen in the NICU include skeletal dysplasias, such as *achondroplasia* (abnormality in the *FGFR3* gene), *osteogenesis imperfecta* (abnormality in *COL1A1* or *COL1A2*), *Apert and Crouzon syndromes* (abnormality in the *FGFR2* gene), *Treacher Collins syndrome* (abnormality in *TCOF1, POLR1C or POLRID* genes – mutations in *TOCF1* are responsible for approximately 93% of cases), and ectrodactyly (Figure 27-9).[1]

AUTOSOMAL RECESSIVE DISORDERS

Autosomal recessive disorders are expressed only in the homozygous state. Thus, to be affected, an individual usually inherits an abnormal gene from each parent. The parent who is heterozygous for a disease-causing gene is usually phenotypically normal and is called a *carrier.* Major characteristics of autosomal recessive inheritance include (1) phenotypically normal parents, (2) affected siblings, (3) both males and females affected, (4) offspring of two carrier parents (25% risk for being affected), (5) unaffected siblings have a two-thirds chance of being carriers, and (6) possibly an increased incidence of consanguinity (mating between blood relatives). Autosomal recessive disorders that may be identified in the neonatal period include many of the metabolic disorders (e.g., *phenylketonuria [PKU], galactosemia,* and isovaleric acidemia) and some of the *multiple-malformation syndromes* (e.g., Meckel-Gruber syndrome), *cystic fibrosis presenting with meconium ileus, Zellweger* (cerebrohepatorenal) *syndrome* (Figure 27-10), and skeletal dysplasias such as achondrogenesis. The specific gene(s) or biochemical defect for many of these disorders is now known.

X-LINKED DISORDERS

X-linked disorders are caused by an abnormal gene (or genes) located on the X chromosome. Most X-linked disorders are recessive. The X-linked recessive disorders are phenotypically expressed in hemizygous males; heterozygous females are generally phenotypically normal and are called *carriers.* Affected fathers do not have affected sons (no male-to-male transmission); however, all daughters of affected males are carriers. A carrier female has a 50% chance of having an affected male offspring.

Occasionally, heterozygous females may be phenotypically affected, although usually less severely than males. If females are severely affected, other mechanisms, including homozygosity for the X-linked gene, may be responsible for the phenotype. X-linked recessive disorders that may be

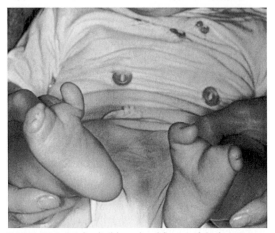

FIGURE 27-9 Ectrodactyly (lobster claw deformity) of the feet. (Courtesy Dr. Eva Sujansky, Genetic Services at The Children's Hospital, Denver, Colo.)

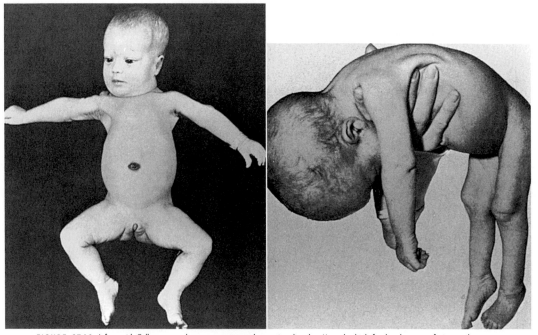

FIGURE 27-10 Infant with Zellweger syndrome, an autosomal recessive disorder. Note the high forehead, narrow facies, and extreme hypotonia. (*Left* from Jan JE, Hardwick DF, Lowry RB, et al: Cerebro-hepato-renal syndrome of Zellweger, *Am J Dis Child* 119:274, 1970. *Right* from Passarge E, McAdams AJ: Cerebro-hepato-renal syndrome: a newly recognized hereditary disorder of multiple congenital defects, including sudanophilic leukodystrophy, cirrhosis of the liver, and polycystic kidneys, *J Pediatr* 71:691, 1967.)

recognizable in the newborn period include factor VIII and IX deficiency (classic hemophilia A and B), X-linked hydrocephalus, and Opitz syndrome.

X-linked dominant disorders occur when the abnormal gene located on the X chromosome is expressed in both the hemizygous and heterozygous states. As in X-linked recessive conditions, there is no male-to-male transmission, because the affected male passes his Y chromosome and not his X chromosome to his sons; however, all of the daughters of an affected male will inherit his X chromosome and thus be affected. Each son and daughter of an affected female has a 50% risk for being affected; males usually are more severely affected than females. Only a few disorders are known to be inherited as an X-linked dominant, such as incontinentia pigmenti, hypophosphatemia (vitamin D–resistant rickets), and ornithine transcarbamylase (OTC) deficiency. Early diagnosis of OTC deficiency is important because, if untreated, it leads to neonatal hyperammonemia and death in affected males. In affected females, the clinical picture can be variable, ranging from an asymptomatic infant to one who presents in the first week of life with lethargy, vomiting, and protein avoidance, ending in seizures and coma.

Complex and Multifactorial Disorders

Complex, common non-Mendelian disorders, often called *multifactorial disorders,* are the result of both environmental and genetic factors.[21] Most isolated single malformations, including congenital heart defects, neural tube defects, cleft lip and palate, pyloric stenosis, and club feet, are inherited in this manner. In addition, the more complex, common familial disorders, such as diabetes mellitus, coronary artery disease, affective disorders, and mild intellectual disability are the result of multifactorial inheritance. In contrast to single-gene inheritance, multifactorial disorders recur within families without a characteristic pedigree pattern and recurrence risks are based on empiric data.[40]

Multifactorial inheritance is explained as a liability model with a threshold effect.[21] The general population as a whole has an underlying genetic predisposition for multifactorial traits and disorders that follow a normal distribution curve; only in those individuals in whom the genetic predisposition

exceeds the threshold will the malformation actually be expressed (Figure 27-11).

Major characteristics of complex/multifactorial inheritance include the following: (1) no consistent pedigree pattern exists between families (i.e., there may be only an isolated occurrence, or the disorder may be seen among siblings, in multiple generations, or scattered throughout the family); and (2) recurrence risks are not constant, as in single-gene disorders, but are influenced by a number of factors. These factors include the following:

- The number of family members affected (i.e., the more family members affected, the higher the recurrence risk becomes)
- The degree of relatedness to those affected (i.e., first-degree relatives are at higher recurrence risk than second- or third-degree relatives)
- The severity of the defect (i.e., the more severely affected an individual is, the higher the recurrence risk)
- The frequency of the disorder, which may vary with ethnic background (e.g., neural tube defects have a higher incidence among English and Irish populations)
- The gender of the individual (for disorders in which one gender is more commonly affected than the other [e.g., pyloric stenosis is more common in males]; if the less commonly affected gender has the defect, then the recurrence risk is higher)

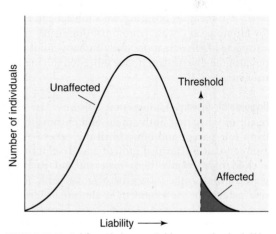

FIGURE 27-11 Multifactorial inheritance. Liability curve with a threshold beyond which the trait is expressed.

With the increasing sophistication of ultrasound diagnosis during pregnancy, a number of these isolated malformations can now be diagnosed before delivery. Moreover, in the case of neural tube defects, it has been shown that folic acid supplements may decrease the incidence of spina bifida by as much as 70% in women of reproductive age.[37]

NONTRADITIONAL INHERITANCE

Germline Mosaicism. Spectacular growth in the field of molecular genetics and its technologies in only the past few years has enabled the clarification of the inheritance patterns of many genetic disorders and birth defects that were previously unknown or unclear. For example, the lethal form of osteogenesis imperfecta (OI) occurring in multiple offspring of unaffected parents was thought to be the result of autosomal recessive inheritance. However, improved molecular techniques have documented that it is an autosomal dominant disorder in which germline mosaicism can result in having more than one affected child. That is to say, the mutation occurs in the gonad of one of the parents, who then has some gametes with and others without the OI mutation. This distinction alters the recurrence risks and is important for genetic counseling.[40]

Genomic Imprinting. In the past, little notice was given to whether the sex of the parent who transmitted an abnormal gene to offspring had any effect on the expression of genes. It is now recognized that maternally and paternally derived genes may function differently, and this is called *genomic imprinting*.[53] For example, offspring who inherit the gene for Huntington disease (autosomal dominant) from an affected father are more likely to have childhood onset of the disease than if they inherited the maternal gene.

Uniparental Disomy. Uniparental disomy is the result of inheriting both copies of a chromosome from one parent and none from the other.[53] It is assumed that for normal growth and development, a child must receive both maternal and paternal genes; if both copies of a gene originate only from one parent, the development is abnormal. Uniparental disomy has been seen in cystic fibrosis with short stature and in the Prader-Willi, Angelman, and Beckwith-Wiedemann syndromes. The parental origin of a child's chromosomes can be identified only by molecular analysis; routine chromosome analysis usually is not helpful.

Trinucleotide Repeat Disorders. Trinucleotide (triple) repeat disorders are disorders that result from an unstable expansion of a segment of DNA that consists of three or more nucleotides adjacent to each other. If a mutation occurs in a gene which contains a segment of repetitive trinucleotide sequences, it can cause the normal number of repeats to increase such that the expansion interferes with the expression or function of the gene.[40] Repeat disorders have been found to be the cause of more than 20 disorders including myotonic dystrophy (an expanded CTG triple repeat in the DMPK gene) and Fragile X syndrome (an expansion of CGG in the FRAXA gene). What is important to note is that the abnormal number of repeats can expand through each generation and lead to a more severe phenotype in the next generation (known as *anticipation*). The sex of the parent who passes on the mutation that causes the abnormal expansion can also affect the phenotype. For example, the repeat expansion in myotonic dystrophy is often larger in offspring of affected mothers.[24]

The possibility of a nontraditional pattern of inheritance makes genetic counseling more complex than previously thought. Thus, it is imperative that health care providers be aware of such complexities and refer families to a geneticist or genetic counselor for a more detailed discussion when appropriate.

INBORN ERRORS OF METABOLISM

Genetic disorders in which defects of single genes cause clinically significant blocks in metabolic pathways are known as *inborn errors of metabolism*. Recognition of disorders caused by inborn errors of metabolism has increased rapidly in recent years, and they are now recognized as important causes of disease in the newborn and pediatric age group.[49] Inborn errors of metabolism include defects of carbohydrate, amino acid, organic acid, and purine metabolism; disorders of fatty acid oxidation; lysosomal storage diseases; and disorders of peroxisomes. Remember that inborn errors can present at any time and may affect almost any organ system. Specific disorders that should be considered in symptomatic newborns include galactosemia, phenylketonuria (PKU), OTC or carbamoyl-phosphate synthetase (CPS) deficiency, maple syrup urine disease, nonketotic hyperglycinemia, propionic and methylmalonic acidemias, isovaleric acidemia, and glutaric acidemia type II.[25]

Although the majority of infants are not found to have an inborn error of metabolism as the etiology of their illness, early recognition is imperative and may be considered a medical emergency if appropriate treatment is to be initiated. Many of these disorders can be treated effectively; if untreated, they can be lethal in the newborn period. Moreover, without the appropriate diagnosis, parents would not be aware of recurrence risks in future offspring.

Inborn errors of metabolism should be included in the differential diagnosis for any critically ill newborn in the following instances: (1) suspicion of neonatal sepsis; (2) recurrent vomiting or altered consciousness; (3) clinical findings of hypoglycemia, seizures, parenchymal liver disease, unusual odor, hyperammonemia, or unexplained acidosis; or (4) a family history of a sibling affected with similar symptoms, mental retardation, or sudden infant death syndrome.[25]

In general, laboratory analysis depends on the presenting symptoms seen in the newborn. Laboratory studies that should be obtained before any treatment is begun are electrolytes, ammonia, glucose, urine pH, urine-reducing substances, and urine ketones. Clues to a possible inborn error are (1) hypoglycemia and ketonuria in the newborn, (2) acidosis with recurrent vomiting and hyperammonemia, and (3) acidosis that is difficult to correct and is out of proportion to the clinical state. If other underlying disorders are not readily apparent, additional laboratory tests that may be appropriate are serum and urine amino acids and urine organic acids.[49] Moreover, molecular (DNA) testing is available for most disorders.[28]

NEWBORN SCREENING

Inborn errors of metabolism, when unrecognized and untreated, may lead to severe consequences, including intellectual disability and death in some instances. Thus, the goal is to identify, treat, and prevent major sequelae whenever possible. Newborn screening accomplishes this goal for a growing number of disorders (Box 27-2). Screening criteria that should be met are relatively high frequency of the disorder, severity of symptomatology in untreated individuals, availability of treatment, simplicity of obtaining tissue for testing,

---

| BOX 27-2 | A PARTIAL LIST OF DISORDERS THAT ARE SCREENED FOR IN NEWBORN SCREENING PROGRAMS |

Defects Identifiable by Tandem Mass Spectrometry (MS/MS)

Amino Acid Disorders and Urea Cycle Disorders

Phenylketonuria
Homocystinuria
Hypermethioninemia
Argininosuccinic acidemia
Citrullinemia
Argininemia
Tyrosinemia types I and II

Organic Acid Disorders

Maple syrup urine disease
Isovaleric acidemia
Methylmalonic acidemia
Propionic acidemia
Glutaric acidemia type I
Isobutyryl-CoA dehydrogenase deficiency
3-Hydroxy-3-methylglutaryl-CoA lyase deficiency
2-Methylbutyryl-CoA dehydrogenase deficiency
3-Methylcrotonyl-CoA carboxylase deficiency

Fatty Acid Oxidation Disorders

Medium-chain acyl-CoA dehydrogenase deficiency
Short-chain acyl-CoA dehydrogenase deficiency
Very-long–chain acyl-CoA dehydrogenase deficiency
Long-chain hydroxyacyl-CoA dehydrogenase deficiency
Glutaric acidemia type II
Carnitine palmityl transferase deficiency type II
Carnitine/acylcarnitine translocase deficiency
Multiple CoA carboxylase deficiency
Trifunctional protein deficiency

Disorders Screened by Other Methodologies

Congenital adrenal hyperplasia
Galactosemia
Sickle cell disease and hemoglobinopathies
Hypothyroidism (congenital)

Data from the National Newborn Screening and Genetics Resource Center; website: http://genes-r-us.uthscsa.edu.

---

and availability of a simple screening test with high sensitivity and specificity and reasonable cost. Recently, there have been major changes in the laboratory technologies available for newborn screening—specifically, the introduction of tandem mass spectrometry (MS/MS).[10] Using MS/MS technology, a single blood spot from a newborn can detect more than 50 inborn errors of metabolism.[39] Although many of the disorders detectable by MS/MS are rare, screening has been instituted in most states because screening remains inexpensive and a variety of disorders can be identified in a single assay. In most instances, additional testing adds approximately $25 to $60 to the cost of the newborn screen.[33]

MS/MS has been used for many years to measure metabolites in blood and urine. The technology is now applied to newborn screening programs. A mass spectrometer is an instrument that separates and quantifies ions based on their mass/charge ratios (m/z). In MS/MS, there are two spectrometers in a series. After sample preparation from the dried blood spot, the process of tandem mass is automated and the analysis is computerized. The process takes only a few seconds, and an entire screen takes less than 2 minutes.[33] The MS/MS system is capable of handling a high volume of samples; thus, it is an excellent technology for use in newborn screening. Currently the false-positive rate is 0.3% for all disorders.[57]

Screening for metabolic disorders is mandated by individual states, and all states require screening for phenylketonuria (PKU), hypothyroidism, congenital adrenal hyperplasia, sickle cell disease, s-beta thalassemia, and galactosemia.[39] However, the Recommended Uniform Screening Panel (RUSP) as noted by the American Academy of Pediatrics (AAP) and the American College of Medical Genetics have recommended that all states screen for a core panel of 31 treatable disorders and an additional 25 conditions that may be detected by screening.[3] The additional disorders most often screened for include amino acid disorders (homocystinuria, maple syrup urine disease), organic acids (glutaric, methylmalonic, and propionic acidemias), disorders of fatty acid metabolism (medium-chain and very-long–chain acyl-CoA dehydrogenase deficiency), hemoglobinopathies, and others such as biotinidase deficiency, congenital adrenal hyperplasia, and cystic fibrosis.[3]

Each state decides individually what will be included in its newborn screening program. Although some states require all of the tests on their list to be mandatory, other states offer a supplemental program in addition to the mandated program, often called *expanded newborn screening.* Testing for disorders listed on the mandated program is necessary, and only parents objecting on religious grounds may decline the mandated screen (e.g., Ohio Revised Code 3701.501). In those states offering a supplemental program, parents can choose whether to screen their child for the disorders listed. The program is optional, and no extra blood or additional tissue is necessary.[27] In most situations, parents are asked to sign a participation form to opt-in to the supplemental program. With states now using MS/MS in their newborn screening process,[39] state legislators are constantly changing and updating their screening practices. It behooves the clinician to periodically check with the state newborn screening program for updates. The National Newborn Screening and Genetics Resource Center (NNSGRC) provides up-to-date information.

Any screening test may give both false-positive and false-negative results; this includes those identified by MS/MS. Thus, a positive screen result must be followed by a confirmatory diagnostic test.[3] Moreover, if there is clinical suspicion of a particular disorder despite a negative screening result, further diagnostic testing is warranted. In addition to confirming positive screens, clinicians may have to deal with the concern for increased parental anxiety based on false-positive screens. Waisbren and colleagues found in a prospective interview study of 254 mothers and 153 fathers that stress levels of parents whose infants had false-positive screening results were significantly higher than those with normal results.[51] Thus, for clinicians in the NICU setting, being cognizant of the potential for an increased number of positive newborn screening results is important for the care of the neonate, as well as for parent teaching. (For an in-depth review of those disorders that may be part of the newborn screening program, refer to the AAP's newborn screening recommendations.)[3]

Newborn Hearing Screening. Newborn hearing screening tests are now available that have high sensitivity when administered properly.[4] Hearing loss is present in approximately 1 to 2 per 1000 infants. Research has demonstrated that there are both genetic and nongenetic causes of deafness. Sixty percent of prelingual deafness has a recognizable genetic etiology, and of these, the most common cause of autosomal recessively inherited nonsyndromic hearing loss results from mutations in the connexin 26

(Cx26) gene, a member of the connexin family of gap junction proteins.[56] Commercial DNA–based screening tests are now available to detect common genetic forms of deafness including **Cx26** and mitochondrial deafness.[5] The AAP has recommended that all newborns be screened for hearing loss before the age of 3 months.[2] The American College of Medical Genetics has recommended, in addition to screening and subsequent confirmation of hearing loss by diagnostic tests, that protocols be developed to ensure that appropriate genetic counseling be provided if diagnostic testing includes genetic testing.[5] This would provide families with accurate information about causes and recurrence risks for parents, siblings, and other family members.

ABNORMALITIES RESULTING FROM ENVIRONMENTAL EXPOSURES

Environmental exposures may have adverse (teratogenic) effects on fetal development, resulting in malformations and functional neurodevelopmental abnormalities in infants and children. The four major prerequisites needed for teratogenic action are as follows[20]:

1. The agent must have the potential to be teratogenic. Few conclusive data are available about the teratogenicity of most chemicals and drugs in humans. Animal studies provide most of the currently available data on the teratogenicity of agents; however, not all are always applicable to human situations. To prove that an agent is teratogenic, a causal relationship between the exposure and presence of a malformation must be documented; just the history of an exposure to an agent is not sufficient. Although very few agents have been documented to be teratogenic in humans, a few stand out, such as alcohol, cocaine, anticonvulsants, and isotretinoin (Accutane) (Figure 27-12).

2. The timing of the exposure during pregnancy is of major importance. For the agent to adversely affect the fetus, it must be present during organogenesis or histogenesis. Exposures occurring within the first 2 weeks after conception, before cell differentiation, will cause no damage or result in fetal wastage. Exposures occurring from 2 to 12 weeks of gestation (period of organogenesis) may result in major malformations. After completion of development of the major organ systems, harmful exposures usually do not result in malformations but can be responsible for organ dysfunction. However, some agents may morphologically disrupt previously intact organs.[11] Conversely, it has been shown that if the harmful exposure to an agent such as alcohol has been discontinued, the damage is less severe than if the exposure continues throughout the pregnancy.

3. Dosage of the teratogen is related to the severity of the teratogenic effect; the higher the dose, the more severe the effect and the higher the frequency of affected fetuses.

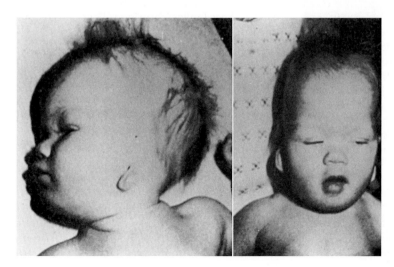

FIGURE 27-12 Infant exposed to Accutane in utero. Note dysmorphic face and auricles with atretic ear canal. (Courtesy Dr. Eva Sujansky, Genetic Services at The Children's Hospital, Denver, Colo.)

4. Finally, genetic makeup or genetic susceptibility of the mother and fetus may affect the
metabolism, as well as tissue sensitivity to the
teratogen.

Teratogenic agents may be divided into four categories: (1) infectious agents, (2) chemical agents
(drugs and environmental agents), (3) radiation, and
(4) maternal factors (such as maternal diabetes or
maternal PKU). Chapter 2 provides excellent overviews of most of these exposures.

Traditionally, only maternal exposures to teratogens have been implicated in malformations. There
has been a concern that some paternal exposures
also may be teratogenic. Theoretically, a teratogen
excreted in the semen could be introduced into the
fetal environment and potentially be teratogenic to
the developing fetus.[12]

Teratogenic exposures should be considered in the differential diagnosis of congenital
malformations and CNS dysfunction if one can
document fetal exposure and the phenotype is
compatible with the known effects of the suspected teratogen. The recognition of exposures
is important for genetic counseling; if they can be
avoided during subsequent pregnancies, recurrence
risk is not increased. Frequently there is phenotypic
overlap between the fetal abnormalities caused by
specific teratogens and other syndromes. The family
should be referred to a genetics clinic to rule out
chromosomal, single-gene, and sporadic syndromes
with overlapping phenotypes.

DATA COLLECTION

A genetic evaluation consists of the same components found in any medical evaluation; however, the
emphasis may be different. Moreover, to make an
accurate diagnosis and assessment, medical information about extended family members may
have to be obtained. An excellent overview of the
evaluation of the neonate with single or multiple
congenital anomalies is published by the American
College of Medical Genetics and available at their
website.[5]

History

Prenatal and perinatal histories, from a genetic
standpoint, should elicit information about potential teratogenic exposures including maternal

disease and acute illness. Fetal growth and behavior
(e.g., fetal movement, swallowing) provide important clues for the assessment of fetal neuromuscular
function. Thus information about fetal position,
movement, and amount of amniotic fluid should
be obtained. Perinatal history should include the
duration of gestation, anthropometric birth measurements including head circumference, and information about perinatal adaptation. In a newborn with
abnormal CNS functioning, it may be difficult to
differentiate between primary maldevelopment
and dysfunction caused by perinatal complications.
An abnormal newborn with a genetic disorder may present with signs suggestive of birth
asphyxia (i.e., hypoxia, acidosis, hypotonia, seizures). Moreover, because many a priori abnormal
newborns have an increased frequency of perinatal
complications, a documented birth injury does not
rule out the presence of a genetic cause.

Family history may be extremely helpful in
clarifying the causes and risk for recurrence. The
information obtained from the parents may have to
be complemented by physical examination of the
parents and other family members and review of
the medical records. This may be necessary because
parents may not be aware that different defects in
family members may be an expression of the same
disorder. For example, an autosomal dominant gene
may cause mild hypoplasia of thumbs in one family
member and complete absence of thumb and radii
in another.

A three-generation pedigree also should be
obtained that includes health information about
parents, siblings, grandparents, aunts, uncles, and
cousins. Specifically, information about miscarriages,
stillbirths, childhood deaths, relatives born with congenital malformations and birth defects, mental retardation, and other disorders that "run in the family"
should be obtained.[6] Information about ethnic background and consanguinity also should be collected.

Physical Examination

A physical examination should enable the examiner to detect major and minor malformations
(dysmorphic features). *Minor malformations* are
defined as structural variations found in less
than 4% of the general population and that
have no significant medical or cosmetic
effect. This is in contrast to structural variations
that are found in more than 4% of the newborn

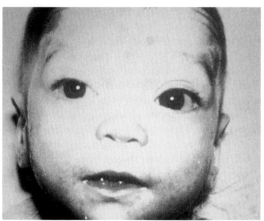

FIGURE 27-13 Dysmorphic feature of hypertelorism. Note wide-spaced eyes. (From Gilbert-Barness E, Kapur RP, Oligny LL, et al: *Potter's pathology of the fetus, infant, and child,* ed 2, St Louis, 2007, Mosby.)

population and represent a normal variation, such as a Mongolian spot and capillary hemangioma on the forehead. Minor malformations may provide important clues to the identification of a specific syndrome. None of the minor malformations as an isolated finding are clinically significant; however, a combination or pattern of minor malformations may indicate a specific disorder. For example, dysmorphic features such as up-slanted eyes, epicanthic folds, hypertelorism (Figure 27-13), and abnormal dermatoglyphic pattern (Figure 27-14) in an infant with a congenital heart defect are suggestive of Down syndrome. Minor malformations also may alert the clinician to the presence of major malformations. For example, preauricular ear tags are associated with an increased frequency of inner ear malformations and hearing impairment. In addition, the greater the number of minor malformations an infant has, the higher the chance of finding one or more major malformations.[30]

If minor malformations are identified, the parents of the infant should be examined. Presence of the same minor malformation in one of the parents may indicate a benign familial feature. Alternatively, finding the same dysmorphic features in other family members may represent an inherited genetic disorder. A mild syndactyly between the second and third toes is frequently an isolated, inherited finding without clinical significance. However, syndactyly associated with craniosynostosis

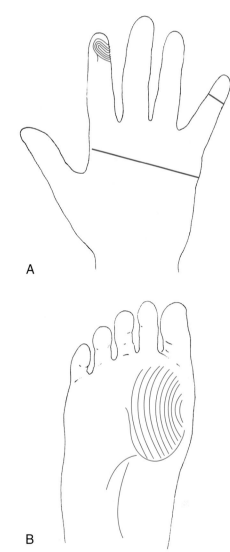

FIGURE 27-14 Dermatoglyphics commonly seen in infants with Down syndrome. **A,** Ulnar loop on the second digit, single flexion crease on the fifth digit, and single palmar crease (simian line). **B,** Tibial arch pattern on hallucal area of foot.

may represent an autosomal dominant disorder with variable expression and significant clinical sequelae.

If an infant looks dysmorphic, documentation of specific features should be recorded. Actual measurements compared with age-related norms should be used to measure body proportions, length of extremities, and such facial features as distance between eyes, length of eye fissures, size of ears, and length of philtrum. Description of the other features, such as the shape of the neck (webbed) or the chest size (widely spaced nipples), or a specific description of any skin lesions including size, shape, location, and color (hyperpigmented or hypopigmented) may provide important clues for a specific diagnosis. Dermatoglyphic analysis—the analysis of the dermal ridges on the digits, palms, and soles—may prove useful for determining the timing of a fetal insult.[54] Development of ridges begins during the thirteenth week of gestation and is complete by the nineteenth week. Thus, many chromosomal and genetic disorders have disruptions of the dermal ridge patterns. For example, an infant with Down syndrome may have a single palmar crease (simian crease), a single flexion crease of the fifth digit, and an open field pattern (tibial arch) on the hallucal area of the foot.[54] Moreover, specific descriptors or, even more useful, photographs, should be used to describe dysmorphic findings (such as noted in Figure 27-13).

Photographs are particularly important if the infant is critically ill and the constellation of findings does not immediately suggest a specific syndrome. Thus, the patient's findings may be more accurately shared with other clinicians in the future.

Smith's Recognizable Patterns of Human Malformation[23] and other texts document a large number of syndromes, some of which are rare and may not be immediately recognized by neonatal staff. It may be helpful and important to consult a clinician who is familiar with dysmorphology and syndromology to help establish a diagnosis.

Laboratory Data

When a genetic disorder is suspected, a number of diagnostic studies may be useful in delineating a diagnosis, including chromosome analysis, CGH array, molecular DNA testing, biochemical studies to rule out inborn errors of metabolism, radiographs, organ imaging, and when appropriate, autopsy. Not all of these studies are routinely used in all patients, but selection of studies is based on clinical suspicion of a particular disorder.

CHROMOSOME ANALYSIS

Routinely, results of chromosome analysis may not be available for 2 or 3 weeks. However, if results of chromosome analysis are urgently needed for clinical management, chromosome analysis from bone marrow can be available within a few hours and preliminary results from blood lymphocyte culture can be obtained in 48 hours. Indications for chromosome analysis have been listed previously. However, chromosome analysis should be obtained in all critically ill infants for whom there is no plausible explanation for their grave clinical course, before death occurs. For postmortem examination, chromosomes also may be obtained from any tissue—in particular, intracardiac blood, thymus, skin, and gonad. Under sterile conditions, these tissues should be obtained as soon as possible after the infant's demise. Tissue should be transported to the laboratory in a tissue culture medium or sterile saline solution, not in formalin.

MOLECULAR DNA ANALYSIS

There is a growing list of disorders for which the gene has been identified, and thus molecular diagnostic tests are commercially available. Although the Genetic Alliance, an international coalition comprising more than 1200 advocacy, research, and health care organizations, has access to databases with more than 1300 conditions at their website *(www.geneticalliance.org),* not all those disorders are amenable to DNA testing. Moreover, often a clinical diagnosis of a recognized syndrome does not require additional diagnostic testing.[5] However, if the diagnosis is not clear, if there is a need to confirm a diagnosis for management issues, or if additional information about a clinically recognized disorder is needed for family planning and genetic counseling, then DNA testing may be extremely helpful.[5]

Whenever the health care professional has a reasonable suspicion of a specific diagnosis based on clinical phenotype, it is reasonable to suggest molecular testing if it is available to confirm the diagnosis and provide appropriate genetic counseling. However, the clinician must remember that mutational analysis is complex and, although it can confirm a diagnosis when the test result is positive, a negative result may not determine conclusively that the neonate is not affected.[1] Some disorders (listed with their gene symbol or chromosomal locus) that might be seen in the neonate for which molecular gene testing is available are listed in Table 27-1.

BIOCHEMICAL STUDIES

A critically ill neonate who has a condition suggestive of an inborn error of metabolism or who

| TABLE 27-1 | PARTIAL LIST OF DISORDERS SEEN IN THE NEWBORN PERIOD WHERE DNA MOLECULAR TESTING IS AVAILABLE CLINICALLY | |

SYNDROME	GENE	CHROMOSOMAL LOCATION
Apert and Crouzon	FGFR2	10q26
Achondroplasia and thanatophoric dysplasia	FGFR3	4p16
Cystic fibrosis	CFTR	7q31
Congenital myotonic dystrophy	DMPK	19q13
Miller-Dieker	Microdeletion	17p13.3
Osteogenesis imperfecta	COL1A1 or COL1A2	17q21.3-q22
Pfeiffer	FGFR1	10q26
Prader-Willi and Angelman	Uniparental disomy, imprinting, deletion	15q11.3-q13
Smith-Lemli-Opitz	DHCR7	11q12-q13
Treacher Collins	TCOF1 POLR1C POLR1D	5q32-q33 6p21.1 13q12.2
22q11.2 deletion syndrome	Microdeletion	22q11.2
Waardenburg type 1	PAX3	2q35
Waardenburg type 2	MITF	3p14.1-p12.3
Williams	ELN (elastin)	7q11.2
Wolf-Hirschhorn	Microdeletion	4p16.3

has no specific diagnosis should have blood and urine sent for appropriate biochemical studies (specified in the "Inborn Errors of Metabolism" section). If such studies have not been obtained, postmortem tissue such as liver should be obtained and frozen for later biochemical analysis. Care providers should request detailed instructions from a laboratory specializing in testing for inherited metabolic disorders about which tissue is appropriate and how it should be obtained, stored, and shipped to the laboratory.

RADIOGRAPHS

X-ray examination should be obtained if a skeletal dysplasia or other skeletal abnormality is suspected or if the differential diagnosis includes a genetic syndrome that has skeletal defects as part of the phenotype. Moreover, if a localized skeletal defect is found, a skeletal survey should be obtained to identify other possible skeletal defects.

ORGAN IMAGING

Organ imaging by ultrasonography, magnetic resonance imaging (MRI), and computed tomography (CT) scan should be used to rule out structural abnormalities of major organs such as the brain, heart, and kidneys. Malformations may be suspected on the basis of clinical symptoms such as anuria or on the basis of known nonrandom associations of certain birth defects, such as the vertebral/anal/tracheoesophageal fistula/renal/radial (VATER) association. In addition, some dysmorphic features are associated with major malformations, and one must rule out these features. For example, there is an increased incidence of underlying midline brain defects associated with some facial dysmorphic features.

AUTOPSY

In the event of a neonate's death, an autopsy may provide crucial information for the establishment of a correct diagnosis. As outlined, chromosome analysis, biochemical studies, x-ray examination, and photographs should all be included. In the absence of a specific, confirmed diagnosis, the family should be strongly encouraged to consent to an autopsy, and a tissue sample should be frozen for further testing. Without this valuable information, subsequent genetic counseling of the parents, including clarification of the causes and recurrence risks, becomes impossible.

TREATMENT AND INTERVENTION

For most genetic disorders and malformations, there are no "cures" and only symptomatic treatment is available; that is, conventional medical and surgical interventions are instituted, although the basic genetic defect is not corrected. Surgical intervention for specific malformations will depend on the malformation, its cause, and prognosis. For example, surgical repair of a cleft lip and palate usually has an excellent outcome, although the underlying genetic cause has not been altered. In other instances, the diagnosis may provide direction and guidance to the health care professionals and family as to the appropriate course of action. An infant born with a hypoplastic left side of the heart may be considered a candidate for a heart transplant. However, if the cardiac malformation is the result of a chromosomal abnormality with an extremely poor prognosis, such as trisomy 13, the management of that infant may be palliative rather than corrective.

With the diagnosis of a metabolic disorder, treatment may be one of a nutritional or pharmacologic approach, such as the restriction of phenylalanine in an infant with PKU or the replacement of a deficient hormone, such as thyroid supplements in hypothyroidism. For some conditions, such as OI, the best approach may be educating the parents on specific techniques of holding and caring for an infant to prevent further fractures. In some disorders, organ or tissue transplantation may be appropriate. Bone marrow transplantation has been found to be effective in treating select genetic disorders, including lysosomal storage disorders[42] and beta-thalassemia.[36] Because specific treatment leading to a cure is not available for most genetic disorders, the use of genetic counseling and available reproductive alternatives, such as prenatal diagnosis, in vitro fertilization, preimplantation diagnosis, and artificial insemination by donor, are acceptable alternatives for some families.

THE HUMAN GENOME PROJECT

The year 2000 marked the announcement that the vast majority of the human genome had been sequenced.[13] This international effort, funded in part by the National Institutes of Health (NIH), began in 1990 with the development of genetic and physical maps of the human genome and completed its initial goals in 2000 with a draft of the sequencing of the 3 billion base pairs of the human genome. Defining the sequence of the human genome is only the beginning of the application of that knowledge to current and future research opportunities that will provide avenues for innovative therapies. With the introduction of massively parallel DNA sequencing (often referred to as NextGen sequencing), the ability to examine the entire genome is now doable. *Whole exome sequencing,* which is available clinically, allows for all the exomes in the genome (the coding portion of DNA) to be examined and to identify disease-causing mutations. *Whole genome sequencing* in which an individual's entire genome (all components of genes) is examined will soon be available clinically as well.[47] New powerful technologies for understanding gene expression are also being applied to designing drugs that will moderate disease pathways. Moreover, the field of genomics is providing opportunities to predict responsiveness to drug therapies, because reactions to drugs often are based on individual genetic variations.[47] With the identification of common gene variants involved in drug action or metabolism, health care professionals might be able to predict an infant's response—good or bad—to a particular drug regimen.[13]

With the numerous advances in molecular genetics, it is predicted that many genetic disorders and malformations may be amenable to treatment in utero or after birth. In utero correction of such birth defects as urinary tract malformations, myelomeningocele, and diaphragmatic hernia has been successful.[7,16,17] In 1990, the first human trial of gene therapy was undertaken at the NIH. The treatment was somatic gene replacement in a 4-year-old child with adenosine deaminase deficiency, a rare inherited disorder that destroys the immune system.[31] Successful efforts using improved gene therapy techniques continue with this disorder.[8] Since that time, a number of gene therapy trials for other genetic disorders have been done. Although the arena of gene therapy in general has been somewhat disappointing, the results have led to new areas of research and experimentation with new promising techniques.[45] The development of safer and more effective vectors based on technologies spearheaded by the Human Genome Project should provide significant improvements in gene therapy, such as that seen in an application of gene therapy with hemophilia B.[26]

PARENT TEACHING

The birth of any infant with a malformation or genetic disorder is a devastating event for any family. Members of the neonatal staff are on the front lines helping families deal with the infant's problems and providing the best environment for both the critically ill newborn and his or her family. In general, the most difficult factor for most parents and families to deal with is the unknown. Thus, once again, the need for an accurate diagnosis becomes paramount (Box 27-3). Moreover, even when the diagnosis carries a very poor prognosis, parents would prefer having the information so they can realistically anticipate and prepare for what is to come.[52] Currently, many parents obtain information about their infant's malformation or genetic disorder through prenatal diagnosis and have already begun the process of anticipatory grief by the time the infant is admitted to the NICU. Parental feelings of disbelief, shock, anger, or despair may have already been replaced with a "sense of relief" about confirmation of the abnormalities and a need to deal with the situation at hand.[32]

Chapter 30 provides an excellent review of the grief and mourning process that parents will experience when their anticipated "perfect baby" is born with a malformation or genetic disorder.

BOX 27-3	PARENT TEACHING
	GENETIC CONSIDERATIONS

- Genetic diagnosis is essential not only for management of the neonate's condition but also for counseling.
- Genetic counseling assists parents and care providers in addressing management issues such as cause and diagnosis, prognosis, treatment and interventions, short-term and long-term care, and follow-up.
- Genetic counseling assists parents in decisions about future pregnancies or the use of assistive reproductive technologies.

From a genetic counseling standpoint, a number of principles should be incorporated into the plan of care for the neonate and his or her family. First—and it cannot be overstated—an accurate diagnosis is essential if genetic counseling is to be provided. Even with what appears to be an isolated malformation, a genetics consultation may be appropriate to rule out other causes, such as single-gene disorders or chromosomal abnormalities. After establishing the diagnosis, one can realistically address the prognosis, treatment, and other management issues with the family. Finally, at the appropriate time for the family, recurrence risks and options for future pregnancies can be addressed (see the American College of Medical Genetics practice guideline regarding when a genetic consult may be helpful).[5]

Certainly, the busy and stressful environment of the NICU is not the most conducive atmosphere for obtaining and providing detailed information. However, it is appropriate for the geneticist to make an initial contact with the family in the NICU, where basic information about the pregnancy and perinatal and family histories can be obtained that will aid in diagnosis and defining the cause. The neonatal staff and geneticist can then address diagnosis and management. Later, at a time appropriate for the family, such issues as recurrence risks can be addressed. Eventually the family should receive a written summary of all the issues discussed for their own documentation.

The genetic evaluation is a complex and multifaceted process that cannot be done in isolation; it requires a team approach. The geneticist can assist the neonatal intensive care staff in determining the diagnosis, cause, and prognosis so that appropriate management of the infant can be implemented and aid in future counseling of the families they serve. The neonatal staff should use the genetics team as a resource for consultation and assistance in providing infants and families with the most appropriate and complete health care available.

REFERENCES

For a full list of references, scan the QR code or visit http://booksite.elsevier.com/9780323320832.

Congenital malformations may be found in up to 3% of all newborns and are an important cause of morbidity, early infant death, and chronic disability. Although overall infant mortality has declined, the mortality attributable to birth defects has increased, and up to 20% of neonatal deaths have been attributed to congenital malformations.[38] In the past decade, improvements in prenatal imaging and perinatology have allowed earlier diagnosis and intervention for surgically correctable malformations. Due to the complexity of accurate prenatal imaging and diagnosis, many anomalous conditions continue to escape early detection and present to the neonatology and surgical teams with advanced developmental consequences. The care of a neonate having a major congenital malformation may therefore be resource-intensive and costly. In a study of one regional neonatal intensive care unit (NICU), newborns having major congenital malformations accounted for 27% of NICU referrals, 32% of total NICU days, and 40% of NICU costs. Moreover, surgery was more frequent in newborns having major malformations, and one-third required ongoing medical support at the time of discharge.[30] Early diagnosis, comprehensive neonatal care, and a multidisciplinary approach are necessary to ensure an optimal outcome for both parent and child. This chapter briefly describes the embryology, clinical history, diagnostic evaluation, and therapeutic intervention of common neonatal surgical conditions.

DIAPHRAGMATIC HERNIA

Physiology and Etiology

Congenital diaphragmatic hernia (CDH) is a defect in closure of the diaphragm that occurs in 1 in 4000 live births. A posterolateral defect, or Bochdalek diaphragmatic hernia (Figure 28-1), accounts for nearly 95% of all CDH and may be left- (95%) or right-sided (5%). Much less common is the Morgagni diaphragmatic hernia (Figure 28-2), which results from a failure of anteromedial closure and resides in a substernal location. Several theories have been proposed to explain the mechanism for how this malformation of the diaphragm occurs, but currently the most widely accepted theory is failure of the pleuroperitoneal canal to close completely during the eighth week of gestation. If a patent pleuroperitoneal canal persists through the 11th week of gestation, a period when the intestine returns from its normal herniation into the umbilical cord, the stomach, bowel, and spleen may be forced into the chest. Resultant compression of the developing lung leads to a variable extent of pulmonary hypoplasia. Despite many studies in both animal models and infants over the past 4 decades, the causes of the pathophysiologic changes that occur in the underdeveloped lung are not well understood and are likely multifactorial. Recognition of the associated abnormal physiologic mechanisms has failed to define these alterations as cause or effect for the malfunctioning lung. In addition to alveolar hypoplasia, abnormal development of the pulmonary vasculature is a major contributor to the clinical challenges in managing CDH and its inherent risk for pulmonary hypertension. Postnatal blood flow through these hypoplastic lungs is compromised by both a reduced total number of pulmonary arterioles and an increased muscularization of the arteriolar bed. As a result, pulmonary vasculature capacitance is reduced and responsiveness to signals for smooth muscle relaxation may be lost. Persistent pulmonary hypertension after birth maintains patency and blood flow through natural fetal shunts. Resultant pulmonary hypoperfusion and systemic hypoxemia may be extreme and is often irreversible and recalcitrant to conventional therapy.

PURPLE type highlights content that is particularly applicable to clinical settings.

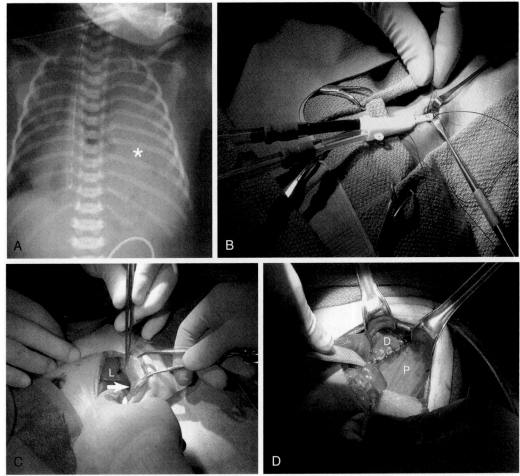

FIGURE 28-1   Newborn with left congenital diaphragmatic hernia, or Bochdalek hernia. **A**, Chest radiograph shows liver herniation *(asterisk)* into the left chest. Note displacement of heart to right and minimally aerated lung on left. **B**, Dual-lumen venovenous cannulation via right internal jugular vein for extracorporeal life support (ECLS). **C**, Four days later, the infant had stabilized on ECLS, so repair was performed in the neonatal intensive care unti on ECLS. Note left lobe of liver (L) herniating beneath a diminutive anterior leaflet of the left diaphragm (in forceps). Left lobe of liver is between forceps and surgeon index finger. **D**, Defect required a biosynthetic patch (P; D, anterior leaflet of diaphragm).

Data Collection

HISTORY

Technological advances in ultrasonography have facilitated earlier and more accurate antenatal diagnosis of diaphragmatic hernias, permitting planning of intervention and counseling of parents, as appropriate. High-quality prenatal ultrasound can diagnose a congenital diaphragmatic hernia early in pregnancy and also identify high-risk infants who have worse outcomes. Prenatal lung-to-head ratio (LHR) is a widely accepted prognostic tool that is

measured at 28 weeks' gestation using ultrasound. A LHR of less than 1.2 can identify infants who have a higher risk of recquiring extracorporeal membrane oxygenation (ECMO) support and death. Identification of the left lateral segment of the liver in the thoracic cavity also identifies infants who have worse outcomes. Recently, fetal MRI to identify lung volumes has been shown to be a useful prognostic tool in infants with CDH. Prenatal identification of high-risk infants with CDH allows the mother to deliver in a high-risk perinatal center with the appropriate level

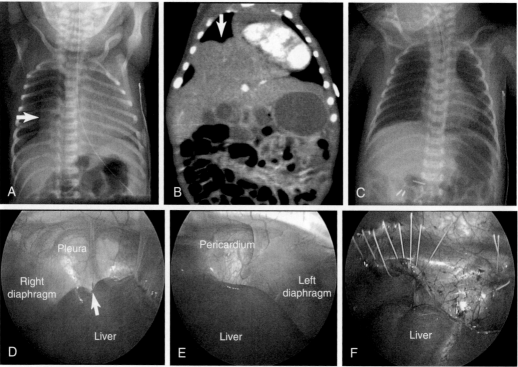

FIGURE 28-2 Newborn with anterior Morgagni diaphragmatic hernia. **A, B,** Chest radiograph and computed tomography (CT) scan, respectively. Arrows show liver herniation. **C,** Postoperative chest radiograph shows complete reduction of liver and correction of hernia. **D-F,** Laparoscopic technique to repair large anterior defect: Right and left diaphragms are sutured to abdominal wall anteriorly; sutures are passed through the entire wall of abdomen and knots are secured below skin level. Arrow shows groove in liver corresponding with CT scan image.

of neonatal and surgical support on standby. Although in utero surgical techniques to promote lung growth and passive reduction of the herniated abdominal contents seemed promising initially, as of this writing, a moratorium has been placed indefinitely on this approach because a demonstrable survival benefit has not been shown largely due to advances made in postnatal care of CDH.[57] Some fetal surgery centers, particularly European, continue to explore minimally invasive means to promote lung growth in utero and thereby reduce the herniated abdominal contents. The Achilles' heel of fetal intervention, however, is the risk of preterm labor and the consequent morbidity of prematurity, risks that must be weighed collectively against a term delivery but with profound compromise in lung development.

SIGNS AND SYMPTOMS

Respiratory distress may develop immediately after birth or after an initial period of relative stability. If significant pulmonary hypoplasia is present and fetal circulation persists, the newborn may become rapidly symptomatic, heralded by profound respiratory distress and circulatory shock. Because much of the bowel is herniated into the chest, the abdomen appears scaphoid and the anteroposterior diameter of the chest may enlarge as the bowel distends with air. Breath sounds are diminished or absent on the affected side, and the mediastinum may be displaced toward the contralateral side. Associated anomalies of the cardiovascular system may include patent ductus arteriosus, aortic coarctation, and hyoplastic left heart syndrome, which require detailed echocardiographic evaluation. Other associated anomalies requiring evaluation include central nervous system (CNS) malformations, genitourinary anomalies, esophageal atresia, omphalocele, cleft palate, and cardiovascular defects.[48]

LABORATORY DATA

A chest radiograph is obtained and shows bowel herniated into the ipsilateral thoracic space with contralateral displacement of the heart. An echocardiogram is necessary to assess cardiac function, degree of pulmonary hypertension, and presence of significant congenital cardiac anomalies. Nonrotation of the intestine is an understood feature of CDH and does not require specific evaluation as a newborn.

Treatment

PREOPERATIVE CARE (STABILIZATION)
As soon as a diaphragmatic hernia is suspected, an orogastric tube should be placed to prevent further distention of the stomach and bowel and to alleviate compression of the lung. The newborn with CDH commonly requires endotracheal intubation and mechanical ventilation to maintain adequate gas exchange. Because cardiac function may also be compromised, a combination of pressor medications such as dopamine, dobutamine, and milrinone may need to be administered. The earlier the infant becomes symptomatic, the more severe the respiratory compromise and the poorer the prognosis may be. Despite the primary defect in the diaphragm, the major determinants of outcome are pulmonary hypertension and lung hypoplasia.

A significant number of CDH newborns may have such severe pulmonary hypertension refractory to conventional or alternative (e.g., high-frequency oscillation or jet) ventilation that extracorporeal life support (ECLS; venovenous and venoarterial) may be required to establish effective gas exchange and end-organ perfusion. The overriding principle in stabilizing CDH newborns is to reduce barotrauma and oxygen toxicity that result in chronic lung disease. Strategies now emphasize *gentle ventilation* and *permissive hypercapnea,* so long as arterial pH does not drift significantly low (<7.25).

OPERATIVE INTERVENTION
Surgical repair does not alter early outcome. Therefore, the baby's condition should be stabilized and efforts directed toward the management of the associated pulmonary hypoplasia and hypertension. Early repair within the first 72 hours of life is indicated only in infants having little or no pulmonary dysfunction. If severe pulmonary insufficiency is present, medical therapies of conventional or high-frequency mechanical ventilation, inhaled nitric oxide, or ECLS are instituted. If these modalities are successful in stabilizing the baby, surgical repair is generally performed between 4 and 14 days of life.[58] If

ECLS has been needed to stabilize the newborn having CDH, some centers advocate herniorrhaphy while on bypass, whereas other centers recommend repair after decannulation (see Figure 28-1).

Most commonly through a subcostal transabdominal approach, the surgeon reduces the stomach, intestine, and spleen from the chest to the abdominal cavity and repairs the diaphragmatic defect. If the defect is large, a prosthetic patch may be required to complete closure of the hernia. Closure of the abdominal wound may be difficult as well because of underdeveloped abdominal wall musculature and loss of abdominal domain. In these circumstances, if abdominal closure is not possible or may result in abdominal hypertension, simple skin closure or prosthetic silo placement may be necessary to cover the abdominal contents, leaving a large ventral hernia for future repair when abdominal domain is more adequate and the baby is more stable. Chest tube placement depends on risk for bleeding, which may be significant if repair is performed on ECLS (because of anticoagulation during extracorporeal membrane oxygenation therapy) or if risk of pneumothorax is anticipated. Minimally invasive techniques to repair CDH may also be utilized in newborns (see Figure 28-2) but may not be well tolerated in fragile neonates. Appropriate patient selection is a premium. Thoracoscopic and laparoscopic techniques to repair CDH have been described and may be better suited for infants who present out of the newborn period and without physiologically significant pulmonary hypoplasia or hypertension.

POSTOPERATIVE CARE
The principal postoperative concern remains effective ventilation and oxygenation while imparting the least amount of barotrauma and toxicity. If conventional mechanical ventilation fails, high-frequency oscillation and inhaled nitric oxide are employed.[26] ECLS is reserved in this setting as a salvage therapy for babies who revert back to fetal circulation and who do not respond to these less invasive modalities.

Complications and Prognosis

The survival rate for newborns having CDH and who require mechanical ventilation in the first 18 to 24 hours of life is approximately 64%. If an infant with a diaphragmatic hernia does not present with respiratory distress in the first 24 hours of life, survival approaches 100%. As improvements in *gentle ventilation* strategies have emerged, a gradual, albeit small, increase in survival has been realized.[48] The primary, early pathophysiologic consequence of CDH is pulmonary hypertension. Late complications include chronic lung disease, recurrent diaphragmatic hernia, gastroesophageal reflux, skeletomuscular deformities (including scoliosis), and growth restriction.[36] Long-term neurologic outcomes have recently become important to evaluate as perinatal mortality has decreased. Survivors of CDH continue to have impaired neurologic development as evidenced by hearing impairment, hypotonicity, and psychomotor dysfunction, affecting collectively 30% to 50% of children with CDH. Basic and clinical research continue in an effort to identify improved therapies for the complex pulmonary dysfunction associated with CDH not only to close the persistent and large survival gap but also to optimize quality of life among survivors.

ESOPHAGEAL ATRESIA AND TRACHEOESOPHAGEAL FISTULA

Physiology and Etiology

Esophageal atresia (EA) occurs between 1 in 3000 to 4500 live births and represents a spectrum of anomalies that arise early in gestation (3–6 weeks) when the trachea normally buds from the primitive foregut. Failure in the normal development of the esophagus and incomplete separation of the trachea from the esophagus gives rise to esophageal atresia (EA) and distal tracheoesophageal fistula (TEF) in 85% of cases, isolated esophageal atresia in 8%, TEF without EA in 5%, or EA with proximal or proximal and distal fistulas in 2%. Etiologies for this collection of defects remain unclear, but it is suspected that genetic alterations in and environmental insults on rapidly proliferating foregut stem cells during this critical period of organogenesis account for such diverse yet predictable esophageal malformations. Aberrations at the cellular level in muscle fibers of the distal esophagus may help explain the nearly universal symptoms of dysmotility and gastroesophageal reflux after operative repair.[29] Because other developing organs are vulnerable to the same insults in this critical period of gestation, associated anomalies are common (50%–70%), particularly vertebral, anorectal, cardiac, genitourinary, limb, and gastrointestinal

(e.g., duodenal atresia).[14,54] In 11% to 33% of infants with EA and distal TEF, concurrent and severe tracheomalacia is present and is manifested by stridorous breathing. Although EA with or without TEF has not been associated with a single gene defect, a high incidence has been observed in children having trisomy 21 (Down syndrome).[38]

Data Collection

HISTORY

Maternal polyhydramnios may suggest EA or other conditions in which the fetus does not swallow amniotic fluid normally.

SIGNS AND SYMPTOMS

Babies with EA are identified soon after birth because of excessive salivary secretions and inability to swallow feedings. Upon feeding, these babies quickly cough and regurgitate undigested formula or breast milk. When attempting to pass an orogastric tube, obstruction is typically encountered between 8 to 12 cm from the lips, and the diagnosis of esophageal atresia is established. If a distal tracheoesophageal fistula is also present, air passes into the stomach and bowel and is present on plain abdominal radiographs. Respiratory distress may arise if gastric secretions reflux through the TEF and into the lungs, which may incite profound chemical pneumonitis. Symptoms of an "H"-type fistula in the absence of esophageal atresia are less obvious and require a high index of suspicion. Coughing and choking with feedings, or recurrent pneumonia over the first months of life, suggest the presence of an occult tracheoesophageal fistula (Box 28-1).

BOX 28-1 CRITICAL FINDINGS

ESOPHAGEAL ATRESIA AND TRACHEOESOPHAGEAL FISTULA

Critical assessment findings for esophageal atresia and tracheoesophageal fistula are as follows:

- Excessive secretions
- Feeding intolerance
- Inability to pass orogastric tube
- Abdominal distention
- Other findings associated with VACTERL (Vertebrae, Anus, Cardiac system, Trachea, Esophagus, Renal (urinary tract), and Limbs)

PHYSICAL EXAMINATION

Once esophageal atresia has been established, the infant should be carefully examined to exclude other anomalies of the VACTERL association, a variable sequence of anomalies affecting the **V**ertebrae, **A**nus, **C**ardiac system, **T**rachea, **E**sophagus, **R**enal (urinary tract), and **L**imbs.[7] Echocardiography permits both the identification of significant cardiac anomalies and the presence of a right- or left-sided aortic arch, which have important implications in the operative approach.

LABORATORY DATA

After obstruction is met with passing of an orogastric tube, a plain radiograph of the chest and abdomen should be obtained with the tube left in place, which is visualized usually at the second or third thoracic vertebra and above the carina. The stomach and intestines may contain luminal air if a distal TEF is present. If no distal fistula exists, the abdomen on radiograph will appear gasless. In the rare setting of EA, distal TEF, and duodenal atresia, the abdominal gas pattern may show the classic "double-bubble" sign, as gas fills the stomach and proximal duodenum only.

Treatment

PREOPERATIVE CARE

Once the diagnosis of EA is established, a 10-Fr Replogle tube is placed in the upper esophageal pouch and set to low continuous suction to prevent aspiration of oral secretions. While awaiting operation, the neonate should be kept in the head-up position and initiated on antireflux medication to minimize gastroesophageal reflux and the consequent risk of acid-induced pneumonitis. Operative repair, in general, is not an emergency procedure. Patients first should be evaluated thoroughly for other associated anomalies by physical examination, echocardiography to delineate the anatomy of the heart and great vessels, abdominal ultrasound of the kidneys and genitourinary tracts, and plain radiographs of the spine and limbs. Newborns having cyanotic congential heart disease may require a palliative cardiac procedure before reconstruction of the esophagus.

If infants with EA and distal TEF are born prematurely and have respiratory distress syndrome (i.e., "stiff lungs"), a significant portion of mechanical tidal volumes, delivered under positive pressure, may be shunted preferentially through the fistula and into the stomach. As a result, effective ventilation is lost and critical gastric distention ensues, further restricting diaphragmatic excursion. Emergent ligation of the TEF with gastrostomy tube insertion is necessary in such instances to restore effective ventilation.

OPERATIVE INTERVENTION

The type of esophageal malformation dictates the surgical approach. Surgical repair of esophageal atresia with or without tracheoesophageal fistula is generally not an emergency but should be carried out as soon as the patient is stable. If the infant is in otherwise good health and the gap between esophageal elements is not too large, primary anastomosis is indicated through a right thoracotomy and retropleural approach. To reduce the pain and potential morbidities associated with a thoracotomy, some surgeons recommend repair thoracoscopically in appropriately selected patients (Figure 28-3).

Unfortunately, in isolated esophageal atresia, the gap distance is generally too long to allow early primary repair. If the gap length is considered too great, with or without TEF, or if the child is too ill, a delayed or staged repair is planned. An early gastrostomy is placed for decompression and feeding, and the TEF if present is divided to prevent reflux into the tracheobronchial tree. After a variable period of time to allow resolution of pneumonitis or maximum growth of the distal esophagus, a second operation completes the repair. To promote lengthening and growth of the distal esophagus in cases of isolated EA, buogienage or balloon dilation may be performed via a mature gastrostomy tract.

If delayed or staged repair is planned, secretions must be controlled. Suction catheters placed in the upper pouch are maintained to reduce the risk of aspiration. In rare cases, reconstruction using the native esophagus is not possible. In these circumstances, esophageal replacement using gastric or colon transposition is necessary. If the infant is not a candidate for early operation because of a lethal chromosomal defect or severe congenital heart disease, cervical esophagostomy and gastrostomy are performed to palliate the infant, and esophageal replacement is performed later, as indicated.

POSTOPERATIVE CARE

Postoperative care includes appropriate pain control and pulmonary care, parenteral nutrition, and a brief

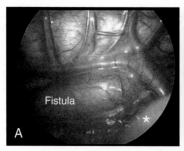
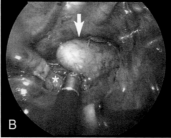
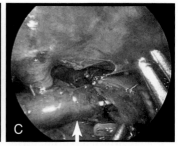

FIGURE 28-3 Thoracoscopic repair of esophageal atresia with distal tracheoesophageal fistula in a newborn. **A,** View of tracheoesophageal fistula, which is distended from ventilation. Azygous vein is obscuring connection to trachea. **B,** After division of azygous vein, one can visualize the fistulous connection *(asterisk)* of the distal esophagus to the posterior trachea. Upper atretic pouch has been mobilized and is being elevated with instrument. **C,** Suturing of upper esophagus to distal esophagus. Replogle tube has been advanced through anastomosis after approximation of posterior row initially. For perspective of small working space, 3- and 5-mm instruments are used for this procedure.

course of systemic antibiotics. Tracheal and esophageal suction catheters should not come in contact with the newly repaired esophagus and trachea, because suture line disruption may cause a leak or recurrent fistula, both potentially catastrophic complications. Antibiotic therapy is continued for 48 to 72 hours. A chest tube and/or retropleural drain is placed to control an anastomotic leak, should it occur. Before initiating oral feedings an esophagram is usually obtained within 7 to 10 days of repair to verify complete anastomotic healing and absence of leak. All EA babies have some degree of esophageal dysmotility and gastroesophageal reflux (GER) after repair. Elevating the head of the bed 30 to 45 degrees, administering histamine H_2 antagonists or proton pump inhibitors, and slow feeding may help to control reflux symptoms.

Complications and Prognosis

Postoperative complications include anastomotic leak and/or stricture, and esophageal dysmotility. Anastomotic leaks may occur in up to 20% of patients and generally are treated conservatively with chest tube drainage, parenteral nutrition, antibiotics, and time for healing. The vast majority of leaks close without operative intervention but tend to heal with some degree of stricture, commonly amenable to dilation. Anastomotic strictures are the most common postoperative complication after EA-TEF repair occurring in 30% to 50% of infants with EA-TEF. In the majority of infants who develop a postoperative esophageal

stricture, esophageal dilation is an effective therapy to maintain esophageal patency, and only a minority of infants (2%–10%) require reoperation and reconstruction of the esophageal anastomosis. Esophageal strictures often are associated with or exacerbated by GER and may be treated successfully by esophageal dilation. If GER is complicated by stricture and is refractory to maximal medical therapy, a fundoplication procedure may rarely be necessary. Some degree of esophageal dysmotility usually exists because of poor peristalsis in the distal esophagus. The child may adapt to a poorly functioning esophagus by altering his or her feeding habits. However, in infancy, gastrostomy feeding may be necessary to prevent vomiting and aspiration. Postoperative airway complications include tracheobronchomalacia and recurrent laryngeal nerve injury with vocal cord dysfunction.

With modern neonatal care and surgical techniques, long-term survival after repair of esophageal atresia and tracheoesophageal fistula is excellent.[14] Prognosis depends on largely two factors: one, the presence and type of cardiac anomalies, and two, the presence of prematurity and respiratory distress syndrome. A useful system to predict survival is the Spitz classification, which stratifies infant survival by birth weight and major cardiac anomaly[50]:

   I: Birth weight greater than 1500 g, no major CHD, survival is greater than 97%
  II: Birth weight less than 1500 g or major CHD, survival is 59%
 III: Birth weight less than 1500 g and major CHD, survival is 22%

CONGENITAL CHEST MASSES

Physiology and Etiology

The most common congenital chest masses requiring surgical intervention in the newborn period are congenital pulmonary airway malformations (CPAMs, also known as cystic adenomatoid malformation), pulmonary sequestrations (both intralobar and extralobar types), bronchogenic cysts, and congenital lobar emphysema. Each of these malformations may exist alone or in combination with other anomalies.

CPAM lesions are believed to arise from focal interruption in coordinated pulmonary progenitor cell growth, resulting in abnormal development of pulmonary tissues and structural distortion. Histologically, CPAM is associated with increased cell proliferation and decreased apoptosis compared with normal lung tissue. The CPAM lesion receives its blood supply from the pulmonary system but does not communicate with normally formed bronchial structures.

Anomalous development of the foregut is the accepted underlying etiology of both the bronchogenic cyst and pulmonary sequestration. Bronchogenic cysts are lined by ciliated columnar and/or cuboidal epithelium. The surrounding tissues resemble those of the normal bronchus and are generally, although not exclusively, located within the mediastinum along the tracheobronchial tree. Extralobar sequestrations are masses of primitive pulmonary parenchyma with no bronchial connection and are supplied by the systemic and not pulmonary vasculature. Congenital lobar emphysema presents in the newborn period as a fluid-filled, overdistended lobe that, under positive-pressure ventilation, may trap air and generate tension physiology. In many cases, although not all, congenital lobar emphysema is associated with the absence or hypoplasia of cartilaginous rings of the major and segmental bronchi. These structurally underdeveloped bronchi are prone to collapse on expiration, thereby trapping air.

Data Collection

HISTORY, SIGNS, AND SYMPTOMS

Although rare, congenital lung malformations may lead to considerable morbidity, such as infection, hemorrhage, respiratory failure, and pulmonary hypoplasia, and may even prove lethal. Some lesions may escape prenatal detection and so appear later in development. Failure to recognize a malformation may lead to inappropriate intervention. For example, placement of a chest tube to manage suspected tension pneumothorax in a baby having congenital lobar emphysema may lead to lung injury and loss of tidal volume through the thoracostomy tube instead of into the remaining healthy lung.

Congenital Pulmonary Airway Malformation. CPAMs are more and more commonly detected prenatally and are nicely characterized on fetal ultrasound, but if not, may be further delineated by fetal magnetic resonance imaging, as indicated. In utero, these lesions may cause a variety of problems, from pulmonary hypoplasia (both ipsilateral and contralateral) to nonimmune hydrops fetalis with congestive heart failure. Polyhydramnios may also be present if the lesion compresses the esophagus and compromises fetal swallowing of amniotic fluid. Fetal intervention may be indicated if the gestation has not yet reached 34 weeks, in which case premature delivery might be planned. Large fluid-filled cystic lesions may be amenable to thoracoamniotic shunt placement while in utero to relieve compression of intrathoracic structures and to restore hemodynamic status. Solid CPAM lesions arising early in gestation and causing similar complications have been resected in fetuses with promising results. If these lesions do not manifest with in utero pathophysiology but are of sufficient size, the neonate may develop respiratory distress shortly after birth. This process is responsible for the cystic appearance on radiographs. Infants may have mediastinal shift and large air spaces, easily confused with a pneumothorax or diaphragmatic hernia. Sonography may be helpful to delineate a solid or cystic mass and should establish the diagnosis. CPAM may result in recurrent infections because mucociliary clearance is poor. Rarely, malignancy may arise in a CPAM in the form of pulmonary blastoma, rhabdomyosarcoma, or bronchoalveolar carcinoma.

Pulmonary Sequestration. Pulmonary sequestration accounts for less than 10% of all congenital lung malformations and mostly occurs in the lower lobes. A sequestration represents a mass of disorganized bronchopulmonary tissue without a normal bronchial communication and may have either a pulmonary or systemic vascular supply. The abnormal sequestered lung tissue may be intralobar or extralobar and is classified according to pleural coverage, either within the pleural investment of the whole lung itself (intralobar) or outside of this normal pleural lining (extralobar). Sequestrations may rarely have some sort of communication with the foregut. Infants having an intralobar sequestration not detected prenatally may present outside of the newborn period and often with recurrent respiratory problems, such as chronic cough, or with recurrent pneumonias, either in the lesion or in the surrounding normal but compressed lung tissue. Plain radiographs may simply show consolidation. Anomalies associated with extralobar sequestration include diaphragmatic hernia and eventration and may share a similar dysregulated embryologic event because approximately 95% of extralobar lesions are left-sided. Extralobar lesions may reside either above or below the left diaphragm. Older children may have exercise intolerance if a large systemic arteriovenous shunt exists. Systemic arterial flow though the lesion may produce a murmur and may lead to congestive cardiac failure. Squamous cell carcinoma, adenocarcinoma, and rhabdomyosarcoma may rarely arise in the sequestration.

Bronchogenic Cyst. Bronchogenic cysts may be considered a foregut duplication, and arise from an abnormal budding of the ventral foregut. Approximately 85% are mediastinal, and 15% are intrapulmonary. Bronchogenic cysts may be filled with air or fluid and may show air-fluid levels on plain radiographs. As a result, bronchogenic cysts may become infected or simply grow over time, and so may behave as a space-occupying and compressive lesion. Many cysts are asymptomatic or have vague symptoms and are discovered on routine chest radiographs. Infection, hemorrhage, and, in rare cases, late malignancy may occur. Associated respiratory symptoms include stridor or wheezing. Chronic air trapping may lead to emphysema, atelectasis, or both. Dysphagia, chest pain, and epigastric discomfort may also occur.

Congenital Lobar Emphysema. Although generally not discovered in utero, congenital lobar emphysema typically manifests in neonates as hyperinflation of one or more lung lobes. Causes include intrinsic absence or abnormality (bronchomalacia) of cartilaginous rings or external compression of

a segmental bronchus by a large pulmonary artery that predispose to air trapping. Hyperinflation of a pulmonary lobe develops after birth because inspired air enters the affected lobe but cannot exit, because the positive pressure of expiration collapses the malacic airway. Congenital lobar emphysema most commonly involves the upper lobes. The left upper lobe is involved in roughly 41% of patients; the right middle lobe in 34%; and the right upper lobe in 21%. Involvement of the lower lobes is rare, occurring in fewer than 5% of patients. Neonates may present with mild-to-moderate respiratory distress. Mediastinal shift may develop with progressive air trapping, and decreased breath sounds are noted on the involved side. Infants who have a milder form of lobar emphysema will present with nonspecific findings, including cough, wheezing, respiratory distress, and cyanosis. Older children may present with recurrent chest infections. On plain radiographs obtained in neonates, the affected lobe may be hyperlucent or slightly opacified if alveoli remain fluid filled. Associated cardiac anomalies may occur in as many as 10% of patients.

LABORATORY DATA

Routine chest radiograph is the initial evaluation tool in distinguishing congenital chest masses and is the principal study to establish the diagnosis of diaphragmatic hernia and congenital lobar emphysema in newborns. Sonography and/or computed tomography (CT) scan of the chest are useful means to evaluate CPAM, sequestrations, bronchogenic cysts, and lobar emphysema in older infants and children. The differential diagnosis of a hyperlucent hemithorax with mediastinal shift on chest x-ray study in the newborn includes tension pneumothorax, cystic CPAM, diaphragmatic hernia with air-filled stomach or intestine in the chest, and congenital lobar emphysema.

Treatment

Surgical resection of these congenital chest masses is curative. Some small, asymptomatic lesions of sequestration or CPAM may be followed expectantly because reports of spontaneous regression may be found in the literature; however, most lesions may be removed with little morbidity in an effort to minimize long-term complications of the various lesions. Operative approach to these lesions

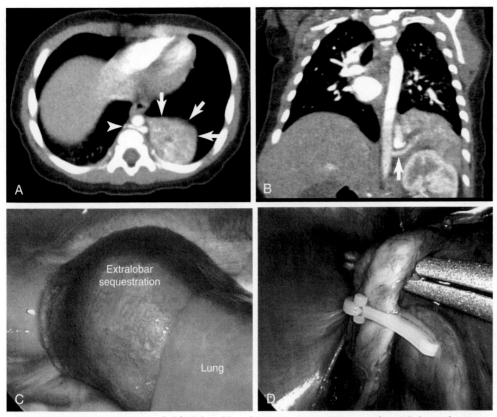

FIGURE 28-4 Thoracoscopic resection of a left-sided extralobar pulmonary sequestration (ELPS) in a newborn. **A, B,** Computed tomography scan shows ELPS at base of left chest (*arrows* in **A**). Note large vein coursing behind aorta in **A** (arrowhead) and large artery supplying lesion directly from aorta in **B** (*arrow*). **C,** Thoracoscopic view of ELPS (looking toward diaphragm). **D,** Clipping of large artery and vein. Lesion is then removed through one of the port sites.

may be either via thoracotomy or thoracoscopy, depending on the suitability of the baby and the skill set of the surgeon (Figures 28-4 and 28-5).

Special consideration to resection of the pulmonary lobe involved with congenital lobar emphysema should be given (Figure 28-6). Extreme caution must be followed upon induction of general anesthesia and endotracheal intubation with positive-pressure ventilation. Because of the malacic airway and the propensity for air trapping in congenital lobar emphysema, rapid development of tension physiology may ensue, compromising the well-being of the baby and necessitating emergent decompressive thoracotomy. Such pathophysiology is possible in any neonate having congenital lobar emphysema and requiring positive-pressure ventilation.

INTESTINAL MALROTATION AND VOLVULUS

Physiology and Etiology

In the fourth week of gestation, the midgut exists as a straight tube deriving its blood supply from the superior mesenteric artery (SMA). The proximal limb of primitive intestine, representing the future duodenum, jejunum, and proximal ileum, lies in the midline and anterior to the SMA. The distal limb, destined to become the terminal ileum, ascending and transverse colon, lies posterior to the SMA. During the sixth week of gestation, these segments of bowel, known collectively as the midgut, are able to lengthen rapidly by herniating through the incompletely closed abdominal wall and into the umbilical stalk. While

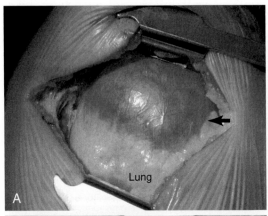

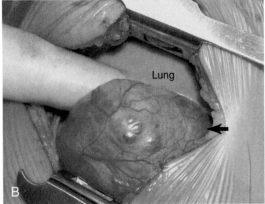

FIGURE 28-5 Thoracotomy in a newborn for congenital pulmonary airway malformations. Views of anterior **(A)** and undersurface **(B)** of cystic lesion *(arrows)*.

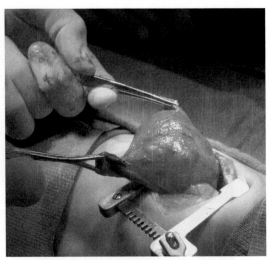

FIGURE 28-6 Thoracotomy in a newborn for congenital lobar emphysema. Note overdistended nature of emphysematous lobe compared with normal lobe just peering out from inferior aspect of wound.

lengthening outside of the coelomic cavity, the midgut undergoes a 270-degree counterclockwise rotation around the SMA axis. On return to the abdominal cavity, the duodenojejunal junction comes to rest in the left upper quadrant and becomes fixed in this location by the ligament of Treitz. At the end of the 11th week of gestation, midgut rotation is completed, and the cecum now resides anterior and to the right of the SMA and is fixed in the right lower quadrant. Because of the counterclockwise nature of this intestinal rotation, the ascending and transverse colon lie to the right of the SMA. The hindgut (splenic flexure of the colon to the rectum) then fixes in the left hemiabdomen and derives its blood supply largely from the inferior mesenteric artery (IMA).

Failure of this rotation and fixation results in the clinical condition termed *malrotation,* which covers a

wide spectrum of rotational anomalies. *Complete nonrotation* is characterized by the entire small bowel existing on the right side of the abdomen and the colon principally to the left. *Partial malrotation* involves the improper fixation of a single segment. *Complete malrotation* is thought to occur from a lax umbilical ring allowing the gut to return en masse to the abdomen. Because proper rotation does not occur, the root of the mesentery is not anchored in the left upper quadrant, and the superior mesenteric artery and vein loosely suspend the entire bowel without fixation. This unfixed, narrow mesenteric pedicle predisposes the midgut and its tenuous blood supply to twisting or volvulus. If volvulus occurs, the blood supply to the midgut may be compromised, leading rapidly to ischemia and bowel infarction. The majority of patients having midgut malrotation are diagnosed in the first month of life but may be seen with decreasing frequency in the older child or rarely the adult.[33]

By definition, malrotation also exists in several anomalies, including gastroschisis, omphalocele, and congenital diaphragmatic hernia, because the midgut is trapped and unable to rotate and fix properly in these conditions.

Data Collection

HISTORY

Malrotation may manifest in the newborn simply as a proximal mechanical bowel obstruction caused by abnormal attachments, or Ladd's bands, between the cecum and porta hepatis. These babies typically show some degree of feeding intolerance early on with or without bilious emesis. A more worrisome presentation of malrotation may arise acutely, should the bowel volvulize around its unfixed, narrow vascular pedicle. These babies present with an acute, high-grade proximal bowel obstruction. In a neonate who develops midgut volvulus, the first few days of life usually are unremarkable, but then the baby develops acute feeding intolerance and bilious emesis in the absence of abdominal distention. If a delay in diagnosis occurs, intestinal ischemia sets in, and the symptoms may progress rapidly to an acute abdomen and profound shock as a result of gangrenous bowel. Abdominal wall erythema and distention are usually present in advanced stages of intestinal ischemia and are ominous findings.[52]

SIGNS AND SYMPTOMS

The symptoms of nonvolvulized malrotation mimic those of duodenal stenosis or atresia, proximal jejunal atresia, or other conditions resulting in proximal intestinal obstruction and result from Ladd's bands compressing the proximal duodenum. These babies develop feeding intolerance followed by bilious emesis and typically have a scaphoid abdomen on examination. Midgut volvulus presents with a more sudden onset of symptoms in a neonate or infant who had been previously feeding normally, suggesting acute proximal intestinal obstruction. If diagnosis is delayed, symptoms of intestinal ischemia become evident and include abdominal distention, lethargy, hypovolemic shock, and anuria. Therefore, any episode of bilious emesis in a neonate should prompt an urgent evaluation for malrotation and volvulus. The presence of bloody emesis or stools suggests intestinal ischemia with mucosal injury or necrosis. In this setting, rapid diagnosis and prompt surgical intervention is essential to avoid extensive bowel loss or death (Box 28-2).

LABORATORY DATA

Plain abdominal radiographs may show a dilated stomach and proximal duodenum, or rarely pneumoperitoneum in the presence of advanced intestinal necrosis. However, the definitive study is an upper gastrointestinal (UGI) series, which shows both abnormal rotation of the duodenum

BOX 28-2	CRITICAL FINDINGS MALROTATION AND VOLVULUS

Critical assessment findings for malrotation and volvulus are as follows:
- Lethargy
- Bilious emesis
- Abdominal distention
- Abdominal radiograph suggestive of intestinal obstruction
- Acidosis, leukocytosis, and shock suggest volvulus

(malrotation) and partial obstruction (from Ladd's bands), or complete obstruction with a bird's beak suggesting midgut volvulus. A contrast enema may show an abnormal location of the cecum but is not diagnostic alone of malrotation, and provides no information about the presence or absence of midgut volvulus.[31] Abdominal ultrasound, although user dependent, can be used to identify a midgut volvulus without the need to expose the infant to radiation and reveals a twisting (i.e., target sign) of the mesentery and an abnormal relationship of the mesenteric vessels. However, this modality is less sensitive for malrotation without volvulus. Laboratory data are generally unremarkable, unless bowel ischemia is present, as suggested by leukocytosis, anemia, and metabolic acidosis.

Treatment

PREOPERATIVE CARE

Although distinguishing between symptomatic malrotation with obstruction (e.g., Ladd's bands) and volvulus in its early stages may be difficult, these conditions should be managed similarly. Gastric decompression, fluid resuscitation, correction of electrolyte and acid–base abnormalities, and parenteral antibiotics are instituted in the preoperative period. Emergent abdominal exploration should be considered in any infant with suspected or confirmed volvulus because the bowel will be irreparably damaged in as little as 4 hours. In this setting, prompt surgical intervention with continued intraoperative resuscitation is indicated to maximize the chances for bowel salvage and survival.

OPERATIVE CARE

Operative correction of malrotation without midgut volvulus includes division of Ladd's bands (to relieve duodenal obstruction), correction of the malrotation (by placement of the small bowel in the right of the abdominal cavity and the colon on the left), broadening the base of the mesentery by dividing its peritoneum and adhesions, and appendectomy (the appendix and cecum will reside in the left upper quadrant). This procedure is best performed via laparotomy, and a laparoscopic approach has limited utility in the newborn. The long-term results of the laparoscopic approach are unknown, and preliminary results are confilcting.[5] Cases of nonrotation in the older child may be amenable to laparoscopic techniques.

If volvulus is present, the bowel is detorsed and allowed to reperfuse (Figure 28-7). Necrotic segments of bowel are resected and stomas created as indicated. In selected instances, substantial resection may result in short bowel syndrome. In these cases, marginal intestine may be left in place rather than removed and a planned reoperation performed within 24 to 36 hours to reevaluate the need for additional bowel resection.

The objective of a second look laparotomy is to allow continued resuscitation and marginally viable intestine the necessary time to recover. Bowel that is nonsalvageable will become more obviously nonviable within this time window but should not have perforated in this short period. This approach is designed to minimize the amount of total intestine resected and the late risk for short bowel syndrome.

Complications and Prognosis

Proximal obstruction related to Ladd's bands is corrected by the Ladd's procedure, and recurrent obstruction is rare. The risk for subsequent volvulus is greatly reduced with Ladd's procedure but is not entirely eliminated. Adhesive small bowel obstruction may occur later in life at the same rare incidence as after any other laparotomy.

The immediate postoperative care from a Ladd's procedure consists of nasogastric decompression and intravenous (IV) fluid therapy until the return of gastrointestinal function (4–6 days on average).[15] Conversely, the outcome after malrotation with midgut volvulus is predicated on the degree of intestinal resection.[32] Midgut volvulus is a leading cause of short bowel syndrome in infants and may render the infant total parenteral nutrition (TPN)-dependent if extensive intestinal necrosis has occurred. Long-term sequelae of

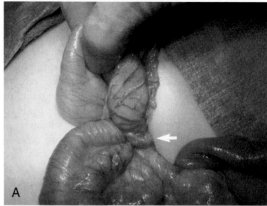

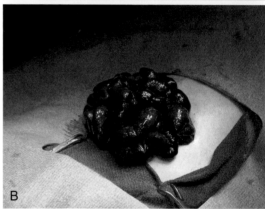

FIGURE 28-7 Two extremes of malrotation with midgut volvulus in newborns. **A,** Volvulus that presented before intestinal ischmuous set in. Arrow shows 720-degree volvulus. Bowel is entirely viable. **B,** Delayed presentation of midgut volvulus with complete necrosis of intestine, a nonsurvivable injury.

a Ladd's procedure, albeit exceedingly uncommon, include the risk of adhesive small bowel obstruction and a failure to prevent recurrent midgut volvulus.

INTESTINAL ATRESIA

Physiology and Etiology

Any segment of the bowel may be narrowed (stenosis) or become discontinuous (atresia). Duodenal atresia is the most commonly involved bowel segment, followed by ileum, jejunum, colon, and stomach.[11]

Duodenal atresia is thought to result from failure of vacuolization (fifth to sixth week of gestation) and recanalization (eighth to tenth week of gestation) of the intestinal lumen. A vascular accident or segmental volvulus occurring later in utero is thought to give rise to jejunal, ileal, or colonic atresia.[44] Because duodenal atresia results from an early in utero event, a high incidence (30%) of anomalies may be associated and include trisomy 21, congenital heart disease, and VACTERL association.[18] Conversely, intestinal atresia occurs later in gestation and so is rarely associated with significant anomalies. Atresias are classified as membranous, fibrous cords, gap defect including mesentery, and "apple-peel" atresia.[56]

Data Collection

HISTORY AND PHYSICAL EXAMINATION

Commonly, a history of maternal polyhydramnios may be provided and the affected neonate may appear small for gestational age (SGA). The more proximal the site of intestinal atresia, the more likely the history of maternal polyhydramnios. Newborns having a proximal atresia (duodenum or jejunum) present with early feeding intolerance and emesis, and also a scaphoid abdomen. Bilious emesis is present when the obstruction is distal to the ampulla of Vater, as is the case in approximately 85% of duodenal atresias. However, in 15% of cases, duodenal atresia occurs proximally to the ampulla of Vater and therefore the baby does not show bile-stained emesis or gastric aspirates.

The more distal the site of atresia and obstruction, the more likely that the infant will manifest significant abdominal distention. Babies having a distal intestinal atresia (ileum or colon) show typical features of a distal intestinal obstruction and develop abdominal distension often with visible intestinal loops. If the atresia occurs early in gestation, the infant fails to pass meconium, and only mucus is passed after birth (Box 28-3).

LABORATORY DATA

Initial evaluation of suspected duodenal atresia begins with a plain abdominal radiograph (flat and left lateral decubitus views), which classically shows a dilated air-filled stomach and proximal duodenum in a pattern called the "double bubble." A contrast study is not indicated unless air is present in the distal bowel, in which case malrotation with midgut volvulus cannot be excluded.

Abdominal x-ray films that show multiple distended loops of bowel suggest a distal intestinal

---

BOX 28-3 CRITICAL FINDINGS — INTESTINAL ATRESIA

Critical assessment findings for intestinal atresia are as follows:

- Maternal polyhydramnios
- Emesis (nonbilious versus bilious depending on location of atresia)
- Abdominal radiograph suggestive of intestinal obstruction
- Abdominal radiograph with "double bubble" suggests duodenal atresia

---

obstruction. In the setting of atresia of the small intestine or colon, abdominal x-ray films demonstrate dilation of intestinal segments proximal to the site of obstruction with absence of air in the distal bowel. For intestinal atresia distal to the duodenum a contrast enema (i.e., per rectum) is generally performed and typically shows a microcolon or unused colon, and no reflux of the contrast agent into the proximal bowel is observed.

Treatment

PREOPERATIVE CARE

Preoperative care includes orogastric tube decompression to reduce the risk of vomiting and aspiration, fluid resuscitation, and correction of electrolyte abnormalities. Preoperative antibiotics are administered to cover enteric organisms.

OPERATIVE INTERVENTION

All forms of intestinal atresia require surgical correction to restore gastrointestinal tract continuity. Duodenal atresia is repaired through a diamond-shaped, end-to-end anastomosis of the proximal and distal duodenum, and care must be exercised to prevent injury to the bile and pancreatic ducts. Repair of duodenal atresia may be performed either through a standard transverse right upper quadrant incision or laparoscopically (Figure 28-8). Other intestinal atresias are generally repaired by a standard end-to-end anastomosis. The size disparity between the dilated proximal loop and the decompressed distal loop may require that the proximal bowel be tapered or partially resected, or the distal bowel may be cut obliquely to allow anastomosis (Figure 28-9). If these methods are not possible because of size discrepancy, then the segments just proximal and distal to the atresia may be brought

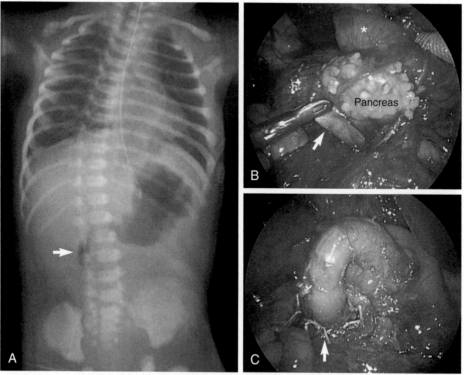

FIGURE 28-8 Duodenal atresia in a newborn. **A,** Abdominal radiograph shows classic "double-bubble" sign. Orogastric tube is in stomach, and arrow shows air-filled proximal duodenum. **B,** Laparoscopic view of duodenal atresia. Asterisk depicts proximal dilated duodeunum (compressed by instrument) and arrow shows small distal duodenum being elevated by a 3-mm bowel grasper. **C,** Completed anastomosis (arrow).

out as stomas and intestinal anastomosis delayed to allow reduction in size of the dilated proximal segment and growth of the distal segment. When the caliber of the bowel becomes more comparable in size, anastomosis is performed.

POSTOPERATIVE CARE

Postoperatively, an orogastric tube remains in place to decompress the stomach until bowel function begins. Stomas must be protected from desiccation by covering with petrolatum gauze or a stoma appliance. Ostomies of the proximal intestine have high output because of a lack of absorptive capacity and therefore require replacement of both fluid and electrolyte losses. The proximal output may be refed into a distal mucous fistula, if present, but this technique may be challenging because of problems intubating the distal stoma and securing the feeding catheter to permit infusion. All infants endure a significant period of bowel dysfunction after surgery, and therefore temporary central venous

access should be established to permit nutritional support.[45] Furthermore, infants with intestinal atresia should undergo screening for cystic fibrosis, which may contribute to both the development of the anomaly and ongoing bowel dysfunction.

Complications and Prognosis

The overall prognosis for these patients is excellent, unless severe associated anomalies are present. Prolonged bowel dysfunction is the primary complication after surgical correction of intestinal atresia. In selected cases, tapering of dilated bowel segments is attempted to enhance the recovery of bowel function.[49] Some infants fail to recover sufficient bowel function and require long-term parenteral nutritional support, either because of dysmotility or inadequate bowel length resulting from long-segment atresia. Fortunately, the majority of patients have no long-term problems after postoperative recovery and return of bowel function.

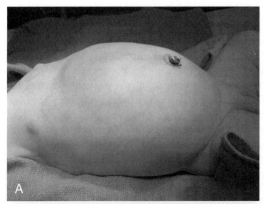

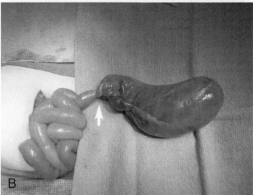

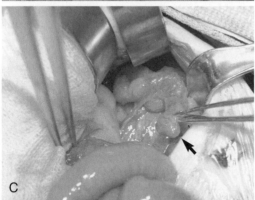

FIGURE 28-9 Newborn having colon atresia. **A,** Markedly distended abdomen. **B,** Atretic colon that has volvulized. *Arrow* shows twist, and note ischemic nature of volvulized colon. **C,** Distal microcolon elevated by forceps *(arrow).*

NECROTIZING ENTEROCOLITIS

Physiology and Etiology

Necrotizing enterocolitis (NEC) is an inflammatory condition of the bowel of uncertain cause

and occurs at a rate of 1 in 1000 live births and in 5% of infants born weighing less than 1500 g (very low birth weight, VLBW). NEC is fatal in 17% of all cases, in 20% of VLBW infants who develop the disease, and as high as 40% to 50% in those infants with a birth weight less than 1000 g. NEC is primarily a disease of premature infants, although approximately 5% of cases occur in term infants. Despite intensive study, major advances in newborn intensive care, and improved survival of the preterm infant in the past 2 decades, the incidence of and mortality associated with NEC has changed little. In fact, the increase in survival of preterm infants has increased the size of the population at risk. Perinatal stressors, an immature intestinal barrier, intestinal ischemia, bacterial colonization of the gut, and nutritional substrate in the gut lumen have all been implicated as contributing factors at play in infants who develop NEC. Other conditions that result in mucosal injury also have been linked to NEC: hypoxia, polycythemia, hyperosmolar feedings, gastrointestinal infection (bacterial or viral), and severe cardiopulmonary disease. Current research using animal models implicates upregulation of multiple inflammatory mediators in the injured intestinal epithelia affected by NEC, and the presence of certain antiinflammatory mediators may be cytoprotective.[8,22,42]

Inflammation and ischemia initially involve the innermost intestinal mucosa, but as the disease progresses, the muscular and subserosal layers of the bowel become involved. The intestinal wall becomes hemorrhagic and attenuated, with evidence of intramural gas (pneumatosis). Histologically, after surgical resection, the intestine shows features of acute and chronic inflammation, with areas of coagulative necrosis. The ileocecal region is most commonly involved (50%), followed by disease limited to the colon (25%) or both large and small intestines (25%). Up to 15% of infants will develop panintestinal necrosis, or *NEC totalis,* which is a nonsurvivable insult. Furthermore, NEC is a significant risk factor for developing short bowel syndrome chronically, if less than 40 cm of small bowel remains in the absence of the ileocecal valve or, in its presence, if less than 20 cm of bowel remains.[2]

There have been significant efforts to prevent the onset of NEC by modifying the feeding regimens in premature infants. One simple measure to decrease the incidence of NEC is feeding with breast milk instead of formula. In a review of several randomized clinical trials, breastfed infants had a lower

BOX 28-4	CRITICAL FINDINGS NECROTIZING ENTEROCOLITIS

Critical assessment findings for necrotizing enterocolitis are as follows:
- Feeding intolerance
- Abdominal distention
- Bloody or hemoccult-positive stools
- Thrombocytopenia, leukocytosis, leukopenia, and metabolic acidosis
- Pneumatosis intestinalis on abdominal radiograph
- Free air on abdominal radiograph in the presence of perforated viscus

incidence of NEC compared with formula-fed infants. It remains unclear, however, whether donor breast milk maintains this protective effect should milk of the infant's mother be unavailable. In addition to breast milk, the addition of probiotics (*Lactobacillus acidophilus* and *Bifidobacterium infantis*) to the feeding regimen seems to decrease the incidence of NEC in 24 randomized trials included in the most recent Cochrane review.[4]

Data Collection

HISTORY AND SIGNS AND SYMPTOMS

The onset of NEC is heralded by the development of feeding intolerance, abdominal distention, and bloody stools in a premature infant receiving enteral feedings. A history of perinatal hypoxia, respiratory distress, congenital heart disease, or indomethacin administration for patent ductus arteriosus (PDA) closure often is elicited. As the disease progresses, the infant develops signs and symptoms of septic shock (lethargy, respiratory distress, temperature instability, hypotension, and oliguria). Examination reveals a distended and tender abdomen that may demonstrate erythema, induration, and pitting edema in severe cases (Box 28-4).

LABORATORY DATA

Complete blood count (CBC) and serum electrolyte evaluations typically reveal thrombocytopenia, leukocytosis or leukopenia, and metabolic acidosis, respectively. C-reactive protein (CRP) levels are being increasingly obtained and appear to be a good marker of onset, persistence, and subsequent resolution of NEC. Stool tests may be positive for

occult blood and reducing substances in more than 50% of cases. The diagnostic test of choice is the three-way abdominal x-ray series (i.e., flat, left lateral decubitus, and in some instances, cross-table views). Plain radiographs are carefully reviewed for the characteristic finding of *pneumatosis intestinalis,* or intramural bowel gas. The radiograph should be assessed for free air (pneumoperitoneum), which would suggest intestinal perforation. Other findings may include dilated bowel, portal venous gas, ascites, or a fixed bowel loop that does not change on repeated studies.

Treatment

PREOPERATIVE CARE

The only absolute and immediate indication for surgical intervention is intestinal perforation, which may be detected radiographically by the finding of pneumoperitoneum. In a clinically stable infant without findings of perforation, medical management consisting of bowel rest, fluid resuscitation, broad-spectrum antibiotic therapy, and TPN are indicated. The infant is monitored carefully (serial abdominal examinations and radiographs every 8 hours) for signs of intestinal gangrene. More than half of infants respond to medical management, but up to 30% of infants treated medically may develop an intestinal stricture requiring surgical management.

A subset of infants continues to deteriorate clinically despite maximal medical therapy, suggesting intestinal gangrene without intestinal perforation. Presence of intestinal gangrene should be considered in infants having persistent metabolic acidosis, thrombocytopenia, leukopenia, refractory shock, erythema of the abdominal wall, or a fixed, dilated intestinal loop on plain x-ray study of the abdomen.[55]

OPERATIVE INTERVENTION

The principle of surgical management is to resect all necrotic bowel while preserving as much of the intestinal length as possible. In cases of extensive bowel involvement, only necrotic segments of intestine are removed and rarely reoperation at 12 to 24 hours may be planned (a second look). After bowel resection, proximal and distal ostomies are created, and the abdomen is thoroughly irrigated to reduce bacterial and fecal contamination. In severely premature infants weighing less than 1000 g, primary peritoneal drainage (PPD) to decompress the abdomen after intestinal perforation may be performed in the NICU as an alternative to laparotomy. PPD and laparotomy may have comparable survival rates, but interestingly, infants treated with PPD have substantial improvement in residual bowel length, which may be in part because up to one-third of these patients do not require further operative therapy.[12] Nevertheless, laparotomy provides more definitive therapy and further aids in establishing the extent of diseased bowel, which if NEC totalis is discovered, may reduce futile care. In most cases, PPD should be considered a temporizing means, or "bridge to laparotomy," to allow complete resuscitation before definitive surgery (Figure 28-10).

POSTOPERATIVE CARE

After laparotomy, supportive care (i.e., resuscitative fluids, TPN, antibiotics) and bowel rest are continued for 10 to 14 days. At 2 weeks postoperatively, low-osmolar elemental feedings may be started once intestinal motility has returned and advanced as tolerated. A stoma closure procedure is planned for 6 to 8 weeks after the initial surgery. All infants should undergo a preoperative contrast enema before ostomy closure to make certain the intestine and colon distal to the ostomy have not strictured.

Complications and Prognosis

Stomal prolapse or retraction, wound infection, intraabdominal abscess, and intestinal obstruction are early complications. Recurrent NEC is uncommon, but may occur in approximately 5% of infants treated medically or surgically. The most significant late complication is that of inadequate intestinal length (short bowel syndrome) and the need for long-term parenteral nutrition. Preservation of the ileocecal valve is critically important to slowing intestinal transit and thereby limiting sequelae of short bowel syndrome. Babies at highest risk for short bowel syndrome have the ileocecal valve but less than 20 cm of small intestine, or have no ileocecal valve and less than 40 cm of small bowel. For infants treated medically, nearly one-third will develop a distal intestinal stricture, most commonly in the colon, that requires operative intervention to resect and to restore intestinal continuity and function. Survival in infants weighing more than 1000 g has improved from 50% to 80% over the last two decades. Severely premature infants weighing less than 1000 g still have a mortality rate in excess of 50%.[28]

MECONIUM ILEUS

Physiology and Etiology

Meconium ileus is an intestinal obstruction caused by hyperviscous secretions from the intestinal glands coupled with an insufficient excretion of pancreatic enzymes necessary to help digest intestinal contents. The result is tenacious, viscous meconium that creates a sticky plug obstructing the lumen of bowel. The obstruction generally occurs within the terminal ileum, mimicking ileal atresia. More than 90% of infants with meconium ileus have cystic fibrosis, a 3 base-pair deletion on chromosome 7. This autosomal recessive gene defect results in alteration of the chloride channel transporter and therefore fluid flow across the apical surface of epithelial cells. Meconium ileus occurs in 10% to 25% of patients with cystic fibrosis; prenatally, 20% of mothers develop polyhydramnios. A family history of cystic fibrosis is present in 10% to 30% of cases.

This ileus of retained meconium is in contrast to meconium plug syndrome, which manifests as a failure to pass stool with obstruction in the colon and is not specific to cystic fibrosis. Meconium plug syndrome is generally recognized as immaturity of the ganglion cells and generally is benign.[25] Rectal dilation and/or contrast enema usually result in passage of the meconium plug(s) and recurrence is uncommon; however, significant obstruction can develop with rare incidences of perforation. Meconium plug syndrome, again in contrast to meconium ileus, is associated with Hirschsprung's disease in 15% of cases.

Data Collection

SIGNS AND SYMPTOMS

Meconium ileus is classified as *simple* (obstruction and obturation) or *complicated* (volvulus, intestinal atresia, perforation, meconium peritonitis). Uncomplicated meconium ileus presents as distal ileal obstruction caused by inspissated meconium (pellets) and proximal intestinal dilation.

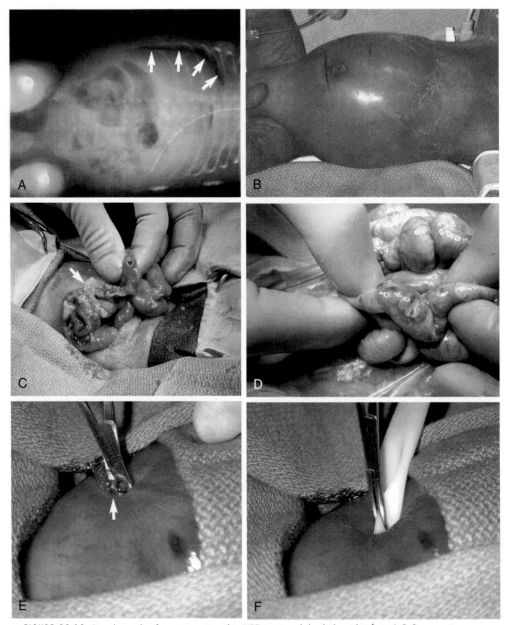

FIGURE 28-10 Several examples of necrotizing enterocolitis (NEC) in extremely low birth weight infants. **A, B,** Pneumoperitoneum on abdominal radiograph (*arrows,* **A**); same baby, **B.** Note abdominal distention and discoloration. **C,** Findings of NEC at laparotomy: perforation is shown between surgeon's fingers. Arrow shows segment of gangrenous bowel. Bowel toward surgeon's middle finger is normal. **D,** Example of pneumatosis intestinalis; this baby had panintestinal necrosis. **E, F,** Placement of peritoneal drain in the neonatal intensive care unit. Arrow shows release of pneumoperitoneum (bubbles).

The onset of symptoms associated with simple meconium ileus begins 24 to 48 hours after birth. Bilious emesis, progressive abdominal distention, and the failure to pass meconium suggest intestinal obstruction. The differential diagnosis in addition to meconium ileus includes ileal atresia, meconium plug, and Hirschsprung's disease. Physical examination shows a patent anus that may express a small amount of gray meconium. Examination of the abdomen reveals moderate distention with a characteristic dough-like sensation on palpation because of the thickened meconium contained in the dilated bowel. *Complicated meconium ileus* often manifests more abruptly and progresses more quickly. Symptoms include abdominal distention within 24 hours of birth, respiratory distress (especially if a postnatal perforation has occurred), and an edematous, erythematous abdomen[43] (Box 28-5).

LABORATORY DATA

Abdominal radiograph demonstrates a "soap bubble" appearance of the bowel caused by trapped gas within the meconium and also shows large dilated (with air) loops of bowel with few air-fluid levels because of the viscous nature of the meconium. A contrast enema shows a microcolon and pellets of inspissated meconium at the site of distal obstruction. If in utero perforation has occurred, microcalcifications may also be present on plain abdominal radiographs.

Treatment

PREOPERATIVE CARE

If meconium ileus is suspected, orogastric decompression, IV hydration, and electrolyte replacement are instituted; once appropriately hydrated, a diluted Gastrografin or CystoConray

enema should be attempted.[24] The infant should be adequately hydrated before the enema because of the hyperosmolarity of the Gastrografin or Cysto-Conray. Intracolonic instillation of these water-soluble agents draws fluid into the bowel lumen, diluting the viscous meconium and facilitating passage, and may be therapeutic to relieve the obstruction. If the Gastrografin enema results in incomplete evacuation, it may be repeated over the next several days.[24] However, if the Gastrografin enema fails to result in passage of meconium, complicated meconium ileus or ileal atresia may be present and operative intervention is indicated.[21]

OPERATIVE INTERVENTION

The goal of operative treatment is to relieve intestinal obstruction. For uncomplicated meconium ileus, several operative approaches are described to eliminate the obstructing inspissated meconium. Techniques include the following: (1) enterotomy with extraction of the tenacious meconium and irrigation of the bowel with saline solution or 2% N-acetylcysteine (Mucomyst), (2) resection of the affected segment with anastomosis, and (3) formation of chimney ostomies just proximal to the obstruction (Bishop-Koop procedure: bowel is divided to create an ostomy of the distal ileum for continued irrigations with an internal anastomosis of the proximal to distal ileum fashioned to maintain intestinal continuity). More commonly now, a *T-tube enterostomy* may be created, in which a soft and small caliber tube is securely placed within the bowel lumen and delivered through a separate wound in the abdominal wall (Figure 28-11). This tube, like the chimney ostomy, allows continued postoperative irrigations with normal saline or diluted Mucomyst to complete or maintain passage of intestinal contents. If complicated meconium ileus is identified, the obstructed segment is resected and ostomies are performed to permit postoperative irrigation. Ostomy closure usually is performed 4 to 6 weeks later.

POSTOPERATIVE CARE

Postoperatively, nasogastric tube decompression, nutritional support, and irrigation of the rectum or ostomies with saline solution or Mucomyst are instituted. After gastrointestinal function returns, feedings using predigested or elemental formula

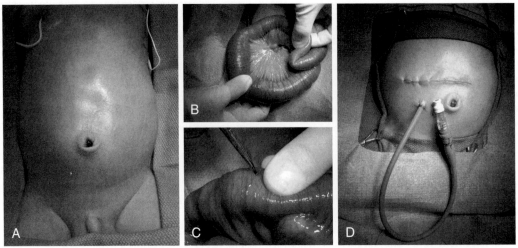

FIGURE 28-11   Newborn with meconium ileus as presenting feature of cystic fibrosis. **A,** Abdominal distention and visible intestinal loops on physical examination. **B,** Equal pressure is being applied to the bowel by both hands of the surgeon. Note how noncompressible the bowel in the right hand is secondary to the inspissated meconium. **C,** Note viscosity of meconium being teased out of the bowel lumen. **D,** After irrigation with Mucomyst and evacuation of the meconium, a tube enterostomy is placed for continued irrigation in the weeks after surgery. Once the infant's bowel is completely cleared of meconium and a full diet is tolerated, the tube may be removed.

and pancreatic enzyme supplements are started. The diagnosis of cystic fibrosis is confirmed with genetic analysis or sweat chloride testing.

Complications and Prognosis

One-year survival for infants with simple or complicated meconium ileus is favorable (greater than 90%), but long-term survival is limited primarily because of the pulmonary complications of cystic fibrosis.[35] Late gastrointestinal complications of cystic fibrosis include distal intestinal obstruction syndrome (meconium ileus equivalent), appendicitis, intussusception, rectal prolapse, intestinal stricture, pancreatitis, and cholestatic liver disease.[16]

HIRSCHSPRUNG'S DISEASE

Physiology and Etiology

Hirschsprung's disease is a congenital intestinal disorder caused by a lack of ganglion cells in the bowel wall, principally the colon, which disrupts and abrogates effective peristalsis. During development, neural crest cells (the progenitor or stem cells of the enteric nervous system) migrate along the intestinal tube to populate the entire gut in a craniocaudal fashion, with the distal colon, rectum, and sphincter being the last to be colonized. These progenitor cells divide, differentiate, and proliferate to form the enteric nervous system, of which the ganglion cells are a critical component. Arrest of migration, proliferation, and differentiation results in the aganglionosis found in Hirschsprung's disease, which is a relatively common cause of distal intestinal obstruction in the newborn. At the site of arrest, a transition from normal to abnormal innervation is present, and all intestine distal to this site will be aganglionic and therefore dysfunctional. The result is a functional obstruction that mimics mechanical intestinal obstruction. In brief, the pathophysiologic consequence of the absence of ganglion cells is failure of the involved rectum and colon to relax, and therefore the fecal stream cannot be passed effectively through the aganglionic region and beyond. Rectosigmoid aganglionosis is most common (85%), with the remainder of patients developing variable lengths of more proximal colonic and, rarely, small intestine disease. Total colonic aganglionosis occurs in roughly 10% of cases.

Hirschsprung's disease occurs in 1 of 5000 live births, having a 4:1 male-to-female predominance. The majority of cases are sporadic

(80%–90%), but familial occurrences are well recognized and multiple genetic alterations have been identified in affected pedigrees. Associated anomalies are rare in sporadic cases but may be seen in as many as 25% of the familial cases. Infants born with Down syndrome also carry a higher incidence of Hirschsprung's disease than the population at large (2%), and between 5% and 10% of Hirschsprung's patients will have Down syndrome.

Approximately 15% of Hirschsprung's neonates will present with meconium plug syndrome (MPS), an obstruction of the colon by inspissated meconium. However, in general, MPS is associated with immature ganglion development and is not indicative of the more serious Hirschsprung's disease.

Data Collection

SIGNS AND SYMPTOMS

Ninety-eight percent of normal infants pass meconium in the first 24 to 48 hours of life. Failure to pass meconium early, feeding intolerance, and abdominal distention suggest a diagnosis of Hirschsprung's disease. In some infants with a short segment of aganglionic bowel, spontaneous evacuation of stool may be noted, and the infant may appear otherwise healthy. If vomiting, abdominal distention, and constipation (or paradoxic diarrhea resulting from watery stool escaping around the obstipated stool) continues, further investigation is indicated. Hirschsprung's disease may rarely escape detection during the newborn period, and in older children, a history of refractory and chronic obstipation may be the only symptom. Approximately 5% to 10% of affected infants will present with a picture of enterocolitis (toxic megacolon), characterized by fever, vomiting, abdominal distention/tenderness, foul-smelling diarrhea, and septic shock. The infant may rapidly deteriorate, with a 50% risk of death if the colon is not rapidly decompressed, either by transanal soft rubber tube irrigations or emergency colostomy. Fortunately, in most cases of Hirschsprung disease, the infant is only mildly ill, allowing time for definitive diagnostic studies before surgical correction is undertaken[9] (Box 28-6).

LABORATORY DATA

The diagnostic evaluation begins with a contrast enema. Surgical practice states that when

---

> **BOX 28-6**
> ## CRITICAL FINDINGS
> ### HIRSCHSPRUNG'S DISEASE
>
> Critical assessment findings for Hirschsprung's disease are as follows:
> - Failure to pass meconium within 48 hours of birth
> - Feeding intolerance
> - Abdominal distention
> - Enterocolitis (fever, abdominal distention, foul-smelling diarrhea, sepsis)
> - Transition zone on barium enema
> - Absent ganglion cells and nerve hypertrophy on rectal biopsy

---

considering the diagnosis of Hirschsprung's, the first enema should be a contrast enema. This study typically shows a contracted or spastic rectosigmoid colon, with contrast material entering the proximal dilated bowel. The area between the contracted and dilated bowel is called the transition zone. If the contrast enema is equivocal, an abdominal x-ray film should be obtained on the next day to evaluate extent of retained contrast material. Significant contrast material retained within the distal colon and rectum suggests the presence of Hirschsprung's disease. Definitive diagnosis is made by performing a bedside suction rectal biopsy, a well-tolerated procedure in neonates that does not require any analgesics or sedatives. On histology, a biopsy diagnostic of Hirschsprung's shows an absence of ganglion cells and the presence of hypertrophic nerve trunks within the submucosal and intermyenteric plexus. Special immunohistochemical staining is commonly performed by the pathologist to corroborate the diagnosis. Conversely, if ganglion cells are observed on histologic examination, a diagnosis of Hirschsprung's disease is excluded.

Treatment

PREOPERATIVE CARE

In infants with Hirschsprung's-associated enterocolitis, orogastric tube decompression, IV fluid resuscitation, broad-spectrum antibiotics, and correction of acid–base deficits and electrolyte abnormalities are promptly initiated. Infants who are less ill with symptoms of obstruction are placed on nil per os (NPO) status, and IV antibiotic therapy and orogastric decompression are instituted, permitting time to complete the diagnostic evaluation. After the diagnostic evaluation is completed,

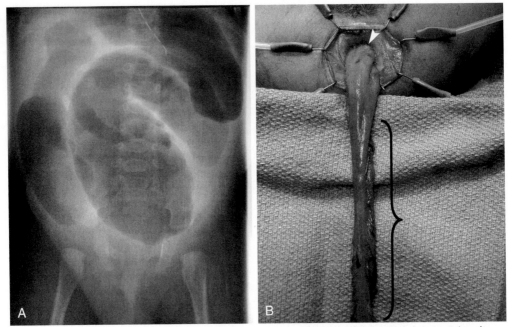

FIGURE 28-12 Newborn with Hirschsprung's disease. **A,** Plain abdominal radiograph shows distal intestinal obstruction 2 days after birth in a neonate who has failed to pass meconium. Note absence of gas in rectum/pelvis. **B,** After laparoscopic mobilization and transanal mucosectomy, the diseased bowel may be delivered through the anus. The bracket denotes the contracted, aganglionic bowel. Arrowhead shows biopsy performed laparoscopically that confirms region of ganglionated bowel. Coloanal anastomosis was performed at this level.

transanal rectal irrigations, not enemas, are performed twice daily until surgery. Infants should have return to normal bowel function with these irrigations and may be fed enterally (so long as rectal irrigations continue) until definitive surgery.

OPERATIVE INTERVENTION

In the presence of profound enterocolitis, an emergency colostomy may be indicated. If necessary, a colostomy is performed at a site of normal bowel (ganglion cells present), as confirmed by a frozen-section histologic examination. In selected cases, the neonate will be too ill, so operative time is minimized by the creation of a right-sided colostomy, because most affected infants have more distal colonic involvement. If the neonate presents with milder symptoms, one of several surgical options may be selected: (1) primary laparoscopically assisted endorectal pull-through (Figure 28-12), (2) primary transanal pull-through, or (3) staged reconstruction (temporary colostomy at the most distal site of ganglion cells, followed by a pull-through in 3–6 months).[47] In all cases, multiple

intestinal seromuscular biopsies are created at the time of operation until the normally innervated bowel is identified. A coloanal anastomosis or colostomy is performed at the site of histologically proven normal bowel. If the anastomosis or colostomy site is missing ganglion cells, the neonate will remain symptomatic—the bowel will not function normally because of aganglionosis.

Several factors influence the decision to perform a primary pull-through procedure in neonates.[47] The neonate should be of sufficient gestational age and size (generally more than 2 kg), have rectosigmoid disease as demonstrated by contrast enema, not have significant proximal bowel distention, and not have evidence of advanced enterocolitis. Neonates who do not meet these criteria should be treated in a staged manner, with an immediate colostomy and a pull-through procedure delayed until later in infancy.[17,51]

POSTOPERATIVE CARE

The recovery period is generally straightforward, and supportive care is provided until the return of

INSTRUCTIONS FOR OSTOMY CARE

Supplies
Dry washcloths
Warm, wet washcloths
Mild soap
Clip or rubber band (if using two-piece appliance)
Skin-prep (United)*
Stoma-adhesive paste (ConvaTec)*
Ostomy set-up (skin wafer and bag)
Pattern for stoma

Application Instructions
1. Measure the diameter of the stoma, using the measuring guide circle enclosed in the wafer box.
2. Trace the appropriate circle onto the white paper backing of the wafer and cut out the hole. Gently bend and slightly stretch the opening with your finger. The goal is to have the hole $\frac{1}{16}$ to $\frac{1}{8}$ inch larger than the stoma. A snug but not constricting fit is needed to prevent stool from leaking onto the skin.
3. Clean and dry the skin around the stoma.
4. Apply a generous coat of Skin-prep (United) on the skin around the stoma.
5. Apply a thin border of Stoma-adhesive paste (ConvaTec) around the stoma.
6. Press wafer firmly to skin.
7. If using a two-piece appliance, snap on the bag and close the end of the bag with a clip or rubber band if it is open-ended. If using a one-piece appliance, the appliance may be applied directly to the skin or to a skin barrier such as Stoma-adhesive (ConvaTec).

Helpful Hints
1. Change the appliance as soon as there is any evidence of leaking.
2. Rinsing the bags with some type of scented soap (peppermint or spice) will help reduce the bag odor.
3. Precut several wafers ahead of time.
4. When traveling, always have an extra set of clothes and a complete set of supplies, as well as a new setup with stoma holes already cut.

*Other products may be used in place of the brand names upon recommendation of medical supplier, physician, or nurse.
Courtesy Kris Altzenbeck, RN, The Children's Hospital, Denver, Colo.

bowel function. For babies treated initially with colostomy, postoperative care includes teaching the parents about stoma maintenance and hygiene (Box 28-7). The pull-through procedure entails resecting abnormal aganglionic bowel and bringing ganglionic bowel to the anus. Several variations of the pull-through operation have been described; each has unique advantages and disadvantages, but in general the results are similar regarding long-term stooling patterns. For neonates having a primary laparoscopically assisted endorectal pull-through, first stool is usually passed within 24 to 48 hours of the procedure, at which time breast milk or Pedialyte may be introduced. Feeds may be advanced to goal (according to tolerance) over the next 24 to 48 hours. Perianal skin care with various barriers is critical in the early postoperative period to prevent excoriation, as defecation is frequent and poorly controlled at this stage of convalescence. Moreover, no transanal manipulation (i.e., temperature probes or suppositories) should be performed until after 4 weeks from the date of surgery.

Complications and Prognosis

Early complications of the pull-through operation include inadequate blood supply to the coloanal anastomosis, anastomotic stricture, anastomotic dehiscence, and cuff abscess. Later complications include Hirschsprung's-associated enterocolitis, perianal skin excoriation, and recurrent constipation. The infant usually thrives postoperatively and grows normally. It is not uncommon for the infant to have frequent stools during the immediate postoperative period, which gradually normalize in frequency. However, some children despite a technically satisfactory operation will experience recurrent constipation requiring some form of bowel management program with or without placement of a colostomy tube (i.e., Chait button) for antegrade enemas.[59]

ANORECTAL MALFORMATIONS
Physiology and Etiology

Anorectal malformations (ARM) encompass a broad spectrum of hindgut anomalies, from isolated imperforate anus in males and females that may include fistulous communications between the urogenital tract and rectum, to the complex persistent cloaca in females. Although the development of the cloaca and its subsequent septation into urogenital and anorectal tracts is not well understood, each organ system is recognizable as a separate entity by the seventh week of gestation. Therefore, persistent cloaca in females arises from an arrest in development of the gut and its complete separation from urogenital tract between the fourth and sixth week of gestation. Cloacal exstrophy arises if disruption of the cloacal membrane occurs before the urorectal septum has separated the urinary bladder from the hindgut. Disruption of the cloacal membrane after septation results in exstrophy of the bladder only. Any insult occurring at this critical period of organogenesis places a number of organ systems at risk and accounts for the fact that 60% of infants with cloaca will have concomitant anomalies.[19]

Imperforate anus is the most common ARM, occurring in 1 in 5000 live births, and predominantly affects males (58%) more than females (42%). Imperforate anus is characterized as low, intermediate, or high, and termination of the rectal fistula varies according to gender. The higher the defect, the more likely the presence of other associated malformations. A high imperforate anus is defined as the end of the rectum terminating above the levator ani muscles. Conversely, in low imperforate anus, the rectum descends below the levator complex. A fistulous connection to the perineum or urogenital tract is almost always present. In high lesions, the rectal fistula enters the membranous urethra in the male or rarely the vagina in the female. In low lesions, the rectal fistula empties on the perineum of both males and females or the posterior fourchette of the introitus, the most common site in females.[40] Congenital VACTERL anomalies and trisomy 21 are common and require further evaluation. Moreover, a high incidence of spinal dysraphism is observed with anorectal malformation; imaging of the spine is indicated.[53]

Data Collection

SIGNS AND SYMPTOMS

Most anorectal malformations are apparent on physical examination of the newborn but may be missed if a careful inspection of the buttocks and anus is not performed. After the diagnosis is made, a fistula should be sought. In low lesions, there may be a thin membrane over the anal orifice, or there may be a fistula along the perineum and scrotal raphe of males. In females, the fistula most commonly terminates in the vestibule or fourchette of the introitus. If meconium passes in the

urine of males, or rarely from the vagina, a high lesion is present. If the condition remains unrecognized, the infant develops signs and symptoms of distal intestinal obstruction. Down syndrome babies having an ARM usually (95%) have a high type variant of rectal atresia without genitourinary tract communication (Box 28-8).

LABORATORY DATA

A plain abdominal radiograph may show features of distal intestinal obstruction without rectal gas, but it will not reliably show termination of the rectum. Perineal ultrasonography may be used to establish the termination of the rectum and its distance from the skin, data that may help operative planning. In males having imperforate anus without a perineal fistula, a contrast study of the urethra should delineate a rectourethral fistula, if present. In females without a perineal or vestibular fistula, contrast genitogram may help define the anatomic relationships of a persistent cloaca. A perineal fistula visible on physical examination does not usually warrant imaging of ARM. However, because of the possibility for VACTERL association, echocardiography and abdominal sonography of the genitourinary tract are indicated, as is a plain radiograph of the spine and limbs.

Treatment

PREOPERATIVE CARE

The infant should be kept NPO while evaluation of ARM is underway, and an orogastric tube should be placed to exclude esophageal atresia and to decompress the stomach. If a fistula is present on the perineum or at the fourchette, an early anoplasty may be performed, assuming the baby has no associated cardiac

---

BOX 28-8	CRITICAL FINDINGS
	IMPERFORATE ANUS

Critical assessment findings for imperforate anus are as follows:
- Absence of anus or presence of anteriorly displaced perineal fistula.
- Signs and symptoms of obstruction if diagnosis not made.
- Perineal ultrasound study will identify the level of defect in the absence of a perineal fistula.

anomaly and is otherwise deemed to be a suitable candidate for a general anesthetic. If early repair is contraindicated, then a perineal fistula tract may be dilated twice daily to promote elimination of fecal contents and until the baby is a more suitable candidate for surgery. If no fistula is visualized and a high lesion or cloaca is present, a divided colostomy is performed, and staged reconstruction is planned for later in infancy.

OPERATIVE INTERVENTION

For low imperforate anus, early reconstruction is performed either in the newborn period or in the first months of life, if the infant can produce stools adequately through the fistulous tract with dilations. After colostomy for high imperforate anus, a formal repair is undertaken when the child is 3 to 6 months of age. Approached most commonly through a posterior sagittal incision (buttock), the fistula is separated from the urethra in males or

vagina in females, and the rectum is mobilized to lie within the center of the sphincter mechanism. The levator muscles and sphincter are closed anteriorly and posteriorly around the rectum, which is then anastomosed to the perineal skin in a procedure known as a posterior sagittal anorectoplasty (PSARP, or Pena procedure).[41] Alternatively, to minimize wound complications and postoperative pain, a laparoscopic-assisted anorectoplasty may be performed (Figure 28-13). A Foley catheter should always be placed in boys at time of the definitive repair to assist in separation of the rectum from the urethra and to facilitate bladder drainage in the postoperative period; this catheter will be in place typically for 7 to 14 days after PSARP.

POSTOPERATIVE CARE

After anorectoplasty, simple skin care is all that is necessary, and a program of anal dilation is instituted 14 days postoperatively, which will

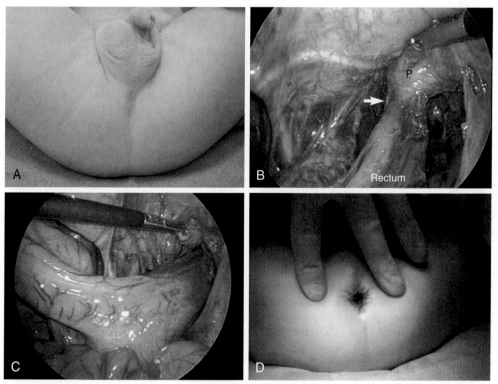

FIGURE 28-13 *Male neonate with an anorectal malformation and rectourethral fistula.* **A,** Flat perineum without cutaneous fistula. **B,** Laparoscopic view of pelvic structures after dissection. Arrow shows rectourethral fistula at level of prostate (P). **C,** Fistula has been divided and ligated (held by 5-mm grasper) and rectum has been delivered through the center of the sphincter complex for colocutaneous anastomosis. **D,** Neo-anus.

continue for 4 to 6 months. After a colostomy, stoma care and teaching are begun with the parents. Colostomy closure will be performed within 6 to 8 weeks of PSARP, assuming the neoanus is of adequate size and not strictured.

Complications and Prognosis

Mechanical complications of the stoma (prolapse, stenosis, and skin breakdown) may arise but generally do not require revision and should be temporized until stomal closure.[39] Urinary tract infection (UTI) or hyperchloremic metabolic acidosis may result from the fistulous connection of the rectum to the urinary tract. Antibiotic prophylaxis is instituted, and selected infants may require bicarbonate supplement until the fistula is divided.

Constipation is the primary long-term problem after correction of low imperforate anus. Stricture of the anoplasty should always be considered and may be treated with anal dilation or rarely revision anoplasty.

High imperforate anus is most often complicated by incontinence (or pseudoincontinence) and frequent soiling. Long-term results are influenced by the degree of sphincter muscle development and innervation. Approximately 25% of infants have good continence, 50% have fair continence, and 25% have poor results. Bowel programs and strategies have been developed to permit some degree of social continence so that permanent colostomy can be avoided.

OMPHALOCELE AND GASTROSCHISIS[27]

Physiology and Etiology

Omphalocele and gastroschisis are distinct defects of the abdominal wall at or near the umbilicus. Omphalocele is characterized by the persistent herniation of the abdominal viscera through the umbilical ring, and the herniated contents are covered by the normal components of the umbilical cord: the peritoneum, Wharton's jelly, and amnion. Omphalocele, also known as exomphalos, is a defect in abdominal wall development which may result from failure of embryonic enfolding as early as the fourth to seventh week of gestation or from failure of closure of the exocoelomic space, which is usually completed by the 12th week of gestation.

Fifty percent of neonates presenting with omphalocele will have an underlying chromosomal abnormality, most often trisomies 12 and 18 but also trisomy 21.[6] Congenital heart lesions, including pulmonary hypertension, are seen in as many as 50% of these affected infants. Congenital syndromes involving an omphalocele are potentially lethal, usually as a result of the associated abnormalities. *Cloacal exstrophy,* occurring in 1 in 200,000 pregnancies and the constellation of defects known as *pentalogy of Cantrell* likely represent the earliest of embryonic failure in the development of this spectrum of anomalies including omphalocele.

Gastroschisis is a full-thickness defect of the abdominal wall that occurs most commonly to the right of the umbilicus and exposes the extruded bowel to the amniotic fluid without a natural covering as seen with omphalocele. It has been hypothesized that this defect results from a weakening of the anterior abdominal wall due to a vascular accident involving the right omphalomesenteric artery, which takes over perfusion of the anterior abdominal wall during the seventh week of gestation. Gastroschisis occurs three to four times more frequently than omphalocele, and its incidence is rising in developed countries for unknown reasons. This increasing incidence seems to be occurring in younger mothers, most frequently in those less than 20 years old, although no clear epidemiology has been correlated with this finding. Gastroschisis typically is not associated with major congenital anomalies or syndromes, although 5% to 10% of affected infants have a concomitant intestinal atresia.[6] This atresia is likely secondary to either the initial vascular accident thought to initiate the defect or compromise of the affected bowel segment arising from a constricting fascial defect.

Nonrotation of the intestine, by definition, is uniformly present in all incidences of these two conditions.

Data Collection

HISTORY

Abdominal wall defects are readily diagnosed by antenatal ultrasonography, which is helpful in planning future delivery and therapy.[27] Spontaneous or induced vaginal delivery should be considered in most cases of gastroschisis, because minimal risk of bowel injury during delivery exists.[1,13,20] Babies having an omphalocele may also be delivered vaginally, but liver herniation or associated anomalies may dictate cesarean delivery.[20]

In cases of gastroschisis, severe serositis resulting from exposure of the bowel to amniotic fluid makes closure more difficult and delays the return of bowel function. Early delivery may be recommended for certain fetuses having gastroschisis, if sonographic evidence reveals progressive bowel distention and thickening, suggesting intestinal obstruction or severe serositis.

In cases of omphalocele, prenatal sonography should thoroughly evaluate the fetus for other potential anomalies and may be supplemented by fetal magnetic resonance imaging (MRI).

SIGNS AND SYMPTOMS

Both anomalies present as a mass of abdominal contents extruding through an anterior abdominal wall defect. Eviscerated bowel without a peritoneal covering characterizes gastroschisis, whereas an omphalocele is defined by a peritoneal covering of herniated bowel and often a segment of liver. Gastroschisis defects are most commonly to the right of the midline and are found adjacent to the umbilical stalk, whereas omphalocele occurs through a central defect at the base of the umbilical cord.

In contradistinction to gastroschisis, omphalocele importantly carries a high incidence of associated anomalies, and cardiac and/or urinary tract malformations are most prevalent. Omphalocele also is a feature of several recognizable syndromes, including Beckwith-Wiedemann, prune belly, cloacal exstrophy, and pentalogy of Cantrell. Chromosomal defects are also identified with greater frequency in cases of omphalocele than gastroschisis and include trisomies 13, 18, and 21. Most babies having an omphalocele will deliver at term.

Gastroschisis in contrast is associated with few anomalies outside of the gastrointestinal tract.[6] Malrotation is understood to exist with gastroschisis, and so the most common associated anomaly is intestinal stenosis or atresia (10%–15%), a rare finding in omphalocele. Infants having gastroschisis are more commonly preterm and small for gestational age (Box 28-9).

LABORATORY DATA

In a neonate having omphalocele, a careful search for associated anomalies is performed before closure is attempted. Echocardiography and an x-ray

---

---

examination of the chest and spine are performed to rule out cardiac, chest wall, diaphragmatic, and spinal anomalies. Abdominal sonography is obtained to evaluate integrity of the urinary tract. Gastroschisis newborns do not require routine radiographic evaluations unless otherwise indicated.

Treatment

PREOPERATIVE CARE

Initial management of gastroschisis includes preservation of body heat and fluid, orogastric decompression, protection of the intestine, and prophylaxis against infection. Covering the exposed viscera minimizes heat and fluid loss. Placing the infant's torso into an impermeable, clear plastic bowel bag is the preferred method to prevent fluid loss. Historically wrapping the bowel in saline-soaked gauze has been advocated. However, if not done properly, this method can result in constriction in the blood supply and ischemia to the intestine. Positioning the infant on his or her side prevents "kinking" of the mesentery at the fascial level and prevents intestinal ischemia.

Intravenous fluids and broad-spectrum antibiotics should be instituted early. Administration of adequate isotonic intravenous fluids is essential to the perioperative care of infants with gastroschisis. Given the insensible fluid losses, these infants may require a minimum of 150 ml/kg/day of total fluids. A Foley catheter to measure accurate urine output in the first 24 to 48 hours of life may be useful to modify the fluid requirements of the infant. To prevent bowel distention, an orogastric tube is placed to low continuous suction. In omphalocele, because the abdominal contents are covered naturally, less evaporative and heat losses are encountered.

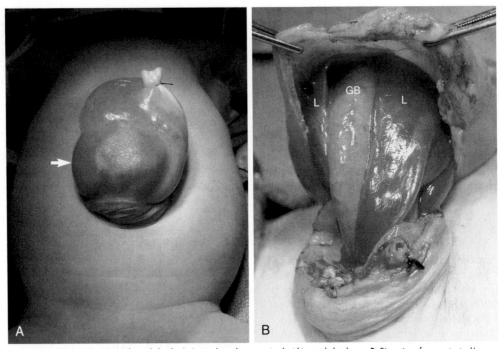

FIGURE 28-14 Neonate with omphalocele. **A,** Arrow shows liver contained within omphalocele sac. **B,** Dissection of sac contents. Liver is adherent to lining of sac (*L,* liver; *GB,* gallbladder). Fascial defect was closed primarily.

OPERATIVE INTERVENTION

Rarely, an infant with omphalocele may be too ill to undergo early abdominal closure, may have other lethal malformations, or may have a "giant omphalocele" defined as the sac containing a significant portion of the liver (Figure 28-14). Under these circumstances, the newborn is given palliative care with a daily application of a desiccant or silver sulfadine to the abdominal sac. The result is eschar formation and subsequent epithelialization in 10 to 20 weeks. A large ventral hernia will remain, and if the patient survives, repair may be performed later in infancy. Infants with omphalocele not having liver herniation or significant associated anomalies may have the sac removed and primary fascial closure accomplished shortly after birth, or at a minimum, simple skin closure may be performed, with ventral hernia repair scheduled for later in infancy once abdominal domain has been restored. Some cases of omphalocele will require biosynthetic fascial substitutes to accomplish visceral coverage.

For infants born with gastroschisis, primary surgical repair entails reduction of the herniated abdominal contents into the peritoneal cavity without increasing abdominal pressure to a point that ventilation, venous return, and intestinal blood supply are compromised. If the amount of eviscerated abdominal contents is small or moderate, primary repair is simple and safe. Before closure of gastroschisis, the surgeon searches carefully for associated atresia but may or may not attempt to restore intestinal continuity during the initial operation. If atresia is identified but inflammation and matting of the intestine will not permit safe anastomosis, the atretic bowel may be placed within a silo or returned to the abdomen primarily, and reexploration may be planned for 4 to 6 weeks later to allow the thickened, edematous bowel wall to normalize, facilitating anastomosis or enterostomy. If atresia is found, but the bowel is not inflamed or matted, intestinal continuity may be restored at the initial operation or an ostomy created, with plans for delayed reconstitution 4 to 6 weeks later.

In selected cases, the fascial defect may have to be enlarged to allow replacement of the herniated organs into the abdomen because of the small size of the fascial ring, loss of abdominal domain, and the amount of intestinal herniation. The inability to perform primary closure necessitates placement of a Silastic

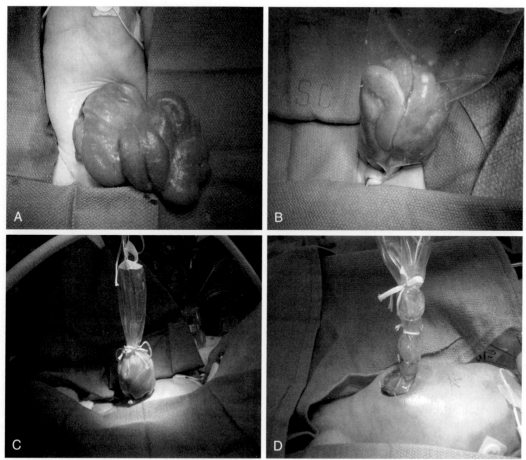

FIGURE 28-15 Neonate with gastroschisis. **A, B,** Note edema, thickening, and matting of bowel. Also, note scaphoid appearance of abdomen (loss of domain). As a result, bowel was placed in a silastic silo. **C,** Postoperative day 1 after placement of silo. Note how the edema has largely drained from the bowel wall (gravity) and how much of the silo contents has reduced spontaneously. The first umbilical tape is placed to prevent bowel from rising in the silo. **D,** Postoperative day 5 (an umbilical tape is applied each day in the nursery) and the bowel has fully returned to the abdomen. The fascia is ready for closure.

silo or patch to permit staged reduction (Figure 28-15). Over the ensuing 2 to 7 days, the herniated viscera are gradually returned to the abdomen on a daily basis by gravity (infant remains supine) and by applying gentle and constant pressure to the silo at the bedside (umbilical tape is tied sequentially along the silo until the intestine has reached the fascial level). Once all of the silo contents have been successfully reduced, the infant is returned to the operating room for removal of the silo and closure of the fascia.[46] While a silo is in place, most neonates will remain on antibiotics and for a short period after definitive fascial closure.

Complications and Prognosis

Bowel injury, respiratory compromise, and diminished venous return caused by abdominal hypertension may complicate recovery after primary fascial closure of abdominal wall defects. In this setting, the infant is returned to the operating room for placement of a silo. Rarely, a silo may become infected or separate from the fascia, complicating closure by this method.

Recovery of bowel function is uniformly delayed, especially in gastroschisis caused by exposure of the bowel to amniotic fluid. A central venous catheter should be placed at the time of initial surgery for long-term total parenteral nutritional support. Intestinal stricture, incisional hernia, and adhesive bowel obstruction are possible short- and long-term complications. The principal long-term morbidity associated with gastroschisis is short bowel syndrome. Morbidity for omphalocele is principally secondary to any associated anomalies and the challenges of abdominal closure. Otherwise, prognosis for both types of abdominal wall defects should be good, unless, again, severe associated malformations are present.

NEONATAL TUMORS

Neonatal tumors are discovered in every 12,500 to 25,000 live births and account for 2% of all childhood malignancies.[34] The majority of affected neonates present with a mass at birth or within the first month of life, which may or may not have been identified on prenatal screening. The two most frequently encountered neonatal tumors are teratoma (principally sacrococcygeal [Figure 28-16] but also cervical [Figure 28-17]) and neuroblastoma. Soft tissue sarcomas, infantile myofibromatosis, renal tumors (benign mesoblastic nephroma and malignant Wilms tumor), hepatoblastoma, and central nervous system tumors follow in frequency. Malignant tumors rarely arise in the newborn, yet some benign tumors encountered at birth may acquire malignant features later in infancy. Nevertheless, although a neonatal tumor may be histologically benign, these tumors may be life-threatening because of size, location, arteriovenous shunts, or rupture with hemorrhage. Some tumors show invasive or infiltrative characteristics, yet these may not have metastatic potential. Furthermore, screening programs have identified potentially malignant tumors earlier in development, such as for neuroblastoma in Japan, but have as yet failed to improve overall survival. Some neonatal tumors even show the potential for spontaneous regression. Taken together, neonatal tumors represent a protean mix of diseases that have a low malignant potential, yet the biological and pathophysiologic behavior may not be entirely predictable.

The etiology of solid malignancies in infants and children is an area of great interest. Many of these "congenital" tumors are classified as embryonal tumors because of retained features of embryonic

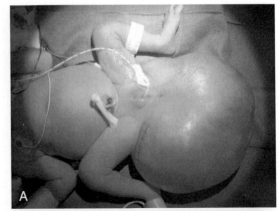

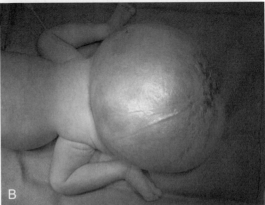

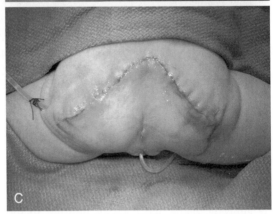

FIGURE 28-16 Female neonate with a huge sacrococcygeal teratoma. **A,** Anterior view. Note anal opening in anterior and just caudal to introitus. **B,** Posterior view. **C,** Immediately after resection. Incision will soften over time.

development within the organ in which each tumor arises. Carcinomas, typical of adulthood, are virtually nonexistent in neonates. Under the microscope, many of these embryonal tumors show a

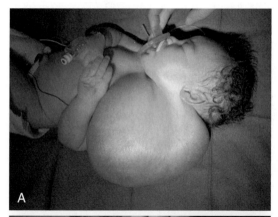

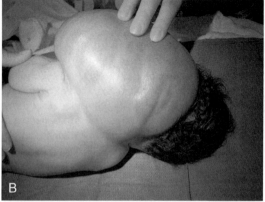

FIGURE 28-17 Huge cervical cystic hygroma. Teratomas show a similar appearance but tend to be more midline than hygromas. **A, B,** Anterior and posterior views.

recapitulation of cell types found in early embryonic development of the particular organ, but terminal differentiation of the progenitor cells has not been completed, and so no functional tissue architecture is appreciated. Associated anomalies may be found in 15% of neonates having congenital tumors, and genetic defects are also relatively prevalent in babies having neonatal tumors.

Routine prenatal ultrasonography has contributed to an increasing diagnosis of fetal and neonatal tumors. Interestingly, several fetal tumors, particularly neuroblastoma, have a unique property to undergo spontaneous regression and involution by 12 months of age. A recent study by the Children's Oncology Group in infants younger than 6 months with small adrenal masses showed that the majority of these lesions will resolve spontaneously without the need for operative intervention.[37]

Commonly, fetuses harboring an embryonal or germ cell tumor will be identified on antenatal screening. Some tumors, in particular sacrococcygeal teratomas, may be so large as to cause dystocia or may present a significant risk for rupture during delivery, and either scenario could be disastrous. Furthermore, a cervical teratoma or cystic hygroma may cause airway obstruction at birth. Fetuses having these occasionally huge cervical tumors should be delivered by cesarean delivery, bronchoscoped, and intubated before clamping of the umbilical cord, referred to as an EXIT procedure (EX-utero Intrapartum Therapy). The tumor may then be resected electively once a full evaluation of the disease extent and the presence of any associated anomalies has been completed.

Most neonatal tumors are benign or of low malignant potential and tend to behave more favorably than the same type of tumor in older children. Neuroblastoma, for example, generally presents as stage I disease in 90% of infants under 1 year of age, and is amenable to observation, if small, or complete resection. And hepatoblastomas presenting in the newborn period also tend to behave more favorably than when presenting later in infancy. Despite a collective rarity, presentation of malignant tumors in the newborn period occurs, and much work remains to identify determinants of tumorigenesis and pathogenesis.

MINIMALLY INVASIVE SURGERY

Laparoscopic or minimally invasive techniques are beginning to supplant many surgical procedures previously performed by laparotomy or thoracotomy. Laparoscopic procedures have been associated with decreased postoperative pain, earlier return to gastrointestinal function, shorter hospital stays, fewer wound complications, and improved cosmetic results, compared with the corresponding open procedures. Laparoscopic techniques have been applied to many of the neonatal procedures described in this chapter. Indeed, laparoscopic Nissen fundoplication for gastroesophageal reflux disease and laparoscopic-assisted pull-through procedures for Hirschsprung's disease are being performed routinely in the neonate and show shorter time to postoperative feeding, decreased hospital stay, and superior cosmesis. Furthermore, thoracoscopic repair of esophageal atresia with tracheoesophageal fistula is beginning to be advocated as an equally effective approach, and supporters claim improved pain management and skeletomuscular benefits. Laparoscopic repair of duodenal atresia is also being performed with good results. Both thoracoscopic and laparoscopic techniques are being increasingly used to repair Bochdalek and Morgagni diaphragmatic hernias with good outcomes in neonates who do not require ECLS. Laparoscopic-assisted endorectal pull-through for Hirschsprung's disease and for anorectoplasty to correct ARM are becoming more and more a part of the neonatal surgeon's armamentarium.[47] However, pathophysiologic effects of pneumoperitoneum or iatrogenic pneumothorax are only recently being analyzed. Such adverse consequences include reduced intraoperative arterial saturation, increased carbon dioxide retention (CO_2 is used for abdominal insufflation and diaphragmatic excursion may be compromised because of increased abdominal pressure), oliguria or even anuria for up to 6 hours postoperatively, hypothermia, and need for extended postoperative intubation, if procedures exceed 100 minutes, which they often may.[23] As experience increases and technical refinements are seen with improved optical systems and smaller instruments, a broader application of laparoscopy inevitably will occur in the neonatal patient population.

PARENT TEACHING

Preoperative

The advent of ever-increasing mechanisms of prenatal diagnosis allows parents to begin adjusting to the presence of certain malformations, some minor and others potentially lethal, before birth.[3] Research shows that parents experience various stages of grief, including shock, denial, anger, and sadness when faced with such news. Although the intensity of the negative emotions associated with the initial diagnosis may lessen by the time of delivery, resolution of these emotions should not be expected. Expressions of fear, anxiety, and guilt are likely.

Because parents' fears and fantasies about their infant's surgical diagnosis are frequently worse than reality, they should see their infant as soon as possible after birth and before surgery. Pictures of the infant should be taken before surgery and should include views with and without the defect if possible. Whenever time and patient condition allow, parents should hold their infant and have pictures taken of the family with their newborn. In the event of a neonate's death, these pictures may be very valuable to the family. In the event neonatal transport from the birth hospital to a referral center is required, the transport team should do everything possible to ensure that the mother, who may be in the early recovery phase from her delivery, sees her infant before departure.[10]

Additionally, the transport staff and the staff at the referral hospital should encourage the mother to begin the process of pumping breast milk soon after delivery. Not only is breast milk almost always best for the surgical neonate but this feeding modality also gives the mother a concrete way of helping her ill newborn The key to successful breast milk establishment is to start early, usually in the labor and delivery suite, and to express milk often, from 8 to 10 times in a 24-hour period (see Table 18-3 in Chapter 18). The more frequently an infant nurses the higher, the mother's milk production, so expression of breast milk is the mother's way of "placing an order in advance" for her infant when he or she is able to eat (http://newborns.stanford.edu/Breastfeeding/PMGs.html#sickbaby).

The planned operative procedure and its expected results, as well as risks and alternatives, are discussed with the parents, ensuring that all questions and concerns are addressed. An informed consent for surgery is signed by the treating surgeon and witnessed by the bedside nurse. The bedside nurse should be present when the physician meets with the family to discuss the operation because the nurse is often the most consistent individual hearing explanations from the neonatologist, surgeon, and anesthesiologist, and must answer questions, interpret information, and reassure an anxious family when these teams leave. The nurse has a further important role to reassure parents about postoperative analgesia and sedation for their infant. Preoperative teaching can involve educating parents to recognize pain cues in their baby, and they should be encouraged to discuss their concerns if they perceive their baby is experiencing discomfort. Care providers' sensitivity to the neonate's pain and advocating for pain relief are comforting for parents (see Chapter 12).

Parents often fear what the infant will look like on return from surgery. Providing written material with simple drawings of the defects and operative procedure may help to prevent postoperative surprises. Seeing another patient who has had a similar procedure and has the postoperative equipment that has been described (e.g., colostomy, orogastric tube, chest tube) may be helpful to the family as well. The nursing staff must be careful, however, to protect the privacy of other patients and should obtain parental consent before using another infant for this purpose.

Intraoperative

Accompanying the infant to the preoperative area and seeing the infant as soon as possible after surgery are comforting to the parents. Progress reports during the surgery, if possible, are helpful for the anxious family members. After the operation, the pediatric surgeon should immediately see the parents to explain the procedure and any unexpected findings or problems that occurred during the operation. It should be clear to both the family and the surgeon where this important communication will take place, and privacy should be protected during the interchange.

Postoperative

After surgery, the nurse should help parents to focus on their infant rather than the surrounding intensive care environment. Although the nursing staff should identify the monitors and equipment in the baby's room and should explain the purpose of each to the family, encouraging parents in ways to comfort their baby will be of greatest benefit to their postoperative child (and to them). Early involvement in caregiving helps the parents to feel that they are essential to their child's recovery. Even in the immediate postoperative period, a parent can quietly sit and hold his or her infant's hand or take an axillary temperature.

Mothers should be encouraged to provide breast milk for use as soon as feedings begin. In the majority of cases it will be the feeding that is best tolerated by the convalescing neonate. The nurse acts as a liaison for consultation with a lactation specialist for coaching and instruction if needed. She should be certain that the mother has access to a pump and supplies and is encouraged to pump every 2 to 4 hours around the clock. Quiet, private accommodations for breast pumping should be available in or adjacent to the patient care area and policies should be in place to ensure expressed breast milk is properly identified and stored at all times. If possible, the mother should also be encouraged to breastfeed her infant as the infant's improvement allows.

If an infant is to be discharged home with an ostomy, parents should begin to participate in stoma care as early as possible. Consultation with an enterostomal therapy nurse is of further benefit. Parents begin by learning to cleanse the skin around the ostomy or to prepare the appliance and peristomal salves. Gradually parents will learn to increase their responsibilities of caregiving as their infant improves. Frequent practice improves proficiency and empowers parents for taking their infant home. Delay until a few days before discharge does not give parents adequate time for practice and familiarity for home care and does not serve the infant or family well. The same is true for infants who are discharged with other types of complicated care, such as home total parenteral nutrition or feedings through a gastrostomy tube and/or on a continuous feeding pump. Parent teaching also includes the possibility of late postoperative complications and recognition of problems that may develop and a plan of action for dealing with them. The importance of follow-up care is emphasized to the parents. It may be helpful for parents to talk with a "graduate" parent who had an infant with similar problems. Contact information about available resources, such as visiting nurses, graduate parents, and parent support groups are provided to parents before discharge. A concise history of hospitalization and the discharge plan is made available to all posthospitalization health care providers and a copy provided to parents at the time of discharge. Encouraging parents to keep a copy of this discharge summary in their diaper bag increases the chances they will have it available should they be required to take their medically complex and vulnerable infant emergently to the hospital.

REFERENCES

For a full list of references, scan the QR code or visit http://booksite.elsevier.com/ 9780323320832.

29

FAMILIES IN CRISIS
Theoretical and Practical Considerations

SANDRA L. GARDNER, KRISTIN VOOS, AND PATTI HILLS

The technical advances in the care of critically ill and premature infants have resulted in decreased morbidity and mortality of the high-risk infant. These developments have been accompanied by a heightened awareness of the psychologic strain and emotional stresses encountered by the family of the sick neonate and the profound effect on family functioning.[7,23,138,148,163] Realization of the need for a family-centered approach to perinatal care has emerged out of an enhanced understanding of individual and family functioning and the challenges in coping and adapting to stress.[8,92,102] It has become essential for perinatal health care teams to be cognizant of the overall psychologic needs of families who are experiencing the painful crisis of the birth of a sick newborn.[148,225] This chapter discusses the complex psychosocial needs of families during this stressful period and offers concrete suggestions for intervention.

NORMAL ATTACHMENT

Emotional connection to an infant begins not at birth but during pregnancy. The terms *attachment* and *bonding*[118] are used to describe this process of relating between parents and their infant. Attachment is characterized by the same qualities used to describe love: care, responsibility, and knowledge. Parental love and romantic love activate the same areas of the human brain, result in

brain processing of infant cues, and elevate the "bonding" hormone, oxytocin.[64,233] Attachment is an individualized process and does not happen automatically.[23,177]

The neonate is totally dependent, both physically and emotionally, on the caregivers, whereas caregivers are not dependent on the infant. Recognition of this unique relationship is evidenced cross-culturally by immediate and prolonged contact with no evidence of separation.[109,177] In most animal species, the mother engages in species-specific behaviors[118] that enable her to become acquainted with and claim the newborn. If there is disruption during this critical period, it can result in rejection by the animal mother and death of the young. Recent studies have shown a relationship between stressful environments, the health of the fetus, and caregiving ability (see Chapter 13). Parental attachment and appropriate caregiving behaviors are crucial for the infant's physical, psychologic, and emotional health and survival. Ultimately, this influence can affect the infant's well-being as an adult and potential parenting ability.

Critical and Sensitive Period

In the period immediately after birth, healthy mothers and infants are physiologically and psychologically ready for reciprocal interaction.[118] Even though labor and birth are tiring, most mothers feel "high" and have an incredible surge of energy after birth. Psychologically, the family is ready to meet

---

PURPLE type highlights content that is particularly applicable to clinical settings.

and interact with the long-awaited newcomer. The first hour of life can be a time of alertness for the newborn. Before the sleep phase, the newborn is alert, makes eye-to-eye contact, fixes and follows, begins to search unassisted for the maternal nipple, and begins to feed. At birth, all five senses are operational and the infant is ready to cue and shape the environment (see Chapters 5 and 13).

The period of mutual readiness between parents and their infant(s) has been compared with the critical period in animals. This human "maternal sensitive period"[118] immediately after birth is an optimal time for attachment to develop. Positive effects of early and extended contact, rather than initial separation, have shown significant differences in caregiving behaviors that persist over time.

Sustained and early contact between parents and their infant gives the family the opportunity for interaction. The presence of the infant enables the parents to understand the reality and individuality of their infant. Early parent-infant contact facilitates parent-infant attachment and contributes to the regulation of the newborn's physiology and behavior.[23,32,148,177,220] Early skin-to-skin contact between mothers and their infants results in significant benefits: (1) better breastfeeding, (2) maintenance of infant body temperature, (3) higher blood glucose, (4) lower respiratory rate, (5) better heart rate stability, (6) more affectionate maternal behavior, (7) lower salivary cortisol levels, and (8) less infant crying.[32,170,220] Unnecessary "routines" and procedures that interfere with initial contact and bonding should be deferred, if possible, until the family has time for this important interaction (see Chapter 5).

Although the delay of immediate contact for medically necessary interventions does not promote attachment, neither does it undermine the entire process of attachment.[51] Fortunately, human mothers do not automatically reject their infant if they cannot interact immediately. During medically necessary interventions, it is important to give parents as much interaction (or at least visual contact) with their infant as is possible.

Crisis Event: Pregnancy and Parenthood

Pregnancy, birth, and parenthood are almost universally defined as a life transition and crisis.[70,109,177] Becoming a parent requires a major adjustment of the roles, lifestyle, and relationships. Because previous ideas and coping strategies may not be helpful, life crisis situations challenge the individual with the potential for growth as new responses and solutions are used for problem solving. Periods of upheaval, change, and vulnerability can provide a time of openness, receptiveness, and readiness for help and support from significant others (including professionals).

Influences on Parenting

Opportunities to experience parenting and observe others in that role are essential learning experiences in developing one's own parenting behaviors and style. The ability to parent is influenced by a multitude of factors that occur before, during, and after the birth of the infant. Previous life events, including degree of life stress/patterns of coping,[141,225,234] genetic endowment, being parented,[78,83,177] previous pregnancies,[113,138] anxiety and distress about parenting role,[★] and interpersonal relationships,[30,78,177] affect the experience of pregnancy and parenthood. The events of the current pregnancy,[†] their significance to the parent, and the availability of support and assistance influence parenting ability.[148,168,177,225]

After birth, infant characteristics (e.g., responsiveness/vulnerability/severity of illness),[57,83,103] appearance,[23,65,168] parental feelings of loyalty and hope, the behavior of health professionals,[‡] separation from the infant,[§] an inability to protect their newborn from pain,[110,168,180] and hospital practices[‖] may positively or negatively influence parents.

Not only the occurrence of these events but also their meaning to the individual and the type of support received influence parenting abilities.

Cultural practices influence maternal and paternal attachment behaviors.[¶] Studies indicate that cultural differences influence (1) parental emotional responses and perceptions of their infant's illness and disability, (2) parental usage of services, and (3) parental interaction with health care providers.[26] Research demonstrates that how parents interact with their newborn varies based on their culture[86] (e.g., Japanese mothers look at their babies more

---

★References 54, 66, 83, 103, 168, 177, 225.
†References 30, 98, 118, 134, 148, 154, 177.
‡References 54, 66, 81, 118, 130, 163, 167, 234.
§References 51, 65, 124, 148, 167, 177, 180.
‖References 23, 51, 54, 80, 83, 98, 103, 119, 130, 148, 163, 177, 236.
¶References 26, 103, 109, 141, 168, 172, 195, 196, 205.

than Brazilian mothers do, who touch and interact more with them).[127] A recent study of Thai mothers in the neonatal intensive care unit (NICU) showed that the most frequent maternal behavior was touching (from infant's extremities to trunk), followed by inspection (of the infant's appearance and recognition of family traits), verbalization (e.g., to the infant and the nurse), and facial expression (e.g., smiling/crying/flat).[226] One must be cautious in viewing parental attachment behavior through one's own cultural filter, because this may result in an incorrect assessment of parent-infant attachment.[226] Differences in parent-infant interaction behaviors reflect cultural differences; therefore health care professionals' observations of these behaviors must be evaluated within the context of the family's culture.[†]

Steps of Attachment

Klaus and Kennell[118] propose nine steps in the process of attachment.

STEP 1: PLANNING THE PREGNANCY

Planning the pregnancy is the initial step of investment and commitment[177] to parenthood. Pregnancies are planned in one of two ways: consciously or unconsciously. Who planned the pregnancy and why this particular time has been chosen are important indicators of the investment of each individual in the decision and in the pregnancy.

Carrying a pregnancy is not assurance that the baby is wanted. Although it may be a legal option, abortion may not be a cultural, moral, financial, or ethical option for the individual woman. Attachment of the mother (or father) to the infant is not ensured merely by the mother remaining pregnant, giving birth, and keeping the infant.

STEP 2: CONFIRMING THE PREGNANCY

Pregnancy confirmation begins the psychologic acceptance of the pregnancy. Delaying confirmation enables the fact of pregnancy to be denied and may influence progression to the acceptance stage.

STEP 3: ACCEPTING THE PREGNANCY

Accepting the pregnancy usually begins early in the pregnancy and is characterized by the emotional changes of primary narcissism, introversion, and passivity. Because the expectant mother is less interested

in the outside world and more interested in her own inner world, the mother can become attuned to her own needs. Although she was previously engaged in active, extroverted behaviors, during the pregnancy she may contentedly participate in quieter, more introspective activities.

At this early stage of pregnancy, the fetus is not perceived by the woman as separate from herself but as an extension of her body. The psychologic changes of pregnancy have survival significance in that caring for herself ensures caring for the fetus as an integral part of herself.[141,177]

During the early months of pregnancy, the man and woman realize that parenting will require a major adjustment of prepregnancy roles, lifestyle, and relationships. The adaptation of parenthood is characterized by upheaval and change, losses and gains. Bombarded with phenomenal lifelong changes, the future parents experience the normal feeling of ambivalence.

STEP 4: FETAL MOVEMENT

Fetal movement, felt by the mother between 16 and 32 weeks of gestation, is the beginning of accepting the fetus as an individual. Fetal movement is the first concrete evidence to the mother of the existence of another person within her. Hearing the baby's heartbeat, seeing the ultrasound images, or experiencing an amniocentesis also confirms the reality of the fetus.[177] Fetal movement is such a significant event that often a pregnancy that began as unplanned and unwanted becomes wanted.

Perception of the first fetal movement is a happy event. When asked "How did you feel when the baby first moved?" most women respond in a happy tone and with a smile. Use of a negative tone or negative words to describe fetal movement is a concern because the individual (fetus) already may be perceived as an intruder.

STEP 5: ACCEPTING THE FETUS

Accepting the fetus as an individual begins with fetal movement. The fetus shows individuality in controlling the movement; the mother can neither start nor stop these movements. With the realization of the presence of another person, parents begin acceptance of the fetus as a separate individual. Love for the fetus as a separate individual occurs as the parents invest a personality in the fetus and start to establish a relationship. Fantasies about how the baby looks, its sex, and the wish for a perfect, healthy infant are common. Women with a history of perinatal loss

[†]References 109, 168, 172, 195, 196, 205, 226.

have been shown to have disturbances in maternal attachment related to differentiating the self from the fetus in a subsequent pregnancy.[159]

Outwardly, preparations are made for the acceptance of an infant into the home; baby clothes and furniture are purchased, and a room is prepared. The fetus may be referred to by a nickname or a term of endearment. The baby's name may be chosen. Choosing a name is a highly personal and significant event. The meaning of the name and who chooses it illustrate the power holder and decision maker within the family. Prenatal questions such as the following may be asked after the birth to elicit information: "Do you have a nickname for the baby?" "Do you have a name picked out for the baby?" "Who picked it out?"

Whether the newborn meets parental expectations for "the right sex" may be crucially important for the parents to attach to the infant. "Do you have a sex preference for the baby?" may be asked before or after the birth to uncover this information. Often parents with a strong sex preference have chosen no names for a baby of the "wrong" gender. "It doesn't matter as long as it's healthy" is often heard and may indicate no conscious gender preference. However, unconsciously, the parents may have a strong gender preference as evidenced by a predominance of dreams about one gender. If dreams are equally divided between male and female children, there may indeed be no gender preference at the unconscious level.

Most parents are fearful of producing a defective child. This fear is experienced as dreams about dead, deformed, or damaged fetuses and babies or dreams with a central theme of destruction. These unconscious contents often are experienced as frightening nightmares that may be imbued with magical ideas such as "If I think (or talk about) it, it will come true." Both before and after birth, it is reassuring for parents to know that this is a common and scary phenomenon, that they aren't "crazy," and that the fears are not magical.

Parental expectations of the newborn are established before birth in the personification and relationship with the unseen, unheard fetus. Research shows that a close, high-quality prenatal attachment to the fetus is associated with fewer depression symptoms in the last trimester and postpartally.[74] Compared with adult women, pregnant adolescents are slower in developing an antenatal emotional attachment to their fetus.[199] After birth, parents often experience the developmental process of working out the potential discrepancy between the wished-for and the actual infant.[216] Before attachment to the actual infant can proceed, the fantasized child must be mourned.

STEP 6: LABOR AND BIRTH

Labor is a physiologic, maturational, and psychologic crisis for the family. Birth is the culmination of pregnancy and the reward for the work of labor. Parents' attitudes about the labor and birth experiences may affect their reactions to the infant.[51] Research shows that continuous physical and emotional support during labor significantly improves birth outcomes for the mother (e.g., shortens labor duration, reduces the need for pain medication and operative vaginal and cesarean section birth) and the newborn (e.g., better Apgar scores, better/longer breast feeding, fewer NICU admissions, fewer complications of obstetric [OB] interventions because fewer OB interventions used). In addition to better physiologic outcomes, improved psychologic outcomes include (1) increase in maternal-infant attachment behaviors, (2) better confidence and ability to cope with labor, (3) better maternal satisfaction and personal control during labor, (4) enhanced maternal self-esteem, (5) positive attitudes toward mothering and family relationships, and (6) easier mothering (i.e., sees baby as less fussy).[201]

Paternal participation in labor and birth is an important issue. Many years ago, health care professionals saw no benefit to the presence of the father and even wished to exclude him because of imagined "horribles" such as increased infection rate, malpractice suits, and disruption of routines. Birth is a powerfully emotional experience; those who attend birth are more attached to the infant than those who do not attend.[118,148] Benefits attributed to a father's participation at labor and birth include use of less analgesia, a more supportive environment, and a deepened relationship[9] between parents and between parents and their infant.[148] Inclusion of the father in perinatal events may engage him for inclusion in parenting activities.[54,148] Rather than just a financial provider, fathering may be perceived as a psychologic necessity for both fathers and children.

Parental behaviors at birth such as the following indicate involvement and investment in the infant[95]:

- How does the mother or father look? At the sound of the infant's cry, parents smile and breathe a sigh of relief at this first breath of life. Support, joy, and happiness are positive feelings shared by couples at birth.

• What does the mother or father say? By speaking in a positive tone with words of affection and endearment, the parents relate to each other and to the new infant.

• What does the mother or father do? When offered the infant, both parents will reach out to take the infant. Spontaneously, parents engage in eye-to-eye contact and touch and explore the infant. Affectionate behaviors such as kissing, fondling, cuddling, and claiming characterize positive parental reactions.

A positive, self-affirming birth experience for the mother enhances her feelings of empowerment and self-esteem and thus her self-concept as a woman and mother.[177,201] A birth experience that does not meet parental expectations may have a negative effect on the self-concept of the mother, her perception of her ability to parent, and her relationship with the infant.[51] In fact, "so intricately are mother and infant entwined in a symbiotic relationship, that what is psychically positive for the mother is positive for the infant. What is psychically negative for the mother will affect the infant."[177]

So powerful is the labor and birth experience that women may be unable to proceed with parenting until psychic closure of the experience has occurred. Even women who experience a normal labor and birth process should recount the experience to others. Maternal perception of the events is obvious in tone and content of the recounting. *Missing pieces*[1] is the term used to describe the aspects of labor and birth that are forgotten or unavailable to recall. Long labor, short labor, or medicated labor can cause missing pieces in the mother's memory of the birth. Labor that did not meet expectations because of difficulty, cesarean section, use of forceps, or episiotomy also could affect the mother.[1] To proceed with parenting, these women should be encouraged to fill in their knowledge gaps by asking questions or looking at pictures or films of the birth to reconstruct the situation.

STEP 7: SEEING

Seeing and touching are the species-specific ways in which humans attach to their young.[118] Immediate attachment is facilitated by (1) positive maternal feelings toward the infant; (2) mother able to see infant immediately after birth; and (3) immediate contact

between mother and infant.[23] Delayed attachment may occur when the infant is ill or premature because he or she does not conform to parental expectations of a healthy full-term baby.[23,51,158,226]

Eye contact between parents and their infant in the initial period after birth may be a positive release of parental feelings of warmth, closeness, and caring. As parents see and inspect the newborn, they begin claiming their infant—"He has my eyes" or "She has your nose." Characteristics of each parent and the family are identified in the infant, and the newborn is claimed as a member of the family.[226]

The term *en face position* is used to describe the mother's (father's) eyes and the infant's eyes positioned in the same vertical plane.[118] This positioning enables the parent and the infant to look directly into each other's eyes, to focus, and to regard each other (Figure 29-1).

The newborn infant is an active participant; he or she cues the mother with eye-to-eye contact. Even minutes-old newborns see and show a preference for the human face (within 7 to 12 inches from their face). The newborn can visually follow the parent's face and voice and signal the parent with facial expressions, movement, and vocalization, including a distress cry when separated from body contact with mother (see Chapter 13).

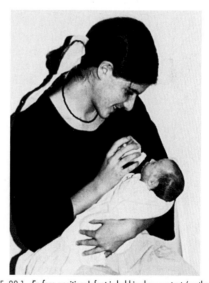

FIGURE 29-1 *En face position:* Infant is held in close contact (mother's body touching infant's); mother is looking at infant *en face;* bottle is perpendicular to mouth; milk is in tip of nipple. (From Klaus MH, Kennel JH: *Parent-infant bonding,* ed 2, St Louis, 1982, Mosby.)

Deterrents to the infant's full participation in this "getting to know you" phase include removal to the nursery, medication (from analgesia), and eye prophylaxis. Unless medically indicated (necessary for physical survival), newborns should remain with their parents after birth.[148] Because eye prophylaxis irritates and interferes with vision, the "routine" instillation immediately after birth (in the delivery room) can be delayed until after the initial acquaintance process is completed. Maternal depression also has been identified as a risk factor for poor mother–infant interaction.[124]

STEP 8: TOUCHING

In exploring the infant, parents systematically use fingertip contact with the infant's extremities. Gradually, there is progression to palm contact with the infant's trunk (Figure 29-2). With the healthy term infant, this progression occurs within minutes of the first contact. After gaining confidence and preliminary knowledge, the parent will hold the infant close in a cuddling position.

With the preterm infant, this characteristic progression may take hours, days, or several visits (see Figure 29-2). Fear of harming the small, fragile preterm infant often prevents parents from feeling at ease in touching him or her.[226] Until the parents feel confident that their actions will not harm the infant, they may be reticent to use palm contact with the trunk. Not only the use of nurturing maternal touch but also the vulnerability of the premature infant affect how touch is perceived by the infant. One study showed that nurturing maternal touch was associated with more secure attachment in robust preterms and with less secure attachment in the most vulnerable infants (see Chapter 13).

Holding and cuddling the infant are significantly different from touching and exploring. The amount of holding influences mother–infant interaction with preterm infants.[125] Mothers who have only seen and touched their infant still experience "empty arms." The species-specific behavior of touch is not completely satisfied until the parent can hold the infant. Most mothers have a preference for holding their infants on the left. Explanations for this preference include hand dominance, importance of maternal heartbeat, left breast sensitivity, and advantages in monitoring the infant. A more recent hypothesis proposes that maternal affective signals (both visual

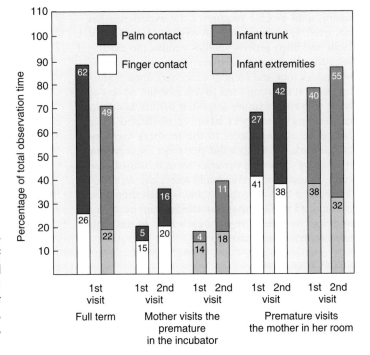

FIGURE 29-2 Fingertip and palm contact on trunk or extremities in three groups of mothers: (1) 12 mothers of term infants at their first visit, (2) 9 mothers who visited their premature infants in incubators in the NICU, and (3) 14 mothers whose premature infants were brought to their maternity rooms and placed in their beds. (From Klaus MH, Kennel JH: *Parent-infant bonding*, ed 2, St Louis, 1982, Mosby.)

and auditory) are given to the infant's free left ear and processed by the more advanced right cerebral hemisphere.[210]

STEP 9: CAREGIVING

The final step of attachment, caregiving, is important for psychic closure of the task of bonding. A metasynthesis of nine qualitative studies found two simultaneous processes necessary in the transition to motherhood: (1) engagement, a commitment to mothering that involves active attachment to the infant, experiencing the infant's presence, and involvement in caregiving for the infant; and (2) growth and transformation, which characterize the change of a woman into the new "self" of a mother.[177] Men also make the transition to fatherhood in the early postpartal period. A qualitative study of first-time fathers indicates that those who wanted to be highly involved in the care of their baby reported not feeling supported by the health care provider/hospital policies to engage in paternal and parental behaviors that favor involvement with their infant.[54] Fathers experienced more negative (63%) than positive (37%) interactions with nurses during the postpartum period.[54] In assisting parental transition, nurses and all health care professionals should support, intervene, and use all encounters with both new parents as "teaching moments and opportunities."[54,145] Empowering new parents with knowledge about how to care for their new baby has been shown to have a significant impact on maternal attachment and self-confidence in first-time mothers.[43]

The relationship between the primary caregiver and the infant is reciprocal. In the caregiving relationship, both care provider and infant give to and receive from each other.[81,177] The physical and emotional needs of the helpless infant are satisfied by parental caregiving behaviors such as feeding, soothing, bathing, grooming, and playing. Based on the infant's ability to perceive and receive care, the infant responds to the care provider. Parental expectations of newborn responses include quieting, sucking, clinging and cuddling, looking, smiling, and vocalizing. The parent's capability to soothe and satisfy the infant provides emotional satisfaction and positive feedback about the parent's competency.

Personal needs for comfort, maintenance of homeostasis, and relief from painful experiences are infant expectations of the relationship with the care provider. Care-eliciting behaviors (e.g., crying, visual following, smiling) are neonatal cues used to signal the care provider that attention is needed. Relief from discomfort enables the infant to respond positively to the care provider. The infant experiences the world through the caregiver and quickly learns that the environment is either nurturing and loving or hostile and nonresponsive. Consistent, predictable nurturing and caregiving enable the infant to develop a sense of trust in the caregiver, the world, and the self (see Chapter 13).

Care by parents is the ideal neonatal care situation, because the infant learns and reacts to one set of cues or caregiving behaviors. Cared for by one or two people, the infant can regulate his or her physiologic behavioral processes (i.e., autonomic, neuroendocrine, behavioral, electrophysiologic) and develop synchrony with the parents.[130,148,177] Single caregiving improves the establishment of biorhythms of the neonate for sleep-wake cycles, feeding, and visual attentiveness. Multiple caregivers confuse the infant, increase distress with feeding, cause irritability, and upset visual attention. Care by parents provides for mutual cuing and acquaintance and a natural setting for observation of parent-infant interaction.[130,148,163]

PSYCHOLOGIC ADJUSTMENTS TO A SICK NEWBORN

The birth of a child is a major life change. Parents of infants requiring NICU care often experience high levels of stress, and as a consequence their ability to interact optimally with their infant(s) is impaired. For many parents this may be the first time they have had to cope with a significant challenge in their lives. This may lead to depression, impaired recall, dysfunctional parenting patterns, and poorer developmental outcomes for their child.[63,165,235] The perinatal health care team is presented with a unique opportunity to practice preventive health care.[225] During this stressful time the families' usual problem-solving mechanisms may not be adequate to cope with the events presented to them.[35] In addition to confronting this situational crisis, the individual or family must master the normal developmental process of parenthood.

Parental behavior and responses are determined not only by preexisting personality factors, social and cultural variables, and interactions with significant others[138] but also by the immediate situation

BOX 29-1	SITUATIONAL FACTORS AFFECTING PARENTAL COPING*

1. The behaviors and attitudes of the hospital staff (physicians, nurses, and allied health professionals)
2. The sensitivity used in the process of separation and transfer of the infant to the intensive care unit or, in some cases, the referral hospital
3. The flexibility of hospital policy concerning parental and sibling involvement and visitation in the nursery
4. The instruction of parents in their infant's individual behaviors and characteristics (thus facilitating appropriate parent-child interaction and reciprocity) (see Chapter 13)
5. The staff's comprehension and appreciation of the psychosocial functioning of families and the family's responses and adaptation to stress and crisis
6. The employment of emotionally supportive intervention programs for parents within the nursery setting
7. The development of appropriate discharge planning to provide adequate follow-up care to the infant and family

*References 23, 28, 66, 81, 82, 92, 98, 100, 103, 138, 167, 180, 234.

in which the parents are placed.* The following six major sources of parental stress in the NICU have been identified:

- Preexisting and concurrent personal and family factors
- Prenatal and perinatal experiences
- Infant illness, treatments, and appearance[†]
- Concerns about the infant's outcome[133]
- Loss of the parental role[‡]
- Health care providers [66,98,103,133]

Situational factors can have an important bearing on the family's ability to cope with the crisis and thus affect the overall outcome (Box 29-1). Uncertainty about their infant's future and separation from their infant are sources of parental stress that can dramatically affect the quality of attachment that develops.[37]

Families are psychologically vulnerable after the birth of a sick infant. During this period of crisis there may be a heightened receptivity to accepting help and being open and responsive to change, because the family is struggling for a way to cope with the crisis. Significant potentialities exist for

individual and family emotional growth and development.[23,34,66,103,214] Parental perception of support by nurses has been shown to be significantly associated with maternal depressive symptoms; as the perception of nursing support decreased, there was a corresponding increase in maternal depressive symptoms.[52] The perinatal health team has an opportunity to influence how the individual and family adapt to the crisis.*

By providing appropriate supportive interventions coupled with enlightened policies and attitudes that reflect family-centered principles (Box 29-2), the team can have a significant positive influence on the family's ability to cope. Supportive interventions enhance the likelihood for successful adjustment and ultimately a healthy parent-child relationship.[†]

Family-centered care (FCC) is a philosophy often strived for in the NICU, but current practice and policies often may lag behind philosophy. NICU staff verbalize acceptance of families being involved in care, but their actions do not always reflect their words.[20,21,27,84]

Studies show a discrepancy between nurses' knowledge about the necessity of and their current practice of FCC.[185] Current practice of FCC scored significantly lower than scores representing necessity. Nurses do not consistently practice what they know to be necessary! NICU nurses scored significantly lower on the necessity scale than did pediatric and pediatric intensive care unit (PICU) nurses; nurses with fewer than 10 years of practice scored higher on the necessary and current use of family-centered principles than did nurses with more practice experience.[185] Organizational barriers to implementation include (1) the design of the health care system; (2) the lack of emotional support, guidance, and direction for the staff; (3) the lack of recognition, confidence, and support for nursing autonomy and skills to perform FCC; and (4) beliefs that dealing with families is stressful, interferes with care of the infant, and is "not part of my job."[6,45,66,185]

FCC principles stress that parents are the most important persons in their infant's life, that they have expertise in caring for the infant, and that their values and beliefs should be central during NICU care.[92,102] FCC demands a change from task-oriented, health care provider–centered care

---

*References 51, 101, 124, 148, 158, 184.
[†]References 23, 51, 65, 83, 133, 168.
[‡]Reference 23, 46, 51, 66, 103, 133, 168, 177, 228, 236.

*References 23, 56, 83, 101, 103, 124, 133, 163, 184, 214, 236.
[†]References 23, 51, 66, 83, 98, 101, 103, 124, 130, 133, 138, 148, 158, 167, 206, 214, 225.

BOX 29-2	PRINCIPLES OF FAMILY-CENTERED NEONATAL CARE

1. Family-centered neonatal care should be based on open and honest communication between parents and professionals on medical and ethical issues.
2. To work with professionals in making informed treatment choices, parents must have available to them the same facts and interpretation of those facts as the professionals, including medical information presented in meaningful formats, information about uncertainties surrounding treatments, information from parents whose children have been in similar medical situations, and access to the chart and rounds discussions.
3. In medical situations involving very high mortality and morbidity, great suffering, and/or significant medical controversy, fully informed parents should have the right to make decisions about aggressive treatment for their infants.
4. Expectant parents should be offered information about adverse pregnancy outcomes and be given the opportunity to state in advance their treatment preferences if their infant is born extremely prematurely and/or critically ill.
5. Parents and professionals must work together to acknowledge and alleviate the pain of infants in the neonatal intensive care unit (NICU).
6. Parents and professionals must work together to ensure an appropriate environment for infants in the NICU.
7. Parents and professionals must work together to ensure the safety and efficacy of neonatal treatments.
8. Parents and professionals must work together to develop nursery policies and programs that promote parenting skills and encourage maximum involvement of families with their hospitalized infants.
9. Parents and professionals must work together to promote meaningful long-term follow-up for all high-risk NICU survivors.
10. Parents and professionals must acknowledge that critically ill newborns can be harmed by overtreatment, as well as undertreatment, and must insist that laws and treatment policies be based on compassion. Parents and professionals must work together to promote awareness of the needs of NICU survivors with disabilities to ensure adequate support for them and their families. Parents and professionals must work together to decrease disability through universal prenatal care.

Modified from Harrison H: The principles for family-centered neonatal care, *Pediatrics* 92:643, 1993.

BOX 29-3	WHAT FAMILIES WANT IN FAMILY-CENTERED CARE[106]

- To be consistently and respectfully involved in decisions about the health care of their family member and their family members to be involved in ways they choose
- Health care providers to listen to the family's observations and incorporate their preferences about treatment into the plan of care
- Useful and understandable information from health care providers
- Personal connection—a relationship with health care providers; need personal connection and to be able to trust those providing care
- Patient comfort and pain control; important to family's (and patient's) perception of the hospital experience
- Information and support for handling transitions in health care

interaction with other allied health professionals and therapists, (5) participant in hospital committees, and (6) as a change agent in health care settings.[59] Box 29-3 contains key components of FCC desired by families; they are remarkably similar to the Principles of Family-Centered Neonatal Care in Box 29-2. A Web-based tool, the Family-Centered Care Map (available at www.fccmap.org), has been developed and studied.[60] This tool is based on 63 potentially better practices and is a joint effort of three NICUs (and their families), Vermont Oxford Network's Neonatal Intensive Care Quality Improvement Collaborative, and the Institute for Family-Centered Care. Use of the "Family-Centered Care Map" results in (1) improved growth for extremely low-birth-weight (ELBW) preterms, (2) decreased length of stay for ELBW preterms by 13 days, and (3) better implementation of FCC principles.[107]

Parenting in the NICU is something most families are not prepared for or expect. Finding their parental role in this situation can be difficult and taxing, especially when their infant is critically ill.[66] Such challenges can have long-lasting effects on parental well-being and family functioning.[221] Fenwick and colleagues' research[66] reports that mothers perceive their relationship with NICU nurses as either facilitating or inhibiting their ability to mother their preterms in the NICU. Actions that facilitate mothering are family-centered. Facilitative nursing actions include fostering the relationship between mother and infant by (1) assisting mothers to gain intimate knowledge and caregiving opportunities, (2) educating parents about their infant's

to a collaborative, relationship-based model of family advocacy and empowerment.[66,92,130,152] Roles for families in FCC include (1) advocate for their infant, (2) peer support to other families, (3) collaboration with and education of clinicians, (4) medical condition, (3) providing ongoing positive feedback to parents, (4) acknowledging the importance of the dyadic mother-infant and father-infant relationship, (5) honoring the mother as the infant's primary caregiver, (6) enhancing mother-infant interaction opportunities, and (7) collaborating with parents and relinquishing control to parents particularly at the bedside.[66,130]

Family-centered nursing care promotes physical closeness and intimacy with premature infants. Inhibitive nursing action can result in (1) patriarchal, authoritarian style of care delivery; (2) focuses on "protecting" the infant (from the parents); (3) maintains the nurse as the "expert" who retains control by directing and "allowing" parent involvement; and (4) dismisses parental worries, concerns, rights, and skills.[66] In the presence of inhibitive nursing actions, mothers are left with the feeling of "struggling to mother" in the NICU.[66] Mothers who are alienated and disaffected by these encounters feel angry, frustrated, distressed, inadequate, unsure, and anxious.[66] These feelings may result in (1) an inability to resume the relationship with the infant that has been interrupted by the stay in the NICU, (2) a delay in the mothering process, (3) feelings of depression or anxiety, (4) an impact on parenting and caregiving after discharge, and (5) affected perceptions of how they see themselves as mothers.[66] Maternal strategies to deal with highly tense NICU relationships include guarding and speaking out about the situation. Guarding strategies include (1) withholding feelings about inhibitive nursing actions and smoothing over the relationship with the nurse(s), (2) withdrawing from the nursery, and (3) blaming oneself to justify the nurse's actions.[66] Mothers who spoke up did so only after tolerating a number of incidents, and often it was the father who complained. The consequences for speaking out may include (1) earning a reputation with the staff as a "troublemaker," (2) recrimination in the form of sanctions and punitive actions that result in a "struggle to mother," or (3) becoming a disenfranchised mother.[66]

Several qualitative studies examining the "lived experience" of parents of a preterm/sick newborn illustrate parental need for a relationship with care providers in the NICU. A prospective, qualitative study from three NICUs in France, about parental expectations from NICU staff, studied 30 mothers and fathers of preterms younger than 32 weeks of gestation.[87] Fathers in the study described the bond with their preterm baby as more fashioned of words and looks involving distance, whereas mothers experienced the bond more physically. Of prime importance in the ability of these parents to form a bond with their preterm in the NICU was their relationship with NICU nurses. Two aspects of NICU nurses' care were cited by parents: (1) a caring attitude by the nurse toward the baby and parents, coupled with (2) caring communication with the parents about their infant, which decreased parental stress and facilitated interactions. The researchers concluded that the creation of a bond between the parents and their preterm infant is "*rooted in their relationship with the caregivers.*"[87] Another study found that relationships with their baby's caregivers enabled parents to (1) trust that their baby was being cared for well, (2) endure the NICU, (3) feel less isolated and more in control, and (4) have hope.[184] A phenomenologic study of parents' experiences with kangaroo care in the NICU illustrated the importance of information, communication, consistency, and individualized knowledgeable support and relationship with staff nurses who give parents the "courage" and confidence to hold and attach to their baby.[133]

Very important in any neonatal illness and subsequent hospitalization is the disruption and stress that is frequently created in the nuclear family system. Just as preterm and sick neonates experience stress in the NICU (see Chapter 13), parents also are stressed when their infant is in a NICU.[46,101,133,163,228] A study of the prevalence of posttraumatic stress disorder (PTSD) in parents with an infant in the NICU found that 35% of mothers and 24% of fathers had acute stress disorder at 3 to 5 days after admission.[132] Thirty days after admission to the NICU, 15% of mothers and 8% of fathers met criteria for PTSD. The severity of parental PTSD was correlated with concurrent stressors and family history of anxiety and depression.[132] A family's functioning and adaptation to stress have important effects on the family's relationship with the infant and the infant's later development. A premature birth places parents at a higher risk for psychologic distress than a full-term birth,[164] and, as a consequence, this can lead to depression, anxiety, and dysfunctional parenting patterns.[63,165,235] A crucial task of the perinatal health care team is to support families and intervene to assist them in adjusting to the unfortunate event of the birth of their sick infant to maximize their own growth, adaptation, and reorganization during this period.★

To assist parents through the difficult experience of having a sick infant, it is helpful to identify the psychologic tasks and emotional reactions they experience. This section describes the six psychologic issues facing families; it discusses the clinical and behavioral indicators that parents are struggling with and then suggests interventions that the perinatal health care team can employ to help families. It is extremely important to remember that these are generalizations and that each family or person must be approached individually.[177] In addition, in assessing families' reactions, it is critical to look at how they cope over time. Initially, there may be a tremendous amount of upset, disruption, and upheaval within the individual or family system. This can eventually lead to improved functioning and a sense of growth and mastery, "adjustment to the new normal." The key is how the individuals or families reorganize, how able they are to return to a state of equilibrium, the coping strategies they are able to develop, and whether the strategies are adaptive or maladaptive. Attachment and parenthood are complex, interactional developmental processes that must evolve and unfold over time.

Kaplan and Mason[113] describe the following four psychologic tasks with which parents of premature infants must deal:

1. Anticipatory grieving and withdrawal from the relationship established during pregnancy
2. Parental acknowledgment of feelings of guilt and failure
3. Resumption of the relationship with the infant that had been previously disrupted
4. Preparation to take the infant home

Two additional tasks also are significant:

5. Crisis events related to labor and delivery
6. Adaptation to the intensive care environment[66]

In general, these six psychologic tasks can be applied to any parent's reaction to a sick infant, with additional specific issues arising, depending on

whether the infant was premature or born with a congenital anomaly.

Labor and Delivery

The first psychologic task involves working through the crisis events surrounding the labor and delivery. Medical problems occurring at any point during the pregnancy or delivery that threaten the health or survival of the fetus or mother can result in the parents delaying their planning and making an emotional investment in the fetus or infant. Parents may psychologically withdraw from the pregnancy as a way of protecting themselves. The parents of an infant born prematurely often do not have the necessary psychologic and physical time to prepare. This deprivation of time may interfere with the parents' ability to complete the final steps of attachment described earlier.

Parents who have been concentrating on themselves in a healthy, narcissistic way may not yet be ready to transfer their investment to the infant, because they have been prematurely thrust into the role of parents.[103,148] There is an overwhelming sense of losing control of the events of the labor and delivery and their timing.[184]

On the other hand, some parents react in the opposite way. They may wish to be rid of the pregnancy as a way of dealing with their fear of the unknown and the uncertainty facing them. Many mothers of premature infants feel that their infants are alien[23,66,103]; they do not feel that the infant is really theirs, making it easier to have feelings of rejection toward the infant. In addition to feeling insufficient and inadequate about their ability to deliver an infant at term, they feel empty inside, as if something is missing. With a premature birth, there is usually a heightened sense of emergency and concern about the health and survival of the infant and, at times, the mother, who herself may have suffered complications.

In the case of a full-term infant born with a problem despite a problem-free pregnancy, there is a sense of overwhelming shock and disappointment.[180] Parents immediately sense the problem; as their apprehension mounts, they frequently imagine the worst. Parents of a newborn with a malformation normally experience lowered self-esteem and view this event as an affront to their reproductive capabilities. The mother specifically views it as a failure of her feminine role. Parents often feel that they

---

★References 23, 51, 66, 83, 98, 101, 124, 138, 148, 158, 168, 180, 225, 236.

have failed and that the infant symbolically represents their own defectiveness. Parents not only fear for the infant, they fear for themselves and what this infant may mean to their future. The reaction of the parents is based on the specific psychologic, social, and cultural meaning of the defect to the parents and the manner in which it is discussed and handled by the health care team.[118]

The emotional reactions and feelings that parents have at and after the delivery of a sick infant range from shock, fright, isolation, panic, anxiety, and helplessness.[148,180,184] Parents may be so overwhelmed by the events that initially they may block any observable emotional response or affect. Staff interventions at this time are extremely important, because they lay the foundations for subsequent interactions between parents and health professionals. Early comments and influential statements during this critical time can have lasting impressions in the minds of parents. This is also an emotionally difficult time for physicians and nurses, because they too are struggling with their own feelings of inadequacy, failure, and helplessness. Unconsciously, in an attempt to deal with their own feelings, staff may withdraw from parents and not be emotionally available to help. This is a normal response but one that needs to be guarded against, because it only perpetuates a breakdown in relationships and communication with parents that are greatly needed at this time. Many helpful interventions can be employed that are sensitive and supportive and that facilitate the emerging relationship between the parents and their infant.

EARLY COMMUNICATION

In the labor and delivery phase, early communication with both parents is essential. Parents normally are apprehensive and extremely sensitive to explicit or implicit cues, such as actual statements by the staff, the atmosphere, looks, or a tone of voice that may indicate how things are progressing. Staff behaviors, as well as wording of parent handouts help set the stage for an FCC unit and build family trust.[84] Because of the emphasis on prepared childbirth, parents are extremely sophisticated in their knowledge of labor and delivery practices and immediately sense some deviation from what they expected. Prompt, direct explanations presented in a calm manner are important and reassuring to parents. This explanation of the process of what is or will be happening can be effective, because it helps organize the parents at a time when they are extremely vulnerable and feeling out of control.

In a review of nursing behaviors identified to assist parents in meeting these needs, emotional support, parent empowerment and education, and a welcoming environment and parent were all key factors.[46]

Although it is normal for the staff to be guarded, members of the health care team should tell the parents the known facts and what actually is being done for their infant without giving any diagnosis, prognosis, or forecast for the future course of the infant. Avoiding or not talking to parents only accelerates parental anxiety and adds to their growing fantasies or distortions. It has been well established and documented that parents' fantasies about their infant's problems are usually worse than the reality. Parents often report that when they actually saw their infant, they were relieved because they had imagined that the infant would appear worse.

SUPPORT OF STAFF

It is also important that one of the staff members stays with the parents through labor, delivery, and recovery to offer continuous support and reassure the parents that communication will continue as soon as more information is known. This, again, is an uncomfortable time for the staff, because they may feel helpless and therefore may avoid the parents or revert to performing more technical activities. Some parents may need someone to be with them,[184] not only to talk to them but also, more important, to listen. On the other hand, some parents may not be able to talk or verbalize their concerns or fears. Others may wish to be alone with each other or any other significant person in their life. Because of the varying responses and needs of people, it is extremely important to be sensitive to individual differences in approaching parents.

Parents have expressed their desire to be together when given "bad news."[92,207] As much as possible, talking to both parents at the same time is helpful when discussing the infant's condition. This decreases their distortions and misconceptions, increases the communication and support between parents, and prevents either parent from feeling excluded. The assumption is commonly made that the father is in a better emotional state to hear about the infant; this misconception leads health professionals to mistakenly exclude or "spare" the mother, which only postpones her ability to begin to cope with the reality of her infant's condition. Sparing the mother may cause the parents to be in different stages of their understanding of the infant's medical condition and in different emotional states. Because emotional support between parents is so critical, the staff should avoid sparing, because it can add to the parents' difficulty in being attuned to each other's needs and creates more opportunities for the parents to be out of synchrony with each other. Both mothers and fathers of critically ill newborns generally find each other to be the greatest source of support in the first 2 weeks of NICU hospitalization.[148,234]

SEEING THE INFANT

The question usually arises about the value of the parents seeing their infant, especially if the infant is very small, not likely to survive, or profoundly malformed. Generally, it is assumed that it is psychologically better for parents to have had the opportunity to see their infant, but this must be individualized for each family and newborn. Seeing the infant helps facilitate attachment,[23,148,158,226] decrease exaggerated fantasies, decrease withdrawal from the infant, and enhance the parents' ability to grasp the reality of the situation. Because of the need to respect individual differences in people, the best approach is to give parents the opportunity to decide whether they together or individually want to see the infant.

Contact between mothers and their preterm infants in the first hours after birth is critical for a secure mother-infant attachment. Mothers who saw their very low-birth-weight (VLBW) preterm infants within 3 hours after birth showed a higher rate (76%) of secure attachment than mothers with no early contact (41%).[158] These researchers concluded that the 3 hours after birth constitutes a "sensitive period" for mothers of preterms to begin a secure attachment to their infant.[158] Another study found that a negative experience for mothers at first sight of their very preterm baby resulted in attachment difficulties at 18 months corrected age.[160] The opportunity to see and touch the infant in the delivery room or before transport may reduce stressful feelings verbalized by parents who see their infant for the first time in the NICU.

Ultimately this decision should be made by the parents with the support of the health care team. It is not uncommon to find a well-meaning family member, physician, nurse, or social worker advising the parents or making the decision himself or herself and concluding it would be in the parents' best interests not to see the infant. The following arguments are given: "It's better not to get attached." or "It would make them cry or upset them to see the anomaly." or "They could not handle it." or "They would lose control." This decision is for the parents, not the professional, to make.

Some parents may know unequivocally what they want to do; others may be ambivalent or indecisive. It is the role of the professional to give the parents assistance (information and support) in making the decision. The parents may need time to think about it or may have to discuss their fear and ambivalence first, before being able to decide. They may need some factual information and preparation from the professional, such as the appearance of the infant and a description of the equipment. They may need assurance that someone will stay with them. Although time often is a factor and a decision must be made quickly, it is important to move at the parents' pace. The professional should still follow as much as possible the principle of facilitating the parents in seeing the infant. If this is not possible for medical reasons related to the mother's condition, a self-developing or digital picture can be taken. If it is medically possible for the parents to touch or hold the infant, the parents should be offered that opportunity. Touching or holding not only facilitates attachment[23,125,148,226] but also can provide parents with an emotional experience that is sustaining and reassuring, helping them proceed through a critical time of separation.

Parents are very sensitive to the staff's attitude toward the infant as reflected by their comments and the manner in which the staff handle the infant. If the infant is regarded with respect and treated as important, the parent is given the feeling that the infant is seen as valued and worthwhile. This is especially important for parents of an infant with a congenital anomaly; the parents could wonder if their infant is viewed as "damaged goods" by society. In describing the infant to the parent, present a balanced picture of both the normal and abnormal aspects of the infant. In discussing the infant with the parents, staff should refer to the infant by name, if they have named the infant; this helps personalize the infant and establish the infant's unique identity.

CAREGIVING

To reinforce the caregiving needs of parents, discuss with them their plans to feed their infant. Support and encouragement should be given whether the parents have decided on breastfeeding or bottle feeding. In most situations, breastfeeding a sick infant is possible, and should be encouraged (see

Chapter 18). Many mothers can pump their breasts for milk that eventually will be given to the infant. There are many psychologic and physiologic reasons why breastfeeding or pumping may be beneficial for mothers and infants alike (see Chapter 18). The breastfeeding or pumping experience helps the mother feel close to her infant and helps her feel that she has some control over what is happening to her infant; she can uniquely contribute to her infant's care in a way no one else can. Fathers, too, can participate in this activity by their support and interest in the actual breastfeeding or the pumping and milk-collection activities. Many mothers can pump and eventually put the infant to breast, but others cannot because of emotional stresses, the condition of the infant, and the length of time until the infant can feed. Regardless of eventual success, the mother should be encouraged to try if she has an interest; then she can feel that she made an attempt to relate to her infant in this way. If a mother does not plan to breastfeed or pump or if she tries but does not continue, she should not be made to feel guilty or that she failed in her role. She is already vulnerable to these feelings.

After the delivery, when the mother is taken to her room without a healthy infant, she usually experiences a void, as though an amputation has occurred.[83,118] She and those around her are beginning to grieve. The interventions of the staff should be flexible and sensitive to the individual needs of the family. Empathy, responsiveness, and an ability to listen to the parents are important at this time.[148]

Encouraging parents to verbalize and express their feelings and concerns (at their own pace), although difficult to do at times, is useful to the parents. Listening is as important to parents as giving them information.[98] Avoiding their grief gives the mother and father the impression that they are "bad parents" for having feelings of sadness, anger, guilt, or loss; this only increases their level of guilt and isolation. Prescribing tranquilizers also gives the message that is it not permissible to talk about what has happened to them and their infant. Tranquilizers only increase the feelings of unreality that normally are experienced. This stifles the parents' coping mechanisms at a time when the parents should begin to come to terms with what has happened.

Room assignments are a very personal matter, and the mother should be given a choice of where she will stay. Some mothers want to stay in a regular maternity unit; for others, this is too painful and they want to be in a separate area. Flexible visiting guidelines[41,80,148] for the father and other significant persons are essential so they can support one another through a difficult, uncertain period.

In talking to parents, bear in mind that the parents do not remember much of what has been said[184]; it is very difficult for them to assimilate all that has happened, both cognitively and emotionally. It is important for the staff to move at the parents' own pace. If the infant has been transferred or the chances for survival are limited, the mother should be discharged or given a pass to visit the infant as soon as possible. It is also important to acknowledge to the mother (and father) that they are parents and that they did give birth to a baby. They need the congratulatory cards, gifts, and attention that they would have received normally.

Anticipatory Grieving

After labor and delivery, parents are struggling with the second psychologic task of anticipatory grieving and withdrawal from the relationship established during pregnancy. This task requires that parents acknowledge that their infant's life is endangered or that the newborn might die. Events surrounding the labor, delivery, and postpartum period may have indicated to the parents that their infant's chances for survival are diminished. Studies have shown that the decision to transfer an infant to a NICU alone is likely to initiate an anticipatory grief reaction.[51,180]

Parents also may experience feelings of grief and sadness over the loss of the expected, idealized child that they had wished for during the pregnancy. For some parents, attaching to a critically ill or malformed infant may be too overwhelming; parents may withdraw from the infant in an attempt to protect themselves from their feelings of hurt, disappointment, and guilt.[23,77,103] Some parents may feel ambivalent[103] about the infant; they may feel they could not love or cope with an infant who might die or who would have significant physical or mental problems. Feeling uncertain about whether they want the infant to survive can cause feelings of guilt that may cause the parents to withdraw from the infant as a way of avoiding confronting these difficult, painful feelings.

During this period, parents may find themselves in a very stressful position; they are faced with the task of balancing the painful realities of a possible loss against their hopes of survival of their infant.[92]

The emotional withdrawal and grieving that parents experience is normal during the critical time that the infant's life is endangered or when parents are faced with the possibility that their infant may have a life-long problem. This withdrawal becomes pathologic only if it continues beyond the time the infant demonstrates definite signs (to the parents) of improvement and survival. In the case of a newborn with a permanent developmental or physical disability, parents who cannot grieve their idealized infant may maintain this withdrawal, which might lead to attachment difficulties and subsequent cognitive and emotional consequences for the infant.[216]

PARENTAL RESPONSES

Parents exhibit many emotional responses and behaviors that indicate they are struggling with the anticipatory grieving and withdrawal. Some parents are very sad, depressed, and teary, and others may be highly anxious, at times bordering on panic states; others react by having a flat affect, withdrawing, and appearing apathetic. Some parents may exhibit very angry, hostile, confrontational behavior as a way of dealing with their distress. Others may deny the situation by optimistically feeling that "everything will be OK."

Parents who typically are verbal may ask questions reflecting their concerns about their infant's survival; this is especially true after the infant has received medical attention and decisions are being made about treatment, including transfer to a NICU. The questions they ask physicians and nurses may include "Will he make it?" "What do you think his chances are?" "He'll be OK, won't he?" "Have you seen other babies with this problem?" "Do other babies make it?" and "How long will he be in the hospital?" Parents struggling with their fears may resist seeing, touching, or visiting the infant. If they do visit the infant in the NICU, they may remain distant by having little or no eye contact with the infant, refusing to touch, standing far from the warmer or incubator, and asking few or no questions of the staff. Parents may be reluctant to name the infant; when they do refer to the infant, they say "it," "she," "he," or "the baby." If the infant has been given a special or treasured family name, they may be reluctant to use it.

A common phenomenon occurs when parents, being protective of each other, discourage each other's involvement with the infant. This is especially true at the time of transport, when the transport nurse may suggest to the father or family members that the infant be shown to the mother before leaving. Many fathers are afraid this will increase the emotional attachment to the infant and thus the feelings of disappointment and loss if the infant should die. The father is usually very apprehensive about how to handle the mother's feelings of grief in addition to his own. This type of behavior also is true with regard to medical information; it is not uncommon for one parent to request that all communication go through him or her. The response is "My spouse is too upset or anxious and couldn't handle hearing any bad news." Many times it is actually the parent making the request who is most anxious and who is dealing with this anxiety by projecting it onto the other partner. Work and childcare responsibilities, transportation difficulties, and financial limitations are all legitimate reasons that parents may be unable to have frequent contact with their infant. However, these factors also may serve as unconscious ways to maintain distance from the infant.

Keep in mind that withdrawal and grieving are part of a necessary and natural process.[22] For parents to develop an attachment to and accept the reality of their infant's condition, they must experience their feelings of grief, sadness, anger, guilt, and disappointment over the loss of the expected infant.[206,216] Maternal grief resolution over premature birth, as well as maternal interaction quality, are necessary for secure infant attachment.[206] This grieving serves to free the parents' emotional energy so they can interact with and become attuned to their infant. Grieving enhances the parents' availability to the infant. This availability aids in their feeling competent to handle their infant. The goal, then, of the perinatal health care team's interventions is to help the family realize their feelings are natural and normal and will be accepted.[23] Parents need permission to have their feelings. It is essential to acknowledge to parents that it is normal to be afraid of attaching to an infant who might die or have a handicap. Giving permission diminishes the guilt that the parents may feel about their behavior being abnormal or about being bad parents because they are afraid. Simple statements such as "Many parents tell us they are afraid of getting close to their baby" or "It's scary to attach when you think the baby may die" are helpful.

Sometimes it is useful for parents to verbalize their actual fears. They may fear their infant dying, being intellectually handicapped, or being paralyzed. Once their fears are clarified in their minds and either confirmed or refuted by the medical staff, it is usually easier for parents to begin to accept their infant's diagnosis and prognosis and begin relating to the infant. Social workers can provide valuable emotional support to families in helping them deal with their realistic and unrealistic concerns.

COMMUNICATING MEDICAL INFORMATION

Most of the foundational work of FCC rests on effective communication.[189,218] Health care provider and patient/parent communication behaviors are associated with improved patient health status, recall, treatment adherence, and satisfaction.[114,139,189,198] The role of the health care professionals in communicating medical information is important. Although the approach should be individualized for each family, some professionals feel a balanced approach is the most beneficial. Parents have stated that information should be accurate, current, and comprehensive but not unduly pessimistic.[98,184] Parents need a realistic assessment of the situation that is honest and direct. Acknowledge the infant's condition and possible problems, but not necessarily every potential problem that can arise.

Parents who hear "brain damage," "retarded," or "the baby will die" are not likely to forget these statements. These statements can linger in the minds of parents and adversely influence how they relate to their newborn.[100] They may believe that some day "brain damage will show up" or that the infant is susceptible and frail and needs to be treated cautiously for fear of a life-threatening condition. These children may become victims of the *vulnerable child syndrome*,[5,72,100] a condition in which a child is overprotected by his or her parents and treated as if he or she had a medical problem when it is no longer the case. Parents who are told their newborn may die may have trouble attaching or becoming emotionally invested. When talking to parents, physicians and nurses should be judicious and careful in making statements of a sensitive nature. Definitive statements should be used only when appropriate and necessary. The long-term emotional implications of such statements should be weighed.

There are several other guidelines in communicating medical information to parents. As discussed, parents' perceptions of their infant's condition are extremely important, remain in parents' minds, and can affect their relationship with the infant. Parents easily misperceive information given to them. They

may believe that a patent ductus arteriosus (PDA) indicates open-heart surgery and therefore worry that their infant has a heart condition. Or perhaps they think a bilirubin problem means their infant has liver disease. Therefore in beginning any discussion with parents, it is essential to determine and address their perceptions. A staff member might say, "Could you tell me what you understand about your baby's condition?" This will give the physician or nurse the opportunity to correct any misinformation or misconceptions and to hear about the parents' concerns. The perceived morbidity of the baby is a source of stress for both mothers and fathers. Parents' perceptions of the severity of their infant's illness are complex, change over time, and are affected by parental anxiety, infant size, amount and type of equipment and treatments, and amount and type of information received from health care providers.[100] A team member might specifically ask about the parents' concerns or worries: "Could you tell me what concerns you have about your baby?" Asking this can make communication between the perinatal health care team and parents more meaningful and helpful; unless the team deals with the parents' anxiety, discussions become one-sided lectures and benefit only the professional. Discussions should be a dialog between parent and professional.

During the course of a discussion and again at the end, it is useful to determine parents' interpretations of what has been said and modify and clarify as needed. The staff should avoid overloading a parent with lengthy explanations that are too technical. It is more productive to move at a pace at which the parent can assimilate the information presented; it is not necessary to describe the entire course of respiratory distress syndrome or bronchopulmonary dysplasia. It is always preferable to use simple language that is understandable. For some parents, the use of statistics is helpful; for others, it is not.[184] Statistics can be confusing, because they do not apply to the individual case and can be misinterpreted easily. When asked about the frequency of brain damage with a grade III intraventricular hemorrhage, a team member might say, "A majority of these babies have some neurologic problem, but some do not." Vivid modifiers such as "This is the worst case of sepsis we have ever had" or "Your baby is the sickest baby in the nursery" are of no real benefit to the parents and only accelerate their anxieties. Finally, if a referring physician and the nursery team are both communicating with the parents, it is essential to coordinate the particular approach. It is very confusing to parents and decreases their trust level for one to be pessimistic and the other optimistic.

CULTURALLY COMPETENT CARE AND COMMUNICATION

Providing culturally sensitive care in a growing multicultural and diverse society is essential and needs to be a constant pursuit in providing perinatal health care to childbearing families and those families who have an infant in the NICU.[108] It is important for the health care team to understand the values, beliefs, customs, and behaviors of the particular group(s) they serve. Culture influences beliefs about what causes illness and how that illness should be treated. The perinatal health care team needs to address cultural, linguistic, and spiritual competencies to provide FCC.[73,86] The National Perinatal Association has published an extensive resource guide that reviews specific cultural practices and beliefs of several ethnocultural and religious groups.[205] Another excellent resource that discusses health and illness in different populations is the book *Cultural Diversity in Health and Illness.*[217]

In the perinatal setting, some common areas that often emerge center around language, folk practices or traditional beliefs, and nonverbal communication.

Use of Language. If a language or educational barrier is encountered, a qualified interpreter who is bilingual and bicultural should be used[108] (Box 29-4). This is especially important in obtaining informed consent. A child or children should not be used as interpreters because they may have inadequate language skills and may be embarrassed by the topics being discussed. Interpreters should be familiar with medical information and terminology. A housekeeper or admissions clerk may be bilingual but have no understanding of the medical issues. Often information that is translated, even by a certified translator, is not understood by families if they are not literate. For example, some undocumented immigrants may have only a second-grade education and may be illiterate in their own native language (and embarrassed about disclosing this to the medical team). However, illiteracy does not mean the family is not intelligent. Some very intelligent parents can comprehend complex information if explained in a relevant manner.

Use of pictures augments what is being explained. Providing a list of common medical terms and

---

BOX 29-4	GUIDELINES FOR THE EFFECTIVE CHOICE OF INTERPRETERS IN CLINICAL SETTINGS

Interpreter Choice
- Unless thoroughly fluent in patient's language, always use trained interpreter.
- Avoid strangers from waiting room or untrained staff as interpreters because of potential problems with accuracy, confidentiality, and medical terminology.
- Children should be interpreters of last resort because of problems with disruption of social roles, sensitive issues, and accuracy.
- Adult relatives or friends brought specifically to translate are acceptable alternatives when trained interpreters are not available, but there may be problems with accuracy, confidentiality, medical terms, and disrupted social roles.
- Always ask patient whether designated interpreter is acceptable.

Interpreter Use
- Clinician, interpreter, and patient or parent should be positioned in equilateral triangle so important nonverbal cues can be appreciated.
- Speak to and maintain eye contact with patient/parent, not interpreter.
- Ask interpreter to translate as literally as possible.
- If mistranslation or misunderstanding is suspected, return to issue later using different wording.
- Emphasize key instructions and explanations by repetition.
- Use visual aids (charts and diagrams) whenever possible.
- To verify quality and comprehension of translation, have patient/parent repeat information through back translation.

At End of Medical Visit
- Interpreter should write lists of instructions for patient or parent, particularly for prescriptions and other therapeutic interventions.
- Indicate to pharmacists that prescription instructions should be printed in the family's language.
- Interpreter should always accompany patient/parent to schedule follow-up appointments with receptionist.

Reprinted from Flores G: Culture and the patient-physician relationship: achieving cultural competency in health care, *J Pediatr* 136:14-23, 2000. Includes information from Perez-Stable, Pachter, and Putsch.

---

educational materials in the native language of the parents is a useful tool. At times, despite numerous discussions about the infant's medical condition, the family may appear unable to comprehend what they have been told. Consider that even if the health care provider and family share the same language, the words may have different meanings depending on core cultural beliefs and values and the families' previous experiences.[11] What is considered an abnormality in our Western culture may not be in another culture.

Folk Practices and Traditional Beliefs. Each culture has their own set of beliefs and traditions about health, illness, and treatment. Many cultures believe that there is a balance between hot and cold forces in nature that are essential for health and harmony. These concepts, which are very prevalent in Latin and Asian cultures, are unrelated to temperature. Pregnancy is seen as "hot," as are vitamins and iron, and should be treated with "cold" products to regulate a proper balance in the system and avoid medical problems. To treat imbalance, one must know what conditions are viewed as hot and cold. There is no general agreement as to what is a hot or cold disease or food. The classification may vary from person to person, so it is imperative to understand the nature of the situation or problem from the perspective of the family.[217] Many of the following beliefs, however, are commonly accepted causes for illness, birth defects, or anomalies:

- *Mal ojo:* A type of magical occurrence caused by a look; the "evil eye" heats up the infant's blood, resulting in fever, crying, diarrhea, vomiting, and aches and pains. This is often treated by a *curandero* (a folk healer), a healing ceremony, or placing an amulet *(azabache)* or leather strap for protection on the infant.
- *Coraje:* Anger or frustration believed to sour breast milk, as well as affect an infant's intrauterine development. It is treated by wearing a good-luck charm in the bra and having a healing ceremony.[73]
- *Mollera caida:* Fallen fontanel is believed to occur when the breast or bottle is removed too quickly. It is believed the soft palate sinks in, causing feeding and swallowing difficulties. Treatment is performed by pushing up the soft palate with the thumb, pulling the hair, and sucking the fontanel.[68]
- *Susto:* A disease or illness resulting from fright. It is treated by relaxation and a cleansing ceremony or other specific actions to counter the *susto.*
- *Lunar or solar eclipse:* A cleft palate, some respiratory ailments, and birthmarks are often associated with an eclipse. It is treated by the pregnant woman wearing a red undergarment or a coin or key over the belly.

Traditional folk healers are multidimensional. In African cultures, they are diviners, herbalists, faith healers, and voodoo practitioners, as well as traditional midwives and birth attendants. Hispanic cultures use a wide range of *curanderos* (*santeros* in the Puerto Rican community), who vary from massage therapists to faith healers and herbalists. Asians rely on medicinal plants or herbology, acupuncture, and moxibustion (heated pulverized wormwood applied to the skin), which restores the proper balance of yin and yang believed to be most helpful during the period of labor and delivery.[217]

In many cultures, decisions are made by a group of elders, removing the responsibility entirely from a new mother and father. Many societies view the whole family as more important than a single individual. Decisions about life and death may be deferred to the elders or the entire family. Ignoring this social structure can result in problems of mistrust and decreased cooperation and communication.

Nonverbal Communication. One must be aware of body language and nonverbal communication and its meaning. Eye contact with the doctor or nurse or authority figures is regarded as disrespectful in some cultures. Loud vocalization also may be considered disrespectful. Rather than openly contradicting a person of authority, a parent will nod as if to communicate agreement but never follow through. Often the parent is viewed as noncompliant. In most societies, touch and space are regulated by rules and social orders. What is acceptable in one group may be forbidden in another; therefore respect personal boundaries and space issues. For example, Southeast Asians typically do not like to be patted on the top of their head or shoulder because this is where the soul resides. In American Indian and Alaska Native populations, note taking is a taboo. Indian history has been passed down by means of verbal storytelling, and note taking is perceived as insensitive.[217]

Becoming culturally competent health care providers is an ongoing developmental process. One should be aware of the dimensions and complexities in caring for individuals from diverse cultural backgrounds. It is important to understand the family's core cultural dynamics, the meaning of the infant's illness, and the social context within which these life events are occurring. Specific customs, traditions, and taboos of each individual group are available in resource materials.[205,217]

COMMUNICATING MEDICAL INFORMATION: EVIDENCE-BASED PRACTICE

The principles of family-centered neonatal care clearly promote family participation in every aspect of their infant's care. The first four principles concern communication, medical information, fully informed parental decision making, and parental advance directives (see Box 29-2). Researchers have confirmed that information given to parents in the NICU is often communicated in euphemisms, vague statements, and half-truths and shields parents from uncertainties and controversies of NICU care.[92] Professional attitudes that may interfere with open, honest communication include (1) assuming that parents are too emotional to assimilate information and make a rational decision, (2) assuming that information about complications and poor outcomes may disrupt attachment to the neonate, (3) assuming that parental guilt and psychologic harm will ensue from decision making (despite research to the contrary), and (4) cultural and language differences.[92,93] A multicenter qualitative study of parental values in decision making about delivery room resuscitation for their extremely preterm infants found that (1) all parents wanted to participate in decision making (although few parents recalled discussing options for delivery room resuscitation; even fewer recalled being offered "comfort care," even though this was documented in the chart), (2) parents did not report that physician predictions of morbidity and mortality were central to their decision making, and (3) religion, spirituality, and hope were the guiding values for most parents in making their decision.[25,184]

Many parents desire and can handle complete, specific, honest, detailed, unbiased, and meaningful information—the same facts and interpretation of those facts as the staff—delivered in a humane and respectful manner.[92,93] Parents have expressed "remarkably uniform and unambiguous requests . . . to receive early, honest, and detailed information in a comprehensible and sympathetic manner and to be together when given bad news."[183,p. 434] Prenatal consultation has been found to be useful by 80% of mothers in one study.[183] These researchers concluded that "in our population of educated mothers, most mothers prefer to be told exact statistics, rather than generalizations, concerning major neonatal morbidities."[183] A nurse-led intervention with 42 high-risk antepartum women expecting their infant to be in the NICU included an educational video, detailed description of prematurity and care requirements, family participation in the NICU, and a tour.[174] Within 48 to 72 hours after NICU admission, mothers were surveyed and found to be significantly less stressed about the sights and sounds of the NICU and their infant's appearance and behavior over time.[174] Another group of researchers uses actuarial data for counseling parents about infants at the limits of viability and for morbidity counseling.[178] Accuracy of prenatal and postnatal counseling of parents is of concern, because information affects practice management and influences parental decision making.[93,122,178,184]

Individuals vary in their desire to be informed and involved in decision making. Individuals also vary in the manner in which they assimilate information. Some parents may want extensive information about their situation, whereas others may not. Some parents may not wish to be decision makers and should be able to delegate decision making to a physician of their choice.[92] However, physicians have an ethical and legal obligation to give parents the facts from which to make an informed choice about their neonate's condition, illnesses, outcomes, and the risks and benefits of various interventions.[93] Proactive risk management strategies include effective communication,[76] because legal action in the form of civil malpractice suits (60%) and criminal action may result from poor communication between parents and physicians. Because language and cultural barriers in medical settings are increasing, federal and state governments have established a number of laws and standards to ensure that providers and health care organizations provide culturally and linguistically appropriate care.

Poor understanding by parents may be the result of poor communication techniques, contradictory messages, poor parental health, inexperience with medical terminology, denial, language barriers, inability to ask questions, shock over the birth of a preterm or sick newborn, or lack of opportunity to review the information.[122,133,184] In one study, parents claimed that a neonatologist had never spoken to them, but, in fact, the conversation did occur and had been recorded.[120] In this study, parents were given a tape recording of their initial conversation with the neonatologist and any subsequent conversations of importance. The audiotape proved useful: 96% of the mothers and 68% of the fathers listened to the tape again an average of 2.5 and 1.8 times, respectively. Eighty-five percent of parents who listened to the tape had forgotten elements of the conversation, and two mothers did not recall that the conversation had ever occurred. Taped conversations were found helpful by 99% of parents and grandparents, 76% of nurses, and 36% of neonatologists. Of the physicians, 40% were not happy about having their conversations taped; "legal implications" was the most frequent reason given. As pointed out in the study, the "legal implications" work both ways; taping encourages precise, organized, clear, and humane communication of information while providing an "alibi" if a legal complication arises. A randomized, single-blind trial found that mothers in the audiotaped conversation group had enhanced recall about their infant's diagnosis, treatment, and outcome (for up to 4 months) compared with the group without audiotapes (6 of the 98 mothers did not recall the conversation with the neonatologist).[123]

Research has documented that postpartum women have transient deficits in cognitive function, particularly in attention and memory function.[61] Because verbal communication may be poorly remembered, augmentation with written instructions is recommended.[61] In addition to relistening to an audiotape, if parents are given written information, such as an evidence-based table of the likely outcomes of babies at different gestational ages, they can look at it again to review it. Such an evidence-based table for infants from 23 to 28 weeks' gestational age has been presented in the literature for use with parents.[120] This table contains information about mortality statistics, need for assisted ventilation, prolonged use of oxygen, length of stay, use of phototherapy, PDA needing treatment, outcomes of brain scans, and long-term neurodevelopmental outcome. A NICU staff member can create a table for parents by using their most recent data.[121] With the advent of computerized databases (e.g., the Vermont Oxford Data Base) that compare statistics from multiple NICUs and a large cohort of infants, parents can be provided with statistical information from multiple NICUs to compare with the outcomes from the NICU in which their baby is hospitalized. Parents may need assistance in interpreting statistics and making them meaningful to their individual

situation. Again, some parents may want and need this type of information, whereas others may not. All communication needs to be culturally and linguistically appropriate.

Ongoing research on the *outcome of gestation table (OGT)* has documented views of parents, nurses, and physicians.[121] The majority of parents and nurses interviewed favored the table; they agreed that the information was frightening but important for parents to know. Parents wanted to keep a copy, and nurses wanted a copy in the medical record. Parents also thought that the information was easy to understand, the table did not contain "too much" information, and although it was frightening, they still would rather have the information. The majority of physicians thought that the table was easy to understand but had "too much" information, and they were ambivalent about using it in their practice. Parents, nurses, and physicians all agreed that the table and its information were not misleading. Of doctors, 21% disagreed about including a copy of the table in the medical record so that other health care providers would know what had been said to the parents. This finding was surprising to the researchers, who thought that inclusion of the table in the medical record would promote consistency in information given to the parents by different members of the perinatal team.

The Neonatal Research Network of the National Institute of Child and Human Development (NICHD) has developed a simple Web-based tool (see Websites for Parents of Premature Infants section at the end of this chapter) to enable clinicians (and parents) to use multiple factors, not just gestational age, in making decisions about intensive care for extremely preterm infants.[131,229] A prospective study of 22 to 25 weeks' gestation preterms (n = 4446) in the NICHD cohort found that the likelihood of favorable outcome of NICU care was best estimated with consideration of gestational age in addition to sex, use of antenatal steroids, single/multiple birth, and birth weight. Calculation of the risk-to-benefit ratio of use of NICU care for the extremely preterm infant provides both care providers and parents with information that is "less arbitrary, more individualized, more transparent and better justified"[229] for informed decision making than use of gestational age alone.[131,229]

The principles of family-centered neonatal care (see Box 29-2) also advocate full and free access to lay and medical literature pertaining to the neonate's condition, proposed treatments, and probable outcomes.[92] A multicenter study was conducted to create an FCC map to enhance the ability of the health care team to work with families to coordinate and deliver care in a holistic manner to meet the developmental, physical, and psychosocial needs of NICU patients and their families. This study led to the development of an innovative Web-based resource to assist individual care providers and family advisors to provide comprehensive FCC to infants and families.[60] Medical literature, articles, books, and videos (in English and Spanish) should be available in the NICU or in the hospital library for the parents' use. A video such as *You Are Not Alone* (see Resource Materials for Parents section at the end of this chapter) is available to help parents understand the impact on the family of long-term handicaps and to support them in making informed decisions. Access to the Internet has proved to be a source of medical information (some accurate; some inaccurate) for families, as well as professionals.

Users report they can receive information, support, relationships, and comfort from their online activities and connections. Although there are many benefits, less is known about the quality of information received and the potential for harm from online communication. Parents may be more comfortable seeking medical advice from anonymous people in cyberspace rather than consulting their own health care providers. When recommending the Internet as a resource, professionals should be aware of its benefits, as well as shortcomings.[56,129]

Acknowledgment of Guilt Feelings

The third psychologic task parents are dealing with simultaneously with anticipatory grieving and withdrawal is confronting and recognizing their feelings of inadequacy and guilt in not delivering a healthy infant. Most parents struggling with these feelings are likely to search for answers to the causes of their infant's situation. The mother may focus on concrete things, such as not eating well, the flu, intercourse, birth control pills, or an unwanted pregnancy. The father also may be concerned about his role in not helping his wife enough, placing too many demands on her, an argument he provoked that precipitated labor, or another family member with the same chromosomal abnormality. Parents search for reasons because they need to find a cause for such an event happening to them. It is harder

for them to feel out of control and helpless than to feel guilty. Some parents place responsibility on themselves; however, some shift the blame to others in their external world, such as their spouse, extended family, doctor, nurses, or God. Often both parents are concerned with the disappointment that they have caused the other. They may withdraw from each other at a time when they both need acceptance and support.

Realistic answers from the medical team are helpful for some parents in diminishing guilt feelings; in other parents, the guilt may be so deeply integrated in their thinking that it is less easily overcome. For example, some parents may focus on irrational, unrealistic factors, such as "This is my punishment for not being a good wife or daughter" or "This is my punishment for running away from home when I was 15." Often the more irrational the parent's thinking, the harder it is to assuage and resolve the guilt. Many feelings of guilt and failure are normal and expected; the feelings are a problem when the parent does not respond to the infant's progress, because the infant may continue to represent the parent's failure.

PARENTAL RESPONSES

Parents demonstrate many behaviors that indicate they are struggling with guilt and failure. Some parents directly verbalize these feelings and attempt to obtain helpful answers and support from the staff. Less obvious are the parents who are markedly depressed and remain so despite any improvement in the infant. These parents demonstrate the classic signs of depression, such as apathy, loss of interest in appearance and self, withdrawal, and loss of self-esteem. They exhibit an overwhelming sense of helplessness, feeling personally responsible for causing their infant's problem and are helpless to remedy the situation. Other parents struggling with guilt are highly anxious about their ability to handle their infant; they feel they have harmed their infant and are uncomfortable coming to the NICU or participating in their infant's care. Another manifestation of guilt is hostility and anger that is usually directed toward others, such as the spouse, the staff, or God. Instead of focusing their anger on themselves like a depressed parent, they direct it outward, projecting the guilt feelings onto others in their life. They may be angry at the physicians, nurses, or social workers for not making their infant healthy (if the infant is premature) or perfect (if the infant has a congenital defect). Unconsciously, they are trying to make the staff feel as guilty, helpless, and responsible as they do.

FACILITATING ADAPTATION

To intervene with parents, it is useful to assist them in acknowledging that their feelings of failure and guilt are a barrier to healthy coping and adjustment. The staff can provide them with appropriate information to modify and clarify the perceptions that may be the source of some of the parents' guilt feelings. Many parents directly ask about the causes of their infant's problem, and the medical team should counsel them with appropriate, honest information. Other parents are not as direct and verbal; they need to have the subject introduced. A staff member might ask, "Have you wondered why this has happened?" or "Many parents find themselves feeling responsible for their baby's problem, as if they failed. Have you had these feelings?" As parents begin to talk about their feelings, they often can test reality and discover the irrationality in their thinking. However, some parents continue to feel guilty even though they have been told they are not to blame. Guilt feelings are very complex and may take a long time to resolve; for some, they may never be completely resolved but at least the intensity of the feelings may diminish. If a child recovers from the illness, guilt can be more easily relinquished. If the child has a chronic problem, the parent has a daily reminder of these feelings of responsibility. The more irrational the source of the guilt, the harder it is to dispel. Because this persistent guilt can cause problems in the parents' relationship with each other and with the child, a referral to a perinatal social worker or other mental health professional may be very helpful.

To facilitate support between parents, it is useful to ask whether they have shared their feelings of guilt and failure with each other. Often a spouse may assume that one is angry at or disappointed with the other. Discussing this may bring a tremendous sense of relief and reassurance. However, if the parents are blaming each other and relationship problems develop, a referral to a perinatal social worker or counselor is appropriate.

In some cases, there may be realistic reasons (either intentional or unintentional) why the parent may feel guilty about the infant's problem. Parental drug or alcohol abuse, domestic violence, an accident, or an inherited genetic problem may be a real reason. In these cases, the staff must acknowledge to the parent that there is a causal relationship and then give the parents support by allowing them to talk about their feelings. If causes were not intentional, it is helpful to acknowledge that fact; if they were, it is important to be nonjudgmental. A judging attitude only reinforces the feelings (e.g., guilt, concern, uncertainty)[208] parents are already experiencing and further alienates them from the infant and staff. When this type of psychosocial issue arises, the involvement of a perinatal social worker or other mental health professional is essential.

POSTPARTUM MOOD DISORDERS

The postpartum period is a time of increased risk for development of mood disturbances in women (and men), that affect the entire family.[44,70,101,136,140] The incidence of postpartum mood disorders is estimated to be 15%; with as many as 50% of mothers still depressed at 6 months and 25% still depressed at 1 year after birth.[136] The incidence of paternal depression is estimated at 4% to 12%, but is underreported, screened, diagnosed, and treated.[175] A recent longitudinal study of paternal mental health during the transition to fatherhood found depressive symptoms scores increased by 68% in the first 5 years of their child's life.[70] The strongest risk factor and predictor of paternal postpartum depression (PPD) is maternal PPD.[175] At a time of individual and family role transition, neither parent receives the support needed from their partner when both are depressed.

Symptoms of postpartum mood disorders may be transient and relatively mild (baby blues) or may be associated with significant impairment of functioning (e.g., postpartum depression and psychosis). Women with a history of mood disorders and those who experience depression during pregnancy are at greatest risk.[4,136] Box 29-5 lists significant predictors of postpartum mood disorders. Evidence suggests that mothers of premature infants or infants with problems and those with multiple births experience a higher rate of PPD than women who deliver a single full-term infant.[15,86,101,153] A study of 111 mothers whose infants were in the NICU found positive depression screens in 52% and 30% received an "at-risk for depression" score.[153] Another study found 20% of mothers of very preterm infants had clinically significant depression and 43% had moderate to severe anxiety.[197] Although anxiety was common,

<table>
<tr><td>

B O X 29-5	SIGNIFICANT PREDICTORS OF POSTPARTUM MOOD DISORDERS

- History of previous depression (before and during pregnancy; bipolar disorder)[4,104,142]
- Present depression and anxiety disorders (panic, posttraumatic stress and obsessive compulsive disorders; phobias)[101]
- Depression and anxiety associated with previous prenatal loss that continues after the birth of a subsequently healthy infant[24]
- Low quality of prenatal attachment[74,199]
- Nonworking women with a history of emesis during pregnancy and depression[75]
- Low self-esteem
- Negative, stressful life events (such as childhood physical abuse[187]; intimate partner violence[104]; mode of delivery that entails maternal lack of control, such as primary[190] or emergency cesarean section[74]; preterm birth[86])
- Marital discord
- Poor social support[4,86]
- Difficult infant temperament
- Childcare stresses
- History of endocrine dysfunction
- Maternity blues
- Single marital status
- Adolescent pregnancy[44,199]
- Unplanned/unwanted pregnancy
- Low socioeconomic status
- Minority racial and ethnic groups (Native Americans, African Americans, Hispanic)[44,142]
- Immigrant women[44,86,146]

</td></tr>
</table>

Data from Beck C: Recognizing and screening for postpartum depression in mothers of NICU infants, *Adv Neonatal Care* 3:37, 2003; and O'Hara M, Gorman L: Can postpartum depression be predicted? *Prim Psychiatry* 11:42, 2004.

the researchers did not find identifiable risk factors but depression was associated with being married, parental role alteration, and prolonged respiratory ventilation for the preterm infants.[197]

PPDs usually are divided into three categories: (1) postpartum blues, (2) nonpsychotic PPD, and (3) postpartum psychosis, although these disorders do exist along a continuum.[16]

Postpartum Blues

Postpartum blues (baby blues) affects approximately 50% to 80% of new mothers. Symptoms may include mood swings, sleep and appetite disturbances with periods of feeling anxious, irritability, and tearfulness interspersed with times of feeling well. Symptoms often begin within a few days of delivery and persist up to several days. Postpartum blues is time-limited and relatively benign. The symptoms worsen by the 5th or 7th day and tend to resolve by the 12th postpartum day. The occurrence of the "baby blues" does not necessarily indicate psychopathology; however, if the symptoms persist longer than 2 weeks, a further evaluation is needed because approximately 20% of women develop postpartum major depression.[7] A study of delivery mode and PPD found higher Edinburgh Postnatal Depression Scale (EPDS) scores at 48 to 72 hours after birth (but not at 6 to 8 months postnatally) in mothers after primary cesarean –section compared with spontaneous delivery.[190]

Postpartum Depression

Postpartum depression is relatively common. Several controlled studies reveal that between 12% and 20% of women experience a postpartum depressive episode and this rate is as high as 26% in adolescent mothers; rates vary by race/ethnic group.[7,142] Most women begin to experience depressive symptoms within the first month after delivery, although some have reported symptoms during the pregnancy. Signs and symptoms include a depressed mood, lack of interest or pleasure in usual activities, guilt, impaired concentration, appetite disturbance, low self-esteem, feelings of hopelessness and worthlessness, and suicidal ideation.[10,16]

Postpartum Psychosis

Postpartum psychosis is a rare but extremely serious mental illness occurring in 1 to 2 per 1000 deliveries. It generally occurs within the first 2 to 3 weeks after delivery and requires immediate attention. The symptoms are crying, irritability, restlessness, sleep disturbances, delusions, hallucinations, and bizarre, irrational behavior. For example, a woman may view the baby as the devil, claim the infant is dead, or accuse the hospital staff of switching babies. There are significant risks for infanticide or suicide.

Paternal symptoms of depression occur after the onset of maternal PPD, are worse during the first 3 to 6 months after birth, and have symptoms similar to those of depressed mothers. However, paternal depression manifests with more subtle symptoms

<table>
<tr><td>

**BOX
29-6**

</td><td>

CRITICAL FINDINGS

**ADDITIONAL FEATURES
OF POSTPARTUM MOOD
DISORDERS**

</td></tr>
</table>

- Overly concerned for the baby or excessive anxiety over the infant's health
- Guilt, inadequacy, worthlessness, especially feeling like a failure at motherhood
- Fear of losing control or "going crazy"
- Lack of interest in the baby
- Fear of harming the baby
- Obsession

that include negative parenting behaviors, withdrawal from social situations, an increase in relationship conflicts, alcohol and drug abuse, and intimate partner violence.[175]

The causes of postpartum disorders are multifactorial. Pregnancy is a complex biologic process that takes place within a psychologic and social context. Some of the determinates are the psychologic makeup of the mother, hormonal changes associated with pregnancy,[62] genetics, socioeconomic issues, stress, the temperament and health of the baby, marital instability, ambivalence toward the pregnancy, culture, and the emotional support system of the new mother.[3,4,86,136] When the features listed in Box 29-6 occur in mothers with a sick infant, it may be hard to differentiate a normal reaction to an adverse situation, a grief reaction, from signs of PPD.

In general, postpartum disorders are often overlooked and not appreciated, thereby putting the mother at risk for development of recurrent depression and altered maternal attachment, which are both associated with deleterious effects on the behavioral, cognitive, emotional, and social development of the infant.* A longitudinal study of first-time mothers (with normal pregnancies and healthy babies) found that 22% who were depressed on day 10 postpartum continued with low mood for the first year of the baby's life and had less closeness, warmth, and confidence in parenting their baby in that first year.[140] Positioned strategically in all

*References 3, 15, 16, 99, 100, 135-137, 224, 227.

aspects of perinatal care, nurses were overwhelmingly supportive of screening women for PPD.[204] Given the inherent stresses and emotional impact the birth of a sick infant(s) has on the mother and her family, it is recommended that universal screening for PPD be a part of every family assessment in the NICU.[15,101,197] "Routine assessment will normalize the process, enhance awareness and increase the health care providers' comfort level and competency."[15]

Assessment Tools

Several assessment tools are designed to identify women with a substantial increased risk for PPD. Ideally it is recommended these assessment tools be administered at each trimester of pregnancy and periodically after delivery to assess a woman's risk status. The literature contains extensive discussion of the various assessment tools, checklists, and their reliability and predictability of PPD.[12,14] Although many tools are available, three seem to be used extensively: (1) the Postpartum Depression Screening Scale (PDSS)[15]; (2) the Postpartum Depression Predictors Inventory–Revised (PDPI-Revised) (Table 29-1) (these tools are also available in Spanish)[14,18,19] based on a meta-analysis of 84 studies published to identify significant risk factors of PPD[13]; and (3) the Edinburgh Postnatal Depression Scale (EPDS) (Table 29-2).[48,49]

The PDSS and PDPI-Revised have different uses. The PDSS is a 35-item self-report Likert scale that assesses seven areas: (1) sleeping/eating difficulties, (2) anxiety/insecurity, (3) emotionality, (4) mental confusion, (5) loss of self, (6) shame or guilt, and (7) thoughts of self-harm.[15,17] The scale measures depressive symptomatology. The total score ranges from 13 to 175. If a mother's score is 80 or greater, this is a positive screen for PPD and a referral for mental health follow-up is indicated. The mother completes the PDSS herself, and then it is scored. The tool is used only after delivery. The PPDS has been found to be reliable as a depression screening scale for mothers in the NICU.[153]

The PDPI-Revised is an inventory that (1) assesses a woman's risk status for developing PPD, (2) can be used during pregnancy and after delivery, and (3) should complement a clinician's professional judgment. It consists of 13 risk factors and is designed for a clinician and the woman

TABLE 29-1	POSTPARTUM DEPRESSION PREDICTORS INVENTORY (PDPI)-REVISED AND GUIDE QUESTIONS FOR ITS USE

DURING PREGNANCY	CHECK ONE	
Marital Status		
1. Single	○	
2. Married/cohabiting	○	
3. Separated	○	
4. Divorced	○	
5. Widowed	○	
6. Partnered	○	
Socioeconomic Status		
Low	○	
Middle	○	
High	○	
Self-Esteem	Yes	No
Do you feel good about yourself as a person?	○	○
Do you feel worthwhile?	○	○
Do you feel you have a number of good qualities as a person?	○	○
Prenatal Depression		
1. Have you felt depressed during your pregnancy?	○	○
If yes, when and how long have you been feeling this way?		
If yes, how mild or severe do you consider your depression?		
Prenatal Anxiety		
Have you been feeling anxious during your pregnancy?	○	○
If yes, how long have you been feeling this way?		
Unplanned/Unwanted Pregnancy		
Was the pregnancy planned?	○	○
Is the pregnancy unwanted?	○	○
History Of Previous Depression		
1. Before this pregnancy, have you ever been depressed?	○	○
If yes, when did you experience this depression?		
If yes, have you been under a physician's care for this past depression?	○	○
If yes, did the physician prescribe any medication for your depression?	○	○
Social Support		
1. Do you feel you receive adequate emotional support from your partner?	○	○
2. Do you feel you receive adequate instrumental support from your partner (e.g., help with household chores or baby sitting)?	○	○

Continued

TABLE 29-1	POSTPARTUM DEPRESSION PREDICTORS INVENTORY (PDPI)-REVISED AND GUIDE QUESTIONS FOR ITS USE — cont'd

DURING PREGNANCY	CHECK ONE	
3. Do you feel you can rely on your partner when you need help?	○	○
4. Do you feel you can confide in your partner?	○	○
(Repeat same questions for family and again for friends)		

Marital Satisfaction

1. Are you satisfied with your marriage (or living arrangement)?	○	○
2. Are you currently experiencing any marital problems?	○	○
3. Are things going well between you and your partner?	○	○

Life Stress

	○	○
1. Are you currently experiencing any stressful events in your life such as:		
Financial problems	○	○
Marital problems	○	○
Death in the family	○	○
Serious illness in the family	○	○
Moving	○	○
Unemployment	○	○
Job change	○	○

After delivery, add the following items:

Child Care Stress

1. Is your infant experiencing any health problems?	○	○
2. Are you having problems with your baby feeding?	○	○
3. Are you having problems with your baby sleeping?	○	○

Infant Temperament

1. Do you consider your baby irritable or fussy?	○	○
2. Does your baby cry a lot?	○	○
3. Is your baby difficult to console or soothe?	○	○

Maternity Blues

1. Did you experience a brief period of tearfulness and mood swings during the first week after delivery?	○	○

Comments

_____

_____

_____

_____

From Beck C: Revision of the Postpartum Depression Predictors Inventory, *J Obstet Gynecol Neonatal Nurs* 31:394, 2002.

TABLE 29-2	EDINBURGH POSTNATAL DEPRESSION SCALE

HEALTH VISITOR	NUMBER

Today's date _____

Baby's date of birth _____

Triplets/twins/single _____

Baby's age _____

Birth weight _____

Male/female _____

How are you feeling?

As you have recently had a baby, we would like to know how you are feeling now. Please <u>underline</u> the answer that comes closest to how you have felt in the past 7 days, not just how you feel today.

Here is an example already completed:

I have felt happy:

Yes, most of the time

<u>Yes, some of the time</u>

Not very often

No, never

This means: "I have felt happy some of the time" during the past week.

Please complete the other questions in the same way.

In the past 7 days:

1. I have been able to laugh and see the funny side of things:
   As much as I always could
   Not quite so much now
   Definitely not so much now
   Not at all

2. I have looked forward with enjoyment to things:
   As much as I ever did
   Rather less than I used to
   Definitely less than I used to
   Hardly at all

3. I have blamed myself unnecessarily when things went wrong:
   Yes, most of the time
   Yes, some of the time
   Not very often
   No, never

4. I have felt worried and anxious for no good reason:
   No, not at all
   Hardly ever
   Yes, sometimes
   Yes, very often

5. I have felt scared or panicky for no very good reason:
   Yes, quite a lot
   Yes, sometimes
   No, not much
   No, not at all

Continued

TABLE 29-2	EDINBURGH POSTNATAL DEPRESSION SCALE—cont'd

HEALTH VISITOR	NUMBER

In the past 7 days

6. Things have been getting on top of me:
   Yes, most of the time I haven't been able to cope at all
   Yes, sometimes I haven't been coping as well as usual
   No, most of the time I have coped quite well
   No, I have been coping as well as ever

7. I have been so unhappy that I have had difficulty sleeping:
   Yes, most of the time
   Yes, some of the time
   Not very often
   No, not at all

8. I have felt sad or miserable:
   Yes, most of the time
   Yes, some of the time
   Not very often
   No, not at all

9. I have been so unhappy that I have been crying:
   Yes, most of the time
   Yes, quite often
   Only occasionally
   No, never

10. The thought of harming myself has occurred to me:
    Yes, quite often
    Sometimes
    Hardly ever
    Never

Edinburgh Postnatal Depression Scale: Scoring Sheet

1. I have been able to laugh and see the funny side of things:	
As much as I always could	0
Not quite so much now	1
Definitely not so much now	2
Not at all	3
2. I have looked forward with enjoyment to things:	
As much as I ever did	0
Rather less than I used to	1
Definitely less than I used to	2
Hardly at all	3

TABLE 29-2	EDINBURGH POSTNATAL DEPRESSION SCALE — cont'd

HEALTH VISITOR	NUMBER
3. I have blamed myself unnecessarily when things went wrong:	
Yes, most of the time	3
Yes, some of the time	2
Not very often	1
No, never	0
4. I have felt worried and anxious for no good reason:	
No, not at all	0
Hardly ever	1
Yes, sometimes	2
Yes, very often	3
5. I have felt scared or panicky for no very good reason:	
Yes, quite a lot	3
Yes, sometimes	2
No, not much	1
No, not at all	0
6. Things have been getting on top of me:	
Yes, most of the time I haven't been able to cope at all	3
Yes, sometimes I haven't been coping as well as usual	2
No, most of the time I have coped quite well	1
No, I have been coping as well as ever	0
7. I have been so unhappy that I have had difficulty sleeping:	
Yes, most of the time	3
Yes, some of the time	2
Not very often	1
No, not at all	0
8. I have felt sad or miserable:	
Yes, most of the time	3
Yes, some of the time	2
Not very often	1
No, not at all	0
9. I have been so unhappy that I have been crying:	
Yes, most of the time	3
Yes, some of the time	2
Not very often	1
No, not at all	0

Continued

TABLE 29-2	EDINBURGH POSTNATAL DEPRESSION SCALE — cont'd	
HEALTH VISITOR		**NUMBER**
10. The thought of harming myself has occurred to me:		
Yes, quite often		3
Sometimes		2
Hardly ever		1
Never		0

to discuss each risk factor that might put her at risk for developing PPD. There is no total score; rather, it is a tool providing detailed information on symptoms.

With some modifications, as reported by a study in Australia, the PDPI-Revised has been used as a checklist that the woman administers herself. The information from the checklist was then used to initiate discussions by midwives and nurses with women about their postpartum depression.[91]

The EPDS is a 10-item screening questionnaire that (1) is completed by mothers (and fathers)[101] and then scored by clinicians, (2) is useful as an inventory to identify parents at risk to initiate an open discussion about PPD, (3) requires minimal training to administer, and (4) is completed in less than 10 minutes. The EPDS is a reliable and valid measure of depression or anxiety disorders in fathers during the perinatal period[151] and can be used by pediatricians in the outpatient setting to help identify and assist mothers at risk.[40] The EPDS can be used at 6 to 8 weeks after delivery and is easy to score. The items are ordered and weighted to reflect severity of symptoms. One study found that the self-administered EPDS and the directed interview EPDS are equal in their ability to screen for PPD, and either technique should be used to screen for PPD.[112] A score of 12+ indicates the likelihood of depression but not its severity, although with this score, further assessment and possible intervention are recommended. If the woman or man scores positive on item 10,

thoughts of harming self, immediate intervention is necessary.[12]

Many studies have demonstrated that mothers of sick or premature infants are at greater risk for psychologic distress than are mothers of full-term infants. These studies have looked at depressive symptoms in mothers during the hospitalization and after discharge. The goal of these studies, by using assessment tools, has been to identify (and ultimately treat) women at risk for depression, thereby decreasing the negative effect on infant development. General themes emerge from these studies.[15,16,86,101,214] Social support was consistently identified as extremely important both during the hospitalization and after discharge when the mother has full responsibility for the infant(s) for the first time. Increased stress at discharge, the isolation, and being disconnected from the NICU support network contribute to the risk for PPD. Therefore social support is necessary and can serve as a buffer to the effects of depression. Logsdon and Usui's work[143] supported what other studies have found—that closeness to one's partner, social support, and self-esteem are important predictors of PPD regardless of ethnic diversity. Stress and uncertainty surrounding the birth of a sick newborn increase the need for support. Support provided by the health care team to a mother's adaptation to the NICU environment, information communicated about the infant and his or her treatment, facilitating maternal self-confidence, accurate knowledge of infant development (at the time of discharge), and self-care knowledge about symptoms of depression and who to contact for help can influence a mother's risk for PPD.[136,144,192] All of these factors indicate the need for enhanced FCC in the NICU and after discharge.

Mothers whose infants have chronic complications and who present long-term management challenges are more likely to experience more severe depressive symptoms. In addition, the role of the hospital environment coupled with the appearance of the infant seems to contribute to maternal symptoms. In a study done in Japan, it was found that close emotional support of the father was much more significant than the existence of other modes of peripheral support.[176] This same study concluded that active intervention for PPD is necessary for the mother to be emotionally available to attach to the infant and cope with the infant's hospitalization and subsequent issues related to discharge. Most investigators believe that chronic exposure to maternal depression has long-term negative effects on a child's emotional, psychologic, and cognitive development.[94,101,135,224,227]

Treatment and Intervention

PPD and its symptoms present themselves along a continuum. Interventions should be guided by the severity of symptoms and the degree of impairment of the individual. Because PPD is a complex biologic and psychologic phenomenon, a comprehensive approach is needed, including reassurance and support (from a doula or telephone-based peer support), comprehensive professional home visits in which nurses screen and counsel for PPD, problem-solving education,[211] psychoeducation, individual or group psychotherapy, and psychopharmacology.[55,71,186]

Fathers identified the need for both professional support and support from family and friends to be supportive to a depressed partner and to deal with their own depression.[137] Parenting classes enable fathers, as well as new mothers, to learn the skills necessary to care for their infant and feel confident, in control, and less frustrated.[176] Education about PPD, its symptoms, and practical coping strategies were also identified by fathers as helpful.[136,137] Depressed fathers are less able to emotionally support the mother and participate in parenting, which negatively affects their relationship, attachment to

the infant, and ultimately the emotional, behavioral, and social development of the infant/child.[99,135,175]

Prior studies have demonstrated that when parents experience less stress they are able to form early attachments to their sick infants.[166,237] Mothers with greater stress have less positive attitudes and interactions with their infants than those with less stress.[50] This lack of parenting confidence has been associated with lower levels of child competence and poorer developmental outcomes.[117,213] Conversely, multiple studies have shown that positive attitudes and parental confidence are associated with secure infant attachments that lead to increased competence and better developmental outcomes.[50,67] Sensitivity training for parents aimed at recognizing signs of infant stress while infants are in the NICU and thereby promoting better mother-infant attachment and improved infant developmental outcomes may be helpful.[29,60]

In childbirth classes, PPD should be addressed with anticipatory guidance discussing risk factors and early symptoms. Information brochures with resources should be available. Support groups often prepare mothers (and fathers) for the reality of parenthood and provide anticipatory guidance and counseling, skill building, validation, and acknowledgment of the concerns and frustrations of caring for a new infant. There are often support groups specifically for PPD available in local communities and at the statewide level. Referral to national organizations such as Postpartum Support International and Depression After Delivery enable mothers and fathers to access many additional resources (see Resource Materials for Parents section at the end of this chapter). Other interventions include visiting nurse services, nurse home visitors, parenting classes, referrals to childcare resources, and mutual aid hotlines. A recent meta-analysis found that *any* psychosocial or psychologic intervention (compared with routine postpartum care) reduced symptoms of depression and the likelihood of continued PPD within the first year after giving birth.[55]

Many psychotherapy modalities are recommended to mothers. Couples therapy may be part of the treatment plan if there is marital discord; however, even when there are no particular difficulties in the relationship, including the father can be useful in providing information and support for the mother. Suggestions for increased help around the home can be of tremendous value, allowing the mother to obtain adequate rest and care for herself. If the symptoms are very severe, psychiatric day treatment or inpatient hospitalization may be necessary. (In England, there are mother/baby inpatient units.) In cases in which the infant's life is in danger, protective services may have to be involved.

The use of medications (selective serotonin reuptake inhibitors, mood stabilizers, antidepressants, and antipsychotics) may be necessary.[53] The use of hormonal manipulation has been investigated. Referral to a clinician who is familiar with PPD is recommended.

Breastfeeding is associated with a reduced risk for PPD that is maintained over the first 4 months of the postpartum period.[89,222] The issue of breastfeeding when considering psychotropic medications needs to be addressed.[31] Parents should be provided necessary information about the effects of these medications on the neonate so that the risks and benefits can be considered on an individual basis. All psychotropic medications enter the breast milk, so careful evaluation with the health care team needs to be undertaken (see Table 18-4).

ADAPTATION TO THE INTENSIVE CARE ENVIRONMENT

The fourth psychologic task involves adaptation to the intensive care environment.[66,83] All of the reactions of guilt, anxiety, fear, anger, and disappointment become heightened when parents attempt to adapt to this unfamiliar and alien environment.[184] They must learn a new language, establish trust in new relationships, and adapt to their role in this setting.[66,152,184] The intense and sometimes chaotic appearance of a high-risk nursery makes it a frightening experience that serves to increase parental feelings of helplessness and anxiety. Parents should gain a sense of security in this environment before initiating a caregiving role with their infant. There may be cultural and linguistic adaptations and geographic obstacles for families who live in small, rural communities and must travel to large, unfamiliar cities and adapt to large hospitals. Locating the hospital and finding accommodations and meals can become overwhelming to parents who have undergone much emotional turmoil. Meeting the infant's care providers, the competent physician and nurse, sometimes can evoke a mixture of positive and negative feelings. Parents may be reassured and grateful for care being given, but their feelings of uselessness, helplessness, and inadequacy can be reinforced.[180] The sophistication of the highly technical care and heroic measures provided to achieve survival for their infant may be met with both awe and uncertainty.[148,184] Family disruption is exaggerated by distance, especially if the infant was transported, and the father must decide whether he is most needed with the infant, the infant's mother, or perhaps other children at home. Decisions must be made about work responsibilities, as well as childcare. The financial concerns related to providing intensive care become an added stress on families and often are compounded by the travel expenditures necessary to visit the infant. In general having an infant in the NICU has wide-reaching effects on the entire family system (parents, grandparents, siblings, employment, finances, childcare). A social worker providing comprehensive services and interventions is imperative to guide the family during this difficult time.

Parental Responses

In comparing the psychosocial adjustments of parents in the NICU, both parents may experience increased levels of emotional distress.[58,184] Mothers have been found to be more anxious, hostile, and depressed than fathers, with poorer adjustments related to work, sexual relations, social environment, and psychologic distress.[58] Mothers and fathers experience the NICU stay differently; mothers found the entire NICU experience and its aftermath more stressful than did fathers.[58,103] It is important to include both mothers and fathers in assessments and interventions and to avoid overlooking the father's needs because he may be less accessible.[58,103,148] Fathers need communication, empathy, and support for the stressful experience of the NICU in a similar fashion as for mothers.[184]

A number of nonverbal and verbal signs indicate that parents are struggling to gain a sense of security in the NICU. Some parents appear frightened, overwhelmed, nervous, and withdrawn, asking few questions or being reluctant to call or visit. Others may be highly anxious and unable to focus on their infant and may instead concentrate on other activities or infants in the nursery. Some parents may ask many questions and become very interested in the technical aspects of their infant's treatment, such as respirator settings and laboratory values, in an attempt to understand and cope with their infant's illness.[57,148] Some parents, uneasy with entrusting their infant to strangers, may initially feel a need to remain at his or her side, maintaining a vigil. Some may wish to read the infant's chart or attempt to read material on their infant's particular condition. Others may become angry or upset at minor differences in the infant's care or the nursery policies, such as a respiratory setting being off a point or discrepancies in enforcing visitation guidelines.[66,80]

Research into the mother's needs in the NICU have found that the mother's priority is to safeguard her infant. Mothers perceive that if they advocate for their own needs (e.g., to mother or care for the infant) in the NICU, they will be labeled as "difficult" or "demanding." Maternal needs in the NICU include information and interaction with their infant, emotional safety, and a supportive NICU environment in which to meet their needs (Table 29-3).[155] When these needs are thwarted, mothers feel helpless, powerless, and emotionally vulnerable and are less able to interact with their infant. A major barrier to implementing FCC is the mother's fear about how her needs, feelings, and actions affect the care of her baby. FCC empowers mothers and fathers through collaboration with health care providers.[184]

For families, the relationship with health care providers progresses through three stages: naïve trust, disenchantment, and guarded alliance.[152,155,184] Naïve trust, the belief that the family will be informed and involved in decision making, becomes disenchantment when unmet expectations, distrust, and anger result in the belief that the sick family member needs to be protected. A guarded alliance develops when families become more able to navigate the health care system and are involved, are in control, and participate in the care of their sick member. Helpful interventions include (1) meeting individual family's needs, (2) providing a welcoming NICU environment, (3) personalizing the infant, (4) teaching parents to interpret their infant's cues and behaviors, (5) fulfilling the continuing need for information, and (6) forming partnerships with families in all aspects of decision making and caregiving,[152,184] including giving them the option to be present during procedures and participate in pain relief for their infant.[110,155,156]

Facilitating Adaptation

Many interventions can be employed to familiarize and orient families.[83] First, the obstetrician, transport team, or any other professional who has initial contact with parents can give them preparatory information and a description of intensive care. A booklet or video[83] in the native language of the parent that includes basic information and illustrative pictures is extremely useful and should include a discussion of the type of care being provided, normal feelings and reactions parents experience, financial information, a glossary of terms, breastfeeding information, available accommodations and meals, calling and visitation policies, the discharge policy, and a city map. Both at the time of transfer and later in the nursery, a self-developing picture or picture from a digital camera can be taken of the infant for the parents. If the infant is being transported, information should be given as to the general length of time of transport and by whom and when the parents will be contacted after the infant has been admitted and evaluated. A personal phone call from the staff with an introduction, information about the infant and unit, and an inquiry about parental visitation plans is useful. Parents feel less anxious when they have an orientation and a name to whom to relate. The staff can then be prepared to be available when the parents arrive.

Certainly, the first visit to the NICU is overwhelming and stressful.[184] Members of the health care team should welcome the parents and stay with them to explain the equipment and procedures, answer questions, review the infant's course, give emotional support, and generally orient the parents to this new experience. Mothers who have not previously seen their baby report more stress in seeing their baby first in the NICU. Seeing the infant is stressful and may evoke shock, fear, guilt, and helplessness.[167] Be attentive to the mother's physical needs; comfortable chairs and perhaps a wheelchair if the mother has had a cesarean section are helpful. The message needs to be conveyed that parents are welcome, that their presence makes a difference, and that they will be partners in the care of their infant.[84,152] Because many parents are uncertain about what questions to ask, it may be necessary at times to help parents construct questions (e.g., "Do you understand why we start IVs in the head?" or "Do you know what blood gases, hood oxygen, and CPAP are?") and repeat explanations using simple, nontechnical language. Relating to the parent's affect or emotional state seems to establish a rapport with the family and helps them feel that the staff is empathetic and understanding.

TABLE 29-3	MATERNAL NEEDS IN THE NEONATAL INTENSIVE CARE UNIT

MATERNAL NEED	RECOMMENDATIONS FOR NICU STAFF
Empowering information	Give information about maternal situation in NICU (e.g., feelings, importance of her role as mother of the baby).
	Give information on how a preterm baby differs from a term baby and how to read/respond to her individual baby's cues/behaviors.
	Facilitate opportunities for parents to provide direct care for their infant.
	Understand parental need for modeling and role-modeling on preterm care tasks (e.g., feeding, bathing).
	Understand parental need for supportive appraisal — give positive feedback and reinforcement of maternal/paternal caregiving (e.g., feeding, diapering) and infant's responses to parental caregiving.
Continuity of care	Understand difficulty or impossibility of mother to negotiate actions with multitudes of caregivers.
	Use primary nursing for continuity of physical and emotional care for mothers, as well as infants.
Vigilant watching over	Understand maternal observations and actions to safeguard their infant and prevent injury or harm.
	Understand that mothers fear being seen as "difficult" by the staff, that voicing their concerns would jeopardize their baby's care.
	Understand mothers' perceptions that the nurse-to-patient ratio/acuity influences her behavior (i.e., mother is hesitant to advocate for her own needs for information, caregiving opportunities, and support). Mothers would shift their priority from interaction with the infant to safeguarding the infant from danger by delaying/rescheduling the activity with the infant. As a result, mothers often become disappointed and frustrated that a meaningful moment with their infant was denied.
Expert knowledge	Understand that, initially, nurses and other health care providers are seen as "experts" in care of the infant.
	With increasing confidence and caregiving, mothers become "expert" in knowing their own infant and what works best and are truly the "constant" in the multiple caregiving system of the NICU.
	Understand that mothers receive conflicting messages from health care providers about respect, acknowledgment, and value of growing maternal expertise.
Emotional safety in the NICU	Understand feelings of extreme emotional vulnerability/exposure experienced by mothers in the NICU. Empathy, emotional warmth, and understanding in interactions with nurses and other health care professionals provide mothers with emotional safety. Feelings of emotional vulnerability were engendered when (1) nurses' actions covertly communicated that the mother was a "bother" or an "intruder,"[155] (2) the mother focused energy on controlling her emotions and behaving so the nurse would approve, (3) the mother attempted to negotiate with the staff for access to her own infant, (4) health care providers were not empathetic about maternal worries, concerns, separation, and distress about their infant and need for frequent information,[155] and (5) there were breaches of confidentiality.

Modified from Hurst I: Mothers' strategies to meet their needs in the newborn intensive care nursery, *J Perinat Neonatal Nurs* 15:65, 2001; and Hurst I: Vigilant watching over: mothers' actions to safeguard their premature babies in the newborn intensive care nursery, *J Perinat Neonatal Nurs* 15:39, 2001.

If parents sense the staff's genuine concern and interest in them and their infant, it is easier for them to leave their infant in the staff's care.[155,167,180,184,216] A team member might say, "You look frightened or scared" or "This can be an overwhelming situation" or "You look like you want to cry." Facilitating the parents' relationship with the infant★ is essential and can be done by offering the parents the opportunity to touch or stroke their infant, hold the infant if possible, or at least remove eye patches. Pointing out

some of the unique personal characteristics of the infant is helpful. A staff member might say, "Your baby is very active," or "He responds well to touch," or "She seems to prefer lying on her side."

Families coming from out of town should be provided with a list of inexpensive housing and restaurants located near the hospital. In many cities, national and local businesses have established nearby homes run by local volunteer organizations for housing parents on a temporary basis. The homes have several sleeping rooms in addition to kitchen and laundry facilities and provide parents with a

★References 148, 155, 184, 216, 225, 234.

comfortable, homelike atmosphere at a nominal charge. A natural support system generally emerges among the parents using the home. A list of apartments, hotels, and boarding rooms reasonably priced and rented by the day or week also can be made available. Social workers often are aware of community resources and support available and can secure food, parking, and cab vouchers to give to families to decrease some of the financial stresses.

Parents usually are concerned with the cost of their infant's hospitalization. Some parents feel that if they cannot pay, their child will receive less attention. Parents should be reassured that their infant's care will not depend on their ability to pay. However, they should be referred to the appropriate funding agencies, such as the Handicapped Children's Program or Health Care Programs for Children with Special Needs, Social Security Disability, Title 19 Medicaid, and state child health insurance programs that provide financial assistance.

Because communication is critical, regular conferences between the family and staff (physicians, nurses, and social workers) should be instituted to give consistent medical information and emotional support; this is especially helpful with both extremely critical and long-term infants. Medical interpreters should be made available if parents do not speak English; the same principle applies for deaf parents. Parents should be given the names of the physicians and nurses taking care of their infant and the personnel's specific role in providing both care to the infant and communication to the family. If the physicians and nurses have a rotation system, this also should be explained from the beginning. At the end of a rotation, the transition can be facilitated by the oncoming physician's participation in even a brief conference with the outgoing physician, primary nurse, and parents.[88]

Primary nursing, especially for long-term infants, can be very helpful in providing for continuity of care.[88] The primary nurse has been identified by parents as the primary source and facilitator of information to parents and between parents and other health care providers and as the link between parents and infant. In a study of maternal values, mothers associated nurses with the human quality of the NICU, a wealth of knowledge about technology, and valuing the personal characteristics of the infants.[188] In the same study, mothers identified the most desirable attributes of care providers as (1) technical skill/competency, (2) caring about or

"really liking" babies, (3) communication abilities, and (4) patience.[188]

Protection of patient privacy and confidentiality is an ethical and legal (state and federal) obligation. Compliance to protect patient privacy, secure private patient information, and protect patient confidentiality is mandatory (in the United States) under the Health Insurance Portability and Accountability Act (HIPAA96). Violations of patient privacy include (1) overheard conversations; (2) failure to identify a telephone caller; (3) failure to obtain written consent to communicate patient information by fax, e-mail, or any other written/electronic format; and (4) leaving patient charts open/accessible to others.[213] HIPAA violations may result in financial penalties ($100 to $250,000) and/or imprisonment. Parental access to the medical record is a legal right (HIPAA96) that cannot be denied by professionals or the hospital. However, institutions must have a specific policy to deal with parent requests for access to the medical record. Many institutions require the presence of a professional to answer questions and interpret medical language for parents as they read the chart. The principles of family-centered neonatal care advocate not only parental access to the complete medical record but also documentation by parents of their own observations in the medical record.[92] All of these activities must be in compliance with the HIPAA regulations.[33,212]

For out-of-town families, the telephone plays a major role in staff-parent communication. The establishment of a telephone calling schedule with families and a toll-free number, if available, can be useful. If the family lives out of town and cannot visit frequently, the local or referring physician can supplement the communication. This physician often knows the family and can talk with them in person. The physician, of course, should communicate regularly with the nursery team to obtain the current medical information and present a consistent approach to the family.

Resumption of the Relationship with the Infant

The fifth psychologic task entails the parents' reestablishment of a relationship with their infant and initiating their caregiving role. Certain medical events may signal to the parents that it is safe to risk a relationship with the infant. These events may be a regular weight gain, changes in feeding patterns or methods, elimination of life support equipment or use of an incubator, the infant crying for the first time or becoming more active and responsive, or the infant's transfer from the NICU to a level II nursery. The parents may begin to read baby books or pamphlets about their infant's condition, buy clothes, set up the baby's room, send out birth announcements, or name the baby. If the infant has a congenital defect, the parents may become involved with genetic counseling and other parents whose infants have similar deficits.

Ideally parents have been involved as partners and caretakers since their infant was admitted to the NICU. If not, parents must begin to shift their level of involvement and activity from that of passive participants to that of active primary caregivers.* This shift includes the parents gaining confidence in their ability to care for their infant. The family who has been disrupted must reestablish themselves and recover from the crisis in an environment that is sensitive and supportive to this essential task.† The transfer of care from staff to parent is influenced by (1) the stability or lability of the infant's condition, (2) the physical health of the mother, (3) the level of parental support, and (4) the staff expectations.[148,180]

Several formalized intervention programs have been developed and tested for efficacy in assisting parents of NICU infants in relating to and parenting these vulnerable infants. An early educational-behavioral intervention program for NICU parents (Creating Opportunities for Parent Empowerment [COPE]) was developed and tested in a randomized controlled trial with 260 families.[162,163] Mothers in the COPE program had significantly less stress in the NICU, more positive interactions with their infants, and less depression and anxiety at 2 months' corrected infant age compared with the control mothers. Other study outcomes included (1) stronger parental beliefs about their role, (2) parents more able to read their preterm's cues and behaviors, and (3) shorter length of both NICU and hospital stays (by 4 days and 8 days for VLBW preterms) compared with the control group.[163] Another randomized study of an early intervention program found that parents who participated had a reduction in parenting stress after birth of their preterm infant.[111] The March of Dimes initiative to encourage FCC

(NICU Family Support [NFS] Program) has been studied at 8 NFS sites by interviewing parents, NICU staff, and administrators. Findings include (1) culture change within the NICU resulting in increased family support; (2) enhanced overall quality of NICU care; (3) less stressed, more informed, and confident parents; and (4) increased receptivity of staff to the concept of FCC and its benefits.[47]

Another formalized and researched intervention program is the Mother-Infant Transaction Program (MITP). Sixty-three mothers in Australia were randomized to intervention with the MITP or a control group.[179] Compared with the control group, mothers in the MITP intervention group were found to be more responsive to their infants, were less stressed at 3 months, and had better mutual interaction with their infants at 3 and 6 months.[179] Infants in the MITP intervention group were more attentive, were perceived by their mothers as "easier" with fewer regulatory problems (i.e., colic, sleep, crying), and had better communication skills.[179] A more recent randomized controlled trial of MITP found a reduction in PPD and longer breastfeeding, but no alteration in maternal stress.[191] A Dutch randomized controlled trial of the Infant Behavioral Assessment and Intervention Program found intervention mothers with higher feelings of social isolation and describing their infants as happier and less distractible and hyperactive than control mothers.[161] Other interventions to relieve parental stress have recently been reviewed.[42]

Involvement in caregiving lessens the parents' feelings of helplessness and frustration and facilitates their identification with their role as parents.* Alteration in their parental role is particularly stressful for mothers in the NICU.[23,98,100,168] The sense of parenthood for both mothers and fathers depends on expectations of the parental role, the infant's state of health, and the environment and professional attitudes in the NICU.[103,148] A study by Jackson and colleagues[103] found that internalization of the parent role with a premature infant occurs over time and often involves initial feelings of alienation and responsibility that change to more confidence (at 3 to 6 months) and familiarity (at 18 months) with the parenting role. For weeks after birth, both parents experience alienation: (1) mothers felt ambivalence about their relationship with the baby and their new role as parent—a concern for the baby's welfare and a need to participate

*References 130, 148, 155, 162, 163, 177, 226.
†References 23, 51, 81, 92, 100, 130, 148, 162, 163, 177, 180, 226, 234.

*References 51, 98, 130, 148, 155, 162, 163, 177, 225, 226.

in and control the infant's care; and (2) fathers shared concern for the baby, felt unprepared for the birth, and were confident in delegating the baby's care to the NICU staff.[103] In this qualitative study, neither parent felt ready for the preterm infant's discharge to home. Taking on total responsibility for the baby's care resulted in both parents feeling insecure, fearful, and worried about the baby and the father taking on more responsibility for infant care. By 6 months of age, both parents had developed more confidence in the care and parenting of their preterm; by 18 months, parents had developed a feeling of relationship with their child.[103] For mothers of the smallest and sickest infants, concerns and worry about the infant remained even at 6 months.[103] Beginning as early as possible in the NICU, health care providers should encourage and facilitate parent participation in their infant's care.[*]

Parents can provide skin care for their infant, learn to read and respond to infant cues, help turn the infant even if a respirator is attached, diaper the infant, and possibly feed the infant. If the parents are separated by distance, they can send family pictures that can be posted at the infant's bed; periodic pictures of the infant taken by the staff can be sent back to the family. Parents can send clothing, mobiles, simple toys, and even cassette tapes or recordings so that the infant can hear the parents' voices. Some mothers who are pumping send frozen breast milk (see Chapter 18). All of these reminders help the nursery staff be aware of the real family, who are genuinely interested. These personal attempts made by parents that help them feel they are important to their infant's development should be encouraged. Sometimes foster grandparents or volunteers can hold, feed, and talk to infants whose parents cannot visit frequently.

A recent prospective cohort study of parental presence and holding in the NICU found significant neurobehavioral benefits for the 81 preterm infants 30 weeks of gestation or younger.[194] Early parenting (i.e., holding) in the NICU resulted in lower arousal and excitability, better quality of movement, less stress, and less hypertonic muscle tone and thus a developmental advantage.[194] Early sensitivity training for parents in the NICU is associated with improved white matter micro-structural development in their preterm infants.[169] Kangaroo care (see Chapter 13), skin-to-skin contact between mother/father and

infant by placing the infant in a vertical position between the mother's/father's breasts, has positive maternal/paternal, as well as neonatal, responses. Use of kangaroo care activates the maternal processes of a search for meaning and adjustment to the experience of preterm birth, a recovery of self-esteem, maternal confidence, and enhancement in the parenting of a high-risk neonate.[28,100,116] Successive sessions of kangaroo care ease the pain and emotional suffering as mothers deal with loss and letting go and develop competence and confidence. Paternal attachment is also facilitated by fathers holding their infants and engaging in skin-to-skin contact.[148] A study by Sullivan[219] indicates that the earlier fathers hold their babies, the sooner they report feelings of love and warmth. The infant may become a reality to the father when he can hold his infant.[148,219] In the same study, fathers reported delaying attachment until they were certain of the infant's survival.[219]

The use of "graduate parents," parents who have had an infant in the NICU and who have successfully dealt with and resolved the crisis of the birth of their infant, can be extremely valuable.[92,100,148,184] They provide support to parents by sharing common feelings, reactions, and experiences about having a hospitalized infant. Graduate parents can provide support and practical assistance for mothers interested in breastfeeding, parents who take their infant home on oxygen, or parents whose infant requires special medical care such as a shunt, tracheostomy, colostomy, or gavage feedings. Organized graduate parent groups in large tertiary settings have become a very popular means of providing support,[36,83,100] but locating one parent or couple to talk with parents in a small community can be just as helpful. Parent classes and Internet resources[100] also can be offered on a variety of topics such as breastfeeding, infant development, premature infant development, sibling and family reactions, discharge, cardiopulmonary resuscitation, coping with the hospitalization, and special medical needs. These classes provide specific, didactic information combined with group discussions that are mutually supportive. Social workers, nurses, and other related health care professionals (e.g., respiratory, occupational, and physical therapists) facilitate the group; graduate parents also participate as a resource.

A third type of support is counseling sessions. The purpose of these sessions is to discuss and deal with common issues among parents arising from the hospitalization of their infant and the effects on their marriage and family life. This type of session also has

---

[*]References 51, 100, 148, 155, 163, 225.

been helpful for parents whose infant has died. The sessions are usually short term and are conducted by the perinatal social worker and another staff member such as a physician, nurse, or chaplain. The focus of the group is not to give specific medical information but, rather, to provide parents with an opportunity to verbalize their feelings about their infant's hospitalization and receive emotional support.

Recently, telemedicine technologies have been used in the NICU to enhance medical, informational, and emotional support for families during and after hospitalization. Baby CareLink[79] is a telemedicine program that incorporates video conferencing and Internet technologies to enhance interactions among families, NICU staff, and community health care providers. The link contains information for families about relevant issues during and after hospitalization. The video conferencing module enables distance learning by the family in their home during the NICU stay and remote monitoring after discharge. A recent survey found that families using this technology were more satisfied with the unit's physical environment and visitation policy, possibly because of the ability to facilitate visitation via teleconferencing when family members could not be present in the NICU.[79] Websites for parents of premature infants, children, and adults in the family are available so that parents can support each other, discuss common problems, and share solutions; caution should be used, however, when recommending the Internet (see Resource Materials for Parents section at the end of this chapter).

Visiting in the Neonatal Intensive Care Unit

VISITING GUIDELINES

Besides their spouse or significant other, parents identify their families and friends as the main source of support through the crisis of having a sick neonate.[155,234] Prohibiting visiting by family and friends or limiting visitors to "two at a time" can isolate parents from a major source of support. NICU visiting policies should be used as guidelines, rather than rules, to facilitate visiting and caregiving by parents and families.[★]

Care providers should use good judgment and discretion about visitation while understanding and respecting the parents' need to be "in charge" of their infant (e.g., make decisions for their infant).[†]

Lack of perceived control by parents is associated with increased anxiety, hostility, depression, and poorer adjustment.[66,148,155,225] A sense of parental control in the NICU is enhanced by parental decision making.[‡] Parents should designate their infant's "guest list"—that is, other family and friends who can visit and perform caregiving activities in their absence.[155]

NICU visiting policies vary within the United States[41] and among European countries. Two thirds of surveyed nurseries "allow" parents to visit during medical rounds, whereas visiting during nurse report was more restricted.[41] When parental visits were restricted, confidentiality was cited as the determinant of the visiting policy.[41] In this same survey, 39% of parents "sometimes" or "often" complained about restricted visitation.[41]

FCC recognizes the family as the constant in the infant's life.[2,21] Liberal visitation policies are accepted as beneficial for patients and families. The American Academy of Pediatrics (AAP) Policy on *Family-Centered Care and the Pediatrician's Role* states that creating 24-hour open unit for policies for families and making a commitment to information sharing are beneficial for families and staff.[8] Specifically, a 24-hour open unit has been shown to decrease length of stay, decrease use of the emergency department, improve parent satisfaction, and decrease parental anxiety.[8,69] A discrepancy exists between parental requests and visitation practices in many NICUs. Before changing to a 24-hour open visitation policy for parents, NICU nurses in one center had reservations and were skeptical.[231] After implementing the 24-hour visiting policy, most nurses were supportive of the change and reported perceived benefits for families. Parent satisfaction increased regarding time spent with their infant.[231] NICU staff should be open-minded and flexible in determining the policy on visitation during rounds, report, and emergencies.[8,80,92]

Many parents are interested in being included in medical rounds to actively participate in the care, discussion, and decision making about their infant.[8,80,92] A qualitative study of 18 NICU parents included in interdisciplinary teaching rounds in a tertiary children's hospital found that parents (1)

[★]References 2, 80, 100, 148, 155, 171.

[†]References 66, 98, 148, 155, 184, 188.
[‡]References 66, 71, 148, 155, 184, 188, 236.

had a positive experience and were "comfortable" being included, (2) preferred rounds in which nurses were included and lay terminology was used, and (3) welcomed the ability to communicate, understand the plan, and participate with the team in decision making about their infant's care.[128] Another study reported that family-centered rounds (FCR) were associated with increased provider satisfaction and collaboration for neonatal nurse practitioners and fellows.[232] In addition, FCR was associated with enhanced communication between providers and parents. Importantly there were no negative aspects to the introduction of FCR.[232] If parents and the NICU staff agree to parental participation in rounds, patient confidentiality can be maintained by moving rounds away from the bedside, speaking quietly, and inviting parents to participate in only their infant's care planning/medical rounds[8,80,92] in this or a separate meeting. Parents may be visitors to the hospital and NICU, but they are not "visitors" to their newborn; parents and family are the constants in the life of a child, whereas health care providers are only temporary "visitors" in the life of the child.[2,28,130,155,171]

Parents may be more comfortable in the NICU if they are accompanied by a family member or friend.[234] A study showed that black teenage mothers establish a relationship with their infant by visiting regularly and learning how to care for him or her.[167] The research states that when these young women bring a friend or family member with them to the NICU, they are more comfortable parenting and caregiving for their infants. Parental visiting patterns may be categorized by care providers as visiting "too much"[80] or "too little."[81] Financial constraints (e.g., transportation and childcare costs, loss of work time), chaotic social situations, or poor physical and mental maternal health may contribute to fewer visits.[100] Parents may fear that the infant will not survive, may feel helpless, or may not think their visits are important for their sick baby. Parents should be taught by example how important their presence and caregiving are to their baby's survival and recovery. In addition, parents need to be taught to interpret their infant's cues and behaviors (see Chapter 13). Maximizing every parental visit by scheduling care by parents★ (e.g., bathing the baby, breastfeeding, kangaroo care, nipple feeding) communicates the importance of parent care and enables

them "to be an expert on how to care for your baby by the time the baby is ready to go home."

SIBLING RELATIONSHIPS

The inclusion of other children in the events surrounding the birth of a sick newborn is important. From a sibling's viewpoint, the anticipated birth of a new infant is a stressful time of noticeable physical and psychologic changes within the family. In preparation for the impending birth, the child is told that the mother will be going to the hospital for a few days and will return with a baby brother or sister. With the birth of a premature or ill infant, the mother may go to the hospital unexpectedly, stay a long time, and not return home with the anticipated playmate. Instead of a celebration of the expected happy event, parents are grieving the loss of the normal newborn and facing the current crisis of their sick infant.

Parents are often unsure about what to tell the other children and whether the children should see the infant. The siblings themselves may feel left out, rejected, or worried that they too may get sick. They may feel they are to blame and that their jealous feelings about their new rival may have caused this tragedy. Confused by their parents' distress, the other children may speculate that it is related to them and their "bad" behaviors. They may be disappointed and angry that they did not get the "playmate" they had wanted. Because parents are unsure about how to manage these issues, it is often helpful for the staff to introduce the topic. Most children's hospitals employ child life specialists who can consult with parents regarding siblings. Child life specialists have extensive knowledge of child development and expertise in talking with children, often using a child's own play in the process of providing support.

Because children will make up an explanation for the infant's illness, it is better to have it based on accurate information. Before explaining the infant's condition to siblings, elicit their ideas and perceptions about "what is the matter." Any fears, fantasies, misconceptions, or accurate information are thus used to begin the explanation of "where the baby is." Explanations must be tailored to the individual child's cognitive and developmental level. The child should be told that the infant is sick but in a way that is different from his or her illnesses, the infant's illness is not "catching," and it is not like any of the illnesses that the child has experienced. To allay the siblings' fears about medical personnel, they should

---

★References 66, 130, 155, 163, 188, 234.

also be told that the nurses and physicians are trying to help the infant "get better." Because children between 2 and 6 years of age are involved in magical thinking, they should be told that they are not to blame and that they did not cause the infant's problem. If the infant is premature, a team member might say to the child, "The baby came out too early or too soon; he needed more time to grow inside." If the infant has spina bifida, a staff member might say, "The baby's spine did not grow right, so he may have trouble lifting his legs or walking."

A child of 3 years of age or younger usually does not understand much about the coming infant. More important to this age group is the separation from parents who are frequently at the hospital. To ameliorate the separation, childcare arrangements should be structured so that the child is cared for by familiar people in a familiar environment. The best care arrangement is with a familiar person in the child's own home; second best would be a familiar person in the caregiver's home; and third best, an unfamiliar person in the child's own home. The least favorable, of course, is an unfamiliar person in an unfamiliar setting. Many hospitals have a childcare facility run by volunteers or child life specialists that allows the child the opportunity to go to the hospital to "see where Mommy and Daddy are going" yet allows the parents the chance to see their infant without having to care for their older child or children. Parents may also choose to include the young child in all or selected visits.

Children ages 3 years and older have more interest in babies and a better grasp of the physical meaning of life. Sometimes a picture of the baby or a look into the nursery through the windows is helpful to the other children. Many children benefit from visits to the nursery to see their brother or sister. The natural curiosity of the child about "what is going on" in the family is answered when the child actually sees the baby. Behavior problems such as bed-wetting, sleeping and eating difficulties, and difficult separations from parents may be prevented or reduced by the reassurance of a visit that decreases the sibling's worry about the baby.[1] Sibling visitation must be individualized for every family.

SIBLING VISITS

The decision to include siblings in the NICU depends to a great extent on the views, beliefs, and attitudes of the hospital staff. Generally, the staff's concerns about and resistance to sibling visitation focus on a fear of an increase in nosocomial infection, disruption of unit routine and order, and potential harm to young children from exposure to the NICU environment. Infection control is the responsibility of parents and professionals. Parents must be educated about the dangers of infection and instructed on how to screen their children for symptoms such as fever, cough, or diarrhea. Professional staff must inquire about the health of visiting siblings, including their exposure to communicable diseases. Both parents and children must wash their hands before entering the nursery; small stools allowing children to reach the sink are helpful. Cover gowns are no longer used by parents, siblings, or professionals. With vigilance, no increased bacterial colonization and no increased incidence of infection occur with sibling visits.[215]

Because sibling visitation may be beneficial, each NICU must evaluate the center's situation and consider instituting a sibling visitation policy.[80] The following general principles may be used in developing this policy:

- Communication and coordination between staff and family are necessary to promote successful sibling visitation, including a review of unit policies and guidelines for parents.
- Children must be prepared, according to their age and development, for what they will see, hear, and feel in the NICU. Language should be simple and honest; pictures of the infant or other infants can be helpful. Dialog with parents before the visit regarding how long they believe the sibling visit should realistically be based on their age and development also can be helpful.
- Parents and staff screen the visiting sibling for signs of illness that would exclude the child from visiting.
- Parents and child must scrub their hands thoroughly.
- The initial visit should be held at a relatively quiet time in the nursery when a care provider can stay with the family. If the infant can be moved to a private room or family room area, this is preferable.
- The presence of a qualified child life specialist can be helpful to families for sibling visits.

At the bedside, the child is introduced to the infant and seated on a chair or stool at eye level with the infant. The care provider then again explains the equipment the child sees and any of the infant's "interesting" behaviors such as crying because of hunger, sucking on a pacifier, or eyes open "looking at you." Children may even be included in age-appropriate caregiving tasks. Choosing clothes, handling diapers and blankets, holding the bottle, and touching and talking to the infant are all ways "to help." The child may bring a present to the infant such as a simple toy, music box, or handmade picture or photograph of the family. After a visit, both parents and staff should be available to talk about the visit or answer any questions. Some children, however, will not discuss the visit or ask questions until some later time. A method for enabling children to express their feelings in a nonverbal way is through play or books. A child who receives a book about physicians and hospitals or a "doctor" or "nurse" doll may "play out" feelings about the brother or sister and the hospital experience.

Creating a comfortable environment in which children feel free to ask questions is essential when siblings visit. Every question deserves an answer, even "I don't know," when appropriate. Children are often quite unrestrained in their remarks and questions. Comments such as "He's sure ugly!" or "Will he die?" or "Why is she tied up (restrained)?" are common. These may be embarrassing to parents who hesitate to make the same remarks or ask the same questions. If the infant is hospitalized for a long time, the other children may lose interest or even wish it were all over. This response may upset parents who themselves may be struggling with the same feelings. The longer the infant is hospitalized, the greater the pressure on time and financial resources. Family routines are disrupted by continuing hospitalization, and the disruption may strain family relationships.

Staff and parent response to sibling visitation has been positive in hospitals in which the policy has been implemented. Such a policy may facilitate family integrity and promotes mutual support during the stressful time of hospitalization. Another advantage of visitation is that the older siblings do not endure repeated separations caused by parental visits to the hospital but are included as important and special family members. The presence of siblings in a nursery can be a rewarding experience for family and staff alike and perhaps is the ideal example of providing safe yet comprehensive FCC.

Although a flexible sibling visitation policy is viewed as the best possible situation, some alternatives such as coloring books and children's books should be considered (see Resource Materials for Parents section at the end of this chapter). Staff should be sensitive to the needs of the siblings and understand that the parents must deal with both time and financial constraints.

Psychosocial Conferences

Psychosocial conferences for staff members to discuss the dynamics of family functioning and the effect of a seriously ill newborn on the family can be quite useful. These conferences, usually led by perinatal social workers or other mental health professionals, can give staff the opportunity to identify current issues of concern by the family and optimal strategies to support the family moving forward. Another function is to enable staff to discuss and better understand their own feelings and reactions to families, infants, and the many stresses related to working in a NICU. In addition, weekly rounds with the entire multidisciplinary team (physicians, nurses, nutritionists, lactation consultants, pharmacists, home health nurse coordinator, social workers, case managers, and financial counselors) are an effective vehicle to discuss and develop medical discharge and psychosocial care plans about each infant and family. Having an infant in the NICU has wide-reaching effects on the entire family system. Families arrive at the doors with their own unique stories and struggles that must be factored into the care and support provided to the family.

The involvement of perinatal social workers to assess and evaluate the psychosocial functioning of families, provide support and counseling services, and coordinate the discharge planning and follow-up care for the infant and family is essential. Social workers should complete a comprehensive assessment at admission for all families with an infant in the NICU. After assessment and discussion with the team, specific focus and interventions for high-risk cases can be identified (Box 29-7), as well as general support needs for all families. Providing support in complicated medical conditions, including the death of the infant, is also extremely important. Programs should be implemented for staff members to increase their competency and comfort level in identifying and intervening with psychosocial issues.[202]

Intimate Partner Violence (Domestic Violence)

Intimate partner violence (IPV) is recognized as a serious risk factor for adverse pregnancy outcomes.[9,157,223]

BOX 29-7   HIGH-RISK FACTORS INDICATING NEED FOR SOCIAL WORK INTERVENTION

1. Teenage pregnancy (ages 11-18 years)[23]
2. Single parent
3. Substance abuse[23]
4. Psychiatric history that interferes with appropriate functioning (including postpartum depression), especially as related to parenting abilities
5. Mother or father with a history of being physically or sexually abused or early deprivation by own family, or history of having abused or neglected own children
6. Intimate partner violence/domestic violence[157]
7. Mental disability, borderline intelligence, or significant physical handicaps
8. History of loss with previous pregnancy or loss of child because of stillbirth, birth defect, prematurity, abortion, custody case, or death
9. Rejection of or ambivalence about current pregnancy as manifested by requests for termination of pregnancy, attempted abortion, or relinquishment
10. No prenatal care with previous or current pregnancies
11. Pregnancy exacerbating extreme depression, anxiety, or suicidal thoughts
12. Stressful home or personal situation because of marital or financial problems or lack of support
13. Long-term hospitalization during pregnancy requiring intervention in helping family adjust by arranging for younger children at home or for financial assistance
14. Other children with physical or mental handicaps
15. Attachment difficulties with the infant
16. Prior history with social services
17. Inadequate housing and living arrangements and homelessness
18. Inadequate food and other essentials
19. Incarceration of mother/father
20. Military families
21. Undocumented immigrants

A recent study of IPV in first-time mothers participating in the Nurse Family Partnership found prevalence rates of (1) 8.1% in the year before pregnancy, (2) 4.7% during the current pregnancy, and (3) 12.4% in the year after the pregnancy.[203] A meta-analysis of 92 studies found prevalence rates of 28.4% for emotional abuse, 13.8% for physical abuse, and 8.0% for sexual abuse.[105] Risk factors for abuse during pregnancy in this meta-analysis included abuse before pregnancy, low education level, unintended pregnancy, low socioeconomic status, and being unmarried.[105]

Injuries resulting from physical abuse increase the risks for low birth weight, preterm birth, intrauterine growth restriction, stillbirth, and neonatal complications.[39,90] Emotional abuse is associated with a 1.6-fold increase in preterm birth; the combination of physical and emotional abuse increases the preterm birth rate 4.7-fold.[200] Poorer maternal outcomes include antepartum hemorrhage, depression (2-fold to 3-fold increased risk for major postpartum depression; 1.5-fold to 2-fold increase for elevated depressive symptoms),[22] inadequate prenatal care, high maternal cortisol, hypertension, early cessation of breastfeeding, poorer parenting behavior, and perinatal death.[90,147,149,173,238] Perinatal violence and stress also are significant risk factors for preterm birth in the teen population.[39] Pregnant women may be victims, perpetrators, or participants in reciprocal violence.[209] In one study, women participating in reciprocal violence had the highest levels of depression, used substances (alcohol, illicit drugs and tobacco), and were not happy about their pregnancy.[209] This finding is consistent with numerous other studies showing depression before, during, and after delivery, a greater prevalence of substance abuse, alcohol misuse in partners, poor nutrition, lower rates of contraception use, and higher repeat pregnancy.[96,97,181,203]

Because IPV is so prevalent and has serious negative effects on the entire family system, protocols and procedures (that are compliant with the policies of the setting [i.e., hospital, outpatient clinic, emergency room] and the reporting laws of the state) should be in place. Legal definitions of IPV vary by state, but IPV is *illegal* in all states. The health care team needs to be educated to recognize the signs and behaviors that may indicate IPV (and child abuse).

Because abuse is so pervasive and too serious to remain unidentified, health care providers should routinely ask all women patients about IPV (although men also can be victims). The AAP and the American Congress of Obstetricians and Gynecologists have position statements and guidelines for routine screening for IPV in all women.[9,223] Battering beginning during pregnancy is a very common phenomenon. Use of standardized screening tools, an anonymous computer-assisted self-interview[193] and recurrent screening results in higher identification rates (i.e., one study found higher disclosure after birth than during pregnancy).[115,182] For a discussion about the benefits and risks of routine screening, refer to the U.S. Preventive Services Task Force recommendation statement.[230]

Pregnancy offers a unique opportunity for health care professionals to intervene in IPV.[150,157,159,182] Once a potentially abusive situation has been identified, culturally and ethnically sensitive interventions should be initiated.[150] Interventions vary depending on the disclosures made by the mother or father (or partner) and the needs identified. Recommendations for interventions include (1) educate the woman about community supports, (2) discuss options with the victim, (3) help identify a safety plan, (4) make appropriate referrals, (5) comply with state statutes about reporting responsibility, (6) document assessments and interventions, and (7) refer for treatment and aftercare (essential). Because of the complexity of issues generated by IPV, a multidisciplinary team approach is recommended.

Transfer Back to the Referring Hospital

Transfer of the infant from a tertiary center back to the referring or local community hospital for convalescent care and discharge is a frequent occurrence. This can help facilitate the relationship between the infant and parents, because the infant will be more accessible. Parents generally view the transfer as positive if the hospital is closer to home and if they feel comfortable with the level of care provided. Transfer is stressful, and there is always an adjustment period any time a transfer occurs.[126] Parents must adapt to different personalities of medical personnel, different procedures and visiting policies. Preparing the parents for the transfer, orienting them to the new hospital, and talking to the staff of the referral hospital about the infant and the parents are important to help ease the transition.[126]

Preparation to Take the Infant Home

The sixth psychologic task for parents concerns preparations for taking the infant home. Parents must understand their infant's individual needs and personality characteristics and must feel a sense of competency in relating to and caring for their infant. Discharge is an anxiety-provoking event and ushers in the "crisis" of homecoming, which parents must face and master.[57,100,103,148,225] The unsuccessful resolution of the previously discussed five psychologic tasks can contribute to maladaptive parenting and

a poor outcome for the infant, including the possibilities of attachment difficulties, overprotectiveness, failure to thrive, vulnerable child syndrome,[118] emotional deprivation, and battering.[38,118,160] To achieve a positive parent-child relationship after the hospitalization and through the transitional period that ensues, provision of appropriate follow-up support through the home adjustment period is crucial.[118,148,225]

Several behaviors demonstrate that parents are trying to understand the infant's care in preparation for discharge. First, parents may ask questions verbalizing a variety of concerns. For a premature infant, they might ask, "Do I need an apnea monitor at home?" or "Can the baby have visitors?" or "Do I have to wash my hands when handling the baby?" For an infant with a congenital defect such as spina bifida, the parents might ask, "Can I lay the baby on his back?" or "Can I bathe him?" or "Do I have to pump the shunt?" For an infant with a heart defect, the staff might be asked, "Do I need oxygen?" or "Do I have to handle him differently?" or "What about going to higher altitudes?" or "Is my baby at risk for sudden infant death syndrome (SIDS)?" All of these questions on the part of parents are typical and normal and represent the parents' working through their fears and anxieties.

On the other hand, parents who are highly anxious,[57] extremely overprotective, or very indifferent should be a concern to the health care personnel. The inability to deal with the task of taking the infant home may indicate some unresolved feelings related to the previous psychologic tasks. Although most parents whose infants have been in a NICU do admit to initially treating their infant differently until they "got to know their child," a group of parents who are excessively overprotective does exist. This type of behavior often stems from parents who are struggling with intense feelings of guilt and failure. These parents either protect their baby from everything because they feel so responsible for having caused the infant's initial problem or they demonstrate an indifference or lack of concern for the infant and the infant's welfare. Such parents may have an ambivalent attachment to their infant, who may continue to represent the threat of death or the parents' personal failure. This group of parents should be considered high risk for potential parent-child relationship difficulties and should be evaluated to determine an appropriate intervention.

At discharge, there are infants whose medical conditions are still fragile, and there is a substantial indication that these infants may not be normal and may have long-term problems. These infants may be temperamentally difficult to manage, and parents understandably treat them differently. These parents and infants need additional support and appropriate intervention (see Chapter 31).

The perinatal health care team can employ many interventions to assist parents with discharge and through the transitional period that follows (see Chapter 31). In the hospital, adequate teaching of caregiving skills that enable the parent to develop a sense of mastery and competence is of paramount importance. Parent education regarding the care and needs of their baby is a learning process that begins at admission and continues throughout the inpatient stay. In addition to tasks of care, parents should participate in planning and providing developmentally appropriate care and be able to read and respond to their infant's cues (see Chapter 13). Maternal concerns about the infant's care center on elimination, feeding/weight gain, the infant's health (breathing, development, or ongoing medical problems),[100] and preparation of medications. If parents do not feel comfortable with their infant, their anxiety can cause adverse interactions with him or her. The parent needs to know the infant's mannerisms and behaviors; otherwise the parent may feel exhausted and resentful and then guilty. Teaching caregiving skills often can be facilitated in an environment that is less intense and crisis oriented than the NICU. Whenever possible, an infant should be transferred to a setting that is more conducive to the parents' initiation of the primary caregiving role, such as a special care or transitional nursery, a level II unit, or a general pediatric ward. Care by parents before discharge enables parents to assume full responsibility for their infant's care, tests the reality of caregiving, helps them learn caregiving activities and their infant's behavioral patterns, and confirms their readiness for independent parenting and the infant's readiness for discharge.[85,100,163,177]

Adequate discharge planning and follow-up arrangements should include general pediatric care; home health care; nurse home visitors; referral for early intervention services, if indicated; and parenting classes, especially for young or psychosocially high-risk parents. Numerous studies document positive effects of home visitation programs. Referrals to county social service departments should be made for single mothers who are eligible for Temporary Assistance to Needy Families; Women, Infants, and Children (WIC) Program; Title 19 Medicaid; and state child health insurance programs. For infants with special problems (e.g., spina bifida, cerebral palsy, Down syndrome), referrals should be made for special programs that provide early intervention services for the infants and support groups for parents. Parents whose infants have special medical needs (e.g., gavage feedings, tracheostomy or colostomy care, oxygen, or ventilators) should be evaluated by the medical and nursing teams to determine helpful community resources (e.g., equipment, supplies, respite, emergency care) and to make appropriate referrals. Home nursing care and homemaker services sometimes are covered by medical insurance and may be necessary to provide actual nursing activities and to relieve parents from the emotional burden inherent in caring for an infant with medical problems. For infants who are developmentally or physically challenged or at risk, participation in developmental intervention programs and other follow-up clinics provided by many hospitals that have NICUs are extremely valuable. These infants are eligible for Part C of the Individuals with Disabilities Education Act (IDEA). Locating babysitters who will care for a child with special problems can be an overwhelming task for parents; cultivating a resource list for parents and suggesting that parents exchange services with each other also can be helpful. Graduate parents, neonatal nurses, or respite care organizations can provide a useful service to parents in this situation. Last, parents should be referred to appropriate funding agencies (e.g., Health Care Programs for Children with Special Needs, Title 19 Medicaid, state child health insurance programs, Social Security Disability) that provide financial assistance.

REFERENCES

For a full list of references, scan the QR code or visit http://booksite.elsevier.com/9780323320832.

As a life passage, pregnancy and birth are associated with hopes, expectations, joy, and happiness for the future. Although pregnancy and birth constitute a developmental crisis and a major life change, expectant parents reasonably believe the gains of a healthy, happy child and family life offset any setbacks. Unfortunately, not all perinatal events have a happy ending. Loss of a healthy infant in the perinatal period when premature delivery occurs also affects the parents' friends, family, and professional care providers.

Perinatal loss may be the first time a young adult has had to cope with the illness or death of a loved one. Perinatal loss is especially significant because (1) it is sudden and unexpected; (2) it is the most difficult loss to resolve[24]; (3) it interrupts the significant developmental stage of pregnancy and the situational crisis of pregnancy[24]; (4) it is the loss of a child who did not have the opportunity to live a full life[45,136]; (5) it prevents progression into the next developmental stage of parenting that has been anticipated and rehearsed (at least mentally) during the pregnancy[87]; (6) it is fraught with ambiguity and disenfranchised grief[82]; and (7) it represents a narcissistic loss, a loss of self, for the parents.[129,159,160] Perinatal loss also often means interpersonal exclusion from the activities of childbearing friends and siblings.

Unfortunately, loss and grief often are thought of only in relation to death. However, as final and irreversible as death is, it is just one form of separation and loss. Although less obvious, other loss situations may have an equally crucial effect. Loss comes in many forms, and during the perinatal period, may occur without necessarily resulting in death.

Circumstances of perinatal loss are parallel and, at the same time, different, because they all entail grief and mourning. Yet each has unique dimensions and characteristics. The process of grief, its stages, and its symptoms are reviewed as a framework for understanding one's own feelings and those of others experiencing a loss. A desire to help and an idea of what is and is not helpful are essential for effective intervention by professionals.

THE GRIEF PROCESS

Grief, the characteristic reaction to the loss of a valued "object"—a person or thing—is not an intellectual and rational response.[48] Rather, it is personally experienced as the deep emotion of sadness and sorrow. To the individual, grief feels overwhelming, irrational, out of control, "crazy," and all-consuming. Mourning occurs in phases over time. After acknowledgment that the person no longer exists, gradual withdrawal of emotion and feeling occurs, so that eventual psychologic investment in a new relationship is possible.

A literature review of the theoretical perspectives of parental grief from the United States and the United Kingdom reveals a change from a traditional to a "newer" model of grief in the Anglo-American culture.[36] Traditional models of grief emphasize the severing of bonds with the deceased, whereas "newer" understandings of parental grief emphasize parents retaining a relationship with their dead child.[166] After reviewing nursing, medical, and social science publications and choosing relevant ones, Davies states: "the concept of continuous bonds challenges the dominant assumption that resolution

---

PURPLE type highlights content that is particularly applicable to clinical settings.

of grief is achieved through severing bonds with the deceased."[36] Parents wish to know that their child's birth and death have meaning and purpose and that their child "mattered" and will be remembered by them and by others who have been "touched" and "changed" by the child.[25] After the death of a child, parents may develop approaches to "make meaning" from their loss in order to maintain a connection to the child, honor and keep the child's memory alive, and to help others facing similar circumstances.[39] Parents in one study said that intergenerational acknowledgment of the ongoing relationship to the deceased child by grandparents was very important, especially during a subsequent pregnancy.[110]

For grief to occur, the individual must have valued the person who is lost so that the loss is perceived as significant and meaningful. Because, prenatally, there is an investment of love in the fetus or newborn, the neonate is a valued person. To the extent that prenatal attachment has occurred, grief should be expected and felt at the loss of the fetus or newborn. Therefore, loss at birth is a significant loss of a valued (although as yet only imagined) person.

Loss, whether real or imagined, actual or possible, is traumatic. The individual is no longer confident in him or herself or in his or her surroundings, as both have been altered. Mourning and grief are forms of separation reactions. Fear of separation and abandonment is the universal of childhood regardless of age or developmental stage. Perhaps loss of a significant other awakens these childhood fears and reminds us of the basic "insecurity of all our attachments."[92]

Life changes are stressful to the individual because they threaten to disrupt continuity and a state of equilibrium.[121] Significant changes in the family configuration, such as accession of a new member, are normally a stressful occasion for family members. Perinatal complication or loss is an even more stressful event for which the family has little or no preparation. The result of this type of crisis may be personal growth, maintaining the status quo, regression, or mental illness.[24,122] Often, outcome depends on a combination of coping skills and the type of help received during the crisis.

Decreasing the element of surprise through preparation for the situation to be encountered may modulate the effect of the event. Anticipatory grief [84,108,135] functions to both prepare and protect the individual from the pain of impending loss. Prenatal diagnostic procedures, such as ultrasonography,[102] amniocentesis, and fetoscopy can detect a variety of severe or lethal birth defects. When there is forewarning that the pregnancy/fetus or the newborn is not healthy, parents may begin a process of anticipatory grief and psychologically prepare for the loss of their baby while at the same time hoping for the child's survival.[10,11]

Parental withdrawal from the relationship established during pregnancy may accompany the intense emotions of anticipatory grief. Detachment protects and defends the parent from further painful feelings associated with the investment of self in a doomed relationship. If anticipatory grief proceeds, the parent may detach to the point of being unable to reattach to the infant if he or she survives. In this situation, the infant survives but the relationship with the parents may be significantly impaired. Maintaining even a remote hope that the fetus or newborn will survive protects the parents from the full experience of grief and total detachment from the baby. Accordingly, antenatal counseling suggesting "the baby will not survive delivery" or "will live only a few minutes," may be detrimental to adjusting to a fairly fluid situation at the time of birth (i.e., a lengthier survival for which some attachment could be anticipated as valuable).

The degree of parental anticipatory grief is correlated with positive feelings about the pregnancy and the mode of delivery but generally not with the severity of the infant's illness. The greater the parental investment and the higher the expectations for the pregnancy, the more anticipatory grief can be expected should perinatal complication ensue. The relative severity of the medical problem itself, however, is not associated with the degree of anticipatory grief.

PERINATAL SITUATIONS IN WHICH GRIEF IS EXPECTED

Loss is a fact of life, not just of death. Every stage of development requires a loss of the privileges of the preceding stage and movement into the unknown of the next stage. Any life event involving change or loss is accompanied by grief work, including moving, divorce, separation, death of a spouse or family member, injury or illness, retirement, job change, menopause, and even success.[121] The concept of loss is even applicable to the physiologic and psychologic events of normal pregnancy and birth. Certainly, when pregnancy fails to produce a live, healthy infant, a perinatal loss situation exists (Box 30-1). These perinatal losses, including stillbirth, loss of the perfect child, and neonatal death, are discussed in detail in this chapter.

Stillbirth

Stillbirth is the demise of a viable fetus that occurs after fetal movement when the parents have often thought of the fetus as having personality and individuality. Because stillbirth occurs later in pregnancy than most pregnancy terminations, there are increased parental expectations about the baby and the birth process. Selective pregnancy termination for genetic indications is often performed in the second trimester of pregnancy and involves the death of a wanted child. Although parents understand the validity of the reason for terminating the pregnancy, sadness, guilt, and self-doubt often accompany the decision to terminate.[81] The anxieties related to termination procedures, which may include labor and birth, and the feelings of helplessness, isolation, and depression should be acknowledged and handled as in a stillbirth.

Fetal demise in utero happens either prenatally or in the intrapartum period. For 50% of stillbirths, death is sudden, without warning, and results from unexplainable causes. The majority of women whose fetus dies in utero spontaneously begin labor within 2 weeks of fetal demise. Carrying the dead fetus while waiting for spontaneous labor or induction is sad and difficult for the woman and her entire family. Feelings such as helplessness, disbelief, guilt, and powerlessness characterize this period. There often is an almost uncontrollable urge to flee and escape the unpleasant situation.

For the family that experiences intrapartum demise, the joyous expectations of labor and birth suddenly change to fear, anxiety, and dread that the "worst" could have possibly happened to them. The suddenness of fetal demise in labor and birth affects both parents and professionals with feelings of shock, denial, and anxiety. Whether the fetal loss is early or late, the woman and her family maintain hope by believing that the professional has made a mistake and that the fetus is still alive.[133] The onset (or continuation) of labor is approached with both hope and dread: hope that the infant may be born alive and dread that the infant's death will soon be a stark reality.

The discomfort of labor and birth is particularly difficult for the woman whose fetus has died because her work will not be rewarded with a healthy infant. However, overly solicitous use of drugs at birth is not recommended because they relegate the experience to unreality and give it a dreamlike quality.[172] Keeping parents together through this crisis is important for mutual support and sharing of the birth.[131] The deafening silence of a stillbirth forces the reality of the infant's death on both the parents and the professionals present at birth.[131]

In the past, at the birth of a stillborn, the mother was heavily sedated or anesthetized and the neonate was hidden and whisked away immediately. These women were often left with fears and fantasies: "Was the baby normal?" "What was the baby's sex?" "What did the baby look like?" Seeing, touching, and holding the infant, when culturally appropriate,

---

BOX 30-1	PERINATAL SITUATIONS IN WHICH GRIEF REACTION IS EXPECTED

1. Pregnancy
2. Birth
   A. Normal
   B. Cesarean delivery
   C. Forceps
   D. Episiotomy
   E. Medicated
   F. Prolonged or short labor
   G. Place of birth
3. Postpartum (see Chapter 29)
   A. "Postpartum blues"
   B. Depression
   C. Psychosis
4. Abortion
   A. Spontaneous[119,148]
   B. Therapeutic[132]
   C. Elective[81]
   D. Selective
   E. Selective reduction (for multiple gestation)[90,113,114]
5. Stillbirth
6. Loss of the perfect child
   A. Premature
   B. Deformed baby or baby with anomaly[50]
   C. Sick newborn[107]
   D. "Wrong" sex
7. Neonatal death
8. Relinquishment

can promote completion of the attachment cycle, confirm the reality of the stillbirth for both parents, and enable grief to begin.[16,133,172]

Because it can be easier to grieve the reality of a situation than a mystical and dreamlike fantasy, contact with the stillborn enables parents to grieve the infant's reality rather than endure their most frightening fantasies about the baby.

After confirming the reality of the infant's death, a search for the cause, characterized by the universal question "Why did the baby die?" begins. Either or both parents may blame themselves or feel guilty about real or imagined acts of omission or commission. An autopsy may determine the cause of death, but most often the cause is unknown, even after an autopsy. However, an autopsy may be useful in reducing parental guilt and uncertainty about future pregnancies, as well as in aiding the recovery from the loss.[97,172] The "empty tragedy" of stillbirth forces the mother to deal with both the inner loss of the fetus and the outer loss of the expected newborn. Fathers who experience stillbirth as a "waste of life," are especially appreciative of the tokens of remembrance from the baby, and need help in expressing their grief.[131]

Loss of the Perfect Child

Although pregnancy ends in the birth of a live newborn, the pregnancy outcome may not be what the parents had anticipated. Birth of an infant who does not meet parental expectations represents the realization of the parents' worst fears: a damaged child. Newborns who are preterm, have an anomaly, are sick, or those with the "wrong" gender or who ultimately die represent the loss of the imagined or hoped-for perfect child.

After the birth of such an infant, parental reactions include grief and mourning for the loss of the loved object (the perfect child), while adapting to the reality and investing love in the defective baby.[52,143] This reaction is analogous to parental mourning at the death of a child.[143] However, unlike the finality of death, birth of a living, but perceivably defective baby entails a persistent, constant reminder of the feelings of loss and grief because of parental investment of time, attention, and care for either a short time (preterm or sick newborn) or a lifetime (physically or mentally impaired child).[124,143]

The psychic work involved in coping with the reality of the imperfect child and the inner feelings of loss is slow and emotionally painful.[50,124] The process is gradual and proceeds at an individual pace that cannot be hurried but can be facilitated and supported. Detachment from and mourning the loss of their fantasized child is necessary before parents are able to attach to the actual child.

Birth of an imperfect infant represents multiple losses for parents. A primary narcissistic injury, a threat to the woman's self-concept as a woman and mother and the father's self-concept as a man and a father, all occur when a less-than-perfect infant is born.[34,35,50,78] Because the child is an extension of both parents, a less-than-perfect (i.e., deformed) child is equated with the perceived less-than-perfect part of the parental self. In the mind of the parent, the imagined inadequate self has failed and caused the birth of the damaged baby.[78]

Prematurity

Every woman expects to deliver a normal, healthy infant at term. Therefore, the onset of premature labor is both physiologically and psychologically unexpected. Premature birth is a crisis and an emergency situation characterized by an increased concern for the survival of the newborn and often the mother. Premature labor and birth are accompanied by feelings of helplessness, isolation, failure, guilt, emptiness, and lack of control.[78,143] The negative and dangerous atmosphere surrounding the premature birth experience may influence the relationship with the premature infant, who also may be perceived as dangerous and negative.

Normal adaptations to pregnancy are abruptly terminated by the birth of a premature infant.[78] Prenatal fantasies about the infant and the new roles of mother and father are interrupted by a premature birth. This forces parents who are "not ready to not be pregnant" to grieve the loss of a term infant and imposes premature parenting on individuals not yet ready for the experience.

As discussed in Chapter 29, anticipatory grief is one of the normal psychologic tasks accompanying premature birth. Anticipatory grief may be decreased by early contact between parents and neonate and, conversely, increased by separation of parents from preterm newborn.[78] Prolonging anticipatory grief with failure to progress through the other tasks results in altered relationships with the parents if the preterm infant survives.

Infants with a Birth Anomaly or Syndrome

In approximately 2 of every 100 births,[78] an infant is born with a congenital anomaly. Because society values physical beauty, intelligence, and success, the birth of a physically or mentally impaired baby is seen as a catastrophe in our culture.[170]

Recent medical advances now make it possible to identify potential fetal problems in utero. As parents receive the information antenatally, they begin the process of anticipatory grief.[11] They experience feelings of shock, anger, guilt, and hope. At the birth of the baby, there usually is the confirmation of the anomaly, and parents must deal with the reality of the situation. Whether anticipated or not, however, the birth of a baby with a congenital anomaly is accompanied by ambivalent feelings for all concerned (parents, relatives, friends, and professionals). The first reactions to the reality of the situation are feelings of disbelief and shock. Feelings of shame, revulsion, and embarrassment at creating a seemingly damaged and potentially devalued child are common.[139] Guilt, self-blame, and a search for a cause or reasons for the tragedy are intermixed with feelings of anger.

The severity of loss and feelings of disappointment heavily burden the parents, a burden they may believe that no one else has experienced.[78] Their loneliness and isolation may be intensified by their self-imposed withdrawal from others. Unlike the birth of a healthy infant, the birth of a sick baby or one with an anomaly is not celebrated with announcements, visits, and gifts from friends and family. The negative responses of society's representatives (family, friends, acquaintances, and professionals) may increase the parents' negative feelings for an impaired child.[170]

The extent of the infant's anomaly cannot be used as a criterion for the degree of parental grief reaction, although a gross, visible anomaly may elicit more emotional reaction than a hidden or minor one.[78] A seemingly "minor" anomaly as defined by a health care professional may represent a severe impairment to individual parents. The professional, who has had more contact with infants with a wide range of anomalies, views the individual infant's anomaly in a different context than that typical for the parents, who may have limited or no experience with such an affected child or adult. The professional also views the infant's anomaly from a less personal, more objective, and less narcissistic position than the new parents.

When the newborn is sick, the degree of mourning and parental feelings of grief and loss are not equated with the severity of the neonate's illness.[10,141] Even seemingly minor illnesses such as jaundice or respiratory difficulty requiring phototherapy or minimal oxygen supplementation are associated with parental concern for survival and feelings of grief and loss.[107] These feelings often are not acknowledged by the parents or professional care providers because of the nonserious medical nature of the condition. In the mind of the care provider, self-limiting and treatable conditions are compared with more serious and often fatal neonatal illnesses. The care provider feels relieved about the minor nature of the neonate's condition and conveys this to the parents: "This is an easy condition to remedy. You don't have anything to worry about. The baby will go home in a few days."

Thus, only the medical aspects of the newborn's illness are dealt with, whereas parental feelings remain unspoken and unresolved.[21] In an altruistic attempt to reassure and comfort the family about the newborn's complete recovery, the professional unwittingly may discount the parents' real feelings. If the care provider is not concerned, parents may feel that they, too, should not be concerned and thus distrust and discount their own feelings.

Neonatal Deaths

The reactions accompanying neonatal illnesses are similar to the grief reactions experienced by parents whose infant dies.[10,165] Failure to acknowledge (even minor) neonatal illness as a loss situation and to work through the associated grief prevents parents from detaching from the image of the perfect child and taking on the sick newborn as a person to love. This may result in an aberrant parent–infant attachment. The liveborn infant who is critically ill or has a severe anomaly will be the focus of a "painful time of waiting"[10] for the family. They must deal with the uncertainty of whether their child will live and be healthy, live and continue to need extensive medical or special care, or die.

More deaths occur in the first 24 hours after birth than in any other period of life. Yet death of a newborn is not the expected outcome of pregnancy. The majority of neonatal losses are caused by congenital anomalies incompatible with life (20%)

and prematurity (17%).[62] Regardless of the cause of death, even infants who live only a short time are mourned by their parents.[73] Prenatal attachment and investment of love in the newborn result in a classic grief reaction at the newborn's death.

Even a short period of life between birth and death gives parents an opportunity to know and take care of their infant.[145] Completion of the attachment process enables parents to psychically begin the next process of detachment. Attachment to the baby's reality encourages detachment from that reality rather than from the parents' most dreaded fears and fantasies about their infant. Parental contact with the child before death enables them to share life for a brief time.

In the case of multiple births, when one or more infants die and the others live, parents simultaneously grieve the loss of the deceased infant or infants while attaching to the survivors.[83,113,114,149,158] In many situations of multiple births, the surviving infant or infants are in an intensive care nursery. The contradictory feelings of love and attachment and grief and detachment, as well as the anxiety associated with the care and well-being of the surviving infant, are emotionally draining for new parents. The process of grief may slow the parents' ability to become intimately involved with their surviving infant(s).[114,115,158,167] They may have ambivalent feelings toward the infant(s) who survives or toward the infant(s) who dies. With the loss of one infant of a multiple birth, there is less support for the grieving parents because the frequent response is that they should be thankful for the survival of one (or more) of their infants. Research shows that the death of a twin (or higher-order multiple) is as great a loss for a mother as the death of a singleton.[113,114,149] Helpful interventions include (1) acknowledging the uniqueness of every baby; (2) viewing, holding, and photographing the babies together—living and dead; (3) private time with each deceased infant; (4) similar mementos and keepsakes from each infant, deceased and living, given to the parents; and (5) reassurance about the health of their surviving child.[113-115,158]

Generally, death of a newborn occurs despite everything done to prevent it. This provides parents with some measure of comfort in knowing that they did everything possible. Yet when the neonate is so severely ill or deformed that a decision about initiating or continuing life support is necessary, the parents have an extra burden. The situation may involve conflicts between physicians, nurses, and family wishes, causing significant personal anguish. Professionals who convey information sensitively, compassionately, and honestly facilitate care transitions toward comfort/palliative care. Such a situation is tenderly conveyed in the article entitled: "Four wishes for Aubrey."[26] Aubrey's parents are asked what they would like to do with their little boy to make lasting memories. Without hesitation, Aubrey's mother states the following wishes for her 5-month-old terminally ill son:

1. Allow more than three visitors in his room at one time.
2. Hold Aubrey to her chest and lie down with him; the mother wanted a bed large enough (in his private room) for her and her son to lie down together (Figure 30-1)
3. The ability to take Aubrey outside so that he can feel the sun and a breeze

All of Aubrey's mother's wishes were made possible by caring, compassionate professionals who actually suggested and accommodated the fourth wish: arranging for special photography of the family with Aubrey, such as *Now I Lay Me Down to Sleep.*[106] Aubrey's family has participated in local and national education for health care providers learning about palliative care and in numerous teaching forums with other parents.[26] The authors enumerate the lessons learned from and with this family: (1) the importance of asking each individual family what is important to them, (2) the caution to never presume that we know what any family needs or wishes, (3) the cruelty of presuming and minimizing

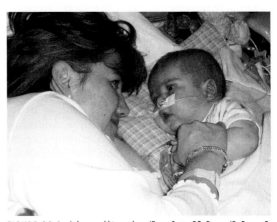

FIGURE 30-1   Aubrey and his mother. (From Carter BS, Brown JB, Brown S, Meyer EC: Four wishes for Aubrey, *J Perinatol* 32(1):10-14, 2012.)

every family's uniqueness, power, and right to their own experience.[26] The article ends with the lesson that fulfilling the family's wishes was profoundly moving and gratifying for the health care providers who were creative, engaged, and caring for Aubrey and his family.

As a consequence of the federal Baby Doe regulations, most hospitals now have ethics committees that address a variety of the medical, legal, and ethical controversies (see Chapter 32). The decision-making process may be collaborative, parent initiated, directive, or nondirective.[113] Regardless of who makes this decision, it is primarily the parents who will live with its ramifications, including feelings of grief, an ongoing void in their lives, and a desire to live better lives to honor their infant.[4] When parents are involved in the decision-making process, they wonder if theirs was the right decision regardless of what it was. Whether the baby lives or dies, they wonder how a different decision would have changed their lives.

STAGES OF GRIEF

The experience of grief is a staged process that occurs over time. To detach both externally and internally from the lost loved object, emotional investment is withdrawn so that it may be invested in new love relationships.[84] Each stage of grief represents a psychologic defense mechanism used to help the individual adapt slowly to the crisis. This slow adaptation is purposeful because it prevents the individual psyche from being overwhelmed by the pain and anguish of loss.[112]

Although the stage of grief is recognizable, the process of grief is dynamic and fluid rather than static and rigid. Parents, families, and professionals progress cyclically through the stages of grief rather than in an orderly progression from beginning to end. However, each person experiences the process of grief uniquely and at an individual pace. Knowledge of each stage is necessary to assess where an individual family member, the family as a unit, and the staff are in their grieving process. This information is then used to support individuals when they are in their particular stage of grief. Rather than attempting to maneuver grieving individuals from stage to stage, contributing to their defense, or stripping individuals of their defenses, knowledgeable professionals are prepared to understand and honor

the individual's grieving process. Regardless of the type of perinatal loss, the experience of that loss through staged grief work closely parallels the grief stages described by Elisabeth Kübler-Ross.[79]

The feelings of disbelief and rejection of the news are reflected in the responses "No! This couldn't happen to me!" "It isn't true! They've made a mistake!" This immediate response protects the individual from the shocking reality of loss by postponing the full effect of reality until the psyche can handle it.[133] By holding on to the fantasy of a positive outcome (e.g., the loss of the heartbeat is only temporary or the dead infant belongs to someone else), facing the awful truth and the grief associated with it is delayed, at least temporarily.[133]

The initial stage of grief is characterized by overwhelming feelings of being stunned and surprised. This often is seen as emotional numbness, flat affect, or immobility.[172] Emotional detachment often is expressed as an inability to cope or respond with activities of daily living, an inability to remember what others have said, and a tendency to repeat the same question.[40,45,61] For the tragedy to be handled in manageable pieces without overwhelming the individual, the mind may acknowledge the event only intellectually and there is a corresponding lack of emotional reaction,[172] or the event may be compartmentalized so that only a part of the situation rather than the whole becomes the focal point of attention.

Anger is the result of a gradually developing awareness of the situation's reality. As the significance of their perinatal loss begins to dawn on them, parents (and significant others) experience the diffuse emotions of anxiety and anger.[78] With the full effect of their loss comes more focused feelings of bitterness, resentment, blame, rage, and envy of those with normal pregnancy outcomes.[79]

Social prohibitions against the expression of anger, especially for women, encourage this powerful emotion to be turned inward toward the self. Anger directed inward results in depression and a deepening sense of guilt. "Why?" and "What did I do wrong or not do right to have caused this to happen?" are the hallmarks of the self-examination and self-blame that accompany perinatal loss.[78,172] Answers often are irrational and have no cause-and-effect relationship with the reality of the circumstances. Irrational, feared causes include sexual intercourse (common worry of both men and women), career (of the mother) outside the home, superstitions, dietary habits, or lifting heavy objects.[172] Ideas of punishment (for past wrongs, for negative or ambivalent feelings, or for an unwanted pregnancy)[12] often are thought to be the reason for the failed outcome. The search for a reason to answer the question "Why me?" requires correct information to dispel unrealistic fantasies of causation. However, the question does not require a literal answer (often no concrete answer exists) but is merely a wish for a change in the situation.[12]

Anger directed outward is usually expressed as overt hostility to those in the immediate environment (family, children, care providers, and infant)[172] or toward God.[112] Fathers exhibit more anger than mothers.[56] Blame and anger may be destructive forces in the relationships among family members and prevent these relationships from being a source of comfort and support. Venting of angry feelings toward professional care providers protects these family relationships for more positive interactions. Anger moves the grieving process along, but persistence of anger may prevent grief work from progressing to subsequent stages.

Bargaining may occur concomitantly with denial and shock as an attempt to prevent or at least delay the loss. Bargaining usually occurs with whoever the parents (family or staff) believe the Supreme Being is. The "Yes, but" of this stage is a form of "conditional acceptance" while still attempting to make the reality other than what it is.[12,79] With an infant who has a congenital anomaly, bargaining may take the form of shopping for a physician or searching for the magic cure.[170]

The onset of depression and withdrawal marks the stage of a greater level of acceptance of the tragedy. With the true realization of the effect of the loss, the individual acknowledges that indeed there is a reason to be sad. The predominant feelings of this stage are overwhelming sorrow and sadness[97] evidenced by tearfulness, crying, and weeping.[133] Feelings of helplessness, worthlessness, and powerlessness contribute to the sense that life is empty and futile. Withdrawal may be evidenced by requests to be left alone, by decreased or complete cessation of visits to the infant, and by silence.[79] The degree of withdrawal may be indicative of the depth of depression and the extent to which there is guilt and self-blame.[133]

Acceptance is the resolution stage of the grief process that is heralded by resumption of usual daily activities and a noticeable decrease in preoccupation with the image of the lost infant.[84] This stage usually is not witnessed by perinatal professionals.

The acceptance stage is characterized by emotional detachment of life's meaning from the lost relationship and reestablishing it independent of the lost object.[79,92] The lost relationship is seen in a new light—as giving meaning to the present.[92] The aggrieved person relinquishes that part of him or herself that was defined in the lost relationship and establishes a new identity that is emotionally free to attach in another relationship.

For the family of an anomalied child, acceptance is not an all-or-nothing proposition but, rather, a daily adaptation and coping with the child and the defect.[138] For the family, periods of frustration and sorrow alternate with periods of delight and enjoyment of the child. Because of the chronic sorrow experienced throughout the life of an anomalied child, the final stage of resolution of the family's grief is possible only after the child's death.[108,170]

The acceptance stage represents the ability to remember both the joys and sorrows of the lost relationship without undue discomfort.[48] With gradual integration of the loss, there are progressively fewer attacks of acute, all-consuming pain.[92] When recalling the lost infant, there are fewer feelings of devastation and more a feeling of sadness. The ability to "celebrate the loss" also identifies grief resolution. Celebration of the loss does not mean recall without sadness and sorrow but with an ability to find some meaning, some good, and some positive aspects in the situation (e.g., "At least we had our child for a time, even though it was a short time").

SYMPTOMS OF GRIEF

Although each person copes with grief in individual ways, there are expected reactions to loss situations. Knowledge of the differences and commonalities of the grief experience enables care providers to understand their own reactions, as well as to share their thoughts and feelings with the grieving family. The professional care provider must learn to "hear" what the family says about how and where each member is in the process of grief resolution. Often the "message" is not a direct reference to the loss or one's feelings but, rather, nonverbal communication. The professional must learn to recognize that individuals often communicate more by what they do and what they omit than by what they say.

The signs and symptoms of acute grief have been well described and include both somatic and behavioral manifestations of the emotional experience of the loss (Box 30-2).[111] The behavior of the bereaved is characterized as ambivalent.[92] In certain perinatal situations, parents simultaneously hope that the infant will live and wish for the infant to die; they want to love and care for the infant and at the same time wish to reject him or her.[78] These feelings are frightening and socially unacceptable and therefore often remain unspoken.

Often the intensity of grief is greater when the relationship with and feelings about the lost person are ambivalent.[76,92] Even with the most positive of pregnancy outcomes, taking a newborn into the family results in ambivalent feelings for all family members. The degree of disruption that a perinatal loss brings to the family is equated with the severity of grief, especially because reproduction and a healthy perinatal outcome are highly valued in our society.[92]

MALE–FEMALE DIFFERENCES

Although members of both genders have the same grief reactions, women express more symptoms (crying, sadness, anger, guilt, and use of medications)[43,64,65,94,126] than men. This difference in symptomatology does not represent a different experience of grief but merely a different expression of it. Understanding these differences and the reasons for them is crucial for care providers working with parents at the time of perinatal loss. Explaining these differences to parents is also crucial so that diverse grief responses do not become divisive in the relationship.[43,126]

The father's degree of investment in the pregnancy, impending parenthood, and the circumstances of birth all affect his feelings of loss. Because the father's body does not directly experience the changes of pregnancy, the pregnancy initially may be

---

BOX 30-2	CRITICAL FINDINGS
	SIGNS AND SYMPTOMS OF GRIEF

1. Somatic (physiologic)
   a. Gastrointestinal system
      Anorexia and weight loss
      Overeating
      Nausea or vomiting
      Abdominal pains or feelings of emptiness
      Diarrhea or constipation
   b. Respiratory system
      Sighing respirations
      Choking or coughing
      Shortness of breath
      Hyperventilation
   c. Cardiovascular system
      Cardiac palpitations or "fluttering" in chest
      "Heavy" feeling in chest
   d. Neuromuscular system
      Headaches
      Vertigo
      Syncope
      Brissaud's disease (tics)
      Muscular weakness or loss of strength

2. Behavioral (psychologic)
   a. Feelings of:
      Guilt
      Sadness
      Anger and hostility
      Emptiness and apathy
      Helplessness
      Pain, desperation, and pessimism
      Shame
      Loneliness
   b. Preoccupation with image of the lost infant
      Daydreams and fantasies
      Nightmares
      Longing
   c. Disturbed interpersonal relationships
      Increased irritability and restlessness
      Decreased sexual interest and drive
      Withdrawal
   d. Crying
   e. Inability to return to normal activities
      Fatigue and exhaustion or aimless overactivity
      Insomnia or oversleeping
      Short attention span
      Slow speech, movement, and thought process
      Loss of concentration and motivation

Data from Colgrove M: *How to survive the loss of a love,* New York, 1976, Lion Publishing; Lindemann E: Symptomatology and management of acute grief, *Am J Psychiatry* 101:144, 1944; Marris P: *Loss and change,* New York, 1974, Pantheon Books.

less of a reality to him than to the pregnant woman. This lag in the physiologic reality contributes to a lag in the psychologic investment of the father in the baby. The father's lag in psychologic investment often contributes to incongruent grieving, a difference in mother's and father's grief reactions. Fathers often comment that the infant became real when he felt the fetus move in the mother or at the first sight of the new infant. Fathers who form an early attachment to the child feel sadness, disappointment, and often anger at being denied the expected son or daughter.[56,72,94,95,131] Conversely, fathers who have been normally ambivalent or overtly negative about the pregnancy may feel guilt and responsibility for the failed outcome.

Participation of the father in the events of labor and birth also influences his attachment and ultimately his feelings of loss. Exclusion decreases his involvement in these life-crisis events, whereas inclusion has many advantages for the mother, infant, and self (see Chapter 29). If the infant is ill, the father may initially have more and closer contact than the mother.[10] In the birth place, the father may see, touch, or hold the infant before the mother does. The father observes the initial resuscitation and stabilization and may accompany the infant to the nursery and on transport to a regional center. Often the father receives the first information and support about the infant's condition and returns to the hospitalized mother with the news. This early, prolonged contact coupled with the father's increased responsibility often contributes to the development of a closer and earlier bond between father and infant than between mother and infant. The initial lag in prenatal investment may be offset after birth by concentrated contact between the father and the baby, so that a loss is highly significant to the father.

Societal expectations about masculinity and femininity markedly influence the expression of grief. Society's message to men starts early in life: "Big boys don't cry" and "Don't cry, you'll be a sissy" (i.e., girl). The preferred male image in our society is the autonomous, independent achiever who is always strong and in control, even in the face of disaster.[56,57] In keeping with this image, the father may feel that he must make all the decisions and have all information filtered through him to protect the mother. However, this altruistic gesture prevents full disclosure to and involvement of the mother. Assuming the role of strong protector also involves a heavy price for the father in suppression of his own feelings and delay of his own grief work.[43,95,126] The role of "tower of strength" often engenders feelings of resentment from the mother. Although he attempts to live up to his (and society's) expectations of himself, the woman views his apparent lack of feelings and emotions, especially crying, as "He doesn't care." A recent study showed that distress experienced by the mother but not by her partner resulted in longer-term marital dissatisfaction for the mother.

Many men have difficulty dealing with irrational behaviors, as well as with the normal ambiguity and conflict of life. This difficulty makes the emotional response of grief and its accompanying ambivalent feelings and conflicts produce discomfort and anxiety in many men. The expression of appropriate human emotions becomes threatening and makes them feel vulnerable. To decrease the anxiety associated with grief and its expression, men often deal with feelings by denying them, increasing their workload, grieving internally, or withdrawing from the situation and refusing to discuss it.[94,126]

The father's attitude and ability to communicate about the loss may help or impede the mother's grief work.[135] Lack of communication between a couple may contribute to intense mourning, psychiatric disturbances, and severe family disruption.[73,126,157] Synchrony of grieving between the mother and the father is important in an ultimate healthy resolution for the family.[29,126] If the father denies and suppresses his own feelings of loss and grief, he may react to the normal signs and symptoms of grief in his partner as if they were abnormal. Often the father can resolve his grief faster than the mother, and he may become impatient with her continual "dwelling" on the loss. Sometimes fearing the woman's prolonged grief, the man decides to "spare her" from his feelings and does not discuss them with her. Instead of being comforting as intended, failure to share grief leads to isolation and alienation within the relationship.[78,126]

In some situations, the man may experience intense emotions several months after the death, not unlike those his partner experienced at the time of the crisis. Because these intense emotions occur so long after the crisis, he may not even associate them with the death.[40,78] A recent study found that at 30 months after the death of a baby, fathers were more distressed than the mothers, who were the more distressed initially after the death.[157]

TIMING OF GRIEF RESOLUTION

Parents

Emotional recovery from the pain of perinatal loss occurs with time. There is no complete agreement on the length of time necessary for the individual to resolve grief. Indeed, a specific timetable for mourning may be impossible to establish.[12] However, some general time frames are available for the duration of a normal grief reaction.

Acute grief reactions are the most intense during the first 4 to 6 weeks after the loss,[84,92,112] with some improvement noted 6 to 10 weeks later. Normal or uncomplicated grief reactions may be expected to last from 6 months to 1[9,48,76,78,112] or 2 years.[76,92] Indeed, significant losses of a spouse or child may never be completely resolved[36,129,159]: "I'll never get over it."

One parameter for differentiating normal from pathologic grief has been the length of time for grief to be resolved. Grief work may still be categorized as normal/uncomplicated even if it lasts longer than a year, especially if the person is working through unresolved grief from the past. Grief work is normally energy draining. Dealing with more than one grief or loss situation compounds the intensity of mourning and may prolong the grief reaction. Because perinatal loss represents more than the loss of the newborn (loss of the perfect child, loss of plans for the future, and loss of self-esteem), feelings of sadness and depression may still be evident for a year or longer.[78,94,157,172] A recent study of white, Hispanic, and black parents (176 mothers and 73 fathers) examined their health and functioning at 1, 3, 6, and 13 months after the death of their infants. At 13 months after the death, one-third of the responding parents had clinical depression and post-traumatic stress disorder (PTSD).[171] At every time period, more Hispanic and black mothers had PTSD symptoms and more moderate/severe depression at 6 months. In the first 13 months, 98 hospitalizations for anxiety, depression, panic attacks, chest pain, and cardiac problems were reported and 29% were stress-related.[171] Chronic illnesses (n = 132) including cancer, angina, hypertension, mental illness, arthritis, and asthma were diagnosed in the surviving parents 13 months after their infant's death.

Sorrow and grief may even last a lifetime. For families of defective children, "chronic sorrow"[40,63,108,124,143] is experienced as long as the child lives. These parents live with the constant reminder of what is not and what the child will never be and can never do. The grief of death is final—parents do the work and go on; chronic sorrow is grieving on a daily basis. Expecting the parents to adjust to or accept their child's defect without any elements of lingering sadness is unrealistic. Although hampered by small sample sizes, research on the gender differences in chronic sorrow show more chronic sorrow in mothers than in fathers.[63,91] Chronic sorrow is a justifiable reaction to the daily stresses and coping necessary when a child is living with a birth defect or major impairment. The final stage of grief resolution is possible only with the finality of the death of the child.

Even when grief has been resolved, anniversary grief reactions are normal.[162] Feelings of sadness, crying, and normal grieving behaviors may be reactivated at certain times. These anniversary reactions may not be limited to the infant's date of death but also may be felt on the expected date of delivery, on the actual birthday, or on seeing an infant of the same age and gender as the lost infant. Holidays may also reactivate grieving behaviors, especially those that bring together family and friends and recall memories of joy and happiness.

Staff

Those sharing a crisis (complication, illness, or death) often become closely attached, so that the loss is felt not only by the family but also by the professional care providers.[*] Repeatedly dealing with death and deformity increases the professional's exposure to personal feelings of grief and loss. This may be perceived either as a threat or a personal opportunity for growth.[46]

The critical variable in the ability to face or assist others in handling loss is the manner in which the care providers have been able to resolve their own personal losses. Unless the care providers can cope with personal feelings of loss and grief, they may not be able to give of the "self" to others. Care given without genuine involvement and responsiveness to the family's feelings does not facilitate and may actually impede the mourning process. Professionals who can deal honestly with their own feelings will be able to help others cope with theirs.[28,114]

---

*References 28, 41, 114, 118, 125, 126, 129.

Helping parents deal with their grief may be difficult for professionals because of their attitudes and feelings about perinatal loss. For professionals trained to preserve life, loss of the best pregnancy outcome or death itself represents both a personal and professional failure.[78] When success is equated with life, the failure of death (or loss) is associated with feelings of guilt, anger, depression, and hostility.[172] Just when professionals are expected to be supportive and therapeutic, they may be overwhelmed with their own feelings. A recent qualitative study of nurses' reactions to being present at a perinatal loss found recurring themes: (1) getting through the shift, (2) symptoms of pain and loss, (3) frustrations with inadequate care, (4) showing genuine care, (5) recovering from traumatic experience, and (6) never forgetting.[118] Professionally, care providers may feel helpless when all efforts inevitably result in no change in the outcome.

The feelings and stages of grief experienced by the family are the same ones felt by the staff who are attached to the parents and their newborn. Many professionals working in perinatal care are of childbearing age, so identifying with the parents and their plight is relatively easy. Because the sick, anomalied, or even dying or deceased infant could easily be that of the staff, they share with the parents the special stress of the loss of a child. The care provider often experiences the same fantasies of blame as the parents: "What did I do (or not do) to cause this?"

Repetitive contact with loss situations and death exposes the staff to recurring feelings of frustration, guilt, self-doubt, depression, anger, classic grief reactions, helplessness, sadness, hopelessness, loneliness, PTSD, and covert relief.[41,96,100] Such uncomfortable feelings often lead to behaviors of avoidance and withdrawal as a means of self-protection; this has been called "compassion fatigue."[28,114,129] Adequate medical care may be given, but psychologic care of the family may be neglected.[87] The involved primary care providers may decrease their attachment to both parents and infant when an unfavorable outcome is inevitable. Withdrawing emotional support and involvement may spare the professional but only adds to parental feelings of isolation, inadequacy, and worthlessness. Professionals who have risked family attachment and shared grief work may be more cautious in future involvements to protect themselves from the pain of loss.

Asynchrony and individual differences in handling grief reactions also may cause problems among the professional staff. Constant exposure to perinatal loss may desensitize some individuals until they are blasé or even callous about the crisis, whereas the grief reactions of others parallel the family's reaction. Some staff members may have reached the stage of acceptance, whereas others who cannot let the infant go persist in the idea of a magical cure, a characteristic of denial. The rationale of prolonging the child's life may in reality be prolonging death, and inevitably one needs to accept death's finality.

Staff members cannot offer support to families experiencing loss unless they receive support in dealing with their own grief reactions.[28,46,49,96] Those who receive support learn about their feelings and how to handle them and so have no need to displace their pain to others. The three most effective ways that neonatal intensive care unit (NICU) nurses have identified to manage their stress after a neonate's death are (1) discussing with co-workers, (2) supporting and comforting the grieving family, and (3) talking with their own families.[41] Various formats are available for meeting staff needs, such as mutual support of colleagues or group sessions involving peer counseling on a long- or short-term basis.[28,41,49,78,125] Group meetings provide a vehicle for support and for sharing information and feelings among staff members.[28,41,49,78,125] Facilitated by an objective person with expertise in group process and the concepts of grief, such "debriefing" meetings have the goal of helping the staff deal with their reactions so they will be better equipped to help the parents.[38,96] Group sessions also serve to decrease stress, increase job satisfaction, and ultimately help prevent burnout and PTSD.[100] Staff members are encouraged to retain their humanity when an environment is created in which emotions are valued and their healthy expression facilitated, both at the time of loss and in its resolution.[38,69,96,125]

Sharing grief work with a family gives the care provider a chance for personal growth, to review past personal losses, and to evaluate the adequacy of their resolution. Helping others with loss or grief provides the professional with the opportunity to contemplate present and future losses, including one's own mortality. By working with those who have suffered a significant loss or death, a health care provider may gain a deeper perspective about life.[68]

INTERVENTIONS

Those in a crisis feel an openness to help and assistance from others, so that they emerge either stronger or weaker, depending on the help they receive.[22,122] This increased openness also makes those in a crisis more vulnerable to the reactions of others—to their facial expressions, tone of voice, and choice of words. Helpful professional interventions provide psychologic assistance during a highly vulnerable period of personal development. The goals of intervention are to maintain the precrisis level of functioning and to improve coping and problem-solving skills beyond the precrisis level (i.e., to facilitate personal growth). Effective intervention is characterized by helping grief work get started, by supporting those who are grieving adaptively, and by intervening with individuals who display maladaptive reactions.[29,44]

For professionals, understanding parental perspectives of the experience of death of a newborn should enable provision of more sensitive and evidence-based care for grieving families. The results of two research studies provide some insight into what is helpful and what is not helpful for grieving families. The first study was a systematic review of 61 studies and more than 6000 parents who suffered neonatal death.[53] This study found that parents valued emotional support, grief education, and attention to mother/baby. Nonhelpful and distressing behaviors from health care providers included avoidance, thoughtlessness, insensitivity, and poor staff communication.[53] Another study conducted semistructured interviews with mothers/fathers (n = 19) a mean of 1.9 years after death of their infant. This exploratory study found a low level of grief, effective coping, and factors important to parents in end-of-life care for their infant.[19] Review of the data from this study in Table 30-1 instructs health care professionals in helpful and nonhelpful interventions during the stressful experience of a dying infant.[25] Because 76% of the dying infants were in the NICU or pediatric intensive care unit (PICU) and 42% of the families had hospice/palliative care team involvement,[19] perhaps the low level of grief and the positive adaptation by this small group of parents were because of the sensitive, helpful interventions of their health care providers. A more recent French survey of parental experiences (after the death of their newborns) found that half of the parents did not think that their feelings and decisions were respected.[47] Parent responders also felt that parental autonomy (in palliative care situations) was difficult for professional caregivers to respect.[47]

Nonhelpful Interventions

Caring for pregnant women and their infants is supposed to be a "happy" job. Birthing and caring for infants are supposed to be times of joy and celebration. Because no one expects death or loss to occur in maternity or nursery areas, when it does, both staff and families are shocked. To protect themselves from the reality of the situation or to "spare" the family, professionals may engage in interventions that do not help themselves or their patients. Such interventions may be meant altruistically but do not have the characteristics of effective intervention.

Maintaining the state of denial arrests grief work by preventing or delaying the acceptance of the reality of the loss situation. Progress toward resolution is not begun until the stage of disbelief is relinquished. Using drugs, not talking or crying about the loss, and using distraction all contribute to maladaptive reactions by maintaining the state of denial. The use of tranquilizers, sedatives, and other drugs does not help the recipient but, rather, benefits the giver. Excessive use of these medications prolongs the denial stage by making the feelings and emotions foggy and dreamlike.[73] The energy needed to begin the grief work is dissipated by the effect of the medications. Avoiding the reality of the situation becomes easier when mind-altering drugs make the tragedy even more unbelievable.

Not talking about the loss is a powerful way of denying that it ever existed.[114,126] The inability of professionals to acknowledge that the loss has occurred and that the family is in pain maintains denial and repression.[21] Not discussing the loss prevents parents from learning the facts and facing their reality. Because a fantasy will be created to substitute for the unknown, the fantasy of what happened and why will be worse than the reality. By receiving truthful, honest communication, parents are not left to spend energy dealing with frightening fantasies.

Professional avoidance and unwillingness to talk with parents after a loss communicate other powerful messages that impede grief work. If the loss is not important enough to discuss, then perhaps it is not important at all. Not talking about the loss serves to reduce it and communicates to the parents, "I don't care; therefore neither should you." Avoidance of the topic or a hurried, businesslike or social communication that skirts the issue tells the parent that grief work is dangerous, that grief emotions are dangerous, and that others are afraid of grief and those

TABLE 30–1	PARENTAL PERCEPTIONS OF GRIEF AND IMPORTANT FACTORS AT THE TIME OF INFANT DEATH: RESEARCH BASIS[19]	

STUDY FINDINGS	COMMENTS
1. Parents scored significantly lower than other parents who had lost a child and other adults with grief experience.	1. Lower levels of grief were measured by the Revised Grief Experience Inventory (RGEI), a 22-item Likert scale.
2. Study investigators viewed parents as positively adapting after loss of their infant.	2. Mean scores were 33.16 (out of a highest possible score of 36) on the Post-Death Adaptation Score, a 10-item scale rated by professionals.
3. Seven important aspects of care:	3. Identified by parents:
A. Honesty	A. Parents expect professionals to be honest in giving information about the infant/condition to them. Parental anger results when (parental) perception is that honest information was not given.
B. Empowered decision making	B. Parents want to be involved in medical decision making, especially about withdrawing life support. Parents who had been involved were glad they had been part of the decision process and felt supported by the medical team. Parents felt anger and abandonment when the decision to withdraw support was not believed to be respected by professionals.
C. Parental care	C. Parents needed care as much as their baby; when staff was insensitive to their needs, parents felt upset.
D. Environment	D. Parents appreciated comforts of sleep/family rooms as well as private, quiet areas where the infant died with family/parents. People present at the death were more important than the place of death. Parents expressed fear when left at home with their dying infant; parents wished they had held the infant longer.
E. Faith/trust in nursing care	E. Parents had greater trust in nurses than other providers; most had positive experiences with their infant's nurses. Parents appreciated nurses personalizing and respecting the infant (using baby's name) as well as providing for the infant's comfort and opportunities for parental care of their baby. Negative experiences included mistakes in care and unprofessional behavior.
F. Physicians bearing witness	F. Parents thought it important that the physician be with them throughout the process, including being present at the time of the infant's death. Parents perceived the absence of the physician at the time of the child's death as negative, especially if they had been told that the physician would be there for them. Parents found it meaningful when the physician and other medical staff had contact with them after they had gone home.
G. Support from other hospital care providers	G. Parents appreciated support that they received from chaplains, social workers, and palliative care and child life workers. Parents also appreciated support and help from these providers in dealing with siblings.
4. Seven coping strategies:	4. Identified by parents:
A. Family support	A. Parents relied on family support to cope with the death, appreciated family presence at the hospital/home when the infant died, and found it helpful to talk to extended family about their infant. When extended family members were not supportive and avoided talking about the infant, parents were distressed.

TABLE 30-1	PARENTAL PERCEPTIONS OF GRIEF AND IMPORTANT FACTORS AT THE TIME OF INFANT DEATH: RESEARCH BASIS[19] — cont'd	
STUDY FINDINGS	**COMMENTS**
B. Keeping the memory alive	B. All parents showed researchers mementoes of their dead infant and emphasized the importance of bringing things home (i.e., photos; plaster castings of hands/feet; blanket/clothes) from the hospital that had been used/belonged to the infant who died. Parents especially appreciated tangible reminders (i.e., garden/tree) and rituals to remember their infant.
C. Spirituality/faith	C. All families were comforted by their religious beliefs and found meaning and purpose in their infant's life and death. No families reported negative spiritual experiences or abandonment of their religious beliefs.
D. Altruism	D. Many parents wanted and did "give back" to the hospitals that had cared for them and their dying infants. These altruistic acts took the form of monetary and equipment donations, volunteering, and becoming resource families to other parents with sick children.
E. Refocusing on life	E. Presence of other children in the family assisted parents in continuing to focus on life and the daily requirements of their surviving children. All parents acknowledged that having another child would never replace the infant who died.
F. Validation of decision	F. Parents were comforted by autopsy results that validated that they had made the correct decision for their infant. Parents also appreciated when physicians communicated to them their support of the parents' decision.
G. Bereavement support groups	G. Bereavement support groups resulted in positive experiences for most families, especially in being able to talk freely about their dead infant with others who understood and were not uncomfortable. However, some parents did not feel validated in their grief/loss of an infant by other parents in the group whose children were "older" when they died.

experiencing it. In essence, not discussing the loss gives a clear nonverbal message to not grieve.

An inability to cry in response to a significant loss is not helpful and impedes grief work. The prohibition against crying may have been learned early in life or may be the result of unresolved grief work. Parents may feel the need to be strong for each other, their family, or the staff and thus do not cry. Sometimes role reversal occurs, so that the grieving person feels the need to support others rather than be the recipient of support. Often the significance of parental loss is neither recognized nor acknowledged by the professional for fear that he or she will cry. Rather than talking about the loss as a technique to facilitate tears, no one says anything so no one will cry, and no one's grief progresses through the grief stages.

Distraction is another way of denying the loss or its significance. Professionals, a spouse, or other family members try to distract parents from the feelings and emotions of acute grief by engaging in light, social conversation or by keeping them busy with work or recreation. Dealing only with the physical care and not the need for psychologic care after birth is a form of distraction used by care providers.[59] Parents are preoccupied with their shattered expectations of the past and the stark reality of the present, and they are not interested in distractions.

After an unfavorable perinatal outcome, the couple is often confused about their status: "Am I a mother or father . . . or not?" This experience has been called the "ambivalent transition into motherhood."[88] Failure to acknowledge the newly acquired role of mother or father (even if the fetus or newborn dies) discounts the parent's psychologic investment in the pregnancy, fetus, and newborn. Quickly removing the infant from the maternity or nursery areas or removing all the baby items from the home negates the infant's existence.[78] This is not helpful for grief resolution and prevents parents from making choices and decisions and thus maintaining control over the reality of the situation.

Isolation of the grieving family prevents the development of dependent relationships with others who might potentially provide support and comfort. Without others, parents cannot share their grief and may thus increase their feelings of guilt, anger, blame, and lack of self-worth at their failed pregnancy. Those directly experiencing a perinatal loss may be isolated from the rest of society, including their families, who do not view loss of a pregnancy or neonate as significant.[16,78,82,126] Empathy with the parents' definition of the loss is important and necessary for society to be supportive. The goal of recent research, professional literature, and education has been to sensitize the care provider to the effect of perinatal loss. Only recently have books and Internet sites specifically about perinatal loss become available to inform and assist parents.

To decrease contact with the grieving mother, the staff may neglect her or perform cursory physical care, or there may be overconcern for providing physical care.[95] Assigning a room at the end of the hall, not going into the room, delaying answering requests, and placing the mother on another floor are ways of avoiding families. Use of private rooms and room assignments off the maternity floor may be helpful but may allow staff to remove themselves from the unpleasant and uncomfortable situation. Early discharge to a supportive environment may be helpful but, without plans for follow-up, may merely be a way to remove the constant, painful reminder.

Keeping the childbearing couple together throughout the perinatal events facilitates a shared experience of the reality of the situation. Separation of the mother and father or of the couple from friends, family, and other children is not helpful. Exclusion of family members from the experience also prevents them from providing support for the mother and the couple. Relaxed visiting policies and as much contact as possible between the hospitalized mother and the father (and other family members) are important.[27,114]

Prohibiting contact between the parents and the infant allows fearful fantasies of the truth that are always more frightening than the reality of the situation. Delayed contact prolongs the state of disbelief and denial.[29] Restrictive visiting policies in the nursery, institutionalizing an infant without looking at all alternatives, or any other policy that separates parents from their infant does not facilitate grief. Especially in the case of an anomalied, stillborn, or dead infant, the message of delayed contact, or none at all, is that the infant is too horrible and unacceptable to be seen or touched. Because parental egos are so symbiotically attached to their offspring, an unacceptable child is equated with an unacceptable and unworthy self. The fantasy that the damaged or dead child is representative of the damaged and defective self is borne out in the behavior and separation policies of the care providers.

In an attempt to offer the grieving family comfort, friends, relatives, and even professionals often make comments that are *nonsupportive* and *nonhelpful*[78,114]:

- "Well, you're young. You can have more babies."
- "Just have another baby right away."
- "Well, at least you have others at home."
- "It's better to lose her now when she's a baby than when she's 4 years old."
- "He never would have been totally normal anyway."
- "He was born dead. You didn't get a chance to know or get attached to him anyway."
- "It's God's will."

Clichés and platitudes such as these do not help because of the message they give about the parents and the infant.[133] These comments at best reduce and at worst negate the effect of prenatal attachment to the fetus. The importance of psychologic investment and attachment by the parents to this fetus or newborn is said to be basically unimportant and essentially nonexistent.[78] Because infants are viewed as an extension of the parent's self, "by a not very subtle process of identification, the parents see a part of themselves in the baby, and nobody likes to be told that part of them is better off dead."[133] Also, comforting parents whose infant has died with the information that the child was not perfect and never would have been normal and healthy reinforces their belief that they are as defective and unsatisfactory as their dead child.[78]

Such comments also convey a message about the importance of an individual life. Essentially, they say that one fetus or newborn is fairly interchangeable with another. They negate the importance of and indeed the existence of the infant for the parents, siblings, family, and society. The life of the individual is devalued, because "another baby" easily replaces him or her. Comparing one infant's illness or deformity with another's is not helpful for parents whose own infant's deformity is certainly more important than any other infant's problem.

The power of words to help during grief is outweighed only by their power to not help. Because parents are increasingly open during a perinatal crisis, they are sensitive not only to what is said and how it is said but also to the nonverbal message. Giving premature or false reassurance may be more for relief of the professionals than for the parents.[22] Comments such as "It's okay" and "Everything will be all right" must be genuine and timed appropriately for the parent. Telling parents that they have a child with Down syndrome and then saying "But everything will be all right" is hardly helpful. Giving reassurance that subsequent pregnancies and infants will be all right or unaffected is not helpful before the parents are ready to think about and project into the future. It is important to remember at these times that in the future these parents may not remember, what specifically you said; but they will remember how you made them feel.[3]

The basic terminology accompanying perinatal grief situations may be upsetting to parents. Instead of *dead,* professionals often substitute less frightening and less final words. The use of *loss* when *death* is appropriate may be misinterpreted (especially by children). The terms *lose, loss,* and *lost* connote misplacing, so that comments such as "I'm sorry you lost your baby" may be responded to by "I didn't lose (misplace) my baby. My child died." Medical professionals skirt the use of the words *dead, died,* and *die.* Care providers are taught as students to use the word *expired* when referring to a patient who has died. Meant to soften the effect of *dead,* the word *expired* may have its own effect, as a mother whose infant son died wrote in a poem: "The baby expired they said, as if you were a credit card."[152]

Other situations that do not facilitate grief work include dealing with multiple losses or stresses and ambivalence or mental illness.[76,172] The reaction to the loss of a significant relationship is intensified in the context of multiple losses, stresses, and problems.[114,172] Because perinatal losses represent not only a loss of the wished-for perfect child but also a threat to the parental self, self-concept, and self-worth, they represent situations of multiple loss.[159,160]

Helpful Interventions

Professionals have an opportunity to make a significant difference in the outcome after the crisis of perinatal loss for the individual, the couple, and the family. A care provider who is knowledgeable about the grief process and comfortable in sharing another individual's grief is equipped to assist the family and its members toward a long-term healthy adjustment rather than a dysfunctional and pathologic adjustment. Interventions that are helpful for family members also assist staff members in their own grief work.

Factors that influence an individual's personal experience of grief (and ultimately appropriate interventions) are outlined in Box 30-3. Care for the grieving is individualized through assessing these factors, planning, and continually evaluating the individual.[43,44,114,129] Eliciting such personal information may not be as difficult as it first seems. Those in crisis often spontaneously share crucial data with little prompting. The importance of active listening to questions and comments or a more formalized therapeutic interview process may provide the needed encouragement and permission to begin communication.

A history of previous losses and their type and timing in the life cycle are important data for the care provider dealing with the current loss. Past experiences with a crisis or loss influence an individual's behavioral and coping style with current problems.[161] Experiencing a previous perinatal loss affects a subsequent pregnancy.[7,31,128] These pregnancies are characterized by guarded emotions, marking the progress of the pregnancy and seeking out or avoiding various behaviors.[30-33,161] A previous perinatal loss may compound the individual's reaction to a current loss. Dealing with problems alone, receiving help and support from others, and withdrawing altogether are possible ways of coping with the loss.

The degree of attachment and the meaning of the pregnancy and impending parenthood to the family define expectations and influence reactions if an optimal outcome does not occur. The experience of grief depends on whether the loss situation was sudden and unexpected or if there was forewarning about a problem or complication. The definition and meaning of the crisis (e.g., the nature and severity of a deformity, the finality of death, or the chronic sorrow of a defective infant) reflect the individual's and

BOX
30-3 FACTORS TO EVALUATE IN INDIVIDUALIZING GRIEF INTERVENTIONS

1. Previous losses
   a. Type
      Separation
      Divorce
      Death
      Spontaneous abortion (miscarriage)
      Elective or selective abortion
      Period of infertility
      Relinquishment of child
      Perinatal loss
   b. Timing in the life cycle
      Distant
      Recent
   c. Coping styles (of each individual and the family as a unit)
   d. Grief work
      Resolved
      Unresolved
2. Prenatal attachment
   a. Degree of psychologic investment in relationship with fetus or newborn
   b. Decision making about pregnancy and infant
      Planned or unplanned
      Wanted or unwanted
   c. Meaning of pregnancy and infant to individual and family
   d. Parental expectation about childbearing

3. Nature of the current loss
   a. Timing
      Sudden and expected
      Anticipatory grief
   b. Definition and meaning of the event (death, deformity) to individual members of the family
   c. Multiple losses
      Self
      Perfect child
   d. Nature and severity
      Of loss
      Of defect
4. Cultural influences (also see Chapter 29)
   a. On experience and the expression of grief
   b. Societal expectations dictate acceptable and unacceptable behaviors of mourning
5. Strengths (individual and family)
   a. Support system (family, friends, religious, community, or social agencies) mobilized when necessary
   b. Stable relationships: couple supportive of each other
   c. Financial stability
   d. Coping abilities: can evaluate, plan for, and adjust to novel situations
   e. Good health
   f. Receptive and intelligent
   g. Realistic expectations about childbearing and childrearing

family's value system and previous crisis experience. The process of grief is affected by the event itself, the previous and current coping mechanisms, and the family's definition of the event. Consideration of all of these factors is crucial in instituting appropriate intervention.

Cultural practices among families and professionals often differ (see Chapter 29).[127] For example, in some cultures, it may not be acceptable to see or hold the baby (as in some Native American cultures). In the Muslim culture, the family is the primary system of support and it is rare to see a Muslim family emote publicly. A phenomenologic study of Muslim women experiencing perinatal loss found them to have experienced a lack of communication and privacy in the hospital during their initial grieving, feelings of confusion, emptiness, anxiety, anger, and guilt and agreement that husbands and families were

the decision makers.[147] It is critical for health care practitioners to recognize cultural and religious differences to minimize misinterpretations and conflicts with families. With increasing immigration, practitioners must be able to respond with a more ethnic and culturally sensitive approach.[27,44,86,104,139] It is essential to be creative and flexible, thus respecting families' cultural and religious belief systems.[1,156,168] Studies show that cultural differences influence (1) parental emotional response to and perception of their infant's illness and disability, (2) parental use of services, (3) parental interactions with health care providers, and (4) the ceremonies and rituals surrounding death.[17,44,86]

A review of published studies over the past 30 years of perinatal grief and loss in Latino parents has been published.[164] Latina women have a 1.5 times higher risk for experience of perinatal loss due to

BOX 30-4 RIGHTS OF PARENTS, INFANT, AND SIBLINGS WHEN AN INFANT DIES

Rights of Parents

1. To be given the opportunity to see, hold, and touch their baby at any time before or after death, within reason
2. To have photographs of their baby taken and made available to the parents or held in security until the parents want to see them
3. To be given as many mementos as possible (i.e., crib card, baby beads or bracelet, ultrasound or other photographs, lock of hair, feet and hand prints, and record of weight and length)
4. To name and bond with their child
5. To observe cultural and religious practices
6. To be cared for by an empathetic staff who will respect their feelings, thoughts, beliefs, and individual requests
7. To be with each other throughout hospitalization as much as possible
8. To be given time alone with their baby, allowing for individual needs
9. To be informed about the grieving process
10. To be given the option to donate their baby's organs for transplant or to donate their baby's body to science.
11. To request an autopsy; in the case of a miscarriage, to request to have or not have an autopsy or pathology examination as determined by applicable law
12. To have information about their baby, including autopsy results, presented in terminology that is understandable by the parents and family.
13. To plan a farewell ritual, burial, or cremation in compliance with local and state regulations and according to their personal beliefs, religion, or cultural tradition
14. To be provided information on support resources that assist in the healing process (i.e., support groups, counseling, reading material, and perinatal loss newsletter)

Rights of the Infant

1. To be recognized as someone who was born and died
2. To be named
3. To be seen, touched, and held by the family
4. To have life ending acknowledged
5. To be cared for and put to rest with dignity

Rights of Siblings

1. To be acknowledged and treated as individuals who have feelings that need to be expressed
2. To be given the choice/opportunity to see and hold the sibling before and after the death with parental input and support
3. To be considered in the choices parents are given—they may have ideas about names, funerals, memorials for their sibling
4. To be informed and educated about grief according to their ages and developmental stages and offered the opportunity/choice to participate in support groups or counseling sessions
5. To be recognized by the family and society that they will always love and miss their sibling

Modified from *SHARE pregnancy and infant loss support.* Available at www.nationalshareoffice.org. Accessed January 14, 2014.

(1) higher teen birth rates, (2) births to unmarried mothers, and (3) receiving no prenatal care or receiving prenatal care late in the pregnancy.[164] Grief responses among Latino cultures vary by country of origin, religious beliefs/practices, and acculturation (i.e., newer immigrants grieve in traditional ways, whereas subsequent generations incorporate the customs of the predominant culture).[164] Emotional expressions of grief, such as crying, are seen as healthy in Latino cultures. Because members of Latino cultures receive the majority of their emotional support from their families, numerous family members may be in attendance. Instead of the Anglo concept of "letting go" after a loss, Latina women believe in the concept of maintaining connections with the dead and are comforted by pictures, seeing/holding their dead infants, naming, and baptizing.

The national association SHARE: Pregnancy & Infant Loss Support, Inc. has revised the "Rights of Parents When a Baby Dies" and "Rights of the Infant" (Box 30-4). These documents serve as guidelines for creation of protocols, checklists, and bereavement programs; affirmation and empowering tools for bereaved parents; and communication points for parents and care providers initiating the grief process.[116]

ENVIRONMENT

The first step in facilitating grief work is to create an ethical environment that is safe, supportive, permissive, and conducive to the expression of feelings.[21,28,114,126,166] This type of environment does not depend on physical surroundings but, rather, is created and maintained by a warm, receptive, accepting, and caring staff. Such an environment centers its concern more on the people giving and receiving care than on the tasks of care.[78] This type of environment is nonjudgmental and is characterized by an attitude of openness and freedom.[25,133] People feel safe enough to ventilate a full range of feelings—sadness, anger, despair, and even humor—without the fear of condemnation or rejection. Staff members become role models of open communication, facing grief, and feeling comfortable in an uncomfortable situation. The safety of such an environment generates feelings of acceptance and understanding so that grieving and healing may proceed.

Professional presence and support are essential to families in crisis because of the increased dependency needs that accompany grief and loss. Yet certain aspects of a conducive environment such as privacy, quiet, and comfort may be difficult to obtain in a noisy and busy perinatal setting. The recommendation to never leave the family alone must be balanced with their need for privacy and personal time alone with their infant (stillborn, ill, or dying). Simply saying "I will stay with you unless you ask me to leave so that you can have some private time alone with your child" or "Would you like me to leave for a while so that you can be alone with your baby?" offers both support and privacy. Many parents later regret not having time alone and not thinking to ask for that alone time.

A quiet place away from the hustle and bustle of the routine may facilitate both attachment and detachment. The mother of a stillborn child who is quickly shown her infant in the delivery room as her episiotomy is being repaired is not in an optimal physical (or psychologic) environment. Attaching to and saying good-bye to her infant are better accomplished in a quieter and more private setting with significant others present.[87,113,149] Active participation of parents at the death of their newborn may not optimally occur in a busy intensive care unit. Rather, adaptation of hospice concepts to neonatal care provides a private, homelike room, with focus on palliative (comfort) care, rather than cure, to the dying newborn and the family (see Chapter 32).[28,129,144,145,166] Optimally, parents are able to hold and comfort their dying infant. A recent phenomenologic study of Scandinavian NICU nurses found a strong belief in offering skin-to-skin care for dying preterm infants and their parents as a way to provide mutual proximity and comfort.[80] When the family is too emotionally drained, they may elect to "say good-bye" and leave the hospital before life support is removed; the nurse then disconnects, holds, and rocks the baby so the infant does not die alone.[20,114] In some situations (e.g., chromosomal anomalies), parents and professionals may opt to provide end-of-life care ideally with hospice care at home.[101]

Supportive, Trusting Relationships. A relationship with a caring individual who offers consistency and support is the foundation of a therapeutic environment.[166] During periods of crisis, when there is a temporary increase in dependency needs and feelings of loneliness, it is an adaptive behavior to seek emotional support from family, friends, and professionals.[21,92,114] Even the crisis of normal childbearing prompts many cultures to provide a doula[123] to teach the new mother and give her emotional support. For a family in mourning, the relationships established with helpful professionals are more important than the physical care received.

Support, "sharing one's ego strength with another in a time of need,"[58] is particularly helpful in perinatal loss because of the threat to self-concept and self-esteem suffered by parents. Support may be as simple as remaining with the parents. "Being there" indicates not only physical presence but also an emotional availability and willingness to share their experience of loss. Often professionals, family, and friends are hampered by not knowing what to say. Usually, words are initially unnecessary or do not adequately describe the moment and silent presence may better convey the message. Often it is not what is said but the mere presence of loving others that conveys empathy and support to parents and colleagues. Yet presence is not enough; meaningful interaction between parents and professionals is also necessary for a trusting relationship to develop.

The initial meeting with the professionals, including verbal and nonverbal cues, leaves a lasting impression on the family. Addressing family members by name personalizes the encounter, and a brief touch or handshake represents an extension of self, a gesture of warmth, concern, and acceptance from professional to parents. An introduction that includes a brief explanation of the professional's role in relation to them and their infant helps orient them: "Good morning, Mr. and Mrs. Black. I'm Sue, your baby's primary nurse. That means that I will be caring for Jason while he is here and working with you." Orientation to the physical surroundings and technical equipment eases the transition to an unfamiliar and often intimidating hospital environment. Providing physical comfort such as rocking chairs, privacy for interaction, and sleeping facilities for parents demonstrates the philosophy of the parents' worth and importance to their infant.

Empathy, an emotional understanding and identification with the plight of another, characterizes a helping relationship. In such a relationship, "How are you?" is asked with the emphasis on you and a genuine interest in the answer—unlike a social inquiry in which an automatic "Fine" is expected. Recognition of verbal and nonverbal cues of parental feelings (e.g., "You look tired" or "I hear that you are frustrated") communicates that these emotions are legitimate, understood, and accepted. A willingness to help, listen, console, and give encouragement and positive feedback establishes the professional as a sensitive, responsive person whom parents will trust.[166] Supporting any and all parental involvement, supporting damaged parental egos, and helping parents succeed in the tasks of attachment and detachment are goals of effective intervention.

A qualitative study examining maternal perceptions and experiences showed that mothers had feelings of both empowerment and powerlessness with professional care after the death of their newborns.[87] Feelings of powerlessness occurred when (1) mothers felt disrespected as a person and a mother; (2) good communication between mother and professionals did not exist; and (3) the mother did not feel treated as an individual.[87] Mothers feel empowered (e.g., more confident, able to ask questions, understood and supported) when they felt that professionals (1) were "near," both psychologically and emotionally; (2) supported their self-esteem and confidence; and (3) provided empathetic, comforting support.[5,53,87]

The nursing staff often determines the tone of in-hospital perinatal settings . Generally, residents, interns, and specialists remain for short periods and the private physician or permanent medical staff are not available on a minute-to-minute basis. Development of a safe, trusting environment depends on viewing parents as essential partners in care of their baby and not as visitors or "disruptors" of the ward routine.[29] Pleasant and relaxed surroundings convey the message of hospitality and "You are welcome here."

Both professional and nonprofessional support systems are available in the crisis of perinatal loss. Yet relating to many people during crisis is difficult

for parents. Primary care (both medical and nursing) uses the same care provider for both the physiologic and psychologic care of the infant and the family. Thus, the family only has to relate to as few professionals as possible. This special caring reassures parents that a few special people love, know, and are invested in their infant. Primary care providers share with the parents the joys of even small gains and the sorrows and tears of complications or death. Professionals and parents benefit from primary care systems in the emotional and psychologic satisfaction of such involvement. Yet this involvement is not without a price of vulnerability to an individual's feelings of loss and grief. Peer support on an individual basis or in a group setting is essential in dealing with the stress of continual attachment and loss.[38,41]

Normal grief reactions may be facilitated by nursing and medical professionals using other professionals (social workers, chaplains, or counselors) when necessary.[10,28,93,114] Interdisciplinary collaboration and consultation helps the staff gain insight into parental and personal behaviors and appropriate intervention strategies.[11,142] The staff also may benefit from the expertise of a trained counselor in dealing with their own feelings of loss and grief.

PATHOLOGIC GRIEF

Maladaptive responses to perinatal loss are indications for referral for specialized care (Box 30-5).[170] Involvement of clergy and religious organizations is often comforting and supportive to the family.[98,113,151,164,168] Religious rituals (i.e., baptism, prayer service, or anointing) may be advocated by certain denominations and provide a measure of comfort and hope. Often parents in crisis do not

---

BOX 30-5	CRITICAL FINDINGS
	INDICATORS OF PATHOLOGIC GRIEF[84]

1. Overactivity without a sense of loss
2. Acquisition of symptoms belonging to the last illness of the deceased
3. Psychosomatic conditions
4. Altered relationships to friends and relatives
5. Furious hostility against specific others
6. Formal manner resembling schizophrenia
7. Lasting loss of social interaction patterns
8. Assuming activities detrimental to social and economic existence
9. Agitated depression

think to request infant baptism or to call their priest, minister, or rabbi. Offering to call a clergy member of their choice or the hospital chaplain may be helpful. A national survey of pastoral care providers noted barriers to providing spiritual care: (1) inadequate numbers of pastoral care staff, (2) inability of health care providers to assess spiritual needs, and (3) being called "too late" to give all the care that could have been provided.[51] Primary care providers who have shared intimately with the parents the experience of their child's life and death may be invited to attend the funeral or memorial service. For both care providers and parents, this may represent the final act of caring for the infant.[41]

Nonprofessional support systems such as the couple, family, friends, and parent groups are often forgotten as sources of potential help to grieving parents. One the one hand, in our society of isolated, mobile, nuclear families, it may be erroneous to assume that a support system exists. On the other hand, it may be unrecognized because it does not fall into a traditional definition, such as the neighbor or other friend who may be more supportive (and available) than the grandparents. Biologic kinship is not the only valid criterion for a support system; an emotional kinship is the most important factor.

Because professional availability and involvement with the parents is not lasting, the professional has a responsibility to identify, foster, and facilitate a nonprofessional (social) support system. Simply identifying supportive others and expecting them to automatically help in a perinatal loss situation may be unrealistic. Unless those who constitute the support system are as well informed and instructed as the parents about the situation, they will not be able to offer emotional comfort. For example, if the parents wish to talk about their loss but the members of the support system empathically want to spare them by not discussing it, no help will be given or received.

The quality and quantity of ties one has with a social network are associated with improved health status and life satisfaction.[40,146,149,168] For parents experiencing a perinatal loss, the quality and quantity of ties with their social network (i.e., extended family, friends, and colleagues) may be profoundly affected. In one study, most families suffered permanent loss of relationships because others were not sure how to react, avoided talking about the baby, or made comments that diminished the intensity of the loss.[37]

Fathers especially receive little personal attention as friends and colleagues focus their attention on the mother's grief.[37,40] Because grandparents grieve for their grandchild and may feel guilt and grief for their own child, they may be emotionally unavailable to support the grieving parents. To prevent social network disruption for grieving families, health care providers can (1) share information with families about reactions to expect and reasons for these reactions, (2) support families and enable them to rebuild their networks, and (3) emphasize and support the family's belief in their strengths and capacities.[37,40,114]

Open communication between the parents is essential in preserving and fostering a close relationship by the giving and receiving of mutual support. Sharing the experience presents the couple with the opportunity for personal growth and growth as a couple. Yet the individual experience of grief within the context of a couple is too often fertile ground for misunderstanding and resentment.[126] One study showed that disruption of a couple's sexual relationship occurred after the death of a child.[137] A national study examining parental relationships after live birth, miscarriage, or stillbirth found an increased risk for dissolution of marriage or cohabitation in couples experiencing loss compared with a live birth.[55]

Parental support groups offer their members an opportunity to discuss their feelings with others who have been through similar traumas.[126,161] Knowing how others who have experienced perinatal loss have felt and dealt with similar situations is emotionally comforting and stabilizing to parents experiencing their own loss. Parents provide each other with validation for their feelings and a sense that they are not alone in their pain. Each individual has different needs, different ways of adapting to crisis, and different ways of giving and receiving support. It is essential that professionals use techniques that are real and spontaneous and not adopt words or actions that are foreign to one's own self. Interventions must also be gauged to the parents' needs and pace.

In one study[159] and from clinical experience, fathers state that they receive most of their support from their spouse. They report that little attention is paid to fathers by hospital staff, causing more denial and difficulty expressing their grief. So that the father's grief is not ignored,[95] it is critical for hospital staff to address the father's feelings when addressing parental grief.[131] Suggestions to assist fathers in their grief include implementation of all-male support groups, validation of their feelings, and asking direct open-ended questions. These may include "What are you feeling right now?" "Tell me how your day is going," and "Tell me about your coping strategies." Health care providers can help a father by reflecting his statements, using his name, and assisting him with expressing his feelings. Fathers should be included and acknowledged in all discussions with staff[160] so that they are not "forgotten mourners."[77] A recent study documented that family adjustment after the NICU experience improved over time for mothers but deteriorated for fathers, especially if the infant had ongoing health problems.[40] Assessing the family as a unit rather than using the mother as a representative of the entire family, being cognizant of and responsive to gender differences in coping, and being supportive of family strengths and resources are recommendations for clinicians.[40]

Information. Information aids in intellectually understanding the crisis, thus facilitating a sense of control over it. Actively seeking and using information enable confrontation and mastery of the crisis. Knowledge about a situation strengthens the ego because it enables "worry work" and psychologic preparation for expected events. Because "the void of the unknown is more frightening than the known; facts are more reassuring than awesome speculations,"[22] a major role of the professional is to provide and clarify facts and information relevant to the perinatal loss situation (Box 30-6).[21,93] In the search for meaning that always accompanies loss, medical facts may help alleviate some parental guilt about causing the tragedy. Repeating to the parents that nothing they did or did not do could have caused this problem is reassuring. Sketchy or no information only serves to contribute to parental denial of the reality or to their fantasies of causation.[133] Confronting the crisis and realizing its real element of danger and trouble starts the process of grief by giving permission for the expression of feelings of fear, sadness, and loss.

　　Because the family as a unit, composed of the individual members, must deal with perinatal loss, professionals should encourage and support open, interfamily communications. Keeping secrets, especially between the parents, should be discouraged because this eventually undermines trust and promotes asynchronous grief work. When parents are

---

BOX 30-6 | **PARENT TEACHING**
GRIEF

1. Grief is a normal reaction and is expected in perinatal situations: pregnancy, abortion, stillbirth, premature birth, when the baby is sick or has an anomaly, death, relinquishment, when the birth process does not meet parental expectations, and when there is postpartal depression.
2. Grief is a staged process that occurs over time and is characterized by stages: shock and disbelief, anger, bargaining, depression and withdrawal, and eventually acceptance.
3. Grief is an individualized process and may be experienced differently by the mother and father.
4. To facilitate grief reactions, the neonatal intensive care unit will provide a safe environment for the expression of feelings, information about the infant and the infant's condition, and supportive, trusting relationships with health care providers.
5. Seeing, touching, and holding the baby are as important to the parents of a sick or dying infant or an infant with an anomaly as they are to the parents of a healthy infant.
6. When an infant dies or is dying, parents and infant(s) have the right to interact with each other, to create memories, to involve extended family and friends, and to engage in specific religious and cultural practices.
7. Parents and families are informed about the grief process, encouraged to support and care for each other, and encouraged to identify and rely on social support systems (e.g., extended family, friends, professional support services).

---

given the same information and talk with each other about their loss and their feelings, more synchronous grief reactions develop.[78] Telling parents together with the infant present prevents misunderstanding, misinterpretations, and "shading" of information to one parent.[113] Informed parents are better able to share their experience with each other and to participate in joint decision making with the professional.[9,19,166] A prospective cohort study found that the quality of the mother's relationship with her partner, secure attachment, and social support affect the course of bereavement after perinatal loss.[134]

　　The questions "When to tell" and "How much to tell" the parents often arise. Parents should be told as soon as possible about perinatal complications or problems.[21,78] Receiving this information at the earliest possible time helps parents establish trust in the care provider, appreciate the reality of the situation, begin the grief process, and mobilize both internal and external support. Information must be given in its entirety because attempts to "spare" parents by staging the truth serve only to undermine their trust in professional credibility. The couple's relationship also may suffer if one parent colludes with the professional in a conspiracy of silence. This is best illustrated by the following incident:

To spare a diabetic mother from the truth about her infant's congenitally absent limbs, the physician and the father decided to tell her about his missing legs but not the missing arm. On arriving to transport the baby, the nurse asked if the mother had been told. "Yes" was the response, so she took the infant to the mother's room before transport. As she uncovered the infant, the mother gasped and looked at the physician and the father and said, "You lied to me. You didn't tell me about his arm, too."

When given the unedited truth, parents can face reality and begin the grief process without fear that there is something else that they are not being told about. The individual's stage of grief influences not when or what will be said but how the information will be given and received. During the initial stage of shock, information, if processed, is processed slowly.[78] Often, events take on a foggy, dreamlike quality so that sensory information remembered is not believed. Yet to give no information only perpetuates this frightening feeling. Communication to those in shock and denial must proceed simply, slowly, and with much repetition and reinforcement. Giving information once does not ensure that it will be retained or understood. Repetition by the professionals is necessary for gradual acceptance of the reality of the situation.[9,19] This may be a nuisance for the professional who has already given the information and wonders why the parents cannot remember it. Parents are so shocked they do not hear what is said, and information must be patiently repeated.[61,166] Although early contact with parents almost ensures they will be in a state of shock, the tone and content of the first meeting are not forgotten.[21,78] Initial information about the infant and his or her condition may have long-term effects on the parents' ability to attach or detach. In the past, parents were given a pessimistic outlook with the belief that "It will be easier for them. They won't get so involved." Negative descriptions and initial pessimism only increase the amount of grief and detachment while effectively blocking attachment behaviors. If the sick or defective infant survives, the parents may have detached to the point

of, at least emotionally, burying him or her. Knowledge of better survival rates and the quality of survival enables a truthfully optimistic outcome for many sick neonates. Therefore, information must be given clearly (not medical jargon) with a minimal focus on possible complications and medical odds.[78,172]

Volunteering information to parents is essential, but encouraging their questions is equally as important. As the normal mechanism for adapting to crisis and gaining mastery over a situation, questions help the professional "start where the parents are" and begin communication with their concerns. Questions and comments unrelated to the discussion may indicate either failure to comprehend or failure to send the information clearly.[172]

Direct questions deserve direct answers because they indicate a readiness and desire for information. Indirect questions or comments by the parents may indicate concern about their own infant that cannot be directly expressed. "Baby Stevie (who died yesterday) had severe respiratory distress syndrome, didn't he?" The parents want to be reassured that their infant will not die, too.

During the crisis of perinatal loss, interpersonal communication is difficult. Therefore, as few professionals as possible should relay information to the parents. Primary care providers (nurse and physician) should coordinate and provide continuity in giving information to parents because individual care providers will supply information about the same topic in different ways.[29,114] The use of varied terms, inflections, and attitudes by a multitude of professionals becomes a monumental source of confusion and anxiety for parents. A trusted relationship[19,21,25] with a primary nurse and physician through whom all communication flows minimizes unnecessary anxiety and concern for parents. It is essential that the nurse (or primary nurse) be present and assists the physician in communication with the parents. Any anxiety-producing information (poor prognosis, complication, or impending death) may not be heard or understood initially by the parents. The nurse must know exactly what and how this information was given to the parents. After the physician departs, the nurse must be able to offer clarification, explanation, and support to the distraught parents. Nothing is more distressing than finding a crying, upset mother who is unable to relate what the physician said, why she is upset, or even if she understood what was said.

No family or parent should have to wonder and worry about a dreaded or feared outcome without being given the proper information. If the primary care physician is unavailable to speak with the family, then someone from the health care team must assume this responsibility. No mother whose infant is ill, deformed, or dead should awaken from an anesthetized birth to find her physician absent and the nurses unable to answer "How's my baby?" A plan of action for telling individual parents must be decided and agreed on by all care providers.

Parents are interested in the daily (or hourly) progress of their infant, including both positive and negative developments. It is important for parents to know about a crisis or negative development in an infant's condition as soon as possible. They are then able to participate and care for their infant through the difficulty and to trust professional communication. Parents should have unlimited access to phone or personal contact with the staff in the perinatal care setting. Phone calls to the hospital from concerned parents should be possible any time of the day or night. The knowledge that information about their infant and access to a caring professional are available at any hour often is enough to comfort parents of a critically ill infant.

Lactation suppression for the mother of a dying newborn often has been a forgotten aspect of care.[103] Engorgement creates a feedback mechanism to the maternal brain that leads to cessation of milk production; however, painful engorgement should be avoided. Using a breast pump to remove enough milk to relieve pressure and discomfort but not enough to empty the breasts will gradually result in a decrease in milk production. If the mother pumps until she is comfortable, gradually prolonging the intervals between pumping, and pumping for shorter periods, lactation gradually is suppressed. Use of a well-fitting and supportive bra relieves the discomfort/pain of heavy breasts. A recent study comparing the use of breast binding to a supportive bra found that the breast-binding group had greater breast pain/tenderness, leakage, and use of other pain relief measures; the study recommendation was to discontinue breast binding for the more comfortable and efficacious supportive bra.[150] Mothers who have pumped and stored breast milk may wish to donate it to a mother's milk bank. A mother also may wish to continue pumping to be a human milk donor. These options should be sensitively discussed with the mother of the dying infant.

ENCOURAGING EXPRESSION OF EMOTIONS

Because grief is an emotional reaction to loss, expression of these emotions is necessary for grief work to begin and proceed. Verbalizing thoughts and feelings provides an outlet for the intense emotions accompanying grief and signifies to others that emotional support is needed.[21] For some, the open expression of emotions may be difficult because of influence from their culture, gender-specific roles, and social status. Yet the containment of intense feelings uses a great deal of emotional and physical energy that could be more productively used in moving on with the grief work. Those who are stoic and non-communicative experience symptoms of grief for a longer period than those who freely express their feelings and emotions.[13]

Experiencing the loss of an infant initiates an "ambivalent transition" into motherhood in a short period.[88] These women often feel totally confused, with broken expectations and elusive grief: "Have I or have I not become a mother?" Supporting families provides them with an opportunity to talk about their infant, confirming the baby's life as important, although short. This process assists parents to attach and subsequently begin the grieving process.[169]

Talking about the loss helps parents validate and assimilate the experience. Timing and events are clarified, including forgotten details, by discussion with each other and with their care providers. Confronting the reality enables them to work through the shock and disbelief, verbalize their fears and disappointments, and begin to cry and grieve. Expression of feelings gradually permits a clarification of the meaning of the loss to the parents. Talking lightens the burden of loss, because every time the experience is shared with another, half of the experience and the accompanying emotions are given away. Telling, retelling, reviewing, and reliving the experience are all necessary ways to understand and gain mastery over a frightening and most often unexpected situation.[21,162]

Verbal and nonverbal cues tell professionals where the parents are in their grief process. To elicit feelings, the professional may verbalize his or her own perceptions and observations:

- "Mrs. Green, you sound tense (upset, tired) today."
- "Mr. Brown, you look worried today."
- "I'm sorry that your baby died."

These statements indicate the listening ear and observing eye of one who cares. They set the stage for communication: "It's okay to talk with me about how you are feeling, because I acknowledge your pain."

Because they feel scared, alone, and out of control, parents often deny their feelings under direct questioning. Thus "Do you think you did or didn't do something to cause your baby's problem?" may be answered negatively, despite parents being consumed with guilt. Direct questioning places parents in an awkward and vulnerable position of revealing their most personal doubts and fears. Direct questions may be reworded with safer and more indirect statements:

- "Most parents feel overwhelmed and sad when their baby is sick."
- "Many parents wonder if the cause of their baby's death is something they did or didn't do."
- "It is helpful to many parents to talk about their doubts and fears. These feelings are common and normal in such a difficult situation."

The professional gives information to the parents about the feelings and emotions commonly felt in similar situations. Because there is safety in numbers, if "most" or "many" parents feel this way and it is expected, then it might be safe to share their feelings. Validating parents' reactions as appropriate reassures them that they are not crazy. With this type of invitation, the feelings may be free to come spilling forth or the parents may need time to establish a relationship with this professional before they are ready to talk about such personal emotions.

Empathetic actions and comments may open communication pathways with parents.[21] A professional presence that is warm and caring may facilitate more communication than any words. Touching or holding grieving parents may help feelings be expressed. Nonverbal cues such as nodding, direct eye contact, uninterrupted attention, and the physical closeness of pulling up a chair and sitting down give positive feedback to verbal communication and indicate active listening by the professional.

Crying is the expression of feelings of sadness, sorrow, and intense longing that accompany the pain of loss.[84,172] A healthy catharsis, crying should be expected and encouraged in any loss situation. Yet the cultural, gender-specific, and professional taboos against crying have defined it as an unacceptable and inappropriate response and one that should be suppressed. Because tears are healing and

therapeutic, professionals must learn to be comfortable with the crying of others. "Don't cry" is often heard from those attempting to comfort grieving parents (or colleagues). This is an admonition against the behavior rather than an empathetic comment. "It's okay to cry" or "Go ahead and cry; let it out" gives permission and acceptance to the behavior and the need for it.

By expecting tears, providing a safe environment for their expression, and encouraging the behavior by words and actions, the professional may facilitate crying in both mothers and fathers. Too often, tears are blocked in a relationship in which one partner (usually the man) is expected to be stoic and in control, whereas the other's (usually the woman's) tears are defined as too upsetting or difficult. Because the ability to cry is a healthy response, the couple must be encouraged to use this outlet together.

In the past, crying in the presence of patients and their families was defined as "unprofessional." Yet the cool, controlled exterior defined as "professional" was seen by others as not caring and not feeling. When the professional cries with the parents, it is an acceptable expression of genuine emotion, a demonstration of empathy, and a role model of the appropriateness of tears given the situation. Parents do not define the tears of care providers as weak or unprofessional. Rather, they feel a special bond of love and care with professionals who have been free enough to share their grief.[4,21,114,126] Instead of relearning that crying is acceptable, many parents and care providers must learn this for the first time.

Talking and crying about the loss are easier to facilitate than the expression of anger.[59] Because of the social expectations of dependency of the patient role and real or imagined consequences of retaliation (against the infant or job status), perinatal care settings are not safe environments for the expression of anger. Parents (and colleagues) will be able to vent anger only in an environment free of punishment or retaliation for their behaviors. It is the responsibility of the professionals to create an environment that allows open expression of negative criticism and anger.

SEEING AND TOUCHING

Seeing and touching are as important to the parents of a sick, deformed, or dead infant as they are to the parents of a normal, healthy one. In the past, fear that seeing a deformed or dead infant would intensify grief and be overly upsetting resulted in a lack of contact between parents and their newborn. Despite the fact that many mothers wished to see their infants, the prevailing practice was to discourage and prevent it. Often no information, including sex or physical characteristics, was given to grieving parents, who were left to fantasize about their newborn's problems or cause of death. Current practice indicates that parental contact with the infant does not cause "unduly upsetting immediate reactions or appear to result in pathologic mourning."[73]

Researchers in the United Kingdom have evaluated mothers and fathers who have seen and held their infants after stillbirth. In several of the studies, researchers correlated posttraumatic stress symptoms in both mothers and fathers[153,154] and disorganized maternal–infant attachment[65] in subsequent pregnancies to seeing/holding the stillborn infant. Although remarking that seeing/holding the dead infant is culturally entrenched and highly valued by parents, these researchers warn that this practice is associated, in their studies, with psychologic sequelae and are based only on clinical impression without empirical evidence of benefit.[9] However, other research cited in Table 30-1 shows how this small sample of well-adjusted and low-grieving parents valued holding their infant, being present at the time of death with family/friends, and keeping mementoes and the memory of their child alive.[19] The sequelae of seeing/holding a stillborn and the sequelae of seeing/holding a live infant who has died may not be similar; clearly more research is necessary.

The British researchers,[9] who found psychologic sequelae of parental contact with their stillborn infant, state that many parents experience great meaning and treasure the memory of time with their dead infant. They concede that some parents would choose to have contact with their dead infants, regardless of potentially harmful outcomes. They also state that parental decision to see/hold the dead infant may be heavily influenced by attending staff who may expose reluctant parents to their dead baby. Clearly, the decision to see and touch their infant is ultimately a parental one.[9,172] Making decisions for parents is not the professional's role; making decisions with parents is the professional's role. Each parent must make the decision for him or herself; neither may decide for the other. Altruistic others, such as professionals, the spouse, or other family members, must not usurp the right to individual decision making. Often, in an attempt

to protect the mother, the father or the professional decides that she should not have contact with her infant. They either actually discourage it or do nothing to facilitate it. Mothers who have not seen their infants always know who prohibited it. The couple's relationship may suffer irreparable damage if one decides for the other, even if the motive is altruistic. The professional's role is to facilitate a healthy decision by each parent so that their individual needs to see or to not see the infant are met.

Parents may not realize that seeing and touching their infant is an option, or they may just be too overwhelmed or afraid to ask if it is possible. Instead of waiting for parents to ask, the professional care provider takes a more active role by offering the possibility to the parents: "Would you like to hold your baby?"

Time is often necessary to make the decision because initially parents are ambivalent about seeing and holding a deformed or dead infant. Most mothers and fathers want to see their child but fear what they might see and how they may feel. The care provider may alleviate the parents' ambivalence by acknowledging that being with the infant will be difficult but that the professional will remain with them unless asked to leave. The emotional support of the physical presence of an empathetic professional may allay the fear of becoming out of control. The professional can reassure the family by explaining what they will see before they hold their infant. Making such a crucial decision in the initial stages of loss is difficult. Giving parents information about the positive aspects of seeing and holding the infant in facilitating their grief process helps make their decision an informed one.[132,172]

Seeing the infant brings the dreaded impossibility of perinatal loss into stark reality.[172] Parents confirm with their own eyes that the infant is alive or dead or normal or abnormal. Contact enables claiming behaviors and identification of the infant as their own. While holding their infant, parents examine it and begin to recognize familiar family characteristics: "She has my long fingers and her father's red hair." Even small, severely deformed, or macerated infants can be recognized and claimed by the parents as part of their family. What is remembered are the normal, endearing characteristics that identify the child as "mine."

Parental contact confirms the infant's own reality and eliminates the prenatal fantasy of the expected child. For the parents of an infant with an anomaly, grief work about the fantasized perfect child may begin so that the actual child may become the object of love. Early and frequent contact between the parents and the infant encourages a realistic perspective of the infant's problems. A stillborn or aborted fetus may be physically normal rather than the deformed infant imagined by the parents. Seeing the infant allays doubts and fears about the infant's normal state and about the parents' ability to subsequently have a normal child.[133] Seeing and touching enable parents to grieve the infant's reality rather than a feared and dreaded, and thus more frightening, fantasy. It is easier to grieve a real infant than a mystical, dreamlike fantasy of the infant.[78]

Whether the ultimate decision is to see or not to see the infant, the professional must honor and respect that choice.[172] Cultural taboos against viewing dead bodies may preclude some parents from seeing and touching their infant. Yet many such cultures support their members by formalizing the grief process in sanctioned ritual and ceremony. For those parents who decide not to see and touch, the professional should reassure them of their infant's normal condition (e.g., "He had 10 fingers and toes."). The infant should be described in as much detail as necessary to give parents a mental picture. Gender, size, hair color, skin, weight, and distinguishing characteristics should be included. A simple, realistic description of any anomaly is also helpful because the fantasy of the defect is worse than its reality.

Adequate preparation for the first encounter with their infant includes a description of everything parents will see, hear, and feel.[172] Verbal preparation for viewing an infant with a congenital anomaly includes not only a simple description of the abnormality but also the infant's normal characteristics. Seeing a picture of the abnormality first may help parents prepare for seeing their infant. Remaining with the parents at the initial visit, the professional should describe the anomaly and point out normal findings. Focusing by parents on the normal familial characteristics helps in attaching to the less-than-perfect baby. Although parents of a dead, deformed infant view the abnormality, they often focus on the normal traits and remember the infant not as "monstrous" but as beautiful.

For those who have never seen a dead body, the mind may invent frightening images and sensations. Certainly, "dead" is associated with the temperature sensation of cold. However, a newborn who has been placed under a radiant warmer or in an incubator may feel warm rather than cold shortly after death, hence the statement by a mother, "You couldn't be dead. You feel so warm." The professional must touch the infant and prepare the parents for the tactile sensation of warm or cold: "The baby will feel warm to you because she (or he) has been under the radiant warmer."

To prepare parents for seeing their infant, the professional must observe the baby. Color, skin condition, and size must all be described and are not shocking with adequate preparation: maceration—"peeling of the skin"; peripheral shutdown—"the blue-white discoloration"; and the small size—"as long as the length of my hand." Any equipment that must remain on the body should be described and explained before viewing. Even an umbilical cord clamp may cause concern in a parent who has never seen one. The reason for not removing equipment also must be explained. Respectful care[5] of the infant's body after death shows respect for the person of the infant and for the grieving parents. Attention to details such as wrapping the infant in a blanket rather than a surgical drape or towel, cleaning the infant, and holding the infant in a cuddling position indicates care and concern.

Parents whose infant has died, has a congenital anomaly, or is ill proceed with attachment behaviors of seeing and touching in the same manner as parents of normal, healthy infants.[78] Touching is important, but the distinction must be made between touching and holding. Cradling one's infant is quite different from merely touching with a hand. Holding the infant, whether healthy, sick, or dead, for the first time is a momentous event. Touching the infant who has died may not be sufficient; parents must be given the opportunity to hold and cuddle the child before, during, and after death. Other parenting behaviors, such as bathing and dressing their infant, also should be offered to parents.[66,72,145]

Parents of a dead infant may need more than one chance to see and touch the infant. The first time they do so, they attach to the reality of their infant. Subsequent encounters allow a final chance to see and hold their child. Parents have described the initial encounter as saying "Hello" and the subsequent one as saying "Good-bye." Some parents may be able to accomplish closure with one visit, whereas others who might benefit from a final visit may not ask or think to ask. Offering another contact with their infant leaves the decision with the parents.

The emotional effect of seeing the infant requires support, time, and permission to cry. Attaching is a process that occurs over time. Providing parents sufficient time with their infant takes precedence over paperwork, ward routine, or taking the infant to the morgue. Parents have indicated a need to hold their infant for a longer time and not feel pushed by care providers.[66,88] Even infants who have been removed to the morgue may be returned if parents need more time and contact for detachment.[87]

When an infant dies, opportunities for memories are limited. Professionals have the responsibility of helping parents make memories so that they will have a tangible person to mourn. Encouraging parents to name their infant gives the infant a separate identity, which helps facilitate the grieving process. Tangible mementos may include photographs, handprints and footprints, a lock of hair, hand/foot castings,[70,114,155] measurements of the infant, identification bands, the blanket the infant was wrapped in, a blessing or baptismal certificate, and birth and death certificates. Parents find most beneficial the interventions that acknowledged the infant (e.g., photographs, holding the infant, and receiving personal mementos).[19,66,72,87,117] Even when parents say they do not want mementos, the mementos should be kept in hospital files and the parents made aware that they will be available to them in the future if they want them.[87] Taking pictures of the infant, obtaining other mementos, and telling the parents that such mementos will be available to them on request not only respects their immediate decision to not see or have information on the infant but also provides a mechanism for them to "know" their infant at a later date if they wish to do so.

Before an infant is transported to a newborn special care unit, photographs should be taken and given to the parents to promote bonding. If the infant remains hospitalized for a long time or requires surgery, pictures taken at weekly intervals or before and after surgery can help confirm the reality of the child's condition and progress and assist with bonding, as well as the grief process. Despite the outcome, parents will appreciate some lasting record of their child's life.

The staff that provides emotional support for parents must also receive support from each other. Expecting staff members to immediately return to work is unrealistic. Such an emotional experience takes time and space for decompression, which is facilitated by the use of exercise, crying, and being alone for quiet time.[41] Interdisciplinary staff often feel inexperienced, anxious, fearful and dread when communicating with families about sensitive end-of-life issues.[5,28,61] Many received inadequate education and support to deal with these families and their own personal pain.[5,28] Just as simulation teaches teamwork in clinical psychomotor skills, simulation of "delivering bad news" enables all members of the health care team to enhance their communication skills with families.[5]

OPEN VISITING AND CAREGIVING POLICIES

Perinatal care settings with open visiting and caregiving policies foster a shared family experience and support from others. Regardless of the type of perinatal loss, no mother should experience it alone—a spouse, friend, family member, or identified supportive other should remain with her.[66,160] Members of the mother's support system will also need an outlet for expression of their grief.

Women suffering the grief of perinatal loss should be given a choice about their room assignment. Arbitrary removal from the obstetric unit may deny the mother's maternity: "Am I a mother or not?" It also may escalate her feelings of failure, guilt, and worthlessness as a woman and a mother. Because she did not produce a normal, healthy infant, she may feel punished and banished from the maternity area by isolation on another floor. Her care may be entrusted to those without expertise in the physiologic and psychologic care of the normal postpartum period, much less a postpartum complicated by loss. Placement at the end of the hall far from the nurses' station, with the door closed and no company from staff and family, only increases her feelings of loneliness and isolation. Yet being on a happy maternity floor with normal, healthy infants and their mothers may be an exceedingly difficult and constant reminder of her loss and even complicate her recovery.[73] Information about the advantages and disadvantages of staying or leaving the maternity ward should be given by the professional. The mother, knowing what will be helpful, can then make the decision.[172]

The alternative to maternal hospitalization is discharge as soon as medically possible so the mother may join her infant when the infant has been transported to another hospital. Early discharge also facilitates an easier mobilization of supportive others in the familiar surroundings of home. Removal from the constant reminder of one's failure (i.e., other healthy infants) may let the grief work begin.[172] Early discharge is not therapeutic when the professional assumes there is a support system to provide care and no one is available. Without a plan for follow-up care and contact, early discharge merely relocates the problem.

Caregiving is as important for the parents of a sick, deformed, or dead infant as it is for the parents of a normal infant. Open visiting and caregiving policies increase interaction between the parents and their infant by actively involving them in the reality of their child's illness, deformity, or impending death. Even if the child lives only a short time, parental access and the ability to take care of the infant complete the attachment process and enable them to begin the detachment of grief work. Even minimal caregiving (i.e., holding, bathing, dressing)[5] helps parents overcome their sense of helplessness and be comforted by "We did all that we could have done. We cared; we made a difference to our baby." Active parental involvement decreases poor outcomes such as aberrant parenting styles, attachment problems, and unresolved grief.[19,78]

The loneliness and isolation of death are decreased for both parents and infant when they are together at the time of death. Parents often are comforted and relieved that their fantasy of the agony of the death scene is not borne out in the quiet, peaceful reality of death.[78] Having experienced the beginning of life together, parents who are present at the ending of life can feel a sense of closure and completion. Parents who can share even a brief life with their baby and the moment of death can face death's finality knowing they did not abandon their infant but provided him or her love and care.[87] Parents who are not present at death may take care of the infant afterward by seeing and holding him or her.

Parents should be given the opportunity to make final plans for their deceased infant.[114] The planning will help them face the death and facilitate the grief process. For many parents, this is their first experience with death and making final arrangements and they are not aware of the options. It is helpful to provide the family with detailed, specific verbal and written information about cremation, burial, funeral, or hospital disposal.[24,66,114]

A funeral may be chosen for religious reasons or as a declaration of the fetus or newborn as a person befitting burial rather than disposal. Burial leaves a specific place of remembrance and recognition that this infant lived. Care for the infant after death may include funeral arrangements, such as choosing the clothes or bathing and even dressing the infant. If parents choose not to have a funeral, they may wish to have a memorial service or do something special, such as plant a rosebush or tree, in memory of their infant. Regardless of their decision, the birth and death of their baby constitute a life event for the family, and one must recognize it.

AUTOPSY

For parents who experience a stillbirth, spontaneous abortion, or neonatal death, knowing why the infant was deformed or died eases their recovery from grief.[78] In the search for a cause, many parents blame themselves for doing too much or too little to favorably influence the outcome. Neonatal autopsies reveal important new information and the cause of perinatal loss in only 10% to 40% of the cases.[120,166] Knowing why the infant died or the converse, that not even the "experts" know why the infant died, may help assuage their personal feelings of guilt and failure.

Primary care providers (physician and nurse) must use the utmost tact and show respect for the family's feelings when approaching them for permission to conduct an autopsy. Too often the permission for autopsy is denied because of the way the subject is broached by professionals. Telling the family about their infant's death in one breath and asking for an autopsy with the next is not appropriate. Parents need time to deal with the reality of the death, including seeing and holding their infant and being with each other and supportive others before they are even ready to think about an autopsy. Consideration of the family's feelings and stage of grief greatly enhances communication with the professional. Reasons for the autopsy, including a possible answer to the question of why their infant died or was deformed, are important to discuss in a relaxed and unhurried manner.[2] Parents may feel rushed to make a decision without clearly understanding the advantages and disadvantages and resist the emotional topic of a postmortem examination. Time for discussion with an empathetic professional, as well as between themselves, facilitates an informed parental decision; sometimes consultation with a religious leader is necessary.

The professional who receives permission for an autopsy is then obliged to discuss with the parents all findings.[2,73,166] This may entail more than one meeting with the parents because they should be informed of the findings as soon as they are available.[113] Therefore, the professional may meet with them within 24 hours of completing the autopsy to discuss gross and preliminary findings and again 2 to 8 weeks later to discuss microscopic results.[78,97] Autopsy data may indicate either a condition that has implications for subsequent pregnancies or one that has little chance of recurrence.[2] The need for genetic counseling for future pregnancies may be evident from autopsy results.[120] Discussing the results with the report in hand and offering parents a copy for future reference are also important.

ANTICIPATORY GUIDANCE

Encounters with parents after the death of their infant give professionals the opportunity for anticipatory guidance/information about what to expect from themselves and from others.[66,72] Reactions to perinatal loss differ markedly, so family, friends, and acquaintances may not act as parents might expect. Some will be supportive and emotionally empathetic, especially if they have suffered a perinatal loss. Others will be uncomfortable and, not knowing what to say or do, may choose to avoid the couple and never mention the loss, even in future conversations. Those who are unaware of the loss may question the newly nonpregnant parents about the new infant. These inquiries are both awkward and painful.

Knowledge of the universal feelings and behaviors associated with grief gives comfort and relief to parents. Knowing what to expect from grief (i.e., how it progresses and how long it takes) is valuable to those who are or will be experiencing it.[53,72,78,114,172] Knowing the stages of grief and that the accompanying behaviors and emotions are normal decreases the feeling of "going crazy." Recovery from the loss takes time and cannot be hurried or ignored. The most difficult time is immediately after birth and the first few months after the loss (2–4 months).[60] The emotions of grief begin to lessen toward the end of the first year.

Parents should be encouraged to support and care for each other in their time of loss. Professionals should advocate mutual support by a free expression of feelings and emotions between the parents. Although parents need each other during grief, they also need an identified support system with whom to talk and cry. Reaching outside of the nuclear family to friends, extended family, and professionals should be encouraged.[19,40,114] Professionals have a responsibility to ask to whom parents turn for help and support in a crisis. If there are no identified supportive others, parents must know whom to call for help in the initial bereavement period.

Anticipatory guidance is also essential at the discharge of an infant with an anomaly, a preterm, or a previously ill newborn. Knowing what to expect when going home with an infant with a defect or an infant who has been hospitalized for months makes the transition from hospital to society easier for parents. Evaluation of the grief process, the attachment level of the parents to a less-than-perfect infant, and the presence or potential for postpartum depression (see Chapter 29) is vital.

LONG-TERM FOLLOW-UP CARE

Assessing the health and functioning of parents over the first year after the death of their infant is essential because of the effect of their loss.[171] Follow-up care and contact with professionals assists grieving parents.* A study of bereaved parents highlighted their needs for follow-up: (1) appointments should be scheduled with the neonatologist soon after the baby's death and certainly within 2 months, even if autopsy results are unavailable; (2) appointments should be held in a setting away from the hospital; (3) families value the professionals' efforts to determine how they are coping; (4) families value full, frank, sensitively delivered information and reassurance that enable them to understand what happened and to assess their future risks; and (5) families do not want false reassurances, half truths, and broken promises.[97] Follow-up meetings function as a catharsis for parents, as well as an opportunity for assessment, counseling (psychologic and genetic), and possibly referral. Primary care providers (physicians, nurses, and social workers) from the perinatal care setting may provide follow-up. One study documented a significant decrease in the intensity of a mother's grief after stillbirth when she received one telephone call from the physician.[112] For the family, relating to providers with whom a relationship has been established may be easier than establishing a new relationship with a stranger.[19,25,114] However, being with those who are associated with the loss event may be uncomfortable for the parents at the height of their grief. For the professional, the ability to continue to be a source of help and comfort to

---

*References 19, 40, 66, 113, 114, 171.

families with whom they have established a relationship may help complete the family's grief reactions. Maintaining contact with the family may be painful as the professional relives the feelings of grief and loss associated with sharing their tragedy. Although painful, this reexperience of intense feelings gives both parents and professionals another opportunity to work toward grief resolution.

When and where to provide continuing care for families are crucial questions. Contact in the perinatal care setting both at the time of death and daily until discharge provides immediate care. However, when discharged, too often the family returns home alone to face weeks and months of unsupported and lonely grief. Without feedback about their normal reaction and society's expectations that they will shortly be "back to normal," they are abandoned to their emotions. They suffer in silence and often drift apart in their misery. With their support system withdrawn but still feeling overwhelmed with grief, parents describe the period between 2 and 4 months after the loss as the most difficult time.[73] At 2 months after perinatal loss, parents show increased symptoms of anxiety and depression that are reduced by 8 months but still higher than in parents not experiencing perinatal loss.[157] Follow-up care from professionals is most meaningful and needed by parents during this period when they feel deserted by previously supportive others.[66] Parents experience a need for spiritual support weeks and months after the loss. Meeting with families sooner (within weeks of their loss) may alleviate the effect of decreasing support as the months go by. The professional who acknowledges the withdrawal of others but can be relied on to be available provides the parents with the emotional anchor of long-term care and support.

Breaking appointments or continually not being available may be resistance to follow-up contact with the professionals but also represents a reluctance to return to the perinatal care setting with its painful memories. A visit from the professional in the home provides a nonthreatening, familiar environment for follow-up care. The more comfortable home environment enables assessment of family interactions and facilitates communication at the "feeling" level.

Each family member and the family as a unit must be assessed for their place in the grief process as follows:

- In what stage of grief is each family member?
- Is anyone "stuck" in a stage of grief?
- Are behaviors appropriate for normal grief reactions, or do altered behaviors represent pathologic grief reactions?
- Do altered behaviors warrant referral for further treatment and evaluation?
- Do the caregiving and attachment behaviors of the parents reflect resolution of grief over loss of the perfect child and adoption of the less-than-perfect child as the love object?

Just because everything was progressing normally at previous encounters does not mean that it should be assumed to still be so. As the flood of initial grief subsides, problems and questions that were not considered suddenly become of great concern. For the first time in months, the regressive behavior of siblings not only may be noticed but also may be extremely annoying to parents. The beginning of grief resolution may allow future projections such as "When can I have another baby?" or the dread of the painful anniversary of the loss.

Referral to public health nurses or visiting nursing services in the community for follow-up care is appropriate. However, a written referral alone is not enough. Involving them in the hospital care and discharge planning is essential for a smooth transition to home care. Having the new professional meet the family in the hospital with the primary care providers facilitates trust transference from the familiar to the unfamiliar. Traditionally, home care providers have been involved in care of normal mothers and infants in the community. Involvement in perinatal loss situations requires knowledge about the process of grief and willingness to share the grief of the parents. Because these may be new skills for many, continuing education programs that teach the theory and skills of effective intervention help the professional be more comfortable with a perinatal loss situation.

Additional expertise may be warranted when the professional recognizes signs and symptoms of pathologic grief, complicated or absent grief, or concurrent multiple stresses or losses. Parents may not be ready for genetic counseling, infant stimulation programs, or financial programs until months later. Between 3 and 6 months after their loss, parents may be ready to reach outside of the nuclear and extended family for help and support for the first time.[126] Suggesting a local hospital support group or the local chapter of a national support organization may at first be met with resistance. Leaving the names and phone numbers of such organizations ensures that the parents have the information at their disposal when they are ready to use it. Until their own support system has withdrawn, parents may not be ready for a support group of other parents.[126]

Throughout this section, examples of what to say and how to say it have been used to illustrate helpful interventions for grieving families. It is essential to state that there are no "scripts." Parents do not say something and the professionals answer with a parroted response. Each encounter is a unique situation consisting of distinct parental and professional personalities. Each situation must be evaluated separately and individual interventions instituted.[66,114] It is recommended that the professional learn by observing an experienced colleague with grieving families and that the professional "practice" with role playing and situation solving before actually attempting to intervene with the parents.[5] Use of formalized education about grief, loss, and bereavement is also recommended for health care providers.[53,93]

Innovative bereavement programs have been developed to provide families and staff with support and follow-up care.[44,66,126,130] Such programs[44,66] provide education and assistance to the health care providers who care for the family at the time of their infant's death. There is follow-up care to the family for up to 1 year after the death of their infant.[66] Perinatal bereavement programs may include intergenerational services in which parents, grandparents, and siblings participate together in education and services.[130] Bereavement programs provide the needed support, education, and help to families, as well as to staff. Use of a couples-oriented program enables the following[126]:

- Participation in the group at 3 to 5 months after the loss when most other support systems have ceased
- Ability of partners to share with the group and each other gender-related differences in grief experiences
- Opportunity for men to share and hear about other men's feelings and coping skills
- Opportunity for couples to learn to tolerate their differences in grief processing and to process their grief together
- Enhancement and preservation of the couple's relationship

Having an evaluation tool to assess and continually change and improve the program is essential.[66,126]

CHILDREN AND GRIEF

Explaining and helping a surviving child to understand the loss of an infant is an enormous task for parents.[145] Facilitating the child's normal feelings of sadness, worry, and anger after a loss may be difficult for parents who fear being flooded with their own emotions. Unresolved grief from the parents' own childhood may prevent the expression of grief by their children.

To maintain the myth of childhood (innocent happiness), children are often shielded from any knowledge about death, even when it is an inevitable event in their lives. Thus, children are prevented from full realization, validation, and expression of their feelings and emotions. They cannot formalize and express their grief over the loss of a significant person, are at increased risk for the development of complicated grief, emotional and behavioral problems, including psychiatric issues, as children and adults and are unable to process their grief into reconciling a future life without their sibling.[23,71,89]

Children are called the "forgotten mourners."[18,162] Although adults are encouraged to cry, talk, and gradually understand and integrate their feelings of grief, no one helps the child deal with the same frightening feelings. No one discusses the loss with the child, because "He might cry" and because of the adult's inadequacy and lack of understanding of how to respond and what to say. No amount of secrecy or denial of the situation will hide the fact that the child is being excluded from an important family event.

Attempts to protect children from feelings of grief and mourning because of death or other important losses isolate the child. Age and developmentally appropriate explanations include the child in the family's experience, rather than separating and excluding him or her from what is happening. Shielding children from the knowledge of death denies them the reality of life and the opportunity for personal growth and mastery of the experience. Often in America, the subject of death, like that of sex, is taboo for children.

A child's grief and mourning in response to perinatal loss depend on his or her cognitive and developmental level, the extent of prenatal attachment and expectation about the infant, the degree of ambivalent feelings, and the response of the parents to the death. Because the child's understanding of death differs from that of adults, knowledge of the stages of growing awareness is essential for both parents and professionals working with children experiencing grief (Box 30-7).[89,162] Regardless of age or developmental stage, the universal fear of childhood is the fear of separation and abandonment. For a young child (younger than 5 years), the loss of the infant is experienced indirectly through parental grief. A young child reacts to the emotional withdrawal of grieving parents and fears loss of them (and their love).

Although children at different developmental stages have their own conceptions of death, adults must provide them with the facts about the situation in language that they can understand. They may benefit from guidance by the nurse, social worker, or other health professional about beneficial approaches to facilitate the child's grief work.[122] The professional serves as a resource, role model, and support system to parents and other family members in caring for their surviving children. Printed and videotaped materials are also available to assist parents in helping their other children understand death (see "Resource Materials for Parents" at the end of this chapter). Age-appropriate storybooks concerning death can facilitate grief

BOX 30-7	CRITICAL FINDINGS
	A CHILD'S DEVELOPING CONCEPT OF DEATH

AGE	COGNITIVE UNDERSTANDING	HOW EXPERIENCED
Infant (to 12 mo)	None	Indirectly through parental grief expressed in: Emotional withdrawal Inability to provide concern and continuity in caregiving behaviors Overconcern for fear of recurrent loss Changes in eating, elimination and sleep patterns; unresponsive to parental holding and cuddling[89]
Toddler (1–3 yr)	Little understanding of cause and effect Death may be confused with sleeping or being away	React to changes in behavior of grieving parents and reflect their feelings and anxiety Changes in sleep, behaviors (shy, aggressive, acting out, attention-seeking, angry), regressive behaviors (enuresis, loss of skills) and complaints of headaches and stomach aches[89]
Preschooler (3–6 yr)	View death as a temporary state and not an inevitable occurrence Believe that they are the center of the universe and can do anything, and that thinking is doing (thoughts have the power of actions)	Expect the dead to return—ask questions about "when?" Changes in sleep, behaviors (shy, aggressive, acting out, attention-seeking, angry), regressive behaviors (enuresis, loss of skills) and complaints of headaches and stomach aches[89]
School age (6–12 yr)	Understand that death is inevitable and irreversible; 6- to 9-yr-olds personify death as a separate person (skeleton; bogeyman) About 8 yrs old: "death phobia," a normal developmental stage characterized by preoccupation with thoughts of own death and that of loved one Reasons concretely with ability to see cause-and-effect relationships	Realize death occurs in adults like parents and even in children; realize death is permanent, not temporary state May show interest in biologic aspects of death and details of funeral Changes in sleep, behaviors (loneliness, isolation, acting-out, sad, unhappy, depressed, anxious and fearful, aggressive, attention-seeking), difficulties with school work as a result of inability to concentrate, headaches and stomach aches, regressive behaviors (enuresis)[89]
Adolescent (12 yr)	Able to think abstractly about death like the adult; philosophic reasoning	Similar to that in adult

Modified from American Academy of Pediatrics, Committee on Psychosocial Aspects of Child and Family Health: The pediatrician and childhood bereavement, *Pediatrics* 105:445, 2000; Gardner SL, Merenstein GB: Helping families deal with perinatal loss, *Neonatal Netw* 5:17, 1986.

discussion and elicit questions and feelings from children.

Just as grieving adults need repetition, children need repeated explanations and discussions about the loss. Constantly in a state of developmental flux, the child attempts to view the loss in new ways as a result of increasing maturation. Asking questions (usually at inopportune times) and making comments about the infant are ways the child continues to process the experience, often long after the parents have completed it. These questions and comments may seem endless and resurrect the parent's own grief. The child's inquiries must be encouraged and supported so that he or she knows that talking about the loss or death is acceptable. Exploring the child's feelings for fears of causation, guilt, or the wonder if "death is catching" enables them to be dealt with appropriately. Truthful discussion with the child dispels the worst fears and fantasies and replaces them with reality that is "not too horrible to discuss" with parents. If the cause of the infant's death is known, it should be explained to the child in simple, direct terms: "Baby Bobby couldn't breathe by himself because his lungs were sick. His sick lungs only happen to little babies."

In one study, bereaved children had more frequent health care contacts for symptoms (e.g., abdominal pain, enuresis, headaches, insomnia) with no organic cause in the year after their loss.[85] Subsequent illness may precipitate worry by the child that he or she, too, will die. Often, this fear is not verbalized but acted out by significant behavioral changes such as withdrawal, clinging, whining, or overactivity that is uncharacteristic for the child. Verbal reassurance that the child will not die and a reminder that "the baby died of a sickness that only little babies get; big boys and girls can't get it" are helpful.

The normal feelings that accompany grief should be acknowledged and explained to the child. "Mommy and Daddy feel sad that Baby Jean died. Sometimes we will cry because we feel sad. It's okay to cry when you feel sad." Permission for the expression of the child's feelings should also be given verbally: "You might feel sad, too. It's okay for you to cry when you're sad. Then we will talk about how you are feeling." Encouraging children to draw or write their feelings is another way of giving them permission to express their grief.

Using words such as "went away," "expired," "lost," or "went to sleep" is dangerous in describing death to children. Because young children are concrete and literal, they think they might die if they "go to sleep" or that anyone who leaves them is in danger of dying. Children also relate current experiences to past ones and interpret "lost" quite literally. In the mind of the child, if the parent only searched well enough, the misplaced (i.e., "lost") child would be found.

Including children at funeral or memorial services facilitates their grief and prevents exclusion from a significant family event.[68,89] Consideration of the family value system, age of the child, and religious customs must enter into the decision to include the child. Adequate preparation includes a discussion of everything the child will see, hear, and feel, including the normal adult emotions of crying and sadness. An adult other than the grieving parents should accompany the child to reiterate what is happening and to meet the child's physical and psychologic needs. Adult support is necessary so that the child can express and deal with his or her feelings.

Helping children with their grief is also therapeutic for parents. Assisting children to master the crisis of loss ultimately augments the parents' self-esteem and restores confidence in their parenting skills.[78] Parents can deal in a healthy way with their own grief when they can facilitate the grief of their other children. Qualitative studies revealed parental spiritual needs and support of siblings after a perinatal loss[67,98]:

- Recognition and acknowledgment of the child's grief, which included listening and answering questions honestly; interpreting and acknowledging the meaning of the child's behaviors; shielding from the insensitivity of others; and knowing when support of the child would be more effectively handled by someone outside the immediate household
- Inclusion of the child in family events, rituals, and practices such as visiting, holding, and touching the baby in the hospital; attending the funeral/memorial service; and visiting the gravesite
- Keeping the baby alive in the family's memory by encouraging questions and comments about the baby; expressing feelings about the loss; including in viewing photos and personal items of the baby; and recognizing the deceased infant in birthday/holiday celebrations

PATHOLOGIC GRIEF

The absence of grief when it would be expected is not a healthy sign but, rather, a cause for concern.[73] The emotions of grief and their expression are healing. Early and full expression of grief is associated with an optimal outcome.[73] However, many people in grief-producing situations attempt to avoid the pain of grief and the expression of emotions, the result of which prolongs mourning, delays a return to the previous lifestyle, prevents the creation of new attachments and relationships, and ultimately results in pathologic grief (see Box 30-5).[73,162]

Not grieving precludes opportunities for growth and change. No new coping styles will be attempted. No novel alternatives to problem solving and adapting to a crisis will be added to the repertoire of behavior for future use. In other words, those who choose not to do grief work say "no" to their own potential and remain frozen in development.[104] Under the stress of not resolving their grief, some may even regress in their development.

Reproductive loss is a blow to self-concept and self-esteem, as well as loss of the infant. Blocking appropriate feelings of loss, grief, and anger results in a significant decrease in one's sense of self-esteem.[35] After death of their neonates, 33% of mothers suffered severe and tragic outcomes (including psychoses, phobias, anxiety attacks, and deep depression; see Chapter 29).[78,172] Those who cannot effectively resolve their grief may suffer lifelong emotional damage[92]; however, some empirical research shows that those who suppress feelings of grief may recover with relatively few difficulties.[9]

Not working through grief associated with repetitive contact with perinatal loss also affects the staff.[46] To cope with feelings, they may hide behind a "professional" demeanor characterized by decreased spontaneity and withdrawal. Such a provider defends against the repeated pain of loss by emotional dissociation from the situation. The real self does not respond; instead, the professional stays in the role of the omnipotent, unemotional physician or nurse. The result, self-alienation, eventually desensitizes the professional to the experience and ultimately prevents any empathy with the experience of others.[69] Emotions that cannot be acknowledged or expressed healthily are vented in ways that may be destructive to relationships in personal and professional life.

Unresolved grief does not disappear and is not dissipated. The emotions accompanying grief may never be expressed but are not forgotten by the unconscious mind. Containment of these emotions through repression or suppression takes psychic energy. A conscious, intentional decision to postpone or dismiss grief to meet others' needs or to meet immediate demands of the loss situation (e.g., funeral arrangements/care of a surviving multiple) is called *delayed grief*.[84,92,114] For a period of time (days, weeks, or longer), there is little or no grief response when such a reaction would be expected and appropriate. Delayed grief also may be the result of repression—the unconscious content seems to have a life and energy of its own that become the sources of later emotional conflict.

Grief that is inhibited and never resolved is called *abortive*.[92] Those who have aborted their grief work often live bereft of *joie de vivre* with no interest, concern, or enthusiasm for life. *Complicated grief*, a failure to transition from acute grief to integrating grief and resuming a fulfilling life, occurs when there is no movement (6 months after the loss) beyond the feelings of acute grief.[105] Inability to function in daily life, accompanied by intense longing and yearning for the deceased, failure to accept the reality of the death, overwhelming guilt, and detaching from family and friends characterize complicated grief and must be distinguished from major depression.[76,105] Complicated grief is more common after the loss of a child, including a perinatal loss.[76,99] One study of parents at 6 and 18 months after the loss of a child in PICU found a decrease in complicated grief symptoms during the studied time period, with some parents still retaining high symptom levels.[99] Although only 10% to 20% of those experiencing grief and loss have complicated grief, referral for intervention from mental health professionals is required.[105,173] Studies of Internet-based cognitive therapy for perinatal loss showed significant reduction in grief, PTSD, and depression in the treated group, thus preventing the development of complicated grief.[74,75]

Grief that is not resolved remains buried in the psyche, waiting for an opportunity to "rear its ugly head." A current loss may remind the psyche of the unmourned grief from a previous loss or losses.[45] As the two (or more) losses become intertwined and are experienced as one and the same, repressed emotions of unresolved grief pour forth. Grieving more than one loss or a lifetime of losses is more difficult and emotionally draining than grieving one event at a time.[45] Cumulative grief work also may be occurring when a current loss of seemingly little importance overwhelms the person with intense emotions.[45,92] This flood of emotions seems disproportionate to the current loss and is only peripherally related to it. The unconscious, unresolved grief is finally uncovered when the individual is flooded with emotions. Thus, aspects of unresolved grief from the past[161] may influence the emotional components of any grief reaction.

Grief and loss events of the perinatal period have been equated only for a relatively short time (about 30 years).[111] Because loss during the perinatal period is a common experience, many childbearing and older women (and men) have never grieved over their spontaneous abortion, stillbirth, or neonatal death, even 10 to 20 years after its occurrence. Parents (or grandparents) in a current perinatal loss situation also may be dealing with unresolved grief from a previous perinatal loss. Unresolved grief (whether from perinatal or other loss events of life) may become available for resolution in subsequent crisis events. A mother who delivers a normal healthy newborn, yet is depressed postpartally, may not have postpartum depression. Instead, she may be grieving the unresolved loss of a spontaneous abortion, therapeutic abortion, or other perinatal loss. The normal grief reaction accompanying relinquishment may persist and often leads to chronic unresolved grief that may present itself during and after a subsequent pregnancy.[8] Her depressed mood could also be resulting from unresolved grief from the loss of a parent, spouse, or child. Depressed menopausal women may be experiencing the cumulative effects of a lifetime of unresolved grief (Box 30-8).

Recognizing unresolved grief has implications for facilitating grief work in a current loss, episodic care, and health maintenance. The energy to keep unresolved emotions restrained could better be used in personal growth and development, grieving, and

maintaining and establishing relationships. The lifelong stress of unresolved grief contributes to both psychologic and physical illness, including increased death rates and an earlier death.[121]

Not grieving a perinatal loss affects the individual involved and the relationships with significant others, including present and future children. Resolution of maternal grief about the infant's prematurity, as well as the quality of maternal interaction, are necessary for secure infant attachment.[140] Asynchronous grief and the absence of grief in one or more family members weaken and strain family relationships.[14,40,78,105] The irritability and preoccupation of normal grief may overly disrupt the family. Differences may be magnified to the extent that major rifts and disruptions in the relationship occur, resulting in increased incidence of strained marital relationships, separation, and divorce.[14,76,78,105]

Exclusive dedication to the care of a malformed or ill infant to the detriment of other family relationships is symptomatic of a pathologic grief reaction.[78,143,170] The parent who neglects other children, the couple's relationship, and social outlets is so overwhelmed with guilt about having caused the baby's defect that nothing else in life matters. This guilty attachment and exclusive dedication are ways of avoiding grief work.[143] Other forms of pathologic reactions include parental rejection and intolerance of the deformed or ill infant.[78]

The parent who is emotionally withdrawn and unavailable to the family because of chronic grief and depression cannot attach to and care for present or subsequent children. Aberrant parenting styles (resulting in a vulnerable, battered, or failure-to-thrive child) may be the result of prolonged separation, unresolved grief, or grief that has progressed beyond the anticipatory phase, so that emotional ties with the infant have been severed.[78] These difficulties with caring and parenting may affect the deformed or ill child and all the children in the family. In turn, these children may grow up unable to parent subsequent generations because of the type of ineffectual parenting they received. Parents who grieve inappropriately may leave their children a legacy of psychosocial problems such as difficulty with separation, independence, and control (e.g., school phobia and toilet training); failure to thrive; and sleep disturbances.

Planning for a new pregnancy and another baby should begin after the grief process for the lost

BOX 30-8	CRITICAL FINDINGS
	SYMPTOMS OF UNRESOLVED GRIEF

1. Vivid memory for the details of the perinatal loss event
2. Flashback to the event
3. Anniversary grief (date of birth or expected date of delivery)
4. Emotions of grief (sadness, anger, or crying) when talking about loss
5. Intense emotions with subsequent loss or crisis

infant is complete (about 6–12 months), so that parents are emotionally ready to invest in a relationship with another fetus/newborn.[78] A national survey of U.S. obstetricians found that two-thirds of the respondents endorsed a waiting time of less than 6 months for subsequent pregnancy after stillbirth.[54] The researchers concluded that this was a "provocative" finding because short interpregnancy intervals are associated with increased fetal risks for poorer outcomes.[54] Because the decision to become pregnant is highly personal and individual, many women are pregnant within 6 to 12 months after a perinatal loss.[64,128] Some women see a subsequent pregnancy as a "cure" for their overwhelming feelings of emptiness and failure,[163] whereas others are averse to a subsequent pregnancy. Pregnancy after a perinatal loss is characterized by (1) increased pregnancy anxiety, a heightened fear, concern, and vigilance about the pregnancy and baby; (2) comparisons of current and previous pregnancies; (3) less attachment to the current versus the previous pregnancy; (4) a desire to see and phone the health care provider more often; (5) a desire for more prenatal testing; and (6) the subsequent pregnancy possibly being the precipitating event for PTSD in both mothers and fathers.* Mothers appreciate being educated by

---

*References 6, 15, 30, 32, 33, 42, 109, 153, 154, 161.

their health care providers about the benefits and risks of subsequent pregnancies so that they can make an informed choice.[42] Benefits of postponing pregnancy include (1) enabling physiologic recovery from pregnancy before another is attempted; (2) enabling psychologic recovery, progression of grief work, and an optimal state to emotionally invest in a new pregnancy and newborn; (3) avoiding anniversary dates with the second pregnancy/child; and (4) improving the maternal-infant relationship—less anxiety, overprotectiveness, overindulgence, and hypervigilance.[109,161] The time necessary for physical and emotional recovery varies widely, and parents may benefit from interconceptual counseling after a perinatal loss.[105,161]

REFERENCES

For a full list of references, scan the QR code or visit http://booksite.elsevier.com/9780323320832.

31 DISCHARGE PLANNING AND FOLLOW-UP OF THE NEONATAL INTENSIVE CARE UNIT INFANT

ANGEL CARTER, LINDA GRATNY, AND BRIAN S. CARTER

Parents with infants in the neonatal intensive care unit (NICU) have immediate worries about whether their newborn infant will survive but soon thereafter start having concerns about how their child will do through infancy and into adulthood. As the infant's convalescence begins, so does discharge planning; this brings to the forefront questions about outcomes. Unfortunately, it is almost impossible to know the outcome of any individual infant at the time of discharge from the NICU. Caregivers within the NICU must be knowledgeable of the latest outcomes literature to respond to these questions and to guide parents in the importance of follow-up care.[145]

Of the many reasons that newborns require neonatal intensive care, the most common one is preterm birth. Numerous publications report the outcomes of very-low-birth-weight (VLBW; birth weights less than 1500 g) and extremely low-birth-weight (ELBW; birth weights less than 1000 g).[4,27,94] Recent studies have focused on the survival and outcome of even more immature infants with birth weights below 750 g, or on infants born at the limits of viability, 22 to 25 weeks of gestation.[27,69,83,96,147] Late-preterm infants have been a topic of renewed interest because they are at risk for a unique set of problems with adverse outcomes.[3,52,82,147] Infants with intrauterine growth restriction (IUGR) are also vulnerable to a wide range of complications requiring neonatal intensive care, especially if they are also preterm and experience extrauterine growth failure.[55,84,112] Full-term infants may also require intensive care due to perinatal or neonatal conditions and are at risk for health and developmental sequelae.[133] Finally, a number of infants with congenital anomalies require surgery and/or neonatal intensive care.

PLANNING FOR DISCHARGE

An organized, well-implemented discharge plan is the beginning of successful follow-up of a NICU graduate. A family-centered multidisciplinary team approach uses the expertise of many disciplines, along with the family, to formulate and implement the discharge and follow-up plan. The team can comprise parents, grandparents, other caregivers, physicians, nurses, case managers, dietitians, therapists, developmental specialists, and social workers.

Integrating family-centered principles into the discharge process as a continuation of family-centered care practiced throughout the NICU stay facilitates better parental adaptation to the transition to home.[65] For many infants, the NICU stay has been lengthy and complex, and families may experience varying degrees of anxiety and stress as they prepare for the infant to come home. In some cases, attachment and bonding may have been affected by a long, complicated medical course.[42] A survey of preterm mothers found

PURPLE type highlights content that is particularly applicable to clinical settings.

that symptoms of psychologic distress (fatigue, depressive mood, anxiety, physical symptoms) persisted up to a year after the birth of their premature baby.[60] Families may need extra attention paid to these issues before they can successfully attend to the discharge process. A thorough assessment of caregiver needs, environmental issues, and knowledge of their infant's care before discharge is an important part of the planning process. Implementation of a parent educational-behavioral intervention program during the NICU stay may be one mechanism to reduce stress, depression, and anxiety and effect more positive interactions of parents with their infant, a shorter NICU stay, and shorter total hospital stay.[89]

Considerations Before Discharge

INSURANCE

Many parents may need assistance to enroll their infant in their existing insurance policy or to identify the procedures necessary to apply for medical assistance. This process can take many weeks and must be accomplished before discharge in order to select a pediatrician for follow-up care and arrange outpatient subspecialty care as needed. Outpatient physician visits, therapies, medical supplies, medications, and nutritional supplements are often reimbursed differently than inpatient services. Out-of-pocket costs can escalate quickly and add additional challenges for families. Social workers, case managers, and financial counselors are valuable resources to assist families in this process.

IDENTIFICATION OF A FOLLOW-UP PROVIDER

A pediatric health care professional to follow the infant after discharge, trained in the care of NICU graduates, should be identified before discharge. Ideally, this provider has been identified early in the admission to facilitate regular communications regarding the infant's medical course. In a 1992 policy statement, the American Academy of Pediatrics (AAP) attempted to define the concept of a medical home for children. Multiple challenges with implementation led to an updated definition with additional designations specific to medical conditions.[5] As defined, a medical home is considered to be the ideal practice for the health care management of children, although challenges

remain with resource allocation, role definitions, and implementation.[5,10]

Immediately before discharge, a written summary should be provided to the provider, with follow-up recommendations regarding nutrition and growth, developmental surveillance, and subspecialty referrals, along with verbal notification of the discharge date. Parents should be advised to keep this summary with the infant at all times because this written documentation of the NICU stay is invaluable if the infant needs to be seen on an emergency basis shortly after hospital discharge. Providing families with a "care notebook" containing specialized forms and organizing tools can be a valuable addition to the discharge process, particularly for those with anticipated complex follow-up needs. Information to compile care plans for children with special health care needs can be found on a number of websites, for example, the National Institute for Children's Health Quality Medical Home, the AAP Medical Home, and others.

CAREGIVER EDUCATION

In a family-centered environment, families have been partners in caring for their infant throughout the hospital stay. Discharge teaching then becomes a process of reinforcing and attending to final details. In some instances, however, this teaching may be limited by the inability of the family to be present because of transportation and family or job constraints. In these cases, readiness of the caregivers and home environment should be thoroughly evaluated (Box 31-1). Infants with complex equipment and care needs at the time of discharge may require skilled nursing support in the home in order to be candidates for discharge from the hospital.

HOME EQUIPMENT

Any necessary durable medical equipment or supplies, such as an apnea monitor, pulse oximeter, feeding pump, ventilator, suction equipment, or oxygen for home use, should be delivered to the hospital before discharge to give parents practice using the equipment. When a home apnea monitor is used, a clear plan outlining the reasons for initiating home monitoring and the indications for discontinuing it should be discussed with the family and the primary care provider before discharge. The company supplying the equipment should provide training in its use and an agreement for maintenance

BOX
31-1 CAREGIVER EDUCATION

- Every encounter with the parents is a teaching opportunity. Assess each individual family's readiness for discharge.
- Inform parents verbally and in writing about the tests included in the newborn genetic screening and how they will receive the results.
- Teach parents the special nutritional needs of preterm infants after discharge, including nutritional supplementation, lactation support and intervention to promote breastfeeding, and use of alternative feeding methods, if necessary.
- Teach parents the importance of maintaining their infant on home oxygen therapy (e.g., for growth and development, sleep, and feeding) at designated pulse oximetry targets until pulse oximetry studies (e.g., awake, feeding, asleep) document that the infant can tolerate weaning and discontinuing the supplemental oxygen.
- Teach parents to dress their infant appropriately to maintain adequate axillary temperature.
- Teach parents appropriate safety precautions:
  - Proper positioning (supine) for sleep: "Back to Sleep."
  - Proper use of car seats.
  - Importance of a smoke-free environment.
  - *NEVER shake the baby!* Dangers of shaking infants include blindness, brain damage, developmental delays, seizures, paralysis, and death.
  - Information, in writing, about all medications for their infant including name, action, dose, route, side effects, schedule.
  - Provide parents opportunity to participate in infant CPR class.
- Teach parents the importance of follow-up care and appointments:
  - Timely follow-up for infants with ROP provided verbally and in writing.
  - Timely follow-up for hearing screen and referral for rescreening.
  - Need for monthly RSV immunizations throughout the RSV season.
- Give parents the newborn immunization record.
- Teach parents the importance of their own self-care, and assist in identifying resources for support.

CPR, Cardiopulmonary resuscitation; *ROP,* retinopathy of prematurity; *RSV,* respiratory syncytial virus.

and service support while equipment is being used in the home. NICU nurses or respiratory therapists should verify the parents' understanding of the purpose of the equipment and its operation and also ensure that home caregivers for the baby have been trained in cardiopulmonary resuscitation (CPR). The family should be provided a clear contact number to the clinician who will be managing the home equipment.

ROOMING-IN

Whether or not an infant is going home with equipment, giving family caregivers the opportunity to provide "independent" care of their infant with professional caregivers nearby for assistance has been shown to increase parental competence and provide confirmation of readiness for independent care at home.[33,102] One intensive care nursery's experience in establishing a step-down unit where mothers provided all basic care for their infant under supervision resulted in earlier discharge to home with no increases in short-term complications or readmissions.[29]

DISCHARGE CRITERIA

Clearly defined discharge criteria provide both the family and the staff a point of reference from which to judge the infant's progress. Discharge criteria should be reviewed in a multidisciplinary team meeting with the family. Setting goals that the infant, parents, and staff must accomplish before discharge helps keep everyone focused and prevents important components of the discharge process from being overlooked.

For preterm infants, the attainment of a minimum weight is no longer the criterion for discharge. Rather, the ability of a preterm or recovering neonate to maintain physiologic stability and the ability of the family to care for the infant's physiologic and developmental needs dictate the infant's readiness for discharge (Box 31-2). There are significant variations across NICUs for specific discharge criteria, with assessment of apnea and feeding behavior significantly influencing the duration of hospitalization in a healthy preterm infant. The AAP policy statement, "Hospital Discharge of the High-Risk Neonate," provides guidance that should minimize such variations.[6]

TRANSFER

Some infants are not discharged home from the regional or tertiary NICU but, instead, are transferred from a regional referral center to a community unit or facility for the duration of their remaining hospital stay. Transfer to a community hospital may be beneficial to families because they are often closer to the parents' home (especially if the NICU is part of a regional referral center). Possible locations for transfer, as well as the criteria for transfer and financial implications to the family, should be discussed with the

Infant
- Sustained weight gain of sufficient duration
- Maintain normal body temperature, clothed in an open bed, at normal room temperature (20° to 25° C)
- Establish and maintain competent breastfeeding or bottle feeding without cardiopulmonary problems
- Nutrition assessment and dietary management provided as indicated
- Hematologic assessment and management provided as indicated
- Documented physiologically mature and stable cardiopulmonary function of sufficient duration
- Parents have been given a report of neurodevelopmental and neurobehavioral status
- Completed metabolic, hearing, and indicated funduscopic screenings
- Appropriately immunized, including respiratory syncytial virus prophylaxis and plan for subsequent injections
- A completed car seat evaluation
- A completed review of the hospital course, pending medical problems noted, and follow-up plans identified
- A home-care plan, individualized to the patient's needs, has been provided by all disciplines

Parents, Family, and Home Environment
- Identify and assess at least two caregivers for home.
- Assess psychosocial and parenting strengths and risks.
- Consider the home environment and on-site visit as indicated.

- Review resource availability (including financial, utilities, and transportation).
- Determine caregiver availability, ability, and commitment to the following:
  - Provide basic infant care: diapering, bathing, dressing, cord and circumcision care.
  - Maintain infant's thermal state: able to take temperature and dress appropriately.
  - Feed infant (breast, bottle, or alternative method—nasogastric tube, gastrostomy, parenteral nutrition), and demonstrate formula preparation if required.
  - Manage home feeding tube, infusion pump, intestinal stoma care, and other devices as indicated.
  - Manage home monitoring, oxygen, and other equipment as indicated; address initial problem solving; demonstrate CPR and initial emergency interventions.
  - Maintain safe environment, car seat, heat, electricity, telephone, transportation, smoke-free, emergency resuscitation.
  - Recognize signs of illness, and identify when to call primary care provider or emergency services.
  - Have support system identified to assist in infant's care.
  - Demonstrate medication administration and recognize signs of medication adverse effects (e.g., toxicity); understand importance of follow-up care, and know whom to call for questions or concerns.
  - Caretakers to obtain influenza vaccine at beginning of influenza season.

Modified from American Academy of Pediatrics, Committee on Fetus and Newborn: Hospital discharge of the high-risk neonate, *Pediatrics* 122:1119, 2008.
CPR, Cardiopulmonary resuscitation.

parents early in the hospitalization if this is an expected possibility. Communication of a comprehensive discharge plan should take place with the receiving hospital before transfer.[70,83] As the capacity for back-transporting convalescing neonates to community hospitals has increased in the United States over the past 20 years, persistent issues of communication, trust, and psychosocial support remain for parents.[47]

EARLY DISCHARGE

Preterm infants are often discharged between 35 and 37 weeks' chronologic age after demonstrating cardiorespiratory stability, thermal stability, and adequate feeding skills.[91] Parental concerns at the time of discharge may include their own ability to have adequate rest, their readiness to learn and assume self-care and newborn care, their readiness to parent, and availability of support systems. Concerns about the newborn may include transition from the intensive care nursery to the home care environment, ability to feed and hydrate adequately, and the early development and recognition of complications.[120]

Late-preterm infants ($34^{0/7}$ to $36^{6/7}$ weeks' gestational age) are often the size of full-term newborns, but are physiologically and metabolically immature.[60] Tomashek and colleagues[132] demonstrated that late-preterm, early-discharged, breastfed infants were 1.5 times more likely to require hospital-related care and 2.2 times more likely to be readmitted than term infants who were breastfed, with jaundice and infection accounting for the majority of readmissions. Timing of discharge of preterm infants should be individualized based on physiologic maturity and feeding competency. Late-preterm infants usually do not meet the necessary competencies for discharge before 48 hours of age.[60] A follow-up visit for medical assessment is recommended for 24 to 48 hours after discharge.[60]

Screening

GENETIC SCREENING

Initial screening of sick or premature infants is performed as soon as possible after birth, before the administration of blood products. Although it is common for these infants to have some relatively abnormal results—especially for thyroid function or amino acid profiles while on parenteral nutrition—early screening is recommended to identify in a timely manner those infants who may have an inborn metabolic disorder, congenital endocrinopathies, or hemoglobinopathies so that early treatment can be initiated.[12,37,45] Subsequent screenings should take place according to established guidelines, depending on state requirements. Recommendations for continued screenings after discharge should be clearly outlined in the discharge summary.

HEARING

All infants should be screened for hearing loss using otoacoustic emissions or auditory brainstem response testing before discharge from the nursery.[100] This initial screening should be performed once the infant is medically stable, and if there are any concerns that warrant a secondary screen, rescreening should occur before 1 month of age. Infants who do not pass (are "referred" after secondary screening) should have a full-scale auditory diagnostic evaluation by 3 months of age. Infants with confirmed hearing loss should receive intervention by 6 months of age from an infant hearing specialist.[11,14,133] Those infants with an increased risk for hearing impairment should be assessed by a pediatric audiologist with a follow-up schedule outlined for the parents (Box 31-3). The goal of early detection and intervention is to maximize language, cognitive, literacy, and social development of the hearing impaired.[127]

VISION

Development of severe retinopathy of prematurity (ROP) may still be a concern at the time of

---

BOX 31-3 CONDITIONS ASSOCIATED WITH INCREASED RISK FOR HEARING LOSS

- Neonatal intensive care unit admission for more than 5 days or any of the following regardless of length of stay: extracorporeal membrane oxygenation, assisted ventilation, exposure to ototoxic medications (gentamicin and tobramycin) or loop diuretics (furosemide [Lasix]), hyperbilirubinemia requiring exchange transfusion
- Syndromes associated with hearing loss such as neurofibromatosis, osteopetrosis, and Usher syndrome
- Family history of hereditary childhood hearing loss
- Craniofacial abnormalities
- Congenital infections such as cytomegalovirus, toxoplasmosis, bacterial meningitis, syphilis, herpes, and rubella
- Physical findings (white forelock) associated with syndromes known to include hearing loss
- Neurodegenerative disorders (e.g., Hunter syndrome) or sensory motor neuropathies (e.g., Friedreich ataxia and Charcot-Marie-Tooth syndrome)
- Culture-positive postnatal infections such as bacterial and viral (especially herpes and varicella) meningitis
- Chemotherapy
- Caregiver concerns regarding hearing, speech, language, or developmental delay

Modified from American Academy of Pediatrics and Joint Committee on Infant Hearing, Year 2007 Position Statement: Principles and guidelines for early hearing detection and intervention programs, *Pediatrics* 120(4):898, 2007.

NICU discharge for infants born prematurely. Infants born at less than 30 weeks' gestation or less than 1500 g birth weight, and selected infants with a birth weight between 1500 and 2000 g or gestational age greater than 30 weeks with an unstable clinical course, should have a retinal screening examination with pupillary dilation.[13] Published tables make recommendations for timing of the initial examination dependent on postmenstrual age and chronologic (postnatal) age.[13] Timing of follow-up examinations should be according to the ophthalmologist's recommendations based on retinal findings. Arrangements for follow-up examinations should be made before discharge. Ophthalmologic follow-up for infants with any stage of ROP (whether they required treatment or not) is recommended at 4 to 6 months after hospital discharge.[13] Current research indicates that the risk to visual development in preterm infants does not end when the risk for ROP has passed. All infants born prematurely, whether or not they develop ROP, are at increased risk for amblyopia/strabismus and refractive errors.[104]

IMAGING

Premature infants are at increased risk for injuries to the brain, potentially causing permanent damage. The most common form of damage and the leading cause of chronic neurologic morbidity is periventricular white matter injury.[25] Identification of infants at high risk for poorer outcomes related to brain injury allows for timely referrals to early intervention therapies. A recent Cochrane review indicates that early intervention can improve cognitive outcomes up to preschool age.[128] Imaging techniques for routine screening for white matter injury have traditionally been the cranial ultrasound, although the ability of ultrasound to predict developmental outcome may be inferior to magnetic resonance imaging (MRI).[92] Woodward and colleagues[147] have reported that abnormal findings of MRI at term equivalent in very preterm infants strongly predict adverse neurodevelopmental outcomes at 2 years of age.[147] A review of MRI screening to identify risks of suboptimal neurologic outcomes suggests the following be considered as indications for screening by MRI at approximately 36 weeks' postmenstrual age[72]:

- Grade III to IV intraventricular hemorrhage
- Periventricular hemorrhagic infarction
- Cystic periventricular white matter damage
- Cerebellar hemorrhage or other abnormalities on ultrasound
- Suspected white matter abnormalities on ultrasound (echodensities/echolucencies)
- Post–hemorrhagic hydrocephalus
- Abnormal neurologic examination
- Other conditions warranting detailed neuroimaging (metabolic disorders or suspected congenital structural abnormality)

Preventive Care

IMMUNIZATIONS

Infant immunizations are recommended for all NICU infants, according to the guidelines issued by the Centers for Disease Control and Prevention (CDC) and approved by the AAP.[38] Immunizations administered in the NICU should appear in the discharge summary. When immunizations have been declined by parents, this should be clearly indicated in the discharge summary, along with follow-up recommendations.

RESPIRATORY SYNCYTIAL VIRUS INFECTION PROPHYLAXIS

Respiratory syncytial virus (RSV) infection poses a risk for serious morbidity or even death for infants who were born prematurely, especially those with chronic heart or lung disease. For qualifying infants, RSV prophylaxis should be initiated with intramuscular palivizumab before discharge into the community setting during RSV season. RSV infection prophylaxis should be coordinated with the follow-up pediatrician for subsequent monthly injections.

Assessments

CAR SAFETY

All 50 states require infants to be restrained in a safety seat while riding in a motor vehicle, although laws vary from state to state. Discharge of smaller infants results in the use of car seat restraint devices that were designed for 7- to 8-pound term infants. In these devices, preterm infants may experience oxygen desaturations and apnea and bradycardia caused by head slouching and airway obstruction.[44,110] Use of rolled diapers/blankets may be necessary to support upright posture, prevent slouching, and enable the preterm to maintain stability while in the car seat. In addition, infants with certain conditions (e.g., Down syndrome, osteogenesis imperfecta, myelomeningocele, Pierre Robin syndrome, cerebral palsy) may benefit from special-needs car restraints.[85]

A car seat challenge before discharge is recommended for all infants born less than 37 weeks' gestation; this includes late-preterm infants (i.e., 34 to 36[6/7] weeks) who are cared for and discharged from level I/normal newborn nurseries.[6,8] Although the car seat challenge has not been standardized, certain components are common: (1) using the car seat purchased by the parents, (2) positioning the infant in the car seat immediately before discharge while on cardiorespiratory and pulse oximetry monitoring, (3) for a prescribed period of time (e.g., 30 to 90 minutes), and (4) recording respiratory/heart rates, oxygen saturations, and apnea/bradycardia events. Although this is a recommended practice, limitations have been identified. First, little objective evidence supports the ability of this challenge to absolutely confirm safe travel for an infant.[63]

A Cochrane review of the literature found no randomized controlled trials that fulfilled eligibility criteria for their review and were unable to recommend or refute a car seat challenge before discharge.[111] Further, common clinical practice has been to recommend the use of a car bed as a safe alternative to infants failing the car seat challenge, although studies have failed to prove any difference in apneic events. A recommendation has been put forth regarding changing the notion of a "test" or "challenge" to a car seat "orientation" in which the emphasis would be on education on proper positioning, limiting duration of automobile travel, and close observation during travel.[63]

NUTRITION AND GROWTH

Before discharge, (1) current growth trends should be reviewed; (2) either breastfeeding, if desired, should be established or guidelines given for increasing and monitoring; and (3) special feeding considerations such as the use of increased calorie formula, vitamin and mineral supplementation, and use of "special" formulas, tube feedings, or home total parenteral nutrition (TPN) should be outlined.[144] In studies of infants who experienced extrauterine growth restriction (EUGR), commonly defined as weight less than the 10th percentile for corrected gestational age (CGA) at discharge, the period from discharge to 30 months is shown to be a critical period for growth.[119] Nutritional intake at this time sets the trajectory for growth and neurodevelopment in childhood and adolescence. VLBW children who have low weight gain in early years of life have a higher probability of cognitive deficits; conversely, those with excessive weight gain have a higher likelihood of obesity, cardiovascular disease, and diabetes.[36]

NEURODEVELOPMENT

Some premature infants may have recognized risks to their later development evident at discharge. For these infants, early evaluation of their functional neurologic status may facilitate referrals to early intervention services soon after discharge.[109] Early intervention has been shown to improve neurobehavioral development with improved cognitive outcomes and parent-child interactions.[31,105]

Technology-Dependent Infants

Infants who rely on long-term technologic support are being discharged home in increasing numbers. In the past, children who were ventilator dependent; who had tracheostomies, gastrostomies, or jejunostomies; and even those who required long-term intravenous (IV) access for medications or parenteral nutrition would remain hospitalized, separated from their families and susceptible to other morbidities associated with long hospital stays (e.g., infection, delayed development, impaired mental health). With this increase of technology-dependent children discharged into the community comes a greater need for support services for the parents, providers, and the infants themselves.[142] Numerous investigators have undertaken projects to understand the impact that caring for these children has on the individual child and the family as a whole. Carnevale and colleagues[35] described the experiences of 12 families with technology-dependent children at home.[35] They identified key themes in this population, including (1) parental responsibility being stressful and, at times, overwhelming; (2) the devotion of significant energy in trying to "normalize" their home life; (3) living in isolation and feeling like strangers in their own communities; and (4) an overall theme of "daily living with distress and enrichment."[35]

In-home nursing care, extensive parent training, and an identified primary care provider comfortable with all aspects of the child's care are essential for successful discharge of technology-dependent children to home.[74] Developing home care plans that contain emergency and resuscitation procedures, as well as parental support and respite services, is vital.[93] Parents need training around all the details of their child's care, including early signs of illness and emergency procedures, whether or not home shift nursing will be provided. Rooming-in with their infant for one or more nights provides an important opportunity to evaluate their abilities and confidence in caring for their child. Communication and care coordination among the subspecialties following these infants are crucial.

NEURODEVELOPMENTAL FOLLOW-UP OF HIGH-RISK INFANTS

Ideally, parents of all NICU infants would be offered comprehensive, coordinated, developmentally based, family-centered follow-up for their child through infancy and childhood

(Figure 31-1). Each infant is unique, as is each infant's family. The following are the primary objectives of follow-up care:

- To counsel the family about their child's development so that they are empowered to optimize the child's health, growth, and development
- To recognize and diagnose (early) significant health conditions and neurodevelopmental disabilities to facilitate appropriate referrals for community services
- To anticipate future difficulties and needs so that optimal development is promoted and secondary complications are avoided or minimized

The ultimate goal is to promote the child's integration into the family, school, and community.

In the current health care environment, follow-up resources are generally limited and both public and private health insurance plans determine how children will access care. Consequently, criteria for developmental follow-up of NICU infants vary widely. Some high-risk infants are routinely referred to early intervention programs for developmental care, but implementation of these programs varies among states. The dynamics of development are such that periodic assessments of the child's health and developmental progress are needed to determine whether current interventions are

Developmental Progress and Monitoring of the Premature Infant

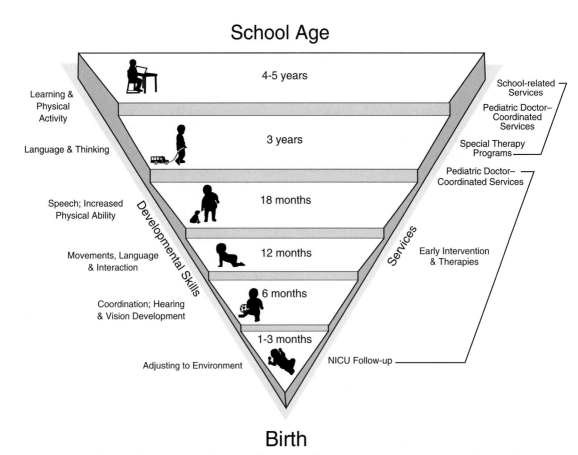

FIGURE 31-1 Developmental progress and monitoring of the premature infant. (Courtesy Angel Carter, Brian S. Carter, and Donna K. Daily, Vanderbilt University Medical Center, 2010.)

effective and sufficient. Parents often need guidance to better understand what to expect from their child, how to interpret their own observations of their child, and how health care and community services can support their child's development. The AAP has emphasized that each child have a "medical home," and especially the child with complex health and developmental needs. Unfortunately, the care of these children often is fragmented among numerous subspecialists and therapists.[9] Well-organized NICU follow-up clinics can facilitate developmental and health care of the NICU infant in coordination with the primary care provider and the family.

Developmental Milestone Attainment

In developmentally based follow-up, much of the information about the child's development comes from a careful interview of the parent about the child's health status and developmental milestone attainment. Noting the age of acquisition of the gross-motor, fine-motor, language, and adaptive-behavioral milestones helps determine a possible developmental delay. Parents are very good historians of their child's current functioning and recent accomplishments, which is why eliciting a history of milestone attainment during serial clinic visits is so useful in assessing a child's rate of development. Sometimes additional explanation may be needed to clearly determine the age of acquisition, especially language milestones.

A number of accurate screening tools are available to monitor general developmental progress or domain-specific evaluation.[61] Early delay in language and self-help milestones raises concerns about cognitive development, language disorder, or hearing impairment.[2] Many NICU developmental follow-up clinics rely on pediatric clinical psychologists to formally evaluate the cognition of high-risk infants, preferably with sequential assessments but sometimes with one assessment at a specific age (e.g., at 18 to 24 months' corrected age). For infants, the *Bayley Scales of Infant and Toddler Development,* third edition, is the most commonly used assessment tool in NICU follow-up programs in the United States.[28] For preschool-age and school-age children, several cognitive tests are available, including the Wechsler Preschool and Primary Scale of Intelligence (WPPSI), the Stanford-Binet Intelligence Scales,

and the Kaufman Assessment Battery for Children (K-ABC II).[81,116,146]

Correction for Degree of Prematurity

One controversy that arises in monitoring developmental scores of preterm infants is whether to correct for degree of prematurity (i.e., whether to use the child's chronologic age, calculated from birth, or to use corrected age for degree of prematurity). The best evidence supports correcting for degree of prematurity, but whether it is best to correct throughout infancy is controversial, and there is no agreement as to when one should stop correcting for degree of prematurity.[137] By convention, most practitioners correct through 2 years of age. It is necessary to be very cautious when interpreting corrected age scores at 12 months or less for ELBW infants. Parental understanding may lead to an overly optimistic outlook that will not be supported by testing at a later date.

Neurodevelopmental Examination

For high-risk infants, the standard pediatric neurologic examination is expanded to include a detailed assessment of posture, muscle tone, reflexes, postural reactions, and functional abilities. Interpretation of the examination requires a thorough understanding of the normal pattern of development over time, the examiner's skill at assessing the infant's performance, recognizing deviations from the norm, and determining the significance of these findings.[2,19,51]

Abnormalities of posture, muscle tone, and reflexes are common in preterm and other high-risk NICU infants during the first year. These abnormalities include asymmetries of movement, marked extensor tone through the neck and trunk with significant shoulder retraction or elevation, hypotonia, and lower extremity hypertonia and hyperreflexia. Cerebral palsy should be considered in infants with persistent abnormalities in tone, posture, movement, and motor delay. Mild delay and neuromotor tone variation suggest transient neuromotor abnormalities.

NICU Follow-Up Guidelines

The issue of how to do NICU developmental follow-up and how to conduct follow-up studies for high-risk infants has been complex. The methodology can lead to inadequate interpretation of published studies. The National Institute of Child Health and Human Development (NICHD), the National Institute of Neurologic Disorders and Stroke, and the CDC convened a workshop in 2002 to address these issues. Their purpose was to provide standardized guidelines for follow-up care, especially for tertiary care centers with neonatal fellowship training programs in the United States. The results of that workshop have been published and address topics such as risk factors that affect outcome, appropriate assessments, correction for prematurity, assessment tools, and research-related subjects.[137]

Again, these criteria may not fit the need or focus of every program. The resources available across states, within communities, and in individual hospitals and the commitment within the NICU strongly drive follow-up programs in different communities. Programs that wish to have developmental follow-up for quality care surveillance and to provide families with information about their high-risk infant can be resourceful in developing partnerships with local early intervention programs and community physicians. Programs that address scientific questions generally need a focused approach or a research network to approach the study.[134]

It is now recognized that survival to the end of the NICU stay is a very short-term outcome. It is generally recommended that NICU graduates be followed until at least 8 years of age, but most programs do not have the resources to do this. Furthermore, it has become apparent that the effects of prematurity may extend throughout the life span.[69] This is important to know but clearly goes beyond the capability of most NICU follow-up programs.

COMPLEX DISORDERS OF BRAIN DEVELOPMENT

Complex disorders of brain development are a group of chronic, nonprogressive disorders of central nervous system (CNS) function that occur as result of malformation of or insult to the developing brain.[2] There is a spectrum of neurodevelopmental impairments, from major disabilities (cerebral palsy) and severe cognitive impairments (formerly referred to as "mental retardation") to sensory impairments and other complex disorders of brain development (Box 31-4).

BOX 31-4   COMPLEX DISORDERS OF BRAIN DEVELOPMENT

Neurodevelopmental Impairment
Major disability
Cerebral palsy
Global developmental delay and severe cognitive impairment

Sensory Impairment
Hearing impairment
Visual impairment

Other Complex Disorders of Brain Development
Language delay or disorder
    Expressive language delay
    Receptive and expressive language delay
Developmental coordination disorder
    Fine-motor incoordination
    Sensorimotor integration problems
Learning disability
    Variable cognitive abilities
    Visual-perceptual problems
Behavior disorders
    Attention-deficit/hyperactivity disorder
    Autism spectrum disorders

Modified from Accardo PJ, editor: *Caputo and Accardo's neurodevelopmental disabilities in infancy and childhood,* ed 3, Baltimore, Md, 2008, Paul H Brookes; Wolraich ML, editor: *Disorders of development and learning,* ed 3, Hamilton, Ontario, Canada, 2003, BC Decker.

Neurodevelopmental Impairment

Preterm infants are at an increased risk for major disabilities and also for other cognitive and behavioral concerns. Both may have a long-term impact on their life.[150] The World Health Organization (WHO) has categorized disability, impairment, and handicap in the *International Classification of Functioning, Disability and Health* (ICF) and places emphasis on the interaction of functioning and disability, health condition of the individual, and factors of the environment.[121,148] The ICF is structured around the following components: (1) body functions and structure, (2) activities and participation, and (3) additional information on severity and environmental factors.[148] This view has aided our thinking not only of the specific disability but also how it affects a child's ability to function physically and socially within his or her home and community.

Cerebral Palsy

Cerebral palsy (CP) "describes a group of permanent disorders of the development of movement and posture, causing activity limitation, that are attributed to nonprogressive disturbances that occurred in the developing fetal or infant brain."[117] Important to this current definition is the recognition of the accompanying disturbances of sensation, perception, cognition, communication, and behavior and by epilepsy and secondary musculoskeletal problems. CP is the most disabling motor impairment found in preterm infants and is difficult to diagnose with any degree of certainty before 6 to 12 months of age. It sometimes takes until the child is 2 years or older before the diagnosis becomes clear.

CP has traditionally been classified by physiologic type (tone abnormality), topography (i.e., muscle groups involved), and severity.[2] Again, the most recent recommendation for definition and classification has been expanded and relates to the WHO ICF.[117,148] Components of the currently recommended classification stress motor abnormalities, accompanying impairments, anatomic and neuroimaging findings, and causation and timing. Because consensus has not been clear on the definition of level of severity, the Gross Motor Classification Scale is now commonly used to address motor function, and scales are being developed to more reliably measure other important areas of functioning, such as hand control, speech, and swallowing.[107,117] Persistently increased muscle tone and increased deep tendon reflexes with persistence of pathologic reflexes (e.g., Babinski) are early signs of spasticity. Variable tone with persistent primitive reflexes, often with involuntary movements, is a sign of extrapyramidal CP. The child may be 2 to 3 years old before involuntary movements are seen. Children who manifest signs of both spasticity and extrapyramidal CP have mixed CP. Extrapyramidal CP is generalized, but spasticity should be further typed according to which limbs are most significantly involved.

Spastic diplegia, the most common form of CP in preterm infants, is characterized by spasticity in both lower extremities, with mild or minimal involvement of the upper extremities.[2,96] *Spastic hemiplegia* is characterized by involvement of one side of the body, with the upper extremity more involved than the lower. Because intrauterine and perinatal strokes are usually unilateral, children who had strokes often demonstrate spastic hemiplegia. *Quadriplegia* is the most severe form of spastic CP, with involvement of both upper and lower extremities and the lower more severely affected than the upper. Children with neonatal encephalopathy (whether caused by hypoxia/ischemia, metabolic disorders, or other causes) who develop CP are most likely to have spastic quadriplegia or severe mixed CP.

Global Developmental Delay and Cognitive Impairments

Developmental delay is used to describe a deficit in any of the five developmental domains (cognition, motor, language, adaptive, social-emotional skills). *Global developmental delay* is used to define deficits in two or more areas of development with scores more than two deviations below norm referenced standards.[125] Currently in the United States, a child may receive services through his or her local school district special education program with a diagnosis of developmental delay until almost 8 years of age before the definition may be switched to mental retardation, again based on standardized testing. Standardized tests, such as the Bayley, third edition, have score groupings and definitions to match, such as low average and borderline, for each domain.[28] It is during this early period of detection that early intervention services become important for the high-risk infant.[31,106,109]

Severe cognitive impairment is a global impairment of cognitive functioning resulting from injury to or malformation of the developing brain that impairs the child's ability to adapt and function in society.[2,150] It frequently manifests with an early delay in language and problem-solving abilities. A diagnosis of severe cognitive impairment requires a comprehensive evaluation of the child, with neuropsychologic testing of intelligence and assessment of adaptive (functional) abilities, which can be reliably done only at school age.

Neuropsychologic testing includes an assessment of a child's intelligence quotient (IQ). Intelligence is not one entity but, rather, many different abilities, including auditory and visual memory, visual–perceptual abilities, and understanding complex language concepts. The older the child is, the greater the number of functions that can be tested and therefore the more accurate the tests are in assessing intelligence. Intelligence and functional ability tests for school-age children and adults consist of a variety of subtests. Most children with severe cognitive impairment have lower abilities for age across all domains of development, so the severity of cognitive impairment is easily classified. Many preterm children have a significant variability in cognitive functions, with high scores on some subtests and low scores on others, which makes them more difficult to classify and appropriate educational services more difficult to determine.

Cognitive impairment is classified in terms of severity, from profound (IQ below 20), severe (IQ 20 to 34), moderate (IQ 35 to 49), to mild (IQ 50 to 70).[2,150] Children with an IQ of 70 to 85 have borderline intelligence, not severe cognitive impairment. They are capable of academic learning but may have trouble keeping up with their class. The most important characteristics of children with cognitive impairments that enhance adult functioning are interpersonal skills and the ability to communicate and relate to other people.

Sensory Impairments

A NICU admission increases the risk of hearing loss. Most states require hearing screening for all newborns using a two-step process: initial screening with otoacoustic emissions, followed by auditory evoked responses if the first test is failed.[11,133] Because of the risk for progressive hearing impairment, infants with congenital cytomegalovirus (CMV) infection, primary pulmonary hypertension, and congenital diaphragmatic hernia and infants treated with extracorporeal membrane oxygenation (ECMO) should have serial hearing evaluations during infancy and early childhood, as should infants with recurrent ear infections.[11,15,57,58]

Neonates demonstrate hearing thresholds similar to those of older children and adults. Even preterm infants as early as 24 to 25 weeks' gestation demonstrate an immature brainstem waveform in response to sound stimuli, although the pattern of the waveform matures to a normal waveform as the infant reaches near-term equivalence. Infants hear and process language throughout their first year, beginning at birth.

Retinopathy of prematurity (ROP) results from injury to the very immature developing retina, which causes abnormal proliferation of blood vessels. Severe ROP, which tends to occur in the most immature and sickest preterm infants, is usually treated with laser to try to prevent retinal detachment and blindness. Recent data indicate that intravitreal bevacizumab monotherapy in infants with stage 3+ ROP showed a significant benefit for zone I disease, but not zone II disease, compared with conventional laser therapy.[13] Preterm infants may develop medically related eye complications (retinal detachment, cataract, glaucoma) and are at increased risk for refractive errors, strabismus, and amblyopia.[103] Infants who have structurally normal eyes, no refractive error, and a history of no or low-level regressed ROP may be dismissed by the ophthalmologist after 12 to 18 months of age but should continue to receive routine childcare eye screening based on the AAP recommendations for routine preventive care.[104] Late-preterm and term infants with other neonatal complications and neurodevelopmental sequelae will often have visual impairments and need ongoing ophthalmologic follow-up.

Infants with congenital CMV infection or toxoplasmosis should be examined by ophthalmologists for chorioretinitis. Neonates symptomatic with congenital infection (e.g., CMV infection, rubella, toxoplasmosis) have a high risk (20% to 30%) of visual and/or hearing impairment.[141] Preterm infants in the NICU with varying types of postnatal sepsis syndromes have also been identified as having an increased risk for neurodevelopmental impairment.[130] If infants with neonatal encephalopathy develop disability, they tend to have severe multiple disabilities, including cortical visual impairment or processing and hearing impairment.[115]

OTHER COMPLEX DISORDERS OF BRAIN DEVELOPMENT

Even if the NICU graduate does not develop major disability or sensory impairment, he or she remains at increased risk for disorders of higher cortical function (see Box 31-4). These disorders may be less evident in infancy and may be associated, initially, with only nonspecific symptoms (e.g., irritability, posturing, feeding problems). Diagnostic criteria, and even nomenclature, for these disorders vary widely, and few reports of preschool and school-age outcome studies have a comparison group evaluated in the identical manner.

Language delay may manifest as early as 6 to 12 months as delay or deviance (i.e., nonsequential) in language milestone acquisition.[2] Expressive language delay, either alone or in combination with receptive language delay, is common in preterm and other NICU infants. Every child who manifests with delayed language should have a hearing test and neuropsychologic testing to distinguish between language disorder, hearing impairment, and cognitive impairment.

Developmental coordination disorder (DCD), also referred to as *minor neuromotor dysfunction,* presents as mild delay or deviant motor milestone acquisition in conjunction with mild or transient neuromotor abnormalities.[43] These are children who sit by 1 year of age and walk by 2 years, although they may have an atypical pattern to their motor progress (e.g., transient low or high tone, toe-walking, persistent wide-base gait). These children generally have typical functioning by 3 to 5 years of age, although they may continue to have some balance or motor planning problems. Fine-motor incoordination, visual–perceptual deficits, and sensorimotor inefficiencies may accompany DCD, but they may not be recognized until preschool or school age.[22,42] *Visual-perceptual deficits,* often in combination with fine-motor incoordination, are manifest by an inability to recognize and copy figures, letters, and numbers; complete puzzles and mazes; or copy block designs; or by some level of difficulty with these tasks. *Fine-motor incoordination* makes it difficult to button, zip, cut with scissors, draw, and write. *Sensorimotor inefficiencies* are characterized by difficulty following directions that include demonstrating an action (e.g., tying shoelaces) and tolerating motion through space (e.g., swinging on a swing) or different tactile sensations (e.g., clothing or food textures). For children with DCD, fine-motor incoordination or sensorimotor inefficiencies and failures in school and on the playground erode self-esteem and peer relationships.

Language disorder, visual-perceptual problems, DCD, transient neuromotor dysfunction, and variable cognitive disabilities are associated with learning disability (LD) and other school problems.[2,22,42] LD means difficulty learning one or more academic subjects (reading, writing, arithmetic) in children with normal intelligence who have had adequate exposure to school. Some children have more of a learning inefficiency, in that they do well in the early grades of school but have a relative inefficiency in reading or writing that causes them trouble as the work becomes more complex. Their intelligence and resiliency help them make adaptations in learning, but they become overwhelmed in situations in which speed and accuracy are viewed as important.

Behavior disorders are more common in preterm and other NICU children.[1,20,79] Some children have attention–deficit/hyperactivity disorder (ADHD), characterized by marked distractibility, short attention span, and impulsivity. ADHD can occur with or without hyperactivity: the child may be restless, always on the move, or constantly busy or may just demonstrate difficulty paying attention and impulsiveness. One must recognize these more subtle concerns as soon as possible. Counseling parents and teachers can prevent the devastating effect these "mild" disabilities have on self-esteem, peer relationships, and performance in school and at home.

Autism Spectrum Disorders

Expanding research indicates that although the causes of autism spectrum disorders (ASDs) likely remain multifactorial, there are key conditions identified in infants that place them at a distinctly higher risk. In an effort to confirm prevalence rates, researchers followed a group of premature infants for 21 years and found the risk to be five times greater for those infants born under 2000 g compared with the general population.[95]

The association between brain injury and the risk of ASD continues to be explored. Following 1105 LBW infants, Movsas and colleagues[95] found strong evidence linking the occurrence of ventricular enlargement in the neonatal period with diagnosed ASD in those children by adolescence or early adulthood. Although any white matter injury significantly increased the risk for a positive screen for ASD, ventricular enlargement increased that risk sevenfold with no associated increase with isolated germinal matrix or intraventricular hemorrhage.[95]

A meta-analysis exploring the relationship between perinatal and neonatal conditions and ASD failed to identify any one causal factor but found evidence to suggest that several complications may be responsible—either alone, or in combination, with some evidence suggesting that these factors may only apply to those who are "genetically vulnerable" to ASD.[59]

As research continues to explore potential explanations for causality, counseling for families and caregivers concerning the risks and prevalence is warranted. Early attention to these risks, and potential, may provide earlier screenings, diagnoses, access to services, and behavioral interventions to the benefit of the child and family.

Diagnosis of Disability

The major disabilities may be recognized and diagnosed in the first 2 years after birth. The more severe the disability, the sooner it may be recognized and diagnosed. Occasionally a child may have significant motor delay initially but seems to "catch up" by 1 to 2 years, with concomitant improvement in neuromotor abnormalities. These are often children with ongoing health problems (e.g., chronic lung disease [CLD]/bronchopulmonary dysplasia [BPD]) and are diagnosed with *developmental coordination disorder* but have a high risk for learning disability at school age. Language disorders, visual-perceptual difficulties, and fine-motor incoordination are generally recognized and diagnosed during the preschool years (ages 3 to 5 years). Specific learning disabilities and attentional difficulties cannot be diagnosed until school age, usually around 7 to 8 years of age. Mild LD or learning inefficiencies may not be recognized until middle school or high school.

Because there is so much overlap among the neurodevelopmental disabilities, whenever abnormality in one area is detected, the child should have a comprehensive, multidisciplinary evaluation of all his or her abilities. Services are now available to all children through the Individuals with Disabilities Education Act (IDEA 2004).[76] Children from birth to 3 years of age receive services through their early intervention program, and after age 36 months receive services through their local public school's special education program.

PERINATAL RISK FACTORS FOR NEURODEVELOPMENTAL IMPAIRMENTS

Many conditions that require neonatal intensive care also increase risk for neurodevelopmental disability. Perinatal risk factors can be used to identify NICU infants with a high risk for neurodevelopmental disability so that they can be followed closely and referred for comprehensive evaluations and early intervention programs when appropriate (Box 31-5). Broad categories of risk include the following:

- Prematurity
- Maternal complications (chorioamnionitis, placental abnormalities)
- Birth complications (asphyxia, need for resuscitation)
- Infant conditions (IUGR, macrosomia, congenital anomalies)
- Neonatal illness (NEC, respiratory conditions, infection)
- CNS-associated conditions (brain hemorrhage, stroke, structural defects)

Multiple risk factors increase an infant's risk for neurodevelopmental impairment, and the effects may be more than additive. As a group, preterm infants or full-term infants with IUGR tend to have lower mean IQ than full-term appropriate for gestational age (AGA) infants.[118,140] Infants with both prematurity and IUGR are vulnerable to the complications of each condition.

SPECIFIC NEURODEVELOPMENTAL OUTCOMES

This section summarizes reported neurodevelopmental outcomes for some of the most frequently encountered conditions in the NICU. A systematic approach (see Box 31-5) allows the clinician to assess the risk factors that may affect developmental outcome. Preterm infants and their medical sequelae are most commonly encountered in neonatal intensive care. However, term infants with pulmonary disease, encephalopathy, or congenital defects also may require intensive care and have significant sequelae. Finally, although we have focused our attention in recent years on smaller and smaller babies in tertiary care centers, it has become

BOX 31–5	PERINATAL RISK FACTORS FOR NEURODEVELOPMENTAL DISABILITIES

- Maternal characteristics
  - Socioeconomic status
  - Education
  - Race/ethnicity
  - Obstetric/prenatal complications
- Maternal illness
  - Chorioamnionitis
  - Maternal ingestions (alcohol, drugs, medications)
  - Congenital infection
  - Multiple gestation
  - Labor or delivery complications
  - Placental abnormalities
- Physical characteristics
  - Prematurity
  - Postmaturity
  - Intrauterine growth restriction
  - Small for gestational age
  - Macrosomia
  - Gender
  - Microcephaly
  - Congenital anomalies
  - Dysmorphic features
- Condition at birth
  - Apgar scores
  - Cord pH
  - Meconium staining
  - Need for and response to resuscitation
- Neonatal complications
  - Hypoxia
  - Acidosis
  - Hypotension/shock
  - Apnea and bradycardia
  - Chronic lung disease
  - Sepsis
  - Meningitis
  - Seizures
  - Hypoxic-ischemic encephalopathy
- CNS structure and function
  - Intraventricular hemorrhage
  - Intraparenchymal hemorrhage or infarction
  - Ventricular dilation
  - Cortical atrophy
  - Periventricular leukomalacia
  - Burst-suppression pattern on EEG
  - Abnormal neurologic examination

Modified from Taeusch W, Ballard R, Gleason C, editors: *Avery's diseases of the newborn*, ed 8, Philadelphia, 2005, Saunders.
CNS, Central nervous system; *EEG,* electroencephalogram.

apparent that we have often neglected issues for larger "late-preterm" infants (see Chapter 5). These infants are more typically followed in level II or transitional nurseries but are not without risk. It is beyond the scope of this chapter to cover congenital malformations or genetic conditions (see Chapter 27), but it is well known that these infants often require complex multidisciplinary care and the principles of follow-up outlined previously apply to them as well.

Prematurity

For more than 50 years, the medical literature has described the neurodevelopmental outcome of preterm VLBW infants (birth weight less than 1500 g). With the beginning of modern neonatal intensive care in the mid-1960s, tertiary care NICUs began reporting the incidence or prevalence of major disability—in survivors. Initially, there was a great deal of variability in reported incidences because of differences in populations studied, neonatal intensive care practices, definitions of disability (e.g., whether they include children with mild CP or children with borderline intelligence), and age at follow-up.[73,138] Because of these issues of study methodology, outcomes are now more frequently reported from large regional studies or research consortiums.

In a review of outcomes studies conducted from 2000 to 2013, Vohr[136] reports that, at 18 to 30 months' follow-up, cognitive impairment (scores greater than 2 standard deviations below the mean) is the most common impairment of preterm infants, with incidences as high as 61% in the smallest survivors.[136] By school age, 50% to 70% of VLBW children exhibit learning difficulties related to executive function, visual-motor skills, and memory, resulting in failed grades and special education requirements.

A study of 6-year-old children who were born at less than 26 weeks' gestational age found that 12% had disabling CP and 21% had moderate to severe cognitive impairment (IQ less than 70).[87] Compared with full-term controls, 41% of these extremely preterm children had moderate to severe cognitive impairments; one quarter had borderline intelligence; 10% had hearing loss (profound in 3%); and 7% had visual impairments (2% were blind). The largest study of infants born at less than 26 weeks' gestation and followed to age 6 years found that 22% had severe disability, 24% had moderate disability, 34% had mild disability, and only 20% were unaffected.[86,87]

In ELBW children, a meta-analysis of the outcomes of infants delivered at 22 to 25 weeks' gestation reports that, when followed at 4 to 8 years of age all survivors have a likelihood of moderate to severe impairment with decreasing severity rates in the higher gestational ages.[94] These authors report this to be a unique analysis of data from nine prospective cohort studies published after 2004 in that it is one of the first meta-analysis of studies reporting impairments from school-age children, rather than in the young toddler, where, because of still developing skills and adaptations, rates of impairment may be overestimated. Compared with full-term controls, ELBW children are three to five times more likely to require special resources in school, and this increases to 8 to 10 times more likely by adolescence.[69]

Although many challenges are possible for the infant born prematurely, particularly the smallest and youngest, the potential also exists to overcome, or adapt to, limitations presented them. Early intervention services, supportive home environments, and access to resources for the families can all help to eliminate or mitigate many of the potential negative outcomes.

Late-Preterm Infants

Larger preterm infants, or *late-preterm infants,* make up 75% of all preterm births and are defined as infants born between 34 and 36 completed weeks. These infants are physiologically and metabolically immature, which predisposes them to special transitional care needs.[53] If these needs are not met or recognized, these infants may be placed at risk for neurodevelopmental sequelae.[3,52] Studies have identified this group of infants to be at a higher risk

for poor neurodevelopment outcomes predisposing them to problems with school performance. Learning and behavioral problems, including ADHD and LDs, occur at a higher rate than in term infants.[71,135,149] Health care utilization during the first year of life is also greater for these infants.[30]

Short-term complications also occur at a higher rate during the first few days of life. These include temperature and glucose instability, apnea, hyperbilirubinemia, and poor feeding.[62] Even with these potential problems identified, early discharge of these infants remains a practice in many centers, whereas elective deliveries of infants less than 39 weeks have been targeted for reduction in the United States.[23,62] This information supports the need for carefully planned discharges, as well as the structuring of appropriate neurodevelopmental follow-up, for this subgroup of premature infants.

Maternal Complications

Maternal complications increase the risk for conditions associated with problematic birth, but also for long-term adverse outcomes for the infant. Placental abruption carries with it the immediate threat of decreased oxygen supply to the fetus potentially resulting in neurodevelopmental impairment.[114] Chorioamnionitis may result in adverse short-term outcomes including need for ventilation, sepsis, intraventricular hemorrhage (IVH) and others.[21] Long-term outcomes associated with exposure to chorioamnionitis include cognitive impairment and death.[108] Finally, other maternal conditions such as infection, preexisting health conditions, mother's weight, age, use of tobacco or other substances, and prior pregnancy and contraceptive history may increase the risk of prematurity or infant compromise. Infant outcomes related to prematurity or birth compromise are detailed in this chapter.

Birth Conditions

NEONATAL ENCEPHALOPATHY

The extent and nature of an initial hypoxic-ischemic event cannot be easily determined for individual infants, leading clinicians to rely on recognizable signs and symptoms of neonatal encephalopathy to predict outcome. These signs and symptoms include the following:

- Poor feeding

- Hypotonia or extensor hypertonia
- Lethargy or hyperexcitability
- Apnea
- Seizures
- Abnormalities on neuroimaging studies, which are far more predictive than low Apgar scores
- The need for positive-pressure ventilation or CPR at birth
- Initial response to resuscitation

Many infants with congenital brain malformations or prenatal brain injury may present with perinatal cardiorespiratory depression. They do not breathe normally at birth and may require positive-pressure ventilation or further resuscitation. It is very difficult to distinguish these infants from those with encephalopathy caused by hypoxia or ischemia. Metabolic problems or neonatal sepsis may also present with these signs. Therefore the term *neonatal encephalopathy* is preferred over the term *hypoxic–ischemic encephalopathy (HIE),* because etiology cannot always be determined with certainty. However, the clinician must evaluate the history and relevant factors in each infant to address the etiology of their encephalopathy. The etiology may be important in decisions about treatment, prognosis, and follow-up, as well as for family planning.

In the absence of a confirmed specific etiology, the stages of encephalopathy described in 1976 by Sarnat and Sarnat remain highly predictive of outcome.[122] Infants with *stage 3 (severe) encephalopathy* and coma, severe hypotonia or increased extensor tone, intermittent decerebration, decreased or absent reflexes, variable pupil reactivity, and abnormal electroencephalogram (EEG) generally will die or have multiple severe disabilities. Only 20% to 30% of infants with *stage 2 (moderate) encephalopathy* with lethargy or coma, mild hypotonia, overactive reflexes, seizures, abnormal EEG, and generalized parasympathetic function (constricted pupils, bradycardia, profuse secretions, and diarrhea) have multiple severe disabilities. The remainder of newborns with stage 2 encephalopathy have lower scores on tests of cognition, vocabulary, reading, spelling, and arithmetic than children with *stage 1 (mild) encephalopathy* (hyperalert state, jitteriness, overactivity and easily elicited reflexes, increased sympathetic function, dilated pupils, and decreased gastrointestinal motility) or healthy control children. Infants with neonatal encephalopathy should be evaluated with both EEGs and neuroimaging studies.

Very-low-voltage EEG patterns (signifying little brain activity) and burst-suppression EEG patterns carry an extremely poor prognosis, as does diffuse encephalomalacia detected by MRI.[115,129] Infants with moderate encephalopathy may benefit from hypothermic treatment, commonly called "cooling" (see Chapter 26), leading to increased survival without disability. The results from all published trials in North America and Europe are most promising for encephalopathies of less than a severe nature, and cooling is considered to be a standard of care in many countries for infants meeting cooling criteria.[24,67,124] Follow-up of infants receiving cooling therapy supports the therapeutic value of hypothermia.[66] Mild encephalopathy with only a subarachnoid hemorrhage carries a good prognosis, although these children should be monitored for later learning difficulties.

Infant Conditions

INTRAUTERINE GROWTH RESTRICTION

Prenatal and postnatal growth can seriously affect neurodevelopmental outcomes of high-risk infants. The neurodevelopmental outcome of IUGR infants is strongly associated with the cause of IUGR; with the timing, severity, and duration of the insult; and with perinatal complications the IUGR infant encounters (see Box 31-5). Early severe IUGR often reflects a chromosomal anomaly, other severe genetic disorder, or congenital infection that occurred early to cause organ malformation or significant injury. Some causes of IUGR result in death (e.g., trisomy 18) or severe disability. Some carry a high risk for neurodevelopmental disability (e.g., fetal alcohol syndrome). Others are associated with only mild disability (e.g., an increased incidence of attention and behavior problems in infants born to mothers who took narcotics or cocaine during pregnancy).

One of the most common causes of IUGR is uteroplacental insufficiency, generally a diagnosis of exclusion. The fetus responds in many adaptive ways when the supply of nutrients or oxygen is limited.[17,18] There is first a decrease in subcutaneous tissue, resulting in lower birth weight, and then a decrease in length, before head and brain growth are affected (symmetric growth restriction). Nevertheless, the problem may be severe enough to overwhelm these adaptations and lead to brain injury. In addition, a chronically compromised fetus, with decreased glycogen and nutrient stores, has more difficulty with the stresses of labor and delivery, leading to perinatal depression, cold stress, hypoglycemia, and hypocalcemia. Polycythemia may result from chronic intrauterine hypoxia but may result in the complications of hyperviscosity.[118]

Prospective studies of full-term IUGR school-age children compared with full-term AGA children showed that more IUGR children had language problems, learning disability, minor neuromotor dysfunction, hyperactivity, and attention and behavior problems. Postnatal growth may also be affected, but this will largely depend on whether the infant has symmetric or asymmetric IUGR. Preterm IUGR children demonstrate the disadvantages of both prematurity and IUGR, but which is more important in determining outcomes is not clear. The degree of IUGR may influence early delivery, either spontaneous or induced, because of concerns of fetal well-being. The most striking findings in studies of preterm IUGR children and preterm AGA controls are the high rates of major disability (7% to 23%) and LDs (36% to 50%).[84]

CONGENITAL ANOMALIES

Cardiac. The presence of congenital heart disease (CHD) places children at increased risks for developmental delays and neurodevelopmental impairment related to cyanosis, cardiac surgery, cardiac surgery with cardiopulmonary bypass, or comorbid conditions such as prematurity.[88,98,101] Accumulated evidence for these risks led to the collaboration between the American Heart Association and the American Academy of Pediatrics to issue policy guidelines for the surveillance, identification, and interventions for these children.[16]

Early assessments of children with CHD show motor deficits as most common with language and cognitive deficits appearing later.[98] The most common indicator of later neurodevelopmental deficit was the failure to achieve full oral feedings without supplemental tube feedings; the presence of comorbidities and poor growth were the next most commonly identified risk factors.[98]

Periodic, longitudinal screening is indicated for children with CHD because evidence shows increased risk for motor, language, and cognitive effects. A management algorithm was developed by the American Heart Association to be used by the primary care provider, within the child's medical home. This algorithm assists with identification,

evaluation, and management of potential neurodevelopmental challenges and allows for earlier access to potential intervention services for the child and family.[16]

Congenital Diaphragmatic Hernia. Congenital diaphragmatic hernia (CDH) increases the risk for poor neurodevelopmental outcomes, likely affected by the severity of CDH (need for ECMO, prolonged ventilation, etc.). Most commonly reported deficits are neuromuscular abnormalities such as hypertonicity or hypotonicity and psychomotor dysfunction.[40,41]

CENTRAL NERVOUS SYSTEM INJURY

Infants with ischemic perinatal stroke are another group of infants with brain injury who are at risk for long-term developmental sequelae. This entity is generally distinctly different from diffuse ischemia seen in the so-called "watershed" injury of perinatal HIE. Timing of the event may also be less easily determined, but the infant may present with focal or generalized seizures or less-defined clinical signs such as poor perfusion ("dusky" or "gray" spells), respiratory distress or apnea, poor feeding, or low neuromotor tone in the first few days of life. MRI is the most reliable method of diagnostic detection in the newborn period if timed appropriately. Neurologic deficits have been reported in 50% to 75% of survivors, and hemiplegic CP is most commonly found. Later difficulties with sensory impairment or learning difficulties are also present, thus requiring long-term follow-up.[113]

HEMORRHAGE

Although intracranial hemorrhages most commonly occur in the preterm infant, they may also occur in the term infant and any concerns need to be carefully investigated with the infant outcomes closely monitored.[68] Impact of intracranial hemorrhage ranges from short-term feeding or state disruptions to severe disability and death (see Chapter 26 for the physiology of these hemorrhages). Attempts to associate the injury with disability have identified that ventricular dilation, as well as grade and laterality, can be predictive of the severity of any deficits, with bilateral grade IV intraventricular hemorrhages having the poorest outcomes.[77,90] Infants may experience cognitive and/or motor disability from the brain injury, as well as the combined effects from risks associated from prematurity, comorbid medical conditions, or illnesses.

ILLNESS

Respiratory. Persistent pulmonary hypertension of the newborn (PPHN) and meconium aspiration syndrome (MAS) often overlap clinically, and many of these infants require neonatal intensive care technologies, including inhaled nitric oxide, high-frequency ventilation, and ECMO. Full-term survivors of this care have an increased risk for major disability, neuromotor dysfunction, borderline intelligence, language delay, and attention problems.[75] Both chronic lung disease (CLD) (seen in 7% to 40%) and hearing impairment (seen in 20% to 50%) are common sequelae of PPHN or ECMO but neurodevelopmental disabilities remain low (less than 20%).[97] Studies of ECMO that include venovenous as opposed to venoarterial flow report a lower incidence (approximately 15%) of developmental disabilities. Inhaled nitric oxide has become a common treatment of pulmonary hypertension in the newborn, and follow-up studies indicate that these infants have a developmental disability rate of 14% to 19%.[39] Because the hearing impairment associated with either PPHN or ECMO may be progressive, serial hearing evaluations during infancy and early childhood are required.[57]

Bronchopulmonary Dysplasia/Chronic Lung Disease. BPD or CLD is the most common morbidity in surviving preterm infants.[56] The etiology of neonatal lung injury appears to have changed over time as methods of treatment of respiratory failure have changed and as an increasing number of extremely immature preterm infants survive.[26,78] Regardless of specific cause, the risk for pulmonary hypertension, postdischarge growth failure, recurrent hospitalizations, and adverse neurodevelopmental outcomes persists in children with BPD.[20,82,126] Many of these infants exhibit low tone and early motor delays, often consistent with developmental coordination disorder.[46] Cerebral palsy is highly associated with infants of extremely low birth weight, as is BPD, but varies in infants with BPD from 11% to 27% based on severity of BPD. Likewise, lower cognitive scores are related to severity of BPD and may be present in 50% of infants with severe BPD.[50,126]

Necrotizing Enterocolitis (NEC). NEC, with or without intestinal perforation, carries with it a high rate of neurodevelopmental impairments, reported to be as much as 82% in infants requiring surgery from NEC.[139] Impairments include cognitive deficits, CP, and severe visual impairment, with rates significantly higher for those infants requiring surgery for the illness.[123]

Infection (Sepsis, Meningitis, and Other Non-NEC Related). The impact on neurodevelopmental outcomes from neonatal infection has primarily been studied by individual insult. A 2012 systematic review, however, attempted to define the burden, on a global basis, of "intrauterine and neonatal insults" with individual sequelae identified per insult.[99] *Sepsis* was identified in five studies reviewed with 40% of the infants affected ($n = 977$). The most commonly identified sequelae were cognitive, general developmental delay, or learning difficulties in 74% of the infants. *Meningitis* was identified in 11 studies, with 42% of the infants affected ($n = 209$) and 100% reporting cognitive deficits as the sequelae. *Cytomegalovirus* identified 377 infants with deafness or hearing loss (67%) and cognitive deficits (66%) as the identified sequelae. *Herpes* affected 116 infants with 94% of them experiencing cognitive sequelae, and *rubella* was a cause of sequelae in 720 infants with deafness or hearing loss reported as the most common impairment (80%).[99]

These data support the need for high surveillance, primary prevention, and close monitoring of follow-up for infants born with or acquiring infection in the neonatal period.

TRACKING HEALTH OUTCOMES: THE PRIMARY CARE PROVIDER

Primary Care Follow-Up

At the time of discharge, the NICU staff must provide the primary care pediatrician and the parents with a complete and accurate history of the child's NICU course, including recommendations for ongoing care (Box 31-6). Special health concerns, specific to the premature infant, should be closely monitored and surveillance of these should supplement the AAP guidelines for preventive, "well-child" care.[32] These additional areas of special concern for the premature infant would include such things as the following:

- Neurodevelopmental follow-up

B O X 31-6	POSTDISCHARGE CARE NEEDS FOR NICU GRADUATES

Central nervous system: IVH/PVL imaging before discharge; consider value of MRI instead of, or in addition to, ultrasound for predicting developmental challenges; plan for ongoing developmental assessment.

Vision: Complete ROP monitoring and treatment in timely fashion as indicated; visual acuity evaluation between 6 and 12 months of age.

Hearing: Universal screening and recurring screening for high-risk groups (CMV, PPHN, HFV, ECMO, CDH); specific evaluation and augmentation, if indicated, by 6 months of age.

Cardiac: Pulse oximetry screening to rule out critical ductal-dependent cardiac lesions (usually completed in first 1-2 days of hospital admission) completed before discharge. Outpatient follow-up of cardiac issues identified during hospitalization (other structural defects, PPHN or other functional problems).

Pulmonary: Evaluation of BPD classification at 36 weeks of corrected age; outpatient management of BPD, management of oxygen and monitor needs; management of additional support, including tracheostomy and ventilators as needed in select patients.

Gastrointestinal: Management of feeding regimens and close attention to growth; managing enteral feeding needs if oral intake inadequate. Referrals for evaluation and management of oral eating problems.

Development: Early referrals for therapies as indicated for speech, motor, and cognitive development.

BPD, Bronchopulmonary dysplasia; *CDH*, congenital diaphragmatic hernia; *CMV*, cytomegalovirus; *ECMO*, extracorporeal membrane oxygenation; *HFV*, high-frequency ventilation; *IVH/PVL*, intraventricular hemorrhage/periventricular leukomalacia; *MRI*, magnetic resonance imaging; *PPHN*, persistent pulmonary hypertension of the newborn; *ROP*, retinopathy of prematurity.

- Visual and hearing outcomes
- Growth, nutrition, and feeding issues
- Osteopenia of prematurity
- Dental enamel defects
- Sequelae related to issues during hospitalization, including pulmonary, gastrointestinal, hematologic, and surgical conditions

Along with the subspecialty medical follow-up, the primary care provider will also need to coordinate other supportive services such as early intervention programs and developmental follow-up through a NICU follow-up program, if available.[34] Recommendations for specialized follow-up of the late-preterm infant have also been proposed with the focus on feeding, sleeping, temperature regulation, jaundice,

and infection in an effort to reduce posthospital morbidities and rehospitalizations of these infants.[52,143]

Growth, Nutrition, and Feeding

Premature infants are at increased risk for growth deficits after discharge—many are discharged below the body weight of their healthy term counterparts. The failure to achieve adequate growth is known as *extrauterine growth restriction (EUGR)* and is defined by weight less than the 10th percentile for CGA at the time of discharge.[119] EUGR also occurs commonly in ill preterm newborns.[36,119] The long-term effects of this early delayed growth have been unclear.[80] However, infants in the lower quartiles of growth in the NICU have higher incidences of neurodevelopmental impairment at 18 to 22 months' follow-up in the NICHD Neonatal Research Network. Although markers of illness severity such as NEC or BPD had a significant effect on outcome, poor postnatal growth itself may exert an independent effect.[49]

Postdischarge growth failure for preterm infants is also a common problem, especially in those with associated CLD. Transitional formulas, occasionally with caloric concentration, may be needed to optimize growth and subsequent development.[48,64] Recommendations from the European Society for Paediatric Gastroenterology, Hepatology and Nutrition (ESPGHAN) Committee on Nutrition support breastfeeding of AGA infants or formula with long-chain polyunsaturated fatty acids for formula-fed, appropriately grown infants.[54] For those infants with evidence of growth deficits present at discharge (EUGR), breastmilk should be supplemented with a human milk fortifier. Formula-fed infants should receive a special postdischarge formula, with increased protein, minerals, and long-chain polyunsaturated fatty acids, for at least the first 9 months.[7] Serial measurements of head circumference, weight, length, and weight/length ratio should be closely monitored.[131]

Some infants do not achieve full breastfeeding before discharge. It is essential, therefore, to provide clear verbal and written instruction to the breastfeeding mother about how to assess her infant's hydration status if the transition from partial to full breastfeeding is to occur at home, along with ensuring that the mother has access to medically sound breastfeeding support from the child's pediatrician or a qualified lactation consultant.

Although premature infants are at an increased risk for childhood obesity and the metabolic syndrome associated with excess weight gain, this risk is thought to be small compared with the risk for growth failure and should be considered with other risk factors such as parental size, adolescent weight, and lifestyle factors.[64] Nutritional status should be monitored closely to intervene for either deficient or excessive weight variations.

Medically Fragile and Chronically Ill Infants

Increasing survival of infants with post-NICU morbidities, including those associated with congenital diaphragmatic hernia (CDH), short bowel syndrome, and others, has increased the need for detailed parent training, home health care arrangements, and comprehensive, coordinated, multidisciplinary follow-up. The AAP has issued extensive follow-up guidelines for infants with CDH, including monitoring neurodevelopment, managing pulmonary morbidities such as pulmonary hypertension and chronic lung disease, assessing hearing function at regular intervals, providing early therapies for feeding difficulties such as oral aversion and gastroesophageal reflux, and monitoring for hernia recurrence, which have been reported in 8% to 50% of CDH infants.[15] Brodsky and Ouellette[34] recommend close monitoring of infants with a history of NEC and/or short bowel syndrome, including neurodevelopmental delays; growth, nutrition, and feeding concerns; dehydration and electrolyte imbalances; and signs of associated complications such as infection, late strictures, and cholestatic liver disease.

LONG-TERM NEURODEVELOPMENTAL FOLLOW-UP

During hospitalization, parents may ask questions about outcome that simply cannot be answered. Although the infant's risk for cognitive and motor impairment should be discussed, parents must understand that the certain diagnosis of developmental delay or disability cannot be made before 12 to 24 months of age. This need to "wait and see" creates an additional burden for families that the NICU staff should help the family anticipate. Referral to a multidisciplinary developmental follow-up clinic should provide the family with ongoing information about their child's progress and give parents the opportunity to speak with professionals about their concerns. These clinics often provide families with concrete, focused tasks to undertake with their child that may optimize infant development and help parents feel they are contributing to their child's success.

An additional concern that has more recently surfaced is even longer-term outcome issues for high-risk children. Because many children may be seen once for a multidisciplinary evaluation (18 to 24 months of corrected age) or may not be followed beyond 3 to 5 years of age in the NICU follow-up clinic, it is important that parents be informed before release from specialty follow-up care about longer-term concerns regarding health and development, especially possible challenges with academics and social-emotional issues.[69,96,150]

Pediatric health care professionals need to be aware also that recent reports delineate some more lifelong effects on the former NICU patient's quality of life as a child and adolescent, daily personal and social functions, and overall experiences with health and disease. Although much of this information may be speculative and studies remain ongoing, it is nonetheless important to inform the family that their child's long-term health and quality-of-life issues may relate to their child with a history of prematurity, regardless of the developmental status of the child when seen in the first few years of life.

REFERENCES

For a full list of references, scan the QR code or visit http://booksite.elsevier.com/9780323320832.

32 ETHICS, VALUES, AND PALLIATIVE CARE IN NEONATAL INTENSIVE CARE

JULIE R. SWANEY, NANCY ENGLISH, AND BRIAN S. CARTER

Clinical decision making is influenced by the values of the individuals involved. In the neonatal intensive care unit (NICU), these values include preserving life, decreasing morbidity, relieving pain and suffering, and, at times, end-of-life care. Sound clinical skills and judgment, combined with societal and personal values, result in the art of clinical practice.

Technologic advances in medicine have benefited many patients. We are better able to prolong life; at the same time, we are more often in a position to make deliberate decisions about when and how death will occur. Concomitantly, it has become necessary for society to reassess whether the value of prolonging life conflicts with other values, such as relieving pain and suffering and enhancing end-of-life care. In such cases, values of society, the family, and the health care professional necessarily enter into and influence the decision-making process.

Ethical reasoning insists that we understand the role of values, as well as medical data, in making decisions.

HISTORICAL OVERVIEW

Historically, ethical concerns in neonatal care focused on the risks and benefits of available technology (Table 32-1). An example is oxygen therapy with the offsetting dilemma that treatment could cause degrees of blindness or residual lung damage, whereas nontreatment might result in death or brain damage (1960s). Treatment of premature infants and those with birth defects became technically possible in the 1950s with development of infant ventilators and refined surgical techniques. Because these new technologies not only failed to eliminate all bad outcomes but also added new problems, controversies developed over when and how much to use them. Care of newborns with spinal cord defects is illustrative.

Zachary[97] and Shurtleff[80] advocated aggressive management, which increased survival rates but offered questionable quality of life for those more severely affected. Lorber[61,62] was less optimistic about the effects of aggressive management of infants with meningomyelocele and is recognized for his selective nontreatment of some of these infants. Today, open neural tube defects are routinely closed in the immediate neonatal period, and research is ongoing to assess the potential for fetal surgery to close these defects to mitigate long-term morbidity in what is clearly acknowledged as a nonlethal condition.[20]

Discussion of treatment of seriously ill newborns was stimulated by the 1973 publication of Duff and Campbell.[35] Their seminal article described the selective nontreatment or withdrawal of treatment for 43 seriously ill newborns at Yale–New Haven Hospital (between 1970 and 1972) whose "prognosis for meaningful life was extremely poor or hopeless." According to Duff and Campbell [35]:

PURPLE type highlights content that is particularly applicable to clinical settings.

TABLE
32-1
SELECTED ISSUES IN PERINATAL/NEONATAL HISTORY OF ETHICAL IMPORT

TIME	FETAL DIAGNOSIS	FETAL THERAPY	NEONATAL THERAPY
1900s (early)			Temperature regulation, nutrition; limited survival in low-birth-weight and anomalous infants Recognition of congenital rubella syndrome Cardiovascular surgery in the newborn period Modern incubator developed Oxygen therapy for respiratory distress
1950s		Tocolysis (ETOH)	Erythroblastosis fetalis (EBF) (Rh) incompatibility recognized Oxygen toxicity recognized: retrolental fibroplasia/blindness in treated infants; cerebral palsy and death in those untreated Other iatrogenic diseases Antibiotic usage broadens
1960s	Placentocentesis Early ultrasonography Fetal heart rate monitoring Fetal scalp pH assessment Amniocentesis Chromosomal analysis	Intraperitoneal blood transfusion for EBF	Birth of "modern" neonatal intensive care units Field of teratology develops after thalidomide disaster Improved outcome for infants <2500 g Surgical management of meningomyelocele becomes an issue
1970s	Fetoscopy Real-time ultrasonography Improved structural, chromosomal, and metabolic diagnostics	Intravascular blood transfusion for EBF Beta-adrenergic agonists for tocolysis Corticosteroids for lung maturation Legalization of abortion	Continuous positive airway pressure, modern neonatal ventilator Improved outcome for infants <1500 g Bronchopulmonary dysplasia recognized Problems of the very-low-birth-weight infant: intraventricular hemorrhage, bronchopulmonary dysplasia, necrotizing enterocolitis Total parenteral nutrition/hyperalimentation (TPN/HAL) becomes available Improved pediatric surgery Newborn metabolic screening
1980s	Chorionic villus sampling Cordocentesis Doppler flow studies of placenta and umbilical vessels New reproductive technology Alpha-fetoprotein monitoring	Fetal surgery Prophylactic penicillin for group B streptococcus infection Treatment of fetal dysrhythmias via maternal medications	High-frequency ventilation Surfactant replacement therapy Improved survival in infants <1000 g Extracorporeal membrane oxygenation Intravenous immunoglobulin
1990s	Fetal cell isolation in maternal blood Polymerase chain reaction and genetic amplification	Treatment of twin-to-twin transfusion syndrome	Liquid ventilation Recombinant erythropoietin Nitric oxide therapy
2000-2010	First-trimester high-resolution ultrasonography	Further advances in fetal surgery (including that for nonlethal anomalies)	Head cooling; total-body therapeutic hypothermia to mitigate HIE
2010-2015	Ever expanding genetic testing (including noninvasive fetal testing from maternal blood) Expanded perinatal, genetic, and metabolic screening	Potential genetic treatments	Prostanoids, endothelin-receptor antagonists, and phosphodiesterase inhibitors for pulmonary hypertension Orphan drug approval for some rare metabolic conditions Erythropoietin to mitigate HIE

ETOH, Alcohol; *HIE,* hypoxic-ischemic encephalopathy.

Both treatment and nontreatment constitute unsatisfactory dilemmas for everyone. When maximum treatment was viewed as unacceptable by families and physicians in our unit, there was a growing tendency to seek early death as a management option,[21] to avoid that cruel choice of gradual, often slow, but progressive deterioration of the child.

They recognized that most survivors of NICUs are healthy; however, they also recognized that some infants remain severely disabled by congenital malformations that, until recently, would have resulted in premature death. They were legitimately concerned about the quality of life for these infants and their families.

The majority of newborns treated in NICUs do grow up to lead active, productive lives, but not all fare well with even the most aggressive treatments.[40,41] Consequently, there is increasing concern over what is "appropriate" treatment of newborns, particularly seriously ill or disabled ones. Recognizing the risks and benefits of technology over 40 years ago, Eisenberg[37] stated, "At long last, we are beginning to ask, not *can* it be done, but *should* it be done."

Baby Doe (1982) and Baby Jane Doe (1983) became the focus of controversy over the issue of withholding treatment and nutrition from handicapped infants.[11,23,65,87] Today, new issues require our attention. Advances in fetal surgery continue to raise the question of whether interventions for nonlethal conditions warrant the attendant risks of preterm birth and treatment postnatally in the NICU.[20] Further, assisted reproduction technologies (ARTs) contribute to increasingly greater numbers of very-low-birth-weight (VLBW) infants born as multiples (twins, triplets, and higher-order multifetal gestations) in NICUs. At what point these well-intended services should be restrained or curtailed to prevent prematurity and its associated morbidities continues to pose new ethical questions.

Throughout this short but focused "history" of ethical issues in neonatal care, it has become increasingly apparent that there are significant issues about appropriate treatment and the limits of treatment.[45,66] Not only numerous issues but also many individuals are involved in the decision-making process about treatment and nontreatment options. More people become involved as technologic advances increase treatment options. Parents have always been presumed to be the best decision makers on their child's behalf. Health care providers also have been committed to providing what is in the best interests of their patients. Historically, decisions were made privately between parents and their physician. In the modern NICU, treatment goals and decisions are made in the context of a health care team composed of professionals from various moral communities who offer specialized input into the care of the neonate and the family. Parents must be included in the team, because their values are of paramount importance in establishing goals and making decisions about their infant's care. Societal concerns generally have focused on protecting infants against decisions that are detrimental to their best interests by statutes on child abuse and neglect. Professional groups such as the American Academy of Pediatrics (AAP),[6,7] the American College of Obstetricians and Gynecologists (ACOG),[9] and the Canadian Pediatric Society (CPS)[22] have now addressed these concerns in published guidelines for care of critically ill infants. Community groups[34,36,93] are addressing limitations of care for high-risk newborns as well. Clinical decision making is affected by parents, the health care team, professional groups, and society. Respect for clinical decision making, preferably made by parents and clinicians together, the appropriateness of care, and the protection of children against harm are constantly being balanced.

DEFINITION OF BIOETHICS

Ethics is the study of rational processes for determining the most morally desirable course of action in view of conflicting value choices. Ethics is a branch of philosophy that considers competing values to obtain the best possible outcome to a given situation. When values conflict and each value is morally justifiable, an ethical dilemma exists. For an ethical dilemma to exist, a real choice between possible courses of action must exist.

Bioethics seeks to determine the most morally desirable course of action in health care given the conflicting values inherent in varying treatment options.[10] Most often, when a conflict of values does not exist, moral conflict does not exist. That is, when the health care providers and parents all agree that it is most beneficial to an infant to not treat the infant aggressively and to allow the infant to die, no dilemma or conflict between them exists. Of course, that they agree does not mean that conflict does not exist with moral views of outside parties or principles. Regardless, the goal is to determine the most morally desirable course of action under a given set of circumstances.

THEORIES OF ETHICS

An ethical theory provides a basis for making morally appropriate decisions. There are many theories or approaches to ethics to consider. *Principle-based ethics* identifies fundamental principles that form the foundation of ethical deliberation. This approach emphasizes the centrality of principles and rules to determine moral duty. Principles commonly recognized are autonomy, beneficence, nonmaleficence, and justice.[14] *Virtue ethics* is character based and, as such, identifies the virtues of the moral agents involved, rather than the applied principles, as essential to ethical outcome. Various views of the moral life emphasize different virtues as more primary than others. In modern bioethics, primary virtues include respect, fidelity, honesty, and benevolence. *Casuistry* is *case-based ethics* in which the claims, grounds, and warrants of a particular case are compared with similar cases. The basic question for moral casuistry is how a general moral precept is to be understood in similar sets of circumstances. *Narrative ethics* is story based, in which the narrative itself is a method of ethical reasoning. Every case has different "narratives" to consider, such as medical knowledge, personal identity, patient experience, and the doctor–patient relationship. Although the medical model may focus on disease, psychopathology, objectivity, and diagnosis, the narrative model may focus correspondingly on illness, "the person," subjective experience, and caring. *Feminist ethics* is relationship based and considers primarily the ethics of care. All of these approaches are important to consider. Deciding which moral theory is operative is important to proceeding.

CLINICAL DILEMMAS IN THE NEONATAL INTENSIVE CARE UNIT

Personhood

Decision making in the NICU often revolves around the concept of personhood. When is one a person? Determining what this means depends on which moral community is consulted. Designation of personhood is morally significant because it determines whether and what duties and obligations are owed to a particular newborn.

Some communities believe personhood is present at the moment of conception; they equate "human" with "person." Shelp[79] refers to this as the "genetic theory of personhood." Others believe personhood depends on the presence or absence of certain basic human qualities. Shelp calls this moral theory "property based." Although with the latter theory there is agreement that the concept of personhood is nongenetic, there are differences about which qualities qualify for "person" status.

Fletcher[44] and Engelhardt[38] support the "property-based" stance. They believe that there are human lives that are "subpersonal." Fletcher states, "It is not what is natural but what is personal which has the first-order value in ethics."[44] Both researchers believe that neocortical function is necessary for personhood. Engelhardt[38] relates qualities such as self-consciousness, rationality, and self-determination to personhood. He distinguishes between persons in a moral sense and persons in a social sense. Infants are deemed persons only in a social sense, not a strict sense by which societal rights are obligatory. The rights of the infant, according to Engelhardt, are held in trust by his or her parents; therefore "decision(s) about treatment belong properly to the parents because the child belongs to them in a sense that it does not belong to anyone else, even to itself."[38]

Tooley[86] suggested that "The ability to see oneself as existing over time is a necessary condition for the possession of a right to life."[55] If Tooley's reasoning is correct, no infant has a right to life, at least not for some time. Although the "pro-life" moral community assigns person status to all with potential life, Tooley denied that potential has anything to do with a right to life. He advocated a quality-of-life standard. When a life is full of intractable pain and suffering, death is seen as a morally acceptable option. In fact, it is sometimes considered a relatively better outcome than continuing life.

Ramsey[74] and Robertson[77] hold a contrasting view. For them, death is never better than life; quality-of-life assessments are not part of their moral reasoning. Life is considered sacred, an absolute good. Both the fetus and newborn are considered persons with a right to live. Therefore "death must always be imposed nonhumanly by God or nature or some other cosmic arbiter."[44] This "pro-life" position supports the moral right of all fetuses and newborns to the same care, implying that abortion and infanticide are morally reprehensible.

If one is deemed a "person," society owes one certain obligations and expects certain duties. If one is not deemed a "person," it is morally reasonable for societal benefits to be withheld or withdrawn. Whatever justification is needed for a particular moral dilemma in the NICU extends from this beginning. Clearly, there is no final definition of personhood, and differing definitions must be considered.

Patienthood

A primary problem confronting a perinatal clinician is this fundamental question: Who is the patient? The adult patient is generally competent and worthy of respect as a moral agent. However, in the case of a newborn, the newborn, the family, and, in some circumstances, society have been variously considered the "patient." The accordance of rights to the newborn as an independent agent is a relatively recent occurrence. Neonatal cases are inextricably bound in the context of varying definitions of personhood and of complicated family and societal situations. This fundamental question remains: To whom is the moral duty owed? To the infant? To the family as "patient"? To society? If there are competing moral obligations, it is essential to determine to whom the primary moral duty is owed.

Professional-Patient Relationship

The importance of the professional-patient relationship cannot be overestimated, because this is the human context in which decision making occurs. With neonates, this includes a relationship between parents as surrogates and the health care team.

When the four major bioethics principles—autonomy, beneficence, nonmaleficence, and justice—are applied to health care relationships, several moral rules can be derived. These moral rules include fidelity, truth telling, and confidentiality. The professional-patient relationship is considerably affected by the meaning and extent of these rules.

Fidelity, or promise keeping, may be derived from the principle of autonomy. The duty to keep promises may promote the greatest good (utilitarian) or be seen as an obligation (formalist). Many relationships between professionals and patients (or surrogates) involve promises or contracts, whether implicitly or explicitly made. For example, once professionals have established a relationship with a patient, their duty of fidelity includes not abandoning or neglecting that patient. An obvious problem in dealing with surrogates may be conflicting duties to the surrogates and the patient. Promises made by professionals are binding except when they are superseded by stronger obligations.

Truth telling, like fidelity, can be derived from the principle of autonomy or respect for persons. It assumes an implicit contract between parties that the truth will be told. At the heart of truth telling is trust, which gives professional-patient relationships their integrity. Lying violates implicit contracts, respect for persons, and trust. It also impedes informed consent.

Utilitarians and formalists may agree on the duty to tell the truth, although they may disagree on the duty not to deceive. Cases have been made for "benevolent deception," when intentional deception is morally justifiable if its primary intent is for the benefit of the patient. In such cases, telling the truth may be a violation of *beneficence and nonmaleficence.* Others argue that deception, benevolent or not, is morally wrong, because it violates respect for persons and trust. Ultimately, the professional-patient relationship erodes. Respect for persons involves acknowledging patient autonomy to know or not to know the truth of his or her particular situation.

It is generally agreed that *confidentiality* should prevail in professional-patient relationships. With minors, confidentiality extends to the parents or legal guardians. Part of the implied contract is that information gained by both parties will be kept confidential. From the earliest days of medicine, protecting the patient's privacy has been a fundamental tenet of clinical practice. There are, of course, instances in which confidentiality is justifiably breached. It is at this point that many ethical dilemmas arise.

Breach of confidentiality may be morally and legally justified to protect the life of a patient or the lives of others who may be endangered. The value of human life overrides the relationship, but the professional should be able to demonstrate clear danger before violating a patient's privacy. This also may be seen as a violation of autonomy. "The health care professional's breach of confidentiality thus cannot be justified unless it is necessary to meet a strong conflicting duty."[14]

Obviously, health care professionals can be torn between conflicting moral obligations, such as between the patient and society. Such instances in which a breach may be justified include child abuse and neglect and certain communicable diseases. However, there is strong justification among both utilitarians and formalists for maintaining the privacy and confidentiality of patient information. Most important, the genuine integrity of the professional-patient relationship will be enhanced and preserved when confidentiality, like fidelity and truth telling, is respected and upheld. This integrity of relationship then becomes the basis of the decision-making process.

Informed Consent

The issue of valid informed consent is repeatedly raised in the environment of the NICU. All relevant information for a decision must be given. Voluntary consent, free of coercion, by competent persons must be obtained. Information given to parents may be poorly understood for many reasons, including the complex nature of the information; the emotional or physical state of the parents after the birth of a sick, premature, or anomalous infant; physical separation of the parents from their newborn; and feelings of bewilderment and intimidation leading to uncontested paternalism. Indeed, there are indications that valid informed consent is an ideal toward which we work but one that, within the realities of practice, may rarely be obtained. Consent should be sought, however, and open lines of communication and parental education established to facilitate some level of understanding and enable more than token participation in decision making by the parents.[3,52,84]

One standard that has been put forth in an effort to accomplish informed consent is the "reasonable person standard." It asks, "What would a reasonable person want in this circumstance?"

There are several ways in which the *reasonable person standard* might be enacted in the NICU, thus ensuring that more valid informed consent is obtained. First, early contact should be made with the parents or family about the expected course of problems and special management needs of the newborn. This consultation may be initiated even before delivery. Advance care birth planning is recognized as vital to delivery room decision making for the at-risk infant. Second, information should be provided by the clinical staff in a factual, compassionate manner. Parents may need continued orientation or

reorientation to the NICU environment. This may be necessary especially for parents who are geographically separated from their infant. Third, phone calls and photographs are important means for parents to maintain emotional involvement with their baby. Fourth, social workers, chaplains, or other support resources should be contacted and used early to manage emotional distress and facilitate communication. Fifth, regular patient care conferences with the parents should be scheduled. This will keep parents apprised of the newborn's status and will keep the staff informed about the parents' level of understanding, perspectives, and values. Additional efforts to communicate must be made at the time of special procedures, tests, or therapies to enhance everybody's understanding and the informed consent process.

An integral part of the informed consent process and one that directly affects decision making is the principle of fidelity, commonly called *truth telling,* as discussed. Issues of what to tell, how and when to tell, and whom to tell become a daily part of the staff's interaction with each other and the families of affected newborns.

In practice, the issue of truth telling is considered an essential component of the professional-patient relationship. Information should be shared among staff members and presented to the family truthfully, compassionately, and without bias. However, it is often best for a single voice (e.g., the attending neonatologist, neonatal nurse practitioner, or primary care clinician) consistently to relate information and interpret facts for families to minimize confusion or misinformation.

Double Effect

The principle of "double effect" asserts that an action may be considered good if the intent of the action is a positive value, even if the secondary effects of the action might be considered harmful if undertaken as the primary goal; further, the good effect should be commensurate with the harm. Double effect is used frequently in the NICU. An example is the use of opioids (morphine or fentanyl) in a newborn for whom there has been a compassionate life-support withdrawal from assisted ventilation: the positive goal is reduction of air hunger and suffering, even at an acknowledged low risk for causing some degree of respiratory depression.

Problems of Uncertainty

A major difficulty in ethical decision making is the uncertainty that exists around medical and prognostic outcomes. It is difficult to determine what may be in the best interest of the child when the prognosis remains unclear. Even when the prognosis may seem clear, there are always those children who confound science, whose developmental outcomes are far from expected.

Some of the most frequent problems in working with perinatal cases arise as a result of this uncertainty. Parents always ask, "Will my baby be okay when he (or she) grows up?" Answers are often unsatisfying or incomprehensible. In most cases with premature infants, truth telling may compel an answer that, when reduced to its simplest form, says, "I don't know." A statistical approach to answering the question may be "Most babies like yours grow up to be normal" or "Some babies like yours have serious problems." These answers are often followed by a litany of statistical probabilities of each morbidity. Neither approach answers the parents' question of what their particular baby will be like. Such approaches serve to complicate the clinician's relationship with parents over issues such as expertise, veracity, and disclosure. The statistical approach may answer the NICU staff's question of quality of care, but few parents understand such statistics or are willing to apply them to a loved one. Nonetheless, uncertainty is a way of life in many perinatal cases, and this observation significantly compromises the resolution of ethical problems in the NICU.

In considering medical uncertainty, it may be helpful to recognize two general classes of perinatal cases. NICU patients can be generally classified as either premature infants without known anomalies or near-term infants with major anomalies, either syndromic or nonsyndromic. Neonatal deaths, by definition occurring in the first 28 days of postnatal life, are principally associated with prematurity or anomalies and account for about two thirds of all infant mortality (death before the first birthday). For infants with known syndromes or major anomalies, prognoses from the literature are describable with reasonable accuracy. This assists with some certainty.

A detailed review of neonatal outcome is beyond the scope of this chapter, but several conclusions appear justified. First, the infant mortality rate has declined rapidly since the establishment of NICUs and the major mortality groups are in lower weight and younger gestational age groups.[2,32,54] Second, coincident with the decline in mortality rate have come major improvements in neonatal morbidity (both neurodevelopmental and pulmonary) from nearly 50% in the pre-NICU era to current figures in the range of 15% from many institutions.[32] Third, the absolute number of normal premature survivors has increased dramatically and the absolute number of moderately and severely affected survivors appears to have increased as well.[32]

Despite this, "extreme prematurity, on the other hand, is characterized by an enormous uncertainty. In these cases predictions of outcome at birth are probabilistic at best."[76] Accordingly, attempts have been made to establish guidelines for treatment of extremely low-birth-weight (ELBW) infants.[9,22,34,36,93] The morbidities in premature survivors are variable in nature, but central nervous system morbidities generally include visual impairment and blindness, speech and hearing impairment, neuromuscular impairment, and serious cognitive impairment.[71] Few premature survivors require long-term institutional care.[32] The combined risk for one or more of these disabilities is in the range of 15% to 20%.[33,48,49,95] Most people agree that these are indeed serious disabilities, with major effect on the patient and family. However, do they justify withholding or withdrawing treatment? If so, under what circumstances?

For perinatal clinicians for whom quality of life is a major consideration, it remains an exceedingly difficult practical problem to predict which particular child will be significantly impaired and in what manner. The predictive value of postnatal evaluations in estimating long-term disability is low.

The intent of raising these questions is to underscore the complexity of ethical discussions as particularly applied to problems in the modern NICU. This in no way reduces the enormity of such problems for the patient, family, health care providers, or society. Technologic advances may resolve old uncertainties but often seem to carry new uncertainties that are equally perplexing.

Setting Goals

Treatment goals should be established so that incremental decisions can be made. Preferably, parents should establish goals based on their values for their child. Parents should be involved, not just informed, in determining the overall goals of treatment. Decisions toward that end then can be made. Goals expressed by parents may be living a "normal" life, living with a debilitating outcome but without persistent pain or suffering, existence without any notable "quality of life," and so on. Accordingly, treatment goals may be to improve an infant's health, help the infant to maintain the current state of health, or help the infant die with supportive palliative care. Too frequently, decisions are made before the treatment goal is established. The parents and health care team members may be working toward different goals. The physician, health care team, and parents all should be guided by established goals so that beneficial treatment can be offered. There should be a model of shared decision making. The AAP Committee on Fetus and Newborn has stated that although the role of parents in goal setting and decision making must be respected[6]:

> The physician is not obligated to provide inappropriate treatment or to withhold beneficial treatment at the request of the parents. Treatment that is harmful, of no benefit, or futile and merely prolonging dying should be considered inappropriate. The physician must ensure that the chosen treatment, in his or her best medical judgment, is consistent with the best interest of the infant.

Treatment and Nontreatment

For parents to be involved in determining overall treatment goals and the decision-making process, they must be fully informed to consent to or refuse treatment for their child. Infants should be treated humanely and with respect in an environment that is conducive to maximum comfort and healing. Humane judgments should be made in determining how infants can most benefit from treatment in any given situation. Palliative care should be provided to all infants at all times.[16] As noted in Chapter 12, sufficient analgesic should be administered to infants having surgery because they can indeed experience physical and psychologic pain. Staff and parents should maximize the development of premature infants and offer every possible benefit to them. The nursery environment should be as free from excessive overstimulation as possible.

Other perplexing ethical questions arise when the benefit of treatment is unclear.[89] Even the most perfunctory of decisions should be based on the patient's best interests, yet "best interests" are often

difficult to determine. Should a baby born with anencephaly be resuscitated or receive life-sustaining interventions solely for the purpose of organ transplantation? Should an ELBW infant receive aggressive ventilatory therapy? Should an infant with trisomy 18 be treated with aggressive life support or surgery? Medical and ethical decisions involve considering not only what kind of treatment serves the patient's best interest but also whether the treatment is appropriate at all. Limited or nontreatment decisions are agonizing and regularly result in ethical discussions. A nontreatment decision is sometimes incorrectly called withholding or withdrawing *care*. Only *treatment* may be withheld or withdrawn. *Care* always should be provided, whether curative or palliative.

"Nonbeneficial" Treatment

The concept of "nonbeneficial" (or futile) medical treatment may be as perplexing as the concept of benefit. It does, however, deserve attention, because there are increasing circumstances in which treatment may be considered to be nonbeneficial and thus withheld or withdrawn. There is no ethical obligation to offer nonbeneficial treatment, yet there is no one definition of "nonbeneficial."

Most often, judgments about benefit are based on medical or physiologic data. It may be medically nonbeneficial to resuscitate an infant under certain conditions, because the treatment cannot alter the course of the illness or problem, yet there are psychologic, social, and religious reasons that such treatment might be offered. If, because of the treatment, the family has time to hold the infant and say good-bye, the resuscitation may not be considered by them to have been nonbeneficial. Of course, the opposite is also true; that is, what may not be physiologically nonbeneficial may be considered to be nonbeneficial by the family or surrogates based on religious or other reasons. Again, there is no ethical obligation to offer nonbeneficial treatment. It is possible to get a medical effect but not a medical benefit.[78] The distinction can be significant. Determination of the appropriateness of treatment should be based on medical benefit as determined by family goals for the patient, which include physiologic, psychologic, social, and religious data.[58] By attending to all of these aspects of care, which include staff and family input alike, a determination of what is nonbeneficial therapy and thus what is beneficial therapy can be made.

Research Ethics

A persistent and controversial issue in neonatal care has been the introduction of new therapies or procedural interventions into the NICU without appropriate research into their safety, efficacy, net benefit, and long-term outcomes for those critically ill infants who receive them. Appropriate studies in animal models ideally are followed by randomized, controlled clinical trials in human newborns (see Chapter 1). Extracorporeal membrane oxygenation, high-frequency ventilation, and recombinant erythropoietin all have been examples of interventions that crept into neonatal care before controlled trials were conducted. In recent years, the use of glucocorticoids either to enhance fetal lung maturity antenatally or to prevent or treat bronchopulmonary dysplasia postnatally is an example worth evaluating.

Although the benefits of a two-dose regimen of antenatal steroids was demonstrated in 1972,[60] the development of recent practice patterns in which multiple doses of steroids were used over successive weeks of pregnancy was unsubstantiated by randomized clinical trials designed to address the efficacy or safety of such practices. Subsequently the National Institutes of Health held a Consensus Development Conference and published a statement advising that repeat courses of steroids not be used routinely.[66] Research conducted after these practice patterns were established demonstrated increased maternal infection and suppression of the normal hypothalamic-pituitary-adrenal axis and both fetal and neonatal decreased somatic and brain growth, adrenal suppression, neonatal sepsis, chronic lung disease, and increased mortality rate. In addition, neurodevelopmental outcome studies suggested an increase in psychomotor delay and behavioral problems.

The acute, seemingly beneficial effects of administering systemic steroids to newborns with lung disease, however, were not met with significantly improved mortality rate or long-term outcome. It is also associated with a number of acute side effects (e.g., gastrointestinal perforation, hypertension, hyperglycemia) and possible long-term harmful consequences on lung and central nervous system function.[13,69,83] Recent studies that caution about the poor postnatal brain growth among some ELBW NICU survivors raise additional concerns about the

wisdom of adding risks associated with steroid treatment to an already at-risk newborn.[69,83] Research into the future use of steroids in premature infants should be well designed and adequately powered to provide answers and should include an evaluation of long-term neurodevelopmental outcome.[42]

Recent concerns have been publicly aired in the lay and professional media over the conduct of neonatal research, the adequacy of the informed consent process for parents of newborns, and the overall safety and conduct of neonatal research.[50] As stated by Lantos, "the clinical judgment of conscientious and knowledgeable physicians is only as good as the evidence on which it is based."[56] This matter is clear, and the requisite evidence-based practices we all seek require carefully acquired evidence from well-conducted and safe studies (see Chapter 1). But there are other lessons in the SUPPORT legacy, not the least of which is the need for transparency and honest communication of what we *do not know*—hence the difficulty in explaining to parents and colleagues alike that the involvement in clinical research may or may not affect the risk of bad outcomes—or good! And that is why the research is being done.[57] Parents are vulnerable, their babies are critically ill, and everyone in the NICU—including clinicians—is hopeful. But these truths can make the informed consent process, and the conduct of research, challenging in seemingly unapparent ways.[63,68] If parents of critically ill children respond to the challenges present in decision making for clinical care by wrestling with multiple influences beyond any simple explanation or exchange of clinical information and attendant risk/benefit analysis, they likely are no less inclined to do the same in the context of clinical research.[24]

DECISION MAKING IN THE NEONATAL INTENSIVE CARE UNIT

In the NICU, decisions of serious proportion are encountered regularly, based on medical facts and nonmedical values.[70] There should be a model of shared decision making aligning values with the expected outcome for the infant. From the moment of birth, and in some cases even earlier, a foremost issue is that of determining the appropriate level of intervention treatment of sick or anomalous newborns. Entire texts have been devoted to this issue.[55,91] Primary concerns are when to treat, when and how to intervene, when to limit intervention, and who should be involved in the decision-making process.

A frequently encountered treatment problem requiring attention, other than the much-publicized anomalous infant, is the extremely premature or VLBW infant whose course is marked by slow or absent progress despite appropriate and seemingly heroic intervention. The development of complications from prematurity is of further concern. In concert, these may portend a guarded or very poor prognosis.

These cases may prompt "quality of life" and "ordinary versus extraordinary treatment" discussions. The President's Commission[73] noted that "there is no basis for holding that whether a treatment is common or unusual, or whether it is simple or complex, is in itself significant to a moral analysis of whether treatment is warranted or obligatory"— a view that had been voiced previously by moral philosophers. The AAP has published a strategy for the initiation and withdrawal of treatment for high-risk newborns.[4] General recommendations include the importance of ongoing evaluation, parental participation, establishing the goals of humane care, and upholding the best interests standard seeking to benefit the infant: "It is inappropriate for life-prolonging treatment to be continued when the condition is incompatible with life or when the treatment is judged to be futile."[4] The AAP Committee on Bioethics further "supports individualized decision making about life-sustaining medical treatment for all children, regardless of age. These decisions should be jointly made by physicians and parents."[4] If we are honest about our professions, we must realize that "quality of life" is what we are all about. Health care professionals are entrusted by society to advance the health and well-being of the mind and body of all persons so that they can lead their lives and function as part of the human family, individually or collectively. No individual is capable of establishing what is an acceptable "quality of life" for all persons in all circumstances. Each case requires our collective efforts to facilitate the best decision for that particular patient.

Steps in Ethical Decision Making

The approach should follow a method that clearly demonstrates the practice of applied clinical ethics.

The goal of applied ethics is to make the best decisions for and with a particular patient. Such a decision requires first that a decision maker be determined. The decision maker, whether a parent, health care provider, or other, must understand his or her own (1) philosophy of relationship to the patient (or family), (2) interpretation of ethical principles and values, (3) theoretic basis of ethics used (e.g., utilitarian, deontologic), and (4) source from which morality is derived.

An ethical "workup" is then undertaken in which substantive issues are identified and worked through, resulting in a decision.[85] Implementing decisions requires determining who shall decide, by what criteria they shall be allowed to do so, and subsequently how the decisions or actions are to be implemented.

Box 32-1 presents the essential steps to decision making in neonatal cases in which a dilemma exists. Consider all involved values and possible solutions to the problem, realizing that alternative solutions may uphold different principles and result in different (positive or negative) consequences. Options that may appear acceptable to the family may be unacceptable to the health care team, or vice versa. There may be societal (legal) constraints on certain actions. In some instances, only one option will be consistent with the rules and principles to which the decision maker subscribes. Other options may

---

BOX 32-1 APPROACH TO ETHICAL DILEMMAS IN NEONATAL CARE

1. Consider who is involved in making and implementing the decision (family, guardians, clinicians, society).
2. Decide who will make the final decision. Is referral to an ethics committee indicated?
3. Clarify all of the medical facts within the case; consider indications, alternatives, and consequences of each action or inaction.
4. Understand significant human factors and values (for patient, family, and health care team).
5. Identify the ethical dilemma or conflict.
6. Make a decision:
   a. List options as solutions to the problem.
   b. Weigh and prioritize values.
   c. Make a decision.
7. Check for moral and rational defensibility.

Data from Brody H: *Ethical decisions in medicine,* Boston, 1981, Little, Brown; and Francoeur RT: From then to now. In Harris CC, Snowden F, editors: *Bioethical frontiers in perinatal intensive care,* Natchitoches, La, 1985, Northwestern State University Press.

present apparent conflicts between competing values or result in unacceptable consequences. In a decision, there will probably be some give and take. A shared decision-making model embraces all parties and viewpoints. Some priority must be assigned to a certain set of values, rules, principles, or resultant effects of any action or inaction. A decision should be made in light of these issues. This process need not always be invoked in full. Often, when the case is carefully dissected and medical facts, values, treatment alternatives, and expected prognoses are revealed, issues that at first seemed in question are clarified and it becomes apparent that no real dilemma exists.

Good ethics, then, starts with good facts and effective communication. A viable patient-professional relationship that clarifies facts (taking into account uncertainties and the difficulties of prognosticating), human values and feelings, and the interests of all relevant parties is essential to ethical decision making. Decisions made should reflect a moral choice that is beneficial to the newborn as determined by the established, informed decision makers.

Although it may be arguable whether the patient is the neonate, family, or another societal group, it is prudent to develop a consensus wherever possible and thus minimize conflict among the interested parties. Efforts should be made to involve the parents early in the care of their child and listen carefully to their values, goals, and dreams. Clinical information should be presented sensitively and thoroughly. These efforts may help minimize the stresses on the parents and prepare them to participate in decision making about the care of their child. These efforts will also assist staff as they participate with the parents in the decision-making process. With careful attention to the needs of patients, families, and staff, many conflicts can be resolved at an early stage before positions are hardened and emotional investment is high.

In most cases, consensus is reached. In a minority of cases, conflict is unavoidable. In some cases, medical care raises issues that are highly controversial either within the group of clinicians providing care or in the broader context of societal problems. In many cases, the family is far from homogeneous in its expression of wishes. Many parents are young and in the process of achieving independent adulthood with well-developed values. Single-parent families are not uncommon. The birth of a critically ill infant may serve as a focus to crystallize disagreements between spouses or may aggravate conflicts between the parent (or parents) and the extended family. In such cases, a more formal process, such as a formal family care conference, appeal to an ethics committee, or even involvement of the legal system, may help resolve or minimize conflicts of values. It is preferable, however, that decisions be made by involved parties as close to the bedside as possible.[81]

Proxy Decision Makers

In dealing with newborns who are, by their very nature, incompetent and cannot make decisions for themselves, value conflicts must be resolved with the input of a proxy or surrogate decision maker acting on the infant's behalf. This may be the parents, a family member, friend, guardian ad litem, or the physician. To be considered a valid surrogate, the person should be competent, knowledgeable of integral values of the patient or family, free from conflicting interests, and without serious emotional conflicts in dealing with the case.

Society has for many reasons allocated to the parents the primary authority role in collaboration with health care providers in making decisions about their newborn's care. In most instances, the parents are best suited for deciding such matters and have the infant's best interests in mind. They are usually present when possible, are concerned for their infant's well-being, and are willing to hear the facts of their infant's condition, as well as learn of needed therapies. Of all people, they also know best the values of the family culture or environment in which the infant will be raised.

Yet parents may be less understandably overwhelmed at times, both physically and emotionally exhausted, and baffled or intimidated by the high-technology environment of the NICU and the complexities of their infant's care. Amid feelings of grief, fear, anxiety, and wonderment over their premature or anomalous infant, they may be uncertain of their proper role and responsibilities as parents. Some parents show signs of acute stress disorder and posttraumatic stress disorder. Health care providers should give daily updates on the infant's condition and anticipated course. Parents' needs for emotional support and avenues to both vent their frustrations and explore their concerns over economic, marital, family or sibling, and career effects of their predicament make resources such as nurses, social workers, and chaplains essential in providing assistance to allow them to participate in goal setting and difficult decision making. Occasionally it will be necessary to assess the level of parental competency in assuming the role of surrogate, recognizing when additional help or support for them is needed to fulfill this role.

Reliance on clinicians as decision makers is yet another option. Clinicians know and understand the complexities of the medical condition and treatment more than parents do and should promote the infant's best interests in advocating treatment. They may be more objective about individual cases and are not emotionally overwhelmed, as the parents might be. Also, based on experience, they offer a perspective of effectiveness of treatments and can be consistent in treating similar cases.

However, clinicians also may encounter problems when they act as the principal decision makers. Although their knowledge of medical facts is the most complete of all persons, it is at the same time, unfortunately, incomplete. Accurate diagnoses and certainty in prognoses are elusive at times. Medical knowledge does have limits. Statistics are helpful for groups of similarly affected patients, but individual outcomes are difficult to predict. Further, while having an advanced degree of specialized information and knowledge, physicians do not necessarily possess any more moral expertise than that of parents or others.

Treatment versus nontreatment decisions are ultimately moral, not simply medical, decisions. These decisions are weightier than most clinical decisions that clinicians make. More is involved than a rote, rational process employed in isolation from the family or health care team. The clinician must contend with his or her own values and emotions, as well as the medical facts, in each individual case. He or she must facilitate parental and health care team communication and interaction and ultimately order the level of intervention.

Fortunately, physicians and nurse practitioners do not work in isolation from the health care team when making decisions about patients. Nurses, child life workers, social workers, and chaplains are vital members of the decision-making team. A potential problem with each of these clinicians as surrogates is that a conflict of interest may exist between them and the infants for whom they are deciding. Members of the health care team may be biased toward the prolongation of life, have preconceived and strong biases about euthanasia, or be influenced by issues unrelated to the infant, including advancement of care, financial issues, or societal issues. Hence they may not fully

consider the best interests of the patient or the values of the involved family. In contrast to parents, they do not live with the results of their decisions and actions. Also, consistency in their application of principles to similar cases may be lacking, and they may give in to strong pressures (real or perceived) exerted by the law or very assertive parents.

Various factors should contribute to minimizing the potential problems in parents and health care professionals reaching morally defensible decisions in the best interest of the premature or anomalous infant. The professionalism of health care team members who are committed to serving the health and interests of their patients is a foremost consideration that serves this purpose. A sense of duty leads these professionals to assist families in achieving their life goals through facilitating open communication and discussion of their varied concerns. A great sense of personal and professional satisfaction may be derived by helping families accept and deal with their emotions, questions, and concerns for their infant and their own circumstances.

For many years, hospital ethics committees have been given an increasing role in facilitating ethical decision making for sick neonates. Generally their roles are to provide education, policy interpretation, and clinical consultation. Clinically, ethics consultants function to clarify the ethical dimensions of various treatment options and serve in an advisory capacity only. They do not make clinical decisions. Clinical decisions are best made at the bedside by parties who are involved with the sick infant. At times, however, clinicians and parents need clarification and support. Ideally, ethics committees facilitate the resolution of any conflicts between parents and clinicians in matters of treatment. They help work through ethical aspects of treatment decisions. One important role they play is to improve effective communication between staff and families. Finally, they may prove to be a safeguard for infants for whom parents and professionals are working toward an end that may be perceived as contrary to the infant's best interests.

Surely, much reflective thinking should be invested in our decisions, as individuals, parents, or members of a committee. However, a small number of cases will proceed beyond institutional review to a court. Every effort should be pursued before going to court. Courts may employ many of the criteria for being proxies. They can ensure that all relevant facts are presented and considered, and judges are capable of exercising unmatched control of data collection, investigation, questioning of experts, and seeking of alternative solutions. A judge also can appoint a guardian ad litem to be the patient's advocate when necessary.

There are at least a few weaknesses in courts as proxies. They are removed from the NICU and have no contact with the case, patient, staff, or family whose problem they are deciding; hence they are more remote than other possible proxy decision makers. Working through cases may be time-consuming, which may result in additional problems, changes in pertinent facts, or prolongation of suffering. Sometimes the consequences of court proxies are that they become the decision maker for the infant instead of the parents and/or clinicians. Although the best interest of the infant may override the rights of the parents, this can result in the rights of the state's legal system overriding the rights of the parents and even the best interest of the infant.

Standard of Best Interest

The best-interest standard has been advocated by the President's Commission and others seeking to accomplish valid moral decision making in difficult neonatal cases.[59,73,74] We are obliged "to try to evaluate benefits and burdens from the infant's own perspective."[59] This standard requires a balance of beneficence, nonmaleficence, and justice. It is accepted in the case of newborns over "substituted judgment." Because newborns are, by definition, never competent, substituted judgment can only be applied hypothetically. The best-interest standard is accepted as the best method available for parents and clinicians to decide on behalf of newborns.

The potential for self-seeking by the decision maker is easy to understand and has been recognized. The interests of parents, siblings, clinicians, hospital staff or administration, and society may all seem to compete with those of the newborn. But the interests of others—be they emotional, economic, or otherwise problematic—cannot justifiably override those of the patient[12,53] based on the actual or potential personhood of the critically ill neonate. Individual or societal problems or perceived burdens generally are not viewed on the same moral plane as a person's claim to life.

Certainly some cases stretch the best-interest standard to its limits. Cases of protracted treatment with uncertain prognoses beg the question of quality of existence (in which nonmaleficence is the principle of concern) and require consideration of

more than mere suffering and pain.[53] Indeed, in the words of Arras,[12] "Sometimes circumstances may be so extreme and the consequences so dreadful that the priority of justice can no longer be maintained." In this sense, we have to find the best balance of beneficence, nonmaleficence, and justice.

We also must consider other morally relevant concerns of neonates who may be doomed to brief lives with less than recognizably "human" existence. Human capacities (e.g., ability to think, be aware of self, relate to other people) may be different from biologic human life. The preservation of biologic human life bereft of the benefit of distinctly human capacities is controversial and has been challenged in quality-of-life decisions.[12,35,55,61,91] Walters[88] has written of the "proximate personhood" model. Arras[12] suggested the "relational potential standard" (Does this child have the ability, or potential, to relate to physical space and time and to communicate to others?) as a means to address these concerns more aptly than the "misapplied best interest standard," calling on society itself to inquire "into the conditions of valuable human life."

Priority should be given to attempts at effecting a cure in these ill infants. Whether or not a cure can be achieved, patient comfort should be sought. Some maintain that life itself may not always be an absolute good; thus it may be morally justifiable to withhold or withdraw futile treatment associated with inhumane risks or harms that would prolong dying. Mitchell, while a member of the American Nurses Association Committee on Ethics, has stated[65]:

Some infants are so premature and underweight, so profoundly impaired, so hopelessly diseased, or so severely asphyxiated that their foreshortened lives are full of misery for them and those around them. For infants who are so impaired that medical therapies are futile or would only prolong suffering, invasive medical procedures and surgery are morally, as well as medically, inappropriate.

She calls on nurses to shift their focus in such cases to "seek primarily to provide comfort, relieve suffering and help a grieving family."

Creating an Ethical Environment

Ethical decisions do not happen in a vacuum. Environments should exist that promote ethical behavior and deliberation. Such environments should be institutional (the nursery, the hospital, the community, social and political structures) and attitudinal. Attitudes include those in which families and staff are empowered to express their opinions and engage in the decision-making process, all voices are valued, information is openly and honestly shared (including uncertainties), respect for all individuals is upheld, and the predominant concern is to benefit the patient, whether that be minimizing overstimulation of patients, administering the appropriate analgesic, or providing appropriate palliative care.[94] Routine ethics rounds or ethics committee and palliative care consultations, along with family care conferences and generally good family communication, are recognized means of enhancing such an environment in the NICU. Yet none of these replace the responsibility of all staff members consistently to promote an overall ethical milieu in the nursery in which ethical practice is the standard of care.

Recent literature has focused on the concept of moral distress, particularly among nursing staff. Moral distress occurs when conflict exists between personal values and treatment being given. The most commonly reported cause of distress is following orders to support patients at end of life with advanced technology when palliative or comfort care would be, from the perspective of the caregivers, more humane.[40]

Some institutions hold weekly staff conferences for education, clarification, and open and informed communication among staff members. Information can be clarified, and family care conferences can be arranged. When the NICU staff enter into these dialogues with parents or when an ethics consultant joins in, the ability to clarify the goals of care and understand the present condition of the patient and potential future concerns of all parties as they view the patient is enhanced.

ETHICS COMMITTEE OR PALLIATIVE CARE CONSULTATION?

Generally in practice, it is preferable to keep the decision-making responsibility within the professional-patient relationship. In the vast majority of cases, members of the health care team and the parents do have the infant's best interests in mind. Yet in view of the vast dimension and difficulties of some of the required decisions, many clinicians will consult with a hospital ethics committee (HEC), infant bioethics committee (IBC), or palliative care team (PCT). Some institutions have all three of these committees—the IBC falling under the HEC—but many do not have an IBC, PCT, or palliative care consultant. For those who have both ethics and palliative care consultation available, it is reasonable to question whom to call, and when, for consultation. These intersecting processes enhance clinical care. When there is agreement about a treatment plan, both the ethics committee and palliative care might be consulted for confirmation of that plan. When there is a dispute about a proposed course of treatment, the HEC (and/or IBC) might be consulted for clarification of ethical principles, values, and various treatment options that would be consistent with ethical and legal standards.[51] The PCT or consultant might also be used for consultation on goals clarification and the development of a comprehensive palliative treatment plan to include comfort measures, specific symptom management, and support to the infant, family, and caregivers. Palliative care provides comprehensive management of physical, psychosocial, spiritual, and existential needs of patients and families facing life-limiting illness.[5,8]

The stimulus to the establishment of IBCs in the United States was the controversy over and death of Baby Doe in Bloomington, Indiana, when society (and government) became acutely aware of the moral issues surrounding what many perceived to be wrongful nontreatment of a handicapped newborn.[72] Resulting government regulations, along with AAP policies, have focused on the importance of ethics consultation to promote quality decisions about treatment of ill newborns. HECs, composed of members from different disciplines, are a resource for consultation and advice. They are not a decision-making body, although some groups are moving toward a consensus model. Different committees have different procedures.[43,59] Ethics consultation should be sought for values clarification and decision making. Committee functions and responsibilities may include (1) offering counsel and ethical review, (2) educating hospital personnel, (3) retrospectively and prospectively reviewing pertinent government guidelines, and (4) developing appropriate institutional policies. In most institutions, *anyone* involved in a particular case may request a consultation from the HEC.

Palliative care is both a philosophy and an approach to care delivery.[6] It focuses on comprehensive, compassionate comfort and support. Many domains of palliative care are appropriate for all patients. Palliative care may, however, be especially important—and become the predominant paradigm of care—when an infant is on the threshold of viability, is gravely ill or has an uncertain outcome, or is dying despite appropriately applied intensive care measures.[16] Palliative care consultation should be sought (1) any time there is a question about comfort or support, (2) any time there is a question about pain and symptom management specific to the realm of comfort and end-of-life, and (3) when an infant has a life-threatening condition or is dying despite life-sustaining interventions. Palliative care services generally work collaboratively with HEC members and the clinical team to ensure maximum comfort and minimal suffering for babies whether their conditions are improving or worsening. Such consultations, along with good family communication, enhance patient care and the ethical environment of the NICU.

COMMUNICATING WITH FAMILIES

The most important element in communicating with families is listening to them. Indeed, consistent, sensitive, and thorough communication of clinicians with families is essential to good patient care. The more complex the medical situation, the more crucial it is that parents receive consistent information, perhaps from a single designated person on the health care team. Parents often are confused by the various prognostications offered by multiple subspecialists and cannot synthesize the data into a "larger picture" of what is happening to their baby. Yet in the urgency to communicate information, clinicians sometimes forget to listen to the grief, fears, and concerns of parents for their child.[47] These feelings can profoundly influence decisions that are made and how they are made. Ethics as a rational process must also consider the range of human emotions involved in life-and-death issues, not just clinical information. What parents would not be distraught over the premature birth of their infant? Overwhelmed by their severely disabled infant?

The prospect of lifetime rehabilitation? The reality or prospect of suffering? The prospect of death of their newborn?

Good communication with parents is essential, because parents play a vital role in the decision-making process. They, along with the infant, are the most affected.[17] No matter what their religious or sociocultural background, almost all parents experience shock and grief over their infant's need for intensive care.[47] They deal with this in better and worse ways. For many parents, the ability to participate in ethical decision making is impaired while they are in such an acute stage of shock. Usually, prenatal diagnosis of anomalies gives parents time to adjust to their baby's condition before birth or before decisions have to be made. This adjustment time can be most valuable. To participate in ethical decision making, particularly decisions about withholding or withdrawing treatment, parents must have achieved some degree of emotional reorganization and acceptance. Staff assistance in helping them move from emotional disorganization to reorganization is crucial to further decisions that should be made. At this point, parents may be better able to absorb medical data, ethical values, and principles. Although a theoretic difference may not exist between withholding and withdrawing treatment, there is a large emotional difference. The sound clinician, as well as the ethicist, must be sensitive to this distinction.

Choices about treatment and nontreatment do affect the grieving process. Questions such as "Am I just prolonging suffering by keeping her alive?" are countered by "Am I not giving her a chance and playing God by allowing her to die?" Duff and Campbell[35] report that families experienced "a normal mourning for their losses" after allowing their seriously ill infants to die. What remains for many parents are doubts that their choice was correct. For some, decisions based on certain religious principles or other value criteria offer moral justification of behavior that assists in the mourning process. For others, the justification may be logically but not emotionally clear. In these instances, grieving can become more complex and difficult.

A valuable role of an ethics committee and/or ethics consultant may be to offer input into, if not confirmation of, the parents' decision in a way that helps allay guilt that can interrupt normal grieving. Ethics, although at once highly theoretic and intellectual, must consider that the situations with which it most intimately deals are highly emotional. For parents, the psychologic trauma will affect their ethical considerations and ethical decisions will have further psychologic effect.

A real value of an interdisciplinary health care team is the particular attention paid to the many complex aspects of a patient's living and dying. When parents are facing the death of their baby, the entire team may be involved in assisting them. Nurses and physicians, social workers, chaplains, and psychologists may all be intimately involved with monitoring the patient's comfort level and deteriorating course and with comforting grieving parents. Baptisms (when appropriate) and especially funerals are important ritualistic ways of organizing the meaning of the traumatic event. The entire staff should encourage parents to offer all that they can to their dying infant. They should provide active palliative care—maximum comfort for the patient and maximum support to the family. Helping patients and families cope with death is a privilege. It can be personally and professionally satisfying, and ultimately immeasurably helpful to everyone involved, to enter emotionally into this process. Often care of the living means care of the dying.

Good communication among staff members is also important. The effect on the health care team members of helping an infant die also should be recognized because their concern and involvement with the infant usually are significant. Helping someone through the dying process can be a difficult, though rewarding, experience. In such instances, professionals may agree with the decision (preferably the parents') to withhold or withdraw treatment. Professionals may also disagree with the decision but may place a higher value on the parents' autonomy to decide than on the decision itself. Respecting this, they may abide by the parents' wishes for their baby. No one should be forced to compromise personal or professional integrity, however, and in cases in which one's ethics or integrity is being violated, the case may be transferred. Catlin and colleagues[31] suggest "conscientious objection" as a potential response to the moral distress experienced by neonatal nurses. Preferably, professionals can learn about the range of ethically defensible options and can support the parents in choices different from their own.

How does the clinician discuss such sensitive issues, especially dying, with parents? In many ways. First and foremost, listen to their thoughts, feelings, and concerns as they express them. Clinicians should consider the vulnerability of parents who are frequently overwhelmed by the delivery, their baby's condition, and other related stressors. Clinicians should be compassionate not only in their listening but also in their communication to parents. What are they feeling, perceiving, wondering about, fearing, hoping for? Box 32-2 suggests some questions to engage in empathic conversation. Such questions are relevant to the parents of the infant whose condition is improving, the infant whose future is uncertain, the infant for whom parents must make agonizing decisions, and the infant who is clearly dying. Empathic communication with families is a critical component of the ethical environment of the NICU.

BOX 32-2 | **SUGGESTED QUESTIONS TO ENGAGE EMPATHIC CONVERSATION**

- What do you understand is going on with your baby?
- Who is your main doctor? What has he or she told you?
- Do you have the medical information you need, or do you want more?
- What kind of information would help you the most right now?
- What are you expecting for your baby?
- What do you think your baby feels?
- What do you see your baby doing?
- Who is your very best support person right now?
- Is he or she available?
- What is your greatest concern about your baby?
- What would give you a sense of peace or comfort in the midst of this, if that is possible?
- What is happening at home?
- Faith and beliefs can be very important in the grief and healing process. Is there anything about your faith or beliefs that we should know to be able to take care of you and your baby?
- Who or what is helping you get through this?
- This may be or is the best condition your baby will ever be in. When this is the case, we usually focus on keeping him or her warm and comfortable until he or she dies rather than on curing. How do you feel about this for your baby?
- Our goals in health care are to (1) improve health, (2) maintain health, and (3) help someone die.
- How can we ease this experience for you?

PALLIATIVE CARE IN THE INTENSIVE CARE SETTING

Palliative care offers families comprehensive, compassionate, and supportive care. Involvement of palliative care clinicians is imperative when their baby's diagnosis has an uncertain outcome or a condition that may end in death.

Families and providers must have access to either a palliative care consultation service or integrated clinical care pathway when the critically ill newborn is admitted into the NICU.[26,27,41,82] Current trends in health care advocate that palliative care be included with *cure-oriented* approaches for all patients who have a serious illness.

In the United States, the majority of infant deaths occur in the NICU after a planned withdrawal of mechanical ventilation. Infant deaths generally occur in two phases. The first phase occurs within the first 24 to 96 hours after birth. These early deaths are a result of multiple causes, including extreme prematurity and life-threatening chromosomal and/or complex congenital anomalies.

The second phase of death occurs from 3 weeks to 3 months. These deaths are characterized by significant prognostic uncertainty at the time of birth.[90] Thus, on admission to the NICU, the newborn is already in critical condition and using all available life-sustaining interventions, without which death may have already occurred.

Multiple professional organizations have published palliative guidelines, clinical pathways, and policy statements urging all maternal and newborn providers to respond to the needs of the seriously ill or dying newborn and their families. (See Resource Materials at the end of the chapter.) The most recent call for increased attention to the needs of the seriously ill child comes from the AAP.[8] In 2013 the AAP issued a policy statement regarding pediatric palliative care (PPC) and pediatric hospice care (PHC). The statement defines the aims of PPC and PHC as relieving suffering, improving quality of life, facilitating informed decision making, and assisting in care coordination between clinicians and sites of care.

PPC includes a team of pediatric providers who have added the specialty of palliative care to their professional practice. These clinicians focus on the palliative care needs of infants and children in the inpatient or ambulatory clinic setting. They offer palliative care in conjunction with cure-oriented approaches in caring for all seriously ill infants and children. The PPC team may be asked to coordinate care with the PHC team when infant care is transitioned to a community hospice where care is provided in the home or a designated hospice setting.

This model of providing children and families with high-quality coordinated care is recognized by a specialized benefit in the Affordable Care Act (2009). The benefit is limited to the infant or child enrolled in the Children's Health Protection Program (Medicaid), and it specifies that cure-oriented therapies can be offered alongside hospice care for the seriously ill infant or child.[15]

Delivery of a Palliative Care Service in the NICU

Two models of palliative care delivery are recognized as effective ways to offer palliative care to patients and their families in an intensive care setting: the Consultation Model and the Integrative Model.[67] In the Integrative Model, palliative care concepts and practice are provided concurrently with cure-oriented care. This model is illustrated in Figure 32-1 and outlined in detail by NICU nurses Gale and Brooks (2006).[46] An interdisciplinary team not only directs care to the infant's needs but also includes the emotional and spiritual needs of the parents and family.

In the Consultation Model, palliative care specialists are available to the NICU staff, as well as to all patients in the acute care pediatric setting. Referrals to a palliative care team are made when deemed necessary by the neonatal team and depend on multiple factors. The neonatal team often refers to the consultation team when the goal of infant care becomes enhanced comfort care and a transition to a community hospice is desired. In this model, parents' grief and overwhelming stress may not be addressed until the approaching death of their infant.

Determining Eligibility for Palliative Care in Life-Limiting Conditions

In the clinical practice of perinatal/neonatal medicine, clinicians encounter four common scenarios in which infant death is a strong possibility when[1,6]

1. A serious or lethal fetal diagnosis is made
2. The prognosis of death is certain at the time of birth

Phase I: Admission to NICU

1. Newborn's status evaluated – information gathered
2. Family conference with neonatal/palliative care team
3. Parents and team agree to goals of infant care
4. Family assessment:
   • Personal values – spiritual/religious
   • Previous losses
   • Family dynamics
   • Support system
   • Financial concerns

Phase II: Ongoing Assessment/Decision-Making

1. Infant's goals of care re-evaluated
2. Family/neonatal/palliative care team discuss all treatment options
3. Intensive support from interdisciplinary team for decisions
4. Beneficial/non-beneficial interventions – Ethics consultation
5. Parents communicate with infant: touch, sound, and voice

Phase III: Transition Care

1. Decision to withdraw ventilation support
2. Enhanced comfort care
3. Increase support to all family, significant others
   a. Create memories, pictures, hand prints
   b. Attention to goal of peaceful death
   c. Family farewells
4. Provide symptom management
5. Death

Phase IV: Bereavement

1. Condolence cards
2. Phone call to family. Attend memorial service if possible
3. Risk assessment (e.g., suicide risks, postnatal depression)
4. Referral to support groups. Child life involvement with siblings

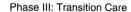

FIGURE 32-1 Integrating palliative care and bioethics in neonatal intensive care: an interdisciplinary approach.

3. There is considerable prognostic uncertainty after the birth
4. Death is certain weeks or months after the birth

In these situations, palliative, maternal, and newborn care specialists join to offer families an integrated care plan for their infant, as well as psychologic, social, and spiritual support.[39]

SERIOUS OR LETHAL FETAL DIAGNOSIS

A palliative care approach can be initiated at the time of the fetal diagnosis to provide support for parental decisions concerning newborn care, grief support, and the creation of an *Advance Care Birth Plan.*[19,30,39] Examples of fetal diagnoses in which parents would benefit from additional support and guidance include certain genetic disorders, as well as complex neurologic, cardiac, and congenital and chromosomal anomalies. Also included are any fetal diagnoses in which a neonatal death could be anticipated if no cure-oriented interventions were offered.

In prenatal birth planning, parents are given time to consider various options of care during the pregnancy and at the time of birth. Crucial decisions concerning newborn care can be discussed (and documented) with maternal-newborn and other pediatric specialists. This process of birth planning is also an opportunity to offer guidance, education, and support to parents regarding their infant's prognosis and how to prepare for their infant's birth or death.

PROGNOSIS OF DEATH IS CERTAIN AT BIRTH

At the time of birth, or soon after, clinicians recognize that the newborn cannot sustain life and that death will occur within minutes or hours, such as in cases of severe neurologic injury or extreme prematurity (less than 23 weeks of gestation or less than 500 g birth weight).[6] Often parents are not prepared for this unexpected outcome to their pregnancy.

At the time of the newborn's birth and imminent death, neonatal and palliative care teams focus their attention on enhanced comfort care for the infant and intense support for the parents. Bereavement support continues for parents, grandparents, and siblings in the postnatal period for as long as needed. Some settings have a designated nurse or social worker to follow up with bereavement support, memory making, and a memorial service.

PROGNOSIS IS UNCERTAIN

The newborn is admitted from the delivery room to the NICU in critical condition. All emergency measures are initiated in order to sustain life until further clarity on the physiologic status is known or the prenatal diagnosis is confirmed. Examples of such conditions are excessive loss of the small intestine, borderline prematurity, pulmonary hypoplasia, and severe congenital anomalies. The neonatal team continues an ongoing assessment of the newborn's response to life outside the womb. Consultations with other pediatric specialists may be necessary in hopes of obtaining a definitive prognosis. Until there is a degree of prognostic certainty, all decisions concerning the newborn's life or death are best deferred.

During this critical time, the neonatal and palliative care teams come together to offer the parents guidance and to clarify information and recommendations. Here, an ethics consultation may be beneficial for the parents. For example, an infant has been diagnosed with a complex cardiac anomaly and the cardiac consultant recommends a series of surgical interventions, which would require a prolonged intensive care stay with the possibility of intense suffering for the infant. The outcome for the life and well-being of the infant remains uncertain. An ethics consultation can help parents clarify the benefits and risks of the proposed interventions.[25,58a] Questions

often arise regarding rates of survival, developmental outcomes, related health issues, and unintended complications related to the suggested interventions.

The palliative care team offers objective guidance to parents in making such critical life-and-death decisions. Furthermore, if the newborn's condition continues to decline during this decision-making period, a palliative care team can initiate a discussion to help parents and the neonatal team clarify the goal of care. These are some of the most difficult cases for parents, as well as the neonatal team. Parents' values and emotional state may determine the decisions concerning the newborn's care.[18]

PROGNOSIS OF DEATH IS CERTAIN— WEEKS TO MONTHS AFTER BIRTH

The infant's diagnosis has been confirmed after birth and the parents agree that the goal of care should be to provide enhanced comfort care for the infant. Often, in these cases, there is not sufficient evidence to know how long the infant will live. For example, in cases of trisomy 18, current evidence suggests that a small percentage of infants may live for weeks or months.[75] In such cases, care coordination with the palliative care/hospice team can offer the infant and family the support needed for the infant's brief life and approaching death. When the home hospice team is unfamiliar with caring for dying infants, the hospital palliative care team may continue to act as consultants.

A Model for the Integration of Palliative Care in the Neonatal Intensive Care Setting

Integration of palliative care in the NICU may present challenges in an environment that emphasizes technical advances directed to saving lives of newborns. We suggest an integrated model of palliative care as the most effective way to ensure the delivery of high-quality family-centered care in the intensive care setting (see Figure 32-1). Before initiating an integrated model, many preparatory steps should be taken to ensure the quality of palliative care delivery. This would include extensive palliative care education of all neonatal intensive care providers. (See Resource Materials at the end of the chapter for a list of palliative care education resources.)

The care team recognizes that each infant and family enter into an intensive care experience with unique needs and expectations. Each phase depends on the neonatal team's prognosis for the infant, as well as the parents' decisions concerning the options of infant care. In the unfamiliar environment of the NICU, parents need time to process, understand, and accept complex information.

Phase I: Admission to NICU. A plan of care is initiated once the newborn's status is stabilized. The neonatal/palliative team meets with the parents to assess their understanding of their newborn's condition, as well as their expectations and hopes for the infant. The team shares with parents what is known and not known about the infant's condition, as well as the current approach to the infant's care. The team and the parents decide on the goals of care emphasizing that goals may change as more information is gathered. Parents and the neonatal/palliative team focus on all available care options considering what is in the best interest of the infant. Parents' values, past experiences, and previous losses, as well as their financial concerns, are explored.

Phase II: Ongoing neonatal assessment and decision making. Parents are given frequent updates concerning their infant's condition. Often, parents find themselves on an "emotional roller coaster," not knowing from day to day if their infant will live or die. Under these stressful circumstances, added support from an interdisciplinary team is essential. If the infant's condition changes significantly, a second family conference is offered where the goals of care are reconsidered. Discussion centers around new information from pediatric specialists and the current status of the infant. All members of the care team who are directly involved with the infant and parents attend the family meeting. Often a member of the ethics committee is also invited to attend. The ethics consultant facilitates a discussion on the risks and benefits of various treatment options. Recommendations for the infant's care could include continuing cure-oriented care or withdrawing of cure-oriented approaches to care.

- In this phase, parents are given time to process often complex information. A series of discussions ensue and family meetings may be reconvened. The care team recognizes parental vulnerability because there is often *no good* decision that can be made. In addition, parents struggle with anxiety and concern in an effort to make the "right" decision.

- Child life specialists are valuable in helping parents find ways to communicate with their infant through touch and other creative ways of bonding. Parents may find guidance and solace with the added spiritual support from the hospital chaplain or a personal religious/spiritual advisor.

Phase III: Transitional care. Parents and the care team have made the decision either to continue with cure-oriented interventions or to withdraw all life-prolonging interventions from infant care.[29] When the decision is to withdraw life-prolonging interventions the goal of care is to offer the infant enhanced comfort care and a dignified death. After withdrawal of support the infant may live for minutes or hours, so active symptom management for pain or distress must continue.[28]

- The care team focuses on ways to create a meaningful experience for parents and extended family as they say good-bye. Memory books, hand/foot prints, a lock of hair, and photographs provide tangible memories of their infant's unique identity. Spiritual providers can facilitate religious or spiritual rituals and a memorial service if requested by the parents.

Phase IV: Bereavement. A designated member of the care team (such as a bereavement coordinator) calls the family within the first week after the infant's death. A brief phone call of condolence often reveals that additional support is needed. Condolence cards are sent from the care team and often one or two members of the care team attend the funeral or memorial service. Parents may benefit from perinatal loss support groups that are available in many communities (see Chapter 30).[64]

This model of palliative care promotes continuity of infant care across care settings, as well as providing support for extreme grief and overwhelming stress of parents when their newborn is seriously ill. This model reflects the AAP policy for pediatric palliative care[8] by incorporating the added support of an interdisciplinary palliative care team in the care of the seriously ill infant. The care team guides parents in making critical decisions concerning the life, and at times the death, of their infant.[92] When necessary, the palliative care team provides coordination of services between hospital and home when the goal of infant care changes.

SOCIAL ETHICS

Moral judgments made in the hospital setting do not occur in isolation from the larger social context of which institutions and individuals are a part. Such judgments can be considerably affected by prevailing social values and perspectives. Further, although decisions in the NICU generally are interpersonal in nature, they also may have a significant effect on the larger community. Technologic advancements have enabled some severely disabled infants to survive and grow, albeit with varying degrees of mental and physical disabilities. Indeed, these are not the majority of newborns, but they often require numerous hospitalizations and costly rehabilitation. Society frequently bears the financial, physical, and social costs of care for these individuals.

Social ethics reflects on the sociocultural aspects of human life. It considers how individuals as moral agents are accountable for their behavior in social structures and public policy issues. It also can refer to shared patterns of moral judgment. Moreover, it focuses on how social contexts influence individual moral behavior and the range of moral responsibility.

In a pluralistic society like the United States, there is no one social ethic. Some believe in rugged individualism; others believe in equality of opportunity, worth, and treatment; still others believe that we bear mutual responsibility for one another. An underlying concern of most socioethical systems is concern for both the individual and the common good.

In NICUs, bioethics and social ethics converge. Treatment decisions have social implications; societal values influence treatment decisions. As described, government regulations highlight the paradox of societal values about the treatment of disabled infants. These federal guidelines advocate the use of "reasonable medical judgment" in treating disabled infants, yet their effect may be seen as increasing the perceived obligation to treat—to the point of "unreasonable." Through government, society expresses the determination to treat, yet societal commitment to the long-term care of special-needs NICU graduates and families is wholly insufficient. Public funds for such care have been reduced while the expressed urgency for treatment of all babies has increased. The values inherent in our public policy decisions about initial and long-term treatment are curiously disparate.

After comparing the health care and social policies of the United States with the seemingly more equitable policies of Great Britain and Sweden, Young[96] concluded, "We need to strive for a better balance between aggressive treatment in the neonatal intensive care units initially, and the resources currently allocated for the long-term care of the disabled." Such a balance might include being more selective about aggressive treatment, as well as learning more about prematurity and trying to prevent it. Young continued, "To the extent that society fails to ensure that seriously ill newborns have the opportunity for an adequate level of continuing care, its moral authority, to intervene on behalf of a newborn whose life is in jeopardy, is compromised."[96]

Recognizing this disparity, various community groups have attempted to establish guidelines for standards of care that are fiscally, morally, and medically responsible to guide parents and clinicians in goal setting and decision making. They have recognized the high cost, in every respect, of neonatal and pediatric intensive care. Their impetus has been to determine community "agreed-upon" values for treatment and nontreatment of disabled infants to effect a standard of care for the extreme premature, severely disabled, and critically ill infant. Managed care organizations are also assessing the ethics of reasonable care and the limits of treatment to be offered. Although not wholly able to determine "agreed-upon" values for treatment and nontreatment standards of care, these community and professional groups have offered important social voices to the complexity of neonatal care.

GLOSSARY

- *Best interest:* A standard used to determine the validity of proxy consent in decision making. Treatment decisions are based on what most "reasonable persons" would assess as the burdens and benefits that would likely accompany the child's life. This standard leads clinicians to seek treatment resulting in a "net benefit" to the child.
- *Casuistry:* Case-based ethics in which the claims, grounds, and warrants of a particular case are compared with similar cases. The basic question for moral casuistry is how a general moral precept is to be understood in similar sets of circumstances.
- *Deontology (formalism):* A theory of ethics that holds that the moral rightness of an act must be decided totally independent of the consequences of that act. Duty is independent of consequential good, and certain moral commands (rules)

operative under fundamental principles must be obeyed under all circumstances.

- *Dilemma:* A situation in which more than one possible course of action exists and differing values are held for each possible course of action by the parties involved. Moral dilemmas arise when an appeal to moral considerations can be made for opposing courses of action—when it is apparent that an act can be considered both morally right and morally wrong, and that on moral grounds there is a sense of "ought" and "ought not" to perform the act.

- *Double effect:* A principle, often viewed within the larger context of nonmaleficence, that claims that an act having a harmful effect is not always morally prohibited. Any harmful effect of an act is viewed as indirect, unintended, or simply a foreseen effect but not as the direct and intended effect (e.g., if an act, as in treatment, brings about death, it is not always to be prohibited). Four conditions are often given to clarify this principle for specific acts:
  - The action itself must be "good" or at least morally indifferent.
  - The agent must intend only the good effect and not the harmful effect.
  - The harmful effect cannot be a means to the good effect.
  - There should be a favorable balance between the good and harmful effects of the action.

- *Ethics:* The study of moral conduct, systems, and ideas.

- *Morals:* The conduct and codes of conduct of individuals and groups. Three popular uses of the term exist: (1) in contrast to immoral (right vs. wrong); (2) in contrast to nonmoral (actions that have no bearing or question of right and wrong); and (3) "morals" (the behavior pattern of an individual or group).

- *Nonbeneficial treatment:* The notion that the efficacy of treatment is very low. There is no ethical obligation to offer nonbeneficial treatment. Non-benefit may best be judged by the overall medical benefit, not just effect, that a given treatment has on a patient. Treatment is nonbeneficial if it is useless. Physiologic, psychologic, religious, and social data should be considered in making a determination of nonbenefit. Determination of nonbeneficial treatment should be based on medical benefit in consort with family goals for the patient.

- *Palliative care:* An approach that improves the quality of life of patients and their families facing problems associated with life-threatening illness, through the prevention and relief of suffering by means of early identification and impeccable assessment and treatment of pain and other problems: physical, psychosocial, and spiritual. Palliative care for children is the active total care of the child's body, mind, and spirit and involves giving support to the family.

- *Personhood:* A characteristic that may be used in decision making that is based on the idea (1) that possession of certain capabilities (typically higher brain functions such as consciousness, rationality, perception of space and time, and the ability to communicate) constitutes personhood and (2) that only "persons" have any moral claim to life, treatment, and so on.

- *"Proxy" (surrogate) decision maker:* A designated person who will act on behalf of an individual who is incapable of making decisions.

- *Reasonable person standard:* A standard by which the validity of informed consent is measured. Information to be disclosed is determined by referring to a hypothetical "reasonable person" and determining whether such a person would see any significance in the information in assessing risk and deciding whether to submit to a treatment or procedure.

- *Rights:* Those things to which people have a just claim; a claim to a condition to which the individual is entitled.

- *Utilitarianism (consequentialism):* A theory in ethics that holds that an act is right when it brings about a good outcome for the greatest number of people, upholds the greatest balance of "good" over "evil," and seeks to effect "utility" or the most useful outcome. "The end justifies the means." This may be developed into rules that are adhered to maximize benefits and minimize harms (rule utilitarian) or simply appealed to in individual actions (act utilitarian).

- *Values:* Those things that have worth or are desirable to an individual or group.

- *Virtues:* A habit, disposition, or trait that a person may possess or aspire to possess; specifically, a moral virtue upholds what is morally right or praiseworthy.

REFERENCES

For a full list of references, scan the QR code or visit http://booksite.elsevier.com/ 9780323320832.

INDEX

Note: Page numbers followed by "b", "f" and "t" indicate boxes, figures and tables respectively.